Eighth Edition

Nancy Caroline's
Emergency
Care in the Streets

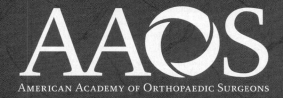

AMERICAN ACADEMY OF ORTHOPAEDIC SURGEONS

Series Editor:
Andrew N. Pollak, MD, FAAOS

Lead Editors:
Barbara Aehlert, MSEd, BSPA, RN
Bob Elling, MPA, EMT-P

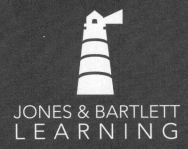

JONES & BARTLETT
LEARNING

World Headquarters
Jones & Bartlett Learning
5 Wall Street
Burlington, MA 01803
978-443-5000
info@jblearning.com
www.jblearning.com

Jones & Bartlett Learning books and products are available through most bookstores and online booksellers. To contact Jones & Bartlett Learning directly, call 800-832-0034, fax 978-443-8000, or visit our website, www.jblearning.com.

Substantial discounts on bulk quantities of Jones & Bartlett Learning publications are available to corporations, professional associations, and other qualified organizations. For details and specific discount information, contact the special sales department at Jones & Bartlett Learning via the above contact information or send an email to specialsales@jblearning.com.

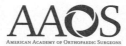
AMERICAN ACADEMY OF ORTHOPAEDIC SURGEONS

Library of Congress Cataloging-in-Publication Data
Names: American Academy of Orthopaedic Surgeons, author. | Pollak, Andrew N.,
   editor. | Elling, Bob, editor. | Aehlert, Barbara, editor.
Title: Nancy Caroline's emergency care in the streets / American Academy of
   Orthopaedic Surgeons ; series editor: Andrew N. Pollak ; lead editors: Bob
   Elling, Barbara Aehlert.
Other titles: Emergency care in the streets
Description: Eighth edition. | Burlington, MA : Jones & Bartlett Learning,
   [2018] | Preceded by Nancy Caroline's emergency care in the streets.
   7th ed. 2013. | Includes bibliographical references and index.
Identifiers: LCCN 2017024835 | ISBN 9781284457278 (casebound)
Subjects: | MESH: Emergency Treatment | Emergency Medical Services |
   Emergency Medical Technicians
Classification: LCC RC86.7 | NLM WB 105 | DDC 616.02/5--dc23
LC record available at https://lccn.loc.gov/2017024835

6048

Printed in the United States of America
22 21 20 19 18   10 9 8 7 6 5 4 3

Brief Contents

Contents: Volume 2

Section 8: Shock and Resuscitation   1941

Section 9: Special Patient Populations · 2023

Section 11: Career Development   2517

Skill Drills: Volume 2

Prepare for Class with Navigate 2 Digital Curriculum Solution Packages

Navigate 2 resources offer unbeatable value with mobile-ready course materials to help you prepare for your paramedic class.

Purchase access to the Advantage, Preferred, or Premier option at 25% off!*

ADVANTAGE PACKAGE
Navigate 2 Advantage Access Includes:

- eBook
- Study Center
- Assessments
- Analytics
- Fisdap Internship Scheduler
- Fisdap Skills Tracker

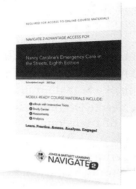

ISBN: 978-1-284-45702-5

PREFERRED PACKAGE
Navigate 2 Preferred Access Includes:

- eBook
- Study Center
- Assessments
- Analytics
- TestPrep
- Fisdap Internship Scheduler
- Fisdap Skills Tracker

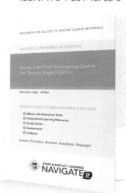

ISBN: 978-1-284-13723-1

PREMIER PACKAGE
Navigate 2 Premier Access Includes:

- eBook
- Study Center
- Assessments
- Analytics
- TestPrep
- Lectures
- Simulations
- Fisdap Internship Scheduler
- Fisdap Skills Tracker

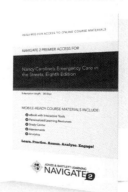

ISBN: 978-1-284-13727-9

Order today at www.psglearning.com

*Prices subject to change. Access codes to Navigate 2 course materials are available at 25% off the cost of the textbook.

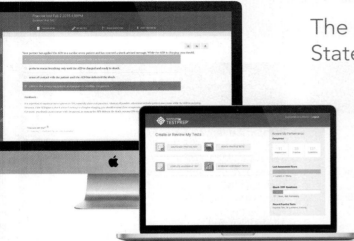
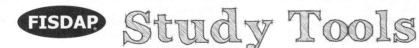

Acknowledgments

The American Academy of Orthopaedic Surgeons and the Public Safety Group would like to acknowledge the editors, authors, and reviewers of previous editions of *Nancy Caroline's Emergency Care in the Streets* who were involved in the development of this textbook.

■ Series Editor

Andrew N. Pollak, MD, FAAOS
The James Lawrence Kernan Professor and Chairman, Department of Orthopaedics, University of Maryland School of Medicine
Chief of Orthopaedics, University of Maryland Medical System
Medical Director, Baltimore County Fire Department
Director, Shock Trauma Go Team
Special Deputy US Marshal

■ Series Editor Designee

Alfonso Mejia, MD, MPH
Program Director, Orthopedic Surgery Residency Program
Vice Head, Department of Orthopedic Surgery
University of Illinois College of Medicine
Medical Director
Tactical Emergency Medical Support Physician
South Suburban Emergency Response Team
Chicago, Illinois

■ Lead Editors

Barbara Aehlert, MSEd, BSPA, RN

Bob Elling, MPA, EMT-P
Educator, Author, and Advocate
High Quality Endeavors, Ltd.
Lake Placid, New York
SMG Events Medic
Albany, New York
Olympic Regional Development Authority Medic
Lake Placid, New York

■ Authors

Matthew Adams, AAS, FP-C, NRP
Chapters 27, 47, 49, 52
Duke Life Flight
Durham, North Carolina

Barbara Aehlert, MSEd, BSPA, RN
Chapters 8, 17, 19, 22, 26, 36, 43, 53, Appendix
President, Southwest EMS Education, Inc.

Leaugeay Barnes, MS, NRP, NCEE
Chapter 23
Tulsa Community College
Tulsa, Oklahoma

Andrew Bartkus, RN, MSN, JD, CEN, CCRN, CFRN, NREMT-P, FP-C
Chapters 13, 45
Sandoval Regional Medical Center
Rio Rancho, New Mexico

Ann Bellows, RN, NR-P, EdD
Chapter 25
Eastern New Mexico University, Ruidoso
Central New Mexico Community College
Outreach Education Opportunities
Las Cruces, New Mexico

Dave Bledsoe, RN, NREMT-P, LNC
Chapter 4
Orlando, Florida

Charles D. Bortle, EdD, NRP, RRT-NPS, CHSE
Chapters 16, 32
Director, Center for Clinical Competency
Einstein Medical Center Philadelphia
Philadelphia, Pennsylvania

Chad E. Brocato, DHSc, JD, REMT-P
Chapter 31
Division Chief
Pompano Beach Fire-Rescue
Pompano Beach, Florida

Bruce Butterfras, MSEd, LP
Chapter 29
Assistant Professor, Director of Bachelor Degree Program
Department of Emergency Health Sciences
The University of Texas Health Science Center at San Antonio
San Antonio, Texas

Derya Caglar, MD
Chapter 43
Associate Professor, Pediatrics
University of Washington School of Medicine
Seattle, Washington
Attending Physician, Emergency Medicine
Seattle Children's Hospital
Seattle, Washington

Julie Chase, MSEd, FAWM, TP-C
Chapter 34
Program Director
Immersion EMS Academy LLC
Berryville, Virginia

Patricia R. Chess, MD
Chapter 42
Professor of Pediatrics (Neonatology) and Biomedical Engineering
Director, Neonatal-Perinatal Medicine Fellowship Program
Vice-Chair for Education, Pediatrics
University of Rochester Medical Center
Golisano Children's Hospital at Strong
Rochester, New York

Stephen John Cico, MD, MEd
Chapter 43
Assistant Dean for Educational Affairs & Faculty Development
Dean's Offices of Educational Affairs and Faculty Affairs & Professional Development (OFAPD)
Associate Professor of Clinical Emergency Medicine & Pediatrics
Fellowship Director for Pediatric Emergency Medicine
Division of Emergency Pediatrics
Department of Emergency Medicine
Indiana University School of Medicine
Indianapolis, Indiana

David L. Dalton, BS, Paramedic
Chapter 3
Captain, Training Officer & AHA TC
   Coordinator
St. Charles County Ambulance District
St Peters, Missouri

Rommie L. Duckworth, LP
Chapters 30, 48, 50, 51
Founder, Director
New England Center for Rescue
   and Emergency Medicine
Sherman, Connecticut

Anne Austin Ellerbee, NRP, AAS
Chapter 46
H.E.R.O. Training Company
Thomaston, Georgia

Bob Elling, MPA, EMT-P
Chapters 11, 12, 39, 40
Educator, Author, and Advocate
High Quality Endeavors, Ltd.
Lake Placid, New York
SMG Events Medic
Albany, New York
Olympic Regional Development
   Authority Medic
Lake Placid, New York

**Wm. Travis Engel, MSc, OMS-IV,
NRP, FP-C**
Chapters 41, 42, 45
Liberty University College of Osteopathic
   Medicine
Lynchburg, Virginia

John Farris, EMT-P, CP-C
Chapter 53
Mobile Integrated Health Paramedic,
   MedStar Mobile Healthcare
Chair, Fort Worth Safe Communities Elder
   Abuse Prevention Task Force
President, Tarrant County Adult Protective
   Services Community Board
Adjunct Clinical Instructor, UNTHSC Texas
   College of Osteopathic Medicine
Fort Worth, Texas

Cullen K. Griffith, MD
Chapter 37
Orthopaedic Trauma
Orthopaedic Specialty Group
Fairfield, Connecticut

Carol Gupton, NRP, BSEMS
Chapter 22
Papillion Fire Department
Papillion, Nebraska

**Seth C. Hawkins, MD, FACEP, FAEMS,
MFAWM**
Chapter 38
Burke County EMS
Wake Forest University Department
   of Emergency Medicine
Morganton, North Carolina

Rhonda J. Hunt, BAS, NRP
Chapter 7
Albany State University
Albany, Georgia

Howard E. Huth III, BA, EMT-P
Chapter 10
Director, SUNY Cobleskill Paramedic
   Program
NYS DOH Bureau of EMS Regional Faculty
Cobleskill, New York

Don Kimlicka, NRP, CCEMT-P
Chapters 1, 2
Executive Director/Critical Care Paramedic
Clintonville Area Ambulance Service
Clintonville, Wisconsin
State of Wisconsin EMS Advisory Board
Adjunct Faculty, MidState Technical College
Wisconsin Rapids, Wisconsin
Adjunct Faculty, Nicolet Technical College
Rhinelander, Wisconsin

Sean M. Kivlehan, MD, MPH, NREMT-P
Chapter 21
Brigham and Women's Hospital
Harvard Medical School
Boston, Massachusetts

Deborah Lardner, DO, DTM&H, FACOEP
Chapter 51
Boarded Emergency Medicine/Family
   Medicine
CityMD—Corporate Offices
New York, New York

Nirupama Laroia, MD
Chapter 42
Professor of Pediatrics/Neonatology
University of Rochester Medical Center
Golisano Children's Hospital
Section Chief, Neonatology & Medical
   Director, Special Care Nursery
Rochester General Hospital
Rochester, New York

Edward "Ted" H. Lee, EdS, NRP, CCEMT-P
Chapter 35
Associate Professor/Program Chair
   Emergency Medical Services
Missouri Southern State University
Joplin, Missouri

Yogangi Malhotra, MD, FAAP
Chapter 42
Assistant Professor of Pediatrics
Division of Neonatology
Albert Einstein College of Medicine
Children's Hospital at Montefiore
Montefiore New Rochelle
New Rochelle, New York

Astra P. Paro, AS, CCEMT-P
Chapter 36
Charleston, South Carolina

**Michael D. Passafaro, DO, DTM&H, FACEP,
FACOEP**
Chapter 51
CarePoint Health
Jersey City, New Jersey

Jason C. Perry, RN, CEN, CFRN
Appendix
Sandoval Regional Medical Center
Rio Rancho, New Mexico

Stephen J. Rahm, NRP
Chapter 15
Deputy Chief, Office of Clinical Direction
Co-Chair, Centre for Emergency Health
   Sciences
Bulverde Spring Branch Emergency Services
Spring Branch, Texas

Becky Ridenhour, PharmD
Appendix
Progress West Hospital
O'Fallon, Missouri

Rob Schnepp
Chapter 49
Division Chief, Special Operations (retired)
Alameda County Fire Department
California

Shadrach Smith, BS Bio, LP, NRP
Chapters 24, 30
Paramedic Advantage
Anaheim, California

**Chuck Sowerbrower, MEd, NRP, NCEE,
CCP-C**
Chapters 18, 20
Sinclair Community College
Dayton, Ohio

**Bryan L. Spangler, DHSc, NRP,
NCEE, CMTE**
Chapter 19
EMS Program Director
Central Ohio Technical College
Newark, Ohio

Chris Stratford, MS, BSN, RN, NRP
Chapter 28
University of Utah Center for Emergency
   Programs
Salt Lake City, Utah

John vonRosenberg, MA, FP-C, NRP
Chapter 9
Air Methods
Edenton, North Carolina

Robert Vroman, MEd, BSNRP
Chapters 33, 34
Associate Professor of EMS
Red Rocks Community College
Lakewood, Colorado

Bryan Ware, EMTP, Fire Chief
*Chapters 4, 6, 30, 31, 32, 33, 35, 36,
   41, 43, 44*
Beulah Fire Protection District
Beulah, Colorado

Katherine H. West, RN, BSN, MSEd
Chapter 26
Infection Control Consultant
Infection Control/Emerging
   Concepts, Inc.
Manassas, Virginia

Keith Widmeier, BA, NRP, FP-C
Chapters 14, 44, Appendix
Director of Education
Good Fellowship Ambulance & EMS
   Training Institute
West Chester, Pennsylvania

Gordon H. Worley, RN, MSN,
FNP, EMT-P, CFRN
Chapter 5
Sutter Amador Hospital
Jackson, California

Matt Zavadsky, MS-HSA, EMT
Chapter 53
Chief Strategic Integration Officer
MedStar Mobile Healthcare
Fort Worth, Texas

■ Contributors

Elyse K. Lavine, MD
Mount Sinai St. Luke's/Mount Sinai West
New York, New York

Jeffrey S. Rabrich, DO, FACEP, EMT-P
Medical Director
Mount Sinai St. Luke's Emergency
   Department
Assistant Professor of Emergency Medicine
Icahn School of Medicine at Mount Sinai
New York, New York

■ Ancillary Authors

Kimberly Bailey, MA, NRP, CHSE, SCCEM
Emerging Infectious Disease Planner
SC DHEC Office of Public Health
   Preparedness
Columbia, South Carolina

Sharon F. Chiumento, BSN, EMT-P
Lead Instructor, Monroe Ambulance,
   University of Rochester
Guest Instructor, Monroe Community
   College
Rochester, New York

Stephen J. Rahm, NRP
Deputy Chief, Office of Clinical Direction
Co-Chair, Centre for Emergency Health
   Sciences
Bulverde Spring Branch Emergency Services
Spring Branch, Texas

Brittany Ann Williams, DHSc, RRT-NPS,
NREMT-P
Professor, Respiratory Care
Director, Clinical Education
Santa Fe College
Gainesville, Florida

■ Reviewers

J. Adam Alford, BS, NRP
Old Dominion EMS Alliance
Richmond, Virginia

Robert Jay Alley, MS, Paramedic
Blue Ridge Community College
Flat Rock, North Carolina

Hector D. Arroyo Jr, EMT-P, CIC
Senior EMT/Paramedic Instructor
FDNY-EMS—Borough of Manhattan
   Community College
New York, New York

Alan M. Batt, MSc, GradCert ICP, CCP
Fanshawe College
Ontario, Canada

Edward Bays, BS, NRP
EMS Education Director
Mountwest Community & Technical
   College
Huntington, West Virginia

Shawn Bjarnson
Advanced Emergency Medical Technician
   and Law Enforcement Officer
Gunnison Valley Hospital
Gunnison, Utah

Mark A. Boisclair, MPA, NRP, US Army
(retired)
Chattahoochee Valley Community College
Phenix City, Alabama

Phillip J. Borum, MPA, RN, CPEN,
Paramedic
Assistant Professor/Lead Paramedic
   Instructor
Santa Fe College Emergency Medical Services
   Programs
Gainesville, Florida

Jason L. Brooks, MA, NRP
University of South Alabama
Mobile, Alabama

Wayne D. Burdette Jr, MS, NRP
Gwinnett County Fire & Emergency Services
Lawrenceville, Georgia

Karen Burns
Clovis Fire Department
Clovis, New Mexico

Aaron R. Byington, MA, NRP
Battalion Chief/Paramedic
Layton City Fire Department
Layton, Utah

Elliot Carhart, EdD, RRT, NRP
Jefferson College of Health Sciences
Largo, Florida

Joshua Chan, BA, NRP, FP-C
Life Link III, Flight Paramedic
Minneapolis, Minnesota
Glacial Ridge Health Systems,
   EMS Educator
Glenwood, Minnesota

Julie Chase, MSEd, FAWM, TP-C
Program Director
Immersion EMS Academy LLC
Berryville, Virginia

Ted Chialtas
Fire Captain/Paramedic, Paramedic Program
   Coordinator
San Diego Fire-Rescue Department
San Diego, California

Sharon F. Chiumento, BSN, EMT-P
Lead Instructor, Monroe Ambulance,
   University of Rochester
Guest Instructor, Monroe Community
   College
Rochester, New York

Glenn Coffin
EMTS-Emergency Medical Teaching
   Services, Inc.
Pembroke, Massachusetts

Jason Lee Collins, BS, NRP
Rockingham Community College
Wentworth, North Carolina

Kevin T. Collopy, BA, FP-C, CCEMT-P,
NR-P, CMTE
Clinical Outcomes Manager
AirLink/VitaLink Critical Care Transport
New Hanover Regional Medical Center
Wilmington, North Carolina

Hiram Colon
Paramedic
FDNY EMS Bureau of Training
Bayside, New York

Helen Compton, NRP
Lifestar Ambulance
Emporia, Virginia
Mecklenburg County Rescue
Clarksville, Virginia

George W. Contreras, MPH, MS, MEP, CEM, EMTP
Associate Professor and Director of Allied Health
Kingsborough Community College
Brooklyn, New York

Scott Cook, MS, CCEMTP
Southern Maine Community College
South Portland, Maine

Bob Coschignano
Lieutenant/Hazmat Technician
City of Orlando Fire Department
Orlando, Florida

Kent Courtney, NREMT-P
EMS Educator, Emergency Specialist
Peabody Western Coal Company
Essential Safety Training and Consulting
Northern Arizona Healthcare
Rimrock, Arizona

Matthew A. Crawford, NREMT-P, UMBC-CCT
CAMC
Sutton, West Virginia

Mark Cromer, MS, MBA, NRP
Jefferson College of Health Sciences
Roanoke, Virginia

Mike Cronin, EMT-P, EMI
Director of Public Safety
Knox Technical Center
Mount Vernon, Ohio

Anthony Cuda, NRP
ALS Program Coordinator
Community College of Allegheny County
Pittsburgh, Pennsylvania

Kevin Curry, AS, NRP, CCEMTP, I/C
United Training Center
Lewiston, Maine

Lyndal M. Curry, MS, NRP
Southern Union State Community College
Opelika, Alabama

Andrew J. Davis, NREMT-P
Gwinnett County Fire Academy
Dacula, Georgia

Lynne Dees, PhD, NRP
UCLA Center for Prehospital Care
David Geffen School of Medicine
Los Angeles, California

James DiClemente, MBA, NRP
Pro EMS Center for MEDICS
Cambridge, Massachusetts

Thomas Dobrzynski, BS, NRP
Sanford Health EMS Education
Fargo, North Dakota

Jeannett Edwards-Banks, NRP, BS, MEd
James City County Fire Department
Williamsburg, Virginia

Wm. Travis Engel, MSc, OMS-IV, NRP, FP-C
Liberty University College of Osteopathic Medicine
Lynchburg, Virginia

Reuben Farnsworth, CCP-C, NRP
RockStar Education & Consulting
Cedaredge, Colorado

Jason Ferguson, BPA, NRP
Central Virginia Community College
Lynchburg, Virginia

David Fifer, NRP
Lecturer, Emergency Medical Care
Eastern Kentucky University
Department of Fire Protection and Paramedic Science
Richmond, Kentucky

Darrell Wayne Fixler, RRT, NRP
Fort Rucker Fire & EMS
Fort Rucker, Alabama

John A. Flora, Paramedic, EMS-I
Columbus Division of Fire
Columbus, Ohio

Charles Foat, PhD, Paramedic
Johnson County Community College
Overland Park, Kansas

Jeffrey L. Foster, CCEMTP, NRP, I/C, EMD
CarolinaEast Health System
New Bern, North Carolina

Lori Gallian, BS, EMT-P
Cascade Training Center
Roseville, California

Scott A. Gano, BS, NRP, FP-C, CCEMT-P
Assistant Professor
Paramedic Program Director
Columbus State Community College
Columbus, Ohio

Fidel O. Garcia, Paramedic
President, Owner
Professional EMS Education
Grand Junction, Colorado

Rodney Geilenfeldt II, BS, EMT-P
Paramedic Coordinator
EMSTA College
Santee, California

Jeffery D. Gilliard, NRP, CCEMTP, FPC, BS
EMETSEEI Institute
Rockledge, Florida

Jamie O. Gray, BS, AAS, FF, NRP (NAEMT/NAEMSE)
Alabama Office of EMS
Montgomery, Alabama
Captain, Elmore Fire Department
Elmore, Alabama

Bill Grayson, NRP
Oklahoma City Community College
Oklahoma City, Oklahoma

James E. Gretz, NRP
Education Center Manager
JeffSTAT—Thomas Jefferson University Hospitals
Philadelphia, Pennsylvania

Jeffrey R. Grunow, MSN, NRP, NCEE
Associate Professor - EMT/Clinical Coordinator
Emergency Care & Rescue Department
Weber State University
Ogden, Utah

Kevin M. Gurney, MS, CCEPT-P, I/C
Delta Ambulance
Waterville, Maine

Jason Haag, CCEMT-P, CIC
Finger Lakes Ambulance
Finger Lakes Regional EMS Council
Wayne County ALS
Geneva, New York

Steven E. Hall Jr, EMT-P
Dabney S. Lancaster Community College
Clifton Forge, Virginia

Kirk Hallett, NREMT-P, CCT
Vital Knowledge Group
Richmond, Virginia

Joseph J. Hamilton, PA-C, NRP
Mt. Nebo Training
Provo, Utah

Jennifer Hannigan, MEd, Paramedic, CLI
Fire Department of the City of New York
Emergency Medical Services Bureau of Training
Bayside, New York

Anthony S. Harbour, BSN, MEd, RN, NRP
Director
Southern Virginia EMS
Roanoke, Virginia

Charles Phillip Head III, BHS, NRP, FP-C, CP-C
Manager of EMS Education
Greenville Health System
Greenville, South Carolina

Greg Helmuth, BA, NREMT-P
Hawkeye Community College
Waterloo, Iowa

Thomas Herron
Roane State Community College
Knoxville, Tennessee

Paul Hitchcock, NRP
Department of Homeland Security
Reston, Virginia

Henry 'Butch' Hoffmann, BA, EMT-P (retired)

Michele M. Hoffman, MSEd, RN, NREMT, AMWAc
James City Volunteer Rescue Squad
Toano, Virginia

James Hood, Paramedic
Lenoir County Emergency Services
Kinston, North Carolina

Troy Hoover, NRP, CCP-C, FP-C
Guardian Flight
Price, Utah

Mark A. Huckaby, NRP
OhioHealth Emergency Medical Services
Columbus, Ohio

James B. Huettenmueller, BSEd, NRP
Tulsa Tech
Tulsa, Oklahoma

Sandra Hultz, NRP
EMS Instructor
Holmes Community College
Ridgeland, Mississippi

Joseph Hurlburt, BS, NREMT-P, EMT-P I/C
Instructor Coordinator/Training Officer
Rapid Response EMS
Romulus, Michigan

Gene Iannuzzi, RN, MPA, CEN, EMT-P
Assistant Professor and EMS Program Director
Borough of Manhattan Community College
New York, NY

Darin Jackson, MDiv, Paramedic
Asheville-Buncombe Technical Community
    College
Asheville, North Carolina

Adam Johnson, NRP
Rhinelander Fire Department
Nicolet Area Technical College
Northcentral Technical College
Rhinelander, Wisconsin

Travis Karicofe, EMS Training Officer
Harrisonburg Fire Department
Harrisonburg, Virginia

Jared Kimball, NREMT-P
Tulane Trauma Education
New Orleans, Louisiana

Timothy M. Kimble, AAS, NRP
Carilion Clinic Life Support Training Center
Craig Co Emergency Services
Roanoke, Virginia

Don Kimlicka, NRP, CCEMT-P
Executive Director/Critical Care Paramedic
Clintonville Area Ambulance Service
Clintonville, Wisconsin
State of Wisconsin EMS Advisory Board
Adjunct Faculty, MidState Technical College
Wisconsin Rapids, Wisconsin
Adjunct Faculty, Nicolet Technical College
Rhinelander, Wisconsin

Mark A. King, MA, EMT-P, MEMS
Instructor Coordinator Paramedic
Kennebec Valley Community College
Fairfield, Maine

Blake Klingle, MS, RN, CCEMT-P
EMS Instructor/Coordinator
Waukesha County Technical College
Pewaukee, Wisconsin

Jim Ladle, BS, EMT-P, FP-C, CCP-C
South Jordan Fire Department
South Jordan, Utah

John F. LeBlanc Jr, AHS, NRP
Greenville Technical College
Greenville, South Carolina

William J. Leggio Jr, EdD, NRP
Creighton University EMS Education
Omaha, Nebraska

Daniel W. Linkins, BHS, NRP, NCEE
John Tyler Community College
Chester, Virginia

Tony Lipari, NREMTP
Operations Administrator
Bolton EMS
Bolton Landing, New York

Joshua Lopez, BS-EMS, NRP, I/C
University of New Mexico School of
    Medicine
Emergency Medical Services Academy
Kirtland Air Force Base Pararescue
    Paramedic Program
Albuquerque, New Mexico

Ricky Lyles, NRP
Southside Virginia Community College
Victoria, Virginia

Patty Maher, MPA, EMTP
Daytona State College
Daytona Beach, Florida

Richard Main, MEd, NRP
College of Southern Nevada
Las Vegas, Nevada

Jeanette S. Mann, BSN, RN, NRP
Director of EMS Program
Dabney S. Lancaster Community College
Clifton Forge, Virginia

Scotty A. McArthur, BS, NRP
University of South Alabama
Mobile, Alabama

Rod McGinnes, Paramedic, MPH
College of Central Florida
Ocala, Florida

Lucian Mirra, MEd, NRP
University of Virginia
Charlottesville, Virginia

Keith A. Monosky, PhD, MPM, EMT-P
Director, EMS Paramedicine Program
Professor, Department of Health Sciences
Central Washington University
Ellensburg, Washington

**Nicholas J. Montelauro, BS, NRP,
FP-C, NCEE**
MHP Education and Training
Terre Haute, Indiana

John Morrissey, NREMT-P
NYS Department of Health Bureau
    of Emergency Medical Services
    and Trauma Systems
Albany, New York

**Gregory S. Neiman, MS, NRP, NCEE,
CEMA (VA)**
Virginia Office of EMS
Richmond, Virginia

C. Jill Oblak, MA, MBA, NRP
Penn State University
Fayette, the Eberly Campus
Uniontown, Pennsylvania

Jim O'Connor, EMTP
Columbus Division of Fire
Columbus, Ohio
Hocking College
Nelsonville, Ohio

**Laurie Oelslager, EdD, NRP, CMPA, AHA
Regional Faculty**
South Central College
Mankato, Minnesota

Danny K. Opperman Jr, MICP, NRP, BS
EMS Educator/Clinical Coordinator
Atlantic Cape Community College
Health Professions Institute
Atlantic City, New Jersey

Kate Passow, NRP
Physicians Transport Service
Herndon, Virginia

Nancy Peifer, PhD, MSN, RN
Palm Beach State College
Loxahatchee, Florida

Jose A. Perez, Paramedic, CLI
Fire Department of New York
New York City, New York

Timothy J. Petreit, MBA, NRP
Montgomery Fire/Rescue
Montgomery, Alabama

Joyce Pettengill
Department Chair EMS
Fayetteville Technical Community College
Fayetteville, North Carolina

Ian Pleet
MedStar/SITEL
Washington, District of Columbia

Jonathan R. Powell, BS, NRP
Department of EMS Education
University of South Alabama
Mobile, Alabama

Lionel Powell, EMT-P, MHEd
An Act of Caring
West Valley, Utah

Dr. Ernest K. Ralston, PG, EMT-P
Center of Asymmetric Emergency
    Medicine and Training, Inc.
Centreville, Virginia

Kevin Ramdayal, NREMT-P
FDNY EMS Academy
Bayside, New York

Kenneth D. Raynor, BS, NRP
Primary Instructor Emergency Medicine
Joint Special Operations Medical Training
    Center, USASWCS
Fort Bragg, North Carolina

William Raynovich, NREMTP, EdD, MPH
Creighton University
Omaha, Nebraska

Curtis A. Rhodes, AAS, NRP, CCEMT-P
Gordon Cooper Technology Center
Shawnee, Oklahoma

Chris Rock, RN, MSN
Paramedic Program Director
City of Tacoma Fire Department
Tacoma, Washington

Hector Roman, RN, EMT-P, TP-C
Reva Air Ambulance
Fort Lauderdale, Florida

Jamie Rossborough, NRP, CCEMT-P, FP-C
Captain/Paramedic
Sunset Fire Department
Sunset, Utah
University of Utah
Salt Lake City, Utah

Jose V. Salazar, MPH, CEMSO, CTO, NRP
Loudoun County Fire and Rescue
Leesburg, Virginia

Keith A. Sharisky, NRP
Aberdeen Fire/Rescue
Aberdeen, South Dakota

Jeb Sheidler, MPAS, PA-C, ATC, NRP
Executive Director, Trauma Services
Lutheran Hospital
Fort Wayne, Indiana
Training Officer Bath Township Fire
    Department
Tactical Paramedic, Allen County Sheriff's
    Office
Lima, Ohio

Karla Short, EMT-P, BBA, MEd
Columbus State Community College
Columbus, Ohio

Warren Short Jr, BS, NRP
Virginia Department of Health, Office
    of EMS
Glen Allen, Virginia

Douglas P. Skinner, MPA, NRP, NCEE
SCS Safety, Health and Security
    Associates LLC
Leesburg, Virginia
Prince George's Community College
Largo, Maryland

Jason P. Smith, MS
Barry University
Miami Shores, Florida

Jeremy Smith, Instructor, NRP
Joint Special Operations Medical Training
    Center
Fort Bragg, North Carolina

**Scott A. Smith, MSN, APRN-CNP,
ACNP-BC, CEN, NRP, I/C**
Yarmouth, Maine

Andrew Snodgrass, NREMT-P, EMSI
Creighton University EMS Education
Omaha, Nebraska

Sandra A. Sokol
Monroe Technology Center/Loudoun
    County Fire Rescue Training Academy
Leesburg, Virginia
Captain, Battalion 4 Station 18
Dale City Volunteer Fire Department
Dale City, Virginia

Mark Spangenberg, CCEMTP/IC
Milwaukee Area Technical College
Milwaukee, Wisconsin

Sara Sproule, NRP, CCEMT-P
Prince William County Department of Fire
    and Rescue
Prince William County, Virginia

Nathan Stanaway, BS, NRP
Greenville Technical College
Greenville, South Carolina

Lieutenant Bruce J. Stark, NRP, TP-C
Fairfax County Fire and Rescue
    Department
Fairfax, Virginia

**Andrew W. Stern, NRP, CCEMT-P,
MPA, MA**
Clinical Instructor
Hudson Valley Community College
Rensselaer, New York

Melissa J. Stoddard, NRP, MPH
Tacoma Community College
Tacoma, Washington

Jonathan C. Stone, MPA, NRP, FP-C
Herriman, Utah

Holly Ann Sturdevant, NRP, CC
Old Dominion EMS Alliance
Richmond, Virginia

**Bruce Swanson, Paramedic,
EMS Captain**
Huntsville Fire & Rescue
Huntsville Fire & Rescue Training
    Academy
Huntsville, Alabama

Benjamin D. Symonds, BA, NRP
Kirkwood Community College
Cedar Rapids, Iowa

Justin G. Tilghman, MS, CEM, EMTP
Lenoir Community College
Kinston, North Carolina

Scott Tomek, MA, Paramedic
Manager, Quality/Safety/Risk
Allina Health EMS
Risk Manager-Allina Corporate Security
St. Paul, Minnesota
Clinical Skills Instructor
University of Minnesota School
    of Medicine
Emergency Medicine Program
Minneapolis, Minnesota
Paramedic
Woodbury Public Safety
Woodbury, Minnesota

Stephen Trala, MPH, BSN, RN, NRP
The University of Vermont Medical Center
    Health Net Transport
Burlington, Vermont

Amy E. Trujillo, NREMT-P, BS
Montana Medical Transport
Helena, Montana

Brian Turner, CCEMT-P, RN
Trinity Medical Center
Rock Island, Illinois

William H. (Bill) Turner, MS, NRP
Program Director-Emergency Medical
    Technology
Shawnee State University
Portsmouth, Ohio

Micheal D. Vance Jr, NRP, LP, BA
Education Coordinator
MedStar Training Academy
Fort Worth, Texas

Scott Vanderkooi, BS, NRP
University of South Alabama
Department of EMS Education
Mobile, Alabama

Leo Vanderpool, EMT-P
Fire Department of the City of New York
New York, New York

Athanasios T. Viglis, NRP
Fire Fighter
Henrico County Division of Fire
Henrico, Virginia

Jimmy Walker, NREMT-P
Midlands EMS
West Columbia, South Carolina

Jon Walker, NRP
Upper Valley Ambulance (retired)
Fairlee, Vermont

Kelly Walsh, RN, BSN, PHRN
Advanced Medical Transport
Peoria, Illinois

Tom Watson, AS, AAS, Paramedic
Adjunct Instructor
Texas A&M University System, Texas
    Engineering Extension Service, EMS/
    Public Health Grant Program
College Station, Texas

Gregory West, EdD, JD, NRP
Waukesha County Technical College
Pewaukee, Wisconsin

Monette Wiedlebacher, BA, EI, Paramedic
Stark State College
North Canton, Ohio

Michael H. Wilhelm, CRNA, APRN
Integrated Anesthesia Associates, School
    of Nurse Anesthesia
Hartford, Connecticut

Dustin Williams, BS, NRP
Deputy Chief
Christiansburg Rescue
Christiansburg, Virginia

**Karen "Keri" Wydner Krause, RN, CCRN,
EMT-P**
Lakeshore Technical College
Cleveland, Wisconsin

**David Yarmesch, BSOL, CSSGB, AAS-EMS,
Paramedic, EMSI**
EMS Coordinator
The MetroHealth System
Adjunct Faculty
Cuyahoga Community College
Cleveland, Ohio

▶ Photoshoot Acknowledgments

We would like to thank the following people and institutions for their collaboration on the photoshoots for this project. Their assistance was greatly appreciated.

Technical Consultants and Institutions

UMass Memorial Paramedics—Worcester EMS
Worcester, Massachusetts

Richard A. Nydam, AS, NREMT-P
Training and Education Specialist, EMS
UMassMemorial Paramedics—Worcester EMS
Worcester, Massachusetts

Centre for Emergency Health Sciences
Bulverde Spring Branch Emergency Services
Spring Branch, Texas

Stephen J. Rahm, NRP
Deputy Chief, Office of Clinical Direction
Co-Chair, Centre for Emergency Health Sciences
Bulverde Spring Branch Emergency Services
Spring Branch, Texas

Scotty Bolleter, BS, EMT-P
Chief, Office of Clinical Direction
Chair, Centre for Emergency Health Sciences
Bulverde Spring Branch Emergency Services
Spring Branch, Texas

Equipment

Jerry Flanagan
Account Manager
BoundTree Medical
Dublin, Ohio

Rachel Jackson, NREMT-P
Paramedic
UMass Memorial Paramedics—Worcester EMS
Worcester, Massachusetts

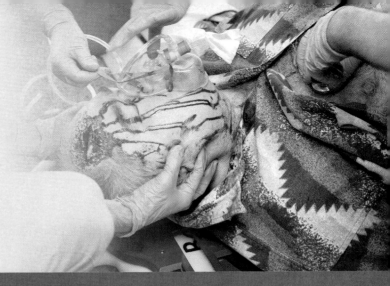

SECTION 7

Trauma

Trauma Systems and Mechanism of Injury

National EMS Education Standard Competencies

Trauma

Integrates assessment findings with principles of epidemiology and pathophysiology to formulate a field impression to implement a comprehensive treatment/disposition plan for an acutely injured patient.

Trauma Overview

Pathophysiology, assessment, and management of the trauma patient
> Trauma scoring (p 1568)
> Rapid transport and destination issues (pp 1566, 1569-1573)
> Transport mode (p 1573)

Multisystem Trauma

Recognition, pathophysiology, assessment, and management of
> Multisystem trauma (pp 1545-1546, 1566-1569)

Pathophysiology, assessment, and management of
> Blast injuries (pp 1561-1564)

Knowledge Objectives

1. Define trauma, including how it relates to energy, kinetics, and biomechanics. (pp 1542-1543)
2. Describe some of the factors that affect types of injuries. (pp 1543-1544)
3. Define mechanism of injury and index of suspicion, including how each one relates to paramedics' assessment of trauma. (pp 1543-1544)
4. Explain multisystem trauma and the special considerations that are required for patients who fit this category. (pp 1545-1546)
5. Define blunt trauma, including an example of the mechanism of injury that would cause blunt trauma. (p 1546)
6. Describe how impact patterns can help paramedics determine or predict injury types following motor vehicle crashes (MVCs). (pp 1546-1548)
7. Name the five types of MVCs and the injury patterns associated with each one. (pp 1548-1552)
8. Describe the benefits of seat belt restraints during a MVC. (pp 1552-1554)
9. Name the four types of impacts in motorcycle crashes. (pp 1554-1555)
10. Describe the three predominant mechanisms of injury during a vehicle versus pedestrian collision. (pp 1555-1556)
11. Explain the five factors to consider when assessing a patient who has been injured in a fall. (pp 1556-1557)
12. Define penetrating trauma, including the mechanisms of injury that would cause low-, medium-, and high-velocity injuries to occur. (p 1557)
13. Explain the factors to consider when assessing a patient who has sustained a gunshot wound. (pp 1558-1560)
14. Discuss primary, secondary, tertiary, quaternary (miscellaneous), and quinary blast injuries, including the damage to the body that is anticipated with each one. (pp 1561-1562)
15. Describe the components that affect the speed, duration, and pressure of the blast shock wave. (p 1562)
16. Explain the special considerations when assessing and managing a patient with a blast injury. (pp 1563-1564)
17. Outline the major components of trauma patient assessment, including special considerations related to multisystem trauma. (pp 1564-1567)
18. Explain trauma management, including special considerations related to multisystem trauma and the trauma lethal triad. (pp 1568-1569)
19. Summarize the American College of Surgeons Committee on Trauma and US Centers for Disease Control and Prevention field triage decision scheme for criteria for referral to a trauma center. (pp 1569-1572)
20. Summarize the American College of Surgeons Committee on Trauma classification of trauma centers and how it relates to making an appropriate destination selection for a trauma patient. (pp 1572-1573)
21. Explain trauma patient management in relation to scene time and transport selection, and the Association of Air Medical Services criteria for the appropriate use of emergency air medical services. (p 1573)

Skills Objectives

There are no skills objectives for this chapter.

Introduction

According to the US Centers for Disease Control and Prevention (CDC), trauma is the primary cause of death and disability in people between ages 1 and 44 years.[1] Improvements in health care and better management of chronic diseases have significantly decreased death rates in younger age groups due to conditions such as heart disease, neoplasms, cerebrovascular events, and respiratory illnesses.

Basic concepts of the mechanics and biomechanics of trauma will help you analyze and manage your patient's injuries. Analyzing a trauma scene is a vital skill because at the scene you are the eyes and ears of the emergency department (ED) physicians. Your documentation is the *only* source available to physicians and surgeons to understand the events and mechanisms that led to your trauma patient's chief complaint. Your documentation is crucial to help visualize and search for injuries that may not be apparent on physical exam.

Trauma, Energy, and Kinetics

Trauma is the acute physiologic and structural change (injury) that occurs in a patient's body when an external source of energy affects the body beyond its ability to sustain and dissipate it **Figure 29-1** .

Words of Wisdom

The top five causes of death from unintentional injury in the United States are poisoning, motor vehicle crashes, falls, choking and suffocation, and drowning.[2]

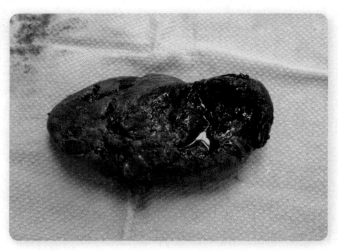

Figure 29-1 Traumatic injury occurs when body tissues are exposed to energy levels beyond their tolerance. Some traumatic injuries may not be visible. This photo shows a ruptured spleen.
© Medical Images RM/Barry Slaven, MD, PhD.

If a body—your patient's body—is in a vehicle that collides into a wall, then the energy of the moving vehicle is released when the vehicle is stopped by the wall. Your patient's body is moving at the same speed as the vehicle, and his or her body does not have bumpers to absorb the energy from stopping. If the energy is not absorbed in other ways, then the patient's body will absorb it, often resulting in broken bones and ruptured internal organs—what you see as traumatic injuries.

Different forms of energy produce different kinds of trauma. These external energy sources can be mechanical, chemical, thermal, electrical, and barometric.

Mechanical energy is energy from motion. Mechanical energy is subdivided into **kinetic energy (KE)**—such as a moving vehicle and **potential energy**—energy stored

---

YOU are the Paramedic   PART 1

You and your partner are enjoying the warm evening breeze, watching people stroll to the nearby mall and amusement park. You see someone running out of a crowd toward the ambulance, waving frantically, just as the dispatcher reports an injury in the amusement park. The person running toward you shouts, "Someone fell! I don't know what happened—in the park—please hurry!" You hear the dispatcher's voice, over the shouts of the people, "Report of a fall from the Ferris wheel at Sixth Avenue Amusements. Park first aid employees on the scene requesting a rush."

As you arrive at the entrance, a man with a radio is waving you into the gate. He runs ahead, clearing people off of the narrow pathway. There is loud music and a large crowd. As you approach, you see a female teenager, supine, contorted, and unmoving, on the ground beneath the Ferris wheel.

1. Looking up at the Ferris wheel, what possible mechanisms of injury (MOIs) should you consider?
2. In addition to determining the trauma sustained in the fall, what other information might you want to elicit from witnesses and friends of the patient?

in an object, such as a brick sitting on a building ledge. KE would be found in the force of two moving vehicles colliding. Potential energy would be present in an object sitting at a height. In that case, gravity would be the *potential* source of energy that converts to KE if the object falls. **Chemical energy** is the energy released as a result of a chemical reaction and can be found in an explosive or an acid or even from a reaction to an ingested or medically delivered agent or drug. **Thermal energy** is energy transferred from sources that are hotter than the body, such as a flame, hot water, and steam. **Electrical energy** comes in the form of high-voltage electrocution or a lightning strike. **Barometric energy** can result from sudden and radical changes in pressure, as can occur during scuba diving or flying.

Biomechanics is the study of the physiology and mechanics of a living organism using the tools of mechanical engineering. Biomechanics provides a way of analyzing the mechanisms and results of trauma sustained by the human body. **Kinetics** studies the relationships among speed, mass, direction of the force, and, for paramedics, the physical injury caused by speed, mass, and force. Knowledge of kinetics can help you predict injury patterns found in your patient.

▶ Factors Affecting Types of Injuries

The kind of injury resulting after trauma is sustained will be determined by the ability of the patient's body to disperse the energy delivered by the traumatic event. The bodies of some patients can adequately stretch and bend to absorb the energy of the traumatic event, while the bones and tissues of other patients cannot absorb the energy. A healthy football player, for example, can absorb a hit on the playing field easier than an older person with diminished bone and muscle mass.

External factors that determine types of injuries include the amount of *force* and *energy* delivered. The amount of injury your patient sustains varies with the size (or mass) of the objects delivering the force, with the velocity of the object (how fast the object is traveling), with acceleration or deceleration (how fast the object speeds up or slows down), and with the body area affected by the force that is being applied. The primary reasons for the extent of trauma your patients sustain are the amount of energy in the object and the mechanism by which the object is delivered to their bodies. The body would experience more widespread trauma from a cannon ball (more surface area and mass) than it would from a bullet (traveling the same speed), although both would likely be lethal.

Duration and direction of the force of application are also important. In motor vehicle crashes (MVCs), you must learn to recognize the directional patterns in injuries from frontal or head-on impacts, side or lateral impacts, and rear-end impacts. The larger the area of force dissipation, the more the pressure is reduced to a specific spot on the body, often without breaking the skin. Injury

from a bullet is less severe if the energy of the bullet is dissipated over the ceramic plate inside a bulletproof vest than if all the force of the bullet is applied at a small location on the skin.

In trauma medicine, this spreading of impact without breaking the skin is defined as **blunt trauma**. Emergency medical services (EMS) providers at all levels learn quickly in the field that blunt trauma is difficult to diagnose because there is often little external damage. Study kinetics to help you recognize this lethal, but almost invisible, trauma.

Words of Wisdom

Suspect a spinal injury when you see a cracked windshield, steering wheel or dashboard damage, intrusion into a vehicle, or an open ankle fracture after a fall. It will make a difference in how you approach the ABCDEs.

The *duration of force application* affects trauma because rapidly applied amounts of energy are less tolerated than an identical amount of energy delivered over a longer period of time. Rapidly delivered energy causes broken wrists, whereas longer term energy delivery might show up as repetitive stress injuries—even though the total amount of energy ultimately might be exactly the same.

The position of the trauma patient—how he or she is positioned—at the time of the event is an external factor. Seat belt use has significantly reduced the number of lethal injuries by keeping occupants in positions less likely to cause fatal injuries.

Injuries sustained when the break point of an organ is exceeded are often easier to identify. In the skin, they include contusions, abrasions, lacerations, punctures, and degloving injuries. Bones will fracture or splinter. The viscera covering structures of internal organs will have ruptures, or disruptions.

The *impact resistance of body parts* will also have a bearing on types of tissue disruptions. Impact resistance is often determined by what is inside your patient's organs: gas, liquid, or solid.

Biomechanical engineers measure the densities of tissues that are traumatized. As a paramedic, you need to know that organs with gas inside, such as in the lungs and intestinal tract, will scatter energy more than liquid or solid boundaries. This means the organ around the gas will be easily compressed, so look for lung and intestinal trauma first. Liquid-containing organs include the vascular system, the liver, the spleen, and muscle. Liquid-containing tissues are less compressible than tissues containing gases. Solid density interfaces occur mostly in bones such as in the cranium, spine, and long bones.

Because many injuries are not obvious on first presentation, having an understanding of the effects of forces and energy transfer patterns will help you in the assessment of the **mechanism of injury (MOI)**, which can also help predict the most likely type of injuries you will

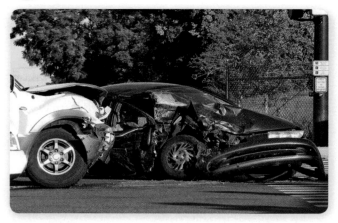

Figure 29-2 The appearance of the vehicle can provide you with crucial information about the severity of the crash and the possible injuries to the occupants.
© jcpjr/Shutterstock.

see when you are in the field Figure 29-2 . You need to learn to have a high **index of suspicion** for injuries that otherwise might be undetected for several hours. Anticipate the possibility of specific types of injuries. If you do, then it will help your patient and the trauma team who depend on your assessment of the scene. Be quick and deliberate with your primary survey and interventions to help prevent further problems for your patient.

▶ Kinetics

Although some drivers of motor vehicles might not obey the community's traffic laws, they must—whether they want to or not—obey the laws of physics that govern all objects. Familiarity with these laws will help you understand more about the mechanisms of trauma.

Velocity (V) is speed at which an object travels in a given unit of time. The difference between velocity and speed is that velocity is also defined by moving in a specific direction. **Acceleration (a)** of an object is the rate of change of velocity that an object is subjected to, whether speeding up or slowing down. **Gravity (g)** is the downward acceleration that is imparted to any object moving toward the earth caused by the effect of the earth's mass. During each second of a fall, the velocity or speed of the falling object increases by 9.8 m/sec^2 (approximately 32 ft/sec^2).

Words of Wisdom

Some situations may have contraindications or relative contraindications for aeromedical transport. These situations include traumatic cardiac arrest, inclement weather conditions, extremely combative patients, morbidly obese patients, patients with barotrauma (diving injuries may necessitate lower flying altitudes), and situations in which ground transport and appropriate level of care are available and would permit quicker care.

As mentioned previously, the KE of an object is the energy associated with the movement of the object. It reflects the relationship between the weight (mass) of the object and the velocity at which it is traveling. It is expressed mathematically as:

$$\text{Kinetic energy} = \frac{\text{Mass}}{2} \times \text{Velocity}^2$$

$$or, \; \text{KE} = \frac{m}{2} \times V^2$$

As you can see, velocity has a much greater effect on KE than mass because velocity is squared while mass (or weight) is divided in half.

In other words, KE increases more by increasing velocity than it does by increasing mass. The KE of an object involved in a crash must be dissipated as the object comes to rest. The KE of a motor vehicle in motion that stops suddenly must be transformed or applied to another object (damaging that object) Figure 29-3 . In a motor vehicle, KE can be dissipated by braking, which transforms the KE into heat (another form of energy). However, if all the energy is not transformed into heat, then the remaining KE will be applied to deform the structure of the motor vehicle, which results in damage to the vehicle and potentially to its occupants. The mechanics of dissipation of energy can easily result in injury. For example, a motor vehicle traveling at 35 mph hits a wall, which stops the vehicle, but the driver is still traveling at 35 mph until restrained by the seat belt or the airbag, or worse (if not wearing a seat belt) the steering wheel, dashboard, or windshield.

Speed affects energy exponentially. Consider what happens when velocity increases by 10 mph versus a 10-pound (6-kg) increase in a person's weight Table 29-1 .

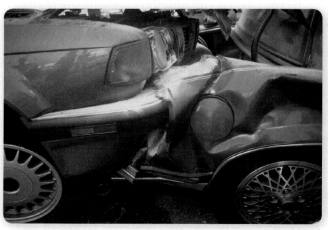

Figure 29-3 The kinetic energy of a speeding vehicle is converted into the work of stopping the vehicle, usually by crushing the vehicle's exterior.
© Terry Dickson, Florida Times-Union/AP Photo.

Table 29-1	Effects of Velocity and Weight	
Miles per hour	**150-lb patient**	**160-lb patient**
10	7,500 KE units	8,000 KE units
20	30,000 KE units	32,000 KE units
30	67,500 KE units	72,000 KE units
40	120,000 KE units	128,000 KE units
50	187,500 KE units	200,000 KE units

Abbreviation: KE, kinetic energy

© Jones & Bartlett Learning.

Note, when weight increases by 10 pounds (6 kg) but velocity remains the same, there is not much change in the KE. However, when the velocity increases from 40 to 50 mph (a difference of only 10 mph), for the 160-pound person, the KE increases by 72,000 KE units!

Modern vehicles are designed with crumple zone areas that maximize the amount of energy absorbed by deformation before the passenger compartment is involved. Because the damaged vehicle will often give you some indication of how fast the vehicle was traveling, you can use the information to help you decide whether to transfer your patient to a trauma center.

In addition to the velocity at which the vehicle, and its occupants, are traveling, the vehicle's **angle of impact** (front impact versus side impact, or how your patient hit the inside of a vehicle), the differences in the sizes of the two vehicles, and the restraint status and protective gear of the occupants will affect the amount of energy dissipation that affects your patients in a crash. Consider, if two vehicles are involved, then each one contributes KE to the crash, so a head-on or frontal crash of two vehicles traveling 60 mph would be the equivalent of one vehicle hitting a stationary object at 120 mph.

Remember the laws of physics that no driver can break? Here's a quick review. The **law of conservation of energy** states energy can be neither created nor destroyed; it can only change form. Energy generated from a sudden stop or start must be transformed to one of the following energy forms: thermal, electrical, chemical, radiant, or mechanical (as discussed earlier).

Energy dissipation is the process by which KE is transformed into one of these forms of mechanical energy. When a vehicle stops slowly, its KE is converted to thermal energy—heat—by friction of the braking action. If the vehicle crashes, KE is converted into mechanical energy as the vehicle body crumples in the crash. Mechanical energy is further dissipated in the form of injury as the occupants sustain fractures or other bodily harm.

Protective devices such as seat belts, airbags, and helmets are designed to manipulate the way in which energy is dissipated. For example, a seat belt converts KE of the occupant into a seat belt-to-body pressure force rather than into a steering wheel deformation against the torso or a windshield shattering against the head.

Newton's first law of motion states a body at rest will remain at rest unless acted on by an outside force. Similarly, a body in motion tends to remain in motion at a constant velocity, traveling in a straight line, unless acted on by an outside force. Most bodies in motion (without the assistance of a motor or other propulsion device) tend to stop eventually due to the action of forces, such as friction, wind resistance, or other force resulting in deceleration.

Newton's second law of motion states the force that an object can exert is equal to the product of its mass times its acceleration:

$$\text{Force} = \text{Mass (Weight)} \times \text{Acceleration (or Deceleration)}$$

The greater an object's mass and/or acceleration, the greater the force that needs to be applied to either change of course of the object or stop the object. Force equals mass × acceleration (or deceleration). **Deceleration** is slowing down or slowing to a stop. Rapid deceleration, as may occur in a MVC, dissipates tremendous force and, therefore, creates the potential for major injuries. Deceleration and acceleration can also be measured in numbers of *g* forces. One *g* force is the normal acceleration due to gravity. A two- or three-*g* acceleration or deceleration force is, two or three times the force associated with the acceleration of gravity. A two-*g* deceleration force would make you feel like you are twice as heavy as you are at rest. Three-*g* acceleration force would make you feel three times heavier. High-speed MVCs can generate decelerations in hundreds of *g*s. The human limit to deceleration is about 30 *g*.

In a head-on collision involving two vehicles traveling in opposite directions, transferred energy is calculated based on the sum of the speeds of both vehicles. If a vehicle strikes an immovable object, forces generated come only from the speed of the moving object. In a rear impact of two vehicles traveling in the same direction, the energy is lower because it is calculated on the difference in speed between the vehicles, also known as the closing speed.

It is important to understand these laws of physics because they help define the types and patterns of trauma you will see in the field. You are the most important witness for the hospital trauma team. The information you learn from physics will help you affect the outcome of your patient's life.

Multisystem Trauma

Multisystem trauma describes injuries that involve several body systems. Examples of these injuries include trauma to the head and spine, chest and abdomen, or chest and multiple extremities. The body can compensate fairly well to an isolated injury, but it has a much harder time dealing with multiple injuries that involve several major body areas. In general, multisystem trauma is caused by events that affect the entire body, such as a MVC or a fall from a height. Often, both blunt and penetrating trauma occur, with a high level of morbidity and mortality. Be alert for multisystem trauma. Assess the patient's entire body if you suspect multiple body systems are affected by trauma. Prioritize how you will treat the injuries and transport multisystem trauma patients without delay.

Blunt Trauma

Injuries are generally described as the consequence of blunt or penetrating trauma. Blunt trauma refers to injuries in which body tissues are not penetrated by an external object Figure 29-4 . Blunt trauma commonly occurs in MVCs, in pedestrians hit by a vehicle, in motorcycle crashes, in falls from heights, in serious sports injuries, and in explosions where the pressure wave is the primary cause of the injuries.

▶ Motor Vehicle Crashes

In 2014, according to the National Highway Traffic Safety Administration, 32,675 people were killed in police-reported motor vehicle traffic crashes and 2.34 million people were injured.[3] That calculates to almost 90 people dying and more than 6,300 people being injured in MVCs every day in the United States.

When a motor vehicle collides with another object, there are five phases tied to the effects of progressive deceleration. The first phase, *deceleration of the vehicle*, occurs when the vehicle strikes another object and is brought to an abrupt stop. The forward motion of the vehicle continues until its KE is dissipated in the form of mechanical deformation and damage to the vehicle and the occupants, or until the restraining force of the object is removed (for example, sheared-off pole, or the yielding of a guard rail). The second phase is *deceleration of the*

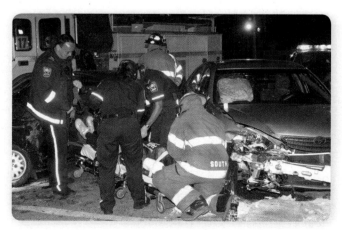

Figure 29-4 Blunt trauma typically occurs in motor vehicle crashes like this head-on collision.

© Jack Dagley Photography/Shutterstock.

occupants, which starts during sudden braking and continues until the occupants' forward motion is stopped by the vehicle. This results in deceleration, compression, and shear trauma to the occupants Figure 29-5 . The effects on vehicle occupants will vary depending on the mass of each occupant, protective mechanisms in the vehicle such as seat belts and airbags, body parts involved, and points of impact. The third phase, *deceleration of internal organs*, involves the body's supporting structures (skull, sternum, ribs, spine, and pelvis) and movable organs (brain, heart, liver, spleen, and intestine) that continue their forward momentum until stopped Figure 29-6 . Energy is absorbed

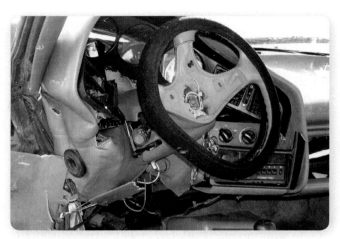

Figure 29-5 Deceleration of the occupant starts during sudden braking and continues during the impact of the crash. The appearance of the interior of the vehicle can provide you with information about the severity of the patient's injuries.

Courtesy of Captain David Jackson, Saginaw Township Fire Department.

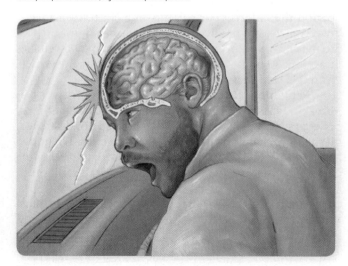

Figure 29-6 Deceleration of internal organs involves the body's supporting structures and movable organs that continue their forward momentum until stopped. In this illustration, the brain continues its forward motion and strikes the inside of the skull, resulting in a compression injury to the anterior portion of the brain and stretching of the posterior portion.

© Jones & Bartlett Learning.

by internal organs, resulting in injury. Moving fixed and suspended organs may result in tears and shearing injuries. The fourth phase is the result of *secondary collisions*, which occur when an occupant inside the vehicle is hit by objects moving within the vehicle, such as unsecured objects, packages, or other passengers. These objects may continue to travel at the vehicle's initial speed and hit an occupant who has come to rest. These types of collisions have been known to cause severe spine and head trauma. The final phase is the result of *additional impacts* that the vehicle

may receive, such as when it is hit by a second vehicle, or is deflected into another vehicle, tree, or other object. This may increase the severity of the original injuries or cause further injury. For example, a frontal impact may cause a posterior hip dislocation and an acetabular fracture via a dashboard mechanism, and a subsequent side impact from another vehicle may add a lateral compression pelvic ring injury, resulting in complex pelvic and acetabular trauma. Table 29-2 shows the structural clues, body clues, and resulting injuries for different types of crashes.

Table 29-2	Mechanism of Injury: Motor Vehicle Crash	
Structural Clues	**Body Clues**	**Potential Injuries**
Head-on or Frontal Impact		
Deformed front end Cracked windshield	Bruised or lacerated head or face	Brain injury Scalp, facial cuts Cervical spine injury Tracheal injury
Deformed steering column	Bruised neck Bruised chest	Sternal or rib fracture Flail chest Myocardial contusion Pericardial tamponade Pneumothorax or hemothorax Exsanguination from aortic tear
Deformed dashboard	Bruised abdomen Bruised knee, dislocated kneecap	Ruptured spleen, liver, bowel, diaphragm Fractured patella Dislocated knee Femoral fracture Dislocated hip
Lateral or Side Impact		
Deformed side of vehicle	Bruised shoulder	Clavicular fracture Fractured humerus Multiple rib fractures
Door smashed in	Bruised shoulder or pelvis	Fractured hip Fractured iliac wing Fractured clavicle or ribs
"B" pillar deformed	Bruised temple	Brain injury Cervical spine fracture
Broken door or window handles	Bruised or deformed arms	Contusions
Broken window glass	Dicing lacerations	Multiple lacerations
Rear-end Impact		
Posterior deformity of the auto	Secondary anterior injuries, especially if the patient was unrestrained	Whiplash injuries Deceleration injuries of a head-on impact
Headrest not adjusted	None detected	Bleeding, bruising, or tearing inside skull

Impact Patterns

Important clues to predict injury types can be obtained by paying attention to details regarding the history of the crash and by examining the scene. Using your knowledge of the physics of trauma, you can make a good estimate of how injured your patients might be by looking at the amount of damage around the scene. How dented and deformed the vehicle looks is a clear indication of the forces involved and of the degree of deceleration sustained by your patient. Dents and deformities on the inside of the vehicle will show you the point of impact on the patient. Do a quick check for injury types visible on your patient: head injury or seat belt marks indicate what parts of the body may have been involved in energy absorption. Tire skid marks at the scene indicate whether significant energy was dissipated by braking before the crash. Debris along the course of the crash may indicate multiple collisions and different force vectors acting on the patient along the course of the crash.

There are primarily five types of impact patterns in MVCs:

- Frontal or head-on impact
- Lateral or side impact
- Rear impact
- Rotational or quarter-panel impact
- Rollovers

Frontal or Head-on Impacts. In frontal or head-on impacts, the front end of the vehicle distorts as it dissipates KE and decelerates its forward motion. Passengers decelerate at the same rate as the vehicle. In a 30-mph crash, the front end of an average American vehicle will crush 2 feet at the rough estimate of 1 inch of deformity for each 1 mph. The forces applied to the driver will differ depending on the vehicle's design, materials, and safety features. The interior will also suggest possible injuries by the damage your patient's body has done to the dash, windshield, or steering wheel, for example.

Abrupt deceleration injuries are produced by a sudden stop of a body's forward motion. Whether from a fall, shaking a baby, or a high-speed MVC, decelerating forces can induce **shearing**, **avulsing**, or rupturing of organs and their restraining fascia, vasculature, nerves, and other soft tissues. These injuries are often invisible during the physical exam, so you need to understand how such injuries are sustained.

The head is particularly vulnerable to deceleration injuries. The brain is a fairly heavy organ that is suspended in fluid inside the skull. Any trauma that jerks the patient's head can cause the brain to strike the inside of the skull, potentially causing bleeding, bruising, or tearing injuries. All of these potential injuries are extremely dangerous and will not show up on a physical exam because they occur within the skull. Your index of suspicion should be on high alert for these injuries.

The chest is vulnerable to aortic injury. The aorta, the largest blood vessel in the body, is the most common site of deceleration injury in the chest. The aorta is often torn away from its points of fixation in the body. Shearing of the aorta due to rapid deceleration can result in loss of the total blood volume and immediate death.

Blunt abdominal trauma results as the forward motion of the body stops and internal organs continue their motion, causing tearing at the points of attachment, shearing injuries, and/or tearing of the abdominal walls. Organs that are commonly affected include the liver, kidneys, small intestine, large intestine, pancreas, and spleen.

Kidneys are injured as forward motion produces tears to the organ or to points of attachment with the abdominal aorta or the renal arteries. Also, as motion is restrained by the large bowel, the small bowel can tear and result in spillage of contents into the abdomen. Trauma can also cause damage without tearing by reducing the supply of blood to the bowel. The spleen can be torn as well, resulting in left upper quadrant pain and life-threatening internal bleeding.

Crush and compression injuries are the result of forces applied to the body by things external to the body at the time of impact. Crush and compression injuries occur at the time of impact. Crush and compression injuries are often caused by dashboards, windshields, the floor, or heavy objects falling on the body. Crush and compression injuries can also occur when the body or one of its parts gets trapped between two objects such as in a machine or the closing of a door.

Compression head injuries may result in skull fracture, and often are associated with cervical spine injury. Therefore, you can assume spinal cord injuries and severe injury to the brain when this mechanism is observed. Brain tissue does not compress well; it swells within the enclosed area of the skull when injured. As the brain swells inside the skull, it is compressed, causing a highly lethal condition.

Words of Wisdom

According to the National Highway Traffic Safety Administration statistics, the overall traffic fatality rate in the United States in 2014 dropped to 1.08 fatalities per 100 million vehicle miles traveled. This still represents a total of 32,675 fatalities in 2014.[3]

Compression injuries of the chest may produce fractured ribs that can lead to internal injuries of the lungs and heart. One of the signs of lung injury is a flail chest, a condition resulting from multiple consecutive rib fractures (two or more adjacent ribs broken in two or more places), in which the chest wall moves paradoxically (opposite of normal) with respirations. Fractured ribs may also cause air or blood to enter the chest cavity, leading to a pneumothorax or hemothorax, which would ultimately require decompression or placement of a chest tube. Blunt cardiac injury can compress the heart between the bones in the chest, causing dysrhythmias and direct injury to the heart muscle. If the lungs are compressed, then acute respiratory distress syndrome may result, requiring intubation and ventilatory assistance to maintain the patient's airway and breathing.

Almost all abdominal organs can be affected by hitting an external object. Organs often injured include the pancreas, spleen, liver, and, occasionally, the kidneys. Compression against the seat belt may result in bowel rupture, urinary bladder rupture, diaphragm tearing, and spinal injuries. The abdomen contains two of the body's largest blood vessels, the abdominal aorta and the inferior vena cava. Rupture of either of these large blood vessels can lead quickly to exsanguination.

Pelvic fractures also result from external compressive trauma, potentially injuring the urinary bladder, vagina, rectum, lumbar plexus, and pelvic floor and leading to severe bleeding from the iliac arteries.

Position at the precise time of impact is very important in determining an occupant's movements and injuries during a crash. Unrestrained occupants usually follow one of two trajectories, a *down-and-under pathway*, or an *up-and-over pathway* **Figure 29-7** .

The down-and-under pathway is traveled by an occupant who slides under the steering column or dash. As the vehicle is decelerating, the occupant continues to travel downward and forward into the dashboard or steering column, led by the knees. The knees hit the dashboard, transmitting the energy of the deceleration up the femurs to the pelvis. With knees locked in the dash and hips in the seat, force vectors go down the tibia and along the femur. If the feet are not locked by folding floorboards or brake pedals, then energy along the tibia will be transferred to the lower leg, with no immediate injury. If the feet are locked in place, then femur fracture can occur. In some cases, the head of the femur will dislocate. If the

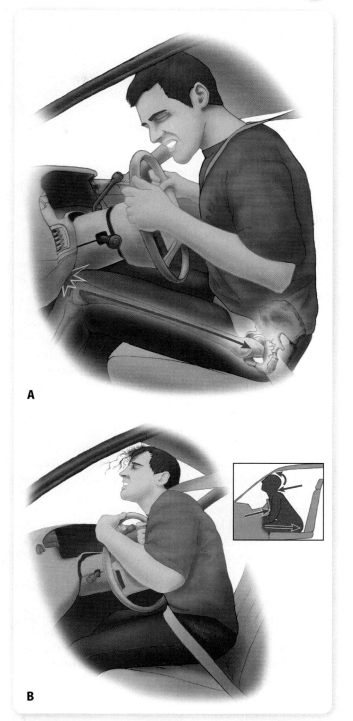

Figure 29-7 A. The down-and-under pathway. **B.** The up-and-over pathway.

© Jones & Bartlett Learning.

occupant's knees hit the dashboard, then anticipate a fracture-dislocation of the knee or other related injuries. Also, look for hip and pelvic fractures or hip dislocation. Your patient's torso can twist in such a way that his or her head hits the steering column. Always consider the possibility of spinal injuries.

The upper torso continues forward until it impacts the vehicle—the steering wheel, the dash, or the seat belt and airbag protection system. Look for rib fractures or pulmonary and cardiovascular injuries caused by internal compression. If your patient is a child, then assume there will be pulmonary or cardiac injuries—children have more flexible ribs but sustain compression injuries more often. Remember how gas-containing organs absorb more of the energy of the crash?

In the up-and-over pathway, the lead point is the head. In this sequence, rotation occurs around the ankles with the torso moving in an upward and forward direction. The head takes a higher trajectory, impacting the windshield, roof, mirror, or dashboard, causing compression and deceleration injuries that can include significant head and cervical spine trauma. The anterior part of the neck may strike the steering wheel, causing laryngeal fracture, serious lacerations, and other soft-tissue injury.

Ejection is possible if the windshield does not stop the body from penetrating through it. Ejection leads to second-impact injuries when the body comes in contact with the ground or objects outside of the vehicle. These injuries can be as severe as initial-impact injuries, and they increase the likelihood of great vessel damage and death. The spine absorbs energy as it is compressed between the stationary head and the moving torso, which leads to injury.

A dangerous lung injury may occur if your patient reflexively takes a deep breath just before impact, hyperinflating the lungs and closing the glottis. The impact of the steering wheel can injure the lungs by generating pressures in the lungs beyond the capabilities of the lung tissue, like a "paper bag being exploded." This often leads to a pneumothorax **Figure 29-8**.

The abdomen, pelvis, or upper thigh contacts the lower aspect of the steering wheel or dash, and lower leg fractures could be present. **Table 29-3** lists the "ring" of chest injuries that can occur from impact with the steering wheel or the dashboard.

Lateral or Side Impacts. Lateral or side (or T-bone) impacts impart energy to the near-side occupant directly to the pelvis and chest **Figure 29-9**. Unrestrained occupants will remain almost motionless, literally having the vehicle pushed out from under them. Seat belts do little to protect these passengers because they are designed to limit forward hinging injuries, not side impacts. As one vehicle makes contact with the side of the other vehicle,

the occupant nearest the impact is hit by the door of the vehicle as the passenger compartment begins to deform and collapse. As the passenger compartment deforms, the passenger's head can strike the impacting vehicle or object. Injury results from direct trauma to the affected side and to tension developed on the far side. Upper extremity trauma depends on the spatial orientation of the arm at impact. The shoulder frequently rotates outward and posteriorly, exposing the chest and ribs to injury. Forces transmitted to the chest may cause rib fractures, lateral flail chest, and lung contusions. If the humerus remains between the door and chest, then the clavicle may absorb side motion and fracture. As the body of the occupant is pushed in one direction, the head moves toward the impacting object, creating a line of tension along the contralateral side of the spine. This may result in ligamentous disruption and dislocation of the spine on the opposite side of the impact. The far-side occupant, if properly restrained, has the advantage of "riding down" with the vehicle, thereby receiving considerably less force. If unrestrained, then he or she may move in a direction parallel but opposite to the impact. This passenger receives forces similar to any unrestrained occupant. Furthermore, because both passengers travel in a direction parallel to impact but in opposite directions, they collide with each other, causing additional injury.

In a lateral crash, if the greater trochanter of the femur is impacted and transmits forces to the pelvis, sometimes it may be driven through the acetabulum into the pelvis. If the force reaches the ilium, then the pelvis may also fracture. The typical pattern of pelvic injury that occurs in this scenario is a lateral compression injury that trauma surgeons call pelvic ring disruption. Lateral compression injuries are less serious than anterior compression injuries. Death in lateral crashes is usually the result of associated torso or head injuries. Remember, the occupants of the other vehicle will most likely be subjected to the forces of a frontal impact.

Rear Impacts. Rear impacts or rear-end impacts have the most survivors, if the driver and passengers are properly restrained **Figure 29-10**. However, if the vehicle coming from the rear is traveling at an excessive speed, then the chance of survival is affected. Most often in this kind of crash, a stationary (or slower moving) vehicle is struck from behind and the impact energy is transmitted as a sudden forward accelerating force. The neck hyperextends as the body moves forward relative to the head. The head does not move forward with the body unless a headrest is in the proper position; if the headrest is not in proper position, the head is snapped back and then forward. Because most seats have some degree of elasticity after the sudden forward acceleration has ended, the stored potential energy in the seat is converted to an energy of forward motion, which can aggravate the hyperextension trauma to the neck and then follow with some rebound forward flexion of the head on the chest resulting in hyperflexion. A third episode of extension may occur as the chest moves forward. This is the so-called **whiplash** injury.

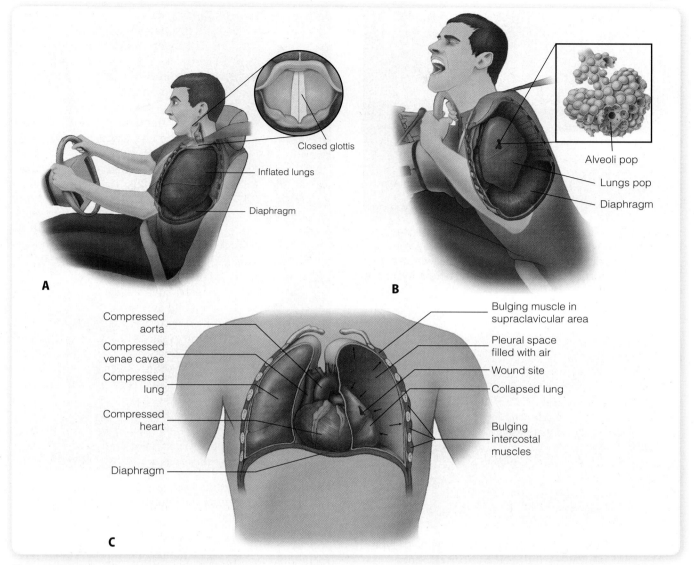

Figure 29-8 The paper-bag syndrome. **A.** The occupant takes a deep breath just before crashing, closing the glottis and filling the lungs with air. **B.** The occupant's chest hits the steering wheel, popping the alveoli in the lungs. **C.** A pneumothorax results.
© Jones & Bartlett Learning.

Table 29-3	**"Ring" of Chest Injuries From Impact With the Steering Wheel or Dashboard**

- Facial injuries
- Soft-tissue neck trauma
- Larynx and tracheal trauma
- Fractured sternum
- Myocardial contusion
- Pericardial tamponade
- Pulmonary contusion
- Hemothorax, rib fractures
- Flail chest
- Ruptured aorta
- Intra-abdominal injuries

© Jones & Bartlett Learning.

In a rear-impact crash, energy is imparted to the front vehicle, which accelerates rapidly, while frontal impact energy to the rear driver is reduced because energy is being transferred to the front vehicle. One concern with rear-impact crashes is the frequency with which seat backs collapse, causing unrestrained occupants to be propelled into the back seat. Head restraints, developed to prevent the head and torso from moving separately, are not always adjusted correctly. Many are placed too low and act as a fulcrum that may actually facilitate the extension injury. They need to be adjusted so they are behind the head and not behind the neck.

Rotational or Quarter-panel Impacts. A rotational or quarter-panel impact occurs when a lateral crash is off center. In this case, rotation occurs as part of the vehicle continues to move and part of the vehicle comes to a stop. The vehicle's forward motion stops at the point of impact,

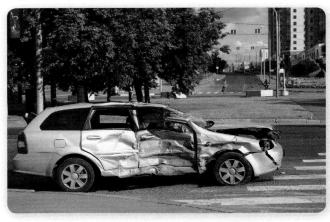

Figure 29-9 In a lateral impact, the vehicle may be struck above its center of gravity and begin to rock away from the side of impact. This causes a type of lateral whiplash in which the passenger's shoulders and head whip toward the intruding vehicle.
© Alexander Gordeyev/Shutterstock.

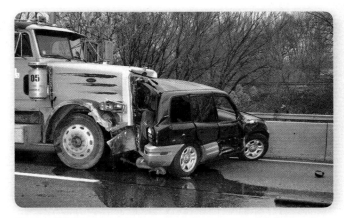

Figure 29-10 Rear-end impacts often cause whiplash-type injuries, particularly when the head and/or neck is not restrained by a headrest.
© Dennis Wetherhold, Jr.

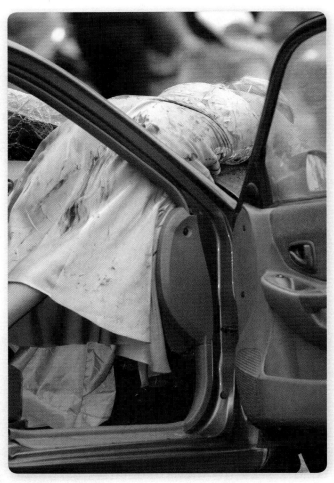

Figure 29-11 Occupants who have been ejected or partially ejected may have struck the interior of the vehicle many times before ejection.
© iStockphoto/Thinkstock/Getty.

but the side continues in rotational motion around the impact point. The point where the vehicle's greatest loss of speed occurs is where the greatest damage to the occupant will occur. The resultant forces act along a vector oblique to the direction of travel. For example, in a ten o'clock impact with twelve o'clock being frontal, the driver would initially move forward and then diagonally as the vehicle rotates, striking the A pillar, the support for the windshield. The front seat passenger would strike the rearview mirror area. The point of greatest deceleration becomes the location of the most severely injured patients. Occupants tend to receive a combination of frontal and lateral injuries. Because rigid objects may be in line with vector forces, head injuries may result. Three-point seat belts are effective in preventing injury in angled crashes of up to 45°.

Rollovers. Rollover scenarios have the greatest potential to cause lethal injuries. Injuries will be serious even if seat belts are worn. However, if your patients did not wear seat belts, they may be ejected, and/or they will have been struck hard against the interior of the vehicle with each change in direction the vehicle makes during the rollover. Even a restrained occupant's head and neck will change direction with each change in the vehicle's position.

The chance of death increase by eight times when an occupant is ejected from a vehicle[4] **Figure 29-11**. A partial ejection can result in injuries to an arm or leg from being caught between the vehicle and the ground.

Restrained Versus Unrestrained Occupants

Seat belts are highly effective because they stop the forward motion of any vehicle's occupant who is traveling at the same speed as the vehicle. The seat belt, although capable of delivering some injury at high speeds, will prevent the serious-to-fatal injuries caused by being unrestrained in the vehicle or being ejected from the vehicle. Many ejected patients sustain major and permanent cervical spine damage. Restrained occupants "ride down" the deceleration with belt elasticity and crush time of the vehicle, with a reduction in fatalities. Restraints limit the contact of the occupants with the interior of the vehicle, prevent ejection, distribute deceleration energy over a greater surface, and prevent the occupants from violently contacting each other. As a result, all types of injuries are decreased, including head, facial, spinal, thoracic, intra-abdominal, pelvic, and lower extremity, and ejection is also limited.

All arguments against seat belt use are unfounded. Every unrestrained passenger poses a hazard to themselves and to other occupants in the vehicle, especially for front seat passengers who are at higher risk for injury in a front-end crash if the back seat occupants are unrestrained.

Specific injuries associated with seat belt use include cervical fractures due to flexion stresses and neck sprains due to deceleration and hyperextension. Most serious injuries occur because the patient did not use the seat belt correctly. If the occupant does not use the shoulder strap, severe upper body injuries, including spinal injuries and decapitation, can occur. If the seat belt is placed above the pelvic bone, then abdominal injuries and lumbar spine injuries may result.

Airbags are another defense device in patient safety. The National Highway Traffic Safety Administration estimates airbags reduce deaths in direct frontal MVCs by about 30%.[5] Front airbags will not activate in side impact crashes or impacts to the front quarter panel, and without the use of a seat belt, they are insufficient to prevent ejection. Airbags are self-deflating and function only for a first impact, not a secondary one. The rapidly

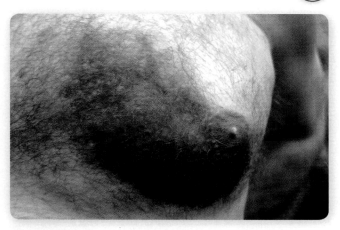

Figure 29-12 Air bags can cause abrasions, contusions, and traction-type injuries to the face, neck, chest, and inner arms.
© crozstudios/Alamy.

inflating bag can also result in secondary injuries from direct contact with the airbag or from the chemicals used to inflate it. Common injuries include abrasions to the face, chest, and arms; minor corrosive effects from irritation of the abrasions by the cornstarch used to load the airbag, chemical keratitis, conjunctivitis, or corneal abrasion, and inhalation injuries **Figure 29-12**.

YOU are the Paramedic   PART 2

The scene appears safe and stable. A park employee is kneeling on the grass beside the patient. You instruct her on how to hold and maintain cervical spine immobilization and call to the patient and try gently squeezing her shoulder. You do not get a response. You ask another employee to find the patient's friends.

You carefully open her mouth with a jaw-thrust maneuver. There is no evidence of blood, broken teeth, or foreign bodies; breathing seems adequate but rapid and shallow. As you attempt to insert an oropharyngeal airway (OPA), she gags and the OPA is removed.

Recording Time: 1 Minute	
Appearance	Unmoving, supine, legs bent to sides
Level of consciousness	U (unresponsive to verbal and painful stimuli)
Airway	Clear, does not tolerate an OPA
Breathing	Rapid, shallow
Circulation	Rapid, weak radial pulse

3. Because the patient is unresponsive with rapid, shallow breathing, you ask your partner to assist ventilations with a bag-mask device. What should you do next to continue your primary survey?
4. The patient's friend comes forward and tearfully explains that her friend, who is a diabetic and was drinking "a few shots of tequila" earlier in the evening, was standing up in the Ferris wheel ride, yelling and waving to her boyfriend, when the ride suddenly jerked to a stop, sending her tumbling out of the car. What important questions will you ask the friend?

Small children can be severely injured or killed if airbags inflate while they are in the front seat. That is why all EMS providers are encouraged to participate in teaching parents how to properly place and secure children's car seats.

Special Populations

Pregnant women in general may wear seat belts less frequently than do nonpregnant women owing to discomfort or the unproven concern that the seat belt may increase damage to the unborn child in the case of a crash. However, no study has reported that seat belts increase fetal mortality. If lap belts are worn alone and too high, they allow enough forward flexion and subsequent compression to rupture the uterus because deceleration forces are transmitted directly to the uterus. Lap belts with shoulder harnesses are essential to provide equal distribution of forces and to prevent forward flexion of the mother. Without the shoulder harness, the protuberant uterus will also receive the impact of the steering wheel or dashboard.

Motorcycle Crashes

In 2014, there were 4,586 motorcyclists killed in the United States compared with 4,692 motorcycle-related deaths in 2013. Although fatalities declined between 2013 and 2014, motorcycle injuries increased by 4.5%. In 2014, an estimated 92,000 motorcyclists were injured in motorcycle crashes compared with 88,000 in 2013.[3]

In a motorcycle crash, any structural protection afforded to the riders is not derived from a steel cage, as is the case in a vehicle, but from protective devices worn by the rider—that is, helmet, leather or abrasion-resistant clothing, and boots. While helmets are designed to protect against impact forces to the head, they transmit any impact into the cervical spine, and as such, do not protect against severe cervical spine injury. Leather and synthetic gear worn over the body were initially designed to protect professional riders in competition, where falls tend to be controlled and result in long sliding mechanisms on hard surfaces rather than multiple crashes against road objects and other vehicles. Leather clothing will protect mostly against road abrasion but offers no protection against blunt trauma from secondary impacts. In a street crash, impacts occur usually against other larger vehicles or stationary objects.

Special Populations

Increased morbidity and mortality, especially chest trauma, is more common in geriatric patients, particularly rib and sternal fractures. Fatalities also increase if child restraint devices are improperly installed or used. Children who have outgrown a car seat but are too small to be restrained by seat belts designed for adults are at risk for hyperflexion and abdominal injury.

When you assess the scene of a motorcycle crash, give attention to the deformity of the motorcycle, the side of most damage, the distance of skid in the road, the deformity of stationary objects or other vehicles, and the extent and location of deformity in the helmet **Figure 29-13** . These findings can help you estimate the extent of trauma in a patient.

There are four types of motorcycle impacts:

- **Head-on impact.** In a *head-on impact*, the motorcycle strikes another object and stops its forward motion while the rider and any parts of the motorcycle that are broken off

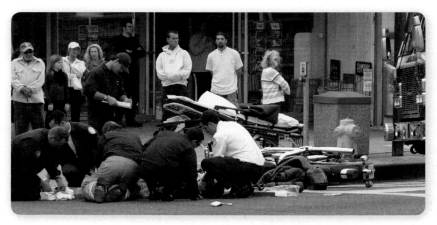

Figure 29-13 At a motorcycle crash scene, attention should be given to the deformity of the motorcycle, the side of most damage, the distance of skid in the road, the deformity of stationary objects or other vehicles, and the extent and location of deformity in the helmet.

© Michael Ledray/Shutterstock.

continue propelling forward until they are stopped by an outside force, such as contact with the road or another opposing force from a secondary crash. Because the motorcycle's center of gravity is above the front axle, there is a forward and upward motion at the point of the impact, causing the rider to go over the handlebars. If the rider's feet remain on the pegs or pedals, then the forward and upward motion of the upper torso is restrained by the femurs and tibias, producing bilateral femur or tibia fractures and severe foot injuries.

For motorcycles with a low riding seat below the level of the gas tank, such as Japanese racing bikes or Italian transalpine style motorcycles, the tank can act as a wedge on the pelvis during the initial phase of the crash. This can result in severe anterior-posterior compression injuries to the pelvis that can cause severe neurovascular compromise. Open pelvic fractures are also common, resulting in severe perineal injuries with loss of the pelvic floor.

- **Angular impact.** In an *angular impact*, the motorcycle strikes an object or another vehicle at such an angle that the rider sustains direct crushing injuries to the lower extremity between the object and the motorcycle. This usually results in severe open and comminuted lower extremity injuries with severe neurovascular compromise, possibly requiring surgical amputation.

Traumatic amputations are also common high-speed injuries. After the initial crush injury to the lower extremity, mechanisms such as those described in a head-on impact also apply. Often the rider is propelled over the hood of the colliding vehicle. Because the impact is at an angle, severe thoracoabdominal torsion and lateral bending spine injuries can result, in addition to head injury and pelvic trauma.

- **Ejection.** An *ejected* rider will travel at high speed until stopped by a stationary object, by another vehicle, or by contact with the road. Severe abrasion injuries (road rash) down to bone can occur. An unpredictable combination of blunt injuries can occur from secondary crashes.

- **Laying the bike down.** A technique used to separate the rider from the body of the motorcycle and the object to be hit is referred to as *laying the bike down*. It was developed by motorcycle racers and adapted by street bikers as a means of achieving a controlled crash. As a crash approaches, the motorcycle is turned flat and tipped sideways at a 90° angle to the direction of travel so that one leg is dropped to the grass or asphalt. This slows the rider faster than the motorcycle, allowing for the rider to become separated from the motorcycle. If

properly protected with leather or synthetic abrasion-resistant gear, then injuries should be limited to those sustained by rolling over the pavement and any secondary crash that may occur. When executed properly, this maneuver prevents the rider from being trapped between the bike and the object. However, a rider who is unable to clear the bike will collide into the vehicle, often with devastating results.

Special Populations

Changes in vision, hearing, posture, and motor ability predispose older people to a greater risk of being struck by a vehicle.

With any type of crash, the helmet should be removed carefully if airway management techniques cannot be performed with the helmet in place or the helmet does not fit snuggly to the head. Assume any dents and abrasions have caused cervical spine fractures until proven otherwise by radiographs. Take precautions when removing the helmet. It should be cut if it cannot be removed without introducing further deformation to the neck.

Bicycles and off-road vehicles, such as four-wheelers and snowmobiles, are capable of producing injuries similar to those from motorcycles, with a few differences. Possibly the biggest difference with injuries from off-road vehicles is that reaching the patients is often a challenge. If the traumatic event happens in a remote location, then you must make immediate decisions about issues such as what medical equipment to take to the location and how you will evacuate the patients. Also, in these types of situations patients are often not wearing helmets or other safety equipment that motorcycle riders often employ. Although bicycle riders who are hit by motor vehicles are more likely to be wearing a helmet, they will sustain injuries similar to those found in pedestrians struck by motor vehicles.

▶ Pedestrian Injuries

In 2014, there were 4,884 traffic fatalities in the United States involving pedestrians, a 2.2% increase from 2013. The largest number of pedestrians killed was in the group age 50 to 54 years; children younger than age 14 years accounted for about 19% of the deaths. The greatest number of deaths (26%) occurred between 1800 and 2059 hours, and an additional 24% died between 2100 and 2359 hours. Of all deaths, 81% occurred in areas other than intersections, and 19% occurred at intersections.[6]

Almost 85% of pedestrians are struck by a vehicle's front end, sustaining a predictable pattern of injuries starting with those caused by direct impact with the bumper.[6] Adult injuries are generally lateral and posterior because adults tend to turn to the side or away from impact, whereas children often turn toward the oncoming vehicle.

There are *three predominant MOIs* during a vehicle versus pedestrian collision. The *first impact*, when the vehicle strikes an adult body with its bumpers, creates lower extremity injuries, particularly to the knee and leg. These injuries are in the form of various patterns of tibia-fibula fractures, often open-knee dislocations and tibial plateau fractures. The tibia is usually fractured on the side of impact; the impact potentially fractures the other leg as well. Knee dislocations are common, with severe multiligamentous injury.

In the field, a dislocated knee should be splinted in the position found if the patient has good distal pulse, motor function, and sensation (PMS). Remember, if the knee reduces spontaneously, then you must communicate this to the trauma team verbally and in your report. Knee dislocation is an indication of possible vascular injury that can be missed by the trauma team if you do not report that you found the knee in a dislocated position initially.

A *second impact* occurs as the adult is thrown on the hood and/or grille of a vehicle, resulting in head, pelvis, chest, and coup-contrecoup traumatic brain injuries. Lateral compression pelvic fractures are common in this mechanism and can cause open fractures with bony punctures in viscera in this area of the body, or in the vagina in women. A *third impact* occurs when the body strikes the ground or some other object after it has been subjected to a sudden acceleration by the colliding vehicle.

Pediatric patterns of pedestrian injury are different from patterns in adults. Small children are shorter, so the vehicle's bumper is more likely to strike them in the pelvis or torso, causing severe injuries from direct impact Figure 29-14 . Although children are less likely than adults to fly over the hood of a vehicle, they are more

likely to be run over by the vehicle as they are propelled to the ground by the impact. Multiple extremity and pelvic fractures and abdominal and thoracic crush injuries are to be expected. Traumatic brain injury often kills young patients.

The **Waddell triad** refers to the pattern of vehicle pedestrian injuries in children and people of short stature: (1) the bumper hits the pelvis and femur instead of the knees and tibias; (2) the chest and abdomen hit the grille or low on the hood of the vehicle (sternal and rib fractures as well as abdominal injuries are likely); (3) the head strikes the vehicle and then the ground (skull and facial fractures, facial abrasions, and closed head injury).

Special Populations

The different MOIs in children and the unique anatomic features of children together produce predictable patterns of injury. Because penetrating injuries are uncommon and because the head (compared with the rest of the body) is larger in childhood, injured children often have blunt injuries primarily involving the head. If the energy impact is severe and involves the entire body, then the child may have a pattern involving the head, chest, abdomen, and long bones.

▶ Falls From Heights

Remember, a fall produces acceleration downward at 9.8 m/sec^2. On contact with the floor or ground, an instantaneous stop occurs that decelerates the person from whatever velocity had been achieved at the end of the fall to zero velocity. If a person falls for 2 seconds, then the speed at impact is nearly 20 m/sec—almost 45 mph.

The severity of injuries you can expect to find in your patient will depend on a number of factors, all of which will be important in your patient assessment:

- **Height.** The height from which the patient has fallen will determine the *velocity* of the fall. A person falling one story (12 feet [4 m]) onto concrete, for example, will fall at about 28 feet per second (fps) and experience an impact force of about 48 g. A person falling from the second story (24 feet [7 m]) will reach a velocity of 39 fps and experience an impact force of 95 g on the same surface. Height plus stopping distance predicts the magnitude of deceleration forces. A fall greater than 15 feet (5 m) or 2.5 to 3 times the height of the patient will have a greater incidence of morbidity and mortality, although it is usually assumed a fall from four stories may be survivable. At five stories, survival is questionable; at six stories, survival is unlikely, and a fall from seven stories or higher is rarely survivable.

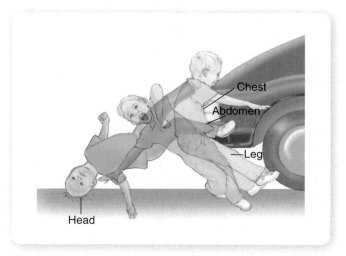

Figure 29-14 In vehicle versus pedestrian collisions, children frequently sustain multisystem injuries involving the head, chest, abdomen, and long bones. This is called the Waddell triad.

- **Position.** The position or orientation of the body at the moment of impact will also determine the type of injuries sustained and the likelihood of survival. Children tend to fall headfirst, owing to the relatively greater mass of a child's head, so head injuries are common in children, as are injuries to the wrists and upper extremities when the child attempts to break his or her fall with outstretched arms. Adults, on the other hand, usually try to land on their feet; thus, controlling their falls. However, adults often tilt backward, landing on their buttocks and outstretched hands. The group of potential injuries from a vertical fall to a standing position is commonly referred to as the *Don Juan syndrome* pattern of injuries Figure 29-15 . Injuries include foot and lower extremity fractures, along with hip, acetabular, and pelvic ring and sacral fractures. Lumbar spine axial loading also results in vertebral compression and burst fractures particularly of T12-L1 and L2. Vertical deceleration forces to organs (liver, spleen, and aorta) and fractures of the forearm and wrist (Colles fracture) are also common.
- **Area.** The area over which the impact is distributed—the larger the area of contact at the time of impact, the greater the dissipation of the force and the lesser the peak pressures generated.
- **Surface.** The surface onto which the person has fallen and the degree to which that surface can deform (degree of plasticity) under the force of the falling body can help dissipate the forces of sudden deceleration. Deep snow, for example, has a relatively large capacity to deform, whereas concrete has scarcely any capacity. Contrary to

what you might expect, water also has very little plasticity at high-speed impacts. The surface of contact may present hazards in the form of irregularities or protruding structures; it is far more dangerous to fall onto a wrought-iron picket fence, for example, than onto the grass beside it. If the surface does not conform, then the unprotected body will.
- **Physical condition.** The physical condition of the patient in the form of preexisting medical conditions may also influence the injuries sustained. Most notably in the case of older patients with osteoporosis, a condition that predisposes to fractures even with minimal falls. Patients with hematologic conditions resulting in an enlarged spleen may also be more prone to ruptured spleen in a fall. Children younger than 3 years have fewer injuries from falls greater than three stories than do older children and adults, most likely because of the more elastic nature of their body tissues and less ossification.

Penetrating Trauma

Unlike blunt trauma, which can involve a large surface area, **penetrating trauma** involves a disruption of the skin and underlying tissues in a small, focused area. Although a variety of objects may cause penetrating injuries in a variety of settings, penetrating trauma is usually interpreted as being more specific to injuries caused by firearms, knives, and other devices used as a means to cause intentional or unintentional harm Figure 29-16 . Penetrating trauma is classified as low, medium, or high velocity. Low-velocity penetrating trauma, such as a stab wound, is caused by the sharp edges of the object moving through the body. In medium- and high-velocity penetrating trauma, the path of the object (usually a bullet) may not be easy to predict because the bullet may flatten out, tumble, or even ricochet within the body before exiting.

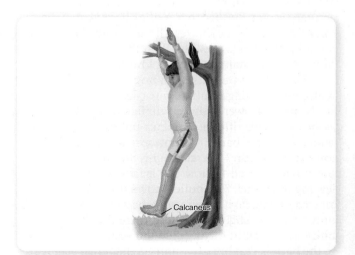

Figure 29-15 When an adult jumps or falls and lands on his or her feet, the energy is transmitted to the spine, sometimes producing a spinal injury in addition to injuries to the legs and pelvis.

© Jones & Bartlett Learning.

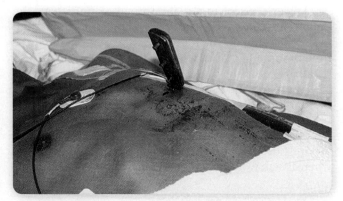

Figure 29-16 Injuries from low-energy penetrations, such as a stab wound, are caused by the sharp edges of the object moving through the body.

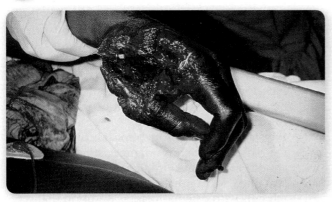

Figure 29-17 Guns are a common cause of penetrating trauma, as shown in this case.

In the United States, the most common sources of penetrating injuries are firearms Figure 29-17 . In 2013, according to US National Vital Statistics Reports, 33,636 people died by gunfire. The number of deaths, while staggering, actually represents a 21% decline in firearm-associated deaths from a peak in 1993. Of the gun-related deaths in 2013, 63% were suicides, 33% were homicides (including justified shootings by law enforcement personnel and gun owners), and 4% were accidental discharge or undetermined.[7]

▶ Stab Wounds

The severity of a stab wound depends on the anatomic area involved, depth of penetration, blade length, and angle of penetration. A stab wound may also involve a cutting- or hacking-type force such as in machete wounds, which not only can result in laceration, but can also cause fractures and blunt injury to underlying soft tissues and bone, and, potentially, amputation.

Neck wounds can involve critical anatomic structures such as the carotid arteries, jugular veins, subclavian vessels, apices of the lung, the upper mediastinum, trachea, esophagus, and thoracic duct. Deep neck wounds of sufficient energy can result in spinal cord involvement and cervical fracture.

Lower chest or upper abdominal wounds have the potential of involving the thoracic and abdominal cavities, depending on the location of the diaphragm at the time of injury—that is, whether the person was taking a breath or exhaling.

The pattern of stab wounds closely relates to the mechanism involved and should be documented in detail because your records may be needed in court proceedings. Ensure you record the directions of the stab wounds. Wounds delivered to the back are generally downward, whereas stab wounds from the front are generally upward.

▶ Gunshot Wounds

Firearms are the primary mechanism resulting in penetrating trauma. The amount of damage a firearm can cause will depend on a number of factors, including the type of firearm, velocity of the projectile, physical design and size of the projectile, the distance the person is from the muzzle of the firearm, and, perhaps most importantly, the exact anatomic location and structures that are struck.

There are hundreds if not thousands of firearm models and designs. They can be classified primarily into three types: shotguns, rifles, and handguns.

Shotguns fire round pellets (referred to as "shot"), from about half a dozen to several dozen at a time, depending on the type of load used. The load denominated 00 or 000 "buckshot" is the larger pellets, and smaller shot such as No. 7 is a common fowl hunting shot or "birdshot." At short range, even the smaller shot can cause devastating injuries. Shotgun shells can also be loaded with a single large and heavy projectile called a sabot, which can cause even worse harm. A shotgun typically has a smooth bore, and its numerous projectiles are not stabilized in flight by spin, as is the single projectile fired from a rifle barrel. The pellets leave the barrel and immediately start dispersing so the shot density (ie, the separation between any two pellets) at the time of impact on a target will be determined by the distance the pellets travel.

At very close range (less than 10 yards [about 1 m]), a shotgun can induce destructive injuries. Entrance and exit wounds can be very large, with shotgun wadding, bits of clothing, skin, and hair driven into the wound that can cause massive contamination, leading to increased infection potential should the patient survive the initial trauma.

Rifles are firearms firing a single projectile at very high velocity through a grooved barrel that imparts a spin to the projectile that stabilizes the projectile's flight for accuracy.

Handguns are of two types: revolvers and pistols. Revolvers have a cylinder holding from 5 to 10 rounds of ammunition, and most pistols have a separate magazine holding as many as 17 rounds of ammunition in some models. Handguns also have rifled barrels to impart spin to a bullet, but their accuracy is more limited than a rifle's because their barrels (and sight radius) are shorter. The ammunition handguns fire is generally less powerful than the ammunition fired from rifles, and handguns fire at lower velocities.

You need some understanding of ballistics to fully realize the damage bullets can cause. **Ballistics** is the study of non-powered objects in flight and is most often associated with rifle or handgun bullet travel. When a bullet leaves the barrel of a gun, gravity begins to pull it towards the earth. The trajectory is the curve of a bullet's travel path related to how fast it falls to the earth after leaving the barrel. As a bullet moves through the air, the air creates drag on it, slowing down its velocity (although only relatively slightly). To minimize the drag and stabilize the bullet in flight, rifles and pistols have grooves in the barrels that impart a spin on the bullet as it leaves the gun. The bullet's shape or profile, with the pointed end to the front, also contributes to its stability in flight. When the bullet contacts with a solid substance, such as body tissue, the drag increases greatly, often causing the bullet to stop.

Most bullets are made of lead, which is a relatively soft metal that deforms easily. When a lead bullet contacts an object, the nose or leading end tends to flatten out, creating a mushroom shape (known as expansion), thereby increasing the diameter of the penetration.

In the beginning of the Twentieth century, automatic weapons were introduced that use the back pressure from the firing of a bullet to eject the spent cartridge (which held the gunpowder). The same mechanism then loads the next round from the magazine into the chamber to be fired. Fully automatic weapons, which are rarely found outside of the military, fire each round as soon as it is loaded into the chamber as long as the trigger is held down and the ammunition holds out. For a semiautomatic weapon to fire, the trigger must be pulled and released each time a new round is loaded. When traditional lead-nose bullets are fired from an automatic or semiautomatic weapon, the mechanism tends to become gummed up by the relatively soft lead, preventing the weapon from operating properly. To prevent this, jacketed bullets were developed. Jacketed bullets have a thin copper or brass coating over the traditional lead bullet. In a full metal jacket bullet, the entire lead bullet is covered with copper. In a jacketed hollow-point bullet, the end of the lead bullet is exposed and hollowed out. When jacketed hollow-point bullets strike, expansion causes the copper coating to spread out and peel away. This fragmentation causes more internal damage to body tissues. Fragmentation of the actual lead bullet can also occur as it passes though body tissue.

The most important factor for the seriousness of a gunshot wound is the *type of tissue* through which the projectile passes. Tissue of high elasticity like muscle, for example, is better able to tolerate stretch (temporary cavitation) than tissue of low elasticity, like the liver. A high-velocity bullet fired through a fleshy part of the leg may do much less damage than a relatively low-velocity bullet that punctures the aorta or the liver. Many bullet wounds of the extremities that are found to have caused no fracture or neurovascular compromise will be treated by the trauma team with splinting and a single dose of antibiotic without a need for wound exploration or bullet retrieval.

An **entrance wound** is characterized by the effects of initial contact and **implosion**. Skin and subcutaneous tissues are pushed in, cut, or abraded externally as missile fragments pass and heat is transferred to the body tissues. At close ranges, tattoo marks from powder burns can occur. At extremely close ranges, burns from muzzle blasts can occur. Heavy wound contamination results from negative pressure generated behind the traveling projectile, which sucks surrounding elements into the wound.

Deformation and tissue destruction sustained in soft tissues and bone are based on a combination of factors, including density, compressibility, missile velocity, and missile fragmentation. The initial path of tissue destruction is caused by the projectile crushing the tissue during penetration. This creates a **permanent cavity** that may be a straight line or an irregular pathway as the bullet is deflected

into a number of angles after initial penetration. **Pathway expansion** refers to the tissue displacement that occurs as the result of low-displacement sonic pressure waves that travel at the speed of sound in tissue (four times the speed of sound in air). These sonic pressure waves push tissues in front of and lateral to the projectile and may not necessarily increase the wound size or cause permanent injury, but they result in **cavitation** (cavity formation). Tissue is compressed and accelerated away, causing injury. The waves of tissue are similar to throwing a rock into a pond. The rock creates a hole in the pond that quickly refills while waves emanate from the penetrating wound, or hole in the pond.

Words of Wisdom

As a general rule, the entrance wound (usually funnel shaped) is always smaller than the exit wound. Assume cavitation involves internal structures that are not readily visible on your clinical exam.

Bowel, muscle, and the lungs are relatively elastic, resulting in fewer permanent effects of temporary cavitation. The liver, spleen, and brain are relatively inelastic, and the temporary cavity may become a permanent defect. **Missile fragmentation** is a major cause of tissue damage as the projectile sends off fragments that create their own separate paths through tissues. Secondary missiles can also be generated by pieces of bone, teeth, buttons, or other objects encountered in the projectile's path as it enters the body. **Exit wounds** occur when the projectile has sufficient energy that is not entirely dissipated along its trajectory through the body. The projectile then exits the patient and can injure others as well (known as secondary impacts).

The size of the exit wound depends on the energy dissipated and the degree of cavitation at the point of exit. Exit wounds usually have irregular edges and may be larger than entrance wounds ⟨ **Figure 29-18** ⟩. There may be multiple exit wounds in the case of fragmentation. The number of exit wounds and the extent of tissue damage encountered must be assessed and carefully documented.

Words of Wisdom

Don't assume a bullet followed a straight path between the entrance and exit sites. It may have ricocheted inside the body, especially off bones, and traveled in many different directions.

Shotgun wounds are the result of tissue impacted by numerous projectiles. As described earlier, the greater the distance from the muzzle to the target, the more

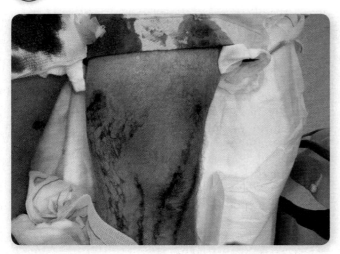

Figure 29-18 Entrance and exit wounds in the leg from a low velocity gunshot wound.

© E.M. Singletary, M.D. Used with permission.

dispersion the multiple projectiles will have and the greater the loss of KE before impact. Thus, shotguns are most lethal when used as short-range weapons. Also, the velocity of each pellet is less than the velocity of any bullet fired from a rifle.

Wounding potential from an injury sustained from a shotgun depends on the powder charge, the size and number of pellets, and the dispersion of the pellets. Dispersion is in turn determined by the range at which the weapon was fired, the barrel length (shorter barrels have more scatter), and the type of choke at the end of the barrel.

To give the trauma team at the hospital as much information as possible, try to obtain the following information if known:

- What kind of weapon was used (handgun, rifle, or shotgun; type and caliber)?
- At what range was it fired?
- What kind of bullet was used? (Ideally, see if the police can find an unfired cartridge.)

What to look for:

- Powder residue around the wound
- Entrance and exit wounds (the exit wound is usually larger and more ragged)

In most cases, the assailant has fled, along with the weapon, so patient care should be your highest priority once you determine the scene is safe. While obtaining the details about the weapon and ammunition may be somewhat beneficial to the hospital, this should take less priority over providing high quality patient care.

YOU are the Paramedic PART 3

The next steps in your primary survey include assessing respiratory status. Palpation of the trachea reveals that it is midline and the chest appears to be expanding equally. Breath sounds are present and no crepitus is noted. A quick look does not reveal any open chest wounds or impaled objects. The radial pulse is present only in her right wrist, but it is very weak and rapid. The left arm is deformed and her hand is cold with no palpable pulse. As you quickly move from head to toe looking for any severe bleeding, your partner reminds you that on-scene time is now approaching 6 minutes. The patient's friend tells you they were just past the top of the ride and the patient initially fell head first, striking the vehicle below them and then tumbled to the ground.

Recording Time: 5 Minutes	
Respirations	12 breaths/min, assisted
Pulse	140 beats/min, weak right radial pulse, absent left radial pulse
Skin	Pale, cool, moist
Blood pressure	140/110 mm Hg
Oxygen saturation (Spo$_2$)	97%
Pupils	Left pupil dilated, nonreactive

5. The patient's rapid, weak pulse and cool, moist skin indicate likelihood of inadequate perfusion, yet the blood pressure does not indicate advanced shock. What are some possible reasons for this finding?
6. According to the friend who witnessed the fall, the patient's initial impact was with her head against the metal car below. What is the significance of a smaller surface area of the body absorbing the initial impact as opposed to a larger body surface area?

Blast Injuries

Although most commonly associated with military conflict, blast injuries are also seen in civilian practice in mines, shipyards, and chemical plants, and, increasingly, in association with terrorist activities. People who are injured in explosions may be injured by any of five different mechanisms, often causing multisystem trauma **Figure 29-19** .

► Categories of Blast Injuries

Primary Blast Injuries

Primary blast injuries are due entirely to the blast itself—that is, damage to the body caused by the pressure wave generated by the explosion. When an explosion occurs, a pressure wave rapidly develops; this tremendous, concentrated pressure results from air displacement and heat originating from the center of the blast. The organs generally affected by primary blast effects are the lungs, eardrums, and other compressible organs. The pressure wave damages air-filled cavities.

Close proximity to the origin of the pressure wave carries a high risk of injury or death. Explosions from a bomb start at the center and move outward, so people closer to the device will be affected to a greater extent. Explosions from fumes or dust involve an entire area, so there is no "safe" region. Underwater blasts have a three times greater range because of the near incompressibility of water. Explosions that occur within a confined space result in more force applied to the body.

Secondary Blast Injuries

Secondary blast injuries result from being struck by flying debris (such as shrapnel from the device or from glass or splinters) that has been set in motion by the explosion. Objects are propelled by the force of the blast and strike the person, causing injury. These objects can travel great distances and can be propelled at tremendous speeds, up to nearly 3,000 mph for conventional military explosives.

A blast wind occurs as the shock wave applies force to air molecules. Although less forceful than the pressure wave, the blast wind is longer lasting and can hurl projectiles at high velocities. Projectiles present serious

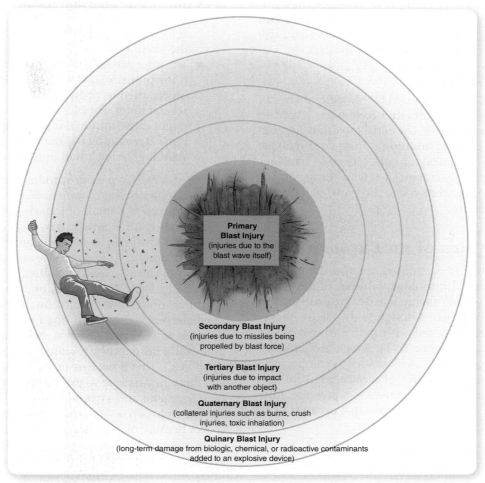

Figure 29-19 The mechanisms of blast injury.

© Jones & Bartlett Learning.

hazards—flying debris may cause blunt and penetrating injuries. With bombs, the casing fragments rip apart with monumental force, spreading in all directions. Structural elements can break apart and travel at high rates of speed. Nails, wood splinters, and glass shards can impale people located in the area of the blast.

Tertiary Blast Injuries

Tertiary blast injuries occur when a person is hurled by the force of the explosion (or blast wind) against stationary, rigid objects, such as the ground, or walls. Physical displacement of the body is also referred to as ground shock when the body impacts the ground. The injuries that result are numerous and result from both blunt and penetrating mechanisms. A blast wind also causes the patient's body to be hurled or thrown, causing further injury.

Quaternary (Miscellaneous) Blast Injuries

Quaternary injuries result from the miscellaneous events that occur during an explosion. For example, the heat generated during an explosion may cause burns, ranging from superficial flash burns to full-thickness burns involving the entire or large areas of the body. These injuries can include burns from hot gases or fires started by the blast, respiratory injury from inhaling toxic gases, and crush injury from the collapse of buildings. There is also a risk for entrapment that may be prolonged for days.

Quinary Blast Injuries

Quinary blast injuries are caused by biologic, chemical, or radioactive contaminants that have been added to a traditional explosive device. The initial explosion disperses these materials, causing additional long-term damage through biologic, chemical, or radioactive mechanisms. This type of blast injury is associated with "dirty bombs" and is of increased concern due to the threat of its use by terrorist organizations.

▶ The Physics of an Explosion

When a substance is detonated, a solid or liquid is chemically converted into large volumes of gas under pressure with resultant energy release. Propellants, like gunpowder, are explosives designed to release energy relatively slowly compared with high explosives (for example, trinitrotoluene, or TNT), which are designed to detonate very quickly. Explosives such as composition C4 can create initial pressures of more than 4 million pounds per square inch. This generates a pressure pulse in the shape of a spherical blast wave that expands in all directions from the point of explosion.

Components of Blast Shock Wave

The leading edge of an explosion pressure blast wave is called the **blast front**. A **positive wave pulse** refers to the phase of the explosion in which there is a pressure front higher than atmospheric pressure. The peak magnitude of the wave experienced by a patient becomes lessened the farther the person is from the center of the explosion. The increase in pressure from a blast can be so abrupt that high-explosive blast waves are also referred to as shock waves. Shock waves possess a characteristic, **brisance**, that describes the shattering effect of the wave and its ability to cause disruption of tissues as well as structures. Tissue damage is dependent on the magnitude of the pressure spike and the duration of force application. The **negative wave pulse** refers to the phase, after the initial positive pressure wave, in which pressure is less than atmospheric. It occurs as air displaced by the positive wave pulse returns to fill the space of the explosion. It can lead to massive movements of air resulting in high-velocity winds.

The speed, duration, and pressure of the shock wave are affected by the following:

- The *size* of the explosive charge. The larger the explosion, the faster the shock waves and the longer they will last.
- The nature of the *surrounding medium*. Pressure waves travel much more rapidly in water, for example, and are effective at greater distances in water than in air.
- The *distance* from the explosion. The farther one is from the explosion, the slower the shock wave velocity, the longer its duration, and the lower the likelihood of injury.
- The presence or absence of *reflecting surfaces*. If the pressure wave is reflected off a solid object, then its pressure may be multiplied several times. For example, a shock wave that might cause minimal injury in the open can cause devastating trauma if the patient is standing beside a wall or similar solid object.

The changes in pressure produced by the shock wave produce transient *winds*, sometimes of very high velocity, that can accelerate small objects to speeds of hundreds of feet per second. A missile traveling at 50 fps can easily penetrate human skin; at 400 fps, a missile can enter any of the major body cavities and cause serious internal injury. Blast winds can also send the human body flying against larger, more stationary objects, or even amputate limbs.

In an underwater explosion, a shock wave travels at greater velocity than in open air, thereby making it possible to receive injuries at three times the distance that would normally be required to receive such injuries in open air. This is because positive pressures are higher and there are no negative pressures or high-velocity wind. Blast fragments and gases move shorter distances in water.

An explosion is significantly more damaging in closed spaces because of a limited dissipation environment for the forces involved and for the generation of toxic gases and smoke. The shock wave is magnified when it comes into contact with a solid surface such as a wall, causing people near a wall to be hit with significantly higher pressure, resulting in increased risk of injury and death.

► Tissues at Risk

Air-containing organs such as the middle ear, heart, lungs, major blood vessels, and the gastrointestinal tract are most susceptible to pressure changes. Junctions between tissues of different densities and exposed tissues such as the head and neck are prone to injury as well. The ear is the organ most sensitive to blast injuries. The **tympanic membrane** (eardrum) evolved to detect minor changes in pressure and will rupture at pressures of 5 to 7 pounds per square inch (about 250–350 Torr) above atmospheric pressure. Thus, the tympanic membranes are a sensitive indicator of the possible presence of other blast injuries. The patient may report ringing in the ears, pain in the ears, or some loss of hearing, and blood may be visible in the ear canal. Dislocation of structural components of the ear, such as the ossicles within the middle ear, may occur. Permanent hearing loss is possible.

> ### Words of Wisdom
>
> When hearing is abnormal after an explosion, look for serious injury to the lungs.

Primary **pulmonary blast injuries** may occur as contusions and hemorrhages. When the explosion occurs in an open space, the side toward the explosion is usually injured, but the injury can be bilateral when the person is located in a confined space. The patient may report tightness or pain in the chest and may cough up blood and have tachypnea or other signs of respiratory distress. Subcutaneous emphysema (crackling under the skin) over the chest can be palpated, indicating underlying pneumothorax. Tension pneumothorax may develop, requiring emergency decompression in the field for your patient to survive. Pulmonary edema may also occur. If there is *any* reason to suspect lung injury in a blast victim, then administer oxygen. Be cautious in giving oxygen under positive pressure as it may create a tension pneumothorax, which may increase the damage to the lung. Use caution administering intravenous (IV) fluids; they may be poorly tolerated in patients with lung injury and lead to pulmonary edema.

One of the most concerning pulmonary blast injuries is **arterial air embolism**, which occurs on alveolar disruption with subsequent air embolization into the pulmonary vasculature. Even small air bubbles can enter a coronary artery and cause myocardial injury. Air emboli in the cerebrovascular system can produce disturbances in vision, changes in behavior, changes in state of consciousness, and a variety of other neurologic signs.

> ### Words of Wisdom
>
> If a blast injury victim has any neurologic abnormalities, then immediately notify the medical control physician!

Solid organs are relatively protected from shock wave injury but may be injured by secondary missiles or a hurled body. Petechiae (pinpoint hemorrhages on the skin) to large hematomas are the dominant form of pathology. Hollow organs, however, may be injured by similar mechanisms as for lung tissue. Perforation or rupture of the bowel and colon is a risk. Underwater explosions result in the most severe abdominal injuries.

Neurologic injuries and head trauma are the most common causes of death from blast injuries. Subarachnoid and subdural hematomas are often seen. Permanent or transient neurologic deficits may be secondary to concussion, intracerebral bleeding, or air embolism. Instant but transient unresponsiveness, with or without retrograde amnesia, may be initiated not only by head trauma, but also by cardiovascular conditions. Bradycardia and hypotension are common after an intense pressure wave from an explosion. This is a vagal nerve–mediated form of shock without compensatory response (similar to vasovagal syncope).

Extremity injuries, including traumatic amputations, are common. Patients with traumatic amputation by blast wind are likely to sustain fatal injuries secondary to the blast. In the global war on terrorism, improved body armor has increased the number of survivors of blast injuries from shrapnel wounds to the torso. However, the number of severe orthopaedic and extremity injuries has increased. In addition, while body armor may limit or prevent shrapnel from entering the body, it also catches more energy from the shock wave, possibly resulting in the person being thrown backward; thus, increasing the potential for spinal cord injury.

Although blast injuries have usually been the domain of military surgeons, they often occur in industrial settings and are, unfortunately, more common today owing to the increased use of explosives as a tool for urban terrorism and, in the United States, from methamphetamine lab explosions. Although civilian blast injuries in an industrial or mining setting were mostly characterized by blast injuries and burns, terrorist bombs often have shrapnel. Modern EMS and trauma services personnel should be fully educated and aware of what to expect in these scenarios.

Assessment and Management of Blast Injuries

When you are at the scene of an explosion, expect significant trauma and multiple patients. The forces generated by the blast have the potential to cover a wide area with devastating effect. If the explosion was intentional, then examine the immediate area for a secondary device. When you cannot ensure scene safety, evacuate to a safe distance until qualified personnel inform you it is safe to approach the patient. Also assess the scene for other hazards that may lead to EMS crew injury, such as exposed electrical wiring, structural instability, and sharp objects.

Pulmonary injuries are common when an explosion occurs and the injuries can be life threatening. Assess breath sounds frequently throughout your care because the pressure wave generated by an explosion can lead to a pneumothorax. Should the air within the chest cavity continue to collapse the affected lung, a tension pneumothorax can develop. Needle decompression is a lifesaving intervention in such a case.

Noncardiogenic pulmonary edema can develop after an explosion. A massive pulmonary contusion can lead to microhemorrhage within the lungs, further compromising ventilation and respiration. Ask the patient about the ease or difficulty of breathing early in your assessment. Rapidly examine the patient for open and closed wounds (abrasions, amputations, avulsions, punctures, penetrations, lacerations, deformities, swelling, burns, contusions, and crush injuries), and manage life threats. Establish a baseline pulse oximetry value, and reassess this measure frequently. Although pulse oximeter readings are important, administer high-flow supplemental oxygen even in the presence of a high reading. Respiratory compromise is likely to develop, even if the initial symptoms are not severe.

A patient injured in a blast commonly sustains abdominal trauma that includes ruptured organs and internal hemorrhage. The pressure wave can cause air-filled cavities, such as the small and large bowels, to burst. Although these injuries can be catastrophic, obvious signs of injury often take time to develop. An absence of overt signs of abdominal injury should not rule out the possibility of these injuries. You must maintain a high index of suspicion.

Ask the patient about the presence of abdominal pain. If he or she reports discomfort, then use the OPQRST mnemonic (Onset, Provocation/palliation, Quality, Region/radiation, Severity, Timing) to guide your history taking. Examine all abdominal quadrants, noting all injuries and tenderness on the patient care report.

During the blast, patients' ears are often adversely affected by the pressure wave. The likelihood of rupture of the tympanic membrane is high. Hearing loss is common when the patient is in proximity to the blast. Because the ears are essential in establishing body position, dizziness can occur when they are affected. Such dizziness can lead to vomiting, which may interfere with airway patency and protection.

Projectiles can produce penetrating wounds during the secondary blast phase. If you discover an impaled object in your patient's body, then follow the management guidelines outlined in Chapter 31, *Soft-Tissue Trauma*. If an object is impaled in the eye, then follow the guidelines outlined in Chapter 33, *Face and Neck Trauma*.

■ General Assessment of Trauma

Managing a trauma scene involves more consideration of external factors than a typical medical emergency scene.

When a trauma patient arrives at the hospital, the staff there will not have the benefit of the scene information; therefore, your observations are critical to them. Trauma patients tend to have visible injuries and an MOI that is fairly easy to identify. At the same time, very few trauma injuries can be truly stabilized on scene, and in some cases there may be hidden traumatic injuries that will not be identified until the patient receives surgical intervention. The way you handle the trauma scene can make a huge difference in the outcome of your patient.

Scene Size-up

As with all calls, determine whether the scene is safe before entering, and don personal protective equipment. Gloves are extremely important because the likelihood of bleeding is much higher in trauma patients than in medical patients. On trauma scenes, it is a good idea to have an extra pair of gloves in your pocket, in case one of your gloves becomes torn and needs to be replaced. In addition to gloves, protective eyewear is important. Blood and bodily fluids from a traumatically injured patient can easily splash into your eyes. Other protective equipment including helmets, heavy coats, and boots may be required based on the MOI.

Anticipate possible scene hazards while en route to the scene. Hazards include weapons, as well as chemical, thermal, atmospheric, electrical hazards. As you identify potential hazards, call for assistance in dealing with them before you move on to patient assessment and care. Fire, rescue, hazardous materials, and police responders require time to travel to the scene; the sooner you call for them, the sooner they will arrive and help you control the scene. Carefully assess your environment.

As you locate and approach your patients, determine the number of patients and consider whether you will need additional medical resources. Be observant as you locate the patients and work to determine the MOI. Obtain the following key information if it is available to you at the scene:

- If the patient fell, then note the height from which the patient fell and the type of surface he or she landed on.
- If the incident was a MVC, then note the extent of intrusion into the vehicle and note whether or not ejection occurred.

This information will be crucial for providers who care for the patient after your handoff.

Primary Survey

The general impression formed when you first approach your patient will often guide how you assess and treat the patient. Patients who look very ill or present with obvious bleeding injuries often have serious injuries, whereas those who appear to be relatively stable may not be as seriously injured. However, do not make major patient care decisions based strictly on your first impression. Use the instincts you have developed throughout your career to anticipate the care and treatment that is appropriate. For example, if you see signs of heavy external bleeding, then immediately investigate and control it.

Keep the MOI in mind as you approach the patient, consider whether cervical spinal immobilization will be necessary and be prepared to protect the patient from *movement-induced* spinal injury. Evaluate the patient's level of consciousness using the AVPU mnemonic (Awake and alert, responsive to Verbal stimuli, responsive to Pain, Unresponsive). If the patient does not appear to be awake, then assess his response to verbal or light painful stimulus. Make a mental note of this status for later reference. Determine the chief complaint and any apparent life threats.

The order in which you present the next steps of the primary survey—ABCDE (Airway, Breathing, Circulation, Disability, and Exposure) or CABDE (Circulation, Airway, Breathing, Disability, and Exposure)—depends on whether the patient has a life-threatening circulatory status (life-threatening bleeding, no pulse). If so, then address these before assessing airway and breathing, as discussed in Chapter 11, *Patient Assessment*.

Assuming the patient does not require cardiopulmonary resuscitation (CPR) and does not have life-threatening hemorrhage, continue your evaluation by assessing the patient's airway status. If your patient is unresponsive, then ask your partner to open the airway using the jaw-thrust maneuver. Remember, if you suspect there is any possibility of a cervical spine injury, then avoid using the head tilt–chin lift maneuver. Observe for obvious oral or facial trauma that may contribute to airway obstruction. Be prepared to remove foreign objects and to suction out blood or vomitus to ensure the airway remains clear. If the patient is unresponsive, then consider the need for an oral or nasopharyngeal airway to maintain the airway once it has been opened. These may be replaced later with an endotracheal tube or a blind insertion airway device if necessary. If you suspect a blockage of the airway due to a foreign object, then apply the appropriate manual airway clearing technique and be prepared to use an advanced technique, such as visualization with a laryngoscope or even a needle or surgical cricothyrotomy.

Once the airway is clear, assess the patient's breathing. Absence of breathing will require you to initiate bag-mask ventilation and to consider a more advanced airway adjunct. If the patient is breathing, then note the relative rate and quality of the respirations as well as the patient's ability to speak. Dyspnea or difficulty breathing may be caused by many traumatic injuries. Note the skin color. Remember, cyanosis is caused by inadequate oxygenation, and observe the chest wall movement with respirations. If you observe a sucking chest injury, then take immediate action to seal the wound to prevent exacerbation of the patient's condition. Assess the thorax and neck for a

YOU are the Paramedic   PART 4

As you place the backboard next to the patient, your partner informs you that it has been almost 9 minutes on the scene. As you cut away the patient's clothing, you see a large contusion on the right lower quadrant and the abdomen appears distended. Her outward-bent legs are gently moved to center. After you apply the cervical collar, you and your partner gently roll the patient and immobilize her on the backboard. You close the buckles over the blanket and load her into the ambulance. As the clock ticks to the 10-minute mark, your partner maneuvers the ambulance out of the park and onto the road to the nearby trauma center.

Recording Time: 9 Minutes	
Respirations	12 breaths/min, assisted
Pulse	88 beats/min, weak right radial pulse, absent left radial pulse
Skin	Pale, cool, moist
Blood pressure	130/116 mm Hg
Oxygen saturation (SpO$_2$)	98%
Pupils	Left pupil dilated, nonreactive

7. What criteria does this patient meet to warrant transport to the trauma center?
8. As you continue your exam and observation of your patient en route to the trauma center, you think about the presentation of your patient to the waiting ED staff. What MOI will you relate to the staff?

deviated trachea, tension pneumothorax, neck and chest crepitation, broken ribs, a fractured sternum, or other conditions that may inhibit breathing. On the basis of all of the information you find, determine how best to support your patient's breathing. Most trauma patients will benefit from application of oxygen even in the absence of dyspnea. Rapid shallow respirations generally do not provide adequate volumes of air to an injured patient, so consider assisted ventilation with oxygen using the bag-mask device for these patients.

Next, evaluate circulation. Check both radial and carotid pulses simultaneously to allow you to estimate the patient's blood pressure as well as the pulse. Note the relative rate and quality of the pulse. If there is no pulse, then begin CPR immediately. Skin condition (color, temperature, and condition) can also be a good indicator of circulation. Quickly scan the patient for any significant external bleeding or other life-threatening injuries. Bleeding that is flowing heavily or spurting should be controlled immediately. Initiate shock management, if needed.

At this time, you should assess for disability. As a part of the general impression, you noted the patient's level of consciousness on the AVPU scale. Now is the time to perform a more complete evaluation of the level of consciousness by evaluating the patient's Glasgow Coma Scale (GCS) score. Note the pupil size, equality, and reactivity to light as part of disability assessment. This is also a good time to evaluate pulse, motion and sensation in all four extremities.

Finally, you should begin to expose the patient for exam if you have not done so already. A quick scan of the exposed patient for life-threatening injuries completes the assessment part of the primary survey. As always, in the primary survey, you should manage any life-threatening injuries as soon as they are identified.

Once you have identified and treated life threats and before you continue the assessment, you should be able to make a *preliminary* transport decision. Patients with altered mental status, airway or breathing problems, multisystem trauma, or significantly compromised circulation should be categorized for immediate transport or "load and go." Patients who do not meet these criteria should be categorized as nonurgent, at least initially, and you should continue your assessment on scene. If a patient is considered "load and go," then continue your assessment en route to the trauma center, and move as quickly as possible to begin transport. In most patients with multisystem trauma, definitive care requires surgical intervention; therefore, on-scene time should be limited to 10 minutes or less. This is sometimes referred to as the "platinum 10 minutes." Spend as little time as possible on scene with patients who have sustained significant trauma. When hemorrhage control in a critically injured patient is achieved within 1 hour after a traumatic injury (referred to as the Golden Hour or Golden Period) the chance of survival is higher than when time to hemorrhage control is more prolonged. Any delay that prolongs time to hemorrhage control will greatly reduce the patient's chance of survival.

History Taking

Gather patient history including a SAMPLE (Signs and symptoms, Allergies, Medications, Pertinent past medical history, Last oral intake, Events leading up to the illness or injury) history as well as OPQRST for any symptoms reported. For trauma patients, obtain a medical history as soon as possible in case the patient's level of consciousness deteriorates. If the patient is unresponsive when you arrive, then gather this information from bystanders or family members who may be present. Identify the patient's symptoms, including where they are feeling the most amount of pain, can be very helpful in the physical exam. Allergies, medications, and past medical history may seem relatively unimportant at this time, but this information will be critical when the patient is treated at the trauma center. The patient's last oral intake is important in case the patient needs to be intubated in preparation for surgical intervention to treat the injuries. Events leading up to the situation may have already been identified, but if not, the last letter of the SAMPLE history should remind you to get more information about what happened.

Secondary Assessment

Trauma patients are classified into two major groups: those with an isolated injury and those with multisystem trauma. From a secondary assessment perspective, the biggest difference between the groups is an isolated injury allows you to immediately focus on the primary condition.

In contrast, with multisystem trauma, you must first find all (or as many as you can reasonably find) of the various conditions (for example, a hematoma on the forehead, a fractured arm, as well as the cause of neck and lower back pain). Then you need to prioritize the injuries by severity and the order in which you plan to treat them. During the assessment, you must continually think about how each injury or condition relates to the others. For example, the mortality rate doubles for a patient with a serious traumatic brain injury who has a single episode of hypotension. In such a case, not recognizing and addressing the hypotension and the lack of adequate perfusion pressure has a huge impact—in some cases, a fatal impact. Another important consideration is the high visibility factor of many injuries, which sometimes creates a visual distraction.

Obtaining a full set of initial or baseline vital signs is critical. The sooner these baselines are established, the better they will serve to help you determine whether your patient's condition is improving or deteriorating. The vital signs should include an accurate assessment of pulse and respirations as well as auscultatory blood pressure. Other measurements that should be considered as part of this assessment include pulse oximetry, blood glucose level, and cardiac monitoring as appropriate. Automatic blood pressure monitoring should be instituted at this time if it is available.

Physical Examination of the Trauma Patient

Trauma patients with an isolated injury such as a sprained ankle or a possible isolated fracture may not require a rapid full-body scan, but most multisystem trauma patients should have a thorough physical exam prior to or during transport. The rapid full-body scan should be done in a systematic manner.

Remember from Chapter 11, *Patient Assessment*: if the patient's injuries are critical, perform the rapid full-body scan during the primary survey, then perform any further physical exam en route if possible. If spinal immobilization is necessary, however, you will need to thoroughly assess the head and neck before applying the cervical collar.

Head and Neck

Begin by palpating and visualizing the head and neck for injuries. Observe for deformities, contusions, abrasions, penetrations, burns, tenderness, lacerations, and swelling in each body area as you examine it. At the head, be sure to inspect and palpate the facial bones, scalp, skull, and jaw. Check the nose, mouth, and ears for evidence of bleeding. Re-examine the pupils for size, equality, and reactivity to light, as this can be a good indicator of head injury. Bleeding from the nose or ears may indicate a head injury, and bleeding from the mouth may obstruct the airway.

At the neck, check for jugular vein distention and tracheal deviation, because these can be signs of a serious internal chest injury. The tracheal position can be checked by pressing a finger down in the notch at the top of the sternum. If the trachea is palpated in this position, then it is midline (normal). If it is off to one side, then it is considered deviated, a fairly reliable sign of an advanced tension pneumothorax. After you complete your assessment of the neck by palpating the cervical spine, consider applying a cervical collar to stabilize your patient while you continue with your assessment.

Words of Wisdom

If you find a life-threatening injury at any point during your assessment, then manage it immediately. As you identify non–life-threatening injuries, ask your partner to treat those as you continue with the physical assessment.

Chest, Abdomen, and Pelvis

As you continue your assessment of the chest, carefully inspect and palpate the chest wall. Fractured ribs are common chest injuries and generally result in rapid, shallow respirations. Look for penetrating injuries and assess for bruising, thoroughly examining the entire chest area. If you have not already done so, then use your stethoscope to listen to breath and heart sounds. As you check breath sounds, auscultate the same area on both sides of the chest so you can compare the sounds. Unequal breath sounds from right to left may indicate a pneumothorax. Ensure you take enough time to carefully evaluate this; overlooking unequal breath sounds can prevent you from providing life-saving treatment to the patient.

After you complete the exam of the chest, proceed to the abdomen and pelvis. Gently palpate the abdomen across the upper and lower quadrants. A rigid and distended abdomen is a serious sign, usually indicating significant internal abdominal bleeding, which may be fatal. Press down on the iliac crests and squeeze them inward to determine pelvic stability. Be careful, as this will cause significant pain in a responsive patient with a pelvic or lower back injury. Palpate the pubic symphysis and examine the patient for signs of incontinence and/or bleeding from the groin area.

Extremities

Palpate the legs from top to bottom while looking for signs of injury. Palpate each leg separately, and note any difference between the legs. Check for distal PMS in both feet. Examine the arms in the same manner. Check for PMS in the hands and wrists.

Back

Prepare to move the patient to a backboard if indicated. If a log roll technique is used, then examine the back for injuries while the patient is on his or her side. Inspect and palpate the entire posterior thorax, as well as the lumbar region and buttocks. Once the back has been examined, the physical exam is completed.

 Reassessment

While en route to the hospital, perform another rapid full-body scan to identify anything you may have missed and to identify any changes in the patient's condition. Repeat the primary survey (ABCDEs), reevaluate vital signs (every 5 minutes for patients in serious condition), and review the status of the interventions you have performed. Notify the hospital staff as quickly as possible, and give them adequate information to prepare for your arrival. Many trauma patients will receive surgical intervention after a quick evaluation in the ED, so early notification can help the hospital prepare for this possibility.

Words of Wisdom

Because traumatic injuries are as varied as the mechanisms that cause them, it is almost impossible to prepare for every possible situation. In all situations, you must remain calm, complete an organized assessment, stabilize life-threatening injuries, and do no harm. Avoid tunnel vision; sometimes the obvious injury is not the critical injury.

Trauma Score

Paramedics must have a strong understanding of trauma scoring systems to appropriately classify patients. Using trauma scoring systems to determine injury severity is a common practice in the health care profession. Trauma scoring systems assist health care providers in rapidly identifying the severity of the patient's injuries.

There are several different trauma scoring systems. The **trauma score** is used to determine the likelihood of patient survival, which is calculated on a scale of 1 to 16, with 16 being the best possible score. It takes into account the GCS score, respiratory rate, respiratory expansion, systolic blood pressure, and capillary refill. As discussed in Chapter 11, *Patient Assessment*, the GCS is an evaluation tool used to determine level of consciousness; scores are assigned for eye opening, verbal response, and motor response. The sum of these scores can be used to predict patient outcomes. However, this scoring system does not accurately predict survivability in patients with severe head injuries because motor and verbal deficits make those criteria difficult to assess; in these instances, the Revised Trauma Score is used.

▶ Revised Trauma Score

The **Revised Trauma Score (RTS)** is a physiologic scoring system used to assess injury severity in patients with head trauma. This system is heavily weighted to compensate for major head injury without multisystem injury or major physiologic changes.

Objective data used to calculate the RTS include the GCS score, systolic blood pressure, and respiratory rate. In addition to assessing injury severity, the RTS is also reliable in predicting the likelihood of survival in patients with severe injuries. The highest RTS a patient can receive is 12; the lowest is 0. An RTS calculation is shown in **Table 29-4**.

Management of Trauma

Managing trauma requires a thorough, accurate assessment of the patient and a good working knowledge of the mechanics

of injury. During transport, begin any interventions that you consider necessary based on your physical exam of the patient. Specific injuries and treatments are discussed in later chapters, but most trauma patients will need to be treated for shock, which may include establishing IV access and administering a fluid bolus, and rapid transport. If the patient is being transported by ground, then IV access may be delayed until the patient is en route to the hospital. Unresponsive trauma patients will most likely need an advanced airway placed; this should be done before transport if possible. However, other treatment, including bandaging minor wounds and splinting fractured extremities, should be done en route if the patient is in critical condition.

Blood loss, fluid shifts, and massive vasodilation all lead to shock. Shock resuscitation techniques are fairly general; however, you need to find the primary cause to treat the patient properly. Most patients who are in shock should be given oxygen, be kept supine if possible, and be transported rapidly to a trauma center. You should also consider fluid resuscitation. If shock is caused by a large fluid shift, which can occur in patients with severe burns, then large quantities of fluid may be required. If shock is caused by blood loss, however, then too much fluid could dilute the blood and increase blood pressure to the point that clots could be dislodged and bleeding can increase. If shock is caused by vasodilation due to a spinal cord injury, then administer medications to constrict the blood vessels instead of adding more fluid through IV boluses. It is important to critically analyze your patient's condition so that you can administer the most appropriate treatment. Contact medical direction.

You should begin fluid resuscitation at volumes that maintain a minimum blood pressure to allow clots to form at sites of bleeding within the body, which will reduce ongoing blood loss. Excessive blood clotting is also a concern in patients with blood loss; clots circulating in blood can be fatal.

How to manage specific trauma injuries is covered in later chapters. Several techniques can be used to treat multisystem trauma. Remember, multisystem trauma patients cannot be stabilized in the field. Use a team approach to rapidly assess and transport your patient.

Table 29-4	Revised Trauma Score Calculation		
GCS Score	**Systolic Blood Pressure (mm Hg)**	**Respiratory Rate (breaths/min)**	**Value**
13 to 15	>89	10 to 29	4
9 to 12	76 to 89	>29	3
6 to 8	50 to 75	6 to 9	2
4 to 5	1 to 49	1 to 5	1
3	0	0	0

Abbreviation: GCS, Glasgow Coma Scale

Data from: Table 1, Triage Revised Trauma Score (T-RTS). *Int Journal Emerg Med.* 2008;1(1):21-26. http://www.ncbi.nlm.nih.gov/pmc/articles/PMC2536180/table/Tab1/. Copyright © Springer-Verlag London Ltd. 2008. Published online March 15, 2008. Accessed April 7, 2016.

Work with emergency medical responders, bystanders, and your partner to get the patient assessed and moved to the ambulance as quickly and safely as possible.

Many tasks can be done simultaneously when you use a team approach; for example, you can administer oxygen while your partner maintains cervical spine control, or your partner can prepare the backboard, if indicated, and stretcher while you perform the physical exam. One team member can obtain vital signs while another can question family members or bystanders to gather more information. The team approach requires extra attention on the part of the lead paramedic, but it can be a very efficient way to treat the patient.

Critical thinking is important when treating a patient with multisystem trauma. When a person sustains many injuries at once, the body tries to resolve all the injuries, resulting in signs and symptoms that are related to different response mechanisms. For example, in a patient with a closed head injury and internal bleeding elsewhere in the body, the body will try to maintain blood flow to the brain by increasing blood pressure and lowering the pulse. However, the body's response to the shock created by blood loss in other parts of the body is to attempt to increase the pulse rate and decrease blood pressure. You must analyze the MOI and the patient's signs and symptoms, and anticipate the injuries that need to be managed. Your ability to critically analyze and choose the best treatment will be a major factor in your patient's chance for survival.

Unfortunately, a few trauma patients may have injuries incompatible with life even though they may have some minimal signs of life when you arrive. Patients with open skull injuries presenting with exposed (or missing) brain tissue might fall in this category. It is critical that you follow your local protocols for these patients, including contacting medical direction. If resuscitation efforts are indicated, then you should give them the same effort that you would any other patient. Half-hearted efforts at resuscitation are highly unethical. If your protocols allow withholding resuscitation efforts, then you should contact medical direction and ensure you follow their instructions precisely. Never consider terminating resuscitation efforts for any trauma patient without approval from medical control.

▶ Trauma Lethal Triad

Recent research has identified what has been termed the trauma lethal triad of hypothermia, coagulopathy (poor blood clotting), and acidosis as a major contributor to death in patients with severe traumatic bleeding[8] Figure 29-20 . It has been well documented that even mildly hypothermic patients have a lower survival rate than normothermic patients. In addition, hypothermia contributes to coagulopathy, which also reduces survival from traumatic bleeding (if the blood cannot clot, the body cannot stop the bleeding). Any factor that interferes with blood clotting will cause the patient more blood loss than would occur. This will lead to poor perfusion and ultimately, death. Finally, acidosis (defined as a blood pH

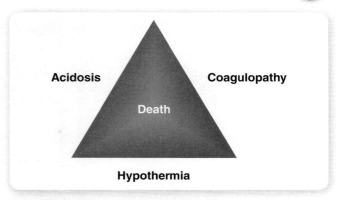

Figure 29-20 The trauma lethal triad.
© Jones & Bartlett Learning.

of less than 7.35) often occurs with excessive bleeding and treatments to compensate for it. For example, normal saline, which is commonly administered via bolus to treat hypotension, is acidic and can increase acidosis. Acidosis contributes to coagulopathy and complicates treatment of these patients.

How should knowledge of this lethal triad of conditions affect your treatment of trauma patients? First of all, you need to aggressively seek to control all bleeding to the best of your ability. Do not hesitate to use a tourniquet to stop bleeding from an extremity if initial attempts are unsuccessful. Next, keep your patients warm; place blankets under them as well as on top of them and ensure IV fluids are warmed to at least normal body temperature. Finally, minimize the volume of acidic IV fluid you administer to prevent interfering with coagulation and contributing to acidosis. If possible, monitor end-tidal CO_2 and ventilations to prevent respiratory acidosis, and consider administering tranexamic acid (TXA), a drug that can help control internal bleeding, if local protocols allow.

▶ Criteria for Referral to a Trauma Center

You are responsible for determining whether your patient should go to a trauma center—and at what level. Before you even get to the scene, you should know the criteria for referral to a trauma center and what hospital resources are available in your area. It is important to transport your trauma patient to the most appropriate facility based on his or her injuries. The National Study on the Costs and Outcomes of Trauma reported a 25% decrease in mortality for severely injured adult patients who received care at a Level I trauma center compared with those treated at a lower level trauma center.[9]

In 2011, the American College of Surgeons Committee on Trauma (ACS-COT) and the CDC published an updated field triage decision scheme Figure 29-21 :

1. **Physiologic criteria:** If one of the following is present, then the patient should be referred to the highest level trauma center:
   • GCS score of 13 or less

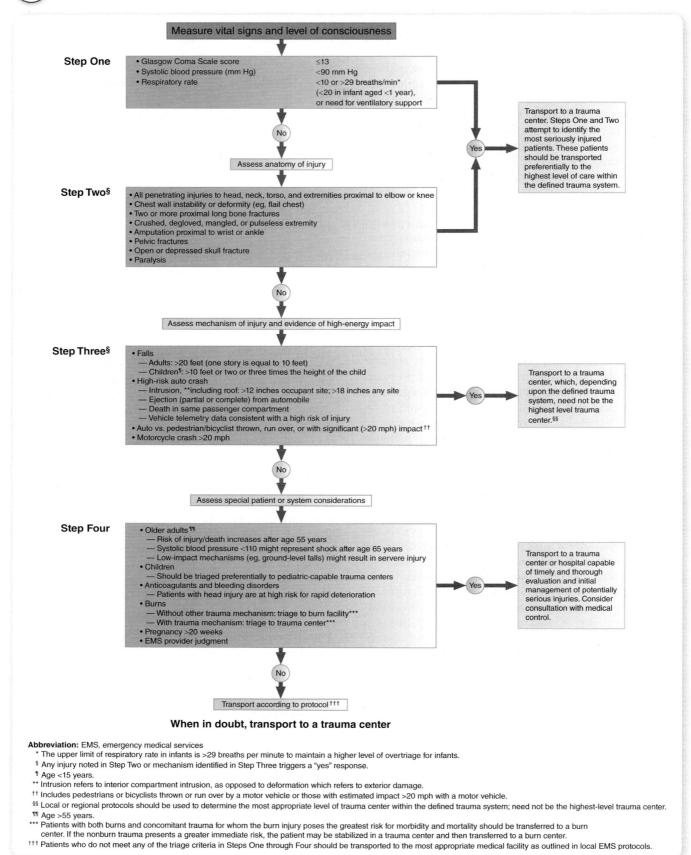

Figure 29-21 2011 decision scheme for field triage of injured patients.

Data from Centers for Disease Control and Prevention. Guidelines for field triage of injured patients: recommendations of the national expert panel on field triage, 2011. Morbidity and Mortality Weekly Report (MMWR), January 13, 2012.

- SBP (systolic blood pressure) of less than 90 mm Hg
- RR (respiratory rate) of less than 10 or more than 29 breaths/min (less than 20 breaths/min in infants younger than 1 year) or need for ventilator support

2. **Anatomic criteria:** If one of the following is present, then transport the patient to the highest level trauma center:
   - All penetrating trauma to the head, neck, torso, and extremities proximal to elbow or knee
   - Chest wall instability or deformity (eg, flail chest)
   - Two or more proximal long bone fractures
   - Crushed, degloved, mangled, or pulseless extremity
   - Amputation proximal to wrist or ankle
   - Pelvic fractures
   - Open or depressed skull fractures
   - Paralysis

3. **MOI criteria:** Evaluate at this point the MOI and examine the trauma scene for evidence of high-energy trauma. If one of the following is present, and depending on the MOI, then transport to the closest appropriate trauma center (may not be the highest level trauma system):
   - Adults: falls more than 20 feet (6 m)
   - Children: falls more than 10 feet (3 m) or two or three times the height of the child
   - High-risk MVC
     - ◆ Intrusion, including roof, into passenger compartment (more than 12 inches [30 cm] occupant site or more than 18 inches [46 cm] any other site)
     - ◆ Ejection (partial or complete) from vehicle
     - ◆ Death of another occupant in same passenger compartment
     - ◆ Vehicle telemetry data consistent with a high risk of injury
   - Pedestrian/bicyclist thrown or run over or vehicle versus pedestrian injury with significant (more than 20 mph) impact
   - Motorcycle crash at more than 20 mph

4. **Special Considerations:** If none of the above criteria are met, then consider transfer to an ED or low-level trauma center if:
   - Patients are older than 55 years
   - Systolic blood pressure of less than 110 mm Hg in adults older than 65 years
   - Children should be triaged to a pediatric-capable trauma center
   - Patients using anticoagulants or with bleeding disorders (patients with

head injuries are at high risk for rapid deterioration)
   - Pregnant patients (more than 20 weeks of gestation)
   - Low-impact mechanism in older adults (ground-level falls) may result in severe injury
   - Burns with other trauma (without other trauma, triage to burn facility)
   - EMS provider judgment

   Note: The criteria, "end-stage renal disease requiring dialysis" and "time-sensitive extremity injury" have been removed from the decision scheme.

Documentation & Communication

Determining the MOI and getting a complete history of the incident can help you to anticipate many injuries. After you ensure your personal safety and maintain the patient's ABCs, the MOI is key information to obtain from the trauma scene Table 29-5. You must relay the suspected MOI by radio and by written report to the receiving trauma center. You are the eyes and ears of the ED trauma team.

Table 29-5	Significant Mechanisms of Injury
Age	**Mechanisms**
Adults	Multiple body systems injured Ejection from a vehicle Death of another person in the same vehicle Fall from height greater than 20 feet (6 m) Vehicle rollover (unrestrained) High-speed (>40 mph) vehicle collision Vehicle versus pedestrian collision Motorcycle crash of greater than 20 mph Auto-pedestrian or auto-bicycle crash of greater than 20 mph Unresponsiveness or altered mental status following trauma Penetrating trauma to the head, chest, or abdomen
Children	All mechanisms in the adult list, with the following additions or modifications: Fall >10 ft (3 m) or two to three times the child's height Fall of <10 ft (3 m) with loss of consciousness Medium- to high-speed vehicle collision (≥25 mph)

Words of Wisdom

The criteria for transport to a trauma center may vary from system to system.

The Field Triage Decision Scheme is intended to help prehospital care providers recognize injured patients who are likely to benefit from transport to a trauma center compared with transport to a lower level ED. It is not intended as a mass-casualty or disaster triage tool; it is intended only for each patient.

The ACS-COT publishes a list of criteria defining four separate levels of trauma centers (Level I, II, III, and IV). The ACS-COT also provides verification for those institutions seeking to achieve and maintain trauma center capabilities. The verification process includes a site visit by experienced reviewers to ensure the centers have appropriately designated resources to care for trauma patients. The guidelines in **Table 29-6** are an overview of the ACS-COT's verification criteria.

In addition, it is important to know which hospitals specialize in neurology, burns, pediatric trauma, cardiac care (centers for heart transplantation, coronary catheter labs), microsurgery (hand and limb reimplantation), or

Table 29-6	Key Elements for Trauma Centers	
Level	**Definition**	**Key Elements**
Level I	A comprehensive regional resource that is a tertiary care facility. Capable of providing total care for every aspect of injury—from prevention through rehabilitation	1. 24-hour in-house coverage by general surgeons 2. Availability of orthopaedic surgery, neurosurgery, anesthesiology, emergency medicine, radiology, internal medicine, and critical care 3. Should also include cardiac, hand, pediatric, and microvascular surgery, as well as hemodialysis 4. Provides leadership in prevention, public education, and continuing education of trauma team members 5. Committed to continued improvement through a comprehensive quality assessment program and organized research to help direct new innovations in trauma care
Level II	Able to initiate definitive care for all injured patients	1. 24-hour immediate coverage by general surgeons 2. Availability of orthopaedic surgery, neurosurgery, anesthesiology, emergency medicine, radiology, and critical care 3. Tertiary care needs such as cardiac surgery, hemodialysis, and microvascular surgery may be referred to a Level I trauma center 4. Committed to trauma prevention and continuing education of trauma team members 5. Provides continued improvement in trauma care through a comprehensive quality assessment program
Level III	Able to provide prompt assessment, resuscitation, and stabilization of injured patients and emergency operations	1. 24-hour immediate coverage by emergency medicine physicians and prompt availability of general surgeons and anesthesiologists 2. Program dedicated to continued improvement in trauma care through a comprehensive quality assessment program 3. Has developed transfer agreements for patients requiring more comprehensive care at a Level I or Level II trauma center 4. Committed to continuing education of nursing and allied health personnel or the trauma team 5. Must be involved with prevention and have an active outreach program for its referring communities
Level IV	Able to provide ATLS before transfer of patients to a higher level trauma center	1. Include basic ED facilities to implement ATLS protocols and 24-hour laboratory coverage 2. Transfer to higher level trauma centers follows the guidelines outlined in formal transfer agreements 3. Committed to continued improvement of these trauma care activities through a formal quality assessment program 4. Involved in prevention, outreach, and education within its community

Abbreviations: ATLS, Advanced Trauma Life Support; ED, emergency department

hyperbaric therapy. Your patient should be transported to the most appropriate facility to receive optimal care. It is essential to give the trauma center early notice of the patient's arrival, including: age, sex, MOI, vital signs, GCS score, intubation and airway status, SAMPLE history, significant comorbidities, and estimated time of arrival. This way all the right people can be in the ED when you arrive.

▶ Mode of Transport

You must decide which mode of transport will offer the greatest benefit to your patient. Should you call for air transport, or is ground transport sufficient? When making the decision to transport by ground, several factors should be taken into consideration. Can the appropriate facility be reached within a reasonable time frame by ground? Ground transportation EMS units are generally staffed by traditional EMTs, advanced EMTs, and paramedics. What is the extent of injuries? If you're in a congested area, can the patient be transported to a more accessible landing zone for air medical transport?

Air transportation EMS units or critical care transport units are generally staffed by critical care transport professionals such as critical care nurses and critical care paramedics **Figure 29-22** . All levels of prehospital providers should recognize the need for and criteria used in making the decision to use aeromedical transport in their service areas.

Words of Wisdom

The National Trauma Data Standard (formerly known as the National Trauma Registry, or NTR) of the National Trauma Data Bank is a reporting system designed to collect standardized trauma-related data in an effort to improve the quality and cost-effectiveness of care and to aid in outcome research. Your contribution as a paramedic is the record of what you found at the scene.

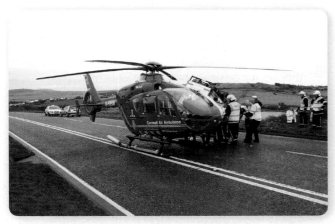

Figure 29-22 A helicopter may be used to transport patients quickly to a trauma center.

Courtesy of Mark Woolcock.

The Association of Air Medical Services and MedEvac Foundation International identify the following criteria for the appropriate use of emergency air medical services for trauma patients in the white paper, *Air Medicine: Accessing the Future of Healthcare*:

- There is an extended period required to access or extricate a remote (eg, injured hiker, snowmobiler, or boater) or trapped patient (eg, in a crashed vehicle) that depletes the time frame to get the patient to the trauma center by ground.
- Distance to the trauma center is greater than 20 to 25 miles.
- The patient needs medical care and stabilization at the Advanced Life Support (ALS)-level, and there is no ALS-level ground ambulance service available within a reasonable time frame.
- Traffic conditions or hospital availability make it unlikely that the patient will get to a trauma center via ground ambulance within the ideal time frame for best clinical outcome.
- There are multiple patients who will overwhelm resources at the trauma centers reachable by ground within the time frame.
- EMS systems require patients to be brought to the nearest hospital for initial evaluation and stabilization, rather than bypassing those facilities and going directly to a trauma center. This may add delay to definitive surgical care and necessitate air transport to mitigate the impact of that delay.
- There is a multiple-casualty incident.

These recommendations serve as a guideline for local decision makers to develop comprehensive protocols for the use of air medical transport. Always follow your local protocols when determining what type of patient transportation is appropriate. If the patient can be transported by ground to definitive care within a reasonable amount of time, then there is no need to call for air transport. The time it will take for the aircraft to lift off, travel, and land, just to reach the scene should be considered as well. By weighing the time frame for air transport against transport by ground, you will be able to make an informed decision. Also, consider the terrain. Is there a safe area for landing? If not, how far will the patient need to be transported to reach a secure landing zone? If the distance is great, then ground transport may be a more reasonable option. Once the decision is made to call for air medical transport, contact your dispatcher to request a unit, or follow local protocols regarding contacting air support. For more information about establishing landing zones, see Chapter 46, *Transport Operations*.

▶ Research and Trauma Care

Trauma patient care has been researched extensively over many years, especially by the military, in an effort to reduce death and disability of soldiers. Civilian trauma care has greatly benefitted from this research; however, occasionally, civilian research shows that what works well in the military does not always work as well in the civilian world. An example of this is the use of pneumatic antishock garments. In the 1980s, civilian research demonstrated that using pneumatic antishock garments for patients with penetrating wounds to the upper body was harmful, even though these devices had been used successfully for many years in the Vietnam war.[10]

Recent military research has shown that the dangers long associated with tourniquet use are not as serious as had once been assumed. This finding greatly increased tourniquet use in the control of extremity bleeding in the civilian population. Other military research has aided in the development of hemostatic materials which, when applied to open wounds, more rapidly control bleeding.[11] In addition, the military has brought the use of TXA to the attention of civilian trauma systems for the evaluation of its use by EMS to control internal bleeding.[12]

As with all aspects of emergency medical care, good research should drive changes in prehospital management of trauma patients. Patient care that is determined to be harmful or non-beneficial in the prehospital setting should be discontinued, and only evidence-based treatments should be adopted for widespread use by EMS. More EMS systems need to be involved in good research to validate the care we provide in every aspect of prehospital medicine.

YOU are the Paramedic   SUMMARY

1. Looking up at the Ferris wheel, what possible MOIs should you consider?

The most obvious consideration is the height from which the patient fell. In addition, the objects that the body may have struck while falling contribute to the index of suspicion of certain injuries. The patient landed on grass. Is the ground wet with some plasticity or dry and hard packed?

2. In addition to trauma sustained in the fall, what other information might you want to elicit from witnesses and friends of the patient?

All of the following information plays a part in helping determine the index of suspicion for possible injury: body position; location on the ride; whether the patient was pushed, fell, or jumped; motion of the Ferris wheel; part of the car from which the patient exited (front, side, back).

3. Because the patient is unresponsive with rapid, shallow breathing, you ask your partner to assist ventilations with a bag-mask device. What should you do next to continue your primary survey?

You need to quickly expose the chest and inspect, palpate, auscultate, seal, and stabilize. Remember, the primary survey is only for identifying and treating life threats.

4. The patient's friend comes forward and tearfully explains that her friend, who is a diabetic and was drinking "a few shots of tequila" earlier in the evening, was standing up in the ride's car, yelling and waving to her boyfriend, when the ride suddenly jerked to a stop, sending her tumbling out of the car. What important questions will you ask the friend?

Did she take her insulin and/or eat? Was she acting strangely prior to the fall? How much alcohol did she have and at what time? Did the patient ingest any other substances, such as drugs?

5. The patient's rapid, weak pulse and cool, moist skin indicate likelihood of inadequate perfusion, yet the blood pressure does not indicate advanced shock. What are some possible reasons for this finding?

Mixed or multisystem trauma will often result in injuries whose signs and symptoms may appear contradictory or confusing. The head injury could be causing development of severe and increasing intracranial pressure. This condition often causes fluctuations in vital signs, most notably, increasing blood pressure with narrowing pulse pressure and an eventual drop in pulse rate. The large contusion and possible pelvic fracture and potential for other internal injuries likely have resulted in hypovolemia. The body is responding to both the decrease in blood volume and the increase in intracranial pressure.

6. According to the friend who witnessed the fall, the patient's initial impact was with her head against the metal car below. What is the significance of a smaller surface area of the body absorbing the initial impact as opposed to a larger body surface area?

Remember, the larger the surface area absorbing energy, the more the energy will be spread out. The witness reports seeing her friend hit her head first before hitting the ground; it is possible that the patient's head experienced a significant impact. Your index of suspicion should be very high for serious head and cervical spine injury.

7. What criteria does this patient meet to warrant transport to the trauma center?

Upon your arrival, you immediately ascertain that the patient's GCS score is less than 13. This score, due to trauma, is all you need to justify transport to the nearest trauma center. Upon noting this, you ask other officials on scene to call the dispatcher and ask them to notify the trauma center of the impending arrival.

YOU are the Paramedic　SUMMARY (continued)

8. As you continue your exam and observation of your patient en route to the trauma center, you think about the presentation of your patient to the waiting ED staff. What MOI will you relate to the staff?

First, it is important to relate the patient's medical history and behavior prior to the fall, because this will greatly assist the staff in evaluating the patient's mental status and determining the course of treatment. Next, relay the height of the ride, possible trajectory, and points of impact while falling; the materials impacted (steel bars, metal cars); the surface on which the patient landed (soft, wet grass as opposed to hard, packed earth or concrete), and the position of body to the staff.

EMS Patient Care Report (PCR)					
Date: 07-02-18	**Incident No.:** 1056		**Nature of Call:** Injury		**Location:** Sixth Ave Amusement Park
Dispatched: 1940	**En Route:** 1941	**At Scene:** 1943	**Transport:** 1953	**At Hospital:** 1959	**In Service:** 2018

Patient Information	
Age: 18 **Sex:** F **Weight (in kg [lb]):** 54 kg (120 lb)	**Allergies:** Unknown **Medications:** Insulin **Past Medical History:** Type I diabetes **Chief Complaint:** Multisystem trauma

Vital Signs				
Time: 1948	**BP:** 140/110	**Pulse:** 140 weak, regular	**Respirations:** 12, assisted	**Spo₂:** 97%
Time: 1952	**BP:** 130/116	**Pulse:** 88	**Respirations:** 12, assisted	**Spo₂:** 98%
Time: 1957	**BP:** 120/112	**Pulse:** 60	**Respirations:** 12, assisted	**Spo₂:** 96%

EMS Treatment (circle all that apply)				
Oxygen @ _____ L/min via (circle one): NC　NRM　**Bag-mask device**	(**Assisted Ventilation**)	**Airway Adjunct**		**CPR**
Defibrillation	**Bleeding Control**	**Bandaging**	(**Splinting**)	(**Other:** Spinal immobilization)

Narrative
Dispatched by 9-1-1 for an injury at Sixth Avenue Amusement Park. Pt reportedly fell from a car near the top of the 30-ft Ferris wheel. Upon arrival, 18-year-old female found supine on wet, grassy area beneath the Ferris wheel. Pt unresponsive to verbal and painful stimuli. Witnesses stated that pt fell forward from a standing position and struck her head while tumbling to the ground. Pt was allegedly drinking tequila earlier in the night, has a history of diabetes, and was acting "crazy" according to friends. Manual stabilization applied immediately upon arrival. Pt airway is open, clear, and maintained. OPA insertion attempted but removed due to patient gag reflex. Breathing was adequate with trachea midline, equal chest rise, no skin breaks, no discoloration, no crepitus noted. Breath sounds present and equal. No severe bleeding noted. Left pupil is dilated and nonreactive. Exposed body shows large hematoma on right lower quadrant extending to pelvic region. Abdominal distention noted. Pt legs both bent outward upon arrival and moved without resistance to midline for immobilization on backboard. Left arm is deformed and cool to the touch. No radial pulse palpable. Immobilized against body and on backboard. No skin breaks or discoloration noted on back. Pt remained unresponsive en route with fluctuating vital signs (see chart). Airway monitored/maintained, ventilation assisted. Blood glucose obtained en route at 1956 hours from right index finger is 73. Trauma center staff notified and waiting for pt arrival—1959 hours. Return to service at 2018 hours.**End of report**

Prep Kit

► Ready for Review

- Trauma is the primary cause of death and disability in people between age 1 and 44 years.
- The amount of force and energy delivered are factors in the extent of trauma sustained. Duration and direction of the force of application are also important.
- Understanding the effects of forces and energy will help in developing a high index of suspicion for the mechanism of injury and the likely types of injuries.
- Kinetic energy of an object is the energy associated with that object in motion. It reflects the relationship between the weight (mass) of the object and the velocity at which it is traveling.
- The law of conservation of energy states energy can be neither created nor destroyed; it can only change form.
- Multisystem trauma describes trauma that involves several body systems. Most trauma affects more than one system, often includes both blunt and penetrating trauma, and has a high level of morbidity and mortality.
- Blunt trauma refers to injuries in which the tissues are not penetrated by an external object, as commonly occurs in motor vehicle crashes (MVCs), in pedestrians hit by a vehicle, in motorcycle crashes, in falls from heights, in serious sports injures, and in blasts when no shrapnel is involved.
- In a MVC, the angle of impact, mechanical characteristics of the vehicle, and the occupant's position at the time of impact will determine types of injuries.
- Trauma in a crash is composed of five phases representing the effects of progressive deceleration: deceleration of the vehicle, deceleration of the occupant, deceleration of internal organs, secondary crashes, and additional impacts.
- There are five primary types of impacts: frontal or head on, lateral or side, rear, rotational, and rollover.
- The front seat occupants of vehicles during a frontal or head-on crash usually follow one of two trajectories, a down-and-under pathway or an up-and-over pathway.
- Vehicle safety devices such as seat belts, airbags, and helmets are designed to manipulate the way in which energy is dissipated into injury.
- In a motorcycle crash, any structural protection afforded to the riders is not derived from a steel cage, as is the case in a vehicle, but from safety devices worn by the rider such as helmets and leather or abrasion-resistant clothing.
- There are four types of motorcycle impacts: head-on collisions, angular collisions, ejected riders, or laying the bike down.
- Adult pedestrians involved in a crash experience three predominant mechanisms of injury: lower extremity injuries from the initial hit, second impact injuries from being thrown onto the hood or grille, and third impact injuries when the body strikes the ground or another object.
- The severity of injuries from falls from heights depends on the height, position, and orientation of the body at the moment of impact; the area over which the impact is distributed; the surface onto which the person falls; and the physical condition of the patient.
- Penetrating trauma involves a disruption of the skin and underlying tissues in a small, focused area, as commonly occurs with stab wounds and gunshot wounds.
- The severity of a stab wound depends on the anatomic area involved, depth of penetration, blade length, and angle of penetration.
- Firearms are the primary mechanism resulting in penetrating trauma. The magnitude of tissue damage depends on the projectile's velocity, the orientation of the projectile as it entered the body, the distance from which the weapon was fired, the design of the projectile, and the type of tissue through which the projectile passed.
- Blast injuries include primary, secondary, tertiary, quaternary (miscellaneous), and quinary injuries.
- A blast wave or shock wave is dependent on many factors including the size of the explosive charge, the nature of the surrounding medium, the distance from the explosion, and the presence or absence of reflecting surfaces.
- Air-containing organs such as the middle ear, heart, lungs, major blood vessels, and gastrointestinal tract are most susceptible to pressure changes and blast injuries.
- Known as the trauma lethal triad, the combination of hypothermia, coagulopathy (poor blood clotting), and acidosis is a major contributor to death in patients with severe traumatic bleeding.
- Managing trauma patients requires a thorough and accurate assessment of the patient as well as a good working knowledge of the mechanisms of injury. In treating multisystem trauma, remember, if a generalized mechanism is present, then you should anticipate multisystem injuries. It is also important to remember that multisystem trauma patients cannot be stabilized in the field.

Prep Kit (continued)

- The criteria for transport to a trauma center vary from system to system. However, there are key variables for transport to a trauma center as defined by the Centers for Disease Control and Prevention National Trauma Triage Protocol.
- There are four categories of trauma centers. Your system may include a Level I, which is the highest level trauma center.
- The Association of Air Medical Services and MedEvac Foundation International identify criteria for the appropriate use of emergency air medical services for trauma patients. The criteria include situations in which there is extended transport time by ground, multiple-casualty incidents, prolonged extrication times, critically injured patients, or when there is a long distance to an appropriate facility.

▶ Vital Vocabulary

acceleration (a) The rate of change in velocity; speeding up.

angle of impact The angle at which an object hits another; this characterizes the force vectors involved and has a bearing on patterns of energy dissipation.

arterial air embolism Air bubbles in the arterial blood vessels.

avulsing A tearing away or forcible separation.

ballistics The study of non-powered objects in flight; most often associated with rifle or handgun bullet travel.

barometric energy The energy that results from sudden changes in pressure as may occur in a diving accident or sudden decompression in an airplane.

biomechanics The study of the physiology and mechanics of a living organism using the tools of mechanical engineering.

blast front The leading edge of the shock wave.

blunt trauma An impact on the body by objects that cause injury without penetrating soft tissues or internal organs and cavities.

brisance The shattering effect of a shock wave and its ability to cause disruption of tissues and structures.

cavitation Cavity formation; shock waves that push tissues in front of and lateral to the projectile and may not necessarily increase the wound size or cause permanent injury but can result in cavitation.

chemical energy The energy released as a result of a chemical reaction.

deceleration A negative acceleration—that is, slowing down.

electrical energy The energy delivered in the form of high voltage.

entrance wound The point at which a penetrating object enters the body.

exit wound The point at which a penetrating object leaves the body, which may or may not be in a straight line from the entry wound.

gravity (g) The acceleration of a body by the attraction of the earth's gravitational force, normally 32.2 ft/sec^2 (9.8 m/sec^2).

implosion A bursting inward.

index of suspicion Anticipating the possibility of specific types of injury.

kinetic energy (KE) The energy associated with bodies in motion, expressed mathematically as half the mass times the square of the velocity.

kinetics The study of the relationship among speed, mass, vector direction, and physical injury.

law of conservation of energy The law of physics that states energy can be neither created nor destroyed; it can only change form.

mechanical energy The energy that results from motion (kinetic energy) or that is stored in an object (potential energy).

mechanism of injury (MOI) The way in which traumatic injuries occur; the forces that act on the body to cause damage.

missile fragmentation A primary mechanism of tissue disruption from certain rifles in which pieces of the projectile break apart, allowing the pieces to create their own separate paths through tissues.

multisystem trauma Trauma caused by generalized mechanisms which affect numerous body systems.

negative wave pulse The phase of an explosion in which pressure from the blast is less than atmospheric pressure.

Newton's first law of motion The law of motion that states a body at rest will remain at rest unless acted on by an outside force.

Newton's second law of motion The law of motion that states the force that an object can exert is the product of its mass times its acceleration.

pathway expansion The tissue displacement that occurs as a result of low-displacement shock waves that travel at the speed of sound in tissue.

penetrating trauma Injury caused by objects that pierce the surface of the body, such as knives and bullets, and damage internal tissues and organs.

permanent cavity The path of crushed tissue produced by a missile traversing part of the body.

Prep Kit (continued)

positive wave pulse The phase of the explosion in which there is a pressure front with a pressure higher than atmospheric pressure.

potential energy The amount of energy stored in an object, the product of mass, gravity, and height, that is converted into kinetic energy and results in injury, such as from a fall.

pulmonary blast injuries Pulmonary trauma resulting from short-range exposure to the detonation of high explosives.

Revised Trauma Score (RTS) A scoring system used for patients with head trauma.

shearing An applied force or pressure exerted against the surface and layers of the skin as tissues slide in opposite but parallel planes.

thermal energy Energy transferred from sources that are hotter than the body, such as a flame, hot water, steam.

trauma Acute physiologic and structural change (injury) that occurs in a person's body as a result of the rapid dissipation of energy delivered by an external source.

trauma lethal triad A combination of hypothermia, coagulopathy (poor blood clotting), and acidosis that is a major contributor to death in patients with severe traumatic bleeding.

trauma score A score that relates to the likelihood of patient survival with the exception of a severe head injury. It is calculated on a scale from 1 to 16, with 16 being the best possible score. It takes into account the Glasgow Coma Scale score, respiratory rate, respiratory expansion, systolic blood pressure, and capillary refill.

tympanic membrane The eardrum; a thin, semitransparent membrane in the middle ear that transmits sound vibrations to the internal ear by means of the auditory ossicles.

velocity (V) The speed at which an object travels per unit of time, in a specific direction.

Waddell triad A pattern of vehicle versus pedestrian injuries in children and people of short stature in which (1) the bumper hits pelvis and femur, (2) the chest and abdomen hit the grille or low hood, and (3) the head strikes the ground.

whiplash An injury to the cervical vertebrae or its supporting ligaments and muscles, usually resulting from sudden acceleration or deceleration.

▶ References

1. Injury Prevention and Control: Data and Statistics. Centers for Disease Control and Prevention website. (WISQARS). http://www.cdc.gov/injury/wisqars/overview/key_data.html. Updated September 19, 2016. Accessed June 29, 2016.

2. Top causes of unintentional injury and death in homes and communities. The National Safety Council website. http://www.nsc.org/learn/safety-knowledge/Pages/safety-at-home.aspx. Accessed June 29, 2016.

3. 2014 motor vehicle crashes: overview. National Center for Statistics and Analysis. National Highway Traffic Safety Administration website. https://crashstats.nhtsa.dot.gov/Api/Public/ViewPublication/8122492. Published March 2016. Accessed January 23, 2017.

4. Esterlitz JR. Relative risk of death from ejection by crash type and crash mode. *Accid Anal Preven*. 1989; 21(5):459-468.

5. Kahane CJ. Updated estimates of fatality reduction by curtain and side air bags in side impacts and preliminary analyses of rollover curtains. National Highway Traffic Safety Administration website. https://crashstats.nhtsa.dot.gov/Api/Public/ViewPublication/811882. Published January 2014. Accessed March 30, 2017.

6. Traffic Safety Facts, 2014 data: pedestrians. National Center for Statistics and Analysis. National Highway Traffic Safety Administration website. https://crashstats.nhtsa.dot.gov/Api/Public/ViewPublication/812270. Published May 2016. Accessed February 27, 2017.

7. Xu J, Murphy SL, Kochanek KD, Bastian BA. Deaths: final data for 2013. *Natl Vital Stat Rep*. 2016;64(2):1-119.

8. Gerecht R. The lethal triad. Hypothermia, acidosis & coagulopathy create a deadly cycle for trauma patients. *J Emerg Med*. 2014;39(4):56-60.

9. MacKenzie EJ, Rivara FP, Jurkovich GJ, Nathens AB. The national study on the costs and outcomes of trauma. *J Trauma*. 2007;63(suppl 6):S54-S67.

10. Bickell WH, Pepe PE, Wyatt CH, et al. Effect of antishock trousers on the trauma score: a prospective analysis in the urban setting. *Ann Emerg Med*. 1985;14(3):218-22.

11. Snyder D, Tsou A, Schoelles K. Efficacy of prehospital application of tourniquets and hemostatic dressings to control traumatic external hemorrhage. National Highway Traffic Safety Administration website https://www.ems.gov/pdf/research/Studies-and-Reports/Prehospital_Applications_Of_Tourniquest_And_Hemostatic_Dressings.pdf. Published May 2014. Accessed February 8, 2017.

12. Morrison JJ, Dubose JJ, Rasmussen TE, Midwinter MJ. Military application of tranexamic acid in trauma emergency resuscitation (MATTERs) study. *Arch Surg*. 2012;147(2):113-9.

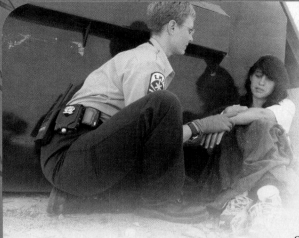

Assessment in Action

You and your partner arrive at the scene of a pedestrian struck by a bicycle. The scene is safe and traffic has been rerouted by police on the scene. As you approach the patient, you see a messenger bicycle on its side. A young man is standing next to the bicycle explaining to a police officer, "I didn't see her. I had no time to even slow down. She walked in front of me like I was invisible." An older adult woman is lying supine on the pavement with her left leg rotated outward. A bystander is holding the patient's hand and talking to her.

Your partner is maintaining manual in-line stabilization and the patient is responding appropriately to your questions. She is shaking and tells you she feels cold. Her airway appears clear and she is maintaining it on her own. Her chest is expanding equally and her respirations are adequate, although rapid. As you carefully inspect the chest, you see some discoloration over the left side. The site is tender to palpation but no crepitus is noted. Breath sounds are equal and clear. She has numerous deep abrasions on her left side, left arm, and left leg, with no severe bleeding. Both radial pulses are present and you notice her hands are very cold. Covering her with a blanket, you continue with your assessment. Her pupils are constricted and nonreactive. She tells you she was diagnosed with cataracts when she was 75 years old and has been using eye drops for treatment for about 5 years. She denies any other medical conditions.

You obtain baseline vital signs. Her blood pressure is 118/60 mm Hg, pulse is 90 beats/min, and respirations are 22 breaths/min. Pulse oximetry shows an SpO_2 of 96% on high concentration oxygen via nonrebreathing mask.

1. The patient's vital signs seem to indicate the patient is stable. At this point, you should:

   A. immobilize the patient on a backboard and rapidly transport.
   B. continue with a secondary assessment.
   C. ask the patient to attempt to sit up.
   D. help the patient onto the stretcher.

2. What information contributes significantly to the potential severity of the patient's injuries?

   A. A history of cataracts
   B. The speed and lack of braking of the bicyclist
   C. The weight of the bicyclist
   D. The angle at which the bicycle struck the patient

3. The type of energy with which the patient was initially hit was:

   A. potential energy.
   B. thermal energy.
   C. kinetic energy.
   D. converted energy.

4. Your patient is approximately 80 years old. The significance of age in terms of being able to disperse the energy is:

   A. important because older adults may not be able to move quickly out of the way.
   B. insignificant.
   C. significant because of reduced bone and muscle mass.
   D. significant due to age-related organ deterioration.

5. During your primary survey, you found a hand-sized discoloration on the left side of the patient's chest. The patient is telling you she feels cold but her vital signs seem normal. You would treat her for shock:

   A. only when her vital signs show significant changes.
   B. based on the injuries you observe.
   C. based on the mechanism of injury.
   D. based on her current vital signs.

Assessment *in Action* (continued)

6. You and your partner decide the patient needs to go to the nearest trauma center. Your decision is based on:

   A. her vital signs.
   B. discoloration over the left side of the chest.
   C. the possible fractured hip.
   D. the impact speed at which the bike hit the patient.

7. Based on your assessment findings, which of the following would you watch closest in your reassessment of the patient while en route to the hospital?

   A. Her blood pressure in case of shock
   B. Her breath sounds in case of pneumothorax
   C. Her pupils in case of narcotics use
   D. Her temperature in case of hypothermia

8. An older patient with multiple injuries presents with a baseline blood pressure of 118/60 mm Hg. You and your partner discuss whether or not this is an important finding. What other information will you need to help you determine whether your patient is experiencing shock?

9. You and your partner responded to a vehicle versus tree collision where you find an unconscious older adult male slumped over the steering wheel. There is minimal damage to the front of the vehicle and no windshield or steering wheel damage. How does this information affect your suspicions of patient injury?

10. You respond to an unconscious victim of a gunshot wound and find three penetrations in the middle back about 0.25 inch (0.6 cm) in diameter and no other injuries. What are your suspicions about the mechanism of injury and what types of injuries would you be most concerned about with this patient?

Bleeding

National EMS Education Standard Competencies

Trauma

Integrates assessment findings with principles of epidemiology and pathophysiology to formulate a field impression to implement a comprehensive treatment/disposition plan for an acutely injured patient.

Bleeding

Recognition and management of
> Bleeding (pp 1585-1587, 1590-1592, 1594-1602)

Pathophysiology, assessment, and management of
> Bleeding (pp 1585-1587, 1590-1602)
> Fluid resuscitation (pp 1589, 1591, 1600-1602)

Knowledge Objectives

1. Discuss the anatomy and physiology of the cardiovascular system. (pp 1582-1585)
2. Discuss the pathophysiology of external and internal hemorrhage. (pp 1585-1587)
3. Describe the body's physiologic response to hemorrhaging. (pp 1586-1587)
4. Describe the types of shock. (pp 1587-1589)
5. Discuss the pathophysiology of hemorrhagic shock. (pp 1588-1589)
6. Discuss the classes of hemorrhage. (p 1588)
7. Discuss the phases of shock. (p 1589)
8. Describe the assessment and management of a bleeding patient. (pp 1590-1593)
9. Describe the assessment and management of a patient with hemorrhagic shock. (pp 1590-1593, 1600-1602)
10. Describe how to assess and manage a patient with external hemorrhage. (pp 1594-1600)
11. Describe how to apply a commercial tourniquet. (pp 1595-1598)
12. Describe how to assess and manage a patient with internal hemorrhage. (pp 1600-1601)
13. Describe how to assess and manage a patient with hemorrhagic shock. (pp 1600-1602)

Skills Objectives

1. Demonstrate the assessment and management of a patient with signs and symptoms of external hemorrhage. (pp 1594-1595, Skill Drill 30-1)
2. Demonstrate how to apply a commercial tourniquet. (pp 1595-1598, Skill Drill 30-2)
3. Demonstrate the assessment and management of a patient with signs and symptoms of internal hemorrhage. (pp 1600-1601, Skill Drill 30-3)
4. Demonstrate the assessment and management of a patient experiencing hemorrhagic shock. (pp 1600-1602)

YOU are the Paramedic   PART 1

On a quiet Friday morning, the dispatcher notifies you that a man is down at a construction site and serious injuries are possible. On your arrival at the scene, a man in a hard hat rushes over to the ambulance. He explains, "I'm Dave, the foreman. One of my guys was up there on the scaffold and was hit by a steel beam that was being lowered into place. His harness lanyard didn't hold. He fell and landed on his back. Hurry! He's hurt bad, I think." The foreman points to a scaffold approximately 15 feet off the ground, on the side of a building under construction.

1. Is there a possibility of more than one mechanism of injury (MOI) in this scenario?
2. This is a high-rise, commercial construction site. What could some of the potential hazards be for you and your partner?

Introduction

"A before B, except after C." This phrase emphasizes the paradigm shift in trauma care from a focus on the airway above all to a focus on circulation when there is evidence, or a high index of suspicion, of severe hemorrhage. Bleeding is one of the most time-sensitive conditions you will face as a paramedic.

The end goal in trauma care is to maintain perfusion. A patient suffering from massive hemorrhage must have his or her bleeding controlled immediately. In such a case, the C of circulation takes priority over airway and breathing (CAB). If you incorrectly place a top priority on airway management in a patient with severe bleeding, you would provide ventilation and oxygenation to the lungs, but by the time that was achieved, there would be inadequate circulation to transport that oxygen to perfuse the tissues. A perfectly secured and managed airway is of minimal consequence if the circulatory system is not able to deliver oxygen to the organs and remove accumulated wastes from them.

Even seemingly inconsequential bleeding may be potentially dangerous, because it may initially cause symptoms as vague as general weakness, but later progress to shock. Uncontrolled bleeding may lead to serious injury and, ultimately, death.

To fully understand the content of this chapter, you should review the anatomy and physiology of the cardiovascular and respiratory systems and their roles in keeping blood flowing between the lungs and peripheral tissues. In this chapter, we will review the cardiovascular and respiratory systems and discuss hemorrhagic shock caused by both internal and external bleeding (Chapter 8, *Anatomy and Physiology*, provides a full review of the cardiovascular and respiratory systems). The control of external hemorrhaging, including the use of tourniquets, splints, and the role of hemostatic agents, is discussed as well.

Anatomy and Physiology Review

The cardiovascular system is designed to carry out one crucial job: keep blood flowing from the lungs to the peripheral tissues, and back to the lungs again. The right side of the heart pumps blood to the lungs, and the left side of the heart receives blood from the lungs and then pumps it around the body. For perfusion to take place, the circulatory system must function efficiently to deliver oxygen to the tissues of the body and transport waste products away from the cells and tissues.

In the lungs, blood unloads the gaseous waste products of metabolism—chiefly carbon dioxide—and picks up life-sustaining oxygen. In the peripheral tissues, this process is reversed: Blood unloads oxygen and picks up wastes. If blood flow were to stop or slow significantly, the results would be catastrophic. The cells of the brain,

heart, and other organs of the body would have no way to eliminate their wastes and would be rapidly engulfed by the toxic by-products of their own metabolism. Oxygen delivery to the tissues would also be disrupted. For a few minutes, the cells could switch to an emergency metabolic system—one that does not require oxygen (anaerobic metabolism)—but that form of metabolism produces even more acids and toxic wastes. Within a few minutes of circulatory failure, cells throughout the body would begin to suffocate and die. In an attempt to survive during this state of widespread inadequate perfusion, or shock, the body would compensate in an organized manner as it sought to maintain the systolic blood pressure and perfusion to the brain and heart, at the expense of other areas such as the skin, muscles, liver, and kidneys.

To keep the blood moving continuously through the body, the circulatory system requires three intact components **Figure 30-1**:

- A "pump": a functioning heart that serves to mechanically push the blood and components around the system

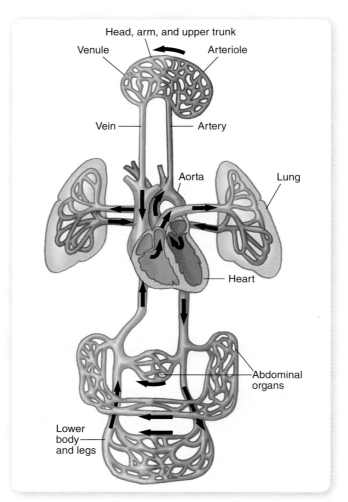

Figure 30-1 The circulatory system requires continuous operation of its three components: the heart, the blood and body fluids, and the blood vessels.

© Jones & Bartlett Learning.

- "Pipes": an intact system of tubing, called blood vessels, capable of reflex adjustments (constriction and dilation) in response to changes in pump output and fluid volume
- "Fluid": adequate fluid volume of the blood to fill the pipes to transport oxygen and nutrients to the tissues and waste products away from the tissues

All three components must interact effectively to maintain life. If any one becomes damaged or is deficient, its failure puts the whole system in jeopardy.

Words of Wisdom

Cellular respiration is a series of metabolic processes that the body uses to make energy. It includes three steps: glycolysis, the citric acid cycle, and the electron transport chain. During glycolysis, glucose is broken down into pyruvic acid and produces two adenosine triphosphate (ATP) molecules. In the citric acid cycle, a sequence of enzymatic reactions occurs to convert pyruvic acid into ATP, water, co_2, acetyl coenzyme A, and high-energy electrons. The electron transport chain converts these high-energy electrons into more ATP, releasing heat and water as by-products. This process is known as the aerobic pathway, so named because oxygen is the final electron donor in this process. A large amount of ATP is produced via this process, which the cells then utilize to do the work of life. In the absence of oxygen, only glycolysis and then fermentation occur; in such a case, the pathway is known as anaerobic. During fermentation, pyruvic acid is converted into ethanol or lactic acid, and in the process regenerates intermediates for glycolysis. This substantially less efficient process yields only a small amount of ATP and will be unable to continue to meet the energy needs of the cells.

▶ The Cardiac Cycle

The cardiac cycle is the repetitive pumping process that begins with the onset of cardiac muscle contraction and ends with the beginning of the next contraction. Myocardial contraction results in pressure changes within the cardiac chambers, causing the blood to move from areas of high pressure to areas of low pressure.

Preload is the amount of blood returned to the heart to be pumped out. It directly affects **afterload**, the pressure in the aorta or the peripheral vascular resistance, against which the left ventricle must pump blood. The greater the afterload, the harder it is for the ventricle to eject blood into the aorta. A higher afterload, therefore, reduces the **stroke volume (SV)**, or the amount of blood ejected per contraction. To a large degree, afterload is governed by arterial blood pressure.

The cardiac cycle is connected to bleeding and shock through its relationship to blood pressure, the level of which is considered the dividing line between the stages of shock. In general terms, blood pressure is represented by the following equation:

$$\text{Blood pressure} = \text{Cardiac output (CO)} \times \text{peripheral vascular resistance (PVR)}$$

where PVR is essentially the resistance in the vessels caused by vasoconstriction or vasodilation. PVR is measured as mean arterial pressure (MAP), which can be estimated using the following equation:

$$\text{MAP} = \text{Diastolic pressure} + 1/3 \text{ pulse pressure}$$

The pulse pressure is calculated by subtracting the diastolic blood pressure (DBP) from the systolic blood pressure (SBP):

$$\text{MAP} = \text{DBP} + 1/3 \text{ (SBP-DBP)}$$

Cardiac output (CO) is the amount of blood pumped through the circulatory system in 1 minute. CO is expressed in liters per minute (L/min). Cardiac output equals the stroke volume multiplied by the pulse rate:

$$\text{CO} = \text{SV} \times \text{pulse rate}$$

Factors that influence the SV, the pulse rate, or both will affect CO and, therefore, oxygen delivery (perfusion) to the tissues.

Increased venous return to the heart stretches the ventricles somewhat, resulting in increased cardiac contractility. This relationship, which was first described by the British physiologist Ernest Henry Starling, is known as the Frank-Starling mechanism or Starling law of the heart. Starling noted that if a muscle is stretched slightly before it is stimulated to contract, it will contract with greater force. Thus, if the heart is stretched, the muscle contracts more forcefully.

Although the amount of blood returning to the right atrium varies somewhat from minute to minute, a normal heart continues to pump the same percentage of blood returned, a measure called the **ejection fraction (EF)**. If more blood returns to the heart, the stretched heart pumps harder rather than allowing the blood to back up into the veins. As a result, more blood is pumped with each contraction, yet the ejection fraction remains unchanged: The amount of blood that is pumped increases, but so does the amount of blood returned. This relationship maintains normal cardiac function when a person changes positions, coughs, breathes, or moves.

If we then connect and expand the two equations presented earlier, we get the following expression:

$$\text{Blood pressure} = \text{SV (includes preload and afterload)} \times \text{heart rate} \times \text{PVR (also known as MAP)}$$

This single formula gives an elegant explanation for shock and indicates where treatment needs to focus. Write it down on a separate piece of paper and, as you read the next section on circulation and perfusion, see where each of these pieces affects each other. For example, as the blood pressure drops, what happens to the heart rate to compensate for it? What do the blood vessels do? How does this affect preload and afterload? Can you see how fluid resuscitation effects blood pressure and, therefore, perfusion? Keep in mind that the loss of blood through hemorrhage reduces the preload, thus, lowering the first part of the equation (SV), triggering an initial compensatory response from the other parts of the equation (HR and PVR).

▶ Blood and Its Components

Blood consists of plasma and formed elements or cells that are suspended in the plasma. These cells include red blood cells (RBCs), white blood cells (WBCs), and platelets. RBCs make up approximately 45% of blood volume, whereas WBCs and platelets account for less than 1% of blood volume.

Words of Wisdom

Red blood cells are about one-third hemoglobin, the protein that gives them their red color. Hemoglobin is responsible for the cells' ability to transport oxygen and carbon dioxide. When hemoglobin binds with oxygen, oxyhemoglobin is formed. Oxyhemoglobin is bright red. When oxygen is released, deoxyhemoglobin is formed. Deoxyhemoglobin is darker red, and blood rich in deoxyhemoglobin may appear blue when seen through blood vessels.

The purpose of blood is to carry oxygen and nutrients such as glucose, proteins, fats, and electrolytes to the tissues, and cellular waste products away from the tissues. In addition, the formed elements serve as the mainstay of numerous other body functions, such as fighting infections and controlling bleeding.

Plasma is a watery, straw-colored fluid that accounts for more than half of the total blood volume. It consists of 92% water and 8% dissolved substances such as chemicals, minerals, and nutrients. (Chapter 8, *Anatomy and Physiology*, provides more information about plasma.) Water enters the plasma from the digestive tract, from fluids between cells, and as a by-product of metabolism.

Platelets are small cell fragments produced from larger cells (megakaryocytes) in the blood that are essential for clot formation. The blood clotting (coagulation) process encompasses a complex series of events involving platelets, clotting proteins in the plasma (clotting factors), other proteins, and calcium. During coagulation, platelets aggregate in a clump and form much of the foundation

of a blood clot. Clotting proteins produced by the liver solidify the remainder of the clot, which eventually includes RBCs and WBCs.

Words of Wisdom

Hematocrit is a blood test that measures the portion of RBCs in whole blood. Normal hematocrit values vary, but in general are as follows:
- Men (any age): 40.7% to 50.3%
- Women (any age): 36.1% to 44.3%

If a patient's hematocrit value is out of range, the patient may have some sort of disease. Many different diseases or conditions could cause an abnormal value, leading to anemia.

▶ Blood Circulation and Perfusion

Arteries are blood vessels that carry blood away from the heart. Veins are blood vessels that transport blood back to the heart. As arteries get farther from the heart, they become smaller. Eventually, they branch into many small arterioles, which themselves divide into even smaller capillaries (microscopic, thin-walled blood vessels). Oxygen and nutrients pass out of the capillaries and into the cells, and carbon dioxide and waste products pass from the cells and into the capillaries in a process called diffusion. To return deoxygenated blood to the heart, groups of capillaries gradually enlarge to form venules. Venules then merge together, forming larger veins that eventually empty into the heart.

Perfusion is the circulation of blood within an organ or tissue in adequate amounts to meet the cells' current needs for oxygen, nutrients, and waste removal. Blood must pass through the cardiovascular system at a speed that is fast enough to maintain adequate circulation throughout the body, yet slow enough to allow each cell enough time to exchange oxygen and nutrients for carbon dioxide and other waste products. Although some tissues, such as the lungs and kidneys, never rest and require a constant blood supply, most tissues require circulating blood only intermittently, but especially when they are active. Muscles, for example, are at rest and require a minimal blood supply when you sleep. In contrast, during exercise, muscles need a large blood supply. As another example, the gastrointestinal (GI) tract requires a high flow of blood after a meal. After digestion is completed, a small fraction of that flow is adequate to meet its needs.

The autonomic nervous system monitors the body's needs from moment to moment, adjusting the blood flow as required. This system is responsible for maintaining homeostasis and is divided into sympathetic and parasympathetic components that oppose each other and keep vital functions in balance.

The sympathetic system is often referred to as the "fight, flight, or freeze" mode and initiates the body's normal response to stress. Such a stressor can be external, such as an immediate danger, or it can be internal, such as having a myocardial infarction or experiencing rapid blood loss. Actions of the sympathetic system include faster and stronger heart contractions, faster and deeper respirations combined with bronchodilation, shunting of blood to vital areas in the core of the body and away from the skin, and slowing and cessation of digestive functions.

The parasympathetic nervous system is often referred to as the "rest and digest" system. The activities of this part of the autonomic nervous system are reparative and restorative. The parasympathetic system's actions include slowing of the heart rate, slowing of the breathing rate, and acceleration of digestive functions.

The vasomotor center in the medulla oblongata helps to regulate blood pressure. If a drop in blood pressure is detected in the aortic arch or the carotid sinus, such as during blood loss, the baroreceptors (stretch or pressure sensors) send stimuli to the brain via cranial nerves IX and X, which causes an increase in sympathetic stimulation. The opposite is true in cases in which blood pressure is rising.

Another important system that responds to blood pressure changes is the endocrine system. For instance, a fall in blood pressure and the resultant changes in plasma osmolality cause the release of aldosterone from the adrenal glands and antidiuretic hormone (ADH) from the pituitary gland. The aldosterone and ADH then cause additional peripheral vasoconstriction as well as a conservation of water in the kidneys.

Thus, the cardiovascular system, working in conjunction with the nervous and endocrine systems, is dynamic and constantly adapts to changing conditions, such as a decrease in circulating blood volume. Sometimes, however, the amount of blood loss is too great and the compensatory mechanisms are insufficient to maintain circulation, resulting in **hypoperfusion** or shock.

The delivery of oxygen to the tissues is dependent on an adequate heart rate, stroke volume, hemoglobin levels, and arterial oxygen saturation. If any of these elements is not adequate, tissues will become ischemic.

Pathophysiology of Hemorrhage

Hemorrhage means bleeding. Hemorrhage can range from a "nick" to a capillary while shaving, to a severely spurting artery from a deep slash with a knife, to a ruptured spleen from striking the steering column during a vehicle crash. External visible hemorrhage from the extremities usually

YOU are the Paramedic PART 2

After grabbing the backboard and trauma kit, you and your partner approach the scene. The foreman assures you that no work is under way and that the site is safe to enter with the appropriate safety equipment.

As you approach the scene, you see a worker crouched next to the injured man. She tells you, "I'm an EMT. I work on a volunteer unit back home. I was down here when he fell. I rushed over and told him not to move."

The EMT is maintaining manual in-line cervical immobilization on the patient, who is supine on the hard-packed dirt and rock ground. As you approach, he looks at you and says, "I'm okay. My back hurts, but I think I'm okay. I'm just a little light-headed." As you communicate with the patient, you check his radial pulse and notice that his skin is cool and his pulse is very rapid and weak.

Recording Time: 1 Minute	
Appearance	Awake, harness and tool belt attached
Level of consciousness	Alert
Airway	Open and clear, self-maintained
Breathing	Rapid, unlabored
Circulation	Rapid, weak radial pulse

3. The patient is alert, is breathing adequately, and has a rapid but weak radial pulse. His coworker is holding proper manual immobilization of the cervical spine. What is your next priority?
4. You and your partner decide that the MOI indicates that this patient has a high risk of serious injury and you want to move quickly. Do you leave the harness and tool belt in place, or do you remove them before completing your assessment?

can be controlled by using direct, even pressure, pressure dressings and/or splints, hemostatic dressings, or tourniquets. Internal hemorrhage is not visible and, if severe, may require rapid surgery to correct. Because internal hemorrhage is not as obvious, you must rely on signs and symptoms to determine the extent and severity of the bleeding.

▶ External Hemorrhage

The extent or severity of external hemorrhage is often a function of the type of wound and the types of blood vessels that have been injured. (Wound types are discussed in detail in Chapter 31, *Soft-Tissue Trauma*.) Hemorrhage from a capillary usually oozes, bleeding from a vein flows, and bleeding from an artery spurts. If the laceration or tear is large enough, the person can exsanguinate in as little as a few minutes. Exsanguination is the loss of the total blood volume, resulting in death.

These descriptions are not infallible. For example, considerable oozing from capillaries is possible when a patient sustains a large abrasion (such as road rash when a cyclist slides along the pavement without protective clothing). Likewise, varicose veins on the leg can produce copious bleeding.

Arteries may spurt initially, but as the patient's blood pressure decreases, often the blood simply flows. In addition, an artery that is incised directly across or in a transverse manner will often recoil and attempt to slow its own bleeding. By contrast, if the artery is cut vertically, along its length, or only partially transected, it does not recoil and continues to bleed.

Some injuries that you might expect to be accompanied by considerable external hemorrhage are not severe. For example, a person who falls off the platform at the train station and is run over by a train may have amputations of one or more extremities, yet experience little bleeding because the wound was cauterized by the heat of the train's wheels on the rail. Conversely, a person who is on the shoulder of the road and removing the jack from his vehicle's trunk when another motorist slams into the rear of the vehicle, pinning him between the two vehicles, may have severely crushed legs. In such a case, hemorrhage may be severe, with the only effective means of bleeding control being tourniquets.

▶ Internal Hemorrhage

Internal hemorrhage as a result of trauma may appear in any portion of the body. A fracture of some appendicular bones, such as the humerus or the tibia, may produce a somewhat controlled environment in which only a relatively small amount of bleeding occurs. By contrast, bleeding in the trunk (ie, the thorax, abdomen, or pelvis), because of its much larger space, tends to be severe and uncontrolled. Nontraumatic internal hemorrhage can occur in cases of GI bleeding from the upper or lower GI tract, ruptured ectopic pregnancies, ruptured aneurysms, or other conditions.

Any internal hemorrhage must be treated promptly. The signs of internal hemorrhage (such as discoloration,

hematoma) do not always develop quickly, so you must rely on other signs and symptoms and an evaluation of the MOI to make this diagnosis. Pay close attention to patient complaints of pain or tenderness, development of tachycardia, and pallor. In addition to evaluating the MOI, be alert for the development of shock when you suspect internal hemorrhage.

▶ The Significance of Hemorrhage

Human adult male bodies contain approximately 0.29 cup of blood per pound (70 mL of blood per kilogram) of body weight, whereas adult female bodies contain approximately 0.27 cup/lb (65 mL/kg). For a typical adult weighing 176 pounds (80 kg), the total blood volume is approximately 10 pints (5 L). The body must compensate for any acute blood loss totaling more than 20% of this total blood volume.[1,2] Thus, if the typical adult has more than approximately 2 pints (1 L) of blood loss, significant changes in vital signs will occur, including increasing heart and respiratory rates and decreasing blood pressure. An isolated femur fracture, for example, can easily result in the loss of approximately 2 pints (1 L) or more of blood in the soft tissues of the thigh.

Because infants and children have less blood volume than adults, they may experience the same effects with smaller blood losses. For example, a 1-year-old child has a total blood volume of approximately 2 pints (~950 mL), so significant symptoms of blood loss may occur after only 3 to 6 ounces (100 to 200 mL) of blood loss. To put this amount in perspective, remember that a soft drink can holds roughly 11 ounces (345 mL) of liquid.

A significant factor is how well people compensate for blood loss is how rapidly they are bleeding. A healthy adult can comfortably donate one unit (1 pint [~500 mL]) of blood in a period of 15 to 20 minutes without experiencing ill effects from this decrease in blood volume. If a similar blood loss occurs in a much shorter period, hemorrhagic shock—a condition in which low blood volume results in inadequate perfusion and potentially even death—may develop rapidly. Consider bleeding to be serious if any of the following conditions are present:

- A significant MOI, especially when the MOI suggests that severe forces affected the abdomen or chest
- Poor general appearance of the patient
- Signs and symptoms of shock (hypoperfusion)
- Blood loss of 20% or more (approx. 2 pints or 1L in a typical 80-kg adult)
- Uncontrollable bleeding

▶ Physiologic Response to Hemorrhage

Typically, bleeding from an open artery is bright red (because of the high oxygen content) and spurts in time with the pulse. The pressure that causes the blood to spurt also makes this type of bleeding difficult to control. As the amount of blood circulating in the body drops, so does the patient's blood pressure. Eventually, the arterial spurting diminishes.

Blood from an open vein is much darker (low oxygen content) and flows steadily. Because it is under less pressure, most venous blood does not spurt, so such bleeding is easier to manage. Blood from damaged capillary vessels is dark red and oozes from a wound steadily but slowly. Venous and capillary bleeding are more likely to clot spontaneously compared to arterial bleeding.

On its own, bleeding tends to stop rather quickly, within about 10 minutes, in response to internal clotting mechanisms and exposure to air. When vessels are lacerated, blood flows rapidly from the open vessel. The open ends of the vessel then begin to narrow (vasoconstrict), which reduces the amount of bleeding. Platelets aggregate at the site, plugging the hole and sealing the injured portions of the vessel, a process called **hemostasis** **Figure 30-2** . Hemostasis proceeds through three steps: (1) vasoconstriction, followed by (2) platelet aggregation, and finally (3) fibrinogen weaving into the clot and forming fibrin to hold the clot together, controlling bleeding. Bleeding will not stop if a clot does not form—that is, unless the injured vessel is completely cut off from the main blood supply. Direct contact with body tissues and fluids or the external environment commonly triggers the blood's clotting factors.

Despite the efficiency of this system, it may fail in certain situations. A number of medications, including anticoagulants such as aspirin and prescription blood thinners, interfere with normal clotting. Beta-blockers can also prevent vasoconstriction, resulting in excessive bleeding. With a severe injury, the damage to the vessel may be so extensive that a clot cannot completely cover the opening. Sometimes, only part of the vessel wall is cut, preventing it from constricting. In these cases, bleeding will continue unless it is stopped by external means. In a situation involving acute blood loss, the patient might die before the body's hemostatic defenses of vasoconstriction and clotting can help.

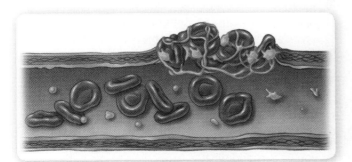

Figure 30-2 The forming blood clot continues trapping blood components until the bleeding, and eventually the plasma secretions, stops.

© Jones & Bartlett Learning.

A small portion of the population lacks one or more of the blood's clotting factors, a condition called **hemophilia**. Several forms of hemophilia exist, most of which are hereditary and some of which are severe. Sometimes, bleeding may occur spontaneously in a person with hemophilia. Because the patient's blood does not clot, all injuries in an individual with hemophilia, no matter how trivial, are potentially serious. A patient with hemophilia should be transported immediately.

Trauma Triad of Death

The trauma triad of death is a combination of hypothermia, coagulopathy, and acidosis that significantly increase mortality in trauma patients. These three conditions work to increase one another in a positive feedback loop, rapidly worsening the patient's condition.

Even mild hypothermia can begin to inhibit the chemical reactions involved in the clotting process. Coagulopathy, the disruption of the body's ability to clot, can lead to further hemorrhage, leading to increasing hypoperfusion. This hypoperfusion causes the cells to use anaerobic metabolism, releasing additional acidic compounds into the blood. This acidosis reduces myocardial performance, further reducing oxygen delivery and body metabolism, leading to increased hypothermia. If this loop continues uninterrupted, the rapidly worsening shock will lead to death of the trauma patient. Thus, paramedics must seek to identify the conditions of hypothermia, coagulopathy, and acidosis in the setting of trauma and intervene where possible.

Hypothermia is often the easiest to identify if looked for and can be the easiest condition to correct. Trauma patients must be kept warm. This is especially true if the patient is also subjected to environmental hypothermia, such as a motor vehicle collision in cold weather. However, you must keep in mind that hypothermia in the trauma triad of death refers to the body's inability to maintain normal operating temperature. This sign may be subtle and easy to overlook.

■ Shock

Shock can result from many conditions, resulting in damage that occurs because of insufficient perfusion of organs and tissues **Table 30-1** . Your early and rapid actions can help to significantly reduce the morbidity and mortality rates from shock.

When shock arises because of inadequate blood volume, it is termed **hypovolemic shock** (*hypo* = deficient + *vol* = volume + *emia* = in the blood). Hypovolemic shock may have either a hemorrhagic or nonhemorrhagic cause. Volume can be lost in the form of blood (internal or external **hemorrhagic shock**), plasma (burns), or electrolyte solution (through vomiting, diarrhea, or sweating—termed nonhemorrhagic shock). When a patient has severe thermal burns, intravascular plasma is lost, as plasma leaks from the circulatory system into the burned tissues that

Table 30-1	**Causes of Shock**

Respiratory Failure

- Obstruction—airway or embolism
- Chest wall movement problems—such as flail chest
- Diffusion failure—acute respiratory distress syndrome (ARDS)
- Toxic exposures—such as carbon monoxide and cyanide

Pump Failure

- Cardiogenic shock
- Intrinsic
- Extrinsic
  - Cardiac tamponade
  - Tension pneumothorax

Poor Vessel Function

- Distributive shock
- Septic shock
- Central nervous system disruption
  - Neurogenic shock
  - Psychogenic shock (vasovagal syncope)
- Anaphylactic shock

Low Fluid Volume

- Hypovolemic shock
  - Hemorrhagic shock, such as internal or external bleeding
  - Nonhemorrhagic shock, such as dehydration
  - Third space loss, such as with some fractures and burns

© Jones & Bartlett Learning.

lie adjacent to the injury. Likewise, crushing injuries may result in the loss of blood and plasma from damaged vessels into injured tissues.

Hemorrhagic shock is the most common cause of shock and is discussed in this chapter. See Chapter 40, *Management and Resuscitation of the Critical Patient*, for information about the other causes of shock, including nonhemorrhagic shock.

▶ Hemorrhagic Shock

The major life threat for most trauma patients is blood loss. Hemorrhage is most likely to occur with blunt or penetrating injuries to vessels or organs, long bone or pelvic fractures, major vascular injuries (as in traumatic amputation), and multisystem injury. Organs and organ systems with a high incidence of exsanguination from penetrating injuries include the heart, thoracic vascular system, abdominal vascular system (eg, abdominal aorta,

Evidence-Based Medicine

A note of caution regarding use of classification systems for shock: different classifications of shock have been available for students and teachers to consider for generations. Like most classification systems, they are sometimes helpful and sometimes not. No classification system of shock presently available is a perfect tool for assessment of blood loss severity or for determination of the most appropriate treatment for patients with shock secondary to hemorrhage. The Advanced Trauma Life Support classification developed by the American College of Surgeons Committee on Trauma, and also used by PreHospital Trauma Life Support, describes four categories of hemorrhage (Class I, Class II, etc.) and associated shock states based on the presumed amount of blood loss. This system describes the stages of progressive physiologic deterioration that are associated with increasing severity of blood loss.

While the progression described seems logical and rational, there is an absence of good clinical evidence that the amounts of blood loss associated with each of the categories described is an actual reflection of the amount of blood loss associated with the clinical presentations described.[3] More commonly in prehospital care, the classification describing **compensated shock**, **decompensated (hypotensive) shock**, and **irreversible shock** has been employed. In the field, it should be possible to distinguish reliably between compensated and decompensated shock based on blood pressure. If the patient has lost the ability to maintain a normal blood pressure, that is an important sign that a significant amount of blood has been lost and that the patient is very likely on the precipice of a significant physiologic crisis that requires urgent intervention.

The term "irreversible" shock has often been used to describe an even later and more dangerous phase in which the patient is no longer able to respond to fluid resuscitation or even vasopressor therapy. There is no clear scientific correlation between a specific level of blood loss and this ominous physiologic state. The determination that the patient does not respond to fluids, transfusions, and vasopressors is made by attempting those therapeutic modalities and noting the lack of response. Such a physiologic condition is a precursor to death.

Never assume that a patient is in irreversible shock. The mere existence of the category in some classification systems should not imply that aggressive prehospital care is not indicated. If there are signs of life present, resuscitate aggressively according to your local protocols and transport the patient as expeditiously as is safely possible to the nearest trauma center. Remember that the goal of all of these classification systems is to help you understand what is happening to the patient as hemorrhage progresses and to help you recognize those patients who are at greatest risk of death as a result of severe and sudden volume loss.

Table 30-2	**Estimated Fluid and Blood Loss for a 154-lb (70-kg) Patient**			
	Class I	**Class II**	**Class III**	**Class IV**
Blood loss (mL)	<750	750–1,500	1,500–2,000	>2,000
% Blood loss	<15	15–30	30–40	>40
Heart rate (beats/min)	Minimally elevated or normal	100–120	≥120, thready	Marked tachycardia
Systolic blood pressure	Within normal limits	Minimal or no change	Significant drop	Significant depression
Pulse pressure	Within normal limits	Narrow	Narrow	Very narrow
Capillary refill	Within normal limits	May be delayed	Delayed	Delayed
Respiratory rate (breaths/min)	14–20	20–24	Markedly elevated	Markedly elevated
Central nervous system/ mental status	Slightly anxious	Mildly anxious	Anxious and confused	Confused and lethargic
Skin condition	Cool, pink	Cool, moist	Cold, pale, moist	Cold, pale
Urine output (mL/h)	>30	20–30	Diminished	Minimal or none
Fluid replacement	Crystalloid	Crystalloid	Crystalloid and blood	Crystalloid and blood

© Jones & Bartlett Learning.

superior mesenteric artery), venous system (eg, inferior vena cava, portal vein), and liver.

Hypovolemic shock caused by hemorrhagic trauma has been organized by the American College of Surgeons Committee on Trauma into four classes, each with its own specific characteristics and treatments Table 30-2.

Shock occurs in three successive phases: compensated shock, decompensated shock, and irreversible shock. Your goal is to recognize the clinical signs and symptoms of shock in its earliest phase and begin immediate treatment before permanent damage occurs Table 30-3.

The initial stage of hemorrhagic shock is characterized by low circulating blood volume with minimal signs of hypoperfusion. However, as the body begins to compensate for low venous return, decreased SV, and low CO, patients begin to exhibit tachycardia, hypotension, and signs of poor tissue perfusion, and including pallor. Patients become more confused and anxious as the oxygen supply to the tissues is compromised and cellular metabolism is altered. Compensatory mechanisms continue to increase systemic vascular resistance (SVR) in an attempt to improve hemodynamics. As SVR increases and CO drops, patients develop cold, mottled, and pulseless extremities and worsening mental status. Left untreated, the shock will eventually progress to decompensated shock that is refractory to any therapy.

Table 30-3	**Compensated Versus Decompensated Shock**
Compensated Shock	**Decompensated Shock**
- Agitation, anxiety, restlessness - Sense of impending doom - Weak, rapid (thready) pulse - Clammy (cool, moist) skin - Pallor with cyanotic lips - Shortness of breath - Nausea, vomiting - Delayed capillary refill in infants and children - Thirst - Normal blood pressure	- Altered mental status (verbal to unresponsive)* - Hypotension - Labored or irregular breathing - Thready or absent peripheral pulses - Ashen, mottled, or cyanotic skin - Dilated pupils - Diminished urine output (oliguria) - Impending cardiac arrest

*Mental status changes are late indicators.
© Jones & Bartlett Learning.

Patient Assessment

Scene Size-up

The assessment of any patient begins with a scene size-up. Once the scene is deemed safe to enter, take standard precautions. Depending on the severity of bleeding and your general impression, these measures may entail use of gloves, a mask, an eye shield, and, when the patient is bloody or blood is spurting, a gown.

A high-energy MOI should increase your index of suspicion for the possibility of serious unseen injuries, such as internal bleeding. See Chapter 29, *Trauma Systems and Mechanism of Injury*, for more information on significant mechanisms of injury. Internal bleeding is possible whenever the MOI suggests that severe forces affected the patient's body, such as with blunt or penetrating trauma. Internal bleeding commonly occurs as a result of falls, blast injuries, and motor vehicle crashes. Also, keep in mind that internal bleeding is not always caused by trauma. Many illnesses—for example, bleeding ulcers, bleeding from the colon, ruptured ectopic pregnancy, and aneurysms—can also cause internal bleeding.

It is often difficult to determine visually the amount of blood loss. You should attempt to determine the amount

Words of Wisdom

Regardless of the type of bleeding—whether hidden in the body cavities or visible on the surrounding surfaces—all patients will proceed through the phases of shock if their bleeding is not controlled. In hemorrhagic shock, the specific phase of shock is a function of the percentage of total blood volume loss. Because internal bleeding is more likely to be uncontrolled, you should stay alert for the subtle signs of shock and be aggressive in your management of its early phase to keep the patient from deteriorating and to avoid shock's later phases.

Words of Wisdom

One method of rapid assessment of a patient's circulatory status has been to check for the presence of a radial pulse, which was long thought to equate to a systolic blood pressure of 80 to 90 mm Hg. This was thought to be significant, as a blood pressure of approximately 90 mm Hg is adequate to perfuse the vital organs. Studies have shown that radial pulses may still be present in patients with a systolic blood pressure of less than 60 mm Hg, leading to a gross over-estimation of the patient's blood pressure.[4]

of external blood loss, but remember that this information is not crucial; instead, the presentation and assessment of the patient must direct patient care and treatment.

For patients who have sustained significant MOIs, scene time should not exceed 10 minutes and the most appropriate transportation destination must be considered.

Documentation & Communication

Just as these data make for thorough written reporting, so taking and recording frequent serial vital signs—and observing perfusion indicators such as skin condition and mental status—will give you a window into the progression of shock. Although a single set of vital signs may be useful, it is the trends in those signs that often signal subtle changes in the patient indicative of progressing shock.

Primary Survey

During the primary survey, you need to determine the patient's mental status using the AVPU scale (Awake and alert, responsive to Verbal stimuli, responsive to Pain, Unresponsive), and locate and manage immediate threats to life involving the airway, breathing, and circulation. This is the point where you would apply the "A before B, except after C" concept. As you approach the patient with an active severe hemorrhage, you may need to address the bleeding prior to initiating airway or respiratory maneuvers, to prevent the patient from bleeding to death. Ensure that the patient has a patent airway and no structural damage. Check the patient's breathing patterns, chest wall integrity, and pulse rate. Assess for signs of hemorrhagic shock. If you observe bleeding from the mouth or facial areas, keep the suction unit within reach.

Special Populations

In older adult patients, dizziness, faintness, or weakness may be the first sign of nontraumatic internal bleeding.

If major external hemorrhage is present, manage it immediately, treat the patient for shock, and transport the patient to the emergency department (ED). Continue with the patient assessment en route to the ED.

Most external hemorrhage can be managed with direct, even pressure, combined with pressure dressings and/or splints, although arterial bleeding may require 5 or more minutes of direct pressure to form a clot. Military experience in Iraq has proven that tourniquets can effectively and safely control hemorrhage without an increase in complications.[5] For this reason, the use of a tourniquet is preferred for external hemorrhage in an

Words of Wisdom

Damage control resuscitation (DCR) is a systematic approach to the management of the trauma patient with severe injuries. This approach begins with the prehospital care provider and continues through the ED, operating room, and intensive care unit. DCR focuses on maintaining circulating volume, controlling hemorrhage, and correcting the deadly triad of coagulopathy, acidosis, and hypothermia.

While some tools of damage control resuscitation such as blood product administration are used by only a few EMS services, many techniques including rapid assessment, minimizing the use of crystalloid fluids, patient warming, and use of tourniquets, pressure dressings, and hemostatic gauze are widely available.

extremity that cannot be controlled with direct pressure and a pressure dressing.

Some evidence supports the use of hemostatic agents to control external bleeding, with these agents being especially helpful for nonextremity wounds where a tourniquet cannot be used.[6] Numerous products are available, each with their positive attributes and drawbacks.

Studies are also examining the use of tranexamic acid (TXA) to aid in the control of internal bleeding in the prehospital setting.[7-9] This medication has been used for years in patients with known bleeding disorders before they undergo surgical intervention. Refer to your local protocol regarding the use of hemostatic agents and TXA.

Because most cases of internal hemorrhage are rarely fully controlled in the prehospital setting, a patient with this type of injury needs rapid transport to the ED. Tachycardia is an early sign of hypoperfusion suggesting internal hemorrhage. Late signs include the following:

- Weakness, fainting, or dizziness at rest
- Thirst
- Nausea and vomiting
- Cold, moist (clammy) skin
- Shallow, rapid breathing
- Dull eyes
- Slightly dilated pupils that are slow to respond to light
- Capillary refill of more than 2 seconds in infants and children
- Weak, rapid (thready) pulse
- Decreasing blood pressure
- Altered level of consciousness

Even if internal bleeding stops, it could begin again at any moment. Therefore, prompt transport is necessary for patients with internal hemorrhage.

If you suspect internal hemorrhage, begin management by keeping the patient warm and administering

YOU are the Paramedic　　PART 3

The patient's breath sounds are clear and equal with full expansion. The patient tells you that his chest hurts a little bit when he breathes. Your partner begins to obtain vital signs as you continue your assessment. As you are cutting away the patient's harness and removing the tool belt, you notice that they are saturated with blood. You see a deep laceration on the right flank where one of the tools penetrated the skin. There is no impalement, but the wound is bleeding heavily.

Recording Time: 5 Minutes	
Respirations	20 breaths/min, unlabored
Pulse	122 beats/min, very weak radial pulses
Skin	Pale, cool, moist
Blood pressure	108/70 mm Hg
Oxygen saturation (Spo$_2$)	97% on oxygen
Pupils	PERRLA

5. The patient has unlabored breathing, normal lung sounds, and high-concentration oxygen in place. His Spo$_2$ reading seems adequate. Could he still be suffering from poor perfusion?
6. If you measure his end-tidal carbon dioxide (ETCO$_2$), would you expect it to be high, low, or normal range? What are some factors that affect the measured levels of ETCO$_2$?

supplemental oxygen by a nonrebreathing mask at 15 L/min en route to the ED.

If the patient has minor external hemorrhage, you should make note of it and move on with the assessment process; management of this problem can wait until the patient has been properly assessed and prioritized. Do not get sidetracked by applying dressings and bandages to a patient who may have more serious problems. Notably, when a patient has signs and symptoms of shock, but only minor visible bleeding, you need to consider that internal bleeding may be occurring.

> ## Words of Wisdom
>
> When you are managing a bleeding patient, take the necessary precautions to protect yourself from splashing or splattering. Wear appropriate personal protective equipment, including gloves, gown, mask, and eye protection. Such precautions are especially essential when arterial bleeding is present. Also remember that frequent, thorough handwashing between patients and after every run is a simple, yet important protective measure.

History Taking

As you continue with the assessment, investigate the chief complaint and obtain a history of the present illness. Ask the patient if he or she has experienced any dizziness or syncope. Ask the patient about current medications that may thin the blood, such as aspirin, warfarin (Coumadin), rivaroxaban (Xarelto), dabigatran (Pradaxa), apixaban (Eliquis), and clopidogrel (Plavix), as well as a history of any excessive bleeding after surgery. Ask about any history of clotting insufficiency. In addition, patients with a history of a previous myocardial infarction may be taking anticoagulants, in which case a "minor" injury such as an extremity fracture can lead to significant blood loss and shock. Ask about use of beta-blockers, calcium channel blockers, antidysrhythmics, and nitroglycerin, because these medications will interfere with the body's ability to compensate for shock. Is there any pain, tenderness, bruising, guarding, or swelling? These signs and symptoms may indicate internal bleeding.

Secondary Assessment

The secondary assessment includes a systematic full-body exam or, if there is less time and the patient is unresponsive or has a significant MOI, a rapid full-body scan. The goal is to identify any injuries or illness that may have been missed during the primary survey.

The most commonly experienced symptom with internal hemorrhage is pain. Significant internal hemorrhage will generally cause swelling in the area of bleeding. Intra-abdominal hemorrhage will often cause pain, distention, and rigidity. Sometimes intra-abdominal bleeding can present at the skin layer. For example, Cullen sign is the appearance of bruising surrounding the umbilicus, whereas Grey Turner sign is bruising in the flanks. A contusion or ecchymosis may also be a sign of internal hemorrhage. It most commonly occurs in head, extremity, and pelvic injuries and can indicate that the patient has experienced significant trauma. It may not be present initially, however, and the only sign of severe pelvic or abdominal trauma may be redness, skin abrasions, or pain. Bleeding into the chest may cause dyspnea in addition to tachycardia and hypotension.

Hemorrhage, however slight, from any body opening is serious. It usually indicates internal hemorrhage that is not easy to see or control. Bright red bleeding from the mouth or rectum or blood in the urine (hematuria) may suggest serious internal injury or disease. Nonmenstrual vaginal hemorrhage is always significant. Note the characteristics of the bleeding and try to determine its source. For example, bright red blood from a wound or the mouth, rectum, or other orifice indicates fresh arterial bleeding. Coffee-grounds emesis is a sign of upper GI bleeding; this type of blood is old and looks like used coffee grounds.

Other signs and symptoms of internal hemorrhage in both trauma and medical patients include the following:

- **Hematoma.** A mass of blood in the soft tissues beneath the skin; it indicates bleeding into soft tissues and may be the result of a minor or a severe injury.
- **Hematemesis.** Vomited blood; a sign of upper GI bleeding. This blood may be bright red or dark red, or, if it has been partially digested, it may look like coffee-grounds vomitus.
- **Hemoptysis.** Coughed-up blood. It is usually bright red.
- **Melena.** Black, foul-smelling, tarry stool that contains digested blood; it indicates lower GI bleeding.
- **Hematuria.** Blood in the urine; it may suggest serious renal injury or illness.
- **Hematochezia.** The passage of bloody stools. If they contain bright red blood, this sign may indicate hemorrhage near the external opening of the anus. Hemorrhoids in the lower colon tend to cause hematochezia.
- Pain, tenderness, bruising, guarding, or swelling. These signs and symptoms may mean that a closed fracture is hemorrhaging.
- Broken ribs, bruises over the lower part of the chest, or a rigid, distended abdomen. These signs and symptoms may indicate a lacerated spleen or liver. Patients with an injury to either organ may have referred pain in the right shoulder (liver) or left shoulder (spleen). You should suspect internal abdominal bleeding in a patient with referred pain.

Assess the respiratory system. Specifically, assess the airway for patency and determine the rate and quality of respirations. In the neck, look for distended neck veins and a deviated trachea, as these could be late signs of a tension pneumothorax. Note, however, that these classic signs may not be present in the patient with hypovolemia; such an individual may have flat—not distended—neck veins due to blood loss.

Assess the cardiovascular system, specifically the rate and quality of pulses. Be careful with the use of a pulse oximeter for patients in shock. When the body uses vasoconstriction to compensate for shock, the pulse oximeter probe, being placed on an extremity, will not be able to give an accurate measurement of the body's oxygen saturation. Use electrocardiography (ECG) to monitor the patient's cardiac rhythm. The presence of pulses is related to perfusion status: As a person's blood pressure begins to drop, the radial pulse will disappear, then the brachial and femoral pulses will disappear, and lastly the carotid pulse will be lost. Blood pressure appears normal in the early stages of shock as the body compensates, and will not drop until the patient begins to decompensate—that is, as the patient moves from Class II to Class III shock.

Normally, in an effort to maintain central perfusion, blood will be shunted away from the periphery and the patient with hemorrhage will present with pale, cool, mottled skin and decreased or absent radial pulses with an increased capillary refill time. However, some medications may alter this process, thereby masking changes in vital signs. For example, beta-blockers interfere with the body's normal sympathetic response and will not allow the heart to speed up or pump harder. Calcium channel blockers can interfere with vasoconstriction and not allow for shunting of blood to vital areas where perfusion is lacking. Patients who have recently taken nitroglycerin or are wearing a nitroglycerin patch may not be able to achieve vasoconstriction because of the vasodilation effect from this medication. Other antidysrhythmics can interfere with the heart's ability to speed up or pump with more force. Thus, obtaining a list of current medications can provide valuable information that allows for correct interpretation of the patient's vital signs.

Assess the neurologic system to formulate baseline data to guide further decisions. This examination should include level of consciousness, pupil size and reactivity, motor response, and sensory response. A trauma patient with an elevated blood pressure and slow pulse may still be in shock, but in the presence of head injury, the patient may be experiencing Cushing reflex owing to increasing intracranial pressure.

Assess the musculoskeletal system. Use your secondary assessment—both physical exam and history—to confirm that you have found all of the patient's problems and injuries quickly.

Assess all anatomic regions. When you are examining the patient's head, be alert for raccoon eyes, Battle sign (bruising over the mastoid process that may indicate skull fracture), and drainage of blood or fluid from the ears or nose. In the abdomen, feel all four quadrants for tenderness or rigidity. In the extremities, note skin pallor, check capillary refill, record the pulse, and assess motor and sensory function. If the patient has bleeding from the extremities, note the level of bleeding and whether the bleeding is arterial, venous, or pulsing.

Reassessment

Reassess the patient, especially in the areas that showed abnormal findings during the primary survey. Be sure to reassess any interventions used to control hemorrhage and ensure they remain adequate. The signs and symptoms of internal hemorrhage are often slow to present because of their covert nature.

In all cases of severe hemorrhage, obtain the patient's vital signs every 5 minutes en route to the ED. Whenever you suspect significant hemorrhage, either external or internal, administer high-flow oxygen. If significant hemorrhage is visible at any time during the assessment process, begin the steps to control the bleeding, discussed next.

Special Populations

Older adult patients are more likely to take medications that interfere with normal compensatory mechanisms, such as beta-blockers, calcium channel blockers, and other antidysrhythmics. The kidneys also atrophy with age and, therefore, are less responsive to fluid conservation; the blood vessels may be affected by atherosclerosis and less able to shunt blood to vital areas. In addition, other medical conditions can be exacerbated during shock states; for instance, ischemia is more likely to interfere with cardiac output in patients with a history of myocardial infarction or angina.

Pediatric patients have underdeveloped kidneys, resulting in an inability to conserve fluid like an adult. Consequently, they have a lower tolerance for volume loss. In addition, children compensate by vasoconstriction better than adults do. This factor tends to allow them to maintain a compensatory state and good blood pressure for a longer period, until the point when their vital signs collapse abruptly, possibly followed by death. An additional complication in small children is their relatively large surface area to weight ratio, when means they feel cold more easily, which in turn results in coagulation difficulties.

Pregnant patients normally will have a faster pulse, greater blood volume, lower blood pressure, and nausea. Manage these patients aggressively according to the MOI and treat for shock; do not automatically assume the altered signs are due to the pregnancy.

Emergency Medical Care of Bleeding and Hemorrhagic Shock

Always take standard precautions when you are treating bleeding patients, and suspect shock if the patient has severe hemorrhage. As with all patients, ensure that the patient with bleeding or shock has an open airway and is breathing adequately. Administer supplemental oxygen as necessary, and assist ventilation if needed, paying special attention to cervical spine control in trauma patients.

Words of Wisdom

Keep in mind that victims of shock may not reliably indicate pain from a spinal or other musculoskeletal injury. These patients should have spinal precautions based on MOI.

▶ Managing External Hemorrhage

To control external hemorrhaging, follow the steps in Skill Drill 30-1.

Skill Drill 30-1 Managing External Hemorrhage

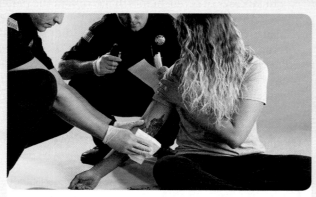

Step 1 Take standard precautions. Maintain the airway with cervical spine immobilization if the MOI suggests the possibility of spinal injury. Apply direct, even pressure over the wound with a dry, sterile dressing.

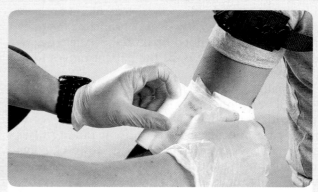

Step 2 If the bleeding stops, apply a pressure dressing and/or splint. Hold the pressure dressing in place using gauze.

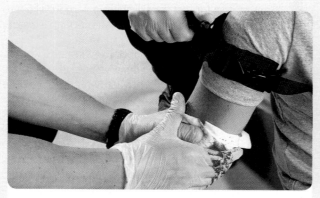

Step 3 If direct pressure does not rapidly control bleeding on an extremity injury, apply a tourniquet above the level of the bleeding.

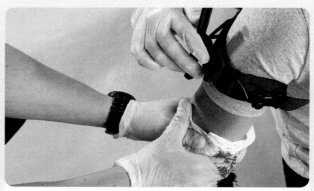

Step 4 Tighten the tourniquet until the bleeding stops. Position the patient supine unless contraindicated. Administer oxygen as necessary. Keep the patient warm, transport promptly, monitor the serial vital signs, and watch diligently for developing shock.

Transport the patient rapidly while providing aggressive management en route. Because a patient in shock is usually emotionally upset, you should provide psychological support as well.

Hemorrhaging From the Nose, Ears, and Mouth

Hemorrhaging from the nose (epistaxis) or the ears following a head injury may indicate a skull fracture. In such a case, you should not attempt to stop the blood flow. Applying excessive pressure to the injury may force the blood leaking through the ear or nose to collect within the head, ultimately increasing intracranial pressure and possibly causing permanent brain damage.

If you suspect a skull fracture, cover the bleeding site loosely with a sterile gauze pad to collect the blood and help keep contaminants away from the site—there is always a risk of infection to the brain with an open skull fracture. Apply light compression by wrapping the dressing loosely around the head. If blood or drainage contains cerebrospinal fluid (CSF), then the dressing will show a staining that resembles a bull's-eye target. Another method that can be used to check for CSF in the blood is the glucometer. Because the CSF has a high glucose content, the glucometer will detect this excess glucose in the blood of a normoglycemic patient.

For a nosebleed from other conditions, such as trauma directly to the nose or bleeding caused by environmental factors such as dry air, apply cold compresses to the bridge of the nose while the patient leans forward. An alternative is to roll gauze and place it under the patient's upper lip. This treatment will generate pressure on the blood supply to the nose and often works within 5 minutes. Check the patient's blood pressure and evaluate for a hypertensive emergency as the cause of epistaxis, especially in older adults.

Hemorrhaging From Other Areas

When the patient has hemorrhaging from other areas of the body, control it through use of direct pressure. Apply pressure dressings, and consider the use of a tourniquet and hemostatic dressings, per your local protocol. In addition, use splints (or air splints) as necessary, always following your local protocols. Air splints can control venous bleeding but will not apply enough pressure to control arterial bleeding until the patient's blood pressure is extremely low (approximately 50 mm Hg systolic).

Once hemorrhaging is controlled and a sterile dressing and pressure bandage have been applied, keep the patient warm and in the appropriate position. Allow the patient's condition to dictate the mode of transport.

▶ Special Management Techniques for External Hemorrhage

Tourniquets

The tourniquet is especially useful if a patient has severe hemorrhaging from an extremity injury below the axilla or groin and when other methods of control, such as direct pressure and pressure dressings, are ineffective or inadequate. The laceration or tear of a large artery can cause a patient to exsanguinate in as little as 2 minutes. To avoid this outcome, you must be able to apply a tourniquet in less than 20 seconds.

For many years, tourniquets were considered a last-ditch effort to be used in patients where the choice was between life or the limb. The consensus was that while the tourniquet could stop the bleeding, the result would be the loss of the patient's arm or leg. This belief was based on the historical use of the tourniquet— these devices were first used to stop the blood flow to the extremity prior to an amputation from battlefield injuries. In World War I, tourniquets were also used to stop bleeding from extremities. However, owing to the long transport times to definitive care, the application of the tourniquet often resulted in the loss of the limb.

Since 2005, tourniquets have proven so efficient and easy to use that the US military has issued tourniquets to all field personnel.[10] A number of commercially available tourniquets are marketed, including the mechanical advantage tourniquet (MAT), the special operations forces tactical tourniquet (SOFT-T), the combat application tourniquet (CAT), the ratcheting medical tourniquet (RMT), and the stretch, wrap, and tuck tourniquet (SWAT-T) **Figure 30-3** . The MAT uses a strap and buckle system with a dial to tension the strap, whereas the CAT uses a strap and buckle system but utilizes a windlass to tighten the strap to control bleeding. The RMT uses a ratchet device to apply mechanical pressure, while the SWAT-T serves as a combination of a pressure dressing, wrap, and tourniquet.

The use of commercial tourniquets generally involves the steps in **Skill Drill 30-2** . A tourniquet is typically released at the hospital, but if instructed by medical control, can be released in the field. Tourniquets differ in their mechanism for being removed; for example, a MAT tourniquet has a release button. Be aware that bleeding may rapidly return upon tourniquet release, so you should be prepared to reapply it immediately if necessary.

If a commercial tourniquet is not available, follow these steps to apply a tourniquet using a triangular bandage and a stick or rod:

1. Fold a triangular bandage until it is 4 inches (6 cm) wide and six to eight layers thick.
2. Wrap the bandage around the extremity twice. Choose an area proximal to the injury to ensure control of the bleeding.
3. Tie one knot in the bandage. Then place a stick or rod on top of the knot, and tie the ends of the bandage over the stick in a square knot.
4. Use the stick or rod as a handle, and twist it to tighten the tourniquet until the bleeding has stopped and distal pulses

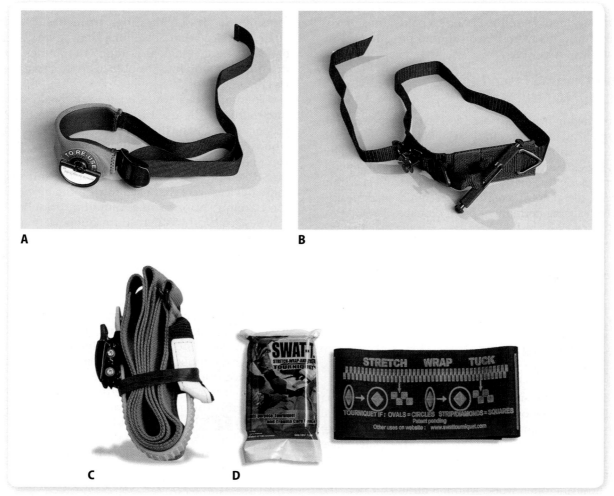

Figure 30-3 Commercially available tourniquets. **A.** Mechanical advantage tourniquet. **B.** Special operations forces tactical tourniquet. **C.** Ratcheting medical tourniquet. **D.** Stretch, wrap, and tuck tourniquet.

A & B: © Jones & Bartlett Learning; **C and D:** Photo by Diane Zahorodny. Courtesy of Chinook Medical Gear.

are no longer palpable; then stop twisting Figure 30-4 .

5. Secure the stick in place, and make the wrapping neat and smooth.
6. Write "TK" (for "tourniquet") and the exact time (hour and minute) that you applied the tourniquet on a piece of adhesive tape. Use the phrase "time applied." Securely fasten the tape to the patient's forehead. Notify hospital personnel on your arrival that the patient has a tourniquet in place. Record this same information on the patient care report form.

As a last resort, you can use a blood pressure cuff as a tourniquet—but keep in mind that blood pressure cuffs with leaks will not hold pressure. Position the cuff proximal to the bleeding point, and inflate it enough to eliminate distal pulses and stop the bleeding. Leave the cuff inflated. Monitor the gauge continuously to ensure the pressure is not gradually dropping, which could allow the bleeding to restart. You may have to clamp the tube leading from the cuff to the inflating bulb with a hemostat to prevent loss of pressure.

Words of Wisdom

There is no evidence that applying the tourniquet closer to the site of bleeding is preferable, and no reason to believe that normal tissue is at risk by placing the tourniquet too high. Keep in mind that there is the possibility of nerve injury by placing the tourniquets at an unsafe site, such as the proximal leg just below the knee or the proximal forearm just below the elbow, where the common peroneal nerve (leg) or the ulnar nerve (forearm) could be at risk.

Skill Drill 30-2 Applying a Commercial Tourniquet (Combat Application Tourniquet)

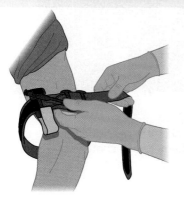

Step 1 Hold direct pressure over the bleeding site and place the tourniquet proximal to the injury, preferably at the groin or axilla. Wrap the band around the limb and fasten it to the buckle.

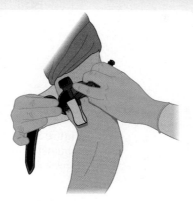

Step 2 Pull the band tightly and secure the band back on itself. Ensure that the tips of three fingers cannot fit between the band and the limb.

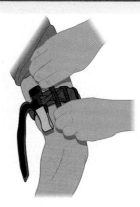

Step 3 Tighten the rod (windlass) until the bleeding stops.

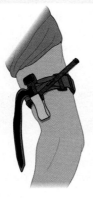

Step 4 Secure the rod inside the clip. Ensure bleeding is still controlled and assess for a distal pulse.

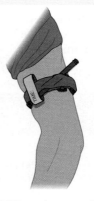

Step 5 Wrap the rest of the band through the clips. Secure the rod with the strap labeled *TIME:* and document the time.

© Jones & Bartlett Learning.

As an alternative to the standard limb tourniquet, another type of tourniquet is used when the hemorrhage is inguinal or axillary. The junctional tourniquet uses a belt system to hold the device in place (either around the hips for an inguinal injury or around the chest for an axilla injury). Using a pump, you then inflate a compression device to put pressure on the deep vessels **Figure 30-5** . The junctional tourniquet, when applied around the hips, can also be used as a pelvic immobilization device, as discussed in the next section.

Whenever you apply a tourniquet, ensure you take the following precautions:

- Do not apply a tourniquet directly over any joint. Ensure it is proximal to the zone of injury, preferably just distal to the groin or axilla.

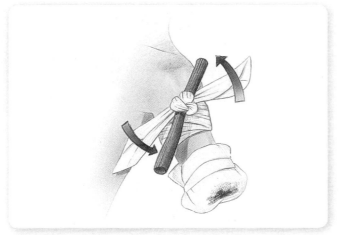

Figure 30-4 Twist the stick or rod to tighten the tourniquet until the bleeding has stopped and distal pulses are no longer palpable; then stop twisting.

© Jones & Bartlett Learning.

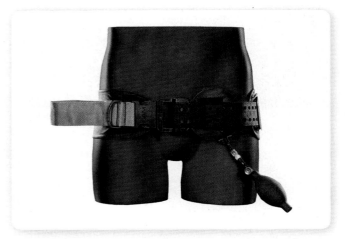

Figure 30-5 SAM junctional tourniquets can be used for inguinal or axillary hemorrhage control.

© SAM Medical Products®.

- Use the widest bandage possible. Ensure it is tightened securely.
- Never use wire, rope, a belt, or any other narrow material as the tourniquet; it could cut into the patient's skin.
- Never cover a tourniquet with a bandage. Leave it open and in full view.
- Inform the hospital both in your radio report and in your verbal report on arrival at the ED that a tourniquet has been applied.

- Do not loosen the tourniquet after you have applied it unless directed to do so by hospital personnel or medical control.

Splints

Bleeding associated with broken bones can occur when the sharp ends of the bones lacerate vessels, muscles, and other tissues. As long as a fracture remains unstable, the bone ends will move and continue to damage tissues and vessels. They may also break up clots that have partially formed, resulting in ongoing hemorrhage. For these

YOU are the Paramedic   PART 4

With proper PPE already in place, you apply direct pressure to the patient's gaping wound and stop the bleeding. The ground has a small puddle of congealed blood on it, and the patient's sweatshirt is soaked with blood. You complete a quick check for any other heavy bleeding but do not find any. This patient is now complaining of feeling cold and tells you that his vision "feels strange."

Recording Time: 8 Minutes	
Respirations	24 breaths/min, unlabored
Pulse	132 beats/min, very weak radial pulses
Skin	Pale, cool, moist
Blood pressure	92/60 mm Hg
Oxygen saturation (Spo$_2$)	98% on oxygen
Pupils	PERRLA

7. Despite you stopping the flow of heavy bleeding, the patient seems to be deteriorating further. What are some of the possible causes of his deteriorating condition?
8. At this point, what is your next priority?

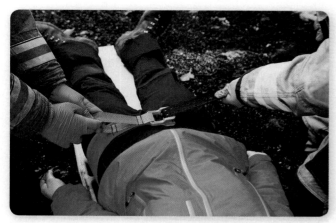

Figure 30-6 Pelvic compression devices or binders are meant to provide temporary stabilization and reduce hemorrhage from pelvic bleeding.
© SAM Medical Products®.

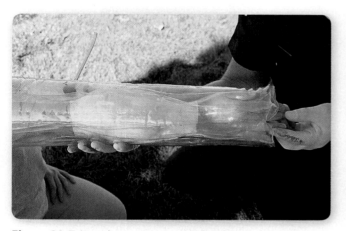

Figure 30-7 Air splints can control bleeding because they act as a pressure bandage for the entire extremity.
© Jones & Bartlett Learning.

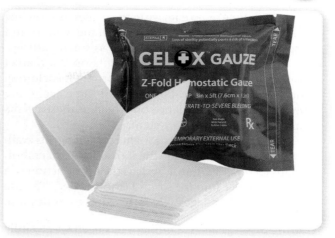

Figure 30-8 Hemostatic agents are being used by some EMS systems to control severe hemorrhage, especially in areas of the body where a tourniquet cannot be placed.
© North American Rescue®, LLC. All rights reserved.

reasons, immobilizing a fracture is a priority in the prompt control of bleeding. Often, simple splints will quickly control the bleeding associated with a fracture. For example, a fractured pelvis should be stabilized using a pelvic binder or sheets used to bind the pelvis and stabilize the area **Figure 30-6**.

Air Splints. Air splints can control the hemorrhage associated with venous bleeding **Figure 30-7**. They also stabilize the fracture itself. An air splint acts like a pressure dressing that is applied to an entire extremity, rather than to a small, local area.

Once you have applied an air splint, monitor circulation in the distal extremity. Because an air splint is typically inflated to a pressure of approximately 50 mm Hg (so you can still dent the splint with your fingertips), it would not be appropriate to use this device on a patient with arterial hemorrhage: The splint would not actually control the hemorrhage until the patient's systolic blood pressure dropped to the pressure of the splint. Use only

approved, clean, or disposable valve stems when orally inflating air splints.

Rigid Splints. Rigid splints can help stabilize fractures as well as reduce pain and prevent further damage to soft-tissue injuries. Once you have applied a rigid splint, be sure to monitor circulation in the distal extremity.

Traction Splints. Traction splints are designed to stabilize femur fractures. When traction is pulled to the ankle, counter-traction is applied to the ischium and groin. This setup reduces the thigh muscle spasms and prevents one end of the fracture from impacting or overriding the other. Be sure to pad these areas well to avoid applying excessive pressure to the soft tissues of the pelvis. Once you have applied a traction splint, be sure to monitor circulation in the distal extremity.

Hemostatic Agents

As noted earlier, the military has successfully used hemostatic agents to control severe hemorrhage, especially to areas where a tourniquet cannot be placed, such as junctional wounds (inguinal and axilla) **Figure 30-8**. These agents work by causing enhanced clot formation in the wound site: They adhere to the damaged tissue and either dehydrate the blood or undergo a chemical reaction that stimulates the natural blood clotting cascade (ie, the intrinsic pathway). Ideally, the bleeding should be stopped in 2 minutes or less.

In general, all hemostatic agents should share a few common attributes. They should be lightweight and easy to store, carry, and deploy in emergency situations. They should be able to conform to the wound itself, allowing the agent to work where it is needed, especially at deep wound sites where direct pressure alone may not be sufficient or be difficult to apply, such as a femoral artery laceration in the groin. Once applied, they should be able to withstand the high pressure or flow of a bleeding wound, cause little or no damage to the tissues surrounding the wound site, be easy to remove from the wound, and not spread into the rest of the system as small particles. As of this writing, the prevalent agents on the market are gauzes impregnated with various proprietary clotting agents. Consult your local protocols if these agents are to be used and seek guidance on which of these agents are approved in your EMS system.

Complications with the use of hemostatic agents available in powder form include the introduction of emboli through open vasculature as well as the introduction of a foreign substance into the wound (the powder). The use of impregnated bandages avoids the latter complication.

Wound Packing. The US military has been successfully using wound packing with standard gauze and hemostatic agents for many years and the techniques are now moving into civilian EMS.[11] The technique is particularly helpful for bleeding in junctional areas, such as the groin and axilla, where tourniquets cannot be used.

Wound packing works by absorbing liquid from the blood and helping to concentrate clotting factors, helping to transfer external direct pressure to deeper blood vessels that are the source of bleeding, and, if using hemostatic dressings, it can also chemically accelerate the clotting process.[11]

Wound packing involves taking standard initial steps to control the bleeding including direct pressure, tourniquets, and other applicable tools and techniques. Simply push the gauze into the wound with an index finger to completely and tightly pack the wound cavity. The goal is to contact the source of the bleeding if possible and to fill the cavity. If extra gauze is left over, place it on top of the wound. Hold firm, direct manual pressure on the wound for at least 3 minutes or secure the wound with a snug pressure dressing over the wound. Consult your local protocols for guidance on wound packing and the use of hemostatic agents.

Words of Wisdom

Hemostatic agents such as Celox, HemCon, and QuikClot are primarily used in the military to promote hemostasis or, in other words, to stop profuse bleeding. These agents may consist of granules poured into a wound or contained in a dressing. The agent absorbs the water component of blood, thereby concentrating the clotting factors, activating platelets, and enhancing the coagulation cascade.

▶ Managing Internal Hemorrhage

Management of a patient with internal hemorrhaging focuses on the treatment of shock, minimizing movement of the injured or bleeding part or region, and rapid transport.

Eventually, the patient may need a surgical procedure to stop the bleeding. In recent years, ultrasound has been used to locate bleeding in the ED before moving the patient to the surgical suite for the ultimate resolution of the problem. Ultrasound is also being used in prehospital environments, particularly the military.

Controversies

In the 1980s, researchers began to question whether use of the military antishock trousers/pneumatic antishock garment (MAST/PASG) and IV fluid infusion were really effective in the treatment of shock.[12,13] At the time of this writing, the MAST/PASG is rarely applied in the treatment of hemorrhagic shock. Consult your medical director and regional protocols if you still carry the device.

Follow the steps in **Skill Drill 30-3** to care for patients with possible internal hemorrhage.

Give the patient nothing by mouth. Insert an 18-gauge IV catheter, and administer a fluid bolus of 250 mL of normal saline or lactated Ringer solution (provided the patient's lungs are clear and the patient's condition warrants such a treatment and to a maximum of four doses before online medical consultation) without delaying patient transport. If IV is access unsuccessful or anticipated to be difficult, utilize IO access if available. Insert an IV line at the scene only if transport is delayed (eg, if the patient is pinned). Establish a second 18-gauge IV line if possible. Whenever possible, use warm IV fluids to prevent the patient from becoming hypothermic.

Keep the patient warm. Consider giving pain medication if the patient's vital signs are stable and after consultation with medical control. Provide immediate transport. Monitor the serial vital signs, and watch diligently for developing shock en route. If the patient shows any signs of shock (hypoperfusion), transport rapidly while providing aggressive management en route. Because a patient in shock is usually emotionally upset, you should provide psychological support as well.

▶ Management of Hemorrhagic Shock

The priorities in treating a patient in hemorrhagic shock are the same as in treating any other patient—with a focus on the sequence of CAB. Always take standard precautions. Identify and try to stop any major bleeding, and quickly evaluate the patient's hemodynamic status with a pulse check. Establish and maintain an open airway while maintaining manual immobilization if necessary, assist ventilation and use airway control adjuncts as needed, and continue to monitor the patient's breathing. Keep suction at hand to clear the mouth and pharynx if the patient vomits. Comfort, calm, and reassure the patient in the supine position. Do not allow the patient to eat or

Skill Drill 30-3 Managing Internal Hemorrhage

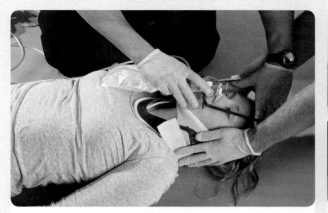

Step 1 Take standard precautions. Maintain the airway with cervical spine immobilization if the MOI suggests the possibility of spinal injury. Administer supplemental oxygen as needed, and assist ventilation if necessary.

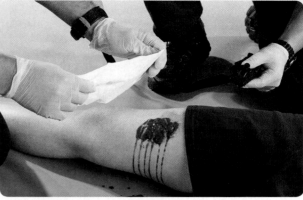

Step 2 Control all obvious external bleeding, and treat suspected internal bleeding using a splint if possible. Apply a tourniquet for severe bleeding from an extremity that cannot be controlled with direct pressure.

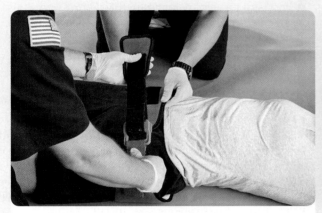

Step 3 Depending on local protocols, if a pelvic fracture is suspected, use a pelvic binder or sheets to bind the pelvic area.

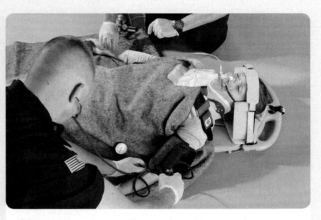

Step 4 Monitor and record vital signs at least every 5 minutes.

© Jones & Bartlett Learning.

drink anything. Splint the patient on a backboard and, unless necessary to control bleeding at the scene, splint individual extremity fractures during transport as opposed to on scene. If the patient exhibits signs or symptoms of shock, administer supplemental oxygen, keep the patient warm, and prepare for transport.

En route to the ED, insert at least one, and preferably two, 18-gauge peripheral IV lines, using an over-the-needle catheter. Obtain IV access at the scene only if transport of the patient is delayed. If allowed by protocol, draw blood (two red-top blood collection [Vacutainer] tubes

Controversies

Many trauma surgeons prefer use of lactated Ringer solution over normal saline because lactated Ringer solution may help decrease acidosis in patients with severe hemorrhagic hypovolemia. This belief remains controversial; however, as lactated Ringer solution may also contribute to hyperkalemia in certain trauma patients.[14]

Controversies

Some prior studies have shown that hypertonic solutions of 7.5% sodium chloride, in 250-mL increments, may optimize blood pressure, cardiac output, intracranial pressure, and microvascular flow without increasing bleeding or volume overloading patients.[14] Nevertheless, no improvement in survival rates has been observed with this practice compared with standard fluid resuscitation.[15] More research in this area may change the face of fluid therapy, but for now, most disciplines in the United States continue to use isotonic crystalloid therapy.

and one purple-top tube) so that hospital personnel may obtain a hematocrit, type and cross-match, and other tests immediately on your arrival.

Unless your local protocol favors a different resuscitation fluid, administer warm isotonic crystalloids of normal saline in 250-mL increments to maintain the patient's systolic blood pressure in the low normal range.

Some evidence suggests that titration of systolic blood pressure to 80 to 90 mm Hg is preferred for hemorrhagic shock. This low pressure (ie, permissive hypotension) may allow the body to clot better and not dislodge clots already formed.[16] However, you must also consider the entire patient before using permissive hypotension. In a patient with multisystem trauma and traumatic brain injury (TBI), the hypotension employed to manage hypovolemia presents severe risks and may potentially lead to a lethal outcome. A retrospective observation study reported in the *Journal of Trauma* showed that a single episode of hypotension (systolic blood pressure <90 mm Hg) in severely brain-injured patients was associated with a doubling of mortality and a parallel increase in morbidity rates among survivors.[17,18] The concern is that the lower blood pressure will not provide for adequate cerebral perfusion pressure. This pressure, which is the difference between the mean arterial pressure and the intracranial pressure, represents the pressure gradient allowing for cerebral blood flow—and with it, oxygen and nutrients into the brain tissue. Without the

oxygen and nutrients, the already damaged and delicate brain tissue will suffer secondary injury.

Blood products should be started early if hemorrhage is suspected. However, blood products will require typing and cross-matching in the ED, which will take some time to accomplish. The American College of Surgeons recommends starting blood products in Class III and IV hemorrhage after an initial 2 L of isotonic solution is administered or immediately in cases of obvious severe hemorrhage with shock.[19] Colloids have not been shown to offer any superior benefit to crystalloids in improving patient outcomes and, therefore, are not typically recommended. For more information about IV therapy and guidance on IV fluid flow rates, refer to Chapter 40, *Management and Resuscitation of the Critical Patient*.

Words of Wisdom

A patient's blood pressure may be the last measurable factor to change in shock. The body has several automatic mechanisms to compensate for initial blood loss and to help maintain the blood pressure. Thus, by the time you detect a drop in the blood pressure, shock is likely to be well developed. This is particularly true in infants and children, who can maintain their blood pressure until they have lost nearly half of their total blood volume.

Do not give the patient anything by mouth because he or she is likely to vomit. Keep the patient at normal temperature, which usually means covering the patient with a blanket—patients in shock are often unable to conserve body heat effectively and are easily chilled. Monitor the ECG rhythm because any critically ill or injured patient is apt to have dysrhythmias. Also monitor the state of consciousness, pulse, and blood pressure. In a patient with substantial vasoconstriction, the blood pressure sounds may be difficult to hear. If you can feel a pulse over the femoral artery but not over the radial artery, for example, the systolic blood pressure is probably between 70 and 80 mm Hg.

YOU are the Paramedic SUMMARY

1. Is there a possibility of more than one MOI in this scenario?

There can be more than one MOI. The foreman reported that the worker was first struck by a steel beam being lowered into place. Where was the patient struck? What does the path through which he fell look like? Are there outcroppings or other obstacles he may have struck during the fall? What about the failed safety harness? Check whether buckles may have struck his body when he hit the ground. What is on the ground under or near the injured worker? Important details—for example, the worker being struck by a steel beam, hitting a concrete outcropping, or landing on tools—will help you determine the extent of the patient's injuries. Multitask and observe the scene while other tasks are being accomplished.

2. This is a high-rise, commercial construction site. What could some of the potential hazards be for you and your partner?

Most construction sites require anyone on the site to be wearing work boots, a hard hat, and a bright reflective vest, and to have specific safety training for that site. Any construction site, but especially a high-rise commercial site, has members of several trades working at the same time. It is important to be sure that all work around the rescue area is stopped and that there is no further risk of falling equipment, moving machines, or other hazards. When you are at a construction site, make sure you are escorted by a supervisor, safety officer, foreman, or another person with the authority to determine whether the scene is safe to enter.

3. The patient is alert, is breathing adequately, and has a rapid but weak radial pulse. His coworker is holding proper manual immobilization of the cervical spine. What is your next priority?

Continue your primary survey. Look for any life-threatening bleeding and bring it under control. Remember, at this point you are identifying and correcting life threats.

4. You and your partner decide that the MOI indicates that this patient has a high risk of serious injury and you want to move quickly. Do you leave the harness and tool belt in place, or do you remove them before completing your assessment?

You should not leave the harness and belt in place. Just as you would do with any trauma patient, you need to inspect this patient's body for any serious injuries. Anything (eg, clothing, harness, tool belt) that gets in the way of a thorough examination needs to be removed. Do not make the mistake of assuming you have corrected all life threats if you have not examined the patient's entire body before you reach the hospital.

5. The patient has unlabored breathing, normal lung sounds, and high-concentration oxygen in place. His Spo₂ reading seems adequate. Could he still be suffering from poor perfusion?

Yes. When hypovolemia is present, a patient's hemoglobin may be saturated with oxygen but because there is so much less hemoglobin, the body's cells cannot be adequately perfused.

6. If you measure his ETCO₂, would you expect it to be high, low, or normal range? What are some factors that affect the measured levels of ETCO₂?

A patient who is hypovolemic may have a deceptively low carbon dioxide level simply because of poor perfusion and the resultant decrease in metabolism. Decreased lung perfusion can also register as a low carbon dioxide measurement. If the patient is hyperventilating because of shock, this factor can also lower his end-tidal carbon dioxide.

7. Despite you stopping the flow of heavy bleeding, the patient seems to be deteriorating further. What are some of the possible causes of his deteriorating condition?

Although the assessment revealed a large contusion over the flank area, this still may not be the whole picture. The patient fell from a significant height and had heavy tools attached to his belt. This added mass increases the likelihood of injury, especially internal injury due to blunt force trauma of hitting the ground. The MOI in this case dictates a decision for high-priority transport, monitoring vital signs, administration of fluids and oxygen, and rapid transfer to a trauma center.

8. At this point, what is your next priority?

Transport! The patient's dropping blood pressure is a late sign of shock. When the blood pressure drops, it signals that the body is beginning to fail at its attempts to compensate for the blood loss. This patient needs the definitive emergency treatment available only at a trauma center.

YOU are the Paramedic SUMMARY (continued)

EMS Patient Care Report (PCR)

Date: 10-01-18	**Incident No.:** 1056		**Nature of Call:** Man down		**Location:** 1425 Church Street
Dispatched: 0930	**En Route:** 0931	**At Scene:** 0936	**Transport:** 0944	**At Hospital:** 0958	**In Service:** 1018

Patient Information

Age: 57 **Sex:** M **Weight (in kg [lb]):** 90 kg (198 lb)	**Allergies:** Denies **Medications:** Denies **Past Medical History:** High blood pressure, diet controlled **Chief Complaint:** Back and chest pain

Vital Signs

Time: 0941	**BP:** 108/70	**Pulse:** 122 weak, regular	**Respirations:** 20	**Spo$_2$:** 97%
Time: 0944	**BP:** 92/60	**Pulse:** 132	**Respirations:** 24	**Spo$_2$:** 98%
Time: 0949	**BP:** 96/66	**Pulse:** 128	**Respirations:** 22	**Spo$_2$:** 98%
Time: 0954	**BP:** 98/60	**Pulse:** 122	**Respirations:** 22	**Spo$_2$:** 100%

EMS Treatment (circle all that apply)

Oxygen @ __15__ **L/min via (circle one):** NC (NRM) **Bag-mask device**	**Assisted Ventilation**	**Airway Adjunct**	**CPR**
Defibrillation	(**Bleeding Control**)	**Bandaging**	**Splinting**	(**Other:** Spinal immobilization)

Narrative

9-1-1 dispatch for a man down at a construction site with possible serious injuries. Upon arrival, pt, a A/0 × 4 57-year-old male, supine and alert on the ground. Witnesses report seeing pt struck by a beam and fall from scaffold approximately 15 feet from the ground. Ground is hard-packed dirt with rocks; pt fall encumbered by tools and tool belt as well as safety harness with large metal buckles. Both still on pt upon arrival. Pt answers all questions appropriately and witnesses deny seeing any loss of consciousness, reporting that pt hardhat stayed on during fall and then bounced off after impact. Coworker/EMT maintained manual cervical spine immobilization within seconds of fall. Pt airway open and clear with no apparent respiratory distress. Trachea midline. Lungs equal and clear with no evidence of limited chest excursion. Radial pulses both palpable but very weak and rapid. Skin pale, cool, and moist.

High-concentration oxygen administered via nonrebreathing mask. Significant blood flow from a deep laceration in the right flank controlled during primary survey. Pt apparently landed on tools (hammer, pry bar, large wrench) upon impact. No other external bleeding noted, although subsequent assessment reveals large area of discoloration over right flank, right buttocks, and right forearm. Pt denies any head pain and remained alert and oriented throughout treatment and transport. No visible discoloration, skin breaks, or deformities noted on scalp, face, anterior/posterior neck. Chest movement normal, with some complaint of discomfort—"pain 5/10"—upon palpation of ribs on both sides upon inspiration. No crepitus noted. Abdomen is soft, nontender. Pelvis is painful to palpation, and pt complains of weakness in both legs. No incontinence or priapism noted. Pt denies any pain in legs; palpation reveals no deformities or skin breaks. Pt unable to push feet against hands due to stated weakness and pain in pelvic area. Distal (dorsalis pedis) pulses palpated (very weak) with equal strength; capillary nail bed refill slightly more than 2 seconds in both feet.

Pt has large (approx 15-cm) laceration to right flank, with bleeding controlled. Some discoloration noted over right buttocks where tools rested as well as across lower back where harness buckle contacted skin upon impact. Large discoloration and abrasions noted on both forearms where patient states that he tried to grab building while falling. Full range of motion noted in both arms with equal but weak radial pulses. Capillary nail bed refill of both hands slightly greater than 2 seconds.

Pt was examined, bleeding controlled with direct pressure and bandaging. Cervical spine immobilization on backboard performed due to MOI plus evidence of shock and suspected pelvic fracture. High-concentration oxygen maintained throughout transport. Two 18-gauge IV lines started (left and right antecubital) for 2 separate 250-mL boluses. Upon arrival at hospital, approximately 500 mL of normal saline infused through each IV line. SpO$_2$ monitored and vital signs measured every 5 minutes throughout transport. Pt remained alert and oriented and stated that he was feeling a little bit better upon arrival at ED. Hospital ED notified of trauma pt en route. Return to service at 1018 hours.**End of report**

Prep Kit

▶ Ready for Review

- The cardiovascular and respiratory systems have distinct roles in keeping blood flowing between the lungs and peripheral tissues.
- Perfusion is the circulation of blood within an organ or tissue in adequate amounts to meet the cells' current needs for oxygen, nutrients, and waste removal.
- Hemorrhage simply means bleeding. Bleeding can range from a "nick" to a capillary while shaving, to a severely spurting artery from a deep slash with a knife, to a ruptured spleen from striking the steering column during a vehicle crash.
- External hemorrhage can usually be easily controlled by using direct, even pressure and pressure dressings and/or splints. For bleeding from extremities, if these methods are not sufficient, use a tourniquet.
- Internal hemorrhage may not be controlled until a surgeon locates the source and sutures it closed.
- Hemorrhagic shock is the most common cause of hypovolemic shock.
- Hypovolemic shock caused by hemorrhagic trauma has been organized by the American College of Surgeons Committee on Trauma into four classes, each with its own specific characteristics and treatments.

- Hypoperfusion (shock) occurs when the level of tissue perfusion decreases below normal.
- Early decreased tissue perfusion may result in subtle changes in the patient's status, such as aberrant mental status, long before a patient's vital signs (ie, blood pressure, pulse rate, respiratory rate) appear abnormal.
- As with any patient, airway and ventilatory support take top priority when treating a patient with suspected shock.
- Stabilizing a serious fracture has a high priority in the control of bleeding. Splinting the fracture helps control bleeding, and splinting should occur before other bleeding control is attempted unless evidence of arterial spurting from the wound.
- Methods for controlling external hemorrhage include direct, even pressure; pressure dressings and/or splints; and tourniquets. Most cases of external hemorrhage can be controlled with direct pressure to the bleeding site.
- If direct pressure fails to immediately stop the hemorrhaging of an extremity, apply a tourniquet above the level of the bleeding. If a commercial tourniquet is not available, a tourniquet can be improvised with a triangular bandage and a stick or rod. Splint after tourniquet.
- If bleeding is present at the nose and a skull fracture is suspected, place a gauze pad loosely under the nose.

Prep Kit (continued)

- Management of a patient with internal hemorrhaging focuses on the treatment of shock, minimizing movement of the injured or bleeding part or region, and rapid transport.
- Patients who have suspected shock, whether compensated or decompensated, can benefit from early surgical intervention and should be transported to a facility with those capabilities.
- Be alert, and search for early signs of shock.

▶ Vital Vocabulary

afterload The pressure in the aorta against which the left ventricle must pump blood; increasing this pressure can decrease cardiac output.

blood The fluid tissue that is pumped by the heart through the arteries, veins, and capillaries; it consists of plasma and formed elements or cells, such as red blood cells, white blood cells, and platelets.

cardiac output (CO) The amount of blood pumped by the heart per minute; calculated by multiplying the stroke volume by the pulse rate per minute.

compensated shock The early stage of shock, in which the body can still compensate for blood loss. The systolic blood pressure and brain perfusion are maintained.

decompensated (hypotensive) shock The late stage of shock, when blood pressure is falling.

ejection fraction (EF) The percentage of blood that leaves the heart each time it contracts.

exsanguination The loss of the total blood volume, resulting in death.

hematemesis Vomited blood.

hematochezia Passage of stools containing bright red blood.

hematocrit The proportion of red blood cells in the total blood volume.

hematoma A mass of blood in the soft tissues beneath the skin; it indicates bleeding into soft tissues and may be the result of a minor or a severe injury.

hematuria Blood in the urine.

hemophilia A bleeding disorder that is primarily hereditary, in which clotting does not occur or occurs insufficiently.

hemoptysis Coughed-up blood.

hemorrhage Bleeding.

hemorrhagic shock A condition in which volume is lost in the form of blood.

hemostasis The body's natural blood-clotting mechanism.

hypoperfusion A condition that occurs when the level of tissue perfusion decreases below that needed to maintain normal cellular functions.

hypovolemic shock A condition that occurs when the circulating blood volume is inadequate to deliver adequate oxygen and nutrients to the body.

irreversible shock The final stage of shock, prior to death.

melena Passage of dark, tarry stools.

perfusion The delivery of oxygen and nutrients to the cells, organs, and tissues of the body.

plasma A component of blood, made of 92% water, 6% to 7% proteins, and electrolytes, clotting factors, and glucose.

platelets Small cells in the blood that are essential for clot formation.

preload The precontraction pressure in the heart, which increases as the volume of blood builds up.

shock An abnormal state associated with inadequate oxygen and nutrient delivery to the metabolic apparatus of the cell.

stroke volume (SV) The amount of blood that the left ventricle ejects into the aorta per contraction.

▶ References

1. Guillermo G, Reines D, Wulf-Gutierrez M. Clinical review: hemorrhagic shock. *Critical Care*. 2004;8:373.
2. American College of Surgeons. *ATLS Advanced Trauma Life Support for Doctors—Student Course Manual*. Chicago, IL: American College of Surgeons; 2012.
3. Mutschler M, Paffrath T, Wolfl C, et al. The ATLS classification of hypovolaemic shock: a well established teaching tool on the edge? *Injury*. 2014;45(3):S35-S38.
4. Rezaie S. Is ATLS wrong about palpable blood pressure estimates? ALiEM: Academic Life in Emergency Medicine website. https://www.aliem.com/2013/is-atls-wrong-about-palpable-blood-pressure/. Published March 31, 2013. Accessed January 23, 2017.
5. Kragh JF Jr, Walters TJ, Baer DG, et al. Practical use of emergency tourniquets to stop bleeding in major limb trauma. *J Trauma*. 2008;64:538-550.
6. Bennett BL. Bleeding control using hemostatic dressings: lessons learned. *Wilderness Environ Med*. 2017;28(1): in press.
7. Roberts I, Perel P, Prieto-Merino D, et al. Effect of tranexamic acid on mortality in patients with traumatic bleeding: prespecified analysis of data from randomised controlled trial. *Brit Med J*. 2012;345:e5839.
8. Morrison JJ, Dubose JJ, Rasmussen TE, et al. Military Application of Tranexamic Acid in Trauma Emergency Resuscitation (MATTERS) Study. *Arch Surg*. 2012;147(2):113-119.

Prep Kit (continued)

9. Ausset S, Glassberg E, Nadler R, et al. Tranexamic acid as part of remote damage-control resuscitation in the prehospital setting: a critical appraisal of the medical literature and available alternatives. *J Trauma Acute Care Surg.* 2015;78(6 suppl 1):S70-S75.

10. Snyder D, Tsou A, Schoelles K. *Efficacy of Prehospital Application of Tourniquets and Hemostatic Dressings to Control Traumatic External Hemorrhage.* DOT HS 811 999b. Washington, DC: National Highway Traffic Safety Administration; May 2014. https://www .ems.gov/pdf/research/Studies-and-Reports /Prehospital_Applications_Of_Tourniquest_And _Hemostatic_Dressings.pdf. Accessed April 12, 2017.

11. Taillac PP, Bolleter S, Heightman AJ. Wound packing essentials for EMTs and paramedics. *J Emerg Med Serv.* 2017;42(4): in press. http://www.jems.com /articles/print/volume-42/issue-4/features/wound -packing-essentials-for-emts-and-paramedics.html. Accessed April 26, 2017.

12. Bickell WH, Pepe PE, Bailey ML, et al. Randomized trial of pneumatic antishock garments in the prehospital management of penetrating abdominal injuries. *Ann Emerg Med.* 1987;16(6):653-658.

13. Pepe PE, Bass RR, Mattox KL. Clinical trials of the pneumatic antishock garment in the urban prehospital setting. *Ann Emerg Med.* 1986;15(12):1407-1410.

14. Martini WZ, Cortez DS, Dubick MA. Comparisons of normal saline and lactated Ringer's resuscitation on hemodynamics, metabolic responses, and coagulation in pigs after severe hemorrhagic shock. *Scand J Trauma Resusc Emerg Med.* 2013;21:86.

15. de Crescenzo C, Gorouhi F, Salcedo ES, Galante JM. Prehospital hypertonic fluid resuscitation for trauma patients: a systematic review and meta-analysis. *J Trauma Acute Care Surg.* 2017;82(5):956-962.

16. Pape HC, Peitzman AB, Rotondo MF, Giannoudis PV. *Damage Control Management in the Polytrauma Patient.* New York, NY: Springer; 2017.

17. Chesnut RM, Marshall LF, Klauber MR, et al. The role of secondary brain injury in determining outcome from severe head injury. *J Trauma.* 1993;34(2):216-222. https://www.ncbi.nlm.nih .gov/pubmed/8459458. Accessed April 12, 2017.

18. Evidence-based EMS: permissive hypotension in trauma. EMS World website. http://www.emsworld .com/article/12163910/evidence-based-ems -permissive-hypotension-in-trauma. Accessed April 12, 2017.

19. American College of Surgeons Committee on Trauma. *Advanced Trauma Life Support Student Course Manual.* 9th ed. Chicago, IL: American College of Surgeons; 2012:72-74.

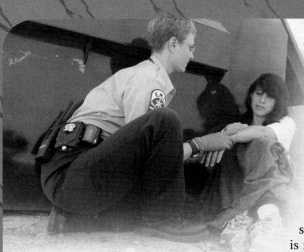

Assessment in Action

You and your partner arrive at the scene of a "motorcyclist down." You assess the scene to be safe and, wearing appropriate PPE, walk toward the police officers who are waving you over. You walk past a large motorcycle on its side. The front wheel is twisted, pieces of red plastic and chrome are scattered on the surrounding pavement, and a white helmet is nearby. About 30 feet away, a man is lying on his back, not moving. A bystander who is kneeling by the man says that the man's name is Jim and he thinks his leg is broken.

A backup crew has just arrived and you instruct one of the crew members to maintain stabilization of the cervical spine. The other crew member administers 15 L/min of oxygen via a nonrebreathing mask.

The patient looks at you as you call to him. He tells you his name, the day, and what happened. His airway is open, and he is maintaining its patency on his own. No blood or other foreign matter is in his mouth. The patient's radial pulse is barely palpable at 130 beats/min. His skin is pale and cool. Blood is oozing steadily from a tear in the right lower leg of his jeans. As you cut the jeans, you see bone protruding from the anterior

Assessment *in Action* (continued)

lower leg. Bleeding is controlled with direct pressure. His right thigh is swollen and deformed. His right foot is twisted in an unnatural angle, and he tells you that he cannot feel his foot.

While one of the EMTs brings the backboard and stretcher, you perform a secondary assessment. During this assessment, you notice that the radial pulses are no longer palpable. The patient is asking if he can get up and find his bike. The EMTs assist you in packaging the patient for transport.

1. To immobilize the patient's right leg, you should:

   A. apply two splints and attach them to the backboard.
   B. manually support the limb.
   C. use a traction splint.
   D. do nothing except strap the patient's leg to the backboard and provide rapid transport.

2. Baroreceptors in the aortic arch and carotid sinus detect a change in pressure as the patient's blood pressure drops. This would most likely result in:

   A. inhibition of the vasomotor center and antidiuretic hormone release.
   B. stimulation of the vasomotor center and antidiuretic hormone release.
   C. inhibition of the vasomotor center and antidiuretic hormone inhibition.
   D. stimulation of the vasomotor center and antidiuretic hormone inhibition.

3. Initially, your primary survey of the patient identified rapid but weak peripheral pulses. In this scenario, this finding is most likely an indication of:

   A. injuries to the arms.
   B. decompensated shock.
   C. compensated shock.
   D. irreversible shock.

4. During your secondary assessment, you once again checked the radial pulses and found them to be absent. In this scenario, you should strongly suspect:

   A. compensated shock.
   B. decompensated shock.
   C. irreversible shock.
   D. injuries to the arms.

5. During your reassessment of the patient, the best early indicator of a significant change in tissue perfusion is:

   A. a decrease in the blood pressure.
   B. a rise in the pulse rate.
   C. a sudden change in mental status.
   D. the amount of visible blood loss from the leg.

6. As the patient's condition deteriorates, you quickly package him for transport to a trauma center. You should attempt to start at least one, and preferably two, 18-gauge IV lines for rapid infusion of normal saline. This action should be taken:

   A. immediately.
   B. en route.
   C. on arrival at the emergency department.
   D. only in the emergency department.

7. The patient weighs approximately 150 pounds (68 kg). He lost 1 L of blood from his femur fracture and another 500 mL from his open tibial fracture. In addition, you suspect that he has other injuries that may be causing blood loss. When fluids are infused, an attempt should be made to:

   A. infuse as much fluid as possible over the shortest time possible.
   B. infuse enough fluid to bring the blood pressure back to normal for that patient.
   C. infuse enough fluid to maintain the systolic pressure at about 80 mm Hg.
   D. infuse enough fluid to maintain the diastolic pressure at about 80 mm Hg.

8. What is the term for shock as a result of inadequate blood volume?

9. Hemorrhaging from the nose (epistaxis) or the ears following a head injury may indicate a skull fracture. In such a case, should you attempt to stop the blood flow?

10. For which reasons is immobilizing a fracture a priority in the prompt control of bleeding?

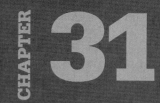
Soft-Tissue Trauma

National EMS Education Standard Competencies

Trauma

Integrates assessment findings with principles of epidemiology and pathophysiology to formulate a field impression to implement a comprehensive treatment/disposition plan for an acutely injured patient.

Soft-Tissue Trauma

Recognition and management of
> Wounds (pp 1613-1615, 1621-1623)
> Burns (see Chapter 32, *Burns*)
  • Electrical (see Chapter 32, *Burns*)
  • Chemical (see Chapter 32, *Burns*)
  • Thermal (see Chapter 32, *Burns*)
> Chemicals in the eye and on the skin (see Chapter 32, *Burns* and Chapter 33, *Face and Neck Trauma*)

Pathophysiology, assessment, and management of
> Wounds
  • Avulsions (pp 1625-1626)
  • Bite wounds (pp 1626-1627)
  • Lacerations (pp 1623-1624)
  • Puncture wounds (pp 1624-1625)
  • Incisions (pp 1623-1624)
> Burns
  • Electrical (see Chapter 32, *Burns*)
  • Chemical (see Chapter 32, *Burns*)
  • Thermal (see Chapter 32, *Burns*)
  • Radiation (see Chapter 32, *Burns*)
> High-pressure injection (pp 1627-1629)
> Crush syndrome (see Chapter 37, *Orthopaedic Trauma*)

Knowledge Objectives

1. Review the anatomy and physiology of the skin, including the layers of the skin. (pp 1611-1612)
2. Understand the functions of the skin, and its role in the inflammatory process. (p 1611)
3. Explain skin tension lines and how they relate to wound healing. (p 1612)
4. Discuss the pathophysiology of soft-tissue injuries, including closed injuries and open injuries. (pp 1612-1613)
5. Discuss the process of wound healing, including hemostasis, inflammation, epithelialization, neovascularization, and collagen synthesis. (pp 1613-1614)
6. Discuss alterations in the wound healing process, including anatomic factors, high-risk wounds, abnormal scar formation, pressure injuries, and wounds requiring closure. (pp 1614-1615)
7. Discuss the pathophysiology of infection. (pp 1615-1616)
8. Describe the assessment process for patients with a soft-tissue injury, with a focus on when to perform a physical exam. (pp 1616-1617)
9. Describe the relationship between airway management and the patient with closed and open injuries. (p 1616)
10. Discuss emergency medical care of a patient with a soft-tissue injury. (pp 1617-1621)
11. Discuss the principles for treating a closed wound. (pp 1617-1618)
12. Discuss the principles for treating an open wound. (p 1618)
13. Describe complications of improperly applied dressings. (p 1618)
14. Understand the functions and types of sterile dressings and bandages. (p 1619)
15. Discuss methods and materials for site-specific dressings. (pp 1621-1623)
16. Discuss the role of pain control when managing patients with soft-tissue injuries. (p 1623)
17. Discuss the pathophysiology, assessment, and management of abrasions, lacerations, puncture wounds, impaled objects, avulsions, amputations, bite wounds, and high-pressure injection injuries. (pp 1623-1629)
18. Discuss the pathophysiology, assessment, and management of soft-tissue injuries to specific anatomic sites, including facial and neck injuries, thoracic injuries, and abdominal injuries. (p 1629)
19. Discuss the pathophysiology, assessment, and management of soft-tissue infections, including myositis, gangrene, tetanus, necrotizing fasciitis, paronychia, and flexor tenosynovitis of the hand. (pp 1630-1631)

Skills Objectives

1. Demonstrate the assessment and management of a patient with signs and symptoms of soft-tissue injury, including:
   a. Contusion (pp 1612, 1617-1618)
   b. Hematoma (pp 1612-1613, 1617-1618)
   c. Blast injuries (pp 1612-1613 and see Chapter 29, *Trauma Systems and Mechanism of Injury*)
   d. Abrasion (p 1623)
   e. Laceration (p 1624)
   f. Puncture wound (pp 1624-1625)
   g. Impaled object (pp 1624-1625)
   h. Avulsion (pp 1625-1626)
   i. Amputation (p 1626)
   j. Animal and human bites (p 1627)
   k. High-pressure injection injuries (pp 1628-1629)

Introduction

The skin is the largest organ of the human body and serves as the interface between the body and the outside world. For that reason, injuries involving the skin are common. A *wound* is any injury to the soft tissues—that is, an injury to the skin with or without involvement of the subcutaneous tissues and muscle.

Most soft-tissue wounds are relatively low-priority injuries. Although they may be the most obvious and dramatic injuries, they are seldom the most serious of the patient's problems unless they compromise the airway or are associated with massive bleeding. Always search systematically and thoroughly for other injuries or life-threatening conditions before tending to soft-tissue trauma. *Do not let dramatic soft-tissue injuries distract you from conducting a thorough primary survey!*

Incidence, Mortality, and Morbidity

The soft tissues of the body can be injured through a variety of mechanisms. A blunt injury occurs when the energy exchange between the patient and an object is more than the tissues can tolerate, as can happen in an automobile crash that leads to the person striking the steering wheel. A penetrating injury occurs when an object, such as a bullet or knife, breaks through the skin and enters the body, creating an entrance wound and possibly an exit wound. Burns (discussed in Chapter 32, *Burns*) may also result in soft-tissue injuries.

Soft-tissue trauma is the leading form of injury. In fact, wound care is one of the most frequently performed procedures in emergency departments (EDs) across the United States. Most of these injuries require basic interventions such as wound irrigation, dressing, bandaging, and limited suturing. Death due to soft-tissue injury is extremely rare. When it occurs, it is typically related to either hemorrhage or infection. Uncontrolled hemorrhage can quickly lead to shock and death. When the skin barrier is breached, invading pathogens—bacteria, fungi, and viruses—can cause local or systemic infection. Infection can be life or limb threatening, especially in people with preexisting medical conditions.

Preventing soft-tissue injuries and their associated complications involves simple protective actions. The use of gloves when working with abrasive materials, for example, can prevent skin injuries. Workplace safety

YOU are the Paramedic — PART 1

You and your partner are dispatched to a call at a factory for an unknown injury. You arrive at the address and see a woman waving frantically from the driveway. "Please come quickly! One of our workers cut his hand very badly. He was working with a saw, and the safety guard was not in place. There is blood everywhere!" She directs you into the work area. As you approach, you see a spray pattern of dark-colored blood and the saw blade that is no longer spinning. A man is sitting on the ground with a dirty shop towel wrapped around his hand, which is saturated with blood. He is pale and appears very anxious. He is rocking back and forth while seated on the ground and says, "My hand hit the blade. It hurts! It hurts! Please do something!" Several workers are gathered around the man.

1. You and your partner continue to assess the scene. After you clear the workers around the injured man, which other scene precautions must be taken?
2. After you ensure the scene is safe, what are your next actions?

measures to reduce injury include use of safety devices to prevent interaction between machine parts and body parts. Teaching children to avoid using sharp objects also helps prevent injury. Plastic scissors, plastic knives, and plastic drinking cups are all designed in part to reduce the risk of cuts and other skin injuries among children.

Anatomy and Physiology Review

The structure and function of the skin are covered in greater detail in Chapter 8, *Anatomy and Physiology*. A brief review that focuses on how the skin is damaged when an injury occurs is presented here.

▶ Skin Structure and Function

The human skin, or **integument**, is a complex organ with a crucial role in maintaining the constancy of the internal environment (**homeostasis**). As discussed in Chapter 8, *Anatomy and Physiology*, the skin performs the following functions:

- **Protection.** The skin protects the underlying tissue from injury and exposure to extremes of temperature, ultraviolet radiation, mechanical forces, toxic chemicals, and invading microorganisms.
- **Temperature Regulation.** The skin aids in temperature regulation (**thermoregulation**), constricting blood vessels to prevent heat loss when the core body temperature starts to fall, and dilating blood vessels to facilitate heat loss when core temperature rises. Sweat is also secreted to the surface of the skin where it can evaporate, causing body temperature to fall.
- **Fluid regulation.** As a watertight seal, the skin prevents excessive loss of water from the body and drying of tissues, thereby helping maintain the chemical stability of the internal environment. Without skin, a person would become waterlogged after the first rain and would resemble a prune after the first hot day of summer.
- **Sensation.** The skin serves as a sense organ, keeping the brain informed about the external environment. Changes in temperature, sensations of pain, and the position of the body are mediated through sensory nerves. The skin also reacts to pressure, pain, and pleasurable stimuli.
- **Inflammatory response.** The skin responds to injuries and wounds with inflammation, which causes redness, increased warmth, and painful swelling. The blood vessels of the wounded area dilate and allow fluids to leak into the damaged tissues. This provides more nutrients and oxygen to the tissues, aiding in healing.

Significant damage to the skin may make the body vulnerable to bacterial invasion, temperature instability, and major disturbances of fluid balance—precisely what happens when an injury results in an opening in the skin.

The skin is composed of two layers—the epidermis and the dermis **Figure 31-1**.

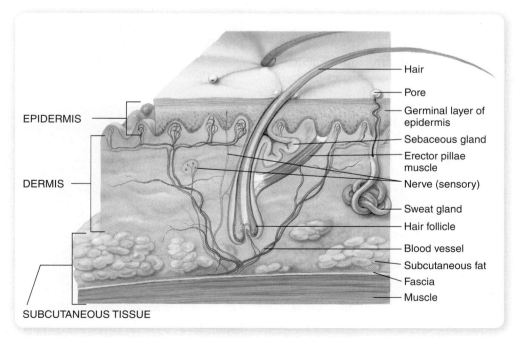

EPIDERMIS

DERMIS

SUBCUTANEOUS TISSUE

Hair
Pore
Germinal layer of epidermis
Sebaceous gland
Erector pillae muscle
Nerve (sensory)
Sweat gland
Hair follicle
Blood vessel
Subcutaneous fat
Fascia
Muscle

Figure 31-1 The skin comprises a tough external layer called the epidermis and a vascular inner layer called the dermis. Between the dermis and the underlying muscle and bone is a thick layer of connective tissue known as subcutaneous tissue, and a layer of fascia.

© Jones & Bartlett Learning.

The **epidermis** is the outer, visible layer of skin. This layer varies in thickness in different areas of the body. The epidermis consists of several layers of cells: an outermost layer (stratum corneum) of hardened, nonliving cells, which are continuously shed through a process called **desquamation**; and four inner layers of living cells that constantly divide to give rise to the cells of the stratum corneum. The stratum corneum are dead cells that have had their cytoplasm replaced with keratin, which is a tough, waterproof substance that further protects the underlying tissues from light, heat, microorganisms, some chemicals, and minor trauma. Because cells of the stratum corneum are dead, they are constantly shed and replaced by new cells that move up through the layers of the epidermis. The deeper layers of the epidermis also contain variable numbers of cells bearing melanin granules. The darkness of a person's skin is directly proportional to the amount of melanin present.

Underlying the epidermis is a tough, highly elastic layer of connective tissues called the **dermis**. The dermis contains specialized structures including nerve endings, blood vessels, sweat glands, hair follicles, and sebaceous glands.

Between the dermis and the underlying muscle and bone is a thick layer of connective tissue known as subcutaneous tissue, or the superficial fascia. The subcutaneous tissue insulates, protects, and stores energy in the form of fat. Subcutaneous injections are given in this layer.

Below the subcutaneous tissue is a thick, dense layer of fibrous tissue known as the deep fascia. Below this layer, tendons connect muscles to the skeleton. In general, the deeper an injury penetrates into the skin, the greater the damage that occurs. A breach of this important anatomic barrier can lead to serious infections.

▶ Skin Tension Lines

The skin is arranged over the body structures in a manner that provides tension. This tautness varies by body region but occurs in patterns known as **tension lines**. *Static tension* develops over areas that have limited movement, such as the scalp. Lacerations occurring parallel to the skin tension lines may remain closed with little or no intervention. Larger wounds may be pulled open by the normal tension and require closure with sutures, staples, or a biodegradable "glue." Even small lacerations that lie perpendicular to the tension lines may result in a wound that remains open. Healing occurs more slowly in an open wound, and abnormal scar formation is more likely.

Dynamic tension is found in areas that lie over muscle. This tension varies according to the contraction of the underlying muscle and subsequent movement of the skin. Open injuries to dynamic tension lines interfere with healing because they disrupt the clotting process and the tissue repair cycle, resulting in slowed healing and a tendency toward abnormal scar formation.

An abnormal scar may prompt the patient to seek **scar revision**—surgery to improve its appearance. The surgeon takes skin tension into account when determining the best procedure for revision. This factor must also be considered when wound debridement is necessary or when hospital personnel must remove an impaled object.

■ General Pathophysiology: Closed Versus Open Wounds

▶ Closed Wounds

In a **closed wound**, soft tissues beneath the skin surface are damaged, but there is no break in the epidermis. A patient with a closed wound may have non-penetrating blunt trauma to organs and other important structures beneath the skin. Always consider underlying injury when a patient has a closed wound, particularly if the wound is located in an area adjacent to a vital organ.

The characteristic closed wound is a **contusion** **Figure 31-2** . In a contusion (bruise), the skin is intact, but damage has occurred beneath the epidermis. Trauma to the tissues produces pain, leakage of fluid into spaces between the damaged cells, and an inflammatory response resulting in redness (**erythema**) and swelling (edema). If small blood vessels in the dermis are disrupted, a black-and-blue mark (**ecchymosis**) will cover the injured area; if large blood vessels are torn beneath the contused area, a **hematoma**—a collection of blood beneath the skin—will be evident as a lump with a blue discoloration **Figure 31-3** .

▶ Open Wounds

An **open wound** is characterized by a disruption in the skin. Types of open wounds include abrasions, lacerations, avulsions, amputations, bites, impaled objects, penetrating blast injuries, high-pressure injection injuries, and puncture wounds. Open wounds are potentially much more serious than closed wounds for two reasons. First, they are vulnerable to infection. An open wound is easily

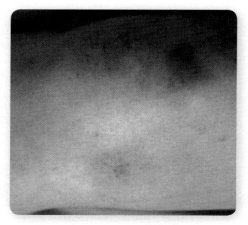

Figure 31-2 Contusions, more commonly known as bruises, occur as a result of a blunt force striking the body. Ecchymosis (blue and black discoloration) signifies bleeding underneath the skin.

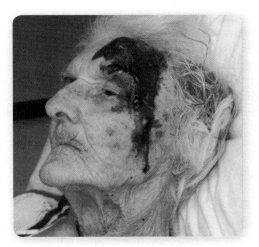

Figure 31-3 A hematoma.
Courtesy of Rhonda Hunt.

Table 31-1	**Conditions That Require Transport**

- Compromise of:
  - Nerves
  - Vessels
  - Muscles
  - Tendons or ligaments
- Foreign body or cosmetic complications
- Heavy contamination

© Jones & Bartlett Learning.

contaminated—that is, microorganisms can readily enter it. Whether the contamination produces infection depends in large measure on how the wound is managed. Second, open wounds have a greater potential for serious blood loss. When the skin is unbroken, bleeding from a disrupted blood vessel is limited. Although a significant volume of blood—up to about two units—can be lost into the soft tissues of the leg, eventually the increasing pressure within the leg will prevent further bleeding. In an open wound, the patient's entire blood volume may be lost.

A physician should always evaluate certain wounds. The injuries in Table 31-1 require transport, even if they appear minor.

▶ Crush Injuries

Crush syndrome occurs because of a prolonged compressive force that impairs muscle metabolism and circulation, and presents following the extrication or release of an entrapped limb.

In a crush injury, the external appearance may not adequately represent the level of internal damage. An upper extremity that merely appears swollen may, in fact, have enough muscle destruction to cause systemic problems, especially if the extremity has been trapped for longer than 4 hours, which is enough time to develop crush syndrome. In other cases, the injured region may be mangled beyond recognition.

Remember that grotesque injuries may not necessarily be the patient's primary injury. Always concentrate on threats to life before addressing injured extremities, no matter how bad the initial appearance. Soft-tissue injuries in this context are almost always less important than the injuries incurred beneath the skin. Crush syndrome is covered in greater detail in Chapter 37, *Orthopaedic Trauma*.

▶ Blast Injuries

Recall that an explosion is a mechanism of injury (MOI) that can result in many types of injuries, including soft-tissue trauma, abdominal trauma, skeletal trauma, and blast lung, among others. Blast injuries as an MOI are covered in detail in Chapter 29, *Trauma Systems and Mechanism of Injury*. Always remember to assess the scene for hazards to yourself and your EMS crew, and do not enter the scene until safety can be ensured.

■ Wound Healing

▶ The Process of Wound Healing

Healing of wounds is a natural process that involves several overlapping stages, all directed toward the larger goal of restoring hemostasis. Ultimately, the goal is for the body to return to a functional state, although the injured area may not always be restored to its preinjury condition.

Hemostasis

Among the primary concerns in wound healing is the cessation of bleeding. Loss of blood, either internally or externally, hinders the provision of vital nutrients and oxygen to the affected area. It also impairs the tissue's ability to eliminate wastes. The end result is abnormal or absent function, which interferes with homeostasis. To stop the flow of blood, the vessels, platelets, and clotting cascade must work in unison (the three phases of hemostasis).

Injury to soft tissue causes chemical mediators of inflammation to be released. Injured blood vessels constrict resulting in less space through which blood can flow and decreased blood loss. The muscular layer in the arteries, arterioles, and some veins constricts to reduce the size of the lumen. Skeletal muscle also has a role in the constriction process. Because capillaries lack smooth muscle, bleeding continues, albeit at a slower rate.

Platelets are also activated by the release of these chemicals. Activated platelets adhere to the affected area and to other platelets. This aggregation of platelets forms a platelet plug. Although not the permanent repair of the wound, the plug temporarily stops the blood loss and is the beginning of blood clot formation.

Inflammation

In inflammation (the next stage of wound healing), additional cells move into the damaged area to begin repair. White blood cells migrate to the area to combat pathogens that have invaded exposed tissue. Chemicals and proteins known as **chemotactic factors** are released and signal repairing cells to migrate to the area of injury. **Granulocytes** and macrophages, which are among the first restoration cells to arrive, engulf bacteria through **phagocytosis**, which involves ingestion of damaged cellular parts. Foreign products and bacteria can also be removed from the body by phagocytosis. Similarly, lymphocytes (a type of white blood cell) destroy bacteria and other pathogens.

Mast cells release histamine as part of the body's response in the early stages of inflammation. Histamine causes dilation of blood vessels, increasing blood flow to the injured area and resulting in a reddened, warm area immediately around the site. Histamine makes capillaries more permeable, and swelling may occur as fluid seeps out of these "leaky" capillaries.

Inflammation ultimately leads to the removal of foreign material, damaged cellular parts, and invading microorganisms from the wound site. Reconstruction of the injured region through epithelialization, neovascularization, and collagen synthesis can then begin.

Epithelialization

In the outer layer of skin, epithelial cells are stacked in layers. To replace the area damaged in a soft-tissue injury, a new layer of epithelial cells must be moved into this region—a process known as **epithelialization**. Cells from the stratum germinativum quickly multiply and redevelop across the edges of the wound. Except in cases of clean incisions, the appearance of the restructured area seldom returns to the preinjury state. For example, large wounds or injuries that result in significant disruption of the skin will often have incomplete epithelialization.

Neovascularization

In **neovascularization**, new blood vessels form as the body attempts to bring oxygen and nutrients to the injured tissue. New capillaries bud from intact capillaries that lie adjacent to the damaged skin. These vessels provide a conduit for oxygen and nutrients and serve as a pathway for waste removal. Because they are new and delicate, bleeding might result from a minor injury. It may take weeks to months for the new capillaries to be as stable as preexisting vessels.

Collagen Synthesis

Collagen is a tough, fibrous protein found in scar tissue, hair, bones, and connective tissue. This vital structural repair unit is synthesized by fibroblasts, repair cells that migrate into damaged tissue. In wound healing, collagen provides stability to the damaged tissue and joins wound borders, thereby closing the open tissue. Unfortunately, collagen cannot restore the damaged tissue to its original strength.

▶ Alterations of Wound Healing

Wound healing does not always follow the pattern described previously. Infection or an abnormal scar may develop, excessive bleeding may occur, or healing may be slow. For example, medications such as corticosteroids, nonsteroidal anti-inflammatory drugs, penicillin, colchicine, anticoagulants, and antineoplastic agents can delay healing. Likewise, a variety of medical conditions, including advanced age, severe alcoholism, acute uremia, diabetes, hypoxia, severe anemia, peripheral vascular disease, malnutrition, advanced cancer, hepatic failure, and cardiovascular disease, may interfere with normal healing.

This section discusses altered wound healing and potential complications.

Anatomic Factors

Areas of the body subjected to repeated motion throughout the day, such as the fingers, tend to heal slowly. One strategy used to speed healing in such cases is to splint the affected part, preventing movement. The positioning of an open wound relative to skin tension lines (static or dynamic) also affects how the wound will heal and determines whether an abnormal scar will form.

High-Risk Wounds

Wounds that carry a high risk for developing infection include human and animal bites. Because the mouth is warm and constantly moist, it offers a hospitable environment for growth of bacteria. Injection of human saliva into tissue can result in significant infection. In particular, rabies is a serious infection that can develop from the bite of an infected animal (such as wild raccoons, dogs, and cats).

If a foreign body or organic matter becomes embedded in an open wound, the wound is considered a high-risk injury because of the likelihood that the material involved is impregnated with microorganisms. Once such material breaches the skin barrier, the pathogen has easy entry into the rest of the body. A foreign body that is in place on evaluation should be left in place because a lacerated blood vessel may not be bleeding freely owing to the foreign body's position. *Do not remove an impaled object in the field unless it interferes with the patient's airway.*

Other high-risk wounds include injection wounds, wounds with significant devitalized tissue, crush wounds (covered in detail in Chapter 37, *Orthopaedic Trauma*), wounds in immunocompromised patients, and injuries to patients with poor peripheral circulation.

Abnormal Scar Formation

Excessive collagen formation can occur if the healing process is not balanced between the building-up and breaking-down phases of healing. A hypertrophic or keloid scar may develop from the excess protein. **Hypertrophic scar** formation occurs in areas subject to high tissue stress, such as the elbow and the knee. Such a scar does not extend past the borders of the wound margins and tends to form in people with lightly pigmented skin. In contrast, a **keloid scar** typically develops in people with darkly pigmented skin. It grows over the wound margins and can become larger than the wound area. Keloid scars tend to form on the ears, upper extremities, lower abdomen, and sternum.

Pressure Injuries

Pressure injuries may occur when a patient is bedridden or when pressure is applied for a prolonged period in an unresponsive patient or a patient immobilized on a backboard. If the involved tissues are deprived of oxygen, localized hypoxia and cell deterioration will develop. Prevention involves determining the risk and providing a mechanism to reduce or release the pressure on the skin.

Wounds Requiring Closure

Many open wounds heal without medical intervention, but some require closure with sutures, staples, or medical glue (octyl-2-cyanoacrylate). Closure involves bringing the wound edges together to allow for optimal healing. Open injuries that require closure include those that affect cosmetic areas, such as the lips, face, and eyebrows. Such injuries should be considered for closure because scarring often has psychological implications. Gaping wounds and those occurring over tension lines also require closure. **Degloving** involves unraveling of the skin from the hand, much like the partial removal of a glove. These injuries require substantial irrigation and debridement before closing. Closure is also indicated for ring injuries and skin tears.

Most open injuries should be closed within 24 hours in most cases, although the scientific evidence to support that recommendation is minimal.[1] Initial hospital management for open wounds involves assessment for foreign material followed by irrigation. The physician can then determine appropriate wound closing options.

Three types of wound closures are performed: primary closure, secondary intention, and delayed primary closure. In primary closure, the wound margins are brought together as primary treatment. Secondary intention entails dressing high-risk wounds and allowing them to heal from inside out. Delayed primary closure involves delayed closure of wounds that were initially managed by secondary intention.

Patients who receive sutures need appropriate follow-up care to determine whether healing is normal or abnormal. Serious complications, including localized or systemic infection, can arise. In some cases, sutures may need to be removed early to allow a wound to drain infectious material.

► Infection

Because the skin serves as an initial barrier against microorganisms, any break in its surface can lead to infection. Larger openings and deeper penetrations result in a higher level of risk for the development of an infection. Not only will there be a delay in healing from the infection, but additional complications or systemic infection can result.

Staphylococcus and *Streptococcus* bacteria account for a majority of bacterial skin infections.[2] Once pathogens have entered the body tissues, they begin to grow and multiply, although clinical signs of infection may not appear for several days. Visible clues of infection include

---

YOU are the Paramedic   PART 2

Your partner asks the bystanders to move back to allow for assessment and treatment of the patient. Based on the amount of blood noted in the area, it was a wise choice for you and your partner to have donned gloves, gowns, masks, and goggles. You now direct your attention to assessing life threats before focusing on the obvious hand injury. The primary survey reveals a patent airway, slightly increased breathing, intact circulation as noted by the presence of bilateral rapid radial pulses, and an alert patient.

Recording Time: 1 Minute	
Appearance	Semi-Fowler position on the floor
Level of consciousness	Alert, oriented
Airway	Open, clear, self-maintained
Breathing	Adequate, slightly increased
Circulation	Pale skin, radial pulses equal/strong, rapid

3. Why was it important to don gowns, masks, and goggles as a supplement to your gloves?
4. While you are assessing your patient, you note that the bystander who assisted the patient before your arrival has blood on his shirt and hands. What should you say to the bystander?

erythema, pus, warmth, edema, and local discomfort. Red streaks adjacent to the wound indicate that the patient has developed **lymphangitis**, an inflammation of the lymph channels. More serious infections can cause systemic signs, such as fever, shaking, chills, joint pain, and hypotension.

Patient Assessment

Although skin trauma is often dramatic, rarely is it immediately life threatening. It is important for you to stay focused on the assessment process discussed in depth in Chapter 11, *Patient Assessment*, and used throughout this book. This process will help you first identify threats to you and your crew using the scene size-up and then identify life threats to the patient using the primary survey.

Scene Size-up

The first aspect to address in any scenario is safety. Once you have determined that the scene is safe, begin evaluating the MOI. Maintain a high index of suspicion whenever a significant MOI is present, even if a patient's external injuries appear minor. Carefully consider the forces involved as you determine the likelihood of internal damage. Remember, the severity of the injury may not be initially apparent, but it will be revealed as you continue the assessment.

Skin injuries typically result in a risk of exposure to blood and other bodily fluids. Significant exposures include contact with body fluids through open wounds or mucous membranes. Less worrisome exposures include body fluid contact with intact skin. Be sure to protect yourself and the patient, and review Chapter 2, *Workforce Safety and Wellness*, and Chapter 26, *Infectious Diseases*, regarding infection control procedures.

Primary Survey

Next, rapidly determine whether any life threats are present. An altered level of consciousness, lack of airway protection or lack of patency, inadequate breathing, uncontrolled bleeding, and a significant MOI indicate serious trauma. Form a general impression as you approach the patient. A patient who is lying prone on the ground in a large pool of blood, for example, is clearly in worse shape than a patient who meets you at the door with a cut finger.

Assess the patient's Airway, Breathing, Circulation, Disability, and Exposure (ABCDEs). Determine whether the patient is alert, responsive to verbal stimuli, responsive to painful stimuli, or completely unresponsive. This is not the time for a thorough mental evaluation; rather, the goal is to determine if there is a potential brain injury or impaired circulation to the brain.

If direct trauma is present, it may severely compromise the airway. Soft-tissue injuries that result in a flow of blood into the airway can also interfere with airway patency. Immediately correct anything that interferes with airway patency; failure to provide a patent airway can quickly lead to the patient's death.

Assess the patient's breathing. During the primary survey, it is not important to obtain an exact rate—just determine whether the patient's breathing is abnormally slow or rapid or excessively deep or shallow. Address a significant alteration in breathing by using a nonrebreathing mask with oxygen at 15 L/min or a bag-mask device and supplementary oxygen.

Assessment of circulatory status involves palpating a pulse and checking the skin signs. If no pulse is present, take resuscitative measures (see Chapter 39, *Responding to the Field Code*). Pale or ashen skin points to inadequate perfusion; cool, moist skin is an early indicator of shock.

Ensure that the patient is adequately exposed during the primary survey. Gunshot wounds and stab wounds, for example, warrant complete removal of the patient's clothing to look for entrance and exit wounds **Figure 31-4**. Remember to preserve the clothing as evidence and cut around, rather than through, knife or bullet holes. If severe hemorrhage from an extremity wound is present, control

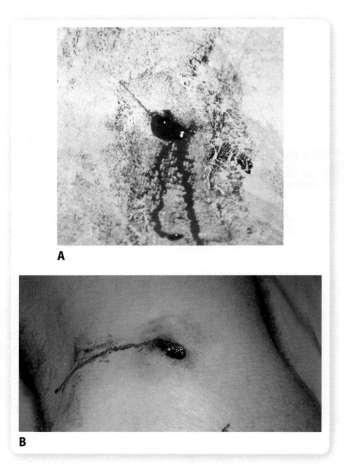

A

B

Figure 31-4 A. An entrance wound from a gunshot may have burns around the edges. **B.** An exit wound is often larger than an entrance wound and is associated with greater local damage to soft tissues.

of that hemorrhage with a tourniquet takes precedence over anything else in the primary survey.

At the conclusion of a primary survey, you must decide whether to rapidly package and transport the patient or remain on scene for more detailed care. Obtain a complete set of baseline vital signs and use the mnemonic SAMPLE (Signs and symptoms, Allergies, Medications, Pertinent past medical history, Last oral intake, Events leading up to the illness or injury) described in Chapter 11, *Patient Assessment*, to obtain a complete past medical history on concluding this assessment.

History Taking

Gathering information is also an important step in determining how the patient was injured. Ask the patient (if responsive and able to respond) or family members and bystanders about the events leading to injury:

- Was the patient wearing a seat belt?
- How fast was the vehicle traveling?
- How high is the location from which the patient fell?
- Was there a loss of consciousness?
- Which type of weapon was used?

When time and patient condition permit, determine when the last tetanus booster was given. Record the information on the patient care report (PCR), and relay it during patient transfer at the hospital. Ask the patient about prescribed and over-the-counter medications, paying particular attention to those that interfere with hemostasis. A higher priority should be given to patients taking warfarin or other anticoagulants. To obtain a pertinent past medical history, use the mnemonic SAMPLE.

Secondary Assessment

After obtaining the history and performing the rapid full-body scan, a more thorough full-body exam should generally be conducted (often en route to the ED) when there is a significant MOI and adequate time and the patient is in stable condition. This detailed assessment examines every anatomic region, looking for hidden injuries and clinical signs. A full-body exam is an excellent way for you to gather information, but it should never delay transport of a patient in critical condition.

For an unresponsive patient with a significant MOI, there may only be time to perform a primary survey prior to transport.

Reassessment

Trauma patients are often critically injured, and life threats evolve over time, so reassessments may reveal problems not found in the initial examination. Frequently reassess the patient's condition en route to the hospital in conjunction with any necessary interventions. As part of this assessment, obtain and evaluate vital signs, check any interventions, and monitor the patient.

Written documentation must be completed for every patient contact. When you are filling out the PCR, in addition to the usual patient and provider information, include all relevant scene findings, such as a severely damaged vehicle or caliber of weapon used. Also record patient findings, the patient's presentation on your arrival at the scene, and the body position on arrival (eg, prone or supine). Describe wounds in terms of size, location, depth, and associated complications. If you performed an intervention, record it, note how the patient responded, and document the patient's level of understanding of the intervention.

Documentation & Communication

Most people charged with shooting another person end up in court at some point, so you may be called to testify in such a case. In incidents involving gunshot wounds, it is especially important that you carefully document the circumstances surrounding the scene, the injury, the patient's condition, and the treatment you provided.

Emergency Medical Care

Management of soft-tissue trauma varies according to the injury present; however, some basic management principles apply to nearly every scenario. These principles will be discussed next. Although attending to clinical issues is important, you must also tend to the patient's feelings about the injury. Be empathetic, because the injury may be perceived very differently in the patient's eyes.

When an extensive closed injury is present, bleeding beneath the skin may reach significant proportions, and swelling may compromise vital structures. In such cases, take steps to minimize the bleeding and swelling by following the RICES mnemonic:

R Help the patient *Rest* by keeping him or her as quiet and comfortable as possible.

I Apply *Ice* or cold packs to the injured area. Cold will stimulate blood vessels to constrict, slowing the bleeding.

C Apply firm *Compression* over the injured area to decrease bleeding. Compression may be manual initially, but is most effectively applied with an air splint thereafter.

E *Elevate* the injured part to a level above the heart, to encourage drainage and decrease swelling.

S Apply a *Splint* to an injured extremity. By preventing motion, a splint decreases bleeding. An air splint provides a double benefit—splinting *and* compression, though an air splint will not control arterial bleeding.

Swelling can be due to blood from a developing hematoma, or can simply be the result of fluid. Use of ice as early as possible (20 minutes on and 20 minutes off to cool the injured tissue) may help to decrease the extent of the swelling and, in turn, speed up the rehabilitation time for the injury.

Two general principles govern the treatment of all open wounds: control bleeding and keep the wound as clean as possible.

▶ Bandaging and Dressing Wounds

Dressing and bandage materials are used to cover the wound, control bleeding, and limit motion. Simple application of a dressing over an open wound will help prevent infection by providing an artificial barrier against microorganisms. Using bleeding control techniques with dressings will stop all but the most serious active blood loss. Correct application of bandage material will limit motion of the affected area, helping the body to recover from the injury.

A variety of materials are used to dress and bandage wounds. A **dressing** directly covers a wound and controls bleeding, whereas a **bandage** keeps the dressing in place. When properly applied, both keep pathogens from entering the open injury. Table 31-2 reviews specific types of dressings and bandages.

▶ Complications of Improperly Applied Dressings

Improper application of dressing and bandage material can result in significant complications. It is important for you to learn how to properly dress a wound in the laboratory, clinical, and field settings to avoid causing harm.

Although it is not always possible to use the sterile technique, you should make every effort to avoid further wound contamination. Irrigate open wounds with normal saline or sterile water to flush out contaminants. If available, apply antibiotic ointment to smaller open wounds to help speed healing and decrease risk of infection. Large open injuries should not have ointment applied but should be dressed. Once the wound is irrigated, apply a dressing over the site. Clean blood around the dressing site, and neatly wrap a bandage over the dressing.

Hemodynamic complications include the possibility for continued bleeding. Once a dressing has been placed, it should not be removed because of the risk of disrupting clot formation. If an extremity wound continues to bleed, consider the use of a tourniquet. Frequent reassessments will help prevent unchecked blood loss and hemodynamic complications. Exsanguination is a possibility when direct pressure does not stop blood loss; the same is true for an improperly applied tourniquet. If a tourniquet occludes only venous flow, bleeding may actually increase. Direct pressure is often sufficient to stop blood loss. If not, do not hesitate to apply a tourniquet to an extremity to achieve bleeding control.

Structural elements—blood vessels, nerves, tendons, muscles, skin, and internal organs—can be damaged when dressings are excessively tight. Prevention of damage entails assessing and readjusting the dressing and bandage as necessary. Assess distal pulses, motor, and sensation when extremity dressings are in place. Tight dressings may cause pain in a patient who already has an injury.

▶ Control of External Bleeding

External bleeding is bleeding that can be seen coming from a wound when the integrity of the skin has been violated. Theoretically, bleeding can be characterized according to the type of blood vessel that has been damaged Figure 31-5 . Capillary bleeding is characterized by a slow, even flow of bright or dark red blood and is present in minor injuries, such as abrasions or superficial lacerations. Venous bleeding is more likely to be slow and steady, and the color of the blood is darker. Venous bleeding can be significant, as in the case of a lacerated lower extremity varicose vein. Arterial bleeding occurs in spurts, and the blood is usually bright red because of the fully saturated hemoglobin. In reality, most large open wounds show a combination of arterial and venous bleeding.

As discussed in Chapter 30, *Bleeding*, several methods are used in the field to control external bleeding. The most commonly used methods include:

- Direct, even pressure
- Pressure dressings and/or splints
- Tourniquets

> ### Words of Wisdom
>
> Direct, even pressure against the bleeding site is the most effective means to control bleeding.

Direct Pressure

Application of pressure over a bleeding wound usually stops blood from flowing into the damaged vessels, allowing the platelets to seal the vascular walls. If possible, use a dry, sterile dressing to exert pressure prior to bandaging. The steps for controlling bleeding are shown in Chapter 30, *Bleeding*.

Splints

Any movement of an extremity, even an uninjured extremity, promotes blood flow within that extremity. When the extremity is also injured, motion may disrupt the clotting process and lacerate more blood vessels. Therefore, attempt to limit motion of an injured extremity. Advise the patient to make every effort to minimize movement. If that is not possible and conditions warrant, apply a splint to prevent motion or immobilize the extremity.

An air splint or padded board works well to keep an upper or lower extremity immobilized. Use of an air splint provides a double benefit—splinting *and* direct pressure.

Table 31-2	Specific Types of Dressings and Bandages
Type	**Considerations**
Sterile	■ Completely free of microorganisms ■ Used when a high probability of infection is present (eg, large open wounds) ■ Sterility is lost when the package is opened; it is important to use quickly
Nonsterile	■ Used when there is a lower risk of infection ■ First dress the wound with a sterile dressing, then apply multiple nonsterile dressings to increase the ability to absorb blood
Hemostatic	■ Used to control serious hemorrhage when application of a tourniquet is not possible (eg, on the chest or pelvis) ■ Contains a hemostatic agent impregnated into the dressing ■ It is important to remove all other dressings before applying a hemostatic dressing
Occlusive	■ Used when it is important to keep air or fluid from entering the wound ■ When applying to an open wound in the thorax, seal on three sides to allow air to escape (helps prevent development of tension pneumothorax)
Adherent	■ Allows exudate from the wound to mesh with dressing material; facilitates clotting and aid in bleeding control ■ Removal of the dressing is painful and may precipitate additional bleeding
Nonadherent	■ Allows the products of wound repair to pass through the material; does not aid in clot formation ■ Applied after wound closure
Dry	■ Most commonly used in prehospital care
Wet	■ Limited use in the field ■ Used in burn care of superficial burns
Roller bandage	■ Self-adherent; overlapping material adheres to itself to keep the bandage in place ■ Used to wrap extremity injuries
Gauze bandage	■ Similar to roller bandage, but nonadherent ■ Used to secure a dressing ■ Does not stretch much; can result in excess pressure to areas that begin to swell
Absorbent gauze sponges	■ Used to create a thicker, bulkier dressing to control heavy bleeding
Elastic bandage	■ Stretches to allow some pressure to be applied ■ Useful in controlling bleeding ■ Used in musculoskeletal trauma to facilitate healing of damaged tendons and ligaments ■ Avoid applying excessive pressure, which could compromise blood flow
Triangular bandage	■ Ideal for making slings and swathes ■ Does not stretch, so it is not ideal if pressure must be applied ■ Can be wrapped into a thin strip to be used as a tourniquet
Medical tape	■ Used to secure a dressing ■ Use caution when applying on patients with skin conditions that might lead to damage upon removal of the tape (such as in older adult patients, who often have thin skin)

© Jones & Bartlett Learning.

Remember to assess distal pulses, motor function, and sensation distal to the splint before and after application. An air splint is not sufficient to stop arterial bleeding, however, because the pressure in the air splint is less than the systolic blood pressure. In the case of arterial bleeding, it is best to use a tourniquet. Sometimes pressure in an air splint is below diastolic blood pressure, and therefore not sufficient to address venous bleeding either.

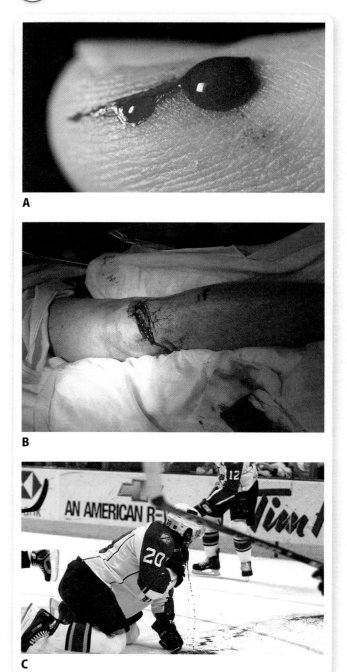

Figure 31-5 A. Capillary bleeding is dark red and oozes from the wound slowly but steadily. **B.** Venous bleeding is darker than arterial bleeding and flows steadily. **C.** Arterial bleeding is characteristically brighter red and spurts in time with the pulse.

A: Sasha Radosavljevic/iStock/Getty; **B:** © E.M. Singletary, M.D. Used with permission; **C:** © Brian Slichta/AP Photo.

Words of Wisdom

Splinting an injury, even when there are no signs of a fracture, can still help control bleeding and pain.

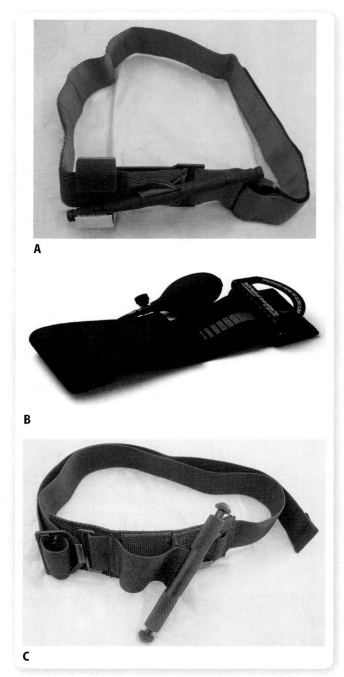

Figure 31-6 If bleeding continues or recurs, apply a tourniquet above the site of bleeding in an extremity—preferably the groin for leg wounds and the axilla for arm wounds. **A.** A combat application tourniquet. **B.** An emergency and military tourniquet. **C.** A SOF-T tourniquet.

A and C: Courtesy of Peter T. Pons, MD, FACEP; **B:** Courtesy of Delfi Medical Innovations, Inc.

Tourniquets

A tourniquet is especially useful if a patient is bleeding severely from an extremity injury below the axilla or groin and other methods of bleeding control are ineffective **Figure 31-6**.

Some commercial tourniquets can be applied with one arm, although you may not have access to them. If a tourniquet is required, follow the guidelines shown in Chapter 30, *Bleeding*.

Hemostatic Agents

Hemostatic agents can be used with direct pressure when direct pressure alone is ineffective, such as with massive chest injuries, or when tourniquet placement is impossible. These dressings are impregnated with agents that are designed to facilitate the coagulation process, thereby assisting with clot formation and controlling bleeding. Unlike with other dressings, it is important to remove *all* other dressings before applying a hemostatic dressing; hemostatic dressings are inserted directly into the wound.

Hemostatic agents were developed for military use but adapted for civilian use, where they are commonly employed. Consult your local protocols for guidance on the use of hemostatic agents.

▶ Managing Wound Healing and Infection

In the prehospital setting, management of altered wound healing and infection entails basic measures. Wounds that are not healing properly or show signs of infection should be dressed and bandaged appropriately. In severe cases, pain control measures may be indicated.

Scalp Dressings

Scalp injuries tend to bleed profusely owing to their rich blood supply. When bleeding is present, application of direct pressure is often effective because of the rigid skull that lies under the scalp. Be careful to accurately determine the extent of the injury because significant trauma may lead to skull damage, such as a fracture. In that case, control of bleeding must be balanced against the issue of not causing additional damage. When the skull has been compromised and bleeding must be controlled, apply pressure to the areas around the break. Use a bulky dressing that assists in stopping blood loss and helps prevent excessive direct pressure on the already damaged cranium.

The shape of the skull is a consideration when you are dressing wounds that involve the scalp. Improperly applied dressings can easily slide up or down the scalp, becoming ineffective. In addition, hair may interfere with securing dressings in place.

Facial Dressings

Facial injuries tend to cause significant anxiety for both patients and family. While you are tending to the clinical needs, take the time to reassure the patient. Application of direct pressure is an effective means to control bleeding from soft-tissue disruption along the face. If an avulsed

YOU are the Paramedic PART 3

The primary survey reveals that the patient's airway is open, breathing is rapid, circulation appears unimpaired, and the patient is alert. Your partner completes the rapid full-body scan and reports no additional injuries. The initial vital signs reveal nothing of immediate concern. You feel confident that the focus must now be the injury to the patient's hand.

As the towel is carefully removed from the hand, you note that the medial aspect of the right palm has a very large jagged laceration with visible subcutaneous tissue, bone, and fascia. The blood flowing from the wound is a combination of bright and dark red colors, though there is no spurting.

Recording Time: 5 Minutes	
Respirations	22 breaths/min, nonlabored
Pulse	96 beats/min, strong radial pulses
Skin	Pale, warm, dry
Blood pressure	142/96 mm Hg
Oxygen saturation (SpO$_2$)	98%
Pupils	PERRLA

5. Why is it important to complete a primary survey and rapid full-body scan when it is obvious that the injury is to the hand?
6. After you determined that the only trauma is the isolated hand injury, you moved on to a focused assessment of the injury, which was covered with a towel. What concerns should you have for this open hand wound that was covered with a dirty shop towel?

piece of tissue is present (the **pedicle**), attempt to replace it to its normal anatomic location as closely as possible. Note that bleeding tends to be quite heavy because of the rich blood supply in this area.

Assess the patient for the presence of or potential for airway compromise early in your encounter. Blood pouring into an unprotected airway is a serious concern, so be prepared to suction and position the patient to facilitate drainage. Do not allow a gruesome facial injury to distract you from attending to life threats.

> ### Words of Wisdom
>
> Patients with soft-tissue injuries will need emotional care. Patients will likely have concerns about how bruising and scarring may look later. Provide emotional support but do not make promises you cannot keep.

Ear or Mastoid Dressings

Trauma to the ear is commonly external, although internal injury is a possibility. Never place a dressing in the ear canal, but rather loosely apply it along the entire length of the external ear. Gauze sponges work well to aid in stopping blood loss. If blood is flowing from the ear canal, do not attempt to control it directly. Cerebrospinal fluid may be leaking, and halting the blood flow may increase pressure within the skull. Place a bulky dressing over the external ear, and transport the patient rapidly.

Neck Dressings

Important anatomic structures in the neck include large blood vessels, the airway, and the cervical spine. There is little room for error when trauma is present in this area. A minor neck laceration can lead to an air embolism, a small puncture can penetrate the spinal canal, and an anterior open wound can disrupt the airway **Figure 31-7** . Pay close attention to the clinical signs that accompany the external trauma.

Open injuries to the neck require use of an occlusive dressing to prevent air from being drawn into the circulatory system through the wound. Apply dressings carefully so that they do not interfere with blood flow or movement of air through the trachea.

Shoulder Dressings

The shoulder is relatively easy to dress and bandage. Apply direct pressure to control external hemorrhage in this region. If immobilization is indicated, a sling and swathe will prevent motion of the shoulder girdle.

Truncal Dressings

Injuries to the torso require vigilant assessment for underlying internal trauma. A seemingly innocuous hole may be the only indication that a gunshot wound is present.

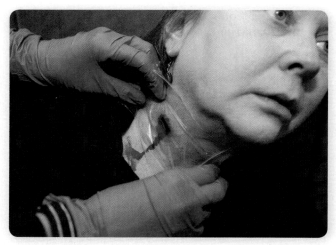

Figure 31-7 Neck wounds can lead to other serious situations such as air embolism and airway problems. Seal these wounds with an occlusive dressing right away.
© Jones & Bartlett Learning. Courtesy of MIEMSS.

Cover open wounds with an occlusive dressing that is taped on three sides. Assessment of breath sounds becomes a high priority when you find an open chest wound because a pneumothorax or hemothorax may develop from penetrating trauma to the thorax. Continually reassess a patient with thoracic soft-tissue injuries.

The best choice for securing a truncal dressing in place is medical tape. Wrapping the entire torso may interfere with air movement.

Groin and Hip Dressings

Soft-tissue injuries to the groin and hip are typically managed with application of a dressing and bandage in combination with direct pressure to control blood loss in this region. Injuries to the genitalia are best managed by a provider of the same gender, whenever feasible. As always, you should remain professional and protect the patient's privacy while you are providing care. There may be times when a patient is averse to allowing a provider to dress a wound located near his or her genital area. In such cases, provide the patient with a dressing and allow self-directed care, if this is the only way the patient will cooperate.

Hand, Wrist, and Finger Dressings

The hands, wrists, and fingers are among the easiest sites to properly dress and bandage. A dressing is applied over any open wound, and bandage material is wrapped completely around the affected area. When possible, the hand should be placed in the position of function. This is accomplished by placing a roll of gauze in the patient's hand **Figure 31-8** . If limited motion is necessary, the hand and wrist can be easily splinted. If possible, leave fingers exposed to access circulation.

Elbow and Knee Dressings

Joints are not difficult to dress and bandage, but movement may cause the materials to shift from their original position.

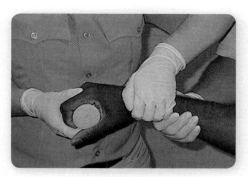

Figure 31-8 The position of function for the hand.
© American Academy of Orthopaedic Surgeons.

It is a good practice to provide immobilization of the elbow or the knee when a larger wound is present. Even smaller wounds may be difficult to manage because of skin tension lines and high tissue stress in these areas. When either of these joints is injured, it is important for you to assess distal neurovascular status. Elbow injuries have a higher risk for neurovascular compromise because of the relatively superficial location of the ulnar nerve and brachial artery.

Ankle and Foot Dressings

The ankle and foot are simple to dress and bandage. Control bleeding with direct pressure. If bleeding is arterial and cannot be controlled by direct pressure, consider applying a tourniquet proximal to the injury. In cases in which bleeding can be readily controlled, application of a bandage must not be so tight that it interferes with circulation or sensation. Always assess distal neurovascular function before and after caring for the wound.

▶ Pain Control

Application of a cold compress will help reduce pain and diminish blood flow to an open wound. Once the dressing is in place, apply the cold pack. Avoid placing the compress directly on the site because excessively cold temperatures may cause further injury.

If basic life support measures fail to relieve pain, consider administering morphine sulfate or other agents as allowed by protocol. As with all medications, carefully assess the patient for allergies, and document pertinent information before and after administration. Consult regional protocols or medical control, especially in burn cases, which often require more pain medication and fluid resuscitation.

■ Pathophysiology, Assessment, and Management of Specific Injuries

▶ Abrasions

An **abrasion** is a superficial wound that occurs when the skin is rubbed or scraped over a rough surface and part

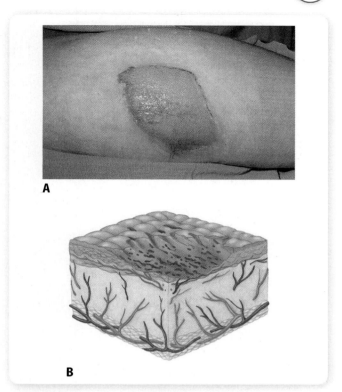

A

B

Figure 31-9 Abrasions usually do not penetrate completely through the dermis, but blood may ooze from the capillaries. These wounds are typically superficial and result from rubbing or scraping across a hard, rough surface.

A: © American Academy of Orthopaedic Surgeons; **B:** © Jones & Bartlett Learning.

of the epidermis is lost **Figure 31-9** . So-called road rash or mat/carpet burns are good examples.

Assessment and Management

Abrasions typically ooze small amounts of blood and may be quite painful. They may also be contaminated with dirt and debris; for example, sliding on the pavement in a motorcycle crash causes road rash. Because the skin has been disrupted, infection is a danger.

Do not attempt to clean an abrasion in the field. Rubbing, brushing, or washing the wound will cause additional bleeding and unnecessary pain. Care should consist of covering the wound lightly with a sterile dressing.

▶ Lacerations

A **laceration** is a traumatic and unintentional cut inflicted by a sharp instrument, such as a knife or razor blade, or by a blunt force that tears the tissue, producing a clean or jagged incision through the skin surface and underlying structures **Figure 31-10** . An **incision** is a clean (linear), intentional cut. Incisions tend to heal better than lacerations because of their relatively even wound margins. Lacerations can injure important structures beneath the skin, including tendons, ligaments, organs, body cavities, and bones.

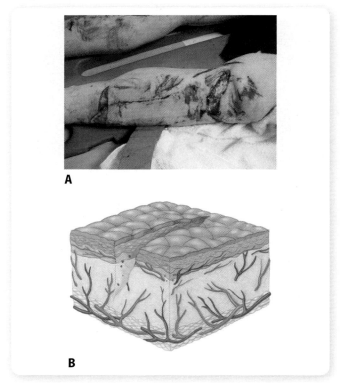

A

B

Figure 31-10 Lacerations can vary in depth and can extend through the skin and subcutaneous tissue to the underlying muscles, nerves, and blood vessels. These wounds can be smooth or jagged as a result of a cut by a sharp object or a blunt force that tears the tissue.

A: Courtesy of Rhonda Hunt; **B:** © Jones & Bartlett Learning.

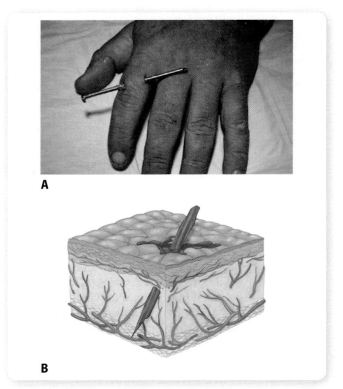

A

B

Figure 31-11 Puncture wounds and impaled objects may cause little external bleeding but can damage structures deep within the body.

© Jones & Bartlett Learning.

Assessment and Management

The seriousness of a laceration will depend on its depth and the structures that have been damaged. Lacerations may be the source of significant bleeding if they disrupt the wall of a blood vessel, particularly in regions of the body where major arteries lie close to the surface (as in the wrist). The presence of lacerations may also be a sign of an underlying fracture.

The first priority in treating a laceration is to control bleeding, initially by applying direct manual pressure over the wound. Laceration of a major artery can be fatal due to the severe bleeding that can occur. Deep lacerations may injure the muscle nerves, or vasculature, so distal pulse, motor, and sensory functions should always be evaluated.

▶ Puncture Wounds

A **puncture wound** (or penetrating wound) is an injury resulting from a piercing object, such as a nail or a knife [**Figure 31-11**]. Technically speaking, a bullet wound is a puncture wound. Puncture wounds can result in injury to underlying tissues and organs; the depth of a puncture wound cannot always be easily determined in the field. Many seemingly superficial wounds are later found to involve vital organs. Always suspect further internal injury, as well as potential shock, in patients with puncture wounds.

Assessment and Management

When you are assessing a puncture wound, consider the potential depth of the wound. The type of object and the speed at which it created the wound are factors that relate to the potential depth and severity of the wound. The location of the puncture wound also relates to its severity. Consider whether the wound could involve important internal organs.

Most puncture wounds do not cause significant external bleeding, but they may produce extensive—even fatal—internal bleeding and cause damage to other structures and systems that cannot be seen from the outside of the body. Treatment of puncture wounds is similar to caring for other types of open wounds. Be sure to look for both entrance and exit wounds. Remember to take measures to prevent infection. Also, should a patient with a puncture wound refuse care, it is important to inform him or her of the potential infection that could result from not seeking care.

With certain puncture wounds, it is possible for air to be injected under the skin, such as in a wound from a gun at close range, or in a wound from an air-pressurized device. In such a case, be alert for edema, and treat swelling with ice.

A special case of the puncture wound is the impaled foreign object [**Figure 31-12**]. When the instrument that caused the injury remains embedded in the wound,

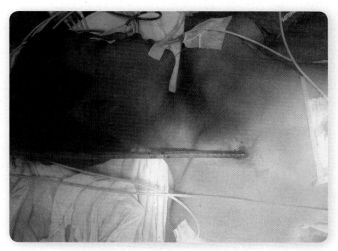

Figure 31-12 An impaled object remains embedded in the wound.
© Barcroft India/Getty.

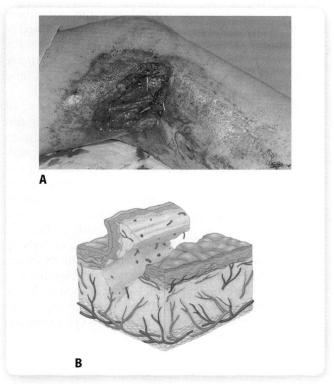

Figure 31-13 Avulsions are characterized by complete separation of tissue or tissue hanging as a flap. Significant bleeding is common.
© Jones & Bartlett Learning.

immobilize the object and transport the patient. Follow these basic points below regarding management of an impaled object:

- Do not try to remove an impaled object. Efforts to do so may precipitate uncontrolled internal hemorrhage, which may lead to exsanguination or further injury to underlying structures.
- Control hemorrhage by direct compression, but do not apply pressure on the impaled object itself or on immediately adjacent tissues.
- Do not try to shorten an impaled object unless it is extremely cumbersome (such as a fence post impaled in the chest); any motion of the object may damage surrounding tissues.
- Stabilize the object in place with a bulky dressing, and immobilize the extremity (if the object is impaled in an extremity) with a splint to prevent motion.

The goal for prehospital care is to limit motion of the impaled object as soon as possible to minimize additional damage. One technique that is effective for thin objects is to use gauze pads cut midway through the center. Stack several pads vertically, and arrange the cut portions so that each stack of pads overlaps. Once it is determined that enough pads are in place for stabilizing the object, tape or bandage them securely. This technique has the dual benefits of providing stabilization and aiding in bleeding control. Larger objects that are impaled in the body can be secured with rolled towels or splinting materials.

Whatever presentation you may encounter, it is important to avoid causing additional harm. Secure the object as best as possible, and be creative in using securing materials. Reassure the patient and family. Constantly assess the risk for developing threats to life, such as airway compromise, breathing inadequacy, and uncontrolled hemorrhage.

On rare occasions, removal of an impaled object may be the best course of action. If the object directly interferes with airway control and the patient's condition is deteriorating rapidly, medical direction may authorize removal. It may also be necessary to remove an object that interferes with chest compressions in a patient who is in cardiac arrest and deemed viable. In severe cases, it may be impossible to leave the object in place, such as when the patient is impaled on an immovable object. Establish direct contact with medical control immediately in such cases, and ask for guidance.

▶ Avulsions

An **avulsion** occurs when a flap of skin is torn loose, either partially or completely Figure 31-13 . The amount of bleeding from an avulsion relates to the depth of injury.

Assessment and Management

Depending on where the avulsion occurs, it may or may not be accompanied by profuse bleeding. The principal danger in this type of injury—besides blood loss and contamination—is loss of the blood supply to the avulsed flap. If the pedicle is folded back or kinked, circulation to the flap will be compromised and that piece of skin will die if the circulation is not restored quickly.

If the wound is contaminated, gently irrigate it with normal saline or sterile water, if available. You may note exudate oozing from the wound. In some cases, there will be serosanguineous drainage, which is composed of a mixture of serum and blood. The discharge is typically thin and has a pink hue. Note the amount of drainage seeping from the wound, document your findings, and relay the information to the receiving facility.

When you are treating a partially avulsed piece of skin, quickly irrigate the wound to wash away any dirt or debris and then gently fold the skin flap back onto the wound so that it is more or less normally aligned. Hold the skin flap in place with a dry, sterile compression dressing. *Never* remove the skin flap, regardless of its size. A surgeon may be able to reattach a flap of skin. Care also includes applying ice packs to the surrounding area to decrease pain and swelling. The cooling effect can also increase the length of time that damaged underlying muscle tissue remains viable. In patients who are in any way unstable or potentially unstable, management of these wounds should never be accomplished in a way that prolongs your on-scene time or otherwise delays your transport time. Become accustomed to managing wounds en route to the hospital.

▶ Amputations

An **amputation** is an avulsion involving the complete or partial loss of a body part, typically one or more of the extremities Figure 31-14 . Hemorrhage from complete or partial amputations can be severe and life threatening. Fractures may also be present with amputations.

In some cases, the body part will be completely detached. In a partial amputation, soft tissues remain attached.

Assessment and Management

Wound edges in an amputation are commonly jagged, and sharp bone edges may protrude. During wound care, be aware of any sharp bone protrusions that may lead to an exposure. Large, thick dressings should be used to cover the site.

When a part of the body is completely avulsed (ie, amputated)—whether a section of skin or an entire

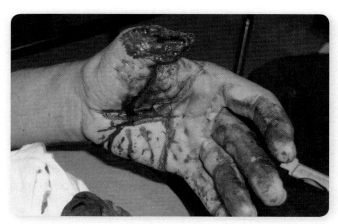

Figure 31-14 An amputation involving the thumb.
© E. M. Singletary, MD. Used with permission.

limb—it is important for you to try to preserve the amputated part in optimal condition to maximize the chances of successful reimplantation. Once the patient's injuries have been stabilized, turn your attention to the amputated part, which will also require meticulous care. Follow these guidelines:

- Rinse off any debris on the amputated part using cool, normal saline or sterile water.
- Wrap the part loosely in saline-moistened sterile gauze.
- Seal the amputated part inside a plastic bag, and place it in a cool container (such as a refrigerator or polystyrene foam cooler). Keep it cold, but do not allow it to freeze.
- Never warm an amputated part.
- Never place an amputated part in water.
- Never place an amputated part directly on ice.
- Never use dry ice to cool an amputated part.

Transport the patient and the amputated part as expeditiously as possible. When the amputated part is a limb or part of a limb, notify ED staff in advance of the type of amputation and your estimated time of arrival so that a surgical team can be mobilized while you are en route. Consider whether transport to the nearest reimplantation center is the best option, and whether air medical support is indicated.

Words of Wisdom

Never place an amputated part directly on ice because this may cause frostbite and make the part unsalvageable.

▶ Bite Wounds

Animal bites and human bites can cause soft-tissue injury. Most people who are bitten by animals do not report the incident to a physician, believing that such bites are not serious; however, in certain instances, they can be very serious, particularly if the animal has certain types of infections. The mouths of dogs and cats are heavily contaminated with virulent bacteria. Cat bites are especially dangerous due to *Pasteurella multocida*, a small gram-negative bacterium that can cause a host of dangerous clinical conditions in humans, including epiglottitis, endocarditis, and brain abscesses. Consider all such bites as contaminated and potentially infected wounds that may require antibiotics and tetanus prophylaxis Figure 31-15 . Occasionally, dog bites result in mangled, complex wounds that require surgical repair.

Bites from humans most commonly occur on the hand. The human mouth—more so than even the dog's or cat's mouth—contains an exceptionally wide range of virulent bacteria and viruses. Multiple types of bacteria can cause infection. For this reason, regard any human bite that has penetrated the skin as a serious injury.

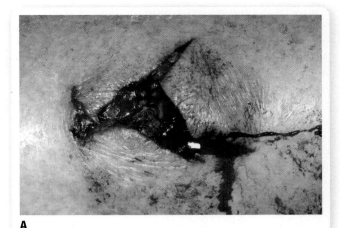

A

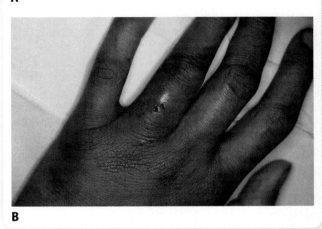

B

Figure 31-15 Animal bite wounds, though small, should be examined at the hospital because these wounds are heavily contaminated with virulent bacteria. **A.** Dog bite. **B.** Cat bite.

A: Courtesy of Moose Jaw Police Service; B: © Charles Stewart, MD, EMDM, MPH.

Infection can occur due to a delay in treatment. Similarly, any laceration caused by a human tooth can result in a serious, spreading infection.

Spiders, insects, and snakes can also cause bites. Such bites are discussed in Chapter 38, *Environmental Emergencies*.

Special Populations

When you are assessing and managing a very young child or older person with an animal or human bite, remember that these patients are more susceptible to infection.

Assessment and Management

In the case of an animal bite, place a dry, sterile dressing over the wound and provide prompt transport to the ED. In case of gross contamination, consider irrigating the wound with sterile water prior to applying a dressing.

If an arm or leg is injured, splint that extremity. Often, the patient will be extremely upset and frightened, a situation that calls for calm reassurance on your part.

In addition, find out and document when the bite occurred, and note the type of animal the bite is from. If the bite is from a human, note that fact as well as what led to the biting incident.

A major concern with dog bites is the spread of *rabies*, an acute, fatal viral infection of the central nervous system that can affect all warm-blooded animals. Although rabies is extremely rare today, particularly with widespread inoculation of pets, it still exists. Once a person shows signs of rabies infection, it is almost always fatal. Stray dogs that have not been inoculated can be carriers of the disease, as can any mammal—for example, squirrels, bats, foxes, skunks, and raccoons. The virus is present in the saliva of a **rabid** or infected animal and is transmitted through biting or through licking an open wound. Infection can be prevented in a person who has been bitten by such an animal only by a series of special vaccine injections that must be initiated soon after the bite. Because animals that have rabies do not always show it immediately in their behavior, a person's only chance to avoid the vaccine is to find the animal and turn it over to the health department for observation, testing, or both. Refer to your local animal control procedures.

Children, particularly young ones, may be seriously injured or even killed by dogs. The dogs are not always vicious or rabid; sometimes, the child unknowingly provoked the animal. However, you must assume that the dog may turn and attack you as well. Therefore, you should not enter the scene until a police officer or an animal control officer has secured the animal. Then you may carry out the necessary emergency care and transport the child to the ED.

Emergency treatment for human bites consists of the following steps:

1. Promptly control all bleeding, and apply a dry, sterile dressing.
2. Immobilize the area with a splint or bandage.
3. Provide transport to the ED for surgical cleansing of the wound and antibiotic therapy.

Most jurisdictions require health care providers to report all animal bites to the appropriate authority, which is typically the ED physician. Human bites may require notification of the authorities because they are a form of battery. It is important to know the local reporting requirements, because you could be fined or face other legal actions for failure to report any type of bite.

▶ High-Pressure Injection Injuries

High-pressure injection injuries occur when a foreign material is forcefully injected into soft tissue. The typical scenario involves a tool or machine failure in which liquid or air was compressed and suddenly released from the hose, tool, or other device. Hydraulic tools used to perform patient extrication from entrapment within a crashed vehicle are an example, with some systems using 10,000 psi (pounds per square inch of pressure or stress) or greater. Other examples include high-pressure systems used to paint automobiles and to clean surfaces. A force as small as 100 psi can break the skin, while 5,100 psi is able to penetrate both clothing and skin.

Injury results directly from the injected material entering the body under great pressure. Sometimes the patient may experience no pain at all and continue to work. Damage arises from the direct insult, chemical inflammation, ischemia from compressed blood vessels, and secondary infection. In addition, acute and chronic inflammation may occur following the injection. Inflammation tends to be most severe when fuel or paint is injected into the soft tissues. In some cases, the product is able to be absorbed into the body, leading to systemic complications.

Assessment and Management

The assessment process for this unique form of injury is similar to that performed for any other type of injury—perform a primary survey, address any life threats, and determine the level of severity. Once the basics are complete and time permits, there are some specific considerations when you are caring for a patient injured by high-pressure machinery or equipment. Question the patient about the nature of the injury. Determine the type of equipment being used and the pressure that the foreign material was under during the circumstances surrounding the injury. An owner's manual may be of assistance if available. Ask about the type of fluid used for the operation. It is important to pass this information on to the receiving ED physician because certain fluids result in a higher rate of amputation.

Carefully inspect the injury to determine the extent of visibly damaged tissue. Often, the greatest amount of injury is under the tissue involved. Palpate the affected area for signs of edema and compare the affected area with the uninjured side. Subcutaneous emphysema may be present as well as crepitus at the site of injury. Because the hand is the most commonly injured site for high-pressure injection, assess capillary refill, ability to move the fingers, and distal sensation to determine whether there is distal neurovascular compromise.

Treatment for high-pressure injection injuries is typically limited in the prehospital setting. Gently irrigate any open wounds with normal saline or sterile water. Dress and bandage open injuries as indicated by patient presentation. In some cases, pain management will be indicated. Consult your local protocols to determine the appropriate medication and dosage on the basis of patient presentation.

Injuries of this type can lead to amputation and, therefore, you should err on the side of caution and transport the patient for further evaluation. Depending

YOU are the Paramedic — PART 4

Your initial care for the patient's hand wound was to place a sterile dressing onto the wound and apply direct pressure. The combination of these actions stopped the flow of blood, but the dressing is now completely saturated with blood. Instead of removing the initial dressing, you place an additional dressing on top of the first dressing. Your partner tightly wraps bandaging material around the patient's hand to help maintain direct pressure.

Recording Time: 10 Minutes	
Respirations	24 breaths/min, adequate
Pulse	110 beats/min, radial pulses
Skin	Pale, warm, dry
Blood pressure	148/98 mm Hg
Oxygen saturation (SpO$_2$)	98%
Pupils	PERRLA

7. Why is it important to not remove the initial sterile dressing that is saturated with blood unless a hemolytic dressing is being applied?
8. Explain, in order, the steps taken to control hemorrhage from an open wound.

on the type of material injected, the injury may require emergent surgery in an effort to prevent limb loss. Gathering adequate information and relaying it to the ED staff can greatly aid the chances for reduced morbidity. Do not underestimate the importance of this aspect of caring for a patient with a high-pressure injection injury.

Pathophysiology, Assessment, and Management of Soft-Tissue Injuries to Specific Anatomic Sites

Soft-tissue injuries that involve the face and neck, thorax, or abdomen deserve special attention. Because the underlying structures in these regions are vital to life, additional concerns arise when they are involved in a traumatic event.

▶ Facial and Neck Injuries

Injuries to the face and neck may involve the airway or large blood vessels. Airway compromise can arise from substantial bleeding or disruption of soft tissue. In such cases, suctioning and patient positioning may become necessary to maintain airway patency. Open injuries involving the jugular or carotid vessels can result in exsanguination if they are not rapidly addressed. These factors, combined with the psychological impact of facial damage, can create challenging scenarios **Figure 31-16** .

Assessment and Management

As always, the airway is high priority. Immediate assessment of patency, protection, and flow of oxygen with removal of carbon dioxide is paramount.

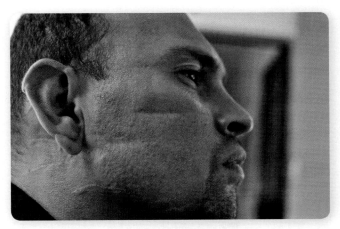

Figure 31-16 In some areas of the United States, paramedics may encounter facial cuttings inflicted as part of gang initiation practices.

© YURI CORTEZ /AFP/Getty.

Suction secretions or blood as indicated by patient presentation. If indicated ensure delivery of high-flow oxygen with a nonrebreathing mask or, if ventilations are compromised, with a bag-mask device. More invasive management may require use of an advanced airway (ie, ET tube, Combitube, King-LT, or other rescue airway). When neither ventilation nor intubation is possible, a surgical airway is indicated.

Control of bleeding can be accomplished while airway control is under way. If only one EMS provider is available, bleeding control should be addressed only after ensuring an open airway. Manage significant bleeding by applying bulky dressings and direct pressure. Open wounds to the neck require occlusive dressings to prevent air emboli. Realign avulsed skin along the face or neck to its original anatomic position, if possible.

▶ Thoracic Injuries

Soft-tissue injuries to the chest may have underlying chest trauma. See Chapter 35, *Chest Trauma*, for more discussion on this topic.

Assessment and Management

Assessment of thoracic injuries includes four steps: inspection, palpation, auscultation, and percussion. Examine the entire chest for signs of visible injury. Listen to breath sounds in at least two sites on each side of the chest. If breath sounds are diminished or absent on one side, suspect a pneumothorax. Palpate the entire chest wall, noting any abnormalities. Subcutaneous emphysema is indicative of a disruption in the tracheobronchial tree.

Open wounds to the thorax may require the application of an occlusive dressing. Tape the dressing on only three sides to allow air to escape.

▶ Abdominal Injuries

Abdominal injuries range from minor abrasions to evisceration. Inspect the abdomen for visible signs of injuries. Palpate the area to identify pain, rigidity, and distention. As the diaphragm travels downward during inspiration, the relative sizes of the thoracic and abdominal cavities change. This process increases the risk of drawing air into the pleural space when an open wound is present.

Assessment and Management

Maintain a high index of suspicion when an abdominal injury is readily evident. Soft-tissue injuries in the abdominal area are typically not the primary concern; rather, focus on any injury to underlying organs and blood vessels. Injury to organs and blood vessels could quickly lead to more serious complications, including death. Specific care of abdominal organ injuries is covered in Chapter 36, *Abdominal and Genitourinary Trauma*.

■ Pathophysiology, Assessment, and Management of Soft-Tissue Infections

▶ Myositis

Myositis, or inflammation of the muscle, can be caused by injury or infection. It can also be caused by overuse of a muscle. In some cases, it is considered to be an autoimmune disorder.

Assessment and Management

Treatment of myositis is based on the patient's complaint and history. Some signs to look for include signs of infection (fever), muscle weakness, and fatigue on exertion. These symptoms generally will not be considered life threatening. Treatment is based on patient presentation. Transport the patient to the hospital for definitive diagnosis.

▶ Gangrene

Gangrene is dead tissue. It is caused when blood supply delivery to tissue is interrupted or stopped. The causes of gangrene include injury, infection, long-term tobacco use, and poor peripheral circulation. *Clostridium perfringens* is an anaerobic, toxin-producing bacterium that leads to the development of gangrene. Once it enters deeply into tissue, it causes the production of a foul-smelling gas.

Gangrene is referred to as "wet" or "dry." Wet gangrene causes sepsis, and the patient can die within hours. Dry gangrene can take months to develop. Diseases such as diabetes and atherosclerotic peripheral vascular disease usually cause gangrene, but traumatic injuries such as burns, frostbite, and wounds can also cause it. Smokers and diabetics are more likely to develop symptoms because their peripheral vasculature is compromised.

Assessment and Management

Suspect gangrene if the patient has chronic risk factors such as diabetes and there is numbness, coolness, or swelling of an extremity. Also, gangrene (particularly wet gangrene) has a very bad odor. Late signs of gangrene will be characterized by discoloration of the limb to black, blue, or red. If the gangrene is not treated, the skin will become necrotic and the infection may lead to sepsis.

Prompt recognition and early, aggressive hospital therapy offer the best chance for reducing morbidity and mortality. Treatment involves transporting the patient to a suitable facility, while being sure to take standard precautions. Treatment in the hospital may involve amputation or surgical debridement of the affected area. Antibiotics are also necessary.

▶ Tetanus

Tetanus is caused by infection with an anaerobic bacterium, *Clostridium tetani* (a member of the same family that causes gangrene). This bacterium causes the body to produce a potent toxin, which results in painful muscle contractions that are strong enough to fracture bones.

Tetanus has become a rare occurrence because of the availability of a vaccine. In the United States, vaccination against tetanus is part of childhood immunization programs. A booster is needed every 10 years, although an inoculation is typically provided to patients who are injured and have not been immunized in the last 5 years. Given the severity of tetanus, you should ask injured patients about the last time they received a tetanus booster.

Assessment and Management

Muscle stiffness associated with tetanus may be noted first in the jaw ("lockjaw") and neck, with progression down the remainder of the body. Early recognition is important because conventional therapy does not result in rapid recovery.

▶ Necrotizing Fasciitis

Fasciitis is inflammation of the fascia. The most serious form of this condition is called **necrotizing fasciitis**, "the flesh-eating disease," which involves the death of tissue from bacterial infection. Necrotizing fasciitis is caused by more than one infecting organism—most commonly group A streptococcus.

Assessment and Management

Recognition of this disease by EMS personnel is particularly difficult but critical because early intervention is crucial. Look for a history of vector transmission, insect bites, or jellyfish stings. Skin at the site may be reddened and warm; additional symptoms include fever, night sweats, chills, vomiting, and diarrhea.

It is important to take standard precautions and properly handle contaminated articles, such as clothing, to limit exposure to the pathogens in necrotizing fasciitis. Transport the patient to the hospital for diagnosis. Antibiotic therapy and surgical debridement are among the available treatments.

▶ Paronychia

Paronychia is the most common infection of the hand in the United States. It is a bacterial infection located near the nail plate. If not recognized and treated, it can spread through the hand and into the circulatory and lymphatic systems.

Assessment and Management

This infection will cause a small pustule or redness, with or without pus, to be present. There may be an abscess at the site. Transport the patient for antibiotic therapy or lancing of the abscess.

▶ Flexor Tenosynovitis of the Hand

Flexor tenosynovitis of the hand is caused by an infection that is usually the result of penetrating trauma to the hand. It involves the sheath of the tendons that flex the fingers.

Assessment and Management

Signs of flexor tenosynovitis include inability to extend the involved finger, pain, and swelling along the path of the tendon. It also occurs chronically in patients with a history of rheumatoid arthritis (RA). It can also occur due to overuse of the hand.

The presentation of this condition may be swelling, redness, and limited mobility in the hand. Pay particular attention to patients with a history of RA. Transport the patient so he or she can receive definitive treatment for the infection and possible orthopaedic intervention.

YOU are the Paramedic   SUMMARY

1. You and your partner continue to assess the scene. After you clear the workers around the injured man, which other scene precautions must be taken?

Have a person with experience in operation of the cutting machine shut off this machine. The scene information revealed that the safety guard was not in place. Also, because the incident occurred in a factory, be aware of your surroundings. There may be forklifts in operation, loud machinery, mechanical hazards, and a host of other industrial elements that present a danger to you and your partner.

2. After you ensure the scene is safe, what are your next actions?

Continue with patient assessment, as usual. It is important not to allow disturbing scenes or grotesque injuries to distract you from your organized approach to patient assessment. Consider body substance isolation as part of your scene safety. If you donned only gloves, it may be prudent to add more protective gear to prevent exposure.

3. Why was it important to don gowns, masks, and goggles as a supplement to your gloves?

The scene size-up provided clues that there was blood spurting from the injury, which heightens the risk of exposure. A gown, mask, and goggles will decrease the likelihood that you will be exposed to the patient's blood, which may harbor dangerous infectious diseases.

4. While you are assessing your patient, you note that the bystander who assisted the patient before your arrival has blood on his shirt and hands. What should you say to the bystander?

While you should focus primarily on patient assessment and care, your overall scene management should include instructing the bystander to wash the blood off and change his shirt. This advice can be given tactfully in way that is not offensive to the patient but helpful to the bystander.

5. Why is it important to complete a primary survey and rapid full-body scan when it is obvious that the injury is to the hand?

You should not allow yourself to become distracted by gruesome injuries. The initial focus for every patient is to ensure that no threats to life exist, which is why the general impression and primary survey are the starting points. It is easy for a layperson to get distracted by an obvious injury, but you are a trained professional who is aware that threats to life can be overlooked when attention is directed to an isolated injury.

6. After you determined that the only trauma is the isolated hand injury, you moved on to a focused assessment of the injury that was covered with a towel. Which concerns should you have for this open hand wound that was covered with a dirty shop towel?

This scenario indicated that the patient had wrapped a dirty shop towel around the injury. You must consider the risk of infection, but controlling the bleeding is top priority. Carefully and quickly apply a pressure dressing, then apply a tourniquet and provide rapid transport to a trauma center.

7. Why is it important to not remove the initial sterile dressing that is saturated with blood?

If you place a dressing on an open wound and it becomes saturated with blood, cover it with a second dressing. Removal of the initial dressing disrupts the blood clotting process and can prolong the time it takes to control bleeding.

8. Explain, in order, the steps taken to control hemorrhage from an open wound.

The steps necessary to control hemorrhage from an open wound may vary based on the severity of the injury and location of the wound. In order, the general approach is direct, even pressure; pressure dressings and/or splints; and if persistent and present on an extremity, a tourniquet. In cases where severe bleeding is present, application of a tourniquet is appropriate at an earlier stage to prevent exsanguination. Your experience and judgment will guide you on when to alter the general order of steps for controlling bleeding.

EMS Patient Care Report (PCR)

Date: 10-15-18	Incident No.: 1061	Nature of Call: Isolated trauma	Location: 639 Trevor Lane

Dispatched: 1310	En Route: 1310	At Scene: 1314	Transport: 1324	At Hospital: 1352	In Service: 1410

Patient Information

Age: 31
Sex: M
Weight (in kg [lb]): 90 kg (198 lb)

Allergies: No known drug allergies
Medications: Denies
Past Medical History: Denies
Chief Complaint: Hand laceration and severe pain

Vital Signs

Time: 1319	BP: 142/96	Pulse: 96, strong, regular	Respirations: 22	Spo$_2$: 98%
Time: 1324	BP: 148/98	Pulse: 110	Respirations: 24	Spo$_2$: 98%
Time: 1329	BP: 146/96	Pulse: 100	Respirations: 24	Spo$_2$: 98%
Time: 1334	BP: 146/94	Pulse: 96	Respirations: 22	Spo$_2$: 99%
Time: 1339	BP: 136/82	Pulse: 102	Respirations: 26	Spo$_2$: 99%
Time: 1344	BP: 138/80	Pulse: 100	Respirations: 24	Spo$_2$: 99%
Time: 1349	BP: 134/78	Pulse: 98	Respirations: 26	Spo$_2$: 99%

EMS Treatment (circle all that apply)

Oxygen @ _____ L/min via (circle one): NC NRM Bag-mask device	Assisted Ventilation	Airway Adjunct	CPR
Defibrillation	(Bleeding Control)	(Bandaging)	Splinting	Other:

Narrative

9-1-1 dispatched to a report of a man injured at a factory. Upon arrival, a female worker directed us to a patient with a severely lacerated hand that was wrapped in a towel. Bystanders reported that the man cut his hand on an unguarded circular saw blade, and a significant amount of blood was noted on the machine and area immediately surrounding it. 31 y/o male is A/O x 4, sitting in semi-Fowler position on the floor with a dirty towel covering the injury. Pt reports that he cut his hand and is in pain. Pt rates pain at a "5" on the 0 to 10 scale. Pt denies any other injuries. Physical exam shows a healthy-appearing physically fit male, pale and anxious but alert. The injury is a jagged laceration to the medial aspect of the right palm with exposed fatty tissue, muscle, and bone.

Treatment included emotional support, bleeding control, dressing, and bandaging. Vital signs remained stable en route, and pt was conscious and alert throughout transport. Arrived at Broward North Trauma Center at 1352. Pt care transferred to the trauma team in room 10. Return to service at 1410 hours.**End of report**

Prep Kit

▶ Ready for Review

- Soft-tissue injuries may be dramatic looking but are not always the most serious injuries. Do not let them distract you from performing a thorough primary survey.
- The skin is a complex organ that fulfills several crucial roles, including maintaining homeostasis, protecting tissue from injury, and regulating temperature.
- The main layers of the skin are the epidermis and the dermis. The epidermis, the outer layer, serves as the principal protective barrier. The dermis, the inner layer, contains nerve endings, blood vessels, sweat glands, and other important anatomic structures.
- Between the dermis and the underlying muscle and bone is a thick layer of connective tissue known as subcutaneous tissue, or the superficial fascia. The skin is arranged in patterns of tautness known as tension lines. Wounds that occur parallel to skin tension lines may remain closed. Wounds that run perpendicular to tension lines may remain open.
- In a closed wound, the skin is not broken but soft tissues beneath the skin are damaged. An example is a bruise. A hematoma (collection of blood beneath the skin) can also form.
- In an open wound, the skin is broken. Such an injury can become infected and can result in serious blood loss. Open wounds include abrasions, lacerations, puncture wounds, avulsions, bites, and amputations.
- The first stage of wound healing is cessation of bleeding. The body uses several mechanisms to control bleeding, such as constricting the size of vessels and releasing platelets to form a blood clot.
- The second stage of healing is inflammation, in which additional cells enter the damaged area in an effort to repair it. Epithelialization (creation of a new layer of epithelial cells) occurs, followed by neovascularization (formation of new vessels) and collagen synthesis (formation of scar tissue).
- Wound healing is affected by factors such as the amount of movement the part is subjected to, medications, and medical conditions. A wound is more likely to become infected if it resulted from a human or an animal bite or if a foreign body has been impaled. Pressure injuries can develop when a patient is bedridden or remains on a backboard for too long.
- Because the skin serves as an initial barrier against microorganisms, any break in its surface can lead to infection. Signs of infection include redness, pus, warmth, edema, and local discomfort.

- Observe scene safety before assessing patients with soft-tissue injuries. Then, regardless of how dramatic a soft-tissue injury looks, assess the ABCDEs first.
- When you are obtaining a patient history, ask about the event that caused the injury, such as whether a weapon was used or whether the patient lost consciousness. Find out when the patient last had a tetanus booster. Pay attention to whether the patient is taking any medications that may affect hemostasis.
- Depending on the mechanism of injury, complete the physical exam en route or at the scene. Direct your attention to the chief complaint and area of injury, and perform frequent reassessments.
- Document scene findings, including vehicle damage or the caliber of weapon used; patient presentation and position; size, location, depth, and complications of injuries; assessment findings; and interventions.
- When you are managing open wounds, control bleeding and keep the wound as clean as possible by irrigating and using sterile dressings. Try to determine the color and type of bleeding and the amount of blood the patient has lost.
- Dressings and bandages are used to cover the wound, control bleeding, and limit motion. Types of dressings include sterile and nonsterile, occlusive and nonocclusive, adherent and nonadherent, and wet and dry. Types of bandages include roller and gauze, absorbent gauze sponges, elastic, and triangular bandages.
- Medical tape may be used to secure a bandage in place, except in patients with thin skin (such as older people), in whom it can cause damage on removal. Do not apply dressings too tightly.
- Methods of external bleeding control include direct, even pressure, pressure dressings and/or splints, and tourniquets.
- Dressing and bandaging techniques vary for different parts of the body. For example, the shape of the skull and the presence of hair make dressing the scalp challenging.
- Cold compresses may help reduce pain. IV medications may be administered if basic measures do not relieve pain.
- Do not remove impaled objects in the field. Instead, stabilize the object in place with a bulky dressing. Control bleeding with direct compression, but do not apply pressure on the object or on the immediately adjacent tissues.
- Management of an avulsion includes irrigation, gently folding the flap back onto the wound, and applying a dry, sterile compression dressing. If the wound is an amputation, preserve the amputated part and transport it with the patient to the emergency department.

Prep Kit *(continued)*

- Animal and human bites can lead to serious infection and must be treated by a physician. Dogs, cats, and other mammals can carry rabies, a fatal viral infection present in their saliva. By law, paramedics must report all animal bites to the appropriate authority.
- High-pressure injection injuries involve the injection of foreign material into soft tissue. High-pressure injection may cause acute or chronic inflammation, even leading to systemic complications or amputation. Gathering and relaying appropriate information to the receiving facility can potentially reduce mortality.
- Soft-tissue injuries of the face, neck, thorax, and abdomen deserve special attention because these areas contain vital structures. Do not underestimate the seriousness of these injuries, and maintain a high index of suspicion.
- Soft-tissue infections include myositis, gangrene, tetanus, fasciitis, paronychia, and flexor tenosynovitis of the hand. It is important to take standard precautions and transport the patient to the hospital for definitive diagnosis and treatment when any of these conditions is suspected.
- Fasciitis is inflammation of the fascia, the most serious form of which is necrotizing fasciitis. Recognition of this condition by EMS personnel is difficult but critical.

▶ Vital Vocabulary

abrasion An injury in which a portion of the body is denuded of the epidermis by scraping or rubbing.

amputation An injury in which part of the body is completely or partially severed.

avulsion An injury that leaves a piece of skin or other tissue partially or completely torn away from the body.

bandage Material used to secure a dressing in place.

chemotactic factors The factors that cause cells to migrate into an area.

closed wound An injury in which damage occurs beneath the skin or mucous membrane but the surface remains intact.

collagen Protein that gives tensile strength to the connective tissues of the body.

contusion A bruise; an injury that causes bleeding beneath the skin but does not break the skin.

degloving A traumatic injury that results in the soft tissue of a part of the body being drawn downward like a glove being removed.

dermis The inner layer of skin, containing hair follicle roots, sweat glands, blood vessels, nerve endings, and sebaceous glands.

desquamation The continual shedding of the dead cells on the surface of the skin.

dressing Material used to directly cover a wound.

ecchymosis Extravasation of blood under the skin to produce a "black-and-blue" mark.

epidermis The outermost layer of the skin.

epithelialization The formation of fresh epithelial tissue to heal a wound.

erythema Reddening of the skin.

fasciitis Inflammation of the fascia.

flexor tenosynovitis of the hand A closed-space infection of the hand.

gangrene An infection commonly caused by *Clostridium perfringens*. The result is tissue destruction and gas production that may lead to death.

granulocytes Cells that contain granules.

hematoma A localized collection of blood in the soft tissues as a result of injury or a broken blood vessel.

high-pressure injection injuries Types of injuries that occur when a foreign material is forcefully injected into soft tissue.

homeostasis The tendency to constancy or stability in the body's internal environment.

hypertrophic scar An abnormal scar with excess collagen that does not extend over the wound margins.

incision A wound usually made deliberately, as in surgery; a clean cut, as opposed to a laceration.

integument The skin.

keloid scar An abnormal scar commonly found in people with darkly pigmented skin. It extends over the wound margins.

laceration A wound made by tearing or cutting tissues.

lymphangitis Inflammation of a lymph channel.

myositis Inflammation of the muscle, usually caused by infection.

necrotizing fasciitis Death of tissue from bacterial infection, caused by more than one infecting organism—most commonly, *Staphylococcus aureus* and hemolytic streptococci; this condition has a high mortality rate.

neovascularization Development of new blood vessels to aid in healing injured soft tissue.

open wound An injury in which there is a break in the surface of the skin or the mucous membrane, exposing deeper tissue to potential contamination.

Prep Kit (continued)

paronychia Infection of the area around the fingernail bed.

pedicle A narrow strip of tissue by which an avulsed piece of tissue remains connected to the body.

phagocytosis The process in which one cell "eats" or engulfs a foreign substance to destroy it.

puncture wound An injury resulting from a piercing object, such as a nail or a knife; also referred to as a penetrating wound.

rabid Describes an animal that is infected with rabies.

scar revision A surgical procedure to improve the appearance of a scar, reestablish function, or correct disfigurement from soft-tissue damage, surgical incision, or lesion.

tension lines The pattern of tautness of the skin, which is arranged over body structures and affects how well wounds heal.

tetanus A disease caused by spores that enter the body through a puncture wound contaminated with animal feces, street dust, or soil or that can enter through contaminated street drugs.

thermoregulation The process by which the body maintains temperature through a combination of heat gain by metabolic processes and muscular movement and heat loss through breathing, evaporation, conduction, convection, and perspiration.

▶ References

1. Brancato J. Minor wound preparation and irrigation. UptoDate website. https://www.uptodate.com/contents/minor-wound-preparation-and-irrigation?source=see_link. Literature review current through March 2017. Accessed April 17, 2017.

2. Causey, WA. Staphylococcal and streptococcal infections of the skin. *Prim Care.* 1979; 6(1):127-139. https://www.ncbi.nlm.nih.gov/pubmed/379890. Accessed April 17, 2017.

Assessment in Action

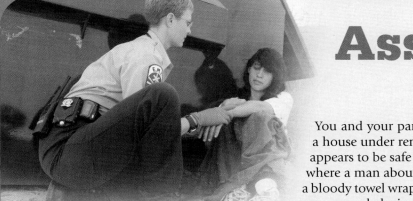

You and your partner are dispatched to a severe injury at a house under renovation. As you pull up to the scene, all appears to be safe and a man is waving you over to the site where a man about 50 years old is sitting on the stairs with a bloody towel wrapped around his lower arm. As he watches you approach, he is shaking his head and pointing to a bag on the ground next to him. He tells you he was using a table saw: "I took the blade guard off because I can't see the cut of the wood with that thing in the way. The blade must have hit a knot and the wood kicked back. Next thing I know, my hand! My hand! It's in the bag, inside the glove."

The patient is very pale and diaphoretic but alert and has an open, clear airway. He is breathing without difficulty and has equal chest movement. No other injuries are noted and he denies having any significant medical history.

Assessment *in Action* (continued)

1. Your next action should be to:

   A. keep the arm wrapped and transport, with the severed hand, to the hospital.

   B. retrieve the severed hand and examine and bandage it right away.

   C. unwrap the injured limb, checking first for severe bleeding.

   D. examine the table saw for additional pieces of his hand.

2. Unwrapping the patient's arm, you see a clean severing of his hand just distal to his wrist. You see some bone exposed, but are surprised to see that most of the bleeding has stopped. This cessation of bleeding is most likely due to:

   A. the pressure he applied to the wound.

   B. the clean cut of the vessels allowing them to retain their ability to contract.

   C. the large amount of blood already lost.

   D. the crushing of the blood vessels.

3. The wound where the hand was severed is barely bleeding. The best way to control the bleeding is by applying:

   A. direct pressure with a dry, sterile dressing.

   B. direct pressure with a moist, sterile dressing.

   C. sterile 4-inch × 4-inch (10-cm × 10-cm) gauze pads bandaged loosely over the wound.

   D. a tourniquet close to the wound.

4. In addition to a pressure dressing, the patient's arm should be:

   A. immobilized at his side.

   B. splinted.

   C. left with a pressure bandage only.

   D. compressed at the site of the brachial artery pressure point.

5. Retrieving the patient's gloved hand, you should first:

   A. gently cut away the glove.

   B. leave the severed hand inside the glove.

   C. cut the glove open, leave the hand inside, and place it on ice.

   D. pack sterile dressings inside the glove to minimize blood loss.

6. In preparation for transport, the patient's arm is bandaged and the hand is prepared by:

   A. placing the entire gloved hand inside a plastic bag and placing it on ice.

   B. placing the hand inside moist, sterile dressings and then on ice.

   C. placing the hand inside moist, sterile dressings and then in a sealed plastic bag, and then inside a cooler or loosely wrapped in cool packs.

   D. placing the hand inside dry, sterile dressings and then in a sealed plastic bag, and then inside a cooler or loosely wrapped in cool packs.

7. After using a stretch gauze to keep the sterile dressing in place on a patient's lacerated forearm, he tells you that his hand feels tingly. His hand distal to the bandage is slightly paler than the noninjured hand and cool to the touch. What is your next action?

8. Explain the difference between nonadherent and occlusive dressings. In which types of injuries would each be the best choice?

9. What is the best choice for securing a truncal dressing in place?

10. What are the two general principles that govern the treatment of all open wounds?

CHAPTER 32

Burns

National EMS Education Standard Competencies

Trauma

Integrates assessment findings with principles of epidemiology and pathophysiology to formulate a field impression to implement a comprehensive treatment/disposition plan for an acutely injured patient.

Soft-Tissue Trauma

Recognition and management of
> Wounds (see Chapter 31, *Soft-Tissue Trauma*)
> Burns
  - Electrical (pp 1659-1663)
  - Chemical (pp 1655-1659)
  - Thermal (pp 1641-1642, 1654-1655)
> Chemicals in the eye and on the skin (pp 1655-1659)

Pathophysiology, assessment, and management of
> Wounds
  - Avulsions (see Chapter 31, *Soft-Tissue Trauma*)
  - Bite wounds (see Chapter 31, *Soft-Tissue Trauma*)
  - Lacerations (see Chapter 31, *Soft-Tissue Trauma*)
  - Puncture wounds (see Chapter 31, *Soft-Tissue Trauma*)
  - Incisions (see Chapter 31, *Soft-Tissue Trauma*)
> Burns
  - Electrical (pp 1646-1651, 1659-1663)
  - Chemical (pp 1646-1651, 1655-1659)
  - Thermal (pp 1646-1651, 1641-1642, 1654-1655)
  - Radiation (pp 1646-1651, 1664-1666)
> High-pressure injection (see Chapter 31, *Soft-Tissue Trauma*)
> Crush syndrome (see Chapter 31, *Soft-Tissue Trauma*)

Knowledge Objectives

1. Describe the anatomy and physiology of the skin, including the layers of the skin. (pp 1639-1640)
2. Describe the anatomy of the surface of the eye. (pp 1640-1641)
3. Summarize the general pathophysiology of burn injuries. (pp 1640-1642, 1644-1646)
4. Discuss the symptoms of hypovolemic shock (burn shock). (p 1641)
5. Describe five types of thermal burns. (pp 1641-1642)
6. Identify some of the warning signs of intentional burns associated with the potential abuse of children, older adults, and people with disabilities. (pp 1641-1642, 1650, 1666)
7. Define and describe the characteristics of superficial, partial-thickness, and full-thickness burns. (pp 1643-1644)
8. Describe the pathophysiology of inhalation burns. (pp 1644-1646)
9. Summarize the safety concerns that must be addressed during the size-up of a burn scene. (pp 1646-1647)
10. Summarize the primary survey and secondary assessment processes for a burn patient. (pp 1647-1651)
11. Compare three different methods for determining the extent of the burn or the total body surface area burned. (pp 1648-1650)
12. Contrast the burn severity classification for patients of different ages. (p 1649)
13. List the referral criteria for transporting a patient to a burn unit. (p 1650)
14. Describe the phases of definitive burn care. (p 1651)
15. Discuss emergency medical care of a patient with a burn injury, including specific airway management techniques, fluid resuscitation techniques, and pain management. (pp 1651-1654)
16. State the Consensus formula, and discuss its use as it pertains to the prehospital environment, including types of solutions to use and amounts to administer during the prehospital phase. (pp 1652-1653)
17. Explain the management of hypovolemic shock. (p 1654)
18. Explain the management of thermal burns. (pp 1654-1655)
19. Explain the management of thermal inhalation burns. (p 1655)
20. Explain the pathophysiology, assessment, and management of chemical burns of the skin. (pp 1655-1657)
21. Explain the pathophysiology, assessment, and management of inhalation burns from other toxic chemicals. (pp 1657-1658)

22. Explain the pathophysiology, assessment, and management of chemical burns of the eye. (pp 1658-1659)

23. Explain the pathophysiology, assessment, and management of electrical burns, including lightning-related injuries. (pp 1659-1664)

24. Explain the pathophysiology, assessment, and management of radiation burns. (pp 1664-1666)

25. Discuss special considerations involved in the treatment of pediatric and geriatric patients. (p 1666)

26. Summarize some of the long-term consequences of burn injury on the patient's quality of life and on the paramedic's psychologic well-being. (p 1666)

Skills Objectives

1. Demonstrate how to care for a burn. (pp 1651-1654)

2. Demonstrate the emergency medical care of a patient with a thermal burn. (pp 1654-1655)

3. Demonstrate the emergency medical care of a patient with a thermal inhalation burn. (p 1655)

4. Demonstrate the emergency medical care of a patient with a chemical burn of the skin. (pp 1656-1657)

5. Demonstrate the emergency medical care of a patient with an inhalation burn from other toxic chemicals. (p 1658)

6. Demonstrate the emergency medical care of a patient with a chemical burn of the eye. (pp 1658-1659)

7. Demonstrate the emergency medical care of a patient with an electrical burn. (pp 1662-1663)

8. Demonstrate the emergency medical care of a patient with a radiation burn. (pp 1665-1666)

■ Introduction

While approximately 450,000 burn injuries require medical attention each year, the United States has seen a significant decrease in burn fatalities through education and stricter building construction codes **Figure 32-1** .[1] Although national trends demonstrate a consistent decrease in fire deaths, more than 3,000 people still die of fire-related causes each year.[1] Children younger than 5 years and older adults are at particularly high risk of dying in fires.[1]

Other effective burn prevention techniques include promoting awareness, reducing domestic water heater temperatures to 120°F (49°C), and making disposable lighters child safe.

Our ability to treat large burns effectively has also steadily improved over the years, with a 97% survival

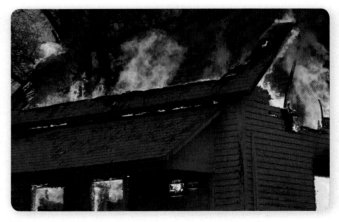

Figure 32-1 The United States has seen a significant decrease in burn fatalities through education and stricter building construction codes.

© Dale A. Stock/Shutterstock.

YOU ▶ are the Paramedic   PART 1

Your patient is standing at the entrance to the office of the gas station. His blistered, reddened arm is stretched out in front of him, and his face and neck appear flushed. The gas station owner walks him over to the ambulance as you slow to a stop, and tells you, "He pulled into the station and before I could say anything, he opened the hood of the car. All of a sudden there was a big burst of steam. I guess a hose blew. It got him pretty good." The scene is safe, and both you and your partner have donned appropriate personal protective equipment. The patient is alert and oriented. Grimacing in pain, he tells you in a quiet raspy voice that he cannot stand the pain in his arm.

1. Your next steps should include which actions?

2. Based on just the information given so far, would this patient's transport be low or high priority at this time?

rate for patients admitted to burn centers.[2] Better understanding of **hypovolemic shock**, sometimes referred to as "burn shock," advances in the use of fluid therapy and antibiotics, improved ability to excise dead tissue, and use of biologic dressings to aid early wound closure have vastly improved burn care. The formation of specialized teams to resuscitate patients from burn shock, delay infection, and achieve wound closure has resulted in impressive gains in survival rates.

Deaths and serious injuries also occur from electrical and chemical burns. In turn, numerous public safety campaigns have sought to reduce these incidents by focusing on the use of smoke detectors and the dangers that surround the use of flammable liquids, petroleum products, solvents, propane, and fireworks.

While you may not see significant burn injuries on a daily basis, you will encounter some serious thermal burn injuries during your career, and you might encounter serious electrical, chemical, and radiation injuries as well. Accurate recognition of the severity of burn injuries can dramatically enhance the care of burned patients by allowing you to institute proper emergency medical care. As a paramedic, it is important to understand the treatment for burn shock. In addition, contacting the receiving facility en route will allow burn specialists to provide triage over the phone and will allow them to prepare for the incoming patient.

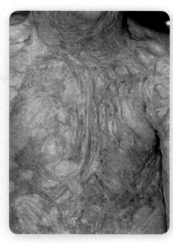

Figure 32-2 People who survive serious burns must live with the ramifications of their injuries.
© Dr. P. Marazzi/Photo Researchers, Inc.

Figure 32-2 . Patients who survive serious burns also have a high rate of depression.[3]

▶ Layers of the Skin

To carry out its functions, the skin has a specialized structure. You may recall that the skin is composed of two principal layers: the epidermis and the dermis **Figure 32-3** .

The **epidermis**, or outermost layer, is the body's first line of defense, constituting the major barrier against water, dust, microorganisms, and mechanical stress. The epidermis is itself composed of several layers of cells.

Underlying the epidermis is a tough, highly elastic layer of connective tissues called the **dermis**. The dermis is a complex material composed chiefly of **collagen** fibers, **elastin** fibers, and a **mucopolysaccharide gel**.

Enclosed within the dermis are several specialized skin structures, including nerve endings, blood vessels, sweat glands, hair follicles, and sebaceous glands **Table 32-1** .

Between the dermis and the underlying muscle and bone is a thick layer of connective tissue known as subcutaneous tissue, or the superficial fascia. The subcutaneous tissue insulates, protects, and stores energy in the form of fat.

■ Anatomy and Physiology Review

As discussed in Chapter 31, *Soft-Tissue Trauma*, the human skin, also known as the **integument**, is the largest and one of the most complex organs in the body. It has a crucial role in maintaining **homeostasis** (balance) within the body. The skin is durable, flexible, and usually able to repair itself. It varies in thickness from almost 0.4 inches (1 cm) on the heel to 0.04 inches (1 mm) on the eyelid. The skin performs the following functions: provides protection from the environment, regulates temperature and fluid, contains sensory nerves that communicate with the brain, and aids in healing by responding to injury with inflammation.

Significant damage to the skin may make the body vulnerable. People who survive serious burns must live with the ramifications of the damage to large portions of the integument:

- Difficulty with thermoregulation
- Inability to sweat from the scarred portions of the skin
- Impaired vasoconstriction and vasodilation in the areas of severe damage
- Little or no melanin (pigment) in the scar tissue, which makes the skin susceptible to sunburn
- Inability to grow hair on the injured site and little or no sensation in the scarred areas

All of these factors may restrict a person's ability to function even many years after the burn trauma has healed

Words of Wisdom

Hair melts when it burns, yet sometimes appears to remain on the patient. When you brush your hand over it, you may find that what you thought was a mustache is now simply a streak of ash. Closely observe nasal hair, eyebrows, and eyelashes in burn patients because damage to them may indicate airway injury. When hair on the arms or legs "falls out" or can be removed without pain, deeper skin structures have been damaged.

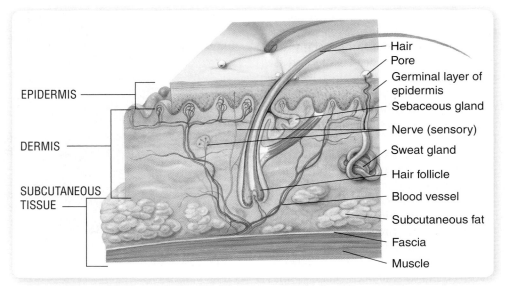

EPIDERMIS

DERMIS

SUBCUTANEOUS TISSUE

Hair
Pore
Germinal layer of epidermis
Sebaceous gland
Nerve (sensory)
Sweat gland
Hair follicle
Blood vessel
Subcutaneous fat
Fascia
Muscle

Figure 32-3 The skin has two principal layers: the epidermis and the dermis.
© Jones & Bartlett Learning.

Table 32-1	Specialized Structures of the Dermis
Structure	**Function**
Nerve endings	These structures mediate the senses of touch, temperature, pressure, and pain.
Blood vessels	These structures carry oxygen and nutrients to the skin and remove carbon dioxide and metabolic waste products. Cutaneous blood vessels also have a crucial role in regulating body temperature by regulating the volume of blood that flows from the warm core of the body to its cooler surface.
Sweat glands	These glands produce sweat and discharge it through ducts passing to the surface of the skin in a process regulated by the sympathetic nervous system
Hair follicles	These small, tubelike structures produce hair and enclose the hair roots. Each follicle contains a single hair. Attached to the hair follicle is a small muscle that, on contraction, causes the follicle to assume a more vertical position. Hairs in each part of the body have definite periods of growth, after which they are shed and replaced.
Sebaceous glands	These glands, located at the neck of each hair follicle, are a specialized secretory mechanism that produce an oily substance (sebum). The secretions of the sebaceous glands empty into the hair follicles and, from there, reach the surface of the skin.

© Jones & Bartlett Learning.

▶ The Eye

The specific anatomy and physiology of the eye are covered in Chapter 19, *Diseases of the Eyes, Ears, Nose, and Throat*, and Chapter 33, *Face and Neck Trauma*. Clearly, the eyes are sensitive to burn injuries—from a flame, superheated gases, light source (such as a welder's torch), or chemicals. The tear ducts and eyelids combine to constantly lubricate the surface of the eyes (Figure 32-4). Unfortunately, intense heat, light, or chemical reactions on the surface of the eye can quickly burn the thin membrane or skin covering the surface of the eye. Ocular damage is a common result of alkali (base) injury: the higher the pH of the substance, the more severe the damage to the eye. When a patient gets a substance such as lime in the eyes, the damage is worsened by repeatedly rubbing the eyes. Damage can be minimized by initiating copious irrigation and providing essential treatment in the emergency department (ED).

■ Pathophysiology

Burns are diffuse soft-tissue injuries created by destructive energy transfer via radiation, thermal, or electrical energy. As noted earlier, the skin serves as a barrier between the

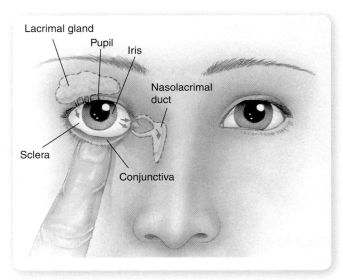

Figure 32-4 Tears act as a lubricant and keep the anterior part of the eye from drying.
© Jones & Bartlett Learning.

environment and the body. When a person is burned, this barrier is destroyed, leaving the individual at high risk for infection, hypothermia, hypovolemia, and shock. Burns to the airway are significant because the loose mucosa in the hypopharynx can swell, leading to complete airway obstruction. Circumferential burns of the chest can compromise breathing. Circumferential burns of an extremity can lead to compartment syndrome, resulting in neurovascular compromise and irreversible damage if not appropriately treated.

▶ Hypovolemic Shock

Burns are not isolated soft-tissue injuries, but rather systemic injuries. They can affect the cardiovascular, respiratory, renal, gastrointestinal, hematologic, and endocrine systems. The most important systemic response to significant burn trauma is hypovolemic shock.

Hypovolemic shock occurs because of two types of injury: fluid loss across damaged skin and a series of volume shifts within the rest of the body. Capillaries become leaky, allowing intravascular volume to ooze out of the circulation and into the interstitial spaces. The cells of normal tissues then take in increased amounts of salt and water from the fluid around them. As blood pressure falls, the body responds with tachycardia and vasoconstriction, which limits blood flow further and continues the shock cycle. A variety of chemical mediators are released that may cause additional damage and worsen the chain of events. Depending on the nature of the burn, coagulation disorders may cause the patient's blood either to clot more easily, resulting in emboli, or to fail to clot, causing excessive bleeding (disseminated intravascular coagulation), as discussed in Chapter 24, *Hematologic Emergencies*.

Hypovolemic shock involves the entire body, not just the area burned. You may have experienced sunburn over a reasonably large surface area, such as your back. In addition to the skin-related discomfort from the sunburn, you may have developed chills and nausea and felt sick as a result of the fluid shifts and electrolyte disturbances. This reaction is a mild form of burn shock. Just as in other forms of shock, these changes limit the effective distribution of oxygen and glucose to the body's tissues and hamper the circulation's ability to remove waste products from both healthy and damaged tissues. Adequate fluid resuscitation is essential to avoid the devastating consequences of burn shock.

▶ Thermal Burns

Thermal burns can occur when skin is exposed to temperatures higher than 111°F (44°C), or when the heat absorbed by the skin exceeds the tissue's capacity to dissipate it. In general, the severity of a thermal injury correlates directly with temperature, concentration, or amount of heat energy possessed by the object or substance, and the duration of exposure. For example, solids generally have higher heat content than gases have, so exposure to a hot solid (such as the rack inside an oven) typically causes a more significant burn than exposure to hot gases (such as those coming out of an oven).

It may be difficult to evaluate the amount of heat energy or the amount of exposure time in many cases involving thermal burns. In a residential fire, for example, the temperature of a fire may vary tremendously from the floor to the ceiling. Although most people reflexively limit the amount of time exposed to such heat, if their clothing is on fire or if the person is trapped or unresponsive, exposure time will be longer. A burn may also be more severe and airway complications more likely for a patient trapped in an enclosed space with accumulating toxins versus an open space.

A thermal burn is sometimes called "trauma by fire." In reality, heat energy can be transmitted in a variety of ways in addition to fire. Many different situations causing thermal burns can pose a safety hazard to responding paramedics.

Flame Burns

Most commonly, thermal burns are caused by open flame. A **flame burn** is often a deep burn, especially if a person's clothing catches on fire Figure 32-5 . The fire is fanned by running—hence the "stop, drop, and roll" technique that is taught in schools as a response to fire on the body. Flame burns may also be associated with inhalation injuries.

Scald Burns

Hot liquids produce scald injuries. A **scald burn** is most commonly seen in children and physically or developmentally challenged adults; however, such a burn can happen to anyone, particularly while cooking. Scald burns often cover large surface areas because liquids can spread quickly. Hot liquids can soak into clothing and

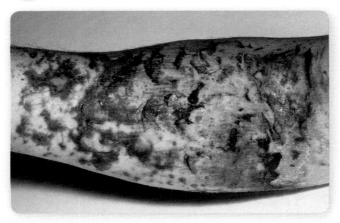

Figure 32-5 Flame burns are often deep burns.
© St. Stephen's Hospital, London/Science Source.

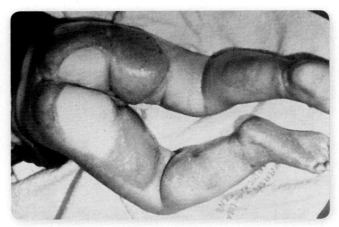

Figure 32-6 Scalds are sometimes associated with child abuse.
Courtesy of Health Resources and Services Administration (HRSA), Maternal and Child Health Bureau (MCHB), Emergency Medical Services for Children (EMSC) Program.

continue to burn until the clothing is removed. Some hot liquids, such as oil and grease, adhere to the skin, causing particularly deep scald injuries.

Approximately 500,000 scald burns occur each year from spilled food and beverages.[4] In such incidents, a child may pull a pot or other container of hot liquid off the stove or counter, a toddler may bump into an adult carrying or holding a hot beverage or food, or a toddler may pull the tablecloth, spilling a hot food or beverage off the table.

Contact Burns

Coming in contact with hot objects produces a **contact burn**. Ordinarily, reflexes protect a person from prolonged exposure to a very hot object. Consequently, contact burns are rarely deep unless the patient was prevented from drawing away from the hot object (eg, if the person was unresponsive, intoxicated, restrained, or impaired). Prolonged contact with something that is just moderately hot can eventually result in a major burn, however. A patient who has a stroke and falls against a household radiator, for example, may end up with major burns.

Scald and contact burns in children, older adults, and people with disabilities may be signs of abuse, especially when they include unusual history patterns. Burns with formed shapes or unusual patterns and burns in atypical places such as the genitalia, buttocks, and thighs are often consistent with abuse **Figure 32-6** .

Steam Burns

A **steam burn** can produce a topical (scald) burn. Minor steam burns are common when microwaving food covered with plastic wrap. When the plastic is peeled away, hot steam escapes directly onto the hand. Steam (ie, gaseous water) is also notorious for causing airway burns. Inhalation of other hot gases may cause **supraglottic** (upper airway) trauma but rarely leads to **subglottic** (lower airway) burns. Steam is unique because the minute particles of hot water can cause significant injury to the lower airway.

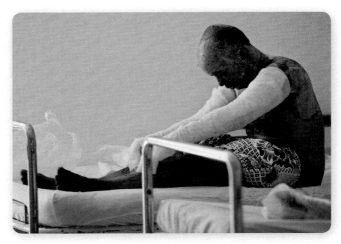

Figure 32-7 Flash burns may be minor compared with the additional trauma inflicted by an explosion.
© Kevin Frayer/AP Photo.

Flash Burns

A relatively rare source of thermal burns is the flash produced by an explosion, which may briefly expose a person to very intense heat. Lightning strikes can also cause a **flash burn**. These injuries are usually minor compared with the potential for trauma from whatever caused the flash **Figure 32-7** .

Burn Zones

Historically, burn wounds have been described by three pathologic progressions, known as zones (a theory referred to as Jackson's thermal wound theory), which radiate from the central zone of greatest damage. Skin nearest the heat source suffers the most profound cellular changes. The central area of the skin that suffers the most damage is called the **zone of coagulation**. There is little or no blood flow to the injured tissue in this area. The peripheral area surrounding the zone of coagulation has decreased blood flow and inflammation; it is known as the **zone of stasis**. This area may undergo tissue necrosis within 24 to 48 hours after the injury, particularly if perfusion is compromised by burn shock. Last, the **zone of hyperemia** is the area least affected by the thermal injury. In this area, cells will typically recover in 7 to 10 days. Similar to the case with a myocardial infarction or stroke, the role of treatment is to salvage as much of the injured tissue as possible by improving perfusion and limiting the secondary changes that turn damaged tissue into dead tissue. Refer to Chapter 31, *Soft-Tissue Trauma*, for a review of the wound healing process (ie, hemostasis, inflammation, epithelialization, neovascularization, collagen synthesis).

Burn Depth

Burn formation is a progressive process: the greater the heat energy, the deeper the wound. Superficial burns may injure only the epidermis, whereas deeper burns extend into or through the dermis, subcutaneous tissue, muscle, and bone.

The severity of burns are classified according to their depth—that is, superficial (first degree), partial thickness (second degree), and full thickness (third degree) **Figure 32-8** . Additional categories exist, such as fourth-, fifth-, and sixth-degree burns, for describing deeper destruction into tissue, muscle, and bone. Do not spend a significant amount of time categorizing burns in the field; the hospital needs to know the approximate type

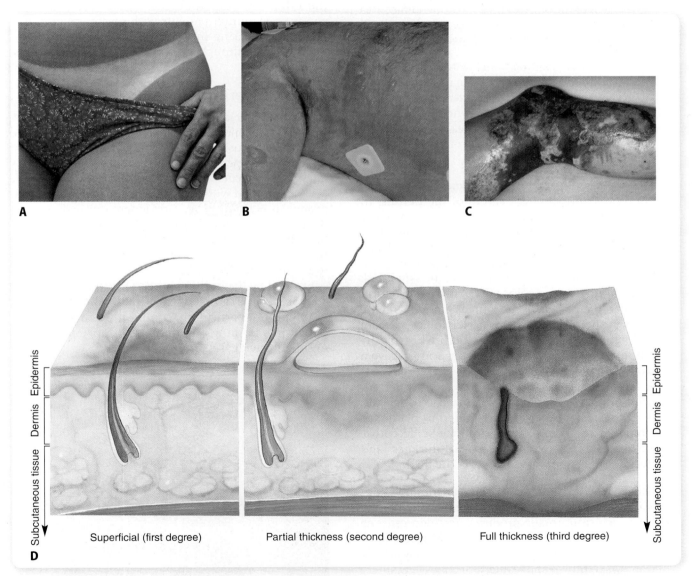

Figure 32-8 Classification of burns according to depth. **A.** Superficial, or first-degree, burns involve only the epidermis. **B.** Partial-thickness, or second-degree, burns involve some of the dermis, but they do not destroy the entire thickness of the skin. The skin is mottled, white to red, and is often blistered. **C.** Full-thickness, or third-degree, burns extend through all layers of the skin and may involve subcutaneous tissue and muscle. The skin is dry, leathery, and often white or charred. **D.** Illustrations of superficial, partial-thickness, and full-thickness burns, showing the extent of internal damage.

of burn, and you need to generally categorize the burn to properly determine the level of care that the patient requires. These burns will look different in a few hours, as the damage evolves, and you should not waste time carefully categorizing something that will rapidly change.

Exposure time is another important factor in determining burn severity. Thermal injury can occur in unresponsive or paralyzed patients from seemingly innocuous heat sources such as heating pads and heat lamps left unattended for long periods. The age of the patient and the thickness of the skin in the involved area will affect the burn severity. Concomitant injuries and preexisting medical conditions also complicate the severity and treatment of burn injuries.

While evaluating the patient's burns, you must approximate the extent of the burn, or the total body surface area (TBSA) burned. This process is discussed in more detail in the Patient Assessment section of this chapter.

Superficial Burns. A **superficial burn** involves the epidermis only. The skin is red and swollen. When it is touched, the color will blanch and return. Usually blisters are not present. Patients will experience pain because nerve endings are exposed to the air. Such a burn will heal spontaneously in 3 to 7 days. The most commonly encountered example of a superficial burn is a sunburn.

Partial-Thickness Burns. A **partial-thickness burn** involves the epidermis and varying degrees of the dermis. In general, the deeper the partial-thickness burn, the more painful it is. The sensation of deep pressure remains intact. Burns in this category can be subdivided into moderate partial-thickness and deep partial-thickness burns.

With a *moderate partial-thickness burn*, the skin is red; when it is touched, the color will blanch and return. Usually there are blisters or moisture is present, and the patient may experience extreme pain. Hair follicles remain intact. A moderate partial-thickness burn will typically heal spontaneously but may develop a scar or have a changed appearance.

A *deep partial-thickness burn* extends into the dermis, damaging the hair follicle and sweat and sebaceous glands. Hot liquids, steam, and grease are often to blame for these injuries. The color of the burn may be deceptive, and distinguishing between deep partial-thickness and full-thickness burns may be difficult in the field.

Full-Thickness Burns. A **full-thickness burn** destroys both layers of the skin, including the basement membrane of dermis, which normally produces new skin cells. As a result of the burn damage, the skin is incapable of self-regeneration. In such an injury, the skin may appear white and waxy, brown and leathery, or charred. Leathery skin is called eschar and is dry and hard. No capillary refill occurs with this type of burn because the capillaries have been destroyed. Sensory nerves are destroyed as well, so there may be no pain in the full-thickness section. Because patients with full-thickness burns usually have mixed depths of burns, they will often experience significant pain in the areas surrounding the full-thickness burns. Treatment of a full-thickness burn will often require skin grafting because the dermis has been destroyed.

▶ Inhalation Burns and Intoxication

Inhalation burns can cause rapid and serious airway compromise. Heat and toxic chemicals can irritate the lungs and the airway, causing coughing, wheezing, and swelling of the upper airway tissues, often evidenced by stridor. Infraglottic (vocal cords and larynx) and lower airway damage is more often associated with inhalation of steam or hot particulate matter, whereas supraglottic (upper airway) damage is more often associated with the inhalation of superheated gases. In rare cases, you may encounter patients with severe upper airway swelling, requiring intervention immediately after a major burn, although this problem may not manifest until transport.

Smoke/Superheated-Gas Inhalation

According to a National Fire Protection Association report, the vast majority of deaths from fires are not caused directly by burns, but rather result from inhalation of toxic gases, upper airway compromise, or pulmonary injury.[5] When materials such as plastic, polyvinyl chloride (PVC) pipes, and synthetic carpets burn, they release toxic chemicals **Figure 32-9**. Firefighters routinely protect themselves from these toxins by wearing self-contained breathing apparatus. Anyone who is exposed to smoke from a fire, however, may experience thermal burns to the airway, hypoxia from lack of oxygen (oxygen is consumed by the burning process), and tissue damage and toxic effects caused by chemicals in the smoke. Such problems are particularly common when a person is caught in a burning building, stands up, and breathes in superheated gases.

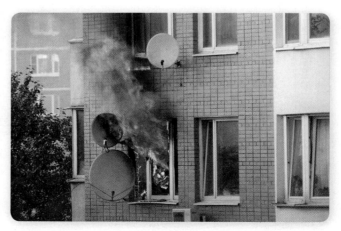

Figure 32-9 Smoke from fires contains many toxins, including particulates, cyanide, carbon monoxide, and other toxic gases.
© Sergey Toronto/Shutterstock.

Words of Wisdom

Hydrogen cyanide is created by the breakdown of hydrogen polymers, which are found in a multitude of products in homes and cars. Polymers are used in such products as PVC pipe, toys, curtains, auto parts, and many more everyday household items. Antidotes for cyanide poisoning are now widely available, but they are expensive. Such antidotes include amyl nitrite, sodium nitrite (Nithiodote), sodium thiosulfate, and the newly approved hydroxocobalamin (Cyanokit).[6] A case can be made that cyanide is a dangerous component in the smoke of residential fires, but it is less clear whether the administration of cyanide antidotes improves survival. Local protocols will dictate whether these agents are available.

Words of Wisdom

The gaseous form of cyanide is hydrogen cyanide. It is generated by the combustion of commonly encountered substances such as paper, cotton, and wool. Hydrogen cyanide is colorless, and although it has a unique odor similar to bitter almonds, it can be difficult to detect at the scene of a fire. Prehospital diagnosis of hydrogen cyanide poisoning is difficult because laboratory studies are necessary. Signs and symptoms involve the central nervous, respiratory, and cardiovascular systems of the body and include faintness, anxiety, abnormal vital signs, headache, seizures, paralysis, and coma.

Carbon Monoxide Intoxication

The combustion process produces a variety of toxic gases. Carbon monoxide (CO) evolves from incomplete combustion of carbon compounds (just about everything that burns). Cyanide is produced by the incomplete combustion of products containing carbon and nitrogen (eg, many plastics, polystyrene, PVC). Hydrogen chloride is a by-product of the combustion of PVC (eg, pipes, insulating materials).

The less efficient the combustion process, the more toxic the gases—such as CO and carbon dioxide (CO_2)—that may be created. When furnaces, kerosene heaters, and other heating devices are in poor repair, they may emit unsafe levels of these toxic gases. Internal combustion engines may emit many of the same gases and, consequently, should always have their exhaust vented to the outdoors. Indeed, a common source of CO exposure is running a small engine in an enclosed space such as a garage or basement. For this reason, many ambulance services and fire departments have added CO detectors to their garages or ambulance bays. Firefighters who are performing an overhaul after a fire may be exposed to high levels of CO, as may people who are exposed to large amounts of car exhaust (eg, toll takers, auto mechanics). Methylene chloride, which is found in some paint removers and bubble lamps and is used as an industrial solvent, is metabolized to CO by the body.

YOU are the Paramedic   PART 2

The patient is attempting to climb into the ambulance even before you get the equipment. He pleads, "Please, give me something for the pain. I can't stand it." He sits on the stretcher and, as you ask questions to determine what happened, he becomes more agitated. While his airway appears open and maintained, the patient's mouth is reddened. His voice is raspy and his lips are red. He tells you, "I can breathe fine, but I'm in a lot of pain. My arm—it hurts so bad." The patient is breathing rapidly with equal chest expansion. His mouth, neck, and chest are bright red. Lung sounds are present bilaterally. There are no adventitious sounds on inspiration or expiration. Both radial pulses are present, strong, and rapid. There is no severe bleeding and no mechanism indicating cervical spine injury.

Recording Time: 1 Minute	
Appearance	Flushed face and neck, walking
Level of consciousness	Alert (oriented to person, place, time, and event); very agitated
Airway	Open, clear, self-maintained with raspy voice
Breathing	Adequate, slightly fast
Circulation	Radial pulses strong and rapid

3. The patient is clearly experiencing significant pain. At which point in treatment should this condition be addressed?

4. How significant is the patient's apparent raspiness as he is speaking to you?

CO can displace oxygen from the alveolar air and the blood hemoglobin. Because CO binds to receptor sites on hemoglobin at least 250 times more easily than oxygen, the patient's hemoglobin may become saturated with the wrong molecule. Being exposed to relatively small concentrations of CO (such as in cigarette smoke) will result in progressively higher blood levels of CO. Most people have approximately 2% CO attached to their hemoglobin, but these levels may be as high as 4% to 8% in heavy smokers. Levels of 50% or higher, however, may be fatal.

CO intoxication should be considered whenever a group of people in the same place all complain of headache or nausea. For example, a malfunctioning furnace or vehicle exhaust being sucked into the air-handling system can cause CO intoxication in groups of people. Similarly, you should be suspicious when people complain of feeling sick at home but not when they go to work or school.

Traditional wisdom tells us that patients with CO intoxication will appear "cherry red." Most practitioners agree that this cherry red skin is most commonly seen in people who have died, not living people. Thus, you should never rule out CO intoxication simply because the patient's skin is not cherry red.

Patients with severe CO intoxication usually present with an oxygen saturation level that appears normal or better. For this reason, you should never trust a pulse oximeter when dealing with a suspected CO poisoning case. New devices that can measure CO levels are available and allow paramedics to identify patients with low-level CO intoxication far more accurately.

Words of Wisdom

Hyperbaric oxygen (HBO) has long been recommended for acute CO intoxication and a variety of other asphyxiants, but this treatment is logistically difficult because the patient needs to be transported to an appropriate chamber in a reasonable amount of time.[7] It still isn't clear if HBO treatment is more effective than oxygen therapy at normal pressure; refer to your local protocol for treatment. The availability of HBO in specific areas and the local medical opinions may result in protocols that differ significantly from place to place.

■ Patient Assessment

Burns can fool paramedics, because we expect critically injured patients to act sick. Most severely injured and dying patients with cardiac and trauma conditions are hypotensive, unresponsive, or in obvious distress. In contrast, patients with an isolated major burn injury may walk up to you at a scene. The chief complaint may be "I'm terribly cold," and the severity of the injuries may not become apparent until you complete your assessment and realize that the person fits the criteria for transfer to a burn center. It is also common for burn patients whose conditions are considered initially stable to be deemed more serious after careful evaluation at the hospital, because the progression of burn-related pathology continues long after the initial incident. Even a patient with moderate burns may ultimately require intubation and transfer to a burn center. Maintain a high index of suspicion even when burn injuries do not initially seem severe.

Burns may occur in remote locations, so that you may not meet the patient until hours after the traumatic burn event. Such patients may present with an entirely different spectrum of problems than you are used to encountering. Sometimes the patient does not realize the ramifications of a burn injury until hours later. Some patients will have additional traumatic injuries from falling debris, explosions, or their attempts to get away from the source of the burn. Seriously burned patients may need to be transferred from tertiary facilities to larger burn centers. Prior to transfer the ED surgical staff may need to deal with complex issues such as an **escharotomy**, a surgical cut through the burned tissue to allow swelling, and begin significant pain and fluid resuscitation for the transport.

The many types of burns, coupled with the many possible presentations of burn patients, can challenge your assessment skills. As with any trauma patient, it is important to address the patient with burns in a consistent, efficient, and systematic manner so that you do not develop tunnel vision for the major burn trauma and miss other occult injuries that could affect the patient's outcome.

Scene Size-up

Safety is a primary concern whenever you are operating near a fire scene. (Non–fire-related scenarios involving burns are discussed in detail later in the chapter.) Stage yourself and others in a place where it is safe to provide patient care. When EMS providers are too close to the hot zone, it is detrimental to their own safety, the care they provide, and the overall medical response to the situation. Remember that your role is to treat victims of the fire—not to become a victim yourself—and potentially to provide rehabilitation for firefighters and other emergency personnel.

When a recently burned patient comes before you, your initial actions must include extinguishing any flames and cooling the burn. That step may seem obvious, but it is remarkable how many patients arrive by ambulance at hospital EDs with clothes still smoldering. A person whose clothing is on fire should not be permitted to run, because running fans the flames. Likewise, the person should not be allowed to remain standing, because inhaling flame and igniting hair are more likely in the upright position. Instead, have the patient stop, drop to the ground, and roll. If the patient cannot roll, lower the patient to the ground, cover him or her with a blanket, and pat the fire out.

Remove all smoldering clothing and any articles that may retain heat. Watchbands, zippers, and rings not only can retain enough heat to continue burning the patient, but also can melt your own gloves and burn you. If the person's hands are burned, they will swell considerably, so that rings may become tourniquets if not removed quickly enough. If bits of smoldering cloth adhere to the skin, do not pull them off; instead, cut around them. Let burn center or hospital personnel deal with materials that are melted to the flesh.

If possible, determine the mechanism of injury (MOI). As mentioned earlier, patients who have been burned also may have sustained other trauma.

As a part of your scene size-up, do not forget to wear the most appropriate personal protective equipment (PPE), perhaps including gloves and a combination mask/eye shield. The burned patient may be "leaking" body fluids and is highly susceptible to infection. Take the most appropriate standard precautions to ensure that you are not exposed and the patient is not exposed to you.

Primary Survey

As you approach a burn trauma patient, simple clues may help you identify how serious the injuries are and how quickly you need to assess and treat the patient. If the patient greets you with a hoarse voice and a chief complaint of "trouble breathing," your general impression might be that the patient has a potential airway or breathing problem. In the absence of hypoxia or other trauma, a patient with a major burn may be responsive and is often able to hold a conversation. Although burns are often painful, the more serious burns may present with little or no pain. Indeed, the chief complaint is often "I'm cold." What may first appear to be tattered clothing could turn out to be sheets of the patient's own skin hanging from his or her burned limbs. Recently burned patients may appear dazed or disconnected from events around them.

Words of Wisdom

Heat loss is a critical problem for burn patients, particularly children. Take immediate steps to prevent hypothermia, such as heating the ambulance until it is uncomfortable for the crew, covering the patient with warm blankets, and administering fluids.

Despite what the injuries may look or smell like, you must use compassion when approaching the patient. Burns are obviously traumatic for the patient; if the person survives, he or she may face significant hospitalization and years of rehabilitation. Burns are also traumatic for you, the provider. Focusing on the basic principles of emergency care—airway, breathing, circulation, disability, and exposure (ABCDEs)—can help you perform properly in this chaotic situation.

Patients with a burn injury may demonstrate varied mental status responses. Combative patients should be considered hypoxic until proven otherwise. Because partial-thickness burns are extremely painful, a patient with this type of injury may be awake and in pain. Even patients with major burns will often be awake and attempting to communicate. Isolated burns do not cause unresponsiveness (although toxic inhalations can). Unresponsive burn patients must be carefully assessed for the presence of other deadly injuries.

As in any other seriously ill or injured patient, airway management is a priority in a patient with a burn. The airway may be in particular jeopardy in such cases because the same heat and flames that caused the external burn may have produced potentially life-threatening damage to the airway. Be prepared to assist ventilations.

The following are signs of airway involvement in a burn patient:

- Hoarseness
- Cough
- Stridor
- Singed nasal or facial hair
- Facial burns
- Carbon in the sputum
- History of burn in an enclosed space

Although rare, laryngeal edema can develop with alarming speed in burn patients, especially in infants and children. Early endotracheal (ET) intubation—before the airway has closed off—could be lifesaving in such cases and should be performed by the most experienced paramedic on your team. To intervene early, however, you need to spot the problem early. Airway management is discussed in greater detail later in this chapter.

Listen to lung sounds, paying special attention to stridor, which may be a sign of impending upper airway compromise. Note if signs and symptoms of edema are present.

Patients with preexisting lung disease may have bronchospasm after even relatively minor exposure to smoke. These patients may respond well to inhaled beta-2 agonists.

Anyone suspected of having a burn to the upper airway may benefit from administration of humidified, cool oxygen. If you do not carry a high-output humidifier (a bubble humidifier is *not* a high-output humidifier), consider using an aerosol nebulizer to administer nebulized normal saline. This approach will not provide a high concentration of oxygen, so you will need to balance the need for a high oxygen concentration against the desire for cool humidity. Keep in mind that the oxygen saturation level may be suspect in patients with carbon monoxide intoxication.

During the first 24 to 48 hours of a patient's burn care, emphasis is placed on fluid resuscitation to prevent burn shock. Burn shock is a result of hypovolemia caused by fluid shifts that typically occur 6 to 8 hours after the burn. Patients with major burns will ultimately require large volumes of fluid, but they do not need it during the first minutes of prehospital care unless their burn injury occurred some time ago. Most patients will ultimately require central venous access, and most intravenous (IV) lines placed in the prehospital setting will be removed owing to tissue swelling and infection risk. Do not delay transport by making multiple attempts at vascular access.

Patients with both burns and other trauma may require immediate vascular access, just like any other trauma patients. Although it is preferable to avoid starting IV lines through burned tissue, this procedure is not contraindicated. Burn patients may challenge your vascular access skills, however. Intraosseous access may provide you with more choices than were available to your predecessors who relied on just IV access.

Once the ABCs are addressed, the severity of the patient's burns should be evaluated to determine which facility the patient should be transported to for the best care. While evaluating the patient's burns, you must approximate the depth of the burn (superficial, partial thickness, or full thickness) and the extent of the burn (the TBSA burned). Most practitioners advocate counting only the areas of partial- and full-thickness burns (not areas with superficial burns). The fastest and most universal mechanism of calculating the TBSA burned is the **rule of nines**, which is based on dividing the body into 11

sections, each representing approximately 9% of the TBSA.[8] The provider adds the portions of the body with burns to obtain the TBSA affected by the burn injury. Because our proportions change as we grow, different rules of nines apply to infants, children, and adults **Figure 32-10**.

Another mechanism of assessing the extent of a burn is the **rule of palms**, also called the rule of ones. This assessment uses the size of the patient's palm (including the fingers) to represent approximately 1% of the patient's TBSA. This calculation is helpful when the burn covers less than 10% of the TBSA or is irregularly shaped.

The **Lund-Browder chart** is an accurate, more time-consuming method used to estimate the burned area.[9] This method divides the body into even smaller and more specific regions and considers TBSA affected by growth **Figure 32-11**.

In the field, providers may disagree on the severity of a given burn, but reaching a consensus is not important enough to justify spending time on the discussion. Hospital personnel need a report that includes an estimate of the severity of burns. **Table 32-2** shows burn severity

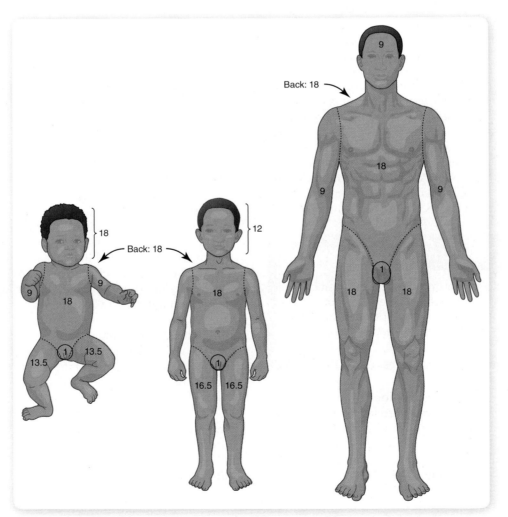

Figure 32-10 The rule of nines is a quick way to estimate the amount of surface area that has been burned. It divides the body into 11 sections, each representing approximately 9% of the total body surface area. The segments differ for infants, children, and adults.

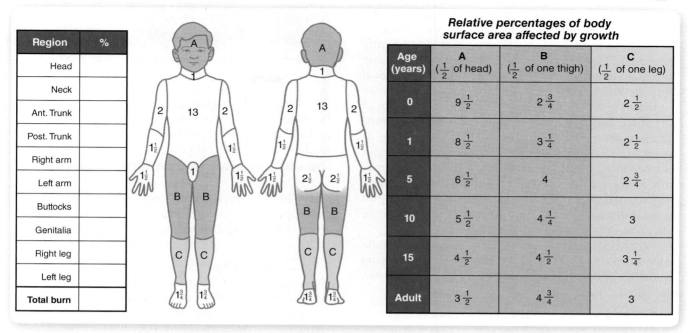

Region	%
Head	
Neck	
Ant. Trunk	
Post. Trunk	
Right arm	
Left arm	
Buttocks	
Genitalia	
Right leg	
Left leg	
Total burn	

Relative percentages of body surface area affected by growth

Age (years)	A ($\frac{1}{2}$ of head)	B ($\frac{1}{2}$ of one thigh)	C ($\frac{1}{2}$ of one leg)
0	$9\frac{1}{2}$	$2\frac{3}{4}$	$2\frac{1}{2}$
1	$8\frac{1}{2}$	$3\frac{1}{4}$	$2\frac{1}{2}$
5	$6\frac{1}{2}$	4	$2\frac{3}{4}$
10	$5\frac{1}{2}$	$4\frac{1}{4}$	3
15	$4\frac{1}{2}$	$4\frac{1}{2}$	$3\frac{1}{4}$
Adult	$3\frac{1}{2}$	$4\frac{3}{4}$	3

Figure 32-11 The Lund-Browder chart. Anterior and posterior, as well as both right and left extremities, must be figured in to equal 100%.

Data from: Lund CC, Browder NC. The estimation of areas of burns. *Surg Gynecol Obstet.* 1944;79:352-358.

Table 32-2   Classification of Burn Severity

Burn Classification	Criteria

Major burns	• Burns involving hands, feet, face, major joints, or genitalia, or circumferential burns of other areas
	• Full-thickness burns covering more than 10% of the TBSA
	• Partial-thickness burns covering more than:
	  • 25% of the TBSA if age 10–50 y
	  • 20% of the TBSA if age younger than 10 y or older than 50 y
	• Burns associated with respiratory injury (smoke inhalation or inhalation injury)
	• Burns complicated by fractures or trauma
	• High-voltage electrical burns
	• Chemical burns
	• Burns on patients younger than 5 years or older than 55 years that would be classified as "moderate" on young adults

Moderate burns	• Full-thickness burns involving 2% to 10% of the TBSA (excluding hands, feet, face, genitalia, and upper airway)
	• Partial-thickness burns covering:
	  • 15%–25% of the TBSA if age 10–50 y
	  • 10%–20% of the TBSA if age younger than 10 y or older 50 y
	• Superficial burns covering more than 50% of the TBSA
	• Low-voltage electrical burns
	• Major burn characteristics absent

Minor burns	• Full-thickness burns covering less than 2% of the TBSA
	• Partial-thickness burns covering:
	  • Less than 15% of the TBSA if age 10–50 y
	  • Less than 10% of the TBSA if age younger than 10 y or older than 50 y
	• Superficial burns covering less than 50% of the TBSA
	• Major burn characteristics absent

Abbreviation: TBSA, total body surface area

Data from: Pappas-Taffer L. Burns. In: Ferri FF, ed. *Ferri's Clinical Advisor, 2017.* Philadelphia, PA: Elsevier; 2017:219-221; and Tintinalli JE, Stapczynski JS, Ma OJ, et al. *Tintinalli's Emergency Medicine: A Comprehensive Study Guide.* 8th ed. McGraw-Hill; 2016.

classifications. These classifications can be used once the depth and extent of the burns have been determined.

During the primary survey, your goal is to identify and manage life threats and to determine the level of care the patient requires (eg, burn center, trauma center, local hospital). This means you will need to estimate the burn's severity to report to the receiving facility. The nature of the patient's burns will evolve during the next 24 hours, and estimations of their severity will inevitably change, so little is to be gained by conducting a comprehensive and time-consuming evaluation of every inch of the patient's body in the field. Nevertheless, a reasonably accurate estimation of the scope of the patient's injuries is helpful for determining both the appropriate destination for the patient and the care to be delivered.

According to the referral criteria identified by the American Burn Association, patients with the following injuries should be transferred to a burn specialty center, also called a burn unit[10]:

- Partial-thickness burns of more than 10% of the TBSA
- Burns that involve the face, hands, feet, genitalia, perineum, or major joints
- Full-thickness burns in any age group
- Electrical burns, including those caused by lightning
- Chemical burns
- Inhalation burns
- Burn injuries in conjunction with preexisting medical conditions that could complicate management, prolong recovery, or affect mortality
- Burns and concomitant trauma (eg, fractures) in which the burn injury poses the greatest risk of morbidity or mortality

- Burns to children in hospitals without qualified personnel or equipment
- Burn injury that requires special social, emotional, or long-term rehabilitation

You must balance the need for accuracy against the time required to make an estimate of the TBSA. The prehospital estimation is used to guide the patient to the correct place for treatment. The ED estimation of the burned area may be used to initiate fluid therapy. The burn center's estimation of injured area will undoubtedly be more accurate and specific.

History Taking

To the degree possible, get a brief history from the patient. Patients with preexisting diseases, such as chronic obstructive pulmonary disease or acute coronary syndromes, may be triaged as severe even if the burn injury is small. As in any other trauma, allergies, medications, and other pertinent medical history may influence the patient's care plan.

Secondary Assessment

When you have finished your brief inspection of the patient's skin, you have only just begun the head-to-toe exam. The secondary assessment is intended to make sure no other injuries have higher priority for treatment. Often, such injuries may be obscured by the burn itself, so you need to pay attention to the circumstances of the burn and the possible MOI. If the patient jumped from a second-story window, for example, there may be fractures beneath the obvious burns on the legs.

Look for injuries to the eyes, and cover injured eyes with moist, sterile pads. Check the neck, chest, and extremities for **circumferential burns**. Progressive edema beneath a circumferential burn—especially when the burned skin has become leathery and unyielding—may act as a tourniquet. In the neck, a circumferential burn may obstruct the airway; in the chest, it may restrict respiratory excursion; and in an extremity, it may cut off the circulation and put the extremity in jeopardy. Patients with circumferential burns must reach a medical facility quickly, because it may be necessary to make an incision into the burned area to decompress it. Check and document the distal pulses in burned extremities often.

Obtaining vital signs may be challenging if the patient has extensive burns on the arms. Standard vital signs for a burn victim should include not only an assessment of blood pressure, pulse, respirations, and oxygen saturation (SpO_2), but also an assessment of end-tidal carbon dioxide and carboxyhemoglobin percentage ($SpCO$), if such technology is available to you. Recall that with burn injuries, often the patient has been exposed to carbon monoxide, carbon dioxide, cyanide, and other caustic agents. Nevertheless, you should try to document vital signs accurately because the management of shock, airway compromise, and pain depends on them to some degree.

Reassessment

If the patient is considered to have a significant MOI, en route to the ED, you should perform a full-body exam and reassessment. Reassessment of vital signs to establish trends is done every 5 minutes for critical patients and every 15 minutes for lower-priority patients (in stable condition).

Emergency Medical Care

Definitive burn care can be divided into four phases: (1) initial evaluation and resuscitation, (2) initial wound excision and biologic closure, (3) definitive wound closure, and (4) rehabilitation, reconstruction, and reintegration **Table 32-3**. Although you will be most heavily

involved in the first phase, it is important to appreciate the magnitude of care that a patient with a major—or even moderate—burn must receive. Your early actions may dramatically affect the patient's long-term outcome. You may also find yourself transporting patients to specialty or rehabilitation facilities at later stages of their care.

Unlike many emergencies you will encounter, burn patient care is measured in weeks, not hours. Burns are devastating multisystem traumatic injuries that dramatically alter a person's life. You should recognize not only the massive physical trauma caused by burns, but also the emotional, psychologic, and financial burdens these horrific injuries impose. Once these costs are appreciated, it is easy to understand the importance of teaching injury prevention strategies to the people we serve.

▶ General Management

Management of a patient with burns begins with the steps taken during the scene size-up and primary survey to extinguish the fire and manage threats to the ABCs. Only when the ABCs are under control should you turn your attention to the burn itself. It is important to have all resuscitative equipment ready for use when treating a burn patient, including advanced airway equipment and an ECG monitor.

Airway Management

Many burn patients will ultimately require intubation, even though they were talking to you and in no distress in the field. Although it is obviously preferable to intubate patients in a controlled environment with a full complement of anesthesia agents available, a few patients will absolutely require an emergency advanced airway in the field. Burn patients fall into four general categories for airway management:

1. **Patients with an acutely decompensating airway who require field intubation.** This group includes burn patients who are in

Table 32-3	**Phases of Definitive Burn Care**	
Phase	**Time Frame**	**Treatment Objectives**
Initial evaluation and resuscitation	First 72 hours	To provide initial resuscitation, secure the airway, achieve accurate fluid resuscitation, and perform a thorough evaluation
Initial wound excision and biologic closure	Days 1 through 7	To identify and remove all full-thickness wounds and obtain biologic closure
Definitive wound closure	Day 7 through week 6	To replace temporary covers with definitive ones and close small, complex wounds
Rehabilitation, reconstruction, and reintegration	Entire hospitalization	To maintain range of motion and reduce edema and to strengthen and prepare the patient for return to the community

cardiac or respiratory arrest and responsive patients whose airways are swelling before your eyes. In these chaotic and difficult situations, you need to plan for the possibility that you may not be able to intubate the patient. Supraglottic swelling or complete obstruction can occur in some burn scenarios. Surgical airways or rescue devices may be necessary if intubation is not possible and bag-mask ventilation fails.

2. **Patients with a deteriorating airway from burns and toxic inhalations who might require intubation.** It is obviously better for the patient to defer treatment of this airway problem to hospital teams with anesthesia, surgery, specialized equipment, and a fully stocked pharmacy. Patients with burns will often be responsive and may become combative with attempts just to place them supine, let alone intubate them. "Awake" techniques, such as nasal intubation, are dramatically more complicated in patients with upper airway burns and should be avoided. Attempt to intubate the burn patient only if left with no other choice. If the patient's airway continues to swell and intubation will become impossible if you wait for arrival at the hospital, you have little choice but to attempt intubation. Try using a tube size smaller than you would usually insert. Consult medical control for advice if there is sufficient time.

The procedure for rapid-sequence intubation is discussed in Chapter 15, *Airway Management*. It is also advised that the "most experienced" intubator perform this procedure, because the swelling can make for a difficult intubation.

An airway compromised by advancing edema represents another classic scenario in which administering a neuromuscular blocker to provide respiratory paralysis may be extremely dangerous. It places you in the worrisome position of having a patient with no gag reflex or ability to breathe and an airway you may be unable to control.

The choice of ET tube may present another conundrum. It would obviously be beneficial to use the largest tube possible: sometimes a smaller ET tube will clog with soot from the patient's airway, causing complete occlusion. At the same time, a smaller-than-usual ET tube may be necessary owing to airway edema. Select the largest ET tube that will not cause additional trauma during insertion.

3. **Patients with a currently patent airway but who have a history consistent with risk factors for eventual airway compromise.**

Administering cool, humidified oxygen from a high-output nebulizer (not a bubble humidifier) is appropriate for this group. Alternatively, you may use an aerosol nebulizer with saline. Such patients will probably *not* require acute interventions in the field, but make sure you report their history to hospital personnel. Many patients will ultimately undergo elective intubation.

4. **Patients with no signs of or risk factors for airway compromise who are in no distress.** While current trends in prehospital care include limiting the aggressive use of oxygen therapy, providing supplemental oxygen to burn patients continues to be considered reasonable treatment, even if patients are not in distress.[11] The potential for carbon monoxide poisoning and the resultant inaccuracy of pulse oximetry and the potential for airway compromise favor the administration of oxygen in this group.

Fluid Resuscitation

Patients with burns covering more than 20% of the TBSA will need fluid resuscitation. Depending on the patient's age and other medical conditions, too much fluid may be as harmful as too little. If fluid resuscitation is delayed more than 2 hours from the time of the burn in patients with major burns, resuscitation is complicated and mortality increases. The goal is to begin to deliver an appropriate amount of fluid to the burn patient as soon as is reasonable.

An IV line may be inserted in the field to administer fluids and pain medications as needed. A 18-gauge IV catheter should be inserted as early as possible in any patient who has major burns. Do not delay transport to do so, but try to get a large-bore IV catheter into a large vein, and administer lactated Ringer solution via this line.[12] You can use the burned extremity for the IV site if you cannot find another site; an IV line in a burned upper extremity is still preferable to an IV line in a lower extremity. Consider establishing IO access if IV access is not possible. Most seriously burned patients will need central venous access, and IV lines placed in the prehospital setting will most often be lost as peripheral swelling begins.

To approximate the amount of fluid the burned patient will need, use the **Consensus formula** (also known as the Parkland formula). The amount of fluids administered in the first 24 hours after injury is typically 2–4 mL of lactated Ringer solution multiplied by the patient's body weight in kilograms (kg) multiplied by the percentage of TBSA burned:

2–4 mL × Body weight (in kg) × Percentage of body surface burned

Half of that amount needs to be given during the first 8 hours, and the other half needs to be given over the next 16 hours in the 24-hour period.

For example, a 70-kg man has sustained burns to 30% of his body. Calculate the amount of **fluid needed during the first 24 hours**:

$$2 \text{ to } 4 \text{ mL} \times 70 \text{ kg} \times 30 = 4{,}200 \text{ to } 8{,}400 \text{ mL}$$

To determine the **amount of fluid needed during the first 8 hours**, divide that number by 2:

$$4{,}200 \text{ mL} \div 2 = 2{,}100 \text{ mL};$$
$$8{,}400 \text{ mL} \div 2 = 4{,}200 \text{ mL}$$

To determine the **hourly rate for the first 8 hours**, divide this total by 8:

$$2{,}100 \div 8 = 262 \text{ mL/hr}; 4{,}200 \div 8 = 525 \text{ mL/hr}$$

Note: The first half of the fluid is administered within 8 hours from the time the patient was injured, not from the time the provider began treatment of the patient. For example, if for some reason you don't reach the patient for 2 hours after the injury occurred, the first half of the calculated total needs to be administered over the next 6 hours. The goal is for the patient to have had the target volume within 8 hours after injury.

Even though the Consensus formula implies that burn patients need enormous amounts of fluid, remember that you should not attempt to deliver the entire initial amount in the field. The large amounts of fluid suggested by this formula often lead providers to give more fluid than necessary prior to the patient's arrival at a burn center—a phenomenon known as fluid creep. (Interestingly, the Parkland formula was devised as a way to limit fluid overload so that burn patients would *not* develop pulmonary edema and acute respiratory distress syndrome.) Ongoing fluid resuscitation at the hospital is based on the patient's urine output and vital signs.

Even though burn patients will need large amounts of fluid, giving it too early or too fast can lead to rapidly increasing peripheral edema that may compromise the effectiveness of airway devices and vascular access and lead to compartment syndrome. It is even more important to monitor older adults and children for fluid overload during this crucial period. In short, you must administer a lot of fluid while simultaneously monitoring the patient to ensure that you are not administering too much.

Pain Management

Initially, all burn injuries are painful. Depending on the depth of the burn, pain can be worsened by clothing rubbing against the burned area, air current moving past exposed tissue, and swelling in response to the body's inflammatory response.

Using a 0 to 10 scale, assess the patient's pain before administering any analgesia. Reassessment should be completed using the same pain scale every 5 minutes. In any patient with burns, pain medication is best given via the IV route. Because of changes in fluid volume and tissue blood flow, absorption of any intramuscular or

YOU are the Paramedic   PART 3

Your partner administers high-concentration oxygen via a nonrebreathing mask and applies cool, moist, sterile dressings to the burns on the patient's arm and neck. Working on his unburned arm, you obtain vital signs and prepare to establish an IV line.

Recording Time: 5 Minutes	
Respirations	22 breaths/min, unlabored
Pulse	120 beats/min, strong radial pulses
Skin	Flushed, warm
Blood pressure	160/110 mm Hg
Oxygen saturation (Spo$_2$)	98% via nonrebreathing mask
Pupils	PERRLA

5. What is the likely cause of the patient's elevated blood pressure?

6. At which point might you consider aggressive airway management including sedation and intubation?

subcutaneous medication may be unpredictable in a burn patient.

It is unlikely that the patient will achieve a completely pain free state while he or she is in your care; however, you should be able to take the edge off his or her pain. As with any patient population, narcotic analgesics should be administered judiciously. Consider factors such as the site of the burn, the presence of shock, concurrent illnesses (eg, hepatitis, cirrhosis), and patient age when administering medications for pain relief. For example, depressing the respiratory drive in a patient with an evolving upper airway burn could be problematic. Similarly, medication clearance may be adversely affected in the presence of shock, hepatitis, or cirrhosis, or in the elderly, and can lead to an unintended buildup of medication. Consult your protocols or contact medical control for guidance in administering analgesics for burn pain.

▶ Hypovolemic Shock

Depending on the TBSA and depth of the burn involved, you most likely will not see the presentation of hypovolemic shock in the field as a direct result of the burn itself. Therefore, if an acutely burned patient is in shock in the prehospital phase, look for another injury as the source of shock. People who are caught in fires may, for example, fall through floors, jump out of windows, and have debris fall on them.

▶ Thermal Burns

While assessing a patient's burns, consider the presence or absence of pain, swelling, skin color, capillary refill time, moisture and blisters, the appearance of the wound edges, the presence of foreign bodies, debris and contaminants, bleeding, and circulatory adequacy. Also assess for concomitant soft-tissue injury. Cool any small burn areas and any large areas that remain hot. Apply dry, clean, nonadherent dressings to help prevent infection and provide comfort. Remember that patients with a large area of the body's surface burned are likely to also have hypovolemia and hypothermia.

Superficial Burns

Although superficial burns can be very painful, they rarely pose a threat to life unless they involve nearly the entire surface of the body. If you reach a patient with superficial burns within the first hour after the injury occurred, immerse the burned area in cool water or apply cold compresses to the burn. Burned hands or feet may be soaked directly in cool water; and towels soaked in cold water may be applied to burns of the face or trunk.

The objectives of this exercise are twofold: to stop the burning process and to relieve pain. Commercial burn dressing products that meet both objectives are available **Figure 32-12**. Regardless of the method used to cool the burn, take care not to cool the whole body; do not let the patient become chilled. A dry sheet or

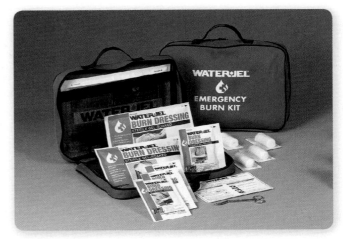

Figure 32-12 Sample burn dressing (Water-Jel).
Courtesy of Water-Jel® Technologies.

blanket applied over the wet dressings will help prevent systemic heat loss. Narcotics are generally not necessary in these patients.

Do not use salves, ointments, creams, sprays, or any similar materials on any type of burn. They will just have to be scrubbed off in the ED or burn unit, causing the patient further pain. Never apply ice to burns, because it can exacerbate the tissue injury.

No further treatment should be necessary in the field for an uncomplicated, superficial burn. Simply transport the patient in a comfortable position to the hospital.

> ### Patient Safety
>
> Never put salves, ointments, creams, or other similar materials on a burn!

Partial-Thickness Burns

Treatment of partial-thickness burns in the field is similar to treatment of superficial burns. Cooling the burned area with water or application of wet or Water-Jel® dressings within the first hour can diminish edema and provide significant pain relief. Burned extremities should be elevated to minimize edema formation.

Do not attempt to rupture blisters over the burn; they initially act as a physiologic burn dressing. Administer IV fluids as dictated by local protocol. Pain in the patient with partial-thickness burns may be severe, so complete a pain assessment and administer pain medication as allowed by your protocols.

Full-Thickness Burns

Although full-thickness burns may not cause pain, most patients will have varying degrees of burns within the affected region of injury. For this reason, you should complete a pain assessment and administer pain medication as described earlier. Usually, dry dressings are used after the fire is out. Check with your burn center or medical center to determine its guidelines on use of wet dressings or analgesia. Begin fluid resuscitation, if possible, preferably within 2 hours of injury.

▶ Thermal Inhalation Burns

Application of cool mist or aerosol therapy may help reduce some minor edema in patients with thermal inhalation burns. Because most ambulances do not carry misters, apply an ice pack to the throat.

More aggressive airway management may be necessary if supraglottic tissue swelling threatens the patient's airway. In addition, heat inhalation may produce laryngospasm and bronchospasm in the lower airway. Patients sometimes experience pulmonary damage from direct thermal injury. Later pulmonary involvement may be from toxic inhalation injury.

■ Pathophysiology, Assessment, and Management of Specific Burns

▶ Chemical Burns of the Skin

Chemical burns occur when the skin comes in contact with strong acids, alkalis or bases, or other corrosive materials Table 32-4. The burn progresses as long as the corrosive substance remains in contact with the skin. The cornerstone of therapy, therefore, is removal of the chemical from contact with the patient's body. Typical management for removal of chemical solutions is copious flushing with water, whereas management of burns caused by powders requires brushing off as much of the substance as possible before washing.

The amount of damage from a chemical burn depends on the nature of the chemical involved as well as the following factors:

- **The concentration and quality of the agent.** Common agents that are not particularly dangerous may be much more reactive in their concentrated or commercial forms. The hydrogen peroxide that you put on cuts, for example, is typically a 3% to 6% solution. By comparison, the hydrogen peroxide being transported in a tanker might be a 70% to 98% solution and is a highly volatile oxidizer.
- **The chemical state or temperature of the agent.** Many gases (nitrogen, oxygen, anhydrous ammonia) are transported in their liquid form, which can cause major burns because they are so cold. Liquid oxygen systems, which are becoming increasingly popular for home use, can cause major burns if their contents are inadvertently released (such as during a building collapse or motor vehicle crash).
- **The length of exposure.** Agents that do not cause significant pain sometimes soak into clothing and are held against the skin for long periods, causing significant injury. Phenol (carbolic acid) causes a painless burn that can result in significant damage before it is identified. Unresponsive patients and patients

Table 32-4	Chemical Burns	
Chemical Type	**Examples**	**Injury**
Acids	Battery acid (sulfuric acid), hydrochloric acid, hydrofluoric acid	Causes immediate pain and **coagulation necrosis**; deeper tissue typically not injured
Bases and alkalis	Potassium hydroxide, sodium hydroxide, lime, drain cleaner, oven cleaner, lye	Causes little pain but extensive damage by **liquefaction necrosis**: breakdown of protein and collagen, saponification of fats, dehydration of tissues, thrombosis of blood vessels
Oxidizing agents	Hydrogen peroxide, sodium chlorate	Exothermic (heat) reaction in addition to tissue destruction; could cause systemic poisoning
Phosphorus	White phosphorus, tracer ammunition, fireworks	Burns when exposed to air; could cause systemic poisoning
Vesicants	Lewisite, sulfur mustard (mustard gas), phosgene oxime	Blister agents; respiratory compromise if inhaled

with paralyzed limbs sometimes sustain significant burns from contact with simple household items such as radiators or cooking grease.

- **The depth of penetration.** One reason that alkaline burns are often worse than acid burns is that acids create a coagulative necrosis that is painful and forms a tough layer of dead tissue, which may prevent deeper burning. In contrast, bases break down protein and collagen, creating a liquefactive necrosis that burns deeper.

Typically, chemical burns react with the skin and tissues quickly. In some cases, however, the injury may take time to develop, as when a person is exposed to cement (calcium oxide). Cement tends to penetrate clothing and can react with sweat on the surface of the skin. Hours later, the patient may notice that a burn injury has occurred.

Acid Burns Versus Alkali Burns

The hydrogen ions formed by an acid are relatively easy to neutralize because they do not form soluble products. Acids cause destruction and coagulation of tissues, resulting in a coagulative necrosis that may actually limit the depth of the burn.

In contrast, the hydroxide ions of an alkaline burn form soluble products that sink into the tissue, carrying the burn deeper and making it more difficult to neutralize. This effect is particularly pronounced in chemical burns of the eye. Flushing—including flushing with the patient's own tears—quickly helps to disperse an acid, whereas alkali burns to the eye are profoundly destructive, often within just a few minutes.

Assessment

Typically, chemical burns are the result of unexpected contact with a caustic substance, so your assessment must begin by ensuring your own safety, followed by appropriate decontamination of the patient. Be careful not to get any of the hazardous chemicals on your own clothing or skin. Consider wearing additional PPE, as your usual nitrile or vinyl gloves may not protect you from many chemicals. Determine the TBSA that is affected.

Management

Speed is essential when treating chemical burns. Begin flushing the exposed area of the patient's body immediately with copious quantities of water **Figure 32-13**. If the patient is in or near the home, using the shower or a garden hose for this purpose is ideal. In an industrial setting, use the decontamination shower or a hose. While flushing, rapidly remove the patient's clothing, especially shoes and socks that may have become contaminated with the offending agent. Removing a patient's clothes removes a majority of the external contamination.

Have the patient bend over when washing the hair and head to avoid having residual chemicals run over the rest of the body. Chemicals can collect in skin

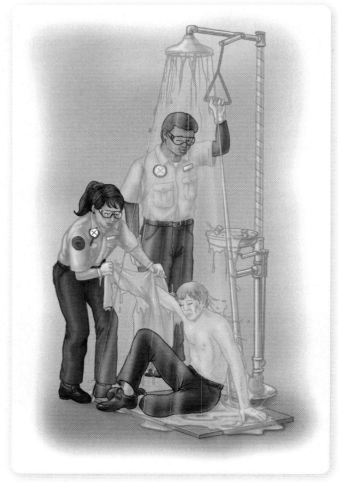

Figure 32-13 Flush the burned area with large amounts of water.

© Jones & Bartlett Learning.

folds, where they remain in contact with the tissue and continue to cause more severe damage. Care must be taken to meticulously wash the skin folds at joints and between fingers and toes. Once you think washing is complete, wash the body again. Some chemicals may adhere to the skin, and a mild detergent (dishwashing liquid) will aid in removal. Rinse and wash gently to avoid abrading the skin and exacerbating the injury or absorption of the chemical.

Do not waste time looking for specific antidotes or neutralizing agents; copious flushing with water is more effective and more immediately available. If the chemical being flushed is determined to be a hazardous material, the patient should not be transported until he or she has been determined by hazardous materials personnel to be clean. If the chemical is not a hazardous material by concentration or quantity, then flushing can be conducted by the paramedic. Paramedics must weigh the realities of flushing on the scene for long periods against the benefits of transport and their ability to continue flushing en route. After flushing, limit hypothermia by keeping the patient covered and warm.

Several types of chemical burns require special management techniques:

- **Dry lime.** In alkali burns caused by dry lime, combination with water will produce a highly corrosive substance. For that reason, when a patient has been in contact with dry lime, *first* remove the patient's clothing and *brush* as much lime as you can from the skin (wear gloves!). *Then* start flushing copiously with a garden hose or shower. Your intention is to completely overwhelm any damaging chemical reaction with a deluge of water.

- **Sodium metals.** Sodium metals produce considerable heat when mixed with water and may explode. Cover this type of burn with oil, which will stop the reaction by preventing the sodium from coming in contact with the atmosphere.

- **Hydrofluoric (HF) acid.** HF acid is used in drain cleaners in the home and for etching glass and plastic in industrial settings. Burns caused by HF acid that exceed 3% to 5% of the TBSA can be fatal. The patient will complain bitterly of pain (caused by the HF acid sucking calcium out of the body), and the pain will not improve even with continuous flushing—a sign that the process of tissue destruction is ongoing. Calcium gluconate gel is the preferred treatment for HF acid burns. If such a gel is not readily available, you can create this gel by combining 25 mL of calcium gluconate 10% solution into 75 to 150 mL of a sterile water-soluble lubricant. If calcium gluconate is not available, calcium chloride (CaCl) jelly may be used. An ampule of CaCl (10 mL of a 10% CaCl solution) can be mixed with a water-based lubricant to make CaCl jelly in an emergency.

- **Gasoline or diesel fuel.** Because we come into contact with these chemicals almost every day, and they are present at almost all vehicle crashes, it is easy to forget the multitude of potential problems that may be caused by gasoline, kerosene, and other hydrocarbons. Prolonged contact may produce a chemical injury to the skin. This condition is managed like contact with any other chemical irritant, with the fuel being washed off as soon as possible. Most hydrocarbons are more effectively removed with a soap solution than with water alone. Hydrocarbons also stimulate gamma-aminobutyric acid receptors and can cause sleepiness and even coma. Many hydrocarbons can also cause a fire or explosion under certain circumstances.

- **Hot tar.** Burns caused by hot tar are, strictly speaking, thermal burns, not chemical burns, although they tend to be classified with chemical burns. The most important step in the prehospital phase is to immerse the affected area in cold water to dissipate the heat from the tar and speed up the hardening process. Once the tar has cooled, it will not do further damage, and there is no need to try to remove it in the field.

▶ Inhalation Burns From Other Toxic Chemicals

A variety of irritant gases can cause local swelling of the airway or a more systemic response. In many cases, the solubility properties of the gas will determine which part of the airway the gas affects Table 32-5 . Highly water-soluble gases such as ammonia and hydrogen chloride will react with the moist mucous membranes of the upper airway and cause immediate irritation and swelling. In contrast, slightly water-soluble gases such as phosgene and nitrogen dioxide will react with tissues over time. Since they are not initially as irritating, the patient will continue to take deep breaths, causing damage at the alveolar level hours or even days after they are inspired. Thus, patients with these types of inhalation burns may present with pulmonary edema long after the exposure took place.

Some other very common irritant gases can be categorized as moderately water soluble, and their site of action will depend on the concentration breathed. For example, chlorine is a common chemical found in powder and liquid forms in homes, in businesses, and on highways. When high concentrations are released, such as after

Table 32-5	Irritant Gases and Their Effects	
Water Solubility	**Examples of Substances**	**Effects**
Highly water soluble	Ammonia Formaldehyde Hydrogen chloride (HCl) Sulfur dioxide	Corrosive local effects upon reacting with water in the upper airways. Effects are usually immediate.
Moderately water soluble	Chlorine	Site of action depends on concentration inhaled. Effects may be immediate or delayed.
Slightly water soluble	Phosgene Nitrogen dioxide	Inflammation and pulmonary edema at the alveolar level. Effects may occur hours or days after exposure.

© Jones & Bartlett Learning.

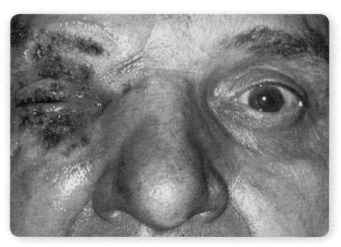

Figure 32-14 The eyes are particularly vulnerable to chemical burns.

a railcar or tanker crash, the evolved gas can be irritating and cause immediate upper airway irritation. The same product in lower concentrations may not be as irritating, resulting in less intense symptoms that do not present until hours or days later.

HF acid is a special case. Fluoride dust can be inhaled in an industrial setting or at the scene of fires or explosions where fluorides are stored. As discussed in Chapter 27, *Toxicology*, HF acid aggressively binds with calcium ions and may require the administration of IV calcium. Significant inhalation frequently results in death.

Assessment

Your usual airway assessment should always include a high index of suspicion for irritant gas exposure if the patient was involved in a fire, explosion, or contaminated environment situation. The irritant gases that affect the upper airway will also usually cause burning of the eyes. Signs of upper airway swelling, such as stridor, are ominous and may signal the potential for acute upper airway obstruction. Signs of lower airway involvement may include wheezing and desaturation or may present as pulmonary edema, ranging from crackles in the lung bases to the expectoration of pink froth.

Management

Maintaining an acceptable oxygen saturation level and monitoring for signs of continued airway compromise are the mainstays of therapy. Aerosolized beta-agonists are usually helpful in maintaining adequate respiration. Be sure to follow your local protocols.

▶ Chemical Burns of the Eye

Chemicals known to cause burning injuries to the eyes include acids (eg, concentrated liquid chlorine), alkalis (eg, cement powder, strong cleaning agents), dry chemicals (eg, lye or lime), and phenols **Figure 32-14**. Always wear eye protection when working with chemicals!

Assessment and Management

If chemicals have splashed into the patient's eyes, flush the eyes with copious amounts of water. It may be most expeditious to simply support the patient's head under a faucet or at an eye-wash station, directing a steady stream of lukewarm tap water into the affected eye **Figure 32-15**. If the patient wears contact lenses and the stream of water does not flush them out, pause after a minute or two of irrigation to allow the patient to remove the contact

Evidence-Based Medicine

When tear gas or pepper spray has been used, the burning sensation may affect you as well as the patient. Take special precautions in such scenarios. Some law enforcement agencies carry an antidote to pepper spray. A study of five commonly recommended neutralizing agents (Maalox, 2% lidocaine gel, baby shampoo, milk, and water) concluded that there was no significant difference in pain relief among these agents.[13]

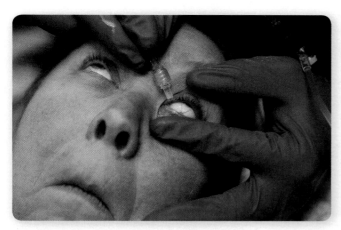

Figure 32-15 Flood the affected eye with a gentle stream of water. Hold the eyelids open—a challenging task because the patient's reflex is to keep the eye shut. Take care to prevent the chemical from getting into the other eye during the flushing.

© Jones & Bartlett Learning.

lenses; if they remain in place, they will prevent water from reaching the cornea underneath. Be sure to irrigate well underneath the eyelids.

Never use chemical antidotes (such as vinegar or baking soda) in the eyes, except possibly in the special case of irritation from tear gas or pepper spray. Irrigate with water only. After irrigating, patch the patient's eyes with lightly applied dressings and begin transport to the hospital for evaluation.

Eye irrigation is extremely important whenever a chemical has gotten into the eye. However, it may be uncomfortable and inefficient to attempt to irrigate an eye by prying it open and rinsing with a standard normal saline IV set. Another option is the Morgan lens, which may make eye irrigation more comfortable, efficient, and effective. This device is discussed in Chapter 33, *Face and Neck Trauma*.

It is important to keep fluid running through the Morgan lens during both its insertion and its removal. Suction can occur between the lens and the eye if the fluid flow is stopped before removal. After flushing, test the pH of the eye with hydrazine paper (pH paper) to determine whether all of an acid or base has been removed; more typically, this step is performed at the hospital with topical anesthetic. Normal pH is between 7 and 7.3.

▶ Electrical Burns and Associated Injuries

The American Burn Association indicates that electrocution causes an average of 400 deaths and 4,400 injuries each year.[14]

This type of burn may result in two injury sites: one at the point where electricity entered the body (entrance wound) and another where it exited (exit wound). The entrance wound may be quite small, but the exit wound can be extensive and deep **Figure 32-16**. The degree of tissue injury is related to the resistance of the body tissues, the intensity of current that passes through the victim, and the duration of exposure. Electrical burns may also

---

YOU are the Paramedic PART 4

You establish an IV line in the patient and administer fentanyl for pain. The patient is quiet during the ride to the hospital, and it seems as though the fentanyl is helping to control the pain.

Recording Time: 9 Minutes	
Respirations	18 breaths/min
Pulse	110 beats/min, strong radial pulses
Skin	Flushed, warm
Blood pressure	150/100 mm Hg
Oxygen saturation (Spo₂)	98% via nonrebreathing mask
Pupils	PERRLA

7. With regard to the patient's respiratory status, what changes should you be particularly alert for en route to the hospital?
8. Explain the steps you would take to identify the cause of a change in respiratory status, and explain how you would correct the problem.

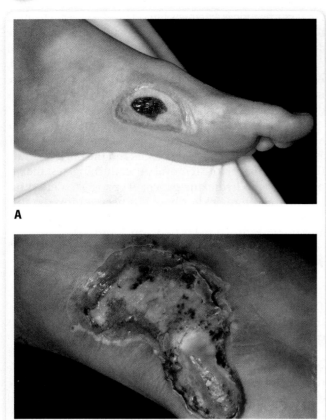

Figure 32-16 Electrical burns have entrance and exit wounds. **A.** The entrance wound is often quite small. **B.** The exit wound can be extensive and deep.

© Charles Stewart, MD, EMDM, MPH.

Table 32-6	The Effects of Electric Current on the Body
Current (milliamps)	**Effect on Body**
1	Tingling sensation/perception.
5	Slight shock felt; not painful. Average individual can let go. Strong involuntary reactions can lead to other injuries.
6-25 (women)	Painful shock, loss of muscular control.[a]
9-30 (men)	The freezing current or "let-go"[a] range. Individual cannot let go but can be thrown away from the circuit.
50-150	Extreme pain, respiratory arrest, severe muscular contractions. Death is possible.
1,000-4,300	Rhythmic pumping action of the heart ceases. Muscular contraction and nerve damage occur; death likely.
10,000	Cardiac arrest, major burns; death probable.

[a]If the extensor muscles are excited by the shock, the person may be thrown away from the power source.

Data from: Kouwenhoven WB. Human safety and electric shock. In: *Electrical Safety Practices*. Monograph 112. Research Triangle Park, NC: Instrument Society of America; November 1968:93. Printed by: Controlling electrical hazards. Occupational Safety and Health Administration website. https://www.osha.gov/Publications/3075.html. Updated 2002. Accessed April 12, 2017.

produce devastating internal injuries with little external evidence.

When a person comes in contact with an electrical source, the amount of current delivered to the inside of the body depends to some extent on the resistance of the skin. Wet, thin, clean skin offers less resistance than does dry, thick, dirty skin; thus, a moist inner surface of the forearm will have much less resistance than a dry, callused palm.

As electric current travels from the contact site into the body, it is converted to heat, which follows the current flow—usually along blood vessels and nerves—causing extensive damage to the tissues in its path **Table 32-6** . The greater the current flow, the greater the amount of heat generated. When the voltage is low (less than 1,000 volts, as in household sources), current follows the path of least resistance, generally along blood vessels, nerves, and muscles. When the voltage is high (as from high-tension lines), current takes the shortest path. The initial damage is usually the greatest at the entry and exit points, because this is where the amperage is concentrated (due to resistance from the skin).

Alternating current is considerably more dangerous than direct current is because the alternations cause

Words of Wisdom

Electricity is the flow of electrons across a potential gradient from high to low through a conductive material. Voltage is the current drop between the entry point and the exit point. **Ohm's law** links voltage and resistance. It tells us that Current (I) = Voltage (V) divided by Resistance (R): I = V/R. Resistance to the flow of current between the entry and exit points across human tissues varies significantly, from as low as a few hundred ohms to as high as a few hundred thousand ohms.

Joule's law describes the relationship between heat production, current, and resistance. One joule is generated when one ampere (amp) flows through one ohm of resistance for one second.

repetitive muscle contractions, which may "freeze" the victim to the conductor until the current source is turned off. Furthermore, alternating current is more likely than direct current is to induce ventricular fibrillation.

The direction of current flow is also significant. For example, current moving from one hand to the other is particularly dangerous because current may then flow across the heart; a current of only 0.1 amp to the heart can provoke ventricular fibrillation. Typical TASER devices deliver 50,000 volts, but only 3 milliamps (0.003 amp) and 0.3 joule of current.

> ## Special Populations
>
> A common cause of electrical injuries in toddlers is chewing on electrical wires **Figure 32-17**.[15] Children 1 to 2 years old have a greater propensity to chew or suck on electrical cords. In turn, they may sustain significant burns to the oral cavity that can result in erosion of the labial and facial arteries, causing life-threatening hemorrhage. The electrolyte-rich saliva completes the circuit between the two wires when they bite the cord.

Electricity can cause several types of injuries:

- **True electrical injury.** This is the most common type of electrical burn. Because the current is most intense at the entrance and exit sites, you may see a characteristic bull's-eye lesion at these sites, with a central, charred zone of full-thickness burns; a middle zone of cold, gray, dry tissue; and an outer, red zone of coagulation necrosis.
- **TASER effects.** Devices such as a conducted electrical weapon (CEW) or TASER incapacitate people via electromuscular disruption. While they are intended to offer law enforcement personnel a nonlethal option for controlling violent people, their use can create injuries that require emergency medical care. If discharged

from a distance, two small darts (electrodes) that puncture the patient's skin are deployed from these weapons. TASER darts can be seen as small impaled objects, with a fishhook-like barb on the end. While the resultant injury is typically minor, reports have cited hits to sensitive areas such as the eyes, major vessels, face, and genitalia. Even innocuous dart placement could potentially result in soft-tissue injury, bleeding, or infection, and dart removal should be done with care and while complying with the appropriate body substance isolation precautions.

Several reports of deaths in people who have been shocked with a TASER have made the use of these devices controversial.[16] In addition, cases exist in which people who have been covered with alcohol-based pepper spray have subsequently caught fire when an electro-shock device was applied.[17] (Water-based pepper spray is typically used in the United States.) Manufacturers now recommend that such devices not be used in potentially flammable environments such as gas stations or near illicit methamphetamine-manufacturing operations.
- **Arc-type or flash burn.** This kind of electrothermal injury is caused by the arcing of electric current. A person who passes close enough to a source of high-voltage current will reach a point at which the resistance of the air between the current source and the person is sufficiently low that the current arcs through the air, from the current source to the passerby. The temperature of this arc may range from 5,400°F to 36,000°F (3,000°C to 20,000°C)—high enough to produce significant charring. When a victim makes contact with a high-voltage source with a tool, the tool is sometimes vaporized, releasing heat, which leaves an imprint or shadow of the tool on the patient's body.
- **Flame burn.** This kind of thermal injury occurs when electricity ignites a person's clothing or surroundings.

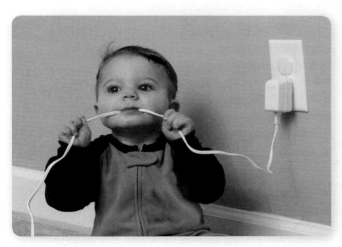

Figure 32-17 Children often sustain electrical burns.
© HKPNC/E+/Getty.

> ## Words of Wisdom
>
> TASERs use a high-voltage (50,000 volts) but low-amperage (0.003 amp) shock to cause neuromuscular incapacitation, demonstrating that even low-amperage electrical shocks can have significant effects on the nervous system.

Electrical burns are most often classified as major burns because there is a strong possibility of severe internal injury between the point of entry and the point of exit from the body. As discussed, in some cases, the electricity may flow across the chest, potentially injuring the cardiac conduction system.

Burns may be only one of the problems experienced by a patient who has come in contact with an electrical source—and not necessarily the most serious. The two most common causes of death from electrical injury are asphyxia and cardiac arrest.

- Asphyxia may occur when prolonged contact with alternating current induces tetanic contractions of the respiratory muscle. It may also result from current passing through the respiratory center in the brain and knocking out the impulse to breathe.
- Cardiac arrest may occur secondarily, from hypoxia, or as a direct result of the electrical shock. Even currents as small as 0.1 amp can trigger ventricular fibrillation if they pass directly through the heart, as when current travels across the body from hand to hand. When cardiac arrest does not occur, cardiac damage may still manifest in various rhythm disturbances on the ECG tracing.

Prompt defibrillation may have good outcomes for these patients. Follow your local protocol.

Electricity can disrupt the nervous system—just ask anyone who has been on the receiving end of a shock from a TASER. A host of neurologic complications have been reported in connection with electrical injury, including peripheral nerve deficit, seizures, delirium, confusion, coma, and temporary quadriplegia. Damage to the kidneys after electrical injury resembles the syndrome seen after a crush injury, which occurs when the breakdown products of damaged muscle (myoglobin) are liberated into the circulation. Electrical contact may affect muscle coordination and strength. Electricity that contacts the eyes may cause cataracts.

Severe, tetanic muscle spasms following contact with electricity may lead to fractures and dislocations, which are often overlooked because of the preoccupation with the electrical injury. Posterior dislocation of the shoulder and fracture of the scapula—otherwise rare injuries—have been reported in several cases of electrocution. Finally, the cervical spine may be injured, especially in a worker who has fallen from a utility pole.

All of the potential injuries that can result from an electrical injury conspire to make the victim of an electrical contact a very complex assessment challenge. Never let obvious injuries distract you from performing a complete assessment, including the neurologic, respiratory, cardiac, and musculoskeletal system assessments. In dealing with a patient who has an electrical injury, the usual priorities apply.

Assessment

The first priority at the scene of an electrical injury is to protect yourself and bystanders from becoming the next victims. Do *not* use a rope, wooden pole, or any other object to try to dislodge the patient from the current source. Do *not* try to cut the wire. Do *not* go anywhere near a high-tension line.

Many parts of the electrical grid are protected by circuit breakers that can automatically reset. When the wind blows a branch into wires or a rambunctious squirrel bridges the gap between two wires, it is desirable to have the breaker reset after a few moments to avoid power outages. As a consequence, a downed wire that "looks dead" can jump back to life, perhaps several times. There is only one safe way to deal with a downed high-tension wire: call the electric company. Wait until a qualified person has shut off the power before you approach the patient. This can be a traumatic event for paramedics, who will feel helpless waiting for the power to be shut down while a possibly critical patient lies on the ground nearby. But remember—*rescuers die in these situations*. You can help the greatest number of people by being cautious and safe in this circumstance.

Once the electrical hazard has been neutralized, assess the patient. Start cardiopulmonary resuscitation (CPR) as indicated, and attach the monitor to identify ventricular fibrillation. Open the airway using the jaw-thrust maneuver, keeping in mind the possibility of cervical spine injury. If the patient is not in cardiac arrest, dysrhythmias remain a risk, and cardiac monitoring is indicated for at least 24 hours after the injury. Make careful note of the patient's state of consciousness, and record his or her vital signs.

Try to determine which path the current took through the body by looking for entrance and exit wounds and by carefully palpating the skin and soft tissues. When deep tissues have been seriously damaged by heat, the surrounding muscle may swell and become rock-hard. Thus, a rigid abdomen or rigid extremity may indicate a serious internal injury. Be alert for fractures or dislocations, and check the distal pulses in all four extremities.

Words of Wisdom

Patients who have been shocked with a TASER will require a cardiac assessment. As soon as your patient is safe and secure, use the 3-lead ECG and pulse oximeter, and consider a 12-lead ECG as part of your secondary assessment.

Management

Management of an electrical burn injury includes prioritizing care of the patient. If the patient has life-threatening injuries, begin related care and prepare to transport the patient as soon as practical. Beyond the basics of care, fluid therapy is the most important aspect during initial care, as electrical burns cause significant fluid shifts. Another common finding in electrical burn injuries is tissue damage and a state of acidosis. If damage to the tissue is suspected based on the injury, sodium bicarbonate 1 to 2 mEq/kg should be administered with the initial fluid bolus. If protocol allows, the administration of mannitol 1 g/kg should be given to facilitate osmotic diuresis.[18]

Early administration of supplemental oxygen is helpful, as is managing the patient for impending shock.

Transport decisions should be made early and take into consideration the regional resources for the care of a patient with a major (electrical) burn. Contact medical control for advice in making a transport decision or regarding the need to use aeromedical evacuation directly to the burn center. These patients will be very anxious and scared, so be sure to talk with them calmly and explain what you are doing and how you plan to obtain the best care for them.

▶ Lightning-Related Injuries

One special case of electrical injury deserves specific mention—the injury sustained from lightning. Approximately 35 people die from lightning strikes in the United States each year.[19] Those who do not die from their injuries are left with varying degrees of disability.

Lightning strikes when a massive discharge of electricity occurs between two bodies that have different charges—for example, between a thundercloud and the ground. The stream of current takes the path of least resistance from its origin to its destination. If any object projects above the surface of the earth that is a better conductor of electricity than the air—such as a building, a light pole, an antenna, a flagpole, or a tree—that object will "attract" the lightning bolt.

A person need not sustain a direct hit from lightning to be injured; in fact, most victims are not struck directly. Much more commonly, the victim is splashed by lightning striking a nearby tree or other projecting object, resulting in an arc-type or flash burn that leaves a characteristic "feathering" pattern on the skin Figure 32-18 . Ground current produced by lightning striking the ground near the victim can also cause severe injury and accounts for incidents in which there are multiple casualties in an extended area, such as on a golf course or in an open field.

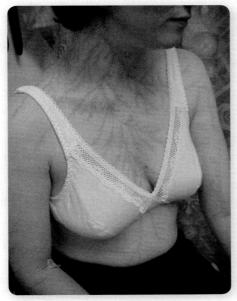

Figure 32-18 An arc-type burn resulting from a nearby lightning strike may leave a characteristic feathering pattern on the skin.
© 2007 British Association of Plastic, Reconstructive and Aesthetic Surgeons.

The best treatment for lightning injuries is prevention, and all health care professionals have a responsibility to educate the public in preventive measures. Clearly, the most effective precaution is to come in out of the storm, but that is not always possible. Bear in mind that a lightning strike may happen before or after the actual storm has passed, and it can strike up to 10 miles (16 km) away from the storm. Lightning tends to strike the tallest objects that are good conductors. The following rules can help avoid lightning injuries:

- **Rule 1: Don't be the tallest object that is a good conductor.** Stay away from the middle of fields, lakes, golf courses, and other large, open areas. If you are stuck in the middle of an open area, try to be as small as you can. Do not hold up an umbrella, golf club, or lightning rod. Do not fly a kite.
- **Rule 2: Don't stand under or near the tallest object that is a good conductor.** Although you do not want to be in the middle of the field, you also do not want to be under the tallest tree, radio antenna, or golf umbrella.
- **Rule 3: Take shelter in the most substantial structure that you can to remain safe if it is hit by lightning.** A large building with a lightning suppression system is the best choice. An enclosed building is better than an open one (eg, shed, lean-to). Close the shelter as much as possible. If in a vehicle, keep the windows rolled up. Lightning tends to flash over the outside of objects (and people). It can travel substantial distances through conductors, however.
- **Rule 4: Avoid touching good conductors during a lightning storm.** Examples of good conductors include plumbing fixtures, fences, and electrical appliances, particularly those connected to wires outside (eg, telephone, TV, computer).

Lightning carries enormous electrical power. Its energy can reach 100 *million* volts, and peak currents can be in the range of 200,000 amps. Unlike other high-voltage electric current, the electricity from lightning is *direct*—not alternating—current, and the duration of exposure is measured in milliseconds. Thus, lightning injuries tend to resemble blast injuries more than they do high-voltage injuries, with damage occurring to the tympanic membranes of the ears and air-containing internal organs. Many reports of lightning strikes indicate victims' clothes were "blown off" of their bodies. Muscle damage may occur, and the release of myoglobin from injured muscle may jeopardize the kidneys.

For the cardiovascular system, lightning acts as a cosmic defibrillator, delivering a massive direct-current countershock that depolarizes the entire heart. The heart may resume beating spontaneously shortly after the shock or after 5 cycles (30:2) or approximately 2 minutes of CPR that is started immediately. Because respiratory arrest is apt to persist in patients who have been struck by lightning, continued ventilatory support may be required. The phenomenon of someone regaining a pulse after a lightning strike and having respiratory arrest is known to lead to a secondary cardiac arrest if left untreated. The central nervous system is almost invariably affected by a lightning strike. Temporary paralysis of the legs has occurred, and permanent paralysis and quadriplegia have been reported in a few cases.

Despite the unique circumstances surrounding a lightning strike, the immediate threats to life are the same as those caused by a high-voltage power line injury: airway obstruction, respiratory arrest, and cardiac arrest.

Assessment

When you reach the scene of a lightning strike, all the usual priorities apply, but there are two special considerations to keep in mind.

First, if the electrical storm is ongoing, your first priority is to get any patients and rescuers to a safe place, preferably indoors, or at least inside the ambulance. Lightning *can* strike twice in the same place. Note that touching the victim of a lightning strike is not hazardous; contrary to what your grandmother may have told you, electricity does not remain within the body of a person who has been hit by lightning.

Words of Wisdom

In a lightning strike with multiple victims, priority goes to the victims who are not breathing.

Second, be aware that a lightning strike is apt to injure more than one person. Therefore, the first thing you need to do on arrival at the scene—before you leave the safety of the ambulance—is to perform a rapid size-up of the entire scene to determine the number of patients.

Start CPR when necessary. Carry out the primary survey as usual. When establishing an airway, bear in mind the possibility of cervical spine injury, and do not hyperextend the neck; instead, use the jaw-thrust maneuver.

Patients with cardiac arrest caused by a lightning strike deserve aggressive, continuing CPR. The chances of a successful resuscitation in such a case are good, even when the patient appears beyond help initially and even when there is a long delay in the return of spontaneous breathing. Minimize the interruption in compressions, and push hard and fast with full chest recoil!

Words of Wisdom

Do not give up quickly on a patient in cardiac arrest due to a lightning strike.

Management

Treatment of lightning injuries is similar to that of injuries sustained from high-voltage lines:

- Make sure the scene is safe. Move the victim to a safer location if necessary.
- Priority for treatment goes to patients who are not breathing.
- Perform CPR as needed. Establish an airway, and take cervical spine precautions.
- Administer supplemental oxygen.
- Monitor cardiac rhythm.
- Insert an 18-gauge IV catheter and run in lactated Ringer solution wide open to keep the kidneys flushed out.
- Cover any surface burns with dry, clean dressings.
- Splint fractures.
- If the patient has fallen, immobilize the cervical spine.

▶ Radiation Burns

Radiation exposure has become more than a theoretical issue as use of radioactive materials increases in industry and medicine, and you must understand it to function effectively in the prehospital arena. Between 1944 and 2010, there were more than 400 radiation accidents worldwide involving significant radiation exposure to more than 3,000 people.[20] More recent events in Japan (the earthquake-triggered tsunami that damaged the Fukushima Daiichi Nuclear Power Plant in March 2011) highlight that radiation accidents continue to be a threat. Other potential threats include incidents related to the use and transportation of radioactive isotopes and intentionally released radioactivity in terrorist attacks. To be effective in treating patients with radiation exposure, you must first suspect radiation and attempt to determine whether ongoing exposure exists. Increasingly, special response units are equipped with pager-sized radiation detectors, or such detection may be provided by other public safety services.

There are three types of ionizing radiation: alpha, beta, and gamma. Alpha particles have little penetrating energy and are easily stopped by the skin. Beta particles have greater penetrating power and can travel much farther in air than alpha particles do. They can penetrate the skin but can be blocked by simple protective clothing designed for this purpose. The threat from gamma radiation is directly proportional to its wavelength. This type of radiation is very penetrating and easily passes through the body and solid materials. Protection from gamma radiation requires either several inches of lead or concrete to prevent penetration.

Radiation is measured in units of radiation equivalent in man (rem) or radiation-absorbed dose (rad).[21] The gray (Gy) is the unit of measure in the International System of Units. One hundred rad equals 1 Gy. Small amounts of everyday background radiation are measured in rads; the amount of radiation released in a major incident may be measured in grays. The average human exposure from natural background radiation is 0.31 rem (310 millirem [mrem]) per year.[22] Mild radiation exposure is considered 1 to 2 Gy (100 to 200 rad), moderate exposure is 2 to 6 Gy (200 to 600 rad), and severe exposure is 6 to 9 Gy (600 to 900 rad). Exposure to more than 10 Gy (1,000 rad) is very severe and rapidly fatal.[23] Keep in mind that this exposure level refers to a total-body dose. For example, radiation therapy is a common treatment for cancer and may expose a very specific part of the body (the tumor) to 8 or 10 Gy of radiation over the course of several treatments.

The vast majority of ionizing radiation accidents involve gamma radiation, or x-rays. People who have suffered a radiation exposure generally pose no risk to the people around them. However, in some types of incidents—particularly those involving explosions—patients may be contaminated with radioactive particulate matter. It is speculated that after a nuclear explosion, most patients will have sustained some type of trauma in addition to the radiation exposure.

Acute Radiation Syndrome

Acute radiation syndrome (ARS), or radiation sickness, is a serious illness that occurs when a person is exposed to very high levels of radiation in a brief period. ARS causes hematologic, central nervous system, and gastrointestinal changes. Many of these changes occur over time and so will not be apparent during contact with EMS providers. The amount of radiation and the duration of exposure will affect how rapidly signs and symptoms present. The onset of vomiting soon after exposure is a predictor of poor outcomes. Consider this fact when triaging patients or considering the risks of entering a high-radiation environment to attempt rescue.

Radiation Contact Burns

A person who handles a radioactive source briefly may sustain a local soft-tissue injury without experiencing much total-body irradiation. This scenario might arise, for example, in a crash involving a vehicle transporting radioactive material or after the detonation of a "dirty bomb." The injury's appearance could range from a superficial sunburn to a chemical burn. Although chemical burns usually become apparent almost immediately after exposure, radiation burns could appear hours or even days after exposure.

Assessment

First and foremost, the assessment of a patient who may have been exposed to radiation involves a scene size-up to determine whether the scene is safe for you to enter. Determine which protective gear you will need to shield yourself from the radiation before you enter the scene **Figure 32-19** . In most cases, it will be appropriate to contact the hazardous materials response team so they may identify the appropriate precautions, including exposure-limiting suits and the most appropriate ED for

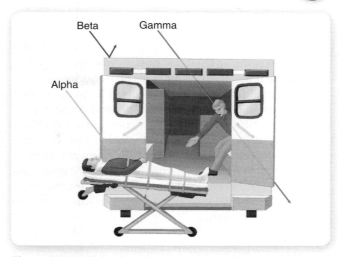

Figure 32-19 Alpha, beta, and gamma radiation shielding.
© Jones & Bartlett Learning.

the patient's treatment. Not all EDs are set up to treat a patient who has been exposed to radiation, so learn the capabilities of your hospitals before an incident occurs! EMS agencies that operate in an area where there is a nuclear power plant or other research facility typically have additional training offered by the facility and regularly practice responding to radiation-related emergencies.

Once the scene is deemed safe, you may proceed with the primary survey of the patient. Assess the patient's ABCDEs, and then prioritize the patient's care. Unfortunately, patients who have sustained significant radiation exposure and a major burn are unlikely to survive, even with major resources expended to keep them alive. A burn over more than 70% of the TBSA is probably fatal by itself; a burn and radiation that together affect more than 30% of the TBSA are probably fatal. When confronted with large numbers of patients who have been exposed to radiation and simultaneously received thermal burns, keep this 30% rule in mind when triaging and making transport decisions. Of course, you should also consult with medical control in these complicated cases. In the field, it is difficult to determine the extent of the patient's internal injuries.

Management

Patients with radiation burns may be contaminated with radioactive material, so they should be decontaminated before transport. The majority of contaminants can be removed by simply disrobing the patient.

Irrigate open wounds. Washing should be gentle to avoid further damage to the skin, which could result in additional internal radiation absorption. The head and scalp should be irrigated the same way. The ED should be notified as soon as practical if you are transporting a potentially contaminated patient. In contrast with other types of contamination, radioactive particulate matter probably poses a relatively small risk to the provider. Consider providing basic care to the patient before undertaking the patient's decontamination if you are wearing protective clothing.

With contact radiation burns, decontaminate the wound as if it were a chemical burn to remove any radioactive particulate matter. You may then treat it as a burn.

Many radioactive isotopes are used in medicine and industry, some of which can be absorbed or have their toxic effects blunted by another substance. Like their radioactive effects, the toxic effects of these isotopes vary. Antidotes may help bind an isotope, enhance its elimination from the body, or reduce the toxic effects on other organs. Such antidotal therapy should be considered only under the guidance of a knowledgeable physician or public health agency.

Potassium iodide is distributed to people who live near a nuclear power plant and may help protect the thyroid gland against the harmful effects of a release from the plant if taken within 6 hours of exposure. Contrary to popular belief, however, this antidote is effective only for radionuclides released from fission products from nuclear power plants and would be of little value for exposure to medical radiation.

Radiation injury follows the "inverse square law": exposure drops exponentially as distance from the source increases. Increasing your (and your patient's) distance from the source by even a few feet may dramatically decrease your exposure, so it is important to identify the radioactive source and the length of the patient's exposure to it. You must try to limit your duration of exposure, increase your distance from the source, and attempt to place shielding between yourself and sources of gamma radiation.

■ Management of Burns in Pediatric Patients

Escaping from a fire can be difficult for children. Although the percentage of fatal outcomes for children younger than 5 years involved in a house fire fell from 18% in 1980 to 6% in 2011,[24] research suggests that young children are not as effectively awakened by smoke detectors, and they are often disoriented immediately after waking. Young children are also more likely to sustain severe scald injuries. Children's thin skin and delicate respiratory structures are more easily damaged by thermal insults than are those of older children and adults.

In children, fluid resuscitation may be more challenging because of their increased body surface–to–weight ratio. As a consequence, children may require more fluid per kilogram compared to adults. You may start by providing fluids based on the Consensus formula in children only to find that medical control orders additional fluids for major burns. Also, because of their relatively poor glycogen stores, children may require dextrose-containing solutions earlier than adults do. Blood glucose monitoring should be routinely performed in seriously burned children.

Burns may raise the suspicion of child abuse. Pay careful attention to the MOI, and relay this information to the hospital staff.

■ Management of Burns in Geriatric Patients

Approximately 1,300 older adults die of fire-related causes each year, which represents a 2.6 times greater likelihood of fire-related deaths in this population as compared to the general population.[25] A significant percentage of older adults smoke (more than 8% of US adults older than age 65 years smoke cigarettes[26]), and smoking is the leading cause of fires that lead to death of older adults. Burns from fires caused by smoking while wearing a supplementary oxygen supply are the leading sentinel event in home care. Cooking fires represent another distinct hazard to older adults, who may be less able to smell a gas leak or a fire in the kitchen. Older adult patients are also particularly sensitive to respiratory insults. Relatively small fires can produce toxic fumes before detection or suppression devices are activated.

Older adult patients may also have poor glycogen stores, so their blood glucose levels should be checked to assess for hypoglycemia. Cardiac monitoring should, of course, be implemented. Although fluid resuscitation is important, pulmonary edema is more likely to develop in older patients. Routinely assess lung sounds in older adults who have burns.

■ Long-Term Consequences of Burns

▶ The Patient

Serious burn injuries are devastating events that leave patients with long-term physical and psychologic challenges. People with major injuries average about 1 day of inpatient treatment for each 1% of the TBSA burned. Extensive rehabilitation may also be necessary to regain function. Survivors of serious burns are left with a host of long-term consequences, including problems with thermoregulation, motor function, and sensory function. Although tremendous improvements in the care of critical burn patients have made long-term survival possible for many who would have died of their injuries one decade ago, large surface area burns remain a serious care challenge on par with other forms of severe multisystem trauma.

▶ The Provider

Caring for patients with major burn emergencies can be one of the most horrifying tasks undertaken by paramedics. Fire scenes are chaotic and dangerous. Patients are often in severe pain. The smell of burned hair and flesh permeates your clothes and equipment. Sheets of tissue may peel off the patient when you perform simple tasks like attempting to take vital signs or moving the patient. Despite the traumatic circumstances, with the proper training and the right mix of confidence and courage, you can make a tremendous impact in the treatment and overall survival of burn patients.

YOU are the Paramedic SUMMARY

1. Your next steps should include which actions?

Continue with the patient assessment. It is up to you, the paramedic, to stay on track so that significant injuries will not be overlooked.

2. Based on just the information given so far, would this patient's transport be low or high priority at this time?

High priority. Airway burns—in this case, inhalation of superheated gases (steam)—can cause serious damage in both the upper and the lower airways.

3. The patient is clearly experiencing significant pain. At which point in treatment should this condition be addressed?

While pain is significant, the primary concern is first to identify and correct life threats. Inhalation burns can cause rapid and serious airway compromise. Although this patient is breathing without difficulty, his reddened face and neck, as well as the raspiness of his voice, indicate the potential for a sudden airway compromise that the paramedic must be ready to aggressively manage with advanced airway techniques and sedation if necessary.

4. How significant is the patient's apparent raspiness as he is speaking to you?

The raspy voice is a red flag that should alert you and your partner that the airway has been injured. Be alert for other developments such as stridor, wheezes, and poor oxygen saturation.

5. What is the likely cause of the patient's elevated blood pressure?

Severe and acute pain leads to increased sympathetic nerve activity and subsequent increased peripheral vascular resistance.

6. At which point might you consider aggressive airway management including sedation and intubation?

Based on the MOI, you should be prepared to perform rapid intubation at any time. The burns on the patient's face and neck are good indications that a significant airway burn may have occurred. Heat can be an irritant to the lungs, and you need to be alert for development of wheezing, coughing, stridor, and other indicators of swelling of airway structures.

7. With regard to the patient's respiratory status, what changes should you be particularly alert for en route to the hospital?

The patient was just given fentanyl to help control pain. Fentanyl acts on the central nervous system and is a respiratory depressant. You must also be alert for the development of airway swelling because of the burns.

8. Explain the steps you would take to identify the cause of a change in respiratory status, and explain how you would correct the problem.

The differences between respiratory difficulty from a central nervous system depressant and respiratory difficulty from airway burns should be fairly clear. If adventitious sounds, such as wheezing or stridor, is absent, the respiratory difficulty is unlikely to be due to burns. To treat such a condition, small doses of naloxone are indicated. Conversely, difficulty breathing with an absence of sounds may be due to external injury. The patient's burns on the neck may be causing a circumferential swelling that may not involve the inner airway, so no abnormal sounds may be heard. Another possibility is that the back of the ambulance is too noisy to hear lung sound changes. In the case in which airway swelling is visible or sounds such as stridor are audible, immediate and aggressive airway management is needed. This patient is most likely experiencing airway compromise due to burns; airway management using a bag-mask device followed by intubation is indicated.

YOU are the Paramedic **SUMMARY** (continued)

EMS Patient Care Report (PCR)

Date: 09-02-18	**Incident No.:** 0930	**Nature of Call:** Man burned		**Location:** 457 Main Blvd. in gas station	
Dispatched: 1530	**En Route:** 1531	**At Scene:** 1534	**Transport:** 1540	**At Hospital:** 1550	**In Service:** 1610

Patient Information

Age: 22 **Sex:** M **Weight (in kg [lb]):** 70 kg (154 lb)	**Allergies:** No known medication allergies **Medications:** Denies **Past Medical History:** Denies **Chief Complaint:** "My arm is burned and it hurts."

Vital Signs

Time: 1539	**BP:** 160/110	**Pulse:** 120, strong, regular	**Respirations:** 22	**Spo$_2$:** 98% NRM
Time: 1543	**BP:** 150/100	**Pulse:** 110, strong radial pulses	**Respirations:** 18	**Spo$_2$:** 98% NRM

EMS Treatment (circle all that apply)

Oxygen @ __15__ **L/min via (circle one):** NC (NRM) **Bag-mask device**		**Assisted Ventilation**	**Airway Adjunct**	**CPR**
Defibrillation	**Bleeding Control**	(**Bandaging:** Clean dressings)	**Splinting**	(**Other:** IV with pain medication)

Narrative

9-1-1 dispatched to a report of a man burned at a gas station. Upon arrival, 22-year-old man found standing at gas station, alert and oriented, and reporting severe pain as indicated by facial grimace and agitation. Gas station owner reports seeing pt drive in to gas station with what appeared to be an overheating car radiator. The pt got out and opened the hood; owner states that he heard him scream and saw large plumes of steam coming from under the opened hood.

Pt walked over to ambulance as we arrived and was able to speak comfortably in complete sentences, although his voice seemed raspy. Initially, he denied any difficulty breathing and reported only pain in right arm. Slight swelling of lips noted. Pt has first-degree burns over face, lips, and anterior neck. Lung sounds are equal and clear. Right forearm (palmar surface) has blistering and redness. Distal (radial) pulse present and strong. Capillary nailbed refill of injured arm is <2 seconds.

Prior to transport, pt given IV fentanyl at 1539 hours. Pt stated decreased pain, reporting an initial pain scale rating of 10/10; after fentanyl, 4/10. ECG monitored en route with sinus tachycardia. Pt delivered to Mercy Hospital and turned over in ED to Dr. Anthony. Return to service at 1610 hours.**End of report**

Prep Kit

▶ Ready for Review

- Although you probably will not see significant burns on a daily basis, you will encounter some serious burn injuries during your career.
- The skin has four functions: to protect the underlying tissue from the environment, to regulate temperature and fluid, to act as a sense organ, and to aid in healing by responding to injury with inflammation.
- Burns are diffuse soft-tissue injuries created from destructive energy transferred via thermal, electrical, or radiation energy.
- Significant burn damage to the skin may make the body vulnerable to bacterial invasion, temperature instability, and major disturbances of fluid balance resulting in burn shock.
- Beyond the visible soft-tissue injury, burns can affect the cardiovascular, respiratory, renal, gastrointestinal, hematologic, and endocrine systems. The most important systemic response to significant burn trauma is burn shock.
- When burn shock occurs, intravascular fluid leaks from capillaries and enters into the interstitial spaces. Cells take in increased amounts of salt and water from the fluid around them. As with other types of shock, the body's ability to distribute oxygen and glucose is hampered. Adequate fluid resuscitation is essential treatment.
- Thermal burns include flame, scald, contact, steam, and flash burns.
- Jackson's thermal wound theory outlines three pathologic progressions of burns: zone of coagulation, zone of stasis, and zone of hyperemia.
- Burn wounds of the skin may be superficial, partial thickness, or full thickness.
- A superficial burn involves only the epidermis, with the skin appearing red and swollen.
- A partial-thickness burn involves the epidermis and part of the dermis. Moderate partial-thickness burns usually are blistered, red, and extremely painful. Deep partial-thickness burns damage the hair follicle and sweat and sebaceous glands.
- A full-thickness burn destroys the epidermis, the dermis, and the basement membrane of the dermis. After this type of burn, skin will not regenerate. Such a burn may appear white and waxy, brown and leathery, or charred.
- Inhalation burns may cause rapid airway compromise when heat and/or toxic chemicals enter the airway and lungs. Signs of irritation include coughing, wheezing, and possible stridor, signifying airway swelling. Carbon monoxide intoxication is also a concern.
- Establishing scene safety should be your first priority in responding to a burn call. Significant threats are likely to remain at the scene of a fire, chemical spill, electrical burn incident, lightning strike, or radiation leak.
- The many types of burns, coupled with the many possible presentations of burn patients, can challenge your assessment skills. Address a burned patient in a consistent, efficient, and systematic manner so you do not develop tunnel vision for the major burn trauma and miss other occult injuries that could affect the patient's outcome.
- Once the ABCDEs are addressed, assess the total body surface area burned, using the rule of palms, rule of nines, or Lund-Browder chart. This is an important step because the extent of the burn relates to the need for transport to a burn unit. Most practitioners advocate counting only the areas of partial- and full-thickness burns (ignoring the areas of superficial burns). When using the rule of nines, different rules apply for infants, children, and older adults.
- The three cornerstones of the emergency medical care of burns are airway management, with the potential need for field intubation; fluid resuscitation to prevent shock; and pain management. Cooling and sterile bandaging are indicated for certain thermal burns. Chemical burns of the skin or eyes generally require copious flushing with water, with certain exceptions.
- Many burn patients will ultimately require intubation, even if during their initial presentation they were able to talk to you. Patients who are in cardiac or respiratory arrest, or whose airways are rapidly swelling, will need field intubation. A deteriorating airway may or may not require field intubation. A patient whose airway is currently patent, but who has a history consistent with risk factors for airway compromise, may or may not need field intubation. Be careful not to do anything to suppress respiratory drive in these patients.
- Patients with burns to more than 20% of their total body surface area will need fluid resuscitation. It is important to give the correct amount of fluid; too much fluid may be as bad as too little. If fluid resuscitation is delayed more than 2 hours from the time of the burn in patients with major burns, resuscitation is complicated and mortality increases. Deliver an appropriate amount of fluid to the burn patient as soon as is reasonable.

Prep Kit (continued)

- The Consensus formula is an equation used to determine the amount of fluid that a burned patient will need during the first 24 hours. Only a small portion of this time will occur in the prehospital environment. Half of the fluid amount must be given during the first 8 hours; the remainder is given over the remaining 16 hours in the 24-hour period.
- Assess the patient's pain using a 0 to 10 scale before administering analgesia. Reassessment should be completed using the same pain scale every 5 minutes. In any patient with burns, pain medication is best given via the IV route. Narcotic analgesics should be administered judiciously.
- Chemical burns may affect the skin, eyes, or airway. Alkali burns are especially devastating. To remove chemical solutions from the skin, implement copious flushing with water; management of powders requires brushing off as much of the substance as possible before washing. If chemicals have entered the eye, flush the eyes with copious amounts of water, and possibly remove the patient's contact lenses. Consider use of a Morgan lens.
- In cases of electrical burn, electric current is converted to heat as it travels through the body, causing extensive damage. Electrical burns generally leave two wounds, an entrance wound and a much larger exit wound. Assessment of electrical injuries includes first ensuring scene safety, then beginning CPR if indicated. Management includes treating life-threatening injuries and potential shock.
- Most radiation burns are caused by gamma radiation, or x-rays. Assessment should begin by addressing scene safety concerns. Management then involves decontamination, irrigation, washing, possibly antidote administration, and transport.
- Compared to other patient populations, pediatric patients can be more readily harmed by thermal injuries, and fluid resuscitation in this population may be more challenging. Children may require dextrose-containing solutions earlier than adults will; consequently, you should perform blood glucose monitoring routinely in seriously ill children. Pay careful attention to mechanism of injury, as some burns may raise the suspicion of child abuse.
- Older adult patients are also particularly sensitive to respiratory insults. They may have poor glycogen stores, so check their blood glucose levels for hypoglycemia. Perform cardiac monitoring. Watch for pulmonary edema if performing fluid resuscitation.

▶ Vital Vocabulary

acute radiation syndrome The clinical course that usually begins within hours of exposure to a radiation source. Symptoms include nausea, vomiting, diarrhea, fatigue, fever, and headache. The long-term symptoms are dose related and are hematopoietic and gastrointestinal in nature.

circumferential burn A burn on the neck or chest, which may compress the airway, or on an extremity, which might act like a tourniquet.

coagulation necrosis Cell death typically caused by ischemia or infarction.

collagen A protein that gives tensile strength to the connective tissues of the body.

Consensus formula A formula that recommends giving 2–4 mL of lactated Ringer solution for each kilogram of body weight, multiplied by the percentage of total body surface area burned; sometimes used to calculate fluid needs during lengthy transport times; formerly called the Parkland formula.

contact burn A burn produced by touching a hot object.

dermis The inner layer of skin containing hair follicle roots, glands, blood vessels, and nerves.

elastin A protein that gives the skin its elasticity.

epidermis The outermost layer of the skin.

escharotomy A surgical cut through the eschar or leathery covering of a burn injury to allow for swelling and minimize the potential for development of compartment syndrome in a circumferentially burned limb or the thorax.

flame burn A thermal burn caused by flames touching the skin.

flash burn An electrothermal injury caused by arcing of electric current.

full-thickness burn A burn that extends through the epidermis and dermis into the subcutaneous tissues beneath; previously called a third-degree burn.

homeostasis A tendency to constancy or stability in the body's internal environment.

hypovolemic shock Also referred to as *burn shock*, the shock or hypoperfusion caused by a burn injury and the tremendous loss of fluids; capillaries leak, resulting in intravascular fluid volume oozing out of the circulation and into the interstitial spaces, and cells take in increased amounts of salt and water.

integument The skin.

Prep Kit (continued)

Joule's law A description of the relationship between heat production, current, and resistance.

liquefaction necrosis A form of necrosis that results from the transformation of tissue into a liquid viscous mass (pus).

Lund-Browder chart A detailed version of the rule of nines chart that takes into consideration the changes in total body surface area that occur with growth.

mucopolysaccharide gel One of the complex materials found, along with the collagen fibers and elastin fibers, in the dermis of the skin.

Ohm's law The formula that describes the relationship between voltage and resistance: Current (I) = Voltage (V) divided by Resistance (R).

partial-thickness burn A burn that involves the epidermis and part of the dermis, characterized by pain and blistering; previously called a second-degree burn.

rule of nines A system that assigns percentages to sections of the body, allowing for calculation of the amount of total body surface area burned.

rule of palms A system that estimates the total body surface area burned by comparing the affected area with the size of the patient's palm, which is roughly equal to 1% of the patient's total body surface area; also called rule of ones.

scald burn A burn produced by hot liquids.

steam burn A burn that has been caused by direct exposure to hot steam exhaust, as from a broken pipe.

subglottic Located below the glottic opening, as in the lower airway structures.

superficial burn A burn involving only the epidermis, which produces very red, painful skin; previously called a first-degree burn.

supraglottic Located above the glottic opening, as in the upper airway structures.

thermal burn An injury caused by radiation or direct contact with a heat source on the skin.

zone of coagulation The reddened area surrounding the leathery and sometimes charred tissue that has sustained a full-thickness burn.

zone of hyperemia In a thermal burn, the area that is least affected by the burn injury; an area of increased blood flow where the body is attempting to repair injured but otherwise viable tissue.

zone of stasis The peripheral area surrounding the zone of coagulation that has decreased blood flow and inflammation; it can undergo necrosis within 24 to 48 hours after the injury, particularly if perfusion is compromised due to burn shock.

► References

1. Centers for Disease Control and Prevention. Trauma statistics. National Trauma Institute website. http://nationaltraumainstitute.org/home/trauma_statistics.html. Updated February 2014. Accessed April 12, 2017.

2. Burn incidence and treatment in the United States: 2016. American Burn Association website. http://www.ameriburn.org/resources_factsheet.php. Accessed April 20, 2017.

3. Alvi T, Assad F, Aurangzeb Malik MA. Anxiety and depressions in burn patients. *J Ayub Med Coll Abbottabad*. 2009;21(1):137-141.

4. Safety facts on scald burns. Burn Foundation website. http://www.burnfoundation.org/programs/resource.cfm?c=1&a=3. Accessed April 12, 2017.

5. Hall JR. Fatal effects of fire. National Fire Protection Association website. http://www.nfpa.org/news-and-research/fire-statistics-and-reports/fire-statistics/demographics-and-victim-patterns/fatal-effects-of-fire. Published March 2011. Accessed April 12, 2017.

6. Hydrogen cyanide (AC): systemic agent. Centers for Disease Control and Prevention website. https://www.cdc.gov/niosh/ershdb/emergencyresponsecard_29750038.html. Updated June 1, 2015. Accessed April 13, 2017.

7. Hyperbaric oxygen therapy for carbon monoxide poisoning. Cigna website. https://www.cigna.com/healthwellness/hw/medical-topics/hyperbaric-oxygen-therapy-for-carbon-monoxide-hw193681. Accessed April 10, 2017.

8. Wachtel TL, Berry CC, Wachtel EE, Frank HA. The inter-rater reliability of estimating the size of burns from various burn area chart drawings. *Burns*. 2000;26(2):156.

9. Lund CC, Browder NC. The estimation of areas of burns. *Surg Gynecol Obstet*. 1944;79:352.

10. American Burn Association. Burn center referral criteria. http://www.ameriburn.org/BurnCenterReferralCriteria.pdf. Accessed March 16, 2017.

11. Rice PL, Orgill DP. Emergency care of moderate and severe thermal burns in adults. https://www.uptodate.com/contents/emergency-care-of-moderate-and-severe-thermal-burns-in-adults. Updated January 2017. Accessed April 12, 2017.

12. Atiyeh BS, Dibo SA, Ibrahim AE, Zgheib ER. Acute burn resuscitation and fluid creep: it is time for

Prep Kit (continued)

colloid rehabilitation. *Ann Burns Fire Disasters.* 2012;25(2):59-65. Published June 2012. https://www.ncbi.nlm.nih.gov/pmc/articles/PMC3506208/. Accessed April 12, 2017.

13. Barry JD. A randomized controlled trial comparing treatment regimens for acute pain for topical oleoresin capsaicin (pepper spray) exposure in adult volunteers. *Prehosp Emerg Care.* 2008;12(4):432-437.

14. American Burn Association. Electrical safety educator's guide. http://www.ameriburn.org/Preven /ElectricalSafetyEducator'sGuide.pdf. Accessed April 12, 2017.

15. Daley BJ. Electrical injuries. http://emedicine. medscape.com/article/433682-overview#a10. Updated February 8, 2017. Accessed April 12, 2017.

16. Associated Press. Justice Department to review TASER deaths. Parker Waichman Alonso LLP website. Published June 14, 2006. Accessed April 12, 2017.

17. Fire is a possibility when using alcohol-based pepper spray with Tasers. Police One website. https://www.policeone.com/police-products/less -lethal/articles/92573-Fire-is-a-Possibility-When -Using-Alcohol-Based-Pepper-Spray-With-Tasers/. Published October 5, 2004. Accessed April 12, 2017.

18. Daley BJ. Electrical injuries treatment and management. http://emedicine.medscape.com /article/433682-treatment. Updated February 8, 2017. Accessed April 13, 2017.

19. Lightning. Centers for Disease Control and Prevention website. https://www.cdc.gov/disasters /lightning/. Updated February 16, 2014. Accessed April 12, 2017.

20. Turai I, Veress K. Radiation accidents: occurrence, types, consequences, medical management, and the lessons to be learned. *Cent Eur J Occup Environ Med.* 2001;7(1):3-14.

21. Rad (radiation absorbed dose). United States Nuclear Regulatory Commission website. https://www.nrc.gov/reading-rm/basic-ref/glossary/rad -radiation-absorbed-dose.html. Updated April 10, 2017. Accessed April 12, 2017.

22. Doses in our daily lives. United States Nuclear Regulatory Commission website. https://www.nrc .gov/about-nrc/radiation/around-us/doses-daily -lives.html. Updated August 30, 2016. Accessed April 12, 2017.

23. Mayo Clinic staff. Radiation sickness: symptoms. Mayo Clinic website. http://www.mayoclinic.org /diseases-conditions/radiation-sickness/basics /symptoms/con-20022901. Published September 19, 2015. Accessed April 12, 2017.

24. Ahrens M. Characteristics of home fire victims. National Fire Protection Association website. http:// www.nfpa.org/news-and-research/fire-statistics -and-reports/fire-statistics/demographics-and -victim-patterns/characteristics-of-home-fire-victims. Published October 2014. Accessed April 12, 2017.

25. US fire deaths, fire death rates, and risk of dying in a fire. US Fire Administration website. https://www .usfa.fema.gov/data/statistics/fire_death_rates.html. Accessed April 12, 2017.

26. Current cigarette smoking among adults in the United States. Centers for Disease Control and Prevention website. https://www.cdc.gov/tobacco /data_statistics/fact_sheets/adult_data /cig_smoking/. Updated December 1, 2016. Accessed April 12, 2017.

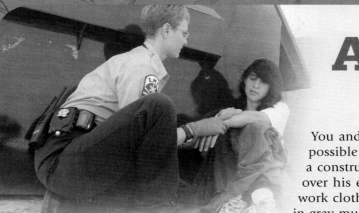

Assessment in Action

You and your partner are dispatched to a patient with possible burns at a construction site. Upon your arrival, a construction worker rapidly leads a man with a cloth over his eyes to the ambulance. The patient is wearing work clothes and heavy boots that appear to be covered in gray mud. He is alert and oriented and readily answers all of your questions appropriately. He tells you that he was working with a special type of concrete—"the kind that sets real fast"—and some splashed into his eyes. His coworker tells you that the pH of the concrete is "very high" and that the concrete "causes nasty burns." The patient removes the cloth from his eyes as he climbs into the ambulance, and you see that his eyes are red, swollen, and tearing with spillover onto his face. He is alert, is breathing adequately with no respiratory compromise, and has no visible skin breaks or bleeding. He denies any other injuries.

1. The coworker tells you that the pH of the substance in the patient's eyes is "somewhere around 13 or so." Immediate treatment should include:

   A. rapid transport to the hospital.
   B. a secondary assessment.
   C. keeping the patient sitting up and flushing his eyes for 30 minutes before transport and while en route.
   D. keeping the patient flat and flushing his eyes for 30 minutes before transport and while en route.

2. Which of the following concurrent situations requires that you take immediate action?

   A. The presence of cataracts
   B. The presence of contact lenses
   C. Blindness in one eye due to an old injury
   D. Recent laser surgery on one of the eyes

3. Your partner hands you a small bottle of eyedrops to numb the patient's eyes. You should:

   A. use them primarily to reduce the pain.
   B. not use them since numbness will mask the extent of injury.
   C. use them to help the patient keep his eyes open.
   D. not use them since you will be holding the patient's eyes open.

4. While irrigating his eyes, you notice that the patient has dried concrete specks on his cheeks and forehead. You should:

   A. remove them from the skin while wearing gloves and flush the skin for 30 minutes.
   B. leave them in place but continue to irrigate the skin for 30 minutes.
   C. do nothing, as they are probably harmless.
   D. make a note of this finding on the patient report and get to it when you can.

5. Following copious irrigation, the patient should first be questioned and examined for:

   A. visual acuity and any vision changes.
   B. redness.
   C. pupillary reaction.
   D. the presence of pain.

Assessment *in Action* (continued)

6. Following delivery of this patient to the ED, you and your partner return to the ambulance. You notice clumps of gray grit and dirt on the floor of the ambulance. The stretcher bar and the overhead rail both have concrete dried on them from the patient's gloved hands. Before going back into service, you should:

   A. sweep the ambulance and wipe away any debris.
   B. clean the ambulance and decontaminate it before returning to service.
   C. wipe the stretcher and overhead bar, not concerning yourself with the floor.
   D. return the ambulance to the station so it can be inspected by your supervisor.

7. Which agent in the concrete is MOST likely the cause of the burning sensation?

   A. Sodium
   B. Lime
   C. Sand
   D. Calcium chloride

8. What are the four phases of definitive burn care?

9. Many construction sites have chemicals unique to the work being performed. When dealing with an injury related to chemical exposure, what are some important considerations?

10. What are some of the similarities between radiation burns and electrical burns?

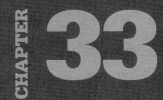
Face and Neck Trauma

National EMS Education Standard Competencies

Trauma

Integrates assessment findings with principles of epidemiology and pathophysiology to formulate a field impression to implement a comprehensive treatment/disposition plan for an acutely injured patient.

Head, Facial, Neck, and Spine Trauma

Recognition and management of
> Life threats (pp 1680-1681)
> Spine trauma (p 1704, and see Chapter 34, *Head and Spine Trauma*)

Pathophysiology, assessment, and management of
> Penetrating neck trauma (pp 1699-1703)
> Laryngotracheal injuries (pp 1699-1703)
> Spine trauma
  • Dislocations/subluxations (see Chapter 34, *Head and Spine Trauma*)
  • Fractures (see Chapter 34, *Head and Spine Trauma*)
  • Sprains/strains (see Chapter 34, *Head and Spine Trauma*)
> Facial fractures (pp 1684-1688)
> Skull fractures (see Chapter 34, *Head and Spine Trauma*)
> Foreign bodies in the eyes (pp 1688-1689, 1692-1694)
> Dental trauma (pp 1698-1699)
> Unstable facial fractures (pp 1684-1688)
> Orbital fractures (pp 1684-1687)
> Perforated tympanic membrane (pp 1697-1698)
> Mandibular fractures (pp 1684, 1686-1687)

Knowledge Objectives

1. Discuss the anatomy and physiology of the head, face, and neck, including major structures and specific important landmarks. (pp 1677-1680)
2. Describe the factors that may cause obstruction of the upper airway following a facial injury. (p 1680)
3. Discuss the general patient assessment process for a patient with a face or neck injury. (pp 1680-1683)
4. Discuss general emergency care of a patient with a face or neck injury, including the importance of airway management. (p 1683)
5. Discuss different types of facial injuries, including soft-tissue injuries, maxillary fractures, nasal fractures, mandibular fractures, orbital fractures, and zygomatic fractures, and patient care considerations related to each one. (pp 1683-1686)
6. Describe the process of providing emergency care to a patient who has sustained face and neck injuries, including assessment of the patient, review of signs and symptoms, and management of care. (pp 1686-1688)
7. Describe the management of a patient who has a foreign body in the throat. (p 1687)
8. List the steps in the emergency medical care of the patient with soft-tissue wounds of the face and neck. (p 1687)
9. Discuss different types of eye injuries, including lacerations, corneal abrasion, foreign bodies, impaled objects, blunt trauma, and burns, and related patient care considerations. (pp 1688-1692)
10. List the steps in the emergency medical care of the patient with an eye injury, including lacerations and corneal abrasion, blunt trauma, foreign object, impaled object, and burns. (pp 1692-1696)
11. Discuss different types of ear injuries, including soft-tissue injuries, foreign body in the ear, and a ruptured eardrum, and related patient care considerations. (p 1697)
12. List the steps in the emergency medical care of the patient with injuries of the ear, including lacerations and foreign body insertions. (pp 1697-1698)
13. Discuss different oral injuries, including soft-tissue injuries and dental injuries, and related patient care considerations. (pp 1698-1699)
14. List the steps in the emergency medical care of the patient with dental and cheek injuries, including how to handle an avulsed tooth. (p 1699)

15. Discuss specific injuries to the anterior part of the neck, including soft-tissue injuries, injuries to the larynx, injuries to the trachea, and injuries to the esophagus. (pp 1699-1703)
16. List the steps in the emergency medical care of the patient with a penetrating injury to the neck, including how to control regular and life-threatening bleeding. (p 1703)
17. Discuss spine trauma that does not involve the spinal cord, including the pathophysiology of sprains and strains, and their assessment and management. (p 1704)

Skills Objectives

1. Demonstrate the care of a patient who has a penetrating eye injury. (p 1693)
2. Demonstrate the stabilization of a foreign object that has been impaled in a patient's eye. (pp 1693-1694)
3. Demonstrate irrigation of a patient's eye using a nasal cannula, bottle, or basin. (pp 1694-1695)
4. Demonstrate how to control bleeding from a neck injury. (p 1703)

■ Introduction

As a paramedic, you will commonly encounter patients with injuries to the face and neck. Violent encounters and motor vehicle crashes are common causes of facial and neck trauma. Preventive measures such as the use of airbags and the creation of laws related to speed limits, seat belt use, and operation of a vehicle while impaired have contributed to a decline in facial bone fractures that result from motor vehicle crashes.

Facial trauma ranges in severity from a broken nose to penetration of the great vessels of the neck. As one of the most exposed regions of the body, the face and neck are frequently subjected to traumatic forces—from the various forces sustained during falls and assaults to the direct blunt forces sustained in a motor vehicle crash. Whereas other regions of the body are often covered with clothing and protective equipment, the face and neck generally do not share this same level of protection. Because the face is the first body part we tend to look at when meeting a person, and, moreover, because injuries to the face and neck can be quite graphic, it is easy to fixate on injuries to this region when arriving at the patient's side. Avoid focusing solely on these distracting injuries at the risk of missing other life threats.

This chapter provides a detailed review of the anatomy and physiology of the face and neck. It also discusses injuries to the face and neck, including their respective signs and symptoms and appropriate prehospital care. The following topics are covered in this chapter:

- Soft-tissue injuries to the region
- Maxillofacial injuries
- Injuries to the eye
- Ear injuries
- Oral and dental injuries
- Injuries to the anterior part of the neck, including penetrating injuries
- Injuries to the spine, not including spinal cord injuries

Chapter 34, *Head and Spine Trauma*, discusses injuries specific to the head and injuries to the spine and spinal cord. These injuries often occur in conjunction with facial

YOU are the Paramedic PART 1

Your unit is dispatched as a second unit for a motor vehicle crash. The first unit at the scene advises you they have two critical trauma patients. Your unit will be responsible for a 21-year-old woman with facial injuries. When you arrive at the scene, you are directed to your patient. The other crew informs you that she was riding with some friends in the bed of a pickup truck when the driver lost control and struck a tree head-on. The patient was not restrained and was thrown forward into the cab face-first. First responders have taken spinal precautions prior to your arrival and the patient is supine on the backboard. The patient has numerous cuts and contusions to her face. She is unresponsive with snoring respirations, and blood is coming from her mouth.

1. What is your primary concern after scene safety is established?
2. What is your first step in controlling the patient's airway?

trauma. Injuries discussed in Chapter 34 include traumatic brain injuries, skull fractures, and spine fractures.

■ Anatomy and Physiology Review

▶ The Facial Bones

Recall that 14 bones form the structure of the face; these bones provide protection and attachment points for a variety of muscles. **Figure 33-1** and **Figure 33-2** provide an overview of these bones and their location. For a detailed review of the facial anatomy, refer to Chapter 8, *Anatomy and Physiology*. Of particular importance to the

paramedic is the highly vascular nature of the face, which can result in significant hemorrhage in the setting of soft-tissue injuries.

The Orbits

The **orbits** are formed by seven thin bones that help reduce the weight of the head. Because of the vulnerable nature of these bones, a **blowout fracture** can occur if enough force is applied to the eye and the bones in the floor of the orbit fracture **Figure 33-3**.

▶ The Eyes, Ears, Teeth, and Mouth

The Eye

The **globe**, or eyeball, is susceptible to a variety of injuries, including foreign objects, impalements, and burns. Movement of the eyes is controlled by the extraocular muscles, which are in turn controlled by several cranial nerves. For example, the **oculomotor nerve** (third cranial nerve) innervates the muscles that cause motion of the eyeballs and upper eyelids. It also carries parasympathetic nerve fibers that cause constriction of the pupil and accommodation of the lens. The **optic nerve** (second cranial nerve) does not control movement but provides the sense of vision **Figure 33-4**.

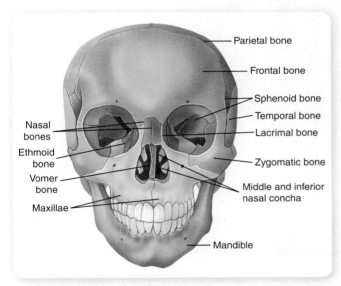

Figure 33-1 The skull and its components (front view).
© Jones & Bartlett Learning.

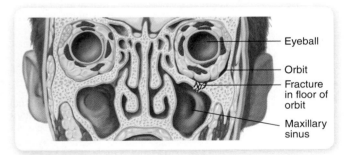

Figure 33-3 A blowout fracture of the left orbit.
© Jones & Bartlett Learning.

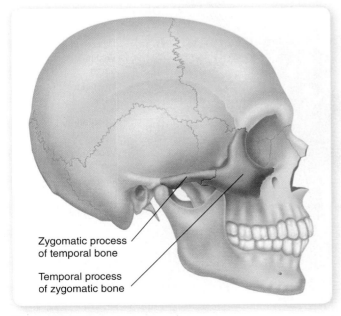

Figure 33-2 The zygomatic arch.
© Jones & Bartlett Learning.

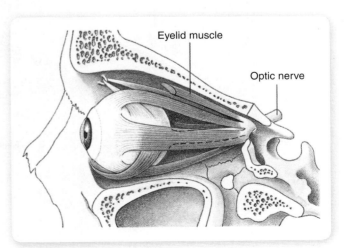

Figure 33-4 The optic nerve.
© Jones & Bartlett Learning.

When assessing for injury of the eye, evaluate the following structures: the **sclera**, the **cornea**, the **conjunctiva**, the **iris**, and the **pupil**. Depending on the clinical setting, you also may use an ophthalmoscope to evaluate the **retina** Figure 33-5 .

The Ear

The ear is divided into three anatomic parts: external, middle, and inner Figure 33-6 . As a paramedic, you will typically treat ear injuries involving the **external ear**. Injuries

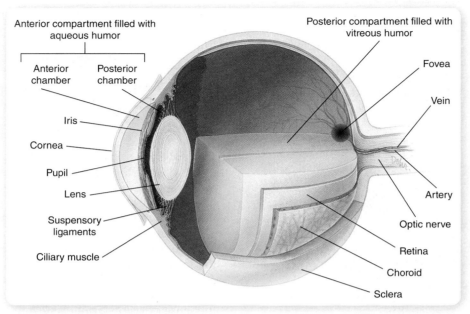

Figure 33-5 The structures of the eye.
© Jones & Bartlett Learning.

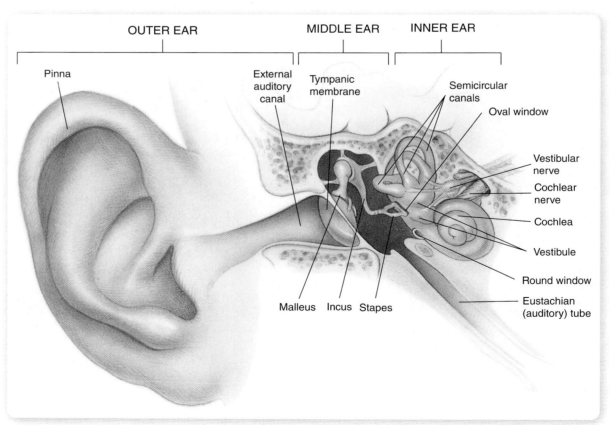

Figure 33-6 The structures of the ear.
© Jones & Bartlett Learning.

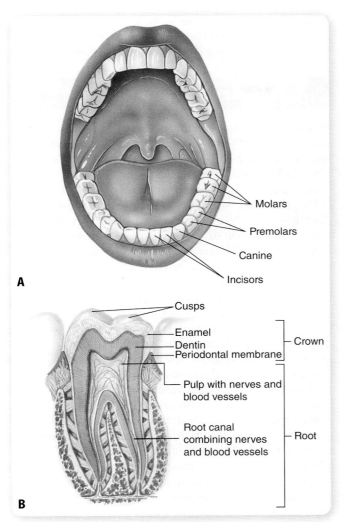

Figure 33-7 The teeth of the adult mouth. **A.** The incisors are used for biting. Canines are used for tearing food. The premolars and molars are used for grinding and crushing. **B.** Each tooth contains nerves and blood vessels.

© Jones & Bartlett Learning.

to the **middle ear** may be visible but are difficult to treat in the field. Injuries to the **inner ear** may be evidenced by complaints of vertigo but generally cannot be treated in the prehospital setting.

The Teeth

The adult mouth normally contains 32 permanent teeth in bony sockets called **alveoli**. When subjected to enough force, the teeth can be dislodged during a traumatic insult to the face. If the loose teeth obstruct the airway, this can be a life-threatening injury. As a paramedic, you should be familiar with the location of the different types of teeth and their various components, including the **crown**, **cusps**, **pulp**, and **dentin** Figure 33-7 .

► The Anterior Region of the Neck

The principal structures of the anterior region of the neck include the thyroid cartilage (often referred to

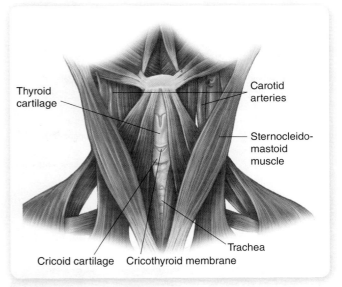

Figure 33-8 Anatomy of the anterior part of the neck.

© Jones & Bartlett Learning.

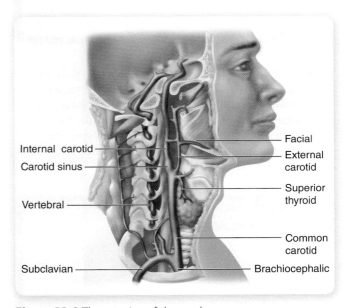

Figure 33-9 The arteries of the neck.

© Jones & Bartlett Learning.

as the Adam's apple), cricoid cartilage, trachea, and numerous muscles and nerves Figure 33-8 . The major blood vessels in this area are the internal and external carotid arteries Figure 33-9 and the internal and external jugular veins Figure 33-10 . The vertebral arteries run laterally to the cervical vertebrae in the posterior part of the neck.

The major arteries of the neck—the carotid and vertebral arteries—supply oxygenated blood directly to the brain and upper spinal cord. Therefore, in addition to causing massive bleeding and hemorrhagic shock, injury to any of these major vessels can produce cerebral hypoxia, infarct, air embolism, and/or permanent neurologic impairment.

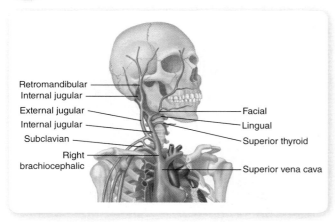

Figure 33-10 The veins of the neck.
© Jones & Bartlett Learning.

Other key structures of the anterior part of the neck that may sustain injury from blunt or penetrating mechanisms include the vagus nerves, thoracic duct, esophagus, thyroid and parathyroid glands, lower cranial nerves, brachial plexus (which is responsible for function of the arm and hand), soft tissue and fascia, and various muscles.

Patient Assessment

Scene Size-up

Your first consideration in any scenario should be safety—your own as well as that of other responders, patients, and bystanders. Chapter 2, *Workforce Safety and Wellness*, covers size-up of the scene for safety issues. On any trauma call, you should also ensure that you and your crew have taken standard precautions, which include, at a minimum, wearing gloves and eye protection. Determine the number of patients, and consider whether you need additional or specialized resources on the scene. Evaluate the mechanism of injury (MOI), and maintain a high index of suspicion for injury whenever a significant MOI is present.

Primary Survey

When responding to incidents involving serious trauma, management of soft-tissue injuries can be distracting but should not take your focus off the ABCDE (Airway, Breathing, Circulation, Disability, and Exposure) approach, recognizing that if there is life-threatening bleeding or cardiac arrest, the order would be CABDE (Circulation, Airway, Breathing, Disability, and Exposure), as you learned in Chapter 11, *Patient Assessment. Do not let soft-tissue injuries distract you from life threats that may not be readily apparent.* However, you must also realize that soft-tissue injuries to the face and neck can cause significant airway issues through the loss of structural integrity or the accumulation of blood and other fluids in the oropharynx.

Form a general impression as you approach the patient and rapidly determine whether threats to life are present. Check for responsiveness even when the patient has a seemingly innocuous soft-tissue injury to the face, as there may be associated head trauma. Listen for obvious respiratory sounds as you approach the patient: sonorous respirations usually indicate a positional problem, whereas gurgling respirations often indicate a need for suction. In a face or neck injury, the oropharynx may become occluded by the tongue, secretions, blood, vomitus, foreign bodies, or improperly inserted airways.

Assess the airway as soon as you arrive at the patient's side. If the patient has a potential neck or spine injury, assign a crew member to perform manual stabilization while the airway is being assessed; maintain that immobilization until it is determined that spinal precautions are not indicated or, if indicated, until full spinal immobilization has been applied. Spinal immobilization is discussed in detail in Chapter 34, *Head and Spine Trauma*. If the patient is unresponsive or has a significantly altered level of consciousness, consider using an airway adjunct.

When blood, vomit, or any other substance is present in the airway, immediately suction it from the airway. If direct airway trauma is present, it may severely compromise the airway. Soft-tissue injuries that result in a flow of blood into the airway can prove extremely challenging. Immediately correct anything that interferes with airway patency; failure to provide a patent airway can quickly lead to the patient's death.

Assess the patient's breathing and its adequacy, employing any corrective measures as needed, which may include supplemental oxygen through an oxygen delivery device.

Closely assess for signs of hypoxia. If possible, monitor the patient's oxygen saturation level, maintaining it at 94% or higher with supplemental oxygen as needed. The administration of oxygen, and assisting with ventilations when indicated, *cannot* be deferred until you are en route for any patient who is exhibiting signs and symptoms of hypoxia. Quickly assess for and treat any life-threatening injuries that may compromise ventilation. Ignoring these injuries until the secondary assessment, or until you are en route, can result in hypoxia and significantly increase the likelihood of mortality and morbidity.

Palpate the pulse for its presence, rate, regularity, and quality, and assess skin CTC (color, temperature, and condition). If no pulse is present, take resuscitative measures. When you are palpating a pulse, determine whether it is abnormally fast or slow. Pale or ashen skin points to inadequate perfusion, whereas cyanotic skin indicates hypoxemia. Cool, moist skin is an early indicator of shock.

If visible significant bleeding is seen, then you must begin the steps necessary to control bleeding, using the appropriate methods.

Reevaluate the patient's mental status and response to stimuli, and note any changes since your initial contact with the patient. Quickly evaluate the presence or absence of pulse, motor function, and sensory function in each extremity, as a baseline assessment of these items is needed prior to placing the patient on a backboard. If the patient is responsive, inquire about any numbness or tingling (paresthesia) to the extremities. Directly observe the back to assess for penetrating trauma. Finally, palpate the patient's spinal column for deformity, step-offs, point tenderness, or crepitus.

At this point you will have enough information to determine if the patient requires spinal immobilization. The criteria for making this decision and the immobilization process are discussed in detail in Chapter 34, *Head and Spine Trauma*.

Provide rapid transport for patients with significant physiologic findings. After any immediate life threats have been addressed, any additional intervention that can be done en route should be delayed until you are in the ambulance. Patients with isolated injuries (no life threats or significant physiologic findings) are often better managed by carefully treating the injuries on scene.

Words of Wisdom

When making your transport decision, do not delay the treatment of threats to the airway, breathing, or circulation in an effort to get off scene quickly. Hypoxia and hypovolemia are major contributors to poor outcomes and can have devastating effects within 4 to 6 minutes of their onset. Such effects can easily occur within the 10-minute on-scene window—and, in fact, they may have been present prior to your arrival. Appropriate airway control measures, ventilatory support, oxygenation, and hemorrhage control must take place on scene while packaging the patient.

History Taking

Gathering information is an important step in determining how the patient was injured. Was there a precipitating factor? For example, did the patient fall because she got dizzy or because she tripped over the cat? Perhaps a medical reason led to the trauma. Ask the patient (if alert

---

YOU are the Paramedic PART 2

Your partner sets up the portable suction unit. When your partner opens the patient's mouth to insert the suction catheter, she reports that she feels crepitus and it seems as if the maxilla is moving. Your partner also notices blood and a clear fluid coming from the patient's nose.

Recording Time: 1 Minute	
Appearance	Facial trauma with bleeding from mouth
Level of consciousness	Unresponsive
Airway	Obstructed with blood
Breathing	Snoring
Circulation	134 thready at carotid, absent radial pulses, skin pale and diaphoretic

3. Which type of facial fracture may this patient have?
4. How will this type of fracture affect the selection of an appropriate airway method?

and able to respond) or family members and bystanders about the injury. For example, you may need to ask the following questions:

- Was the patient wearing a seat belt?
- Was there airbag deployment?
- How fast was the vehicle traveling?
- How high is the location from which the patient fell?
- Was there a loss of consciousness?
- Which type of weapon was used?

Record the information on the patient care record, and relay it during patient transfer at the hospital.

Make every attempt to obtain a SAMPLE (Signs and symptoms, Allergies, Medications, Pertinent past medical history, Last oral intake, Events leading up to the illness or injury) history from the patient. Using the mnemonic OPQRST (Onset, Provocation/palliation, Quality, Region/radiation, Severity, Timing) may provide some background information on isolated extremity injuries. You have the opportunity to interview the patient well before the emergency department (ED) physician's examination. Any information you receive will be valuable if the patient loses consciousness.

If the patient is unresponsive and bystanders or family members cannot provide information, the scene and any medical alert jewelry may be your only sources of information for a SAMPLE history.

 ## Secondary Assessment

The secondary assessment is a more systematic head-to-toe or focused examination of the patient that is used to reveal injuries that may have been missed during the primary survey. In some cases, such as with a critically injured patient or a short transport time, you may not have time to conduct a secondary assessment.

For critical patients, physical examinations typically will be performed en route to the hospital, and they should result in reconsidering or reconfirming your initial transport decision. In noncritical patients with isolated injuries, you may choose to perform the secondary assessment while on scene.

The secondary assessment of the head and neck is performed using the techniques of inspection and palpation. Although you may have been called for a traumatic injury to the face or neck, you must evaluate for the presence of any medical conditions that could have led to the injury (eg, a stroke or a seizure). Findings during the assessment of the face and neck may provide clues to an underlying cause of the traumatic incident. As you inspect these areas, observe for the following:

- Drainage from the ears or nose, noting if it is bloody or clear
- The presence of periorbital ecchymosis (raccoon eyes)

- The presence of retroauricular ecchymosis (Battle sign)
- The symmetry of the face, including the eyes, ears, skull, and ability to smile
- Any deformity, soft-tissue injuries, lumps, or hemorrhage to the head or neck
- Swelling, occlusion, and asymmetrical narrowing at the ear openings
- Lacerations, bite marks, missing teeth, and evidence of dehydration (even though the oropharynx was evaluated for obstructions during the primary survey)

Additional assessment items include the following:

- Look at the position and condition of the uvula, the posterior pharynx, and the condition of the mouth, oral mucosa, teeth, gums, and tongue. Recall that poor dental health is associated with several medical conditions, as well as poor nutrition, pain, abscesses, and both localized and systemic infections.
- Evaluate the patient's gaze, noting if it is focused, distant, conjugate, or disconjugate. Ask about visual disturbances such as diplopia.
- Observe the position and coloration of the eyes, and look for any evidence of trauma or infection.
- Evaluate the size, shape, and symmetry of the pupils. Assess the direct and indirect pupillary reflexes, and assess the extraocular movements and for the presence of a nystagmus.
- Assess the visual fields and for the presence of any visual field defects such as a hemianopsia (also called a hemianopia).
- Inspect the neck for jugular venous distention.
- Note the presence of any enlarged lymph nodes on the neck.

Palpate the face and neck, asking the patient to report any pain or tenderness during palpation. Note any of the following findings:

- Palpate the skull for any deformities, bony instability, lumps, or depressions.
- Part the hair and look for deformities or evidence of soft-tissue injury.
- Palpate the face for any deformities or bony instability.
- Palpate the mandible and the temporomandibular junction.
- Palpate the lymph nodes, noting any enlargement or tenderness.
- Palpate the neck for tracheal deviation. Recall that in the setting of a tension pneumothorax, tracheal deviation, if present, is a late finding.

Recall that many of the cranial nerves are evaluated by visualization and palpation of the eyes, face, mouth, and tongue. These assessment techniques may be incorporated into your exam of the face and neck, or the cranial nerves may be evaluated all at once as a separate part of your assessment.

Reassessment

Frequent reassessments of the patient's condition should be made en route to the hospital and in conjunction with any necessary interventions. A patient in stable condition should be reassessed every 15 minutes; a more serious condition warrants reexamination every 5 minutes. As part of this assessment, vital signs should be obtained and evaluated, any interventions checked, and the patient's condition monitored.

Repeat the primary survey and confirm whether the treatments you provided are still effective. Identify and treat changes in the patient's condition. Reassessing a patient with an open soft-tissue injury is extremely important. Frequently, other emergency care personnel may have dressed and bandaged the wound before your arrival. Therefore, you should regularly reassess the injury; you may need to add more dressings over the original dressing or bandages.

Special Populations

In the older adult population, poor skin tone and loss of body fat can produce significant soft-tissue injury in the presence of even a simple MOI. Anticoagulation therapy in older patients can lead to significant blood loss from minor insults. Additionally, normally trivial physical findings such as bruises and minor lacerations can belie severe underlying trauma such as traumatic brain injury.

Your communication and documentation must include a description of the MOI, the position in which you found the patient, the location and description of injuries, and an accurate account of how you treated these injuries. In patients who have open injuries with severe external bleeding, it is important to recognize, estimate, and report how much blood has been lost and how rapidly that loss occurred.

Emergency Medical Care

General emergency care of face and neck injuries must focus on protection of the airway. Airway issues are the most dangerous of the results of injuries to both the face and the neck.

Assess all bandaging frequently. If blood continues to soak through bandages, use additional methods to control bleeding as discussed later in the chapter.

Although most open soft-tissue injuries are not serious, if not appropriately treated, they can lead to substantial blood loss and even shock. By appropriately treating open soft-tissue injuries, you can minimize the common complications such as bleeding, shock, pain, and infection. You should expose all wounds, control bleeding, and be prepared to treat the patient for shock.

Closed soft-tissue injuries can be life threatening if not appropriately treated. Evaluate all patients to see if they need supplemental oxygen to maintain an oxygen saturation level of 94% or greater.

The next sections cover assessment and treatment of specific injuries, but regardless of the injury type, always constantly manage the airway of any patient with face or neck injuries.

Pathophysiology, Assessment, and Management of Face Injuries

▶ Pathophysiology

Soft-Tissue Injuries

Although open soft-tissue injuries to the face—lacerations, abrasions, and avulsions—by themselves are rarely life threatening, their presence, especially following a significant MOI, suggests the potential for more severe injuries (eg, closed head injury, cervical spine injury). Furthermore, massive soft-tissue injuries to the face, especially if associated with oropharyngeal trauma and bleeding, can compromise the patient's airway and lead to ventilatory inadequacy.

Maintain a high index of suspicion when a patient presents with closed soft-tissue injuries to the face, such as contusions and hematomas **Figure 33-11**. These indicators of blunt force trauma suggest the potential for more severe underlying injuries.

Impaled objects in the soft tissues or bones of the face may occur in association with facial trauma. Although

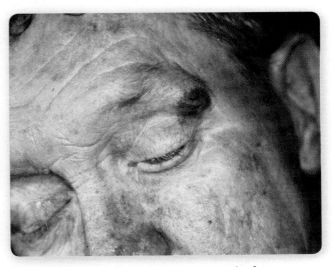

Figure 33-11 Closed soft-tissue injuries to the face may indicate more severe underlying injuries.
Courtesy of Rhonda Hunt.

these objects can damage facial nerves, the risk of airway compromise is of far greater consequence. An impaled object that penetrates the cheek is of particular concern, because massive oropharyngeal bleeding can result in airway obstruction, aspiration, and ventilatory inadequacy. In addition, blood is a gastric irritant and its ingestion may lead to vomiting, further increasing the likelihood of aspiration.

Maxillofacial Fractures

Maxillofacial fractures commonly occur when the facial bones absorb the energy of a strong impact. The forces required to fracture the maxilla are extreme; a force of that magnitude is also likely to produce traumatic brain injuries and cervical spine injuries. Therefore, when you are assessing a patient with a suspected maxillofacial fracture, you should evaluate the need to protect the cervical spine and monitor the patient's neurologic signs, specifically the patient's level of consciousness.

The first clue to the presence of a maxillofacial fracture is usually ecchymosis; therefore, a black-and-blue mark on the face should alert you to this possibility. However, it is important to realize that ecchymosis takes time to develop. If the injury just occurred, there may be no discoloration or only a slight reddening of the skin. A deep facial laceration should likewise increase your index of suspicion that the underlying bone may have been fractured, and pain over a bone tends to support the suspicion of fracture. General signs and symptoms of maxillofacial fractures include ecchymosis, swelling, pain to palpation, crepitus, dental malocclusion, facial deformities or asymmetry, instability of the facial bones, impaired ocular movement, and visual disturbances.

Nasal Fractures. Nasal fractures are characterized by swelling, tenderness, and crepitus when the nasal bone is palpated. Deformity of the nose, if present, usually appears as lateral displacement of the nasal bone from its normal midline position.

Nasal fractures, like any maxillofacial fracture, are often complicated by the presence of an anterior or a posterior nosebleed (**epistaxis**) that can compromise the patient's airway.

Mandibular Fractures and Dislocations. Fractures of the **mandible** typically result from massive blunt force trauma to the lower third of the face; they are particularly common following an assault injury. Because of the shape of the mandible and the force required to fracture it, this structure may be fractured in more than one place and, therefore, unstable to palpation. The fracture site itself is most commonly located at the angle of the jaw.

Mandibular fractures should be suspected in patients with a history of blunt force trauma to the lower third of the face who present with dental **malocclusion** (misalignment of the teeth), numbness of the chin, and inability to open the mouth. Other findings include swelling and ecchymosis over the fracture site (eg, on the floor

of the mouth), and teeth may be partially or completely avulsed. As the patient moves his or her jaw to speak and answer your questions, take note of symptoms of pain, such as decreased normal range of motion. You may elicit tenderness by palpating specific locations on the mandible such as near the joints or specific impact points. This "point tenderness" and pain on motion can help you identify injuries that patients might not have otherwise reported because they may be distracted by other injuries.

Temporomandibular joint (TMJ) dislocations may occur as the result of blunt force trauma to the lower third of the face, but this outcome is rare. These dislocations are most often the result of exaggerated yawning or otherwise widely opening the mouth. The patient commonly feels a "pop" and then cannot close his or her mouth; it is locked in a wide-open position. The jaw muscles eventually go into spasm, causing severe pain.

Maxillary Fractures. Maxillary fractures are most commonly associated with mechanisms that produce massive blunt facial trauma, such as motor vehicle crashes, falls, and assaults. They produce massive facial swelling, instability of the midfacial bones, malocclusion, and an elongated appearance of the patient's face.

Le Fort fractures **Figure 33-12** are classified into three categories:

- **Le Fort I fracture.** A horizontal fracture of the maxilla that involves the **hard palate** and inferior maxilla, separating them from the rest of the skull.
- **Le Fort II fracture.** A fracture with a pyramidal shape, involving the nasal bone and inferior maxilla.
- **Le Fort III fracture** (**craniofacial disjunction**). A fracture of all midfacial bones, separating the entire midface from the cranium.

Le Fort fractures can occur as isolated fractures (Le Fort I) or in combination (Le Fort I and II), depending on the location of impact and the amount of trauma.

Patients with Le Fort fractures report severe facial pain, anesthesia or paresthesia of the upper lip, and some visual disturbances. Facial swelling, subconjunctival hemorrhage, deformity of the face, ecchymosis, periorbital or orbital swelling, facial asymmetry, epistaxis, and malocclusion will be evident. Also look for cerebrospinal fluid (CSF) leaking from the patient's nose; this sign may indicate an open skull fracture. You can assess the maxilla by gently, but firmly, grasping the front gum and teeth and trying to move it. If the palate moves, suspect a Le Fort fracture.

Orbital Fractures. An orbital blowout fracture involves the bones of the orbital floor. A typical MOI involves a fist, dashboard, or baseball striking the globe of the eye and surrounding soft tissues. Larger objects are unable to compress the globe because of the protection afforded by the orbital rim surrounding the globe. The impact pushes the globe into the orbit, compressing its contents.

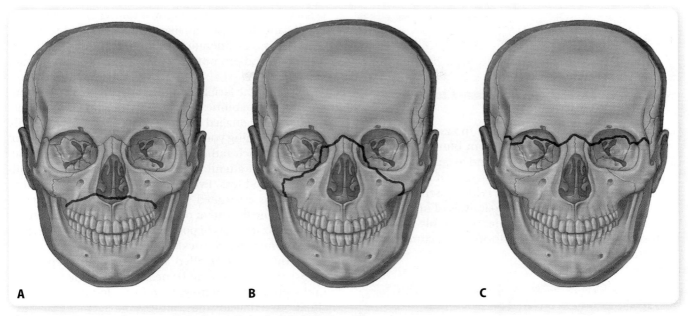

Figure 33-12 Le Fort fractures. **A.** Le Fort I. **B.** Le Fort II. **C.** Le Fort III.
© Jones & Bartlett Learning.

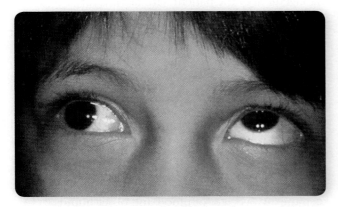

Figure 33-13 In a patient with a blowout fracture, the eyes may not move together because of muscle entrapment, so the patient sees double images of any object.

The sudden increase in pressure causes a fracture at the weakest point of the orbit, which is usually the orbital floor. The fragments of fractured bone can entrap some of the muscles that control eye movement **Figure 33-13** .

The patient with an orbital fracture may report double vision (**diplopia**) and lose sensation above the eyebrow or over the cheek secondary to associated nerve damage. The injury may cause the patient to have reduced sensation to areas that are innervated by the infraorbital nerve—a symptom called *infraorbital hypoesthesia*. The affected area extends from the tip of the nose, including the nares, and follows the margin of the maxilla, curving up to meet the temple. Also, the eyeball may retract posteriorly into the space created when the cavity is enlarged; this symptom is called *enophthalmos traumaticus*.

Massive nasal discharge of blood and possibly CSF may occur with an orbital fracture, and vision is often impaired. Fractures of the inferior orbit are the most common type and can cause paralysis of upward gaze (the patient's injured eye will not be able to follow your finger above the midline).

Most orbital fractures are isolated injuries resulting in discharge from the ED for follow-up by a specialist; however, it is possible that the entrapped extraocular muscles can stimulate the oculocardiac reflex. The oculocardiac reflex generally occurs when the patient attempts to look upward. The stretching of the trapped muscle causes stimulation of the vagus nerve. This stimulation results in bradycardia, which may be associated with nausea and syncope. In some cases, the bradycardia can be severe and asystole can even occur. Knowledge of this condition has direct applicability to the paramedic because the resulting bradycardia, especially if persistent, can be confused with the bradycardia associated with traumatic brain injuries. Therefore, assess a patient with orbital trauma and bradycardia for the presence of other findings indicating traumatic brain injury.[1-5]

Treatment of an isolated orbital fracture is primarily supportive. If the globe has been ruptured, place a rigid eye shield over the affected eye and bandage both eyes. The application of ice packs will help reduce pain and swelling. Consider medications for pain relief. If the oculocardiac reflex has been stimulated, the bradycardia will usually be relieved by having the patient return his or her gaze to the normal position; doing so relieves the stretching of the entrapped muscle and stops the vagal stimulus. In cases of persistent and symptomatic bradycardia, atropine may be required.

> ### Words of Wisdom
>
> Check eye movements in all planes in the patient with possible facial fractures.

Zygomatic Fractures. Fractures of the zygomatic bone (cheekbone) commonly result from blunt trauma secondary to motor vehicle crashes and assaults. When the zygomatic bone is fractured, that side of the patient's face appears flattened, and there is loss of sensation over the cheek, nose, and upper lip; paralysis of upward gaze may also be present. Other injuries commonly associated with zygomatic fractures include orbital fractures, ocular injury, and epistaxis.

> ### Words of Wisdom
>
> Any patient with significant head injury should be evaluated for the presence of a cervical spine injury.

▶ Assessment

Table 33-1 summarizes the characteristics of various maxillofacial fractures. It is not important to distinguish among the various maxillofacial fractures in the prehospital setting; this determination requires radiographic

Table 33-1	Summary of Maxillofacial Fractures
Injury	**Signs and Symptoms**
Multiple facial bone fractures	Massive facial swelling Dental malocclusion Palpable deformities Anterior or posterior epistaxis
Zygomatic and orbital fractures	Loss of sensation below the orbit Flattening of the patient's cheek Paralysis of upward gaze
Nasal fractures	Crepitus and instability Swelling, tenderness, lateral displacement Anterior or posterior epistaxis
Maxillary (Le Fort) fractures	Mobility of the midface Dental malocclusion Facial swelling
Mandibular fractures	Dental malocclusion Mandibular instability

© Jones & Bartlett Learning.

evaluation, usually via computed tomography, in the ED. Rapid patient assessment, management of life-threatening conditions, consideration of spinal immobilization if indicated, and prompt transport are far more important considerations.

Because the facial region is difficult to assess without radiologic capabilities and because the underlying structures can be damaged easily, your assessment is primarily clinical, meaning you will use your observation skills of sight and touch rather than use diagnostic equipment. Pay particular attention to swelling, deformity, instability, and blood loss. Evaluate the cranial nerve function; subtle signs associated with its alteration can help you to determine the extent of the injury. Visually inspect the oropharynx for signs of posterior epistaxis, including frank blood continuing to trickle down the back of the throat after you have controlled a simple anterior epistaxis. A posterior epistaxis can be nearly impossible to control in the prehospital setting; therefore, alert the ED to this situation so that advanced airway management can be in place on your arrival.

▶ Management

Management of the patient with facial trauma begins by protecting the cervical spine. Because many severe facial injuries are complicated by a spinal injury, you must evaluate for this possibility. This topic is discussed in detail in Chapter 34, *Head and Spine Trauma*.

Open the airway with the jaw-thrust maneuver while simultaneously maintaining manual stabilization of the head in the neutral position; if, however, the patient reports severe pain or discomfort upon movement, the head and neck should be immobilized in the position found. Inspect the mouth for fragments of teeth, dentures, or any other foreign bodies that could obstruct the airway, and remove them immediately. Suction the oropharynx as needed to keep the airway clear of blood and other liquids.

Insert an airway adjunct as needed to maintain airway patency. However, remember that *nasal airways and blind nasotracheal intubation are relatively contraindicated in the presence of midface trauma.* Thus, such a maneuver should not be performed in any patient with suspected nasal fractures or in patients with CSF or blood leakage from the nose or with any evidence of midface trauma, unless it is absolutely necessary. If necessary, such maneuvers must be performed using extreme caution and in some systems may require the approval of medical direction.

After establishing and maintaining a patent airway, assess the patient's breathing and intervene appropriately. Administer oxygen as needed to maintain an oxygen saturation level of 94% or greater if the patient is breathing adequately. Patients who are breathing inadequately (ie, fast or slow rate, inadequate tidal volume [shallow breathing], irregular pattern of inhalation and exhalation) should receive bag-mask ventilation with 100% oxygen. Maintain the patient's oxygen saturation level at greater than 94%. Airway management can be

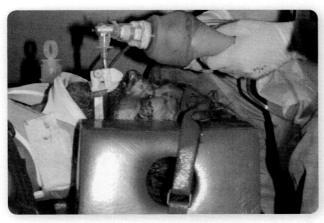

Figure 33-14 In patients with massive facial injuries, bleeding poses a threat to airway management.

© Eddie M. Sperling

especially challenging in patients with massive facial injuries Figure 33-14 . Oropharyngeal bleeding poses an immediate threat to the airway, and unstable facial bones can hinder your ability to maintain an effective mask-to-face seal for bag-mask ventilation. Therefore, perform endotracheal (ET) intubation of patients with facial trauma, especially those who are unresponsive, to protect their airway from aspiration and to ensure adequate oxygenation and ventilation. Remember that the forces that produce the insult to the victim are often transferred to the spinal column; therefore, it is imperative for you to provide in-line stabilization while attempting ET intubation. Cricothyrotomy (surgical or needle) may be required for patients with extensive maxillofacial injuries when ET intubation is extremely difficult or impossible to perform (ie, in patients with unstable facial bones, massive swelling, or severe oral bleeding).

Foreign Bodies in the Throat

Foreign bodies lodged in the mouth should alert you to the potential for airway obstruction and aspiration. It is paramount to keep the patient calm and positioned such that if the object becomes dislodged, gravity will allow it to fall out. Patients who have an object lodged in their throat often panic, thinking they cannot breathe. As the patient speaks to you, comfort him or her by explaining, "By the sound of your voice, I can tell your airway is open. The object lodged in your throat may be very uncomfortable, but you seem to be breathing fine." Transport the patient in a position of comfort.

Soft-Tissue Injuries

Treat facial lacerations and avulsions as you would any other soft-tissue injury. Control all bleeding with direct pressure, and apply sterile dressings. If you suspect an underlying facial fracture, apply just enough pressure to control the bleeding. Leave objects impaled in the face in place and appropriately stabilize them, unless they pose a threat to the airway (such as an object impaled through

the cheek). When you are removing an object from the cheek, proceed carefully, preferably in the same direction that it entered. Next, pack the inside of the cheek with sterile gauze and apply counterpressure with a dressing and bandage firmly secured over the outside of the wound. If profuse bleeding continues, position the patient on his or her side—while maintaining stabilization of the cervical spine—to facilitate drainage of secretions from the mouth, and suction the airway as needed.

For severe oropharyngeal bleeding in patients with inadequate ventilation, suction the airway for 15 seconds and provide ventilatory assistance for 2 minutes; continue this alternating pattern of suctioning and ventilating until the airway is cleared of blood or secured with an ET tube. Monitoring the pulse oximeter during this process can further serve to keep the patient from becoming hypoxic.

Words of Wisdom

In some cases, no matter what the recommendations are, time guidelines are exceeded because it is simply not possible to ventilate if the airway is full of blood or keeps refilling with blood despite suctioning. Other recommendations for suctioning time limits may be based on clinical presentations such as SpO_2 and ECG monitoring.

Epistaxis following facial trauma can be severe and is most effectively controlled by applying direct pressure to the nares. Some emergency medical services (EMS) agencies allow the use of nasal sprays containing oxymetazoline hydrochloride or phenylephrine hydrochloride. These medications stimulate alpha-adrenergic receptors, causing localized vasoconstriction in the nasal mucosa. If the patient is responsive, and spinal immobilization is not indicated, instruct the patient to sit up and lean forward as you pinch the nares together. Unresponsive patients should be positioned on their side, unless contraindicated by a spinal injury. Proper positioning of the patient with epistaxis is important to prevent blood from draining down the throat and compromising the airway either by occlusion or by vomiting and then aspirating gastric contents. If the responsive patient with severe epistaxis is immobilized on a backboard, discourage the patient from swallowing the draining blood and aid him or her with suctioning as needed. Consider drug-assisted intubation (eg, rapid-sequence intubation [RSI]) to gain definitive control of the airway.

Although facial lacerations and avulsions can contribute to hemorrhagic shock, they are rarely the sole cause of this condition in adults. Severe epistaxis, however, can result in significant blood loss. To counter this problem, you should carefully assess the patient for signs of hemorrhagic shock and administer intravenous (IV) crystalloid fluid boluses as needed to maintain adequate perfusion.

Maxillofacial Fractures

If the facial fracture is associated with swelling and ecchymosis, cold compresses may help minimize further swelling and alleviate pain. Do not apply pressure to the eyeball (globe) if you suspect that it has been injured following an orbital fracture; doing so may increase the intraocular pressure and further damage the eye. Additionally, it may stimulate the oculocardiac reflex. Other than protecting the airway, there is little you can do to treat instability resulting from facial fractures.

Special Populations

In contrast to younger, healthy adults, older adult patients are at high risk for severe epistaxis following even minor facial injuries, especially in those patients with a history of hypertension or anticoagulant medication use (such as warfarin [Coumadin]). This bleeding often originates in the posterior nasopharynx and may not be grossly evident unless you look in the patient's mouth.

Pathophysiology, Assessment, and Management of Eye Injuries

Each day in the United States, there are approximately 2,000 work-related eye injuries that require medical treatment.[6] Because trauma to the eyes is so common and the potential consequences are so serious, you must know how to assess and manage ocular injuries.

Blunt trauma, penetrating trauma, or burns frequently cause eye injuries. Blunt MOI may include motor vehicle crashes, motorcycle crashes, falls, and assaults. Penetrating injuries often occur secondary to foreign bodies on the surface of the eye (such as sand) or an object impaled in the globe. Burns to the eye can result from a variety of corrosive chemicals or during industrial accidents.

▶ Pathophysiology

Lacerations, Foreign Bodies, and Impaled Objects

Lacerations of the eyelids require meticulous repair to restore appearance and function. *If there is a laceration to the globe itself, apply no pressure to the eye;* compression can interfere with the blood supply to the back of the eye and result in loss of vision from damage to the retina. Furthermore, pressure may squeeze the **vitreous humor**, iris, lens, or even the retina out of the eye and cause irreparable damage or blindness Figure 33-15 .

The protective orbit prevents large objects from penetrating the eye. However, moderately sized and smaller foreign objects can still enter the eye and, when

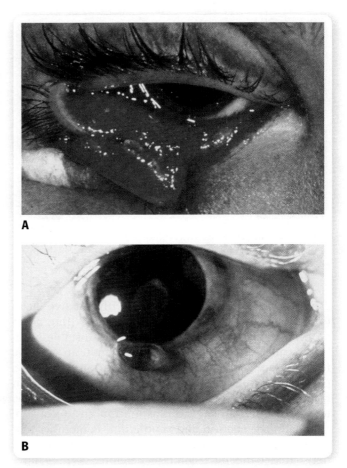

A

B

Figure 33-15 Eye lacerations are serious injuries that require prompt transport. **A.** Although bleeding can be heavy, never exert pressure on the eye. **B.** Pressure may squeeze the vitreous humor, iris, lens, or retina out of the eye.

lying on the surface of the eye, produce severe irritation Figure 33-16 . The conjunctiva becomes inflamed and red—a condition known as **conjunctivitis**—almost immediately, and the eye begins to produce tears in an attempt to flush out the object Figure 33-17 .

Corneal abrasions are common. They result from superficial trauma to the cornea, often from a foreign body, but may also be due to excessive rubbing, chemical burns, or being poked in the eye by a finger or makeup brush. Irritation of the cornea or conjunctiva causes intense pain. The patient may have difficulty keeping the eyelids open because the irritation is further aggravated by bright light. When interviewing the patient, attempt to determine what the patient thinks the object may be. Most objects are easily flushed out; however, rust and metal cannot be removed by flushing and require removal by a physician. In this case, the patient may have also developed a rust ring in the eye around the embedded metal Figure 33-18 , especially if he or she did not promptly call for help. This ring is removed with a drill and corneal burr. The longer it remains in the eye, however, the more damage it causes. For this reason, the patient needs to be evaluated by a physician as soon as a rust ring is recognized.

Dust, dirt, splinters, and other particles are commonly involved in eye injuries. Although most do not threaten the patient's ability to see, they can cause significant pain. Most foreign objects in the eye occur as a result of occupational injury; however, you may also treat patients whose injury is hobby related. The use of grinders, sanders, nailers, weed whackers, and other machines commonly cause these injuries, notably in the absence of personal protective equipment. As the machinery is working, it can dislodge and eject particles a long distance, and if safety glasses are not worn, foreign objects can enter the eyes. Foreign objects in the eye can also be due to auto crashes, firearm use, and recreational activities.

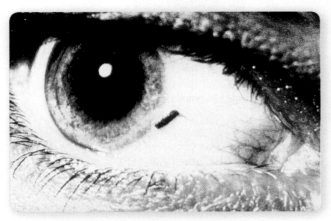

Figure 33-16 A foreign object on the surface of the eye.

Words of Wisdom

Large and small foreign bodies, particularly small metal fragments, can become completely embedded in the globe. The patient may not even be aware of the cause of the problem. Suspect such an injury when the history includes metal work (eg, hammering, exposure to splinters, use of grinders, vigorous filing) and when you observe signs of ocular injury (eg, redness, irritation, inflammation).

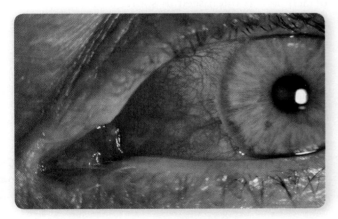

Figure 33-17 Conjunctivitis is often associated with the presence of a foreign object in the eye.
Courtesy of John T. Halgren, M.D., University of Nebraska Medical Center.

Blunt Eye Injuries

Blunt trauma can cause serious eye injuries, ranging from swelling and ecchymosis **Figure 33-19** to rupture of the globe. **Hyphema** is bleeding into the **anterior chamber** of the eye that obscures vision, either partially or completely **Figure 33-20**. It often follows blunt trauma and may seriously impair vision. An "eight-ball hyphema" is a dark-colored clot that covers the entire anterior chamber. Because an acute injury usually leads to the collection of bright red blood in the anterior chamber, the presence of dark blood suggests a nonacute injury. To visualize the hyphema clearly, shine a penlight from an angle through the anterior chamber. This light will exaggerate the height of the blood in the chamber, allowing it to be differentiated from blood on the corneal surface. The patient with hyphema usually will report photophobia, pain, and

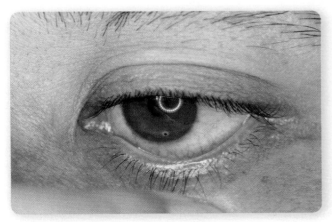

Figure 33-18 A rust ring in the eye.
© ARZTSAMUI/Shutterstock.

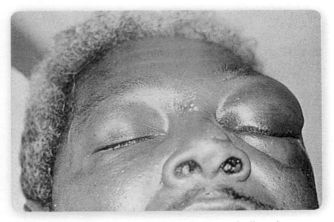

Figure 33-19 Swelling and ecchymosis are hallmark findings associated with blunt trauma to the eye.

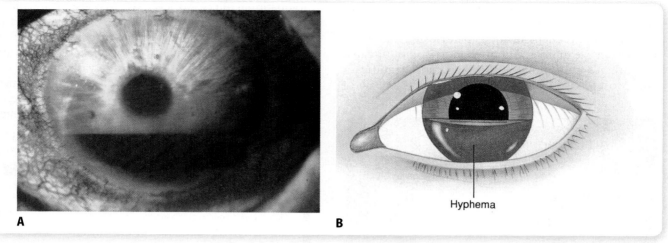

Figure 33-20 A hyphema, characterized by bleeding into the anterior chamber of the eye, can occur following blunt trauma to the eye. This condition should be considered a sight-threatening emergency. **A.** Actual hyphema. **B.** Illustration.
B: © Jones & Bartlett Learning.

blurred vision. Such patients are often drowsy, although the cause of this finding is unclear. Assess the patient with hyphema for associated injuries, such as a ruptured globe. If a patient with a hyphema has an altered level of consciousness, suspect and treat for a head injury.

Another potential result of blunt eye trauma is **retinal detachment**, or separation of the inner layers of the retina from the underlying choroid (the vascular membrane that nourishes the retina). Without a blood supply, the outer retinal tissue layer becomes ischemic and the cells can eventually die. Because of this risk, the time to treatment is a significant factor in the patient's outcome. Retinal detachment is often seen in sports injuries, especially boxing, but can also be spontaneous. It can occur at any age but is more common in people older than 50 years.[7] This painless condition produces flashing lights, specks, or "floaters" in the field of vision and a cloud or shade over the patient's vision. Because it can cause devastating damage to vision, retinal detachment is an ocular emergency and requires urgent medical attention.

YOU are the Paramedic PART 3

You set up your equipment in preparation for performing ET intubation on this patient. Your partner is attempting to insert an oral airway that is not properly seating because of the free-floating maxilla injury. You direct one of the first responders to start ventilating the patient using a bag-mask device. Your partner returns to suctioning blood from the airway.

Recording Time: 5 Minutes	
Respirations	8 breaths/min
Pulse	130 beats/min
Skin	Cool, pale, moist
Blood pressure	90/60 mm Hg
Oxygen saturation (Spo$_2$)	92% on room air
Pupils	PERRLA, but slow to react

5. Which challenges do facial fractures present during ventilation with a bag-mask device?
6. Which precautions will you need to take when you attempt ET intubation?

Although not a traumatic eye injury, another time-sensitive eye condition you may encounter as a paramedic is central retinal artery occlusion. This condition causes ischemia and necrosis of the retina; if blood flow is not restored quickly, it can result in permanent damage to vision. Patients who experience such an occlusion will complain of sudden, painless loss of vision in the affected eye, which can range from mild to complete loss. Patients who develop central retinal artery occlusion are commonly in their early 60s, with males being slightly more likely to be affected than are females.[8]

Burns of the Eye

Chemicals, heat, and light rays can all burn the delicate tissues of the eye and **adnexa** (the surrounding structures and accessories), often causing permanent damage. Your role is to stop the burning process and prevent further damage.

Chemical burns, which are usually caused by acid or alkali solutions, require immediate emergency care Figure 33-21 . The individuals at greatest risk for chemical burns include laboratory technicians and hazardous materials technicians. However, anyone who works with or around chemicals should be considered at risk and receive proper training on how to handle the product and what to do in case of an emergency.

A patient who has a chemical burn to the eye usually has a loss of vision and shows evidence of facial skin burns. An acid burn generally causes immediate epithelial damage to the cornea. The cornea will appear white and opaque. After the initial damage, no further changes are noted in the cornea because proteins in the tears of the eye act as a barrier to further penetration of the acid. Acidic injuries still cause permanent visual changes.

Alkaline substances are not easily neutralized by the body, but instead penetrate deep into the eye as a result of emulsification. Such substances can have devastating effects on the eye. Alkalis can pass into the anterior chamber of eye rapidly, exposing the iris, ciliary body, lens, and other structures to further damage. Alkalis are most commonly found in concrete, lye, and drain cleaners. These substances damage each tissue layer of the eye they touch until the substance is removed. The damage to these tissues stimulates an inflammatory response, which further damages the tissues through the release of proteolytic enzymes, resulting in liquefactive necrosis. Alkaline burns cause permanent scarring of the cornea and sometimes permanent vision loss.[9]

When the patient has a chemical burn to the eye, flush the eye with water or a sterile saline solution. If sterile saline is not available, you can use any clean water for this purpose. Specific techniques for irrigating the eyes are discussed later in this section.

Thermal burns occur when a patient is burned in the face during a fire, although the eyes usually close

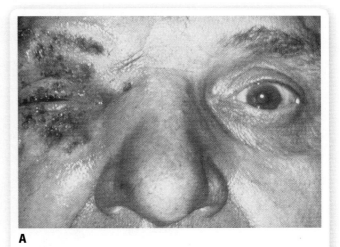

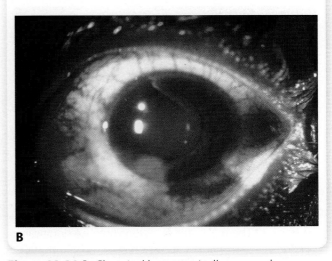

Figure 33-21 A. Chemical burns typically occur when an acid or alkali is splashed into the eye. **B.** A chemical burn from lye, an alkaline solution.

rapidly because of the heat. This reaction is a natural reflex to protect the eyes from further injury. However, the eyelids remain exposed and are frequently burned Figure 33-22 .

Infrared rays, eclipse light (if the patient has looked directly at the sun), and laser burns can cause significant damage to the sensory cells of the eye when rays of light become focused on the retina. Retinal injuries that are caused by exposure to extremely bright light are generally not painful but may result in permanent damage to vision.

Superficial burns of the eye can result from ultraviolet rays from an arc welding unit, prolonged exposure to a sunlamp, or reflected light from a bright snow-covered area (snow blindness). This kind of burn may not be painful initially but may become so 3 to 5 hours later, as the damaged cornea responds to the injury. Severe conjunctivitis usually develops, along with redness, swelling,

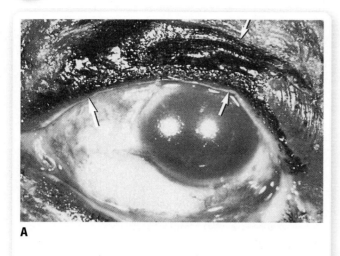

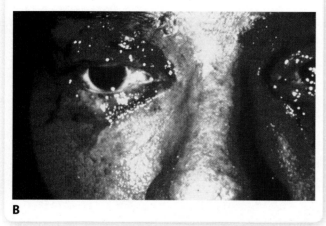

Figure 33-22 Thermal burns occasionally cause significant damage to the eyelids. **A.** Arrows show some full-thickness burns. **B.** Burns of the eyelids require immediate hospital care.

photophobia, the sensation of a foreign object in the eye, and excessive tear production.

► Assessment

Eye injuries can be a distracting injury. If the MOI suggests a high index of suspicion for a spinal injury, all spinal precautions must be followed. Spine and head immobilization may be necessary, and any life threats must be addressed. Ensure a patent airway and adequate breathing, and control any external bleeding. If the MOI is significant, or if the patient's clinical status dictates it, perform a rapid full-body scan.

When you are obtaining the history, determine how and when the injury happened, when the symptoms began, and which symptoms the patient is experiencing. Were both eyes affected? Does the patient have any underlying diseases or conditions of the eye (such as glaucoma)? Does the patient take medications for his or her eyes? Does the patient have any systemic conditions that are known to affect the eyes, such as hypertension or diabetes mellitus?

A variety of symptoms may indicate serious ocular injury:

- *Visual loss* that does not improve when the patient blinks is the most important symptom of an eye injury. It may indicate damage to the globe or to the optic nerve.
- *Double vision* usually points to trauma involving the extraocular muscles, such as a fracture of the orbit.
- *Severe eye pain* is a symptom of a significant eye injury.
- A *foreign body sensation* usually indicates superficial injury to the cornea or the presence of a foreign object trapped behind the eyelids.

Treatment for specific eye injuries begins with a thorough examination to determine the extent and nature of any damage. Always perform your examination using standard precautions, taking great care to avoid aggravating the injury. Assessment may be difficult because the patient may be forcibly keeping his or her eyelids closed. You will need to gain the patient's trust and open the lid to irrigate the eye with sterile water or saline solution. You may not be able to adequately assess the patient's eye until the pain has been managed.

When full examination is possible, assessment should include checking whether the eye can move to the following six cardinal positions of gaze: right, right up, right down, left, left up, and left down (following in a pattern). Assessment should include checking pupil dilation to light and checking the patient's vision when he or she looks to the left and to the right. Peripheral vision can be checked by having the patient look straight ahead and indicate whether he or she can see an object placed at the extreme left and extreme right of the normal field of vision. One method is to move your hand into the field of vision, starting beyond the normal field of vision, asking the patient to acknowledge when he or she sees your hand.

During the physical examination of the eyes, evaluate each of the visible ocular structures and ocular function:

- **Orbital rim.** Check for ecchymosis, swelling, lacerations, and tenderness.
- **Eyelids.** Check for ecchymosis, swelling, and lacerations.
- **Corneas.** Check for foreign bodies.
- **Conjunctivae.** Check for redness, pus, inflammation, and foreign bodies.
- **Globes.** Check for redness, abnormal pigmentation, and lacerations.
- **Pupils.** Assess size, shape, equality, and reaction to light.
- **Eye movements in all directions.** Assess for paralysis of gaze or discoordination

between the movements of the two eyes (**dysconjugate gaze**).

- **Visual acuity.** Make a rough assessment by asking the patient to read a newspaper or a handheld visual acuity chart; test each eye separately and document the results.

Although isolated eye injuries are usually not life threatening, they should be evaluated by a physician. More severe eye injuries often require evaluation and treatment by an ophthalmologist.

▶ Management

Lacerations and Blunt Trauma

Injuries to the eyelids—lacerations, abrasions, and contusions—require little in the way of prehospital care other than bleeding control and gentle patching of the affected eye. No eyelid injury is trivial, however, so every patient with eyelid trauma should be transported to the hospital. Bleeding from lacerations to the soft tissue of the eye, such as the eyelids, may be heavy, but it usually can be controlled by gentle, manual pressure. Remember not to apply pressure to the globe even when attempting to control bleeding of the soft tissues surrounding it, as doing so could ultimately result in loss of vision.

Patients with corneal abrasions will likely experience significant pain, sensitivity to light (photophobia), and excessive tearing. Examining the eye by inverting the upper and lower eyelids can expose the source of the corneal abrasion. It is important to carefully look for a foreign body in the eye. Close examination of the cornea may reveal a line or scratch. Abrasion sensation may vary, from the sensation of having a grain of sand in the eye to a stabbing sensation. It is usually more painful when the injury is exposed to the air.

Supportive care in the prehospital setting may include irrigation, which may help remove the object. A topical anesthetic like tetracaine can relieve some symptoms of corneal abrasion, and a lubricant can resolve some of the pain. If movement of the eye causes severe discomfort, you may need to cover both of the patient's eyes to prevent **sympathetic eye movement**, the movement of both eyes in unison. Taping the eyelid closed with paper tape can allow the patient to relax without forcibly holding the injured eye shut and keeps the eye from drying out. These injuries, especially those involving metal fragments, may need to be examined under a special microscope. If the cause of the abrasion is still present, it may need to be removed at an appropriate facility. In-hospital treatment consists of removing the fragment (if still present), treating the eye with topical antibiotics, and patching the eye. The cornea heals quickly.

Most injuries to the globe—including contusions, lacerations, foreign bodies, and abrasions—are best treated in the ED, where specialized equipment is available. Rigid eye shields (not gauze patches) applied over *both* eyes are generally all that are necessary in the field. Follow these three important guidelines in treating penetrating injuries of the eye:

1. Never exert pressure on or manipulate the injured globe in any way.
2. If part of the globe is exposed, gently apply a moist, sterile dressing to prevent drying.
3. Cover the injured eye with a protective rigid eye shield, cup, or sterile dressing. Apply soft dressings to both eyes, and provide prompt transport to the hospital.

If hyphema or rupture of the globe is suspected, take spinal immobilization precautions. Such injuries indicate that a significant amount of force was applied to the face and, therefore, suggest the presence of a spinal injury. Elevate the head of the backboard approximately 40° to decrease intraocular pressure, and discourage the patient from performing activities that may increase intraocular pressure (eg, coughing).

If there are no other contraindications, transport should be performed with the patient in Fowler position, and both eyes should be patched.

On rare occasions following a serious injury, the globe may be displaced (avulsed) out of its socket **Figure 33-23**. Do not attempt to manipulate or reposition it in any way! Cover the protruding eye with a moist, sterile dressing and stabilize it along with the uninjured eye to prevent further injury due to sympathetic eye movement. Place the patient in a supine position to prevent further loss of fluid from the eye, and provide prompt transport to the hospital.

Foreign Bodies and Impaled Objects

When the patient reports a foreign body in the eye, the paramedic, using a light, should carefully evaluate the entire eye. Note any blood or discoloration of the sclera.

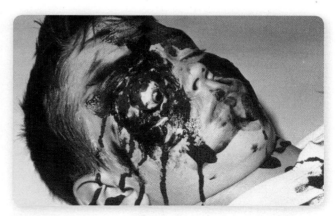

Figure 33-23 Do not attempt to manipulate or reposition a globe that is displaced (avulsed) out of its socket.
© American Academy of Orthopaedic Surgeons.

Gentle irrigation usually will not wash out foreign bodies that are stuck to the cornea or lying under the upper eyelid. To examine the undersurface of the upper eyelid, pull the lid upward and forward. If you spot a foreign object on the surface of the eyelid, you may be able to remove it with a moist, sterile, cotton-tipped applicator. *Never attempt to remove a foreign body that is stuck or imbedded in the cornea.*

To relieve pain and assist with dislodging the foreign body, begin by irrigating the eye with a sterile saline solution. Irrigation will frequently flush away loose, small foreign objects lying on the surface of the eye. Always flush from the nose side of the eye toward the outside to avoid flushing material into the other eye. After its removal, a foreign body will often leave a small abrasion on the surface of the conjunctiva, which leads to continued irritation; for this reason, you should transport the patient to the hospital for further assessment and treatment.

When a foreign body is impaled in the globe, *do not remove it!* Prehospital care involves stabilizing the object and preparing the patient for transport. The greater the length of the foreign object sticking out of the eye, the more important stabilization becomes in avoiding further damage. Cover the eye with a moist, sterile dressing; place a cup or other protective barrier over the object, and secure it in place with bulky dressing **Figure 33-24** . Cover the unaffected eye to prevent further damage that could occur from movement as the patient tries to use the uninjured eye to compensate for the loss or limited vision of the injured eye. Promptly transport the patient to the hospital.

Words of Wisdom

After covering the patient's eyes, keep him or her constantly reassured and oriented to your location and what you are doing.

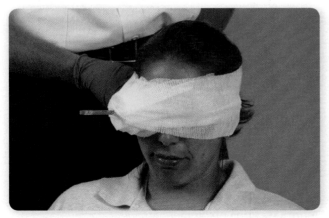

Figure 33-24 Secure an impaled object in the eye with a protective barrier and bulky dressing.
© Jones & Bartlett Learning.

Burns of the Eye

Burns to the eye that are caused by ultraviolet light are most effectively treated by covering the eye with a sterile, moist pad and an eye shield. The application of cool compresses *lightly* over the eye may afford the patient pain relief if he or she is in extreme distress. Place the patient in a supine position during transport, and protect the patient from further exposure to bright light.

Chemical burns to the eye—acid or alkali—can rapidly lead to total blindness if not immediately treated. The most important prehospital treatment in such cases is to begin immediate irrigation with sterile water or saline solution. *Never use any chemical antidotes (such as vinegar or baking soda) when you are irrigating the patient's eye; use sterile water or saline only.*

Words of Wisdom

Patients may have difficulty keeping their eyelids open during irrigation or the removal of foreign objects. In such cases, many services allow for the administration of 0.5% tetracaine hydrochloride drops to anesthetize the eye, thereby making the procedure more comfortable for the patient.

When you are irrigating the eye, the goal is to direct the greatest amount of solution or water into the eye as gently as possible. Because opening the eye spontaneously may cause the patient pain, you may have to force the lids open to irrigate the eye adequately. Ideally, you should use a device designed to irrigate the eye, such as a Morgan lens. This device is placed much like a contact lens and attached directly to a standard IV drip set **Figure 33-25** . If such a device is not available, you can use a bulb or irrigation syringe, a nasal cannula attached to an IV drip set, or some other device that will allow you to control the flow **Figure 33-26** . In some circumstances, you may have to pour water into the eye by holding the patient's head under a gently running faucet. You can have the patient immerse his or her face in a large pan or basin of water and rapidly blink the affected eyelid. If only one eye is affected, take care to avoid contaminated water getting into the unaffected eye.

Irrigate the eye for at least 5 minutes. If the burn was caused by an alkali or a strong acid, irrigate the eye continuously for 20 minutes because these substances can penetrate deeply.

One type of eye injury you may encounter occurs from the use of anhydrous ammonia, which is used during the process of cooking methamphetamine. If the patient's eyes are not irrigated promptly and efficiently, permanent damage is likely.

Whenever you have to irrigate the eye or eyes, continue irrigation en route to the hospital if possible, while being sure to control any contaminated runoff. Local protocol will direct you to specialized treatments for burns to the eyes.

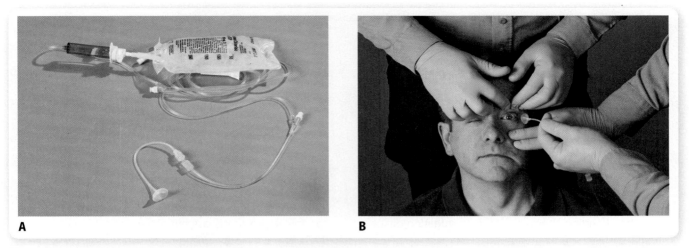

Figure 33-25 A. A Morgan lens. **B.** Morgan lens being inserted.
© Jones & Bartlett Learning.

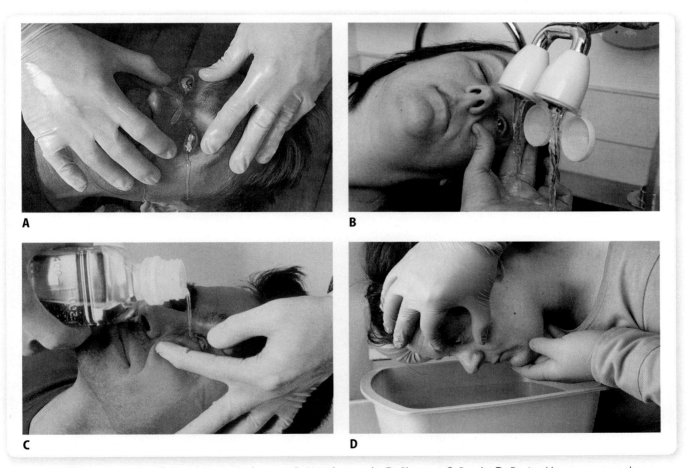

Figure 33-26 Four ways to effectively irrigate the eye: **A.** Nasal cannula. **B.** Shower. **C.** Bottle. **D.** Basin. Always protect the uninjured eye from the irrigating solution to prevent exposure to the substance.

A & C: © American Academy of Orthopaedic Surgeons; B & D: © Jones & Bartlett Learning.

Words of Wisdom

There are three types of contact lenses: hard, rigid gas-permeable, and soft (hydrophilic). Small, hard contact lenses usually are tinted, making them relatively easy to see. Large, soft contact lenses are clear and can be difficult to see, especially if they "float" up or down under an eyelid.

In general, you should not attempt to remove contact lenses from a patient with an eye injury because removal could further aggravate the injury. The only indication for removing contact lenses in the prehospital setting is a chemical burn of the eye. In this situation, the lens can trap the offending chemical and make irrigation difficult, thereby worsening the injury.

To remove a hard contact lens, use a small suction cup, moistening the end with saline solution **Figure 33-27A**.

To remove a soft contact lens, place one to two drops of saline solution in the eye **Figure 33-27B**, gently pinch the lens between your gloved thumb and index finger, and lift it off the surface of the eye **Figure 33-27C**. Place the contact lens in a container with sterile saline solution. Always advise ED staff if a patient is wearing contact lenses.

Occasionally, you may care for a patient who is wearing an eye prosthesis (artificial eye). You should suspect that an eye is artificial when it does not respond to light, move in concert with the opposite eye, or appear quite the same as the opposite eye. If you are unsure as to whether the patient has an eye prosthesis, ask the patient about it. Although no harm will be done if you care for an artificial eye as you would a normal one, you need to clearly understand the patient's eye function.

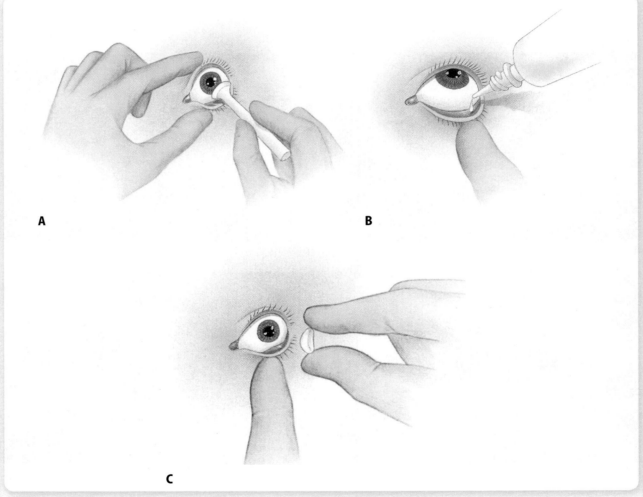

A

B

C

Figure 33-27 Contact lenses should be removed only when treating patients with chemical burns to the eye. To remove hard contact lenses, use a specialized suction cup moistened with sterile saline solution **(A)**. To remove soft contact lenses, place one or two drops of saline solution in the eye **(B)**, and pinch and lift the lens with your gloved thumb and index finger **(C)**.

Pathophysiology, Assessment, and Management of Ear Injuries

Injuries to the ear may be isolated, or they may occur in conjunction with other injuries to the head or face. Although isolated ear injuries are typically not life threatening, they can result in sensory impairment and permanent disfigurement.

▶ Pathophysiology

Soft-Tissue Injuries

Lacerations, avulsions, and contusions to the external ear can occur following blunt or penetrating trauma. The **pinna** can be contused, lacerated, or partially or completely avulsed. Trauma to the earlobe can result in similar injuries.

The pinna has an inherently poor blood supply, so it tends to heal poorly. Healing of the cartilaginous pinna is often complicated by infection.

Foreign Bodies in the Ear

Foreign bodies in the ear are most common in the pediatric population. The majority of the objects are solid, such as beads, stones, or even erasers. However, it is possible for an insect to crawl into the ear canal or for a child to put organic matter in the ear.

Assessment of a foreign body in the ear canal should determine the nature of the object and the urgency of treatment. The assessment of a foreign body in the ear in the prehospital environment is limited to visual clues if the object can be seen. Look for bleeding, redness or inflammation, and symptoms associated with infection. Some objects, such as organic matter and food, will swell from moisture and may become more entrapped as they swell. Small batteries such as those found in watches can leak chemicals and cause burns if left untreated. Serious symptoms or discomfort, as well as inserted objects that may cause harm or damage if left untreated, must be considered an emergency.

Ruptured Eardrum

Perforation of the **tympanic membrane** (ruptured eardrum) can result from direct blows, foreign bodies in the ear, pressure-related injuries, such as blast injuries resulting from an explosion, or diving-related injuries that result in barotrauma to the ear. Blast injuries are covered in detail in Chapter 50, *Terrorism Response*, and diving injuries are covered in Chapter 38, *Environmental Emergencies*.

Signs and symptoms of a perforated tympanic membrane include loss of hearing and blood drainage from the ear (hemorrhagic otorrhea). Although the injury is extremely painful for the patient, the tympanic membrane typically heals spontaneously and without complication. Nevertheless, a careful assessment should be performed to detect and treat other injuries, some of which may be life threatening.

▶ Assessment and Management

Assessment and management of the patient with an ear injury begin by ensuring airway patency and breathing adequacy. If the MOI suggests the need for spinal immobilization, apply full spinal immobilization precautions.

An adequate assessment of the external ear canal and middle ear cannot be performed in the field. In general, the ears' poor blood supply limits the amount of external bleeding. If manual direct pressure does not control this bleeding, first place a soft, padded dressing between the ear and the scalp, because bandaging the ear against the tender scalp can be extremely painful. Then apply a roller bandage to secure the dressing in place **Figure 33-28** . An ice pack can help reduce swelling and pain.

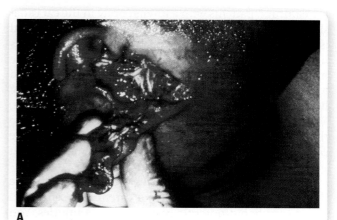

A

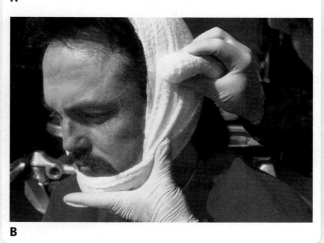

B

Figure 33-28 A. A major laceration of the ear. **B.** Place a soft, sterile pad behind the ear, between it and the scalp. Then wrap a roller gauze bandage (ie, Kling, Kerlix) around the head to include the entire ear.

B: © Jones & Bartlett Learning.

If the pinna is partially avulsed, carefully realign the ear into position and gently bandage it with sufficient padding that has been slightly moistened with normal saline. If the pinna is completely avulsed, attempt to retrieve the avulsed part, if possible, for reimplantation at the hospital. If the detached part of the ear is recovered, treat it as any other amputation; wrap it in saline-moistened gauze, place it in a plastic bag, and place the bag on ice.

If a chemical ice pack is used, it is recommended to shield the avulsed part with several 4-inch × 4-inch gauze pads to diffuse the cold, because chemical ice packs are actually colder than ice and inadvertent freezing of the part can occur. If blood or CSF drainage is noted, apply a loose dressing over the ear—taking care *not* to stop the flow—and assess the patient for other signs of a basilar skull fracture.

Do not remove an impaled object from the ear. Instead, stabilize the object and cover the ear to prevent gross movement and minimize the risk of contamination of the inner ear.

Because of the potential for infection and damage to the eardrum, patients with a foreign body in the ear canal should be seen by a physician in the ED. The ear canal is narrow and angulated, so probing for foreign bodies in the ear is discouraged. In some areas, the paramedic may use an otoscope to look farther into the ear if trained to do so and it is permitted based on local protocols; however, this is not a common practice in most regions. Management of both adults and children is to transport to the appropriate facility in the position of comfort. Severe pain or anxiety can be treated with pain management medication and/or mild sedation.

Because isolated ear injuries are typically not life threatening, you must perform a careful assessment to detect or rule out potentially more serious injuries. You may then proceed with specific care of the ear, provide emotional support, and transport the patient to an appropriate medical facility.

▮ Pathophysiology, Assessment, and Management of Oral and Dental Injuries

Oral and dental injuries are commonly associated with trauma to the face. Blunt mechanisms are commonly the result of motor vehicle crashes or direct blows to the mouth or chin. Penetrating mechanisms are commonly the result of gunshot wounds, lacerations, and punctures.

The primary risk associated with oral and dental injuries is airway compromise from oropharyngeal bleeding, occlusion by a displaced dental appliance such as a bridge or partial plate, or possibly occlusion by the aspiration of avulsed or fractured teeth. Any patient with significant facial trauma should be carefully assessed for injuries to the mouth and teeth.

▶ Pathophysiology

Soft-Tissue Injuries

Lacerations and avulsions in and around the mouth are associated with a risk of intraoral hemorrhage and subsequent airway compromise. Therefore, your assessment of any patient with facial trauma should include a careful examination of the mouth, including the teeth. Fractured or avulsed teeth and lacerations of the tongue may cause profuse bleeding into the upper airway **Figure 33-29** . A responsive patient with severe oral bleeding is often unable to speak unless he or she is leaning forward; this position facilitates drainage of blood from the mouth.

Patients may swallow blood from lacerations inside the mouth, so the bleeding may not be grossly evident. Because blood irritates the gastric lining, the risks of vomiting and aspiration are significant. Objects that are impaled in or through the soft tissues of the mouth (such as the cheek) can also result in profuse bleeding and, once again, the threat of vomiting with aspiration.

Dental Injuries

Fractured and avulsed teeth—especially the anterior teeth—are common following facial trauma. Dental injuries may be associated with mechanisms that cause severe maxillofacial trauma (such as motor vehicle crashes), or they may occur in isolation (such as a direct blow to the mouth from an assault).

You should always assess the patient's mouth following a facial injury, especially in cases of fractured or avulsed teeth. Teeth fragments (or even whole teeth) can become

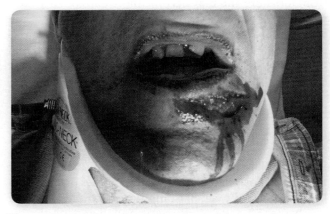

Figure 33-29 Soft-tissue injuries around the mouth can be associated with profuse oral bleeding and airway compromise.

© E. M. Singletary, MD. Used with permission.

an airway obstruction and should be removed from the patient's mouth immediately. In an unconscious patient with missing teeth that cannot be located, you must assume that the teeth are in the airway. Direct visualization with a laryngoscope may be necessary to ensure they are not, or to remove them if they are.

Words of Wisdom

When you are assessing a patient with fractured or avulsed teeth following an assault, you should also assess the person who struck the patient, *if it is safe to do so*. The human mouth is filled with bacteria and other microorganisms, and lacerations to the person's hands or knuckles can easily become infected without proper care. Occasionally, you may encounter fragments of broken teeth impaled in a person's knuckles!

▶ Assessment and Management

Ensuring airway patency and adequate breathing is the priority of care when you are managing patients with oral or dental trauma. Suction the oropharynx as needed, and remove fractured tooth fragments to prevent airway compromise. Apply spinal immobilization precautions if indicated by your physical exam. If profuse oral bleeding is present and the patient cannot spontaneously control his or her own airway (such as with a decreased level of consciousness), pharmacologically assisted intubation (such as RSI) may be necessary.

Impaled objects in the soft tissues of the mouth should be stabilized in place unless they interfere with the patient's breathing or your ability to manage the patient's airway. In those cases, remove the impaled object from the direction that it entered, if possible, and control bleeding with direct pressure.

An avulsed tooth may be successfully reimplanted even if it has been out of the mouth for as long as 1 hour. Medical control may sometimes ask you to reimplant the tooth in its original socket. Carefully place the tooth in its socket, and hold it in place with your fingers or have the patient gently bite down. If prehospital reimplantation of a tooth is not possible, follow the guidelines established by the American Association of Endodontists and the American Dental Association Table 33-2 .

Retrieval and reimplantation or storage of an avulsed tooth is a low priority if the patient is in a clinically unstable condition (such as a compromised airway or shock). In such cases, aggressive airway management, spinal precautions, and rapid transport of the patient are obviously more important, with the dental problem being addressed at a later time.

Table 33-2	Care for an Avulsed Tooth

Handle the tooth by the crown only. Avoid touching the root surface of the tooth so you do not compromise the periodontal ligament.

Gently rinse the tooth with sterile saline solution or water. Avoid the use of soap or chemicals, and do not scrub the tooth!

Do not allow the tooth to dry. Place it in one of the following:
- Emergency tooth preservation system (such as EMT Tooth Saver, 3M Save-a-Tooth): a break-resistant storage container with soft inner walls and a pH-balanced solution (such as Hanks' Balanced Salt Solution) that nourishes and preserves the tooth
- Propolis
- Egg white
- Coconut water
- Ricetral
- Cold whole milk
- Sterile saline solution (only if no other option is available and for storage periods of less than 1 hour)

Transport the tooth with the patient, and notify the hospital of the situation.

Data from: Patil S, Dumsha T, Sydiskis R. Determining periodontal ligament (PDL) cell vitality from exarticulated teeth stored in saline or milk using fluorescein diacetate. *Int Endodontic J.* 1994;27(1):1-5; and Poi W, Sonoda C, Martins C, et al. Storage media for avulsed teeth: a literature review. *Braz Dent J.* 2013;24(5):437-445.

■ Pathophysiology, Assessment, and Management of Injuries to the Anterior Part of the Neck

The neck is a vulnerable stretch of anatomy because it houses a critical portion of the airway (ie, larynx, trachea), the major blood vessels to and from the head, and the spinal cord. Other structures contained within the neck that are also vulnerable to injury include portions of the upper gastrointestinal system, such as the esophagus, and other muscles, nerves, and glands located in the region. Any injury to the anterior part of the neck—blunt or penetrating—must be considered critical until proved otherwise.

One method used to identify the structures within the neck and assist in classification of neck injuries divides the neck into zones Table 33-3 and Figure 33-30 . Injuries in zone I can extend into the chest and may not

Table 33-3	Zones of the Neck	
Zone	**Boundaries**	**Important Anatomic Structures**
I	Area between the cricoid cartilage and the clavicles and sternum	Carotid and vertebral arteries Subclavian veins Brachiocephalic veins Jugular veins Aortic arch Lungs Trachea Esophagus Thoracic duct Cervical spine Spinal cord
II	Area between the angle of the mandible and the cricoid cartilage	Carotid and vertebral arteries Jugular veins Pharynx Larynx Trachea Esophagus Cervical spine Spinal cord
III	Area above the angle of the mandible	Carotid and vertebral arteries Jugular veins Salivary and parotid glands Esophagus Pharynx Trachea Cranial nerves IX through XII Cervical spine Spinal cord

© Jones & Bartlett Learning.

be easily recognized on physical examination. Injuries in this area are associated with the highest mortality rate. Injuries in zone II are the most common, are usually the most obvious, and have a lower mortality rate than do zone I injuries. Injuries in zone III often are difficult for a surgeon to access and repair because many of the structures enter the base of the skull.

▶ Pathophysiology

Soft-Tissue Injuries

Blunt and penetrating mechanisms can damage the soft tissues of the anterior part of the neck and its associated structures. In both cases, you must be alert for the possibility of cervical spine injury and airway compromise.

Common mechanisms of blunt trauma include motor vehicle crashes, direct trauma to the neck ("clothesline"-type injury), and hangings. Such injury often results in swelling and edema; injury to the various structures, such as the trachea, hyoid bone, larynx, epiglottis, or esophagus; or injury to the cervical spine. Less commonly, blunt injuries damage the vasculature of the anterior part of the neck. Because blunt trauma to the neck is associated with a high incidence of airway compromise and ventilatory inadequacy, you must carefully assess the patient and be prepared to initiate aggressive management.

Common mechanisms of penetrating trauma include gunshot wounds, stabbings, and impaled objects. The lacerations or puncture wounds produced may be superficial and involve only the fascia or fatty tissues of the neck, or they may be deep and involve injury to the larynx, trachea, esophagus, nerves, or major blood vessels.

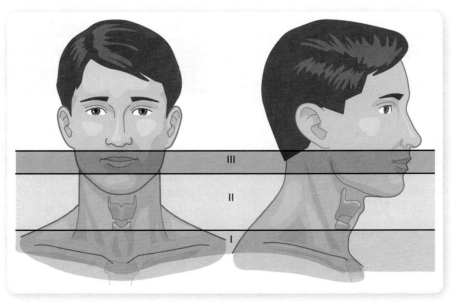

Figure 33-30 The zones of the neck.
© Jones & Bartlett Learning.

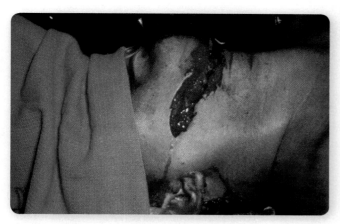

Figure 33-31 Open injuries to the neck can be dangerous. If veins are exposed to the environment, they can suck in air, resulting in a potentially fatal air embolism.

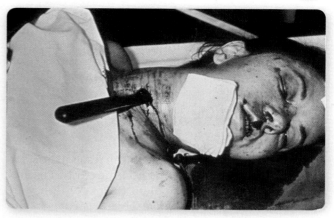

Figure 33-32 Impaled objects in the neck can cause profuse bleeding if the major blood vessels are damaged and can cause direct injury to the larynx, trachea, esophagus, or cervical spine.

The primary threats from penetrating neck trauma are massive hemorrhage from major blood vessel disruption and airway compromise secondary to soft-tissue swelling or direct damage to the larynx or trachea.

A special danger associated with open neck injuries is the possibility of a fatal air embolism. If the jugular veins of the neck are exposed to the environment, they may entrain (suck) air into the vessel during inspiration, creating a venous embolism **Figure 33-31** . Such an embolism can lead to right ventricular dysfunction and failure, which will reduce cardiac output and can lead to cardiovascular failure. To prevent these complications,

open neck wounds should be sealed with an occlusive dressing immediately. Use caution to avoid constricting the vessels and structures of the neck, and be alert for swelling and expanding hematomas because they can turn the occlusive dressing into a constricting band.[10-12]

Impaled objects in the neck can present several life-threatening problems for the patient—namely, injury to major blood vessels with massive hemorrhage; damage to the larynx, trachea, or esophagus; or injury to the cervical spine **Figure 33-32** . Impaled objects should not

YOU are the Paramedic PART 4

Your partner assists the first responder by gently holding the mask of the bag-mask device in place while the bag is squeezed. When you are ready to intubate the patient, you instruct your partner to gently hold the mandible and sides of the patient's face to provide stability. You gently lift your laryngoscope and visualize the vocal cords. You successfully watch the ET tube slide through the vocal cords.

Recording Time: 10 Minutes	
Respirations	12 breaths/min, assisted
Pulse	126 beats/min
Skin	Cool, pale, moist
Blood pressure	90/60 mm Hg
Oxygen saturation (Spo₂)	95% via bag-mask device at 15 L/min
Pupils	PERRLA, but slow to react

7. Describe the steps in determining proper placement of an ET tube.
8. How will you secure the ET tube in place with this type of facial fracture?

be removed, but rather should be stabilized in place and protected from movement. The *only* exception is if the object is obstructing the airway or impeding your ability to effectively manage the airway. In some cases, an emergency cricothyrotomy may be necessary to establish and maintain airway patency.

Injuries to the Larynx, Trachea, and Esophagus

A variety of life-threatening injuries can result if the structures of the anterior part of the neck are crushed against the cervical spine following blunt trauma or if they are penetrated by a knife or similar object. The larynx and its supporting structures (ie, **hyoid bone**, thyroid cartilage, and cricoid ring) may be fractured, the trachea may be separated from the larynx (**tracheal transection**), or the esophagus may be perforated. Many injuries to the larynx, trachea, and esophagus are occult; because they are not as obvious and dramatic as penetrating neck injuries, they can be easily overlooked. Therefore, you must maintain a high index of suspicion and perform a careful assessment of *any* patient with blunt trauma to the anterior part of the neck.

Significant injuries to the larynx or trachea pose an *immediate* risk of airway compromise due to disruption of the normal passage of air, soft-tissue swelling, or aspiration of blood into the lungs. In addition, esophageal perforation can result in **mediastinitis**, an inflammation of the mediastinum often due to leakage of gastric contents into the thoracic cavity. Mediastinitis has a very high mortality rate, particularly without rapid surgical treatment.

Patients with injuries to the anterior part of the neck may experience concomitant maxillofacial fractures, which can make bag-mask ventilation difficult (usually because of an inadequate mask-to-face seal). Likewise, ET intubation may be extremely challenging, if not impossible, owing to distortion of the normal anatomic structures of the upper airway.

If basic and advanced techniques to secure the patient's airway are unsuccessful or impossible, a surgical or needle cricothyrotomy may be your only means of establishing a patent airway and ensuring adequate oxygenation and ventilation. Prior to deciding to perform a surgical airway, using a lighted stylette or a gum bougie may allow you to secure the airway in a timely fashion while avoiding riskier procedures.

▶ Assessment

Bruising, redness to the overlying skin, and palpable tenderness are common signs associated with all injuries to the anterior part of the neck. **Table 33-4** summarizes the signs and symptoms of specific injuries.

Begin your assessment by noting the MOI and maintaining a high index of suspicion, especially if the patient has experienced blunt or penetrating trauma between the

Table 33-4	Signs and Symptoms of Injuries to the Anterior Part of the Neck
Injury	**Signs and Symptoms**
Laryngeal fracture, tracheal transection	Labored breathing or reduced air movement Stridor Hoarseness, voice changes **Hemoptysis** (coughing up blood) Subcutaneous emphysema Swelling, edema Structural irregularity
Vascular injury	Gross external bleeding Signs of shock Hematoma, swelling, edema Pulse deficits
Esophageal perforation	**Dysphagia** (difficulty swallowing) Hematemesis Hemoptysis (suggests aspiration of blood)
Neurologic impairment	Signs of a stroke (suggests air embolism or cerebral infarct) Paralysis or paresthesia Cranial nerve deficit Signs of neurogenic shock

© Jones & Bartlett Learning.

Words of Wisdom

Any force that is powerful enough to disrupt the larynx, trachea, or esophagus has the potential to injure the cervical spine. Carefully assess the patient for signs of a spinal injury—for example, vertebral deformities (step-offs), paralysis, paresthesia, and signs of neurogenic shock (hypotension, normal or slow pulse rate, lack of diaphoresis). If your exam reveals signs of spinal injury, implement spinal immobilization precautions.

upper part of the chest and the head. Fractures of the first rib are associated with nearly 50% mortality—not because of the rib fracture, but rather because fracturing such a short, stout bone takes so much force that significant face, head, and neck trauma are often present as well. Remember that obvious and dramatic-appearing soft-tissue injuries may mask occult injuries to the larynx, trachea, or esophagus. Also, the patient may have experienced trauma to multiple body systems, especially following a significant MOI.

As you begin your primary survey, manually stabilize the patient's head in a neutral in-line position and simultaneously open the airway with the jaw-thrust maneuver if the patient is unresponsive. Use suction as needed to clear the airway of blood or other liquids. Assess the patient's breathing—rate, regularity, and depth—and intervene immediately. If the patient is breathing adequately, apply a nonrebreathing mask at 15 L/min. If breathing is inadequate (ie, reduced tidal volume, fast or slow respirations), assist with bag-mask ventilation and 100% oxygen.

▶ Management

Your primary focus when caring for a patient is always to treat the injuries that will be the *most rapidly fatal*. Because death following trauma to the anterior part of the neck is usually the result of airway compromise or massive bleeding, aggressive airway management and external bleeding control are the highest priorities of care.

After addressing any life-threatening or other serious problems during the primary survey, you may perform a rapid exam to detect and treat other injuries. To control bleeding from an open neck wound and prevent an air embolism, immediately cover the wound with an occlusive dressing. In the case of one or more small wounds, use of electrocardiography electrodes can be a fast and effective way to seal the small hole or holes. Apply manual direct pressure over the occlusive dressing with a bulky dressing. To secure a pressure dressing over the wound, wrap roller gauze loosely around the patient's neck and then firmly through the opposite axilla **Figure 33-33**. *Do not* circumferentially wrap bandages around the neck to secure the dressing in place. This practice is contraindicated and could even be fatal: It may impair cerebral perfusion by occluding both carotid arteries or interfere with the patient's breathing. Monitor the patient's pulse for reflex bradycardia, which indicates parasympathetic nervous stimulation due to excessive pressure on the carotid artery.

If signs of shock are present, administer oxygen as necessary to maintain an oxygen saturation level of 94% or higher, control any external hemorrhage, and keep the patient warm. Establish vascular access with at least one 18-gauge IV catheter and infuse an isotonic crystalloid solution (such as lactated Ringer solution or normal saline) as needed to maintain a systolic blood pressure of 80 to 90 mm Hg.

Many patients with serious laryngeal trauma have airway obstruction and may require a surgical or percutaneous airway. ET intubation may be hazardous in these patients because you cannot see the tip of the ET tube once it passes between the vocal cords; it may pass straight

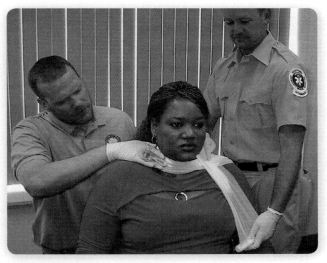

Figure 33-33 Cover open neck wounds with an occlusive dressing, and apply manual pressure to control bleeding. *Do not* compress both carotid arteries simultaneously; doing so may impair cerebral perfusion.
© Jones & Bartlett Learning.

through a defect in the laryngeal or tracheal wall or could result in the complete transection of the trachea. Signs of this complication include increased swelling of the neck and worsening subcutaneous emphysema during assisted ventilation.

If the patient has experienced an open tracheal wound, you may be able to pass a cuffed ET tube directly through the wound to establish a patent airway. However, you must use caution because the trachea may be perforated both anteriorly *and* posteriorly, thereby increasing the risk of false passage of the ET tube outside the trachea. It is critical to use *multiple* techniques for confirming correct ET tube placement: frequently monitor breath sounds, directly measure the expired carbon dioxide (waveform capnography is preferred for this purpose), assess for adequate chest rise, and assess for vapor mist in the ET tube during exhalation.

Documentation & Communication

Whenever injury to the anterior part of the neck (specifically the larynx) is recognized or suspected, it is prudent to advise the patient to refrain from speaking to allow the vocal cords to rest and recuperate. To keep the patient from speaking, you will need to ask questions that can be answered with a simple yes or no. Alternatively, you may ask the patient to write answers for you. Keep in mind that if the larynx is injured, the incidence of cervical spine involvement is relatively high; therefore, the patient should avoid shaking his or her head when answering.

Pathophysiology, Assessment, and Management of Spine Trauma

▶ Pathophysiology

The neck, because of its relative exposure to forces both directly applied and referred, is subject to injury that does not necessarily result in a specific bony injury such as fracture or dislocation. Most of these nonpenetrating injuries are ultimately classified as **sprains** (stretching or tearing of ligaments) and **strains** (stretching or tearing of a muscle or tendon).

In response to strains in the neck, the muscles contract as they attempt to support the neck. It is believed that this response is the result of injury to the facet joint. This injury can be difficult, if not impossible, to identify in the prehospital setting. As a result, you should maintain a high index of suspicion of cervical involvement and thoroughly assess the need for cervical spine immobilization.

The most common form of cervical strain is often called **whiplash**. Whiplash can be difficult to differentiate from unstable spine fracture or dislocation. If the paramedic's scope of practice involves clearing the spine after injury, findings of point tenderness and pain on movement often preclude "ruling out" a spinal injury, and cervical precautions should be taken and maintained throughout contact and transport. Although mortality from whiplash is rare, morbidity can occasionally develop in the form of persistent and chronic cervical pain, with some patients experiencing prolonged spasms and exacerbation.

▶ Assessment

Because the evaluation of complaints of neck pain can be difficult, it is recommended that you transport patients to the ED for radiologic studies. Conduct a visual inspection for signs of soft-tissue injury, which may indicate muscular and bony involvement. If the patient is symptomatic and has pain (either with or without movement and palpation), maintain spinal immobilization. If the MOI dictates that the **spinal clearance** protocol be used and your examination produces any pain or resistance, most protocols require that the provider stop the examination, maintain spinal immobilization, and transport the patient for further evaluation in the ED.

▶ Management

Because of the risk of orthopaedic and central nervous system involvement, most specialists recommend that patients reporting neck pain after injury should be evaluated in the ED. You should address any airway, ventilation, and oxygenation considerations and ensure there is no major circulatory compromise. Prehospital management should focus on preventing further injury with provision of motion restrictions, typically with application of an extrication collar and placement of the patient on a long backboard, scoop stretcher, or vacuum mattress, if indicated. In critical patients, it may be necessary to perform these tasks simultaneously. If the patient requires advanced airway control, it is acceptable to open the extrication collar while providing in-line stabilization to facilitate the intubation. During application of a backboard, scoop stretcher, or vacuum mattress, as in all splinting procedures, it is essential for you to check distal circulation and sensory and motor function before and after the full-body splint (backboard or vacuum mattress) is applied and to document those findings in your patient care report.

If your examination and questioning of the patient reveal no obvious MOI, you may consider treatment of the suspected strain as you would for any other muscular strain. This can include rest, ice, and elevation. A soft collar may help to gently support the head and decrease the workload on the strained muscles. An extrication collar can provide limited similar benefit. It is still recommended that patients reporting neck pain be evaluated for occult injuries and prevention of long-term consequences. For full coverage of this topic, see Chapter 34, *Head and Spine Trauma*.

Injury Prevention

Because injuries to the face and neck in all of their varying degrees can be life altering and permanent, many improvements and advancements have been made in providing protection to these regions of the anatomy. This is especially true in the area of organized events such as contact sports and wheel-borne sports. Helmets, face shields, mouth guards, and safety glasses help to prevent injury during activities in which the risk of being hit with objects that are in motion is proportionately high. The same holds true for advances in motor vehicle safety. Better occupant safety restraints and airbags help to prevent contact with the interior of the vehicle, and improvements to the headrests, if they are used properly, are reducing the number of neck strains.

YOU are the Paramedic   SUMMARY

1. What is your primary concern after scene safety is established?

Your immediate concern is the condition of the patient's airway. The patient is unresponsive and has snoring respirations. Without conducting any further assessment, you know the patient has an incomplete airway that needs immediate management.

2. What is your first step in controlling the patient's airway?

You know the patient sustained a significant impact to her face, but you do not know how extensive the damage is at this point. You can suction the patient to remove blood as you begin the assessment of facial structures.

3. Which type of facial fracture may this patient have?

The crepitus, the free-floating feel of the maxilla, and the clear fluid coming from the patient's nose lead to the suspicion of a Le Fort fracture. Whether it is a type I, II, or III fracture will be determined in the clinical setting. What is important is for you to understand that a Le Fort fracture is an unstable facial fracture. The instability will require extra caution when you are ventilating the patient or using invasive airway techniques.

4. How will this type of fracture affect the selection of an appropriate airway method?

Le Fort fractures are unstable and will move with manipulation. Movement will cause further injury, which in turn will cause more damage and swelling. A definitive airway needs to be placed immediately. In this case, ET intubation, if possible, would be best.

5. Which challenges do facial fractures present during ventilation with a bag-mask device?

When you think of the method used to perform bag-mask ventilation on a patient with normal facial features, you can imagine how unstable facial fractures will complicate the process. If an adequate number of care providers are present on scene, use two people to operate the bag-mask device. The provider responsible for placement of the mask needs to use extreme caution to not press inward to maintain a seal. Care should also be taken to not move the mask laterally.

6. Which precautions will you need to take when you attempt ET intubation?

Because blood has already been noted in the patient's upper airway, be ready to perform suctioning when you are inserting the laryngoscope. There may be more blood, tissue, bone, or teeth in the airway on visualization. Have your forceps ready should you need them. Have a second provider gently hold the patient's face to maintain its stability while you visualize and insert the airway.

7. Describe the steps in determining proper placement of an ET tube.

Proper placement of the ET tube begins with visualizing the tip of the tube passing through the vocal cords. If you did not see the tube, you cannot be certain where it is. After inflating the cuff (if supplied), auscultate starting with the epigastrium. If you hear air movement, the ET tube is not in the trachea. If there is no air movement in the stomach, auscultate over both lungs to ensure equal inflation. Repeat the listening process after securing the ET tube in place. Finally, apply capnography and monitor the readings.

8. How will you secure the ET tube in place with this type of facial fracture?

As with the bag-mask device, securing the ET tube in place may be challenging because of the injury to the maxilla. Commercially available devices may still work as long as you use caution when tightening the straps. Alternatively, tape may be used.

YOU are the Paramedic   SUMMARY *(continued)*

EMS Patient Care Report (PCR)

Date: 03-27-18	Incident No.: 23542		Nature of Call: MVC		Location: Hwy 12/River Rd
Dispatched: 1115	**En Route:** 1116	**At Scene:** 1121	**Transport:** 1135	**At Hospital:** 1142	**In Service:** 1200

Patient Information

Age: 21
Sex: F
Weight (in kg [lb]): 55 kg (120 lb)

Allergies: Unknown
Medications: Unknown
Past Medical History: Unknown
Chief Complaint: Facial trauma

Vital Signs

Time	BP	Pulse	Respirations	Spo$_2$
Time: 1126	BP: 90/60	Pulse: 130	Respirations: 8	Spo$_2$: 92% RA
Time: 1131	BP: 90/60	Pulse: 126	Respirations: 12	Spo$_2$: 95% bag-mask device
Time:	BP:	Pulse:	Respirations:	Spo$_2$:

EMS Treatment (circle all that apply)

Oxygen @ __15__ L/min via (circle one): NC NRM (Bag-mask device)	(Assisted Ventilation)	(Airway Adjunct: 7.5 ET tube)	CPR
Defibrillation	Bleeding Control	Bandaging	Splinting	(Other: Spinal immobilization, suction, IV)

Narrative

Arrived to find a 21-year-old female who was riding in the bed of a pickup that hit a tree head-on. This pt was unrestrained and was projected forward, striking her face on the cab. Pt was placed in spinal precautions prior to our arrival by Engine 21 crew. Pt is unresponsive with snoring respirations. Attempted oral airway w/o success. Pt has what appears to be a free-floating maxilla with associated blood and clear fluid coming from nose. Suction applied and bag-mask device used with two providers so as to not push in on the maxilla. ET tube 7.5 mm inserted with visualization of the tube passing the cords. No epigastric sounds and positive equal lung sounds noted on ventilation with ET tube. Tube secured using a commercially manufactured device and ET tube placement reassessed. Capnography applied. IV NS established with 12-gauge left AC. Transported emergency without incident to the trauma center and no change in pt condition. Report to Dr. Sterrett on arrival.**End of report**

Prep Kit

► Ready for Review

- A strong working knowledge of anatomy and physiology of the face, head, and brain is essential to accurately assess and manage patients with injuries to these locations.
- Personal safety is your initial primary concern when you are treating any patient with head or face trauma.
- When responding to incidents involving serious trauma, management of soft-tissue injuries should wait until you have achieved control of the airway, breathing, and circulation.
- Trauma to the face can range from a broken nose to more severe injuries, including massive soft-tissue trauma, maxillofacial fractures, oral or dental trauma, and eye injuries.
- Your primary concerns when assessing and managing a patient with facial trauma are ensuring a patent airway and maintaining adequate oxygenation and ventilation. Trauma to the face or neck can compromise the patient's airway, and foreign bodies lodged in the mouth should alert you to the potential for airway obstruction and aspiration. Airway management is crucial in managing these injuries.
- Any patient with head or face trauma should be suspected of having a spinal injury. Apply spinal immobilization precautions as indicated.
- Nasal airways and blind nasotracheal intubation are relatively contraindicated in the presence of midface fracture; such maneuvers should not be performed unless absolutely necessary and with approval of medical control.
- Remove impaled objects in the face or throat only if they impair airway patency or breathing or if they interfere with your ability to effectively manage the airway. Otherwise, stabilize them in place and protect them from further movement.
- Injuries to the eye can be varied, including lacerations and corneal abrasion, blunt trauma, impaled objects, or burns. Never exert pressure or manipulate an injured globe in any way.
- Never remove impaled objects from the eye; stabilize them in place and put a protective cone (such as a cup) over the object to prevent accidental movement. You should also bandage the unaffected eye to prevent sympathetic movement.
- Chemical burns to the eye should be treated with gentle irrigation using sterile water or saline.
- Ear injuries should be realigned and bandaged. If a part is avulsed, transport it with the patient if possible. Stabilize an object that is impaled in the ear. Probing for foreign bodies in the ear is discouraged.
- The primary threat from oral or dental trauma is oropharyngeal bleeding and aspiration of blood or broken teeth. Keep the airway clear, and ensure adequate oxygenation and ventilation. Endotracheal intubation may be required.
- Aggressively manage injuries involving the anterior part of the neck, ensuring that airway management and external bleeding control remain the top priority. Treat for shock if signs are present, and transport rapidly.

► Vital Vocabulary

adnexa The surrounding structures and accessories of an organ; for the eye, these parts include the eyelids, lashes, and lacrimal structures.

alveoli Small pits or cavities, such as the sockets for the teeth.

anterior chamber The anterior area of the globe between the lens and the cornea, which is filled with aqueous humor.

blowout fracture A fracture to the floor of the orbit, usually caused by a blow to the eye.

conjunctiva A thin, transparent membrane that covers the sclera and internal surfaces of the eyelids.

conjunctivitis An inflammation of the conjunctivae that usually is caused by bacteria, viruses, allergies, or foreign bodies; should be considered highly contagious if infectious in origin; also called pinkeye.

cornea The transparent anterior portion of the eye that overlies the iris and pupil.

craniofacial disjunction A Le Fort III fracture that involves a fracture of all of the midfacial bones, which separates the entire midface from the cranium.

crown The part of the tooth that is external to the gum.

cusps Points at the top of a tooth.

dentin The principal mass of the tooth, which is made up of a material that is much denser and stronger than bone.

diplopia Double vision.

dysconjugate gaze Paralysis of gaze or lack of coordination between the movements of the two eyes.

dysphagia Difficulty swallowing.

epistaxis Nosebleed.

external ear One of the three anatomic parts of the ear; it contains the pinna, the ear canal, and the external portion of the tympanic membrane.

globe The eyeball.

Prep Kit (continued)

hard palate The bony anterior part of the palate that forms the roof of the mouth.

hemoptysis Coughing up blood.

hyoid bone A bone at the base of the tongue that supports the tongue and its muscles.

hyphema Bleeding into the anterior chamber of the eye; results from direct ocular trauma.

inner ear One of the three anatomic parts of the ear; it consists of the cochlea and semicircular canals.

iris The colored portion of the eye.

Le Fort fractures Maxillary fractures that are classified into three categories based on their anatomic location.

malocclusion Misalignment of the teeth.

mandible The movable lower jaw bone.

mediastinitis Inflammation of the mediastinum, often a result of the gastric contents leaking into the thoracic cavity after esophageal perforation.

middle ear One of the three anatomic parts of the ear; it consists of the inner portion of the tympanic membrane and the ossicles.

oculomotor nerve The third cranial nerve; it innervates the muscles that cause motion of the eyeballs and upper eyelid.

optic nerve Either of the second cranial nerves that enter the eyeball posteriorly, through the optic foramen.

orbits Bony cavities in the frontal part of the skull that enclose and protect the eyes.

pinna The large outside portion of the ear through which sound waves enter the ear; also called the auricle.

pulp Specialized connective tissue within the cavity of a tooth.

pupil The circular opening in the center of the eye through which light passes to the lens.

retina A delicate 10-layered structure of nervous tissue located in the rear of the interior of the globe; it receives light and generates nerve signals that are transmitted to the brain through the optic nerve.

retinal detachment Separation of the inner layers of the retina from the underlying choroid, the vascular membrane that nourishes the retina.

sclera The white part of the eye.

spinal clearance The act of declaring that a spinal injury is not present.

sprain Stretching or tearing of ligaments.

strain Stretching or tearing of a muscle or tendon.

sympathetic eye movement The movement of both eyes in unison.

temporomandibular joint (TMJ) The joint between the temporal bone and the posterior condyle that allows for movements of the mandible.

tracheal transection Traumatic separation of the trachea from the larynx.

tympanic membrane A thin membrane that separates the middle ear from the outer ear and sets up vibrations in the ossicles; also called the eardrum.

vitreous humor A jellylike substance found in the posterior compartment of the eye between the lens and the retina.

whiplash An injury to the neck in which hyperextension occurs as a result of the head moving abruptly forward or backward; it can be difficult to differentiate from injuries that involve cervical bony structures and the spine.

▶ References

1. Fahling JM, Mckenzie LK. Oculocardiac reflex as a result of intraorbital trauma. *J Emerg Med.* 2016.
2. Jurdy L, Malhotra R. White-eyed medial wall blowout fracture mimicking head injury due to persistent oculocardiac reflex. *J Craniofac Surg.* 2011;22(5):1977-1979.
3. Kasi SK, Gorovoy IR, Vagefi MR, Kersten RC. The oculocardiac reflex in an adult with a non-displaced orbital floor fracture. *Orbit.* 2014;33(4):286-288.
4. Kim BB, Qaqish C, Frangos J, Caccamese JF. Oculocardiac reflex induced by an orbital floor fracture: report of a case and review of the literature. *J Oral Maxillofac Surg.* 2012;70(11):2614-2619.
5. Worthington J. Isolated posterior orbital floor fractures, diplopia and oculocardiac reflexes: a 10-year review. *Br J Oral Maxillofac Surg.* 2010;48(2):127-130.
6. Centers for Disease Control and Prevention website. https://www.cdc.gov/niosh/topics/eye/default.html. Accessed March 21, 2017.
7. Mayo Clinic: Retinal detachment. http://www.mayoclinic.org/diseases-conditions/retinal-detachment/symptoms-causes/dxc-20197292. Accessed March 21, 2017.
8. Graham R, Ebrahim S. Central retinal artery occlusion: background, pathophysiology, epidemiology. Medscape website. http://emedicine.medscape.com/article/1223625. Updated August 1, 2016. Accessed March 15, 2017.
9. Solano J, Rosen C. Ocular burns: background, pathophysiology, etiology. Medscape website.

Prep Kit (continued)

http://emedicine.medscape.com/article/798696. Updated April 7, 2015. Accessed March 15, 2017.

10. Natal B, Doty C. Venous air embolism: background, pathophysiology, etiology. Medscape website. http://emedicine.medscape.com/article/761367. Udpated October 19, 2016. Accessed June 7, 2016.

11. Palmon S, Moore L, Lundberg J, Toung T. Venous air embolism: a review. *J Clin Anesthes*. 1997;9(3):251-257.

12. Platz E. Tangential gunshot wound to the chest causing venous air embolism: a case report and review. *J Emerg Med.* 2011;41(2):e25-e29.

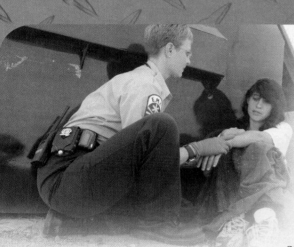

Assessment in Action

Your unit is dispatched to a local baseball field for a player hit by a baseball bat. When you arrive on scene, you are directed to a man who was hit in the neck by a broken bat. The patient is responsive, alert, and oriented. The patient reports difficulty swallowing, and his voice sounds raspy. There is no visible bleeding, but a hematoma is developing on the right lateral neck.

1. An understanding of the neck's anatomy is crucial to this patient assessment. In any neck trauma, you must consider injury to the trachea, which is made of several cartilaginous rings. Which cartilaginous ring is commonly referred to as the Adam's apple?

   A. Cricoid
   B. Thyroid
   C. Hyoid
   D. Laryngeal

2. Your patient suffered an injury to the right side of his neck and is now presenting with a hematoma. Vascular injury must be considered as you evaluate the patient. What is the large vein that runs laterally on both sides of the neck?

   A. Carotid
   B. Thyroid
   C. Jugular
   D. Esophageal

3. If the patient had a penetrating injury to the neck, which type of dressing would be applied?

   A. Bulky dressing, lightly bandaged in place
   B. Bulky dressing, tightly bandaged in place
   C. Occlusive dressing, sealed on all sides
   D. Occlusive dressing, sealed on three sides

4. What should also be considered in this patient as a result of the symptoms and mechanism?

   A. Partial airway obstruction
   B. Lower airway swelling
   C. Cervical spine involvement
   D. Likelihood that the patient is a chronic smoker

Assessment *in Action* (continued)

5. You start to provide spinal immobilization to the patient using a cervical collar and a long backboard. The patient is unable to tolerate lying supine and reports increased shortness of breath. What is the most suitable alternative treatment?

 A. Provide supplemental oxygen and elevate the head of the backboard to facilitate breathing.

 B. Force the patient to comply with the protocols in place.

 C. Provide spinal immobilization with a short backboard or extrication vest to allow the patient to sit upright and control his airway.

 D. Provide nasal tracheal intubation to bypass the laryngeal fracture.

6. If the patient had a foreign body impaled in the globe, which type of dressing would be applied?

 A. Bulky dressing, lightly bandaged in place for both eyes

 B. Bulky dressing, tightly bandaged in place for the affected eye

 C. Moist, sterile dressing and protective cup for the affected eye

 D. Moist, sterile dressing; protective cup for the affected eye; and bandage for the unaffected eye

7. Upon further assessment, you find that the patient has unequal pupils, but his teammates tell you this is normal for him. What is the medical term for a person with normally unequal pupils?

 A. Dysconjugate

 B. Glaucoma

 C. Anisocoria

 D. Diplopia

8. Describe each of the three types of Le Fort fractures.

9. Your patient was cutting metal with an angle grinder when the cutting wheel shattered and struck him in the left side of the neck halfway between the clavicle and the angle of the mandible. He now has moderate hemorrhage from the laceration caused by the shrapnel. What are your concerns about an open wound to the lateral neck? How would you manage an open wound to the lateral neck?

10. A 22-year-old man was struck in the left eye with a fist during a fight. He is experiencing heavy discharge from the left nostril and is complaining of numbness over the left side of the upper lip. He also states that he has double vision. When you ask him to look up, the upward gaze of his left eye is paralyzed. What is your diagnosis of this patient's injury? What is your treatment plan?

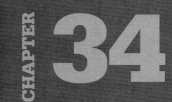

Head and Spine Trauma

National EMS Education Standard Competencies

Trauma

Integrates assessment findings with principles of epidemiology and pathophysiology to formulate a field impression to implement a comprehensive treatment/disposition plan for an acutely injured patient.

Head, Facial, Neck, and Spine Trauma

Recognition and management of
> Life threats (pp 1721-1723)
> Spine trauma (pp 1719-1721, 1725-1727, 1729-1732, 1747-1752, 1755-1773)

Pathophysiology, assessment, and management of
> Penetrating neck trauma (see Chapter 33, *Face and Neck Trauma*)
> Laryngotracheal injuries (see Chapter 33, *Face and Neck Trauma*)
> Spine trauma
  • Dislocations/subluxations (pp 1748, 1750, 1752, 1755-1773)
  • Fractures (pp 1747-1749, 1755-1773)
  • Sprains/strains (pp 1774-1775)
> Facial fractures (see Chapter 33, *Face and Neck Trauma*)
> Skull fractures (pp 1734-1735)
> Foreign bodies in the eyes (see Chapter 33, *Face and Neck Trauma*)
> Dental trauma (see Chapter 33, *Face and Neck Trauma*)
> Unstable facial fractures (see Chapter 33, *Face and Neck Trauma*)
> Orbital fractures (see Chapter 33, *Face and Neck Trauma*)
> Perforated tympanic membrane (see Chapter 33, *Face and Neck Trauma*)
> Mandibular fractures (see Chapter 33, *Face and Neck Trauma*)

Nervous System Trauma

Pathophysiology, assessment, and management of
> Traumatic brain injury (pp 1719-1725, 1727-1729, 1730-1733, 1736-1742)
> Spinal cord injury (pp 1725-1727, 1729-1732, 1747-1752)

> Spinal shock (pp 1751-1752)
> Cauda equina syndrome (pp 1718, 1751)
> Nerve root injury (pp 1717-1718, 1751)
> Peripheral nerve injury (pp 1717-1718, 1723)

Knowledge Objectives

1. Differentiate head trauma, head injury, and traumatic brain injury. (p 1713)
2. Review key points of head and spine anatomy and physiology. (pp 1713-1719)
3. Explain patient assessment for a person with a suspected head or spine injury, including variations that may be required for specific injuries. (pp 1719-1732)
4. Discuss general signs and symptoms of a head injury. (pp 1719-1720)
5. Discuss mechanisms of head and spine injury that paramedics should consider when assessing a patient. (pp 1720-1721)
6. Describe cases in which paramedics would use advanced airway techniques to gain definitive airway control in a patient with a head injury versus a spinal cord injury (SCI). (p 1721)
7. Describe the circumstances in which paramedics should establish intravenous access in a patient with a head or spine injury, including the importance of judicious fluid administration. (pp 1722-1723)
8. Discuss specific assessments used with a patient with possible SCI, including a neurologic exam. (pp 1724-1725, 1727-1732)
9. Discuss patient assessment and management of scalp lacerations. (p 1733)
10. Discuss types of skull fractures, including linear, depressed, basilar, and open skull fractures. (pp 1734-1735)
11. Explain the difference between a primary (direct) injury and a secondary (indirect) injury, giving examples of mechanisms of injury (MOIs) that could cause each injury. (p 1736)
12. Discuss the pathophysiology of intracranial pressure and posturing that can appear with brain injury. (pp 1736-1739)
13. Discuss diffuse brain injuries, including cerebral concussion and diffuse axonal injury, and their corresponding signs and symptoms. (pp 1738-1743)

14. Discuss focal brain injuries, including cerebral contusion and the various types of intracranial hemorrhage, and signs and symptoms of each. (pp 1742-1746)
15. Describe management of head and brain injuries, including thermal management, treatment of associated injuries, and pharmacologic therapy. (pp 1746-1747)
16. Discuss MOIs that may damage the cervical, thoracic, or lumbar spine, including flexion, rotation with flexion, vertical compression, and hyperextension. (pp 1747-1750)
17. Differentiate primary SCI and secondary SCI, including complete versus incomplete cord injury. (pp 1750-1751)
18. Discuss various cord syndromes and the signs and symptoms, including anterior cord syndrome, central cord syndrome, posterior cord syndrome, cauda equina syndrome, and Brown-Séquard syndrome. (p 1751)
19. Discuss the signs and symptoms of neurogenic shock and spinal shock. (pp 1751-1752)
20. Discuss the evolution of spinal care. (pp 1753-1755)
21. Describe the sequence of emergency medical care for a patient with a spinal injury and the steps for performing manual in-line stabilization, including immobilizing a supine patient, a seated patient, and a standing patient. (pp 1755-1767)
22. Discuss when and how to perform rapid extrication. (pp 1766-1770)
23. Explain how to remove and package a patient with a possible spinal injury from a water incident. (pp 1770-1771)
24. Explain the various circumstances in which the helmet of a patient with a possible head or spinal injury should be left on or removed; include the steps paramedics must take to remove a helmet, including the alternative method for removing a football helmet. (pp 1770-1772)
25. Describe prehospital pharmacologic treatment of patients with SCI. (pp 1772-1773)
26. Discuss possible complications of SCI, including autonomic dysreflexia, requiring prehospital management. (p 1773)
27. Discuss nontraumatic spinal conditions, including causes of low back pain and conditions requiring prehospital treatment. (pp 1774-1775)

Skills Objectives

1. Demonstrate how to immobilize to a long backboard a supine patient with a suspected spinal injury. (pp 1758-1763, Skill Drill 34-1)
2. Demonstrate how to immobilize with a scoop stretcher a supine patient with a suspected spinal injury. (p 1764, Skill Drill 34-2)
3. Demonstrate how to immobilize a patient with a suspected spinal injury who was found in a sitting position. (pp 1765-1767, Skill Drill 34-3)
4. Demonstrate how to perform rapid extrication. (pp 1767-1770)
5. Demonstrate how to immobilize a patient who is found in the water. (pp 1770-1771)
6. Demonstrate how to remove a helmet from a patient with a suspected head or spinal injury. (pp 1771-1772)

■ Introduction

In this chapter, you'll learn about central nervous system injury. Recall from Chapter 8, *Anatomy and Physiology*, that the central nervous system (CNS) consists of the brain and the spinal cord, both of which are encased in and protected by bone. The brain, located within the cranial cavity, is the largest component of the CNS. It contains billions of neurons that serve a variety of vital functions. You must understand the form and function of spinal anatomy and have a high level of suspicion for spinal cord injury (SCI) to decipher the often subtle findings associated with an SCI.

The two primary divisions of insult are head trauma and spinal cord injury. *Spinal cord injury* refers to any injury

YOU are the Paramedic   PART 1

It is 0130 hours when you are dispatched to a public swimming pool. While en route to the scene, dispatch tells you the police were called after a neighbor heard screams. You arrive to find a teenage boy lying on his back next to the pool. Even with the dim lighting, you immediately notice that he is having difficulty breathing.

1. What should you consider doing?
2. What safety concerns do you have?

of the spinal cord, such as ischemia, bruising, fracture, or severing, that disrupts normal spinal cord functions. However, the definitions of *head trauma*, *head injury*, and *traumatic brain injury* may not be as simple[1,2]:

- **Head trauma** is a general term that includes both head injuries and traumatic brain injuries. The medical community began to differentiate between these two types of injury only in the last decade or so. Before that, the terms *head trauma*, *head injury*, and *brain injury* were used interchangeably, making it difficult to track specific injuries and epidemiologic studies. Differing definitions of traumatic brain injury and variation in inclusion criteria among studies further complicated this issue. Over time, however, the definitions of these injuries have become relatively consistent.
- A **head injury** is a traumatic insult to the head that may result in injury to the soft tissues of the scalp or bony structures of the head and skull, not including the face.
- A **traumatic brain injury (TBI)** is an impairment of brain function caused by an external force that may involve physical, intellectual, emotional, social, and vocational changes.

Generally speaking, this chapter covers head and spine topics separately. You must realize, however, that although head injury and TBI can occur in isolation, these injuries often occur in association with each other. Remind yourself to look for coexisting injury.

Anatomy and Physiology Review

As a paramedic, you must have a strong working knowledge of anatomy and physiology. This knowledge will enable you to anticipate and recognize signs and symptoms in your patient, as well as formulate appropriate treatment plans. Chapter 8, *Anatomy and Physiology*, offers an overview of anatomy and physiology; you should refer to that chapter as needed while reading this chapter. Several other topics are also worth reviewing because they apply to your assessment and treatment of patients with head and spine injuries.

▶ The Scalp

Recall the scalp is composed of multiple layers. The subcutaneous tissue contains the major vessels supplying the scalp. These vessels are attached to the superficial fascia. Laceration or other compromise of these vessels can prevent vasospasm. This interruption of vasospasm can lead to profuse hemorrhage. Although this hemorrhage is generally not life threatening, it can distract you from other life-threatening injuries. At the same time, you cannot underestimate the potential for blood loss from scalp hemorrhage, particularly in patients who take blood thinners or have clotting disorders.

▶ The Skull

The skull is composed of 28 bones that make up the cranium, the auditory ossicles, and the face. Eight of these bones make up the **cranial vault** and are flat, irregular bones. They are one of the primary sites at which blood cells are generated, a process called *hematopoiesis*.

Recall the parietal and temporal bones are paired, while the rest, such as the frontal and occipital bones, are single. The cranial vault not only protects the brain by directing impacts around it, rather than through it, but it also creates a nondistensible container for the brain, **cerebrospinal fluid (CSF)**, and blood. With an expanding mass, such as a hematoma, the skull cannot expand, and **intracranial pressure (ICP)** (the pressure within the cranial vault) increases Figure 34-1 .

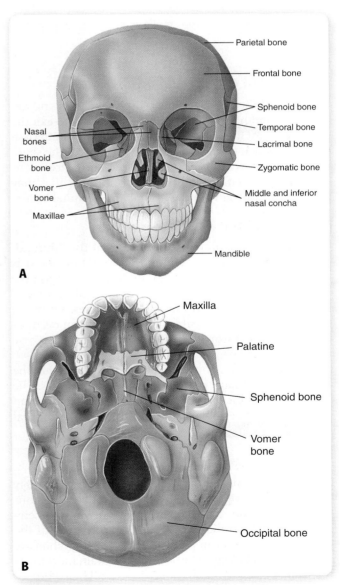

Figure 34-1 The skull and its components. **A.** Front view. **B.** Bottom view.

© Jones & Bartlett Learning.

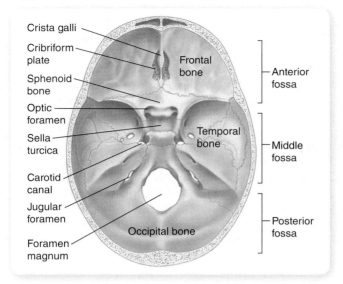

Figure 34-2 The floor of the cranial vault and its anatomy.
© Jones & Bartlett Learning.

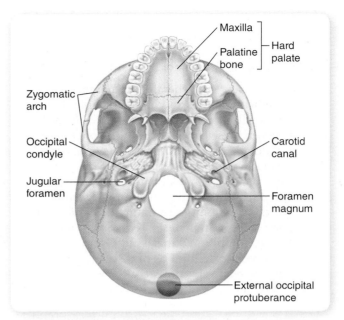

Figure 34-3 The base of the skull from below.
© Jones & Bartlett Learning.

The Floor of the Cranial Vault

The floor of the cranial vault has several ridges and depressions and has openings that allow nerves to exit the skull **Figure 34-2** . In an injury such as a **coup-contrecoup injury**, in which the brain impacts two sides of the skull, the brain slides across the skull floor, leading to lacerations of the brain itself, in addition to contusions that may result from contact with the frontal and occipital bones.

The Base of the Skull

The base of the skull consists of parts of the ethmoid, sphenoid, occipital, frontal, and temporal bones. It is divided into the anterior fossa, middle fossa, and posterior fossa. The concern for the patient, and ultimately for you, is a fracture of any of these bones, termed a **basilar skull fracture**. Basilar skull fractures can occur in the anterior fossa or the middle fossa, or can involve the temporal bone.

Basilar skull fractures are most often revealed in the field by the drainage of CSF from the nose or ears. The most common location of this drainage is the nose, and it usually indicates fracture of the ethmoid or temporal bone **Figure 34-3** .[3]

▶ The Brain

The brain contains billions of neurons that serve a variety of vital functions **Figure 34-4** . The major brain regions are the cerebrum, diencephalon, brainstem, and cerebellum. When you know the areas each region of the brain controls, you can perform a more comprehensive assessment and identify the areas of the brain most likely to be affected in a TBI. This knowledge will help you not only treat the patient, but also track the progress of the injury and deliver valuable information and insight to the next level of care.

The brain accounts for only 2% of total body weight, but it is the most metabolically active and perfusion-sensitive organ in the body. Because the brain has no mechanism for storing oxygen or glucose, it is completely reliant on cerebral blood flow provided by the carotid and vertebral arteries for a constant flow of both fuels.

The brain will continually manipulate the physiology as needed to ensure a ready supply of oxygen and glucose to the brain. Therefore, maintaining perfusion to the brain is paramount in the treatment of a patient with a TBI or other head trauma. A loss of blood flow to the brain for 5 to 10 seconds will result in unconsciousness. In the setting of a TBI, hypotension increases mortality significantly.

The Cerebrum

The largest portion of the brain is the **cerebrum**, which is responsible for higher functions, such as reasoning. The falx cerebelli, a crescent-shaped fold, divides the cerebrum into right and left hemispheres.

The largest portion of the cerebrum is the **cerebral cortex**, which regulates voluntary skeletal movement and level of awareness. Injury to the cerebral cortex may result in paresthesia, weakness, and paralysis of the extremities.

Each cerebral hemisphere is divided functionally into specialized areas called lobes **Figure 34-5** . The **frontal lobe** is important to voluntary motor action and personality traits. Injury to the frontal lobe may result in seizures or placid reactions (flat affect). Recall the frontal lobe filters the raw emotional impulses from the **limbic system**. Therefore, any injury to the frontal lobe may result in personality changes in the patient. For instance, he or she might become aggressive, have an emotional outburst, or use inappropriate language **Figure 34-6** .

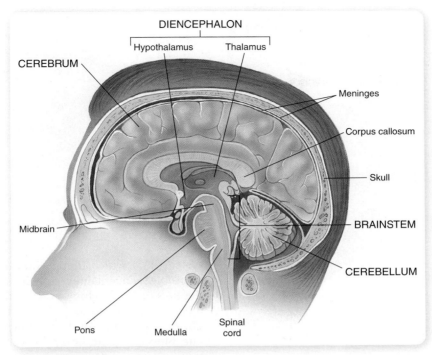

Figure 34-4 The major regions of the brain.
© Jones & Bartlett Learning.

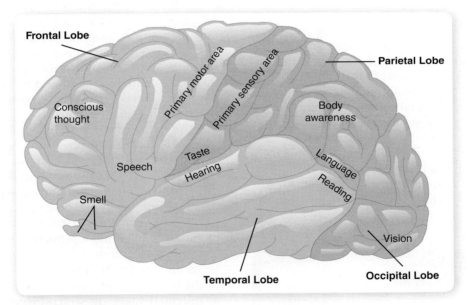

Figure 34-5 Lobes of the cerebrum.
© Jones & Bartlett Learning.

The **parietal lobe** processes information from sensory receptors in the skin and joints. For example, this lobe governs the perception of pain, temperature, and vibration. The parietal lobe is also responsible for **proprioception** (the ability to perceive the position and movement of one's body or limbs—for example, determining whether the elbow is flexed or extended, or how far above the ground the foot is during ambulation) and enables people to make mathematical calculations. Patients with injury to this lobe may not be able to calculate 2 + 2 or tell you how many dimes are in a dollar. Posteriorly, the optic nerve originates in the **occipital lobe**. This lobe, then, is responsible for processing visual information. A blow to the back of the head may hurl the occipital poles of the brain (the vision centers) against the skull, causing the person to see flashes of light, sometimes referred to as "seeing stars."

The speech center is located in the **temporal lobe**. In most patients, speech is processed in the left temporal

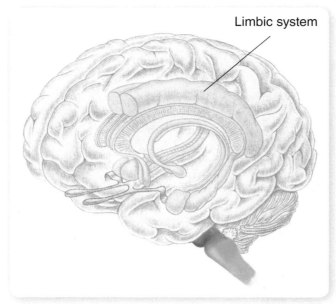

Figure 34-6 The limbic system is the seat of emotions, instincts, and other functions.

© Jones & Bartlett Learning.

lobe. This lobe also controls long-term memory, hearing, taste, and smell.

The Cerebellum

The **cerebellum** is located beneath the cerebral hemispheres in the inferoposterior part of the brain. It is sometimes called the "athlete's brain" because it is responsible for maintaining posture and equilibrium and coordinating skilled movements. Cerebellar injury can prevent the patient from performing rapid alternating movements, such as placing the back of the hand on the thigh and turning it over rapidly, hitting the same part of the thigh, or bringing the thumb and forefinger together rapidly and repeatedly. Cerebellar dysfunction may also impair the patient's ability to touch the finger to the nose or walk a straight line.

Words of Wisdom

Consider the roadside sobriety tests that law enforcement officers administer. Many of these tests measure cerebellar function because alcohol affects the cerebellum as well as the rest of the brain.

The Brainstem

The **brainstem** consists of the midbrain, pons, and medulla. It is located at the base of the brain and connects the spinal cord to the remainder of the brain. The brainstem houses many structures that are crucial to vital functions. High in the brainstem, for example, is the **reticular activating**

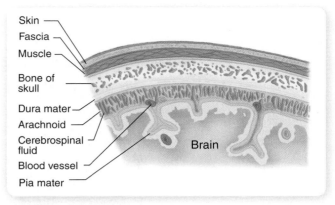

Figure 34-7 The meninges.

© Jones & Bartlett Learning.

system (RAS), which, along with the cerebral cortex, is responsible for maintaining consciousness. Damage to either the RAS or the cerebral cortex will affect consciousness to some degree, up to and including unconsciousness. The centers that control basic but vital functions—heart rate, blood pressure, and respiration—are located in the lower brainstem. Damage to this area can easily produce cardiovascular derangement, respiratory arrest, or death.

▶ The Meninges

The **meninges** are protective layers that surround and enfold the entire CNS—specifically the brain and spinal cord **Figure 34-7**. The outermost layer is a strong, fibrous wrapping called the **dura mater**. The dura mater covers the entire brain, folding inward to form the **tentorium**, a structure that separates the cerebral hemispheres from the cerebellum and brainstem.

The dura mater is firmly attached to the internal surface of the skull. Just beneath the suture lines of the skull, the dura mater splits into two surfaces and forms venous sinuses. When those venous sinuses are disrupted during a head injury, blood can collect beneath the dura mater to form a subdural hematoma.

The second meningeal layer is a delicate, transparent membrane called the **arachnoid**. The third meningeal layer, the **pia mater**, is a thin, translucent, highly vascular membrane that firmly adheres directly to the surface of the brain. Between each of the meningeal layers is a "potential space" in which bleeding can occur. The location of the hemorrhage is described by its location within the meninges:

- An epidural hematoma, for example, occurs between the dura mater and the skull and is usually caused by a rupture of the middle meningeal artery.
- A subdural hematoma occurs between the dura mater and the arachnoid membrane and is usually caused by a rupture of the bridging veins in this space.
- A subarachnoid hemorrhage occurs below the arachnoid membrane.

As discussed later in this chapter, each of these injuries is possible in head trauma. Although they will all increase ICP, their presentations differ depending on the vessels involved.

▶ The Spine

Recall the structure of the spine **Figure 34-8**. Both ligaments and muscle stabilize the skeletal components of the spine. Together, these components support and protect neural elements while enabling fluid movement and erect stature.

The **vertebral body**, the anterior weight-bearing structure, is made of bone that supports and stabilizes the body. Vertebral components include the **lamina**, **pedicles**, and spinous processes. Each vertebra is unique in appearance and, with the exception of the atlas and axis (C1 and C2) **Figure 34-9**, shares basic structural characteristics with other vertebrae.

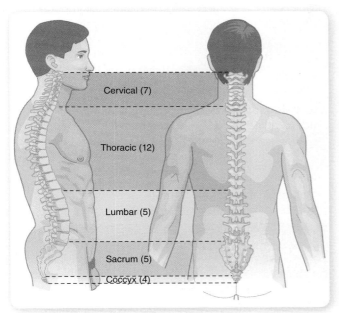

Figure 34-8 The spinal column consists of 33 bones divided into five sections—the cervical, thoracic, lumbar, sacral, and coccygeal vertebrae. Each vertebra is labeled with a letter corresponding to its section of the spine, along with its number. For example, the fifth thoracic vertebra is referred to as T5. Recall there are 7 cervical vertebrae, 12 thoracic vertebrae, 5 lumbar vertebrae, 5 (fused) sacral vertebrae, and 4 (fused) coccygeal vertebrae.

© Jones & Bartlett Learning.

Words of Wisdom

The lumbar spine is a common site of injury. Many of these injuries involve muscle spasm and do not threaten the integrity of the spinal cord and its roots. Nonetheless, low back pain is a common medical condition, as well as a frequent cause of impairment and disability.

There are intervertebral disks that separate and cushion each vertebra to limit bone wear and act as shock absorbers. As the body ages, these disks lose water content and become thinner, causing the loss of height linked with aging. Stress on the vertebral column may cause a disk to herniate into the spinal canal, resulting in an injury to the spinal cord or a **nerve root injury** **Figure 34-10**. Nerves can also be injured at the peripheral level (anywhere in the body outside the spinal cord). This is called **peripheral nerve injury**.

The muscles, tendons, and ligaments that connect the vertebrae allow the spinal column a degree of flexion and extension limited by the need for these soft tissues to stabilize the spinal column. The vertebral column can flex and extend 60% to 70% without stressing the spinal cord. Flexion or extension beyond those limits may damage structural ligaments and allow excess vertebral movement that could expose the spinal cord to injury.

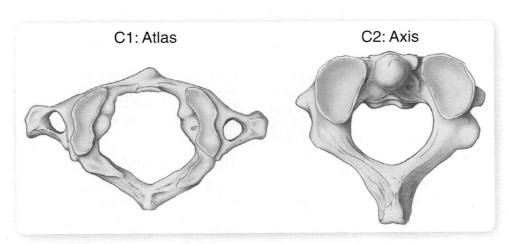

Figure 34-9 Structure of the atlas and axis.

© Jones & Bartlett Learning.

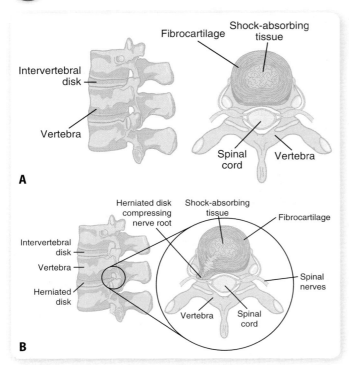

Figure 34-10 A. Normal, uninjured vertebral disk.
B. Herniated disk.

© Jones & Bartlett Learning.

Table 34-1	Major Spinal Tracts
Anterior Spinal Tracts	**Function**
Anterior spinothalamic tracts (ascending)	Sensation of crude touch and pressure sensation to the brain
Lateral spinothalamic tracts (ascending)	Sensation of pain and temperature
Spinocerebellar tracts (ascending)	Coordination of impulses necessary for muscular movements by carrying impulses from muscles in the legs and trunk to the cerebellum
Corticospinal tracts (descending)	Voluntary motor commands
Reticulospinal tracts (descending)	Muscle tone and sweat gland activity
Rubrospinal tracts (descending)	Muscle coordination and posture
Posterior Spinal Tracts (Dorsal Column)	**Function**
Fasciculus gracilis and cuneatus tracts	Proprioception—the ability to perceive the position and movement of one's body or limbs

© Jones & Bartlett Learning.

The Spinal Cord and Spinal Nerves

The spinal cord transmits nerve impulses between the brain and the rest of the body. Starting at the base of the brain, the spinal cord is the continuation of the CNS. This bundle of nerve fibers leaves the skull through a large opening at its base called the foramen magnum. In most adults, the spinal cord extends from the base of the skull to L2; here it separates into the **cauda equina**, a collection of individual nerve roots. Here, 31 pairs of spinal nerves arise from the different segments of the spinal cord. Each pair of spinal nerves is named for the vertebral level at which they arise. Spinal nerves C1 to C7 exit the spinal cord above their respective vertebrae, spinal nerve C8 exits below the C7 vertebra, and all other spinal nerves exit the spinal column below the respective vertebrae for which they are named.

The names of nerve groups are based on their source of origin and point of termination. As we have seen, ascending tracts carry information to the brain, and descending tracts carry information from the brain to the body **Table 34-1**. Knowing these tracts and their functions will help you understand the signs and symptoms of conditions such as anterior cord syndrome, central cord syndrome, and Brown-Séquard syndrome.

In five areas of the body, the spinal nerves converge in a **plexus** that enables several spinal nerves to control one area of the body **Figure 34-11**. For example, the cervical plexus includes vertebral levels C1 through C5; the phrenic nerve (C3 through C5) also arises from this plexus and contains nerves that supply, or innervate, the diaphragm.

The brachial plexus (C5 through T1) joins nerves controlling the upper extremities. The main nerves arising from this plexus are the axillary, median, musculocutaneous, radial, and ulnar. The lumbar plexus (L1 through L4) supplies the skin and muscles of the abdominal wall, external genitalia, and part of the lower limbs. The sacral plexus (L4 through S4) gives rise to the pudendal and sciatic nerves and supplies the buttocks, perineum, and most of the lower limbs. Trauma to any of these areas affects multiple nerves and can therefore have widespread consequences.

The Sympathetic Nervous System

Recall from Chapter 8, *Anatomy and Physiology*, the autonomic nervous system contains the sympathetic and parasympathetic divisions. The **sympathetic nervous system** mobilizes the body for activity and is responsible for our fight-or-flight responses. The brain transmits information through the brainstem and the cervical spinal cord.

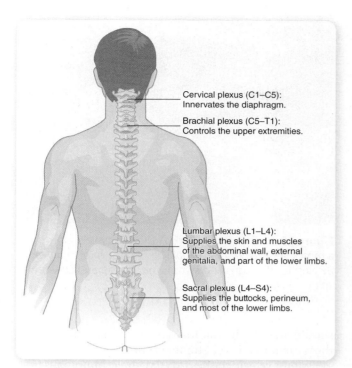

Cervical plexus (C1–C5):
Innervates the diaphragm.

Brachial plexus (C5–T1):
Controls the upper extremities.

Lumbar plexus (L1–L4):
Supplies the skin and muscles
of the abdominal wall, external
genitalia, and part of the lower limbs.

Sacral plexus (L4–S4):
Supplies the buttocks, perineum,
and most of the lower limbs.

Figure 34-11 Nerve roots originating from groups of vertebrae along the spine converge in plexuses, enabling them to function as a group.

© Jones & Bartlett Learning.

The short preganglionic fibers then exit at the thoracic and lumbar levels of the spine, ending at the paravertebral ganglia.

The long postganglionic fibers of the sympathetic nervous system (also called the thoracolumbar system) stimulate the periphery largely through alpha and beta receptors. Alpha receptor stimulation induces smooth muscle contraction in blood vessels and bronchioles. Beta receptors respond with relaxation of smooth muscle in blood vessels and bronchioles and have chronotropic and inotropic effects on myocardial cells. The sympathetic nervous system is also responsible for sweating, pupil dilation, temperature regulation, and shunting of blood from the periphery during the flight-or-fight response.

SCI at or above the level of T6 may disrupt the flow of sympathetic communication. Loss of sympathetic stimulation can disrupt homeostasis and leave the body poorly equipped to deal with changes in its environment. Stimulation of sympathetic nerves without parasympathetic input can cause sympathetic overdrive, producing autonomic dysreflexia, a complication of SCI discussed later in this chapter.

The Parasympathetic Nervous System

The **parasympathetic nervous system** is responsible for conserving energy and maintaining organ function. Its fibers arise from the cranial nerves and sacral nerves, and it is often called the craniosacral nervous system. It carries signals via long preganglionic fibers and short

postganglionic fibers to the organs of the abdomen, heart, lungs, and skin. The vagus nerve travels from its origins outside of the medulla to the heart posterolateral to the carotid arteries within the carotid sheath; thus, vagal tone is unaffected by a spinal injury.

When the sympathetic nerves are stimulated and produce autonomic dysreflexia, the parasympathetic nerves attempt to slow the rapidly increasing blood pressure by slowing the heart rate. Parasympathetic nerves that supply the reproductive organs, pelvis, and leg begin at the sacral level (S2 through S4). Disruption of the lower parasympathetic nerves in the sacrum results in loss of bowel/bladder tone and sexual function.

Special Populations

In older adult patients, SCI can result from even seemingly minor falls. Decreased bone density or osteoporosis, arthritis, and general weakening of the ligaments and musculature of the neck in older adults contribute to the increased risk of SCI. For example, a fall down a small flight of stairs may be enough to cause significant injury to the spine.

Similarly, infants and children are more susceptible to direct brain injury because their skull formation along suture lines is not complete. This flexibility of the skull may also mask injuries that would be obvious in adolescents or adult patients. A force that compresses an adult skull and readily fractures it will not necessarily fracture a pediatric skull because the sutures may allow that same force to compress the pediatric brain without causing fracture. Skull bones are also thinner and softer in infants, and only a fibrous sheath covers the fontanelles.

■ Patient Assessment of Head and Spine Injuries

When you care for patients with head and spine injuries, remember that identifying the type of brain injury may be impossible. It is more important to recognize the presence of a brain injury and begin immediate care than it is to identify the type. Also, remember, a patient with TBI is presumed to have a cervical spine injury until proven otherwise.

Table 34-2 lists the signs and symptoms of head injuries.

Words of Wisdom

The single most important sign in the evaluation of a patient with head injury is a change in the state of consciousness.

Table 34-2	**Signs and Symptoms of Head Trauma**
Head Injury	
Lacerations, contusions, or hematomas to the scalp	
Soft area or depression noted on palpation of the scalp	
Visible skull fractures or deformities	
Battle sign or raccoon eyes	
CSF rhinorrhea or otorrhea	
Traumatic Brain Injury	

Pupillary abnormalities
   • Unequal pupil size
   • Sluggish or nonreactive pupils	

A period of unresponsiveness	
Confusion or disorientation	
Repeatedly asks the same questions (perseveration)	
Amnesia (retrograde and/or anterograde)	
Combativeness or other abnormal behavior	
Numbness or tingling in the extremities	
Loss of sensation and/or motor function	
Focal neurologic deficits	
Seizures	
Cushing triad: hypertension, bradycardia, and irregular or erratic respirations	
Dizziness	
Visual disturbances, blurred vision, or double vision (diplopia)	
Seeing "stars" (flashes of light)	
Nausea or vomiting	
Posturing (decorticate and/or decerebrate)	

Abbreviation: CSF, cerebrospinal fluid
© Jones & Bartlett Learning.

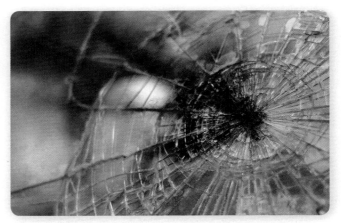

Figure 34-12 The classic "star" on the windshield after a motor vehicle crash is a significant indicator of injury. Be alert for the signs and symptoms of head and cervical spine injury.
© Kristin Smith/Shutterstock.

should activate the trauma system (eg, air evacuation of the patient to a Level I trauma center).

Motor vehicle crashes (MVCs), direct blows, falls from heights, assaults, and sports-related injuries are common causes of head injury and TBI. When your patient has experienced any of these events, you should immediately elevate your index of suspicion and search for signs and symptoms of these types of injuries. A deformed windshield or dented or cracked helmet indicates a major blow to the head **Figure 34-12**.

The following high-risk mechanisms of injury (MOIs) suggest possible spinal injury.[4] Whenever you suspect a spinal injury, you should assess for spinal injury to determine whether the patient should be placed in full spinal immobilization.

- High-velocity crash (greater than 40 mph) with severe vehicle damage
- Unrestrained occupant of moderate- to high-speed MVC
- Vehicular damage with compartmental intrusion (12 inches [30 cm]) into the patient's seating space
- Fall of an adult from a height greater than 20 feet (6 m)
- Fall of a child from a height greater than 10 feet (3 m), or a height two to three times the child's height
- Penetrating trauma near the spine
- Ejection from a moving vehicle
- Motorcycle crash of greater than 20 mph
- Auto-pedestrian or auto-bicycle crash of greater than 20 mph
- Death of occupant in the same passenger compartment
- Rollover crash (unrestrained)

Diving is also considered a high-risk MOI,[5] especially when it involves injury to the head or a witness who saw a deep dive in the shallow end of a swimming pool.

Scene Size-up

After you have taken standard precautions, the initial step of any assessment is to assess the scene safety and identify the need for additional resources. Decide if you

MOIs with uncertain or low risks for spinal injury include the following:

- Moderate- to low-velocity MVC (less than 40 mph)
- Motor vehicle crash in which the patient has an isolated injury without positive assessment findings for spinal injury
- Isolated minor head injury without positive mechanism for spinal injury
- Syncopal event in which the patient was already seated or supine
- Syncopal event in which the patient was assisted to a supine position by a bystander

Words of Wisdom

Any patient with significant head injury is presumed to have a cervical spine injury until proven otherwise.

Primary Survey

As you begin your primary survey of a patient with a head injury, ensure manual stabilization of the cervical spine in a neutral, in-line position. With the head and neck in a neutral position through manual stabilization, identify the level of consciousness and conduct your primary survey as described in Chapter 11, *Patient Assessment*. You may apply a cervical collar during the primary survey if your findings require it. However, take care not to skip elements of the airway, breathing, and circulation when sizing and applying a cervical collar. Avoid moving the neck unnecessarily and continue manual stabilization until you determine spinal immobilization is not indicated, or, if indicated, spinal immobilization has been applied. Application of the cervical collar is considered a treatment intervention. Failure to assess pulse, motor, and sensory function prior to application of this medical device could potentially alter your baseline assessment. There will be no way for you to know if neurovascular compromise was present prior to your intervention or if you, in fact, worsened the patient's injury.

Prior to measuring the patient for proper cervical collar size, the cervical and thoracic spine must be in a neutral position. If the patient is seated with a slouching posture, then cervical collar measurement may be inaccurate, which may not be noticed until the patient has been transferred to the backboard.

Remember during your airway assessment, patients with head injuries often vomit; thus, after you open their airways, you must be prepared to roll patients onto their sides—while stabilizing their spines—to prevent aspiration. *Mortality increases significantly with aspiration.*

Facial fractures and physical findings or suspected basilar skull fractures are possible contraindications for a nasopharyngeal airway. *If your local protocols allow you to insert a nasal airway, then use caution if CSF or bloody rhinorrhea is present or if you suspect a nasal fracture. If you meet resistance at any point during insertion, then abandon the attempt and establish control of the airway through other methods.*

Patient Safety

Because of the nature of spinal immobilization, especially in the presence of head trauma, the patient is at risk for aspiration. Therefore, be diligent in monitoring the patient's airway, and be prepared for immediate airway management as needed.

Advanced Airway Management in Patients With Head or Spine Injury

You must maintain manual stabilization during all airway management procedures. As with any nasal procedure in the presence of facial trauma or a possible basilar skull fracture, nasotracheal intubation carries risk and is generally contraindicated. When possible, use another method to manage the airway.

The patient may be awake with an unmanageable airway or may not tolerate advanced airway management—for example, because of combativeness or clenched teeth (**trismus**). In such circumstances, your protocols may allow you to perform pharmacologically assisted intubation (ie, rapid sequence intubation). This procedure is described in detail in Chapter 15, *Airway Management*.

Your authority to perform rapid sequence intubation (RSI) in the setting of head trauma varies with local protocols. According to the Brain Trauma Foundation's *Guidelines for Prehospital Management of Traumatic Brain Injury*, the routine use of RSI is not recommended in patients who are breathing spontaneously and maintaining an oxygen saturation above 90% on supplemental oxygen.[6] The foundation classifies this recommendation as weak, because it is based primarily on evidence from Class III studies. You must know your local protocols and be familiar with the available airway management options.

Controversies

Patients with potential head injury or TBI historically have been administered 1 to 1.5 mg/kg of lidocaine via intravenous push before intubation. This technique was believed to blunt an acute increase in ICP that may occur during intubation. This procedure is controversial, however, and the current view is that evidence is insufficient to support or refute its use during intubation in these patients.[7-12] Thus, your local protocols may or may not include it.

Ventilation in the Context of Head or Spine Injury

Cerebral edema (an increase in cerebral fluid) and ICP are aggravated by hypoxia and hypercapnia; thus, you must constantly ensure adequate oxygenation and ventilation in any patient with a head injury. As such, in any patient exhibiting signs and symptoms of hypoxia, the administration of oxygen (and assisting with ventilations when indicated) *cannot* be deferred until you are en route.

Administer 100% oxygen via a nonrebreathing mask if the patient is breathing adequately (ie, adequate rate and depth [tidal volume], regular respiratory pattern). An injured brain tolerates hypoxia even less than a healthy one. Research has demonstrated that prompt administration of supplemental oxygen can reduce brain damage and improve neurologic outcome.

Words of Wisdom

When you assess and manage an adult with a severe head injury, remember the Brain Trauma Foundation's "90-90-9 rule"[13,14]:

- A *single* drop in the patient's oxygen saturation (Spo$_2$) to less than 90% significantly increases his or her chance of death.*
- A *single* drop in the patient's systolic blood pressure to less than 90 mm Hg significantly increases his or her chance of death.*
- A *single* drop of 2 points or more in the patient's prior best Glasgow Coma Scale score of less than 9 increases his or her chance of death.

*The chance of death increases exponentially if both hypoxemia and hypotension occur compared with occurrences of only one of these conditions.

If the brain's respiratory center (pons, medulla) has been injured, then the rate, depth, or regularity of breathing may be ineffective. Ventilation may also be impaired by concomitant chest injuries or, if the spinal cord is injured, by paralysis of some or all of the respiratory muscles. The phrenic nerve (C3 through C5) innervates the diaphragm. Thus, lesions occurring at or above C3 and C4 may lead to diaphragmatic paralysis that is seen clinically as use of the accessory muscles of the neck and possibly some spastic movement of the abdominal muscles. An injury involving the lower cervical or upper thoracic spinal cord (T2) may result in paralysis of the intercostal muscles, leaving the patient dependent on the diaphragm and accessory muscles of the neck for breathing.

Regardless of the cause, patients with inadequate ventilation should receive bag-mask ventilation and 100% oxygen flowing at a rate of 12 to 15 L/min. Monitoring end-tidal carbon dioxide (ETCO$_2$) and avoiding hypocapnia or hypercapnia are crucial during the ventilation, especially in patients with a TBI. Ventilate the patient at

Table 34-3	Signs of Cerebral Herniation

Unresponsive patient with two or more of the following:

- Asymmetric (unequal) pupils *or* bilaterally fixed and dilated pupils
- Decerebrate (extensor) posturing *or* no motor response to painful stimuli
- Original Glasgow Coma Scale score of less than 9 that decreases by 2 or more points from the patient's best score

© Jones & Bartlett Learning.

the rate needed to maintain an ETCO$_2$ of 35 to 40 mm Hg. If you cannot monitor ETCO$_2$, then a respiratory rate of 10 to 12 breaths/min in the adult patient generally achieves the target range. *Avoid routine hyperventilation of patients with brain injury.* Although hyperventilation causes cerebral vasoconstriction, which will shunt blood from the cranium and lower the ICP, this shunting also results in a drop in **cerebral perfusion pressure (CPP)** (the pressure of blood flow through the brain).[15] This drop in CPP may reduce oxygen delivery to the brain and cause cerebral ischemia.

The Brain Trauma Foundation recommends hyperventilation *only* if signs of cerebral **herniation** are present Table 34-3 , because brief periods of hyperventilation may be beneficial. If the findings of cerebral herniation resolve, then the patient should be ventilated as described previously. Monitoring ETCO$_2$ is the ideal method of determining the appropriate ventilatory rate when hyperventilating the patient with signs of cerebral herniation. You should ventilate the patient to maintain the ETCO$_2$ between 30 and 35 mm Hg.[15,16]

Recall from Chapter 15, *Airway Management*, that increasing the respiratory rate will decrease the ETCO$_2$, and decreasing the respiratory rate will increase the ETCO$_2$. Under no circumstances should the ETCO$_2$ be allowed to drop below 25 mm Hg, because the subsequent vasoconstriction will almost certainly result in brain death due to anoxia and cerebral ischemia.[15] If you do not have ETCO$_2$ monitoring, then the recommended rates of hyperventilation are as follows:

- Adult: 20 breaths/min
- Child: 25 breaths/min
- Infant (younger than 1 year): 30 breaths/min[6]

Circulation and Volume Resuscitation in a Patient With Head or Spine Injury

After you have secured the patient's airway and ensured adequate oxygenation and ventilation, and while your partner continues to maintain manual in-line cervical stabilization, you must turn your attention to supporting the patient's circulation. In the absence of a pulse, initiate

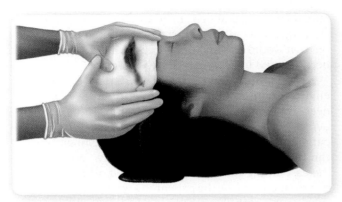

Figure 34-13 If you suspect a depressed skull fracture, then do not apply excessive pressure to the fracture to control bleeding; rather, apply direct pressure around the suspected fracture site.

© Jones & Bartlett Learning.

CPR, consider correctable causes of arrest such as tension pneumothorax, and follow your local protocol.

Recall from Chapter 11, *Patient Assessment*, that you must control life-threatening bleeding even before you address airway and breathing concerns. Control major bleeding with direct pressure, gauze, hemostatic agents, or pressure dressings, as appropriate.

Take care not to apply excessive pressure to scalp lacerations in which an underlying fracture is present or suspected. When you apply direct pressure digitally to injuries that suggest **depressed skull fractures**, you may need to apply pressure around the suspected fracture site rather than directly on the injury site **Figure 34-13** . Active bleeding will cause or worsen hypoxia and will decrease CPP and increase cerebral ischemia by reducing both blood flow and oxygen delivery to the brain.

Patients with significant sensory loss from SCI may take on the surrounding environmental temperature because of the lack of input from the peripheral nerves for temperature control. In **neurogenic shock**, the skin is usually warm, dry, and flushed because of vasodilation (dilated blood vessels) and the absence of sweating. These findings should be correlated with the patient's mental status.

Words of Wisdom

A patient can have a significant SCI and associated sensory loss with or without neurogenic shock. The skin will present differently based on whether neurogenic shock is present.

Volume resuscitation may be necessary in patients with absent or diminished pulses, especially in patients with multisystem trauma with hypovolemic shock. The skull does not have enough room to accommodate a large volume of blood. As a result, an isolated closed head injury will not cause hypovolemic shock in an adult. If signs of

shock are present (ie, persistent hypotension, tachycardia, diaphoresis), then carefully assess for (and suspect) occult bleeding, such as intra-abdominal or intrathoracic hemorrhage. Also consider the possibility of neurogenic shock in patients with a spinal injury with hypotension and bradycardia.[17]

Intravenous (IV) therapy is often used to support circulation; however, if your patient is critical, you should defer this therapy until you are en route. Establish at least one 18-gauge IV line with normal saline or lactated Ringer solution. Do not administer dextrose-containing solutions (such as 5% dextrose in water [D_5W]) because they may worsen cerebral edema. The *only* indication for administering glucose to a patient with head injury is confirmed hypoglycemia (eg, a glucometer reading of 45 mg/dL or lower), in which case dextrose would be the medication of choice.

Administer IV fluids based on the patient's blood pressure. Patients with a severe closed head injury may become hypertensive—a sign of the body's autoregulatory response. Limit your use of IV fluids, typically to 30 to 50 mL/h, for these patients to minimize cerebral edema and ICP.[18]

You must prevent hypotension, usually defined as a systolic blood pressure of less than 90 mm Hg for adults, in the patient with a TBI; some sources define it as high as 100 or 110 mm Hg.[19] Hypotension is one of the five most powerful predictors of poor outcome in such patients.[20,21] You must continuously monitor the patient's blood pressure to quickly identify any downward trend in the systolic blood pressure and respond before hypotension develops.

If you notice systolic blood pressure dropping in a patient with a suspected TBI, or if your patient is hypotensive upon initial contact, then infuse fluids as needed to maintain a systolic blood pressure of at least 90 mm Hg. Hypotension in a patient with brain injury can be lethal because it may decrease the CPP, with resultant cerebral ischemia, permanent brain damage, and death. This topic will be explored further later in the chapter.

Patients with SCI in pure neurogenic shock might not require large amounts of volume resuscitation, but they might need vagolytic drugs (eg, atropine) and vasopressors (such as dopamine) to reverse the uninhibited vagal stimulation and alpha receptor blockade associated with this type of shock. You may also consider transcutaneous pacing for refractory symptomatic bradycardia. Again the goal is to maintain a systolic blood pressure of 90 mm Hg or greater with a combination of fluids and medications, but you must take care to avoid hypervolemia, because it can lead to fluid overload and pulmonary edema.[22]

Finally, severe head injuries, especially those involving the lower brainstem, can cause a variety of cardiac rhythm disturbances, so use a cardiac monitor with every critically injured patient. If the patient experiences cardiac arrest, then follow the advanced cardiac life support (ACLS) cardiac arrest algorithm shown in Chapter 17, *Cardiovascular Emergencies*.

Assessment of Disability and Exposure

As you learned in Chapter 11, *Patient Assessment*, the next step of the primary survey is assessing for disability. This assessment is a cursory baseline evaluation of the CNS, but it is especially important in the patient with a potential spinal injury, head injury, or TBI.

Reevaluate the patient's mental status and response to stimuli, and note any changes since your initial contact with the patient. Quickly check for presence of pulse and evaluate motor and sensory function in each extremity, because you need a baseline assessment of these signs before the patient is moved in any way. If the patient is responsive, then ask about any numbness or tingling (paresthesia) in the extremities. Directly observe the back to assess for penetrating trauma. Finally, palpate the patient's spinal column for deformity, step-offs, point tenderness, and crepitus.

Words of Wisdom

Always palpate over the spinous process before concluding that a patient "has no neck tenderness." You must perform a physical exam, not simply ask the patient.

At this point, you will have enough information to determine whether the patient needs spinal immobilization. (Spinal immobilization techniques are discussed in detail later in this chapter.) If the patient meets the criteria for spinal immobilization, then place a properly sized cervical collar while continuing to maintain in-line manual stabilization. If your assessment reveals that treatment for a spinal injury (which may include a cervical collar alone or a cervical collar and an immobilization device) is not indicated, and your protocols allow it, then stabilization measures may be released.

Words of Wisdom

Pupil assessment is important when you check for indicators of a head or spine injury. Recall from Chapter 11, *Patient Assessment*, that asymmetric pupils are normal in about 19% of the population.[23] Correlate the finding to the patient's overall condition.

Pupil assessment is often deferred until the secondary assessment, especially in critical patients. However, with head trauma and TBI, the pupils can reveal valuable information about the patient and his or her condition. You may elect to perform a quick baseline assessment during the disability portion of your primary survey.

The patient has likely been exposed to the waist for the first steps of the assessment. You should expose any remaining areas that need to be assessed. Also remove any clothing that would obstruct your secondary assessment but that would be difficult to remove once the patient has been secured to an immobilization device.

As you make your exposure decisions, consider the environment and cover the patient with a blanket as needed to maintain normal body temperature. Remember, hypothermia in the trauma patient will impair the patient's ability to unbind oxygen from hemoglobin and can result in acidosis and coagulopathy, leading to an increase in the risk of mortality and morbidity. In cold environments, move the patient to a warmer environment, such as the ambulance, as quickly as possible without further compromising the spine.

Level of Consciousness

Whenever you suspect a head injury, you should perform a baseline neurologic assessment using AVPU (Awake and alert, responsive to Verbal stimuli, responsive to Pain, Unresponsive) and record the time. In addition to evaluating responsiveness with AVPU, you should obtain a Glasgow Coma Scale (GCS) score (outlined in Chapter 11, *Patient Assessment*), because it gives more specific clinical

Documentation & Communication

A single GCS score cannot reliably capture the clinical progress of a patient with head injury. Obtain a baseline GCS score, and repeat the assessment at least every 5 minutes if possible. Document all GCS scores and the time of each assessment on the patient care report. The physician will compare his or her neurologic assessment with those you performed in the field. Report the GCS score by category, not just by the total score.

Special Populations

When responding to an incident involving a shaken baby, you may encounter a child with an abnormal appearance but no external signs of injury. Shaken baby syndrome occurs when a caregiver violently shakes a child, often when the child is crying inconsolably, producing a severe brain injury in the child. Given that few caregivers will admit to having hurt the child, be alert for a history that is inconsistent with the clinical picture. Note whether the infant has **petechial hemorrhages**. These are pinpoint red dots in the sclera of the eye and represent the rupture of tiny vessels. This finding indicates that the baby was shaken, although this finding may not be present in every case of shaken baby syndrome. Be sure to document the presence or absence of this finding; this information could be significant if law enforcement investigates the case.

information. A change in the level of consciousness is the single most important sign that you can detect when you assess the severity of brain injury. The level of consciousness usually indicates the extent of brain dysfunction. The GCS score is a reliable predictor of outcome for a patient with brain injury. An adjusted GCS scoring system is used to assess infants and children, as discussed in Chapter 43, *Pediatric Emergencies*.

Formulating a Plan

Prompt transport to a definitive care facility (ie, a trauma center) is crucial to the survival of a patient with brain injury. Consider air transport if your transport time will be long. If you are transporting the patient by ground, do so quickly but cautiously.

Many patients with severe brain injuries and increased ICP require neurosurgic intervention. The extra time needed to move the patient from one medical facility to another could be the difference between life and death. Therefore transport the patient *directly* to a trauma center that has neurosurgic services, even if you must bypass the nearest facility.

Placement on the Backboard

Based on the findings of your primary survey and your local protocols, you may need to apply some degree of spinal immobilization to your patient, which may involve a backboard, scoop stretcher, or similar device. The timing of this action is based on the condition of your patient. In the critical patient, you will apply the immobilization at the end of your primary survey to enable rapid transport to

an appropriate medical facility. In the noncritical patient, you may apply the immobilization after you complete your secondary assessment. Current considerations and controversies in spinal immobilization will be discussed in depth later in this chapter.

Most patients can be log rolled while you watch for deformity or injury and palpate over each posterior spinous process for pain, deformity, or step-offs. In a reliable patient, the absence of pain or tenderness along the spine, coupled with a normal neurologic exam and absence of distracting injuries, may eliminate the need for spinal immobilization in select patients.[24-26] A patient is considered *reliable* if he or she is alert and oriented, there is no language barrier, there is no evidence of brain injury or intoxication by drugs or alcohol, and the patient is not so emotionally upset as to impair his or her ability to make decisions or adequately recognize pain and injury. In addition, patients with severe injuries to other body parts (eg, femur fracture) may have such significant pain that it sufficiently distracts them from being able to discern spinal pain or tenderness, rendering them effectively unreliable.

You should always protect paralyzed limbs with appropriate restraint and stretcher immobilization. The specific techniques for immobilizing patients found in various positions are taught later in this chapter.

Patients in severe pain may require an alternative method of transfer to a long backboard. Using a scoop stretcher often requires less patient movement than is required for a log roll. When the scoop stretcher is in place and the patient has been lifted, another crew member can slide the backboard, air mattress, or vacuum mattress under the patient. Although you can still palpate the patient

YOU are the Paramedic — PART 2

As you begin to manage the patient's airway and breathing, your partner asks the bystanders, "What happened?" A young woman tells you that she and a group of friends, all of whom appear to be in their teens, were drinking when they decided to sneak into the pool for a skinny-dip. The young man dove into the shallow end of the pool and did not come up. Several of his friends jumped into the water and pulled him out.

Recording Time: 1 Minute	
Appearance	Wet, naked, and lying on his back
Level of consciousness	U (unresponsive)
Airway	Snoring
Breathing	Rapid and shallow
Circulation	Slow, weak radial pulse

3. What injuries do you suspect?
4. What interventions are required?

with this method, a disadvantage of this procedure is that you cannot visually inspect the area. You may also choose to use the scoop stretcher alone without transferring the patient to a backboard or other device.

Time on a backboard should be kept to a minimum, because skin breakdown can be a complication of SCI. This condition is caused by excessive pressure over the bones of the buttocks, the two scapular ridges, and the base of the occiput. These five areas are the primary supports for the patient's weight. The initial stages of pressure lesions may begin in a matter of hours. In a study, after 30 minutes of immobility on a nonpadded backboard, the skin overlying the sacrum of a healthy adult showed evidence of tissue hypoxia.[27] Tissue oxygenation was measured using near infrared spectroscopy. These findings emphasize the importance of proper padding in the prehospital setting followed by prompt removal of the backboard in the emergency department (ED). Failure to do so will increase the patient's pain and the probability that the patient will develop pressure sores over the bony prominences of the body.[27,28] Blood distribution shifts to the skin and subcutaneous tissues, and decreased muscle tone and sensation predispose a patient with SCI to these injuries.

Several devices have been developed to improve patient comfort. If you have a high suspicion of spinal injury or a long transport time, then consider using a vacuum mattress to help prevent pressure ulcers **Figure 34-14** . Use of a vacuum mattress may also be wise if the patient exhibits diaphragmatic breathing or if you note **dermatome** changes. In these cases, the patient may need to remain immobilized longer, until he or she can be seen by a neurosurgeon.

The Back Raft is a device that takes pressure off specific areas of the back and fills voids that might otherwise allow patient movement. This low-profile air mattress fits under the patient from the shoulders to the waist **Figure 34-15** . Slightly flexing the patient's knees with towel rolls or a blanket and slightly separating the legs with a pillow or blanket increases patient comfort and reduces the risk of postimmobilization complications while adequately immobilizing the patient **Figure 34-16** .

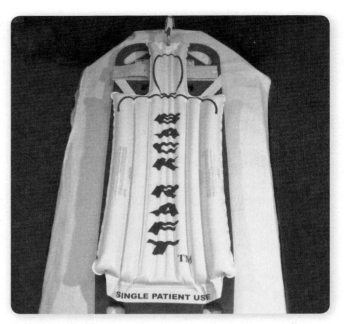

Figure 34-15 The Back Raft.

Courtesy of Thomas E.M.S.

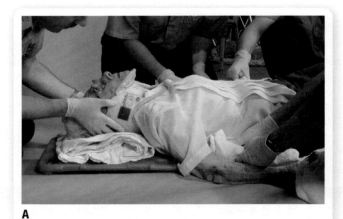

A

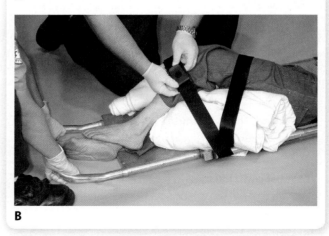

B

Figure 34-16 Use towel rolls or blankets to pad voids between the patient and the backboard to increase patient comfort and minimize complications resulting from immobilization of the older adult patient. Some examples of voids include beneath the neck **(A)** and beneath the knees **(B)**.

© Jones & Bartlett Learning.

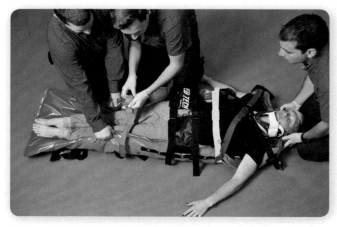

Figure 34-14 A vacuum mattress.

© Jones & Bartlett Learning.

Concave backboards also conform more closely to a patient's anatomy than do flat backboards. Use five straps to properly immobilize a patient.

History Taking

An accurate history and physical exam are crucial for directing management of patients with possible neurologic trauma. The history of the present illness typically provides most of the information needed to reach a diagnosis.

You must always assess the patient's reliability as a historian before you perform a secondary assessment. The patient should appear calm, cooperative, and unimpaired and should be able to perform cognitive functions appropriately. Patients who present with an acute stress reaction, distracting injuries (eg, long bone fractures, rib fractures, pelvic fractures, or clinically significant abdominal pain), or an alteration in mental status caused by brain injury or intoxication from drugs and/or alcohol must be considered unreliable as a source of information in the neurologic exam. These patients should have continuous spinal protection until an appropriate radiographic evaluation at the receiving facility can exclude injury.

As a paramedic, you must remember your decision regarding the likelihood of SCI is based on your physical exam, which also guides your treatment decisions.

You should maintain a high index of suspicion in any patient for whom the MOI suggests a possible SCI. Associated injuries, especially those that suggest involvement of massive forces, may also provide clues to the presence of SCI.

All patients found unresponsive after trauma must be treated as if they have a spinal injury, because many cervical spine injuries are associated with head injury. Patients with evidence of major trauma above the clavicle should be considered at risk for an associated spinal injury.

When possible, obtain a SAMPLE (Signs and symptoms of current complaint; Allergies; Medications; Pertinent past medical history; Last oral intake; and Events leading up to current injury or illness) history from the patient or bystanders. Try to learn what the patient was doing. What happened? What is wrong now? What does not seem right? Did the patient lose consciousness? If so, did it happen immediately before or after the event or later? Determine as precisely as possible the circumstances of the incident and the forces to which the patient was subjected, including the intensity, speed, and trajectory (direction) of the impact. Was there blunt or penetrating trauma? Was it a flexion injury, such as the classic diving accident? Was there torsion on the neck? In the case of a fall, estimate the height of the fall. Determine whether the patient struck anything on the way down, how he or she landed, and the surface on which he or she landed. In vehicular crashes, note the use and positioning of restraints, the patient's position in the vehicle, and the degree of damage to the vehicle. Learn the exact time of the initial injury, and record any times and changes in the patient's presentation throughout the prehospital phase.

Secondary Assessment

Perform the secondary assessment as described in Chapter 11, *Patient Assessment*. Modify the physical exam of any patient with suspected SCI based on the patient's level of consciousness, reliability as a historian, and MOI. In cases of high- or intermediate-risk mechanisms, when the patient has not already been immobilized, complete the physical exam with the patient in a neutral position without moving the spine. Apply manual stabilization while asking the patient not to move unless specifically asked to do so. The neck and trunk must not be flexed, extended, or rotated.

For a combative patient, sedation or RSI procedures may be required, depending on the patient's ability to protect his or her airway and local protocols.

Thoroughly assess the head and face for soft-tissue injuries, bony instability, depression, drainage from the ears or nose, retroauricular ecchymosis (bruising behind the ears, often called **Battle sign**), and **periorbital ecchymosis** (bruising under the eyes, often called **raccoon eyes**). Remember, you assessed the anterior and posterior neck during the primary survey before you placed the cervical collar. If a cervical collar is not in place, then you can reevaluate these areas.

Frequently monitor the pupil size, shape, equality, and reactivity. The nerves that control pupil dilation and constriction are sensitive to ICP. Assess both the direct and consensual response to light. A pupil that is slow (sluggish) to constrict is a relatively early sign of increased ICP; a sluggish pupil also could indicate cerebral hypoxia. Unequal or bilaterally fixed and dilated ("blown") pupils are later, more ominous signs of increased ICP; in the context of other evidence of severe TBI, they indicate pressure on one or both oculomotor nerves **Figure 34-17** .

If the patient is conscious, then evaluate the extraocular movements, identify any nystagmus, and evaluate the ability of the pupils to accommodate changes in focal length. The pupils should constrict and the eyes should turn medially as the patient focuses on an object moving toward the nose. The acronym PERRLA (Pupils Equal,

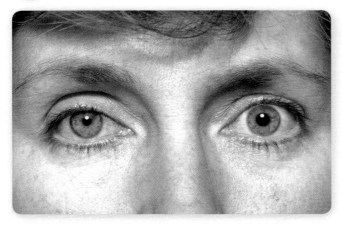

Figure 34-17 Unequal or bilaterally fixed and dilated pupils in a patient with a head injury are ominous signs and indicate a significantly increased intracranial pressure.
© Mediscan/Alamy.

Round, and Reactive to Light and Accommodation) often is used to document these findings.

Evaluate the chest and abdomen for both internal and external injuries. Fractures of the ribs, sternum, clavicle, scapula, or pelvis are often associated with SCI in patients with multisystem trauma. Remember, the physical exam in the SCI patient could be skewed by decreased sensation below the level of the spinal injury. Inadequate ventilation or use of accessory muscles may indicate diaphragmatic impairment resulting from SCI.

Continually monitor the cardiovascular system for signs of shock. Neurogenic shock may require pharmacologic management, volume replacement, and/or transcutaneous pacing (for symptomatic bradycardia), as described previously.

Examination of the gastrointestinal system may be unreliable in the presence of a neurologic deficit. Remember, patients may be insensitive to pain, and, because muscle tone may be absent, they may not develop a rigid abdomen. Lower abdominal distention with or without suprapubic tenderness may be due to urinary retention. In male patients, assess the urethral meatus for evidence of blood, scrotal swelling, and scrotal ecchymosis, which may occur with pelvic fractures. Also assess for priapism.

Look for abnormal posturing, and assess the patient for potential long bone injury or other significantly distracting, painful injuries that may mask a spine or cord injury.

Finally, obtain a glucose level if possible in patients who show evidence of alterations in sensation.

Assessing ICP

Although you cannot quantify ICP (ie, you can't assign a numeric value) in the prehospital setting, you can estimate the severity of increase based on the patient's clinical presentation Table 34-4. You will base important treatment decisions for patients with brain injury on the presence or absence of certain key findings: posturing,

Table 34-4	Levels of Intracranial Pressure
Elevation Level	**Clinical Indicators**
Mild elevation	• Increased blood pressure; decreased pulse rate • Pupils still reactive • **Cheyne-Stokes respirations** (gradually increasing rate and depth of respirations followed by a gradual decrease of respirations with intermittent periods of apnea) • Patient initially attempts to localize and remove painful stimuli; this is followed by withdrawal and extension • Vomiting (often without nausea) • Headache • Altered level of consciousness • Seizures • Effects are reversible *with prompt treatment*
Moderate elevation (indicates middle brainstem involvement)	• Widened pulse pressure and bradycardia • Pupils are sluggish or nonreactive • **Central neurogenic hyperventilation** (deep, rapid respirations; similar to Kussmaul, but without an acetone breath odor) • Decerebrate posturing • Survival possible but often with significant permanent neurologic deficit
Marked elevation (indicates involvement of lower portion of brainstem/medulla)	• Unilaterally fixed and dilated ("blown") pupil • **Biot (ataxic) respirations** (irregular pattern, rate, and depth of breathing with intermittent periods of apnea) or absent respirations • Flaccid paralysis • Irregular pulse rate • Changes in the QRS complex, ST segment, or T wave • Fluctuating blood pressure; hypotension common • Many patients do not survive this level of intracranial pressure

Data from: Stiver SI, Gean AD, Manley GT. Survival with good outcome after cerebral herniation and Duret hemorrhage caused by traumatic brain injury. *J Neurosurg.* 2009;110(6):1242-1246.

hypotension or hypertension, and abnormal pupil signs. Use serial GCS and pupillary assessments to monitor the progression of ICP.

Words of Wisdom

The most important aspect of neurologic assessment is whether the patient's findings are changing and the direction of change. Be sure to document the area in which the patient's GCS score changed.

Neurologic Exam

The focused neurologic evaluation in the field is intended to establish a baseline level of the lesion for later comparison—that is, to determine the completeness of the lesion and to identify cord syndromes if the lesion is incomplete. A normal neurologic exam does not rule out the possibility of SCI. The neurologic assessment is intended not only to determine whether the patient should be immobilized, but to also furnish data about the patient's precise initial presentation so that medical facility personnel can measure any changes and determine whether immediate surgery is necessary.

Words of Wisdom

A normal neurologic exam does not rule out the possibility of SCI.

The initial step of any neurologic assessment is to determine the level of consciousness. You first note the patient's AVPU in the primary survey, and then you address the GCS level during the secondary assessment.

When you assign the GCS score, do not score the patient as having no motor response if the patient's limbs are paralyzed. Ask the patient to blink or move some facial muscles that would be innervated by a cranial nerve. Remember, an unresponsive patient is always at risk for having a spinal injury.

Motor components of spinal nerves supply specific tissues and muscles in regions called **myotomes** Table 34-5. You should examine these myotomes in the typical head-to-toe fashion, beginning with the cranial nerves. Cranial nerve assessment is especially important in circumstances suggesting a high cervical injury. Observe the patient for drooping of the upper eyelid and a small pupil (Horner syndrome), which would indicate an interruption in the sympathetic nervous pathways to the eye.

Bilaterally assess each major motor group from the top down to identify the lowest spinal segment associated with normal voluntary motor function. Because incomplete spinal cord lesions are possible, you must determine the extent of function in segments below this level. Monitor for possible ascending lesions, paying special attention to alterations in respiratory patterns resulting from cervical lesions.

Ask the patient to flex (C5) and extend (C7) both elbows and then both wrists (C6). Have the patient abduct the fingers and keep them open against resistance, and then adduct the fingers and attempt to close them against resistance (T1) Figure 34-18. As an alternative maneuver, have the patient curl all four fingers while the examiner applies opposing pull with his or her fingers

Table 34-5	Myotomes			
Nerve Root	**Muscle Group**		**Nerve Root**	**Muscle Group**
C3-C5	Diaphragm		L2	Hip flexors: iliopsoas
C5	Elbow flexors: biceps, brachialis, brachioradialis		L3	Knee extensors: quadriceps
C6	Wrist extensors		L4	Ankle dorsiflexors: tibialis anterior
C7	Elbow extensors: triceps		L5	Long toe extensors: extensor hallucis longus
C8	Finger flexors: flexor digitorum profundus to middle finger		S1	Ankle plantar flexors (gastrocnemius, soleus)
T1	Hand intrinsics: interossei, small finger abductors		S4-S5	Anus, bowel, urinary bladder
T2-T7	Intercostal muscles			

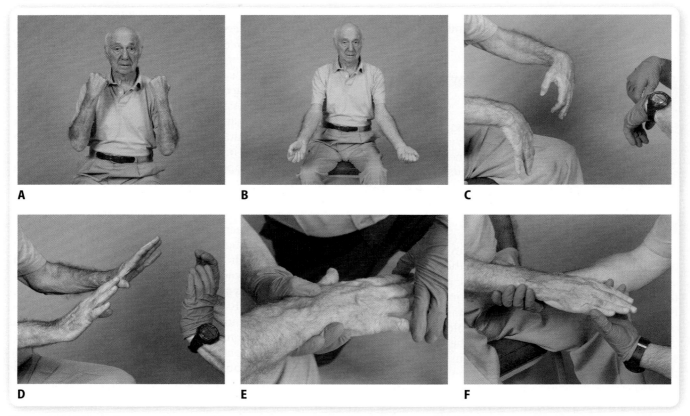

A   **B**   **C**

D   **E**   **F**

Figure 34-18 Neurologic evaluation of the upper extremities. Ask the patient to flex **(A)** and then extend **(B)** both elbows. Ask the patient to flex **(C)** and then extend **(D)** both wrists. Have the patient abduct the fingers and keep them open against resistance **(E)**. Have the patient try to curl four fingers against resistance **(F)**.

© Jones & Bartlett Learning. Courtesy of MIEMSS.

to determine strength against resistance. This maneuver tests the finger flexors (C8).

To evaluate the lower extremities, ask the patient to bend and extend the knees. Next, ask the patient to plantar flex the feet and ankles as if pressing down on the gas pedal of a car (S1 to S2) and to dorsiflex the toes to gravity and against resistance (L5) **Figure 34-19**.

Assessment of motor integrity in an unresponsive patient is based mostly on the patient's response to a painful stimulus. Spinal injury with loss of motor function is likely if an unresponsive patient grimaces, vocalizes, or opens his or her eyes to a painful response above the level of the neurologic deficit but does not move the limbs. Test pain responses at several locations before assuming an absence of response. If the motor exam cannot be completed because of local injury, then the exam is considered unreliable, and spinal immobilization is necessary.

Sensory components of spinal nerves supply specific, well-defined areas of the body surface called dermatomes **Table 34-6** **Figure 34-20**. In addition to testing for a general loss of sensation, ask the patient whether he or she has abnormal sensations in these areas, such as "pins and needles," electric shock, or hyperacute pain to touch (**hyperesthesia**). As with the motor exam, sensory integrity must be assessed bilaterally, but from the feet up. Identify the lowest level of normal sensation and any areas below

this level in which the patient retains sensation. In the responsive patient, a thorough assessment will include his or her perception of light touch, temperature, and position (proprioception).

Reflexes can produce valuable information about sensory input, especially in the unresponsive patient. In significant SCIs, reflexes are usually absent but return several hours to several weeks after injury. If reflexes are intact, the preservation of motor and sensory activity in the same spinal cord segments is likely. In the patient older than 2 years, the **Babinski reflex** is positive when the toes move upward in response to stimulation of the sole of the foot. Under normal circumstances, the toes move downward. Refer to Chapter 11, *Patient Assessment*, for a discussion of reflexes.

Reassessment

You must reassess the patient frequently to determine whether the patient is stabilizing, improving, or deteriorating. Monitor vital signs every 5 minutes (unstable patients) to 15 minutes (stable patients), with special attention to the patient's cardiovascular status. Watch for hypotension without other signs of shock. The combination of hypotension with a normal or slow pulse and

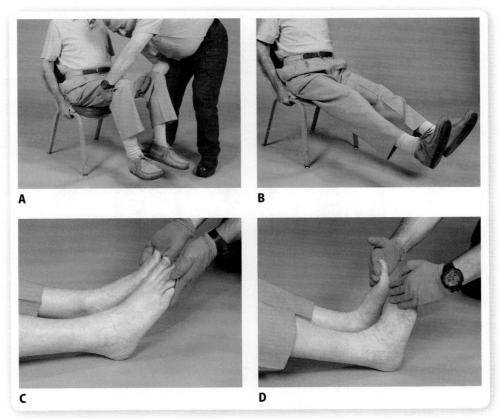

Figure 34-19 Neurologic evaluation of the lower extremities. Ask the patient to bend **(A)** and extend **(B)** the knees. Ask the patient to flex the feet and ankles downward **(C)** and flex the toes upward **(D)**.

© Jones & Bartlett Learning. Courtesy of MIEMSS.

Table 34-6	**Dermatomes**			
Nerve Root	**Anatomic Location**		**Nerve Root**	**Anatomic Location**
C2	Occipital protuberance		T10	Umbilicus
C3	Supraclavicular fossa		L1	Inguinal line
C5	Lateral side of antecubital fossa		L2	Mid anterior thigh
C6	Thumb and medial index finger (six-shooter)		L3	Medial aspect of the knee
C7	Middle finger		L5	Dorsum of the foot
C8	Little finger		S1-S3	Back of leg
T2	Apex of axilla		S4-S5	Perianal area
T4	Nipple line			

© Jones & Bartlett Learning.

warm skin is highly suggestive of neurogenic shock. The SCI responsible for neurogenic shock also usually produces a flaccid paralysis and complete loss of sensation below the level of injury. In contrast to neurogenic shock, hypovolemic shock is associated with pale, cold, clammy skin and tachycardia.

Check interventions such as oxygen flow and spinal immobilization to ensure they are still effective. Some

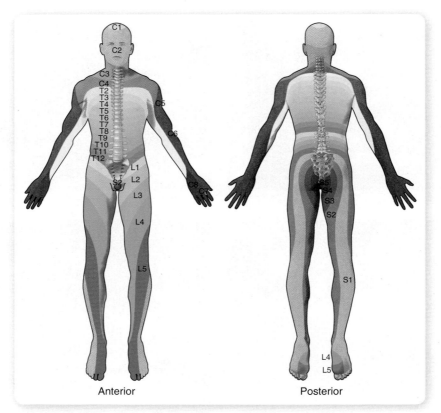

Figure 34-20 Dermatomes.

© Jones & Bartlett Learning.

EMS organizations may administer an antiemetic or corticosteroid per medical control. Repeat the physical exam and reprioritize the patient as necessary.

Document suspected SCI, note the area involved, sensation, dermatomes, motor function, and areas of weakness.

The Incidence of Head Trauma

Recall, *head trauma* comprises both head injury and TBI. The term *head injury* describes a traumatic insult to the head with injury to the scalp or skull, not including the face or brain. TBI is impairment of brain function brought about by an external force, such as a fall. A person can have head injury and TBI at the same time, a situation captured by the term *head trauma*.

According to the Centers for Disease Control and Prevention (CDC), TBI is a significant cause of death and disability and is responsible for about 30% of trauma-related deaths each year.[29,30] In 2013, TBI resulted in approximately 2.8 million visits to EDs, was diagnosed in 282,000 hospitalizations, and contributed to 50,000 deaths.[30] From 2007 to 2013, TBI-related ED visits increased by 50%, but the number of deaths decreased by 7%.

Falls are the most common MOI, accounting for 47% of all TBIs each year.[30] Other common causes of TBI are unintentional blunt trauma (such as being struck by or against an object or person, as occurs in sports-related incidents), which accounts for 15% of TBI-related ED

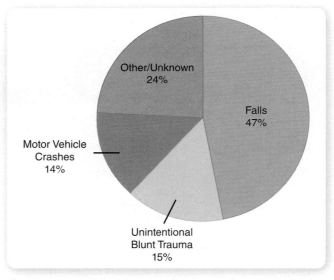

Figure 34-21 Leading causes of traumatic brain injury.

Data from TBI: Get the Facts. Concussion. Traumatic Brain Injury. CDC Injury Center. (2016). www.cdc.gov/traumaticbraininjury/get_the_facts.html.

visits, and MVCs, which account for 14% of TBI-related ED visits **Figure 34-21** .[30]

TBI is most likely to result in death in people 75 years and older.[30] Leading causes of death relating to TBI vary by age group[30]:

- Falls: 65 years and older
- Intentional self-harm: 25 to 64 years

- Motor vehicle crashes: 5 to 24 years
- Assault: 0 to 4 years

There are two general types of head injuries: open and closed. A closed head injury, the most common type, is usually associated with blunt trauma. Although the dura mater is undamaged and brain tissue is not exposed to the environment, closed head injuries may result in skull fractures or TBIs. Such brain injuries may be either focal or diffuse. Focal injuries are limited to a focused area. Diffuse injuries are literally diffused—in other words, spread out and not focused on a central, easily defined area. These injuries are often complicated by increased ICP.[31]

With an open head injury, the dura mater and cranial contents are penetrated, and brain tissue is open to the environment. Gunshot wounds—the most common penetrating MOI—have a high mortality rate, and those who survive almost always have significant neurologic deficits and a decreased quality of life.[31]

Pathophysiology, Assessment, and Management of Head Injuries

▶ Scalp Injuries

Recall from Chapter 8, *Anatomy and Physiology*, that the scalp comprises five layers. Its role is to protect the head from outside organisms, to provide thermal regulation, and to control the loss of extracellular fluid through evaporation.

Scalp injuries can vary from minor injuries to serious lacerations and scalp avulsions. The scalp's rich blood supply means that even small lacerations can quickly lead to significant blood loss **Figure 34-22**. Because these injuries typically produce a large amount of blood, you must avoid becoming distracted or overly focused on the scalp injury and remember to conduct a thorough evaluation to avoid missing a more significant underlying injury.

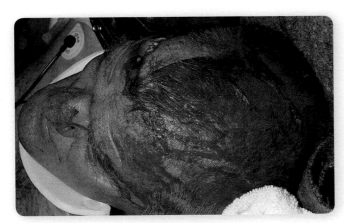

Figure 34-22 The scalp has a rich blood supply, so even small lacerations can lead to significant blood loss.

Scalp lacerations alone in adults rarely cause hypovolemic shock; this result is more common in children. However, bleeding from the scalp can contribute to hypovolemia in any patient, especially one with multiple injuries.[32] If the adult patient is exhibiting signs of hypovolemic shock, and the shock persists after you treat the scalp laceration, then continue to search for other possible causes of the volume loss. In addition, because scalp lacerations usually result from direct blows to the head, they often indicate deeper, more severe injuries.

Assessment and Management of Scalp Injuries

When you assess the laceration, consider the mechanism as a key piece of information in choosing the course of treatment. If you were to apply direct pressure to a laceration that overlies a skull fracture in which the bone ends can be moved, the resulting injury to the brain or meninges could be devastating and have long-term consequences. Inspect the laceration for indications of missing tissue (avulsions) and possible impaled objects or residual contaminants.

Remember, some types of hematomas may mask a depressed skull fracture, so identifying the mechanism will be paramount. Evaluate the wound for signs of continued bleeding. Reevaluate the wound often as the vital signs return to normal, because bleeding may recur when sympathetic stimulation has receded. If you cannot determine the primary mechanism, then you should assume the skull is involved.

In isolated lacerations without possible skull fractures, stopping the bleeding is your primary concern. Apply direct pressure with minor to moderate lacerations. With significant lacerations, direct pressure may be insufficient to control blood loss. You may need pressure dressings and hemostatic agents to control the bleeding. When you suspect your patient has skull instability, your protocol may allow you to move directly to the use of hemostatic agents.

In the prehospital setting, if time and other injuries allow, give a quick cleansing rinse, preferably with sterile saline, to help reduce the incidence of significant infection. Exploring the injury is not recommended because doing so may disrupt clot formation and restart bleeding, and you may disturb bone fragments in patients with skull involvement.

Words of Wisdom

The hypotensive patient may have minimal bleeding from the scalp. As the pressure increases, however, so can the severity of the hemorrhage. Reassess any scalp hemorrhage throughout your time with the patient. If the laceration has been bandaged, then the increased hemorrhage can be easily missed.

► Skull Fracture

There are four types of skull fractures: linear, depressed, basilar, and open **Figure 34-23**. The significance of the skull fracture directly relates to the type of fracture, the amount of force applied, and the area of the head that sustained the blow. Skull fractures are seen most often after MVCs and significant falls. These fractures may or may not occur with soft-tissue scalp injuries. Some potential complications of skull fracture are intracranial hemorrhage, cerebral damage, and cranial nerve damage, among others.

Linear Skull Fractures

Linear skull fractures (nondisplaced skull fractures) account for the majority of all skull fractures.[33] Most linear fractures occur in the temporal-parietal region (see Figure 34-23A).[31] Diagnosing a linear skull fracture requires radiographic evaluation because the skull often displays no gross physical signs (eg, deformity, depression). If the brain is uninjured and the scalp is uninjured, then linear fractures cause relatively little damage. However, a scalp laceration that occurs in conjunction with a linear fracture—making it an open fracture—carries a risk of infection. In addition, if the skull fracture occurs over the temporal region, injury to the middle meningeal artery may result in epidural bleeding.

Depressed Skull Fractures

Depressed skull fractures result from high-energy direct trauma to a small surface area of the head with a blunt object (such as a baseball bat to the head) (see Figure 34-23B). The bones in the frontal and parietal regions of the skull are relatively thin compared with other bones of the skull. Thus, they are the areas most susceptible to these types of fractures.

These fractures are generally secondary to an assault and are the regions an attacker will usually strike.[33] Such a strike may drive bony fragments into the brain, resulting in underlying injury. The overlying scalp may or may not be injured.

If there is an associated scalp laceration, the fracture is considered to be open, and contamination of the cranial vault is a risk. Of depressed skull fractures, 75% to 90% are open fractures.[33] Patients with depressed skull fractures often present with neurologic signs (such as loss of consciousness) because they have greater associated brain injury than is seen with other skull injuries. Thus, this type of fracture has the greatest association with patient death compared with other types of skull fractures.

Basilar Skull Fractures

Basilar skull fractures generally result from the extension of a linear fracture into the base of the skull. They are also associated with high mortality rates and occur secondary to high-energy trauma. They usually occur after diffuse impact to the head, as may occur in a fall or a MVC, for example. Trauma to any part of the head can produce a basilar skull fracture. Impacts to the back and side of the head are the most common cause of fracture, however. Fracture of the temporal bone represents 75% of basilar skull fractures.[33] Such injuries generally result from extension of a linear fracture to the base of the skull and cause a tear in the dura mater. As with linear skull fractures, temporal fractures can be difficult to diagnose with radiography (see Figure 34-23C).

Open Skull Fractures

Open fractures of the cranial vault result when severe forces are applied to the head and are often associated with trauma to multiple body systems (see Figure 34-23D). Brain tissue may be exposed to the environment, significantly increasing the risk of a bacterial infection (eg, bacterial meningitis). Open cranial vault fractures have a high mortality rate.

Assessment and Management of Skull Fractures

During the secondary assessment, use the pads of your fingers to apply pressure over the entire skull, noting any

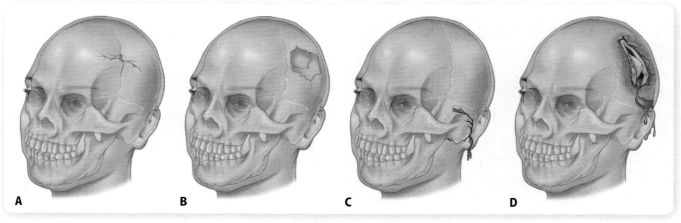

Figure 34-23 Types of skull fractures. **A.** Linear. **B.** Depressed. **C.** Basilar. **D.** Open.
© Jones & Bartlett Learning.

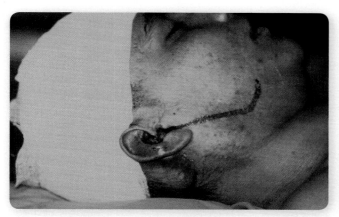

Figure 34-24 Blood or cerebrospinal fluid draining from the ear after a head injury suggests a basilar skull fracture.

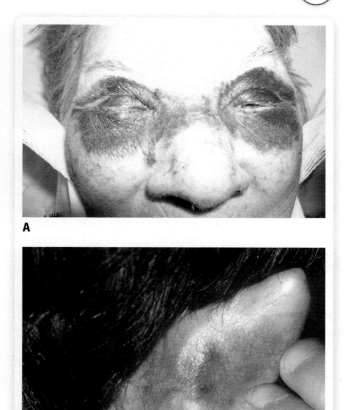

Figure 34-25 Suspect a basilar skull fracture if ecchymosis is present in a patient with head trauma. **A.** Ecchymosis under or around the eyes (raccoon eyes). **B.** Ecchymosis behind the ear over the mastoid process (Battle sign).

A: © E.M. Singletary, M.D. Used with permission; **B:** © Mediscan/Alamy.

swelling, edema, deformity, depressions, or crepitus. Palpation of linear skull fractures often produces no external findings. Therefore, an injury may be located under a hematoma and you may not be able to find it until the patient undergoes radiography at the medical facility. Thus, your index of suspicion is paramount in patients who have a mechanism consistent with this type of fracture.

In depressed skull fractures, you may or may not feel a depression or crepitus because a hematoma often develops over the fracture site. If you do feel a depression, do not press into the area, because you will likely drive bone fragments into the brain. Note the finding and move on with your assessment. Don't palpate the depression again when you reassess the patient, because doing so poses a risk of further brain injury.

Signs of a basilar skull fracture include CSF drainage from the ears or nose. Such drainage indicates a tear in the dura mater **Figure 34-24**. Patients with leaking CSF are at risk for bacterial meningitis. Depending on the site of the fracture, patients may also experience a loss of hearing or sense of smell, have balance disorders, and exhibit weakness in the facial muscles.

Other signs of a basilar skull fracture include periorbital ecchymosis (raccoon eyes) **Figure 34-25A** and ecchymosis behind the ear over the mastoid process (Battle sign) **Figure 34-25B**. Depending on the extent of the damage, raccoon eyes or Battle sign may appear relatively quickly, but in many cases, they may not appear until up to 24 hours after the injury. Their absence in the prehospital setting, then, does not rule out a basilar skull fracture.

The presence of raccoon eyes or Battle sign may also indicate a prior injury that may be the cause of the current incident. Thus, you must perform a comprehensive history and physical exam. For example, the patient may have been in a fight the night before and now have an altered level of consciousness. Or, you might respond to a MVC and find either of these signs.

Treating skull fractures is secondary to identifying and treating any life threats you find during the primary survey. Because these patients may have associated brain injury, airway depression, and vomiting may occur. Carry airway adjuncts and suctioning in anticipation of such complications.

Because of the high energy required to cause skull fractures, consider the possibility of a spinal injury and evaluate the patient to determine whether spinal motion restriction is indicated. Until you complete that evaluation and make a decision, provide manual in-line stabilization of the cervical spine.

Linear skull fractures generally require only supportive care. If the patient has an open skull fracture with exposed brain tissue, then *lightly* cover it with a sterile dressing that has been moistened with sterile saline. Likewise, for leakage of CSF from the ears or nose, apply loose sterile dressings to keep the area clean, but do not attempt to stop the flow. Objects impaled in the skull should be stabilized in place and protected from movement.

Pathophysiology, Assessment, and Management of Traumatic Brain Injury and Diffuse Brain Injuries

Traumatic brain injuries are divided into two broad types: primary (direct) injury and secondary (indirect) injury. **Primary brain injury** is injury to the brain and its associated structures that results instantly from impact to the head. **Secondary brain injury** is a consequence of the primary injury; it includes abnormal processes such as cerebral edema, intracranial hemorrhage, increased ICP, cerebral ischemia and hypoxia, hypoglycemia, hypotension, and infection. Secondary brain injury can last from a few minutes to several days after the initial injury.

Preventive programs are the only avenue for reducing brain injuries, but you can and must prevent the development of secondary brain injuries, or immediately treat these injuries when you find the patient. The Brain Trauma Foundation defines hypoxia in the setting of TBI as an oxygen saturation level of less than 90%.[13] Hypoxia and hypotension (systolic blood pressure less than 90 mm Hg) are among the five most powerful predictors of poor outcome in the patient with a TBI. If the patient has a single incident of hypotension, regardless of the amount of time, then mortality increases from two to four times that of patients who did not experience hypotension. Hypoxia has similar effects, and the combination of hypotension and hypoxia has exponential effects on mortality. As a paramedic, you must remember secondary brain injury, especially hypotension and hypoxia, *must be avoided*.

The brain can be injured directly by a penetrating object, such as a bullet, knife, or other sharp object. More often, brain injuries occur indirectly, through external forces exerted on the skull.

Consider the most common cause of brain injury, the MVC. When the passenger's head hits the windshield (impact with a fixed object), the brain continues to move forward until it stops abruptly by striking the inside of the skull. This rapid deceleration produces compression injury (or bruising) to the anterior portion of the brain along with stretching or tearing of the posterior portion of the brain **Figure 34-26** .

As the brain strikes the front of the skull, the body begins its path of moving backward. The head falls back against the headrest and/or seat, and the brain slams into the rear of the skull, resulting in a coup-contrecoup injury. The same type of injury may occur on opposite sides of the brain in a lateral crash.

The injured brain starts to swell, initially because of dilated cerebral vessels. An increase in cerebral fluid (cerebral edema) then contributes to further brain swelling. Cerebral edema, however, may not develop until several hours after the initial injury.

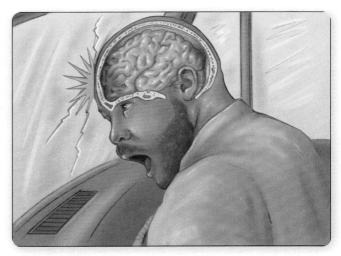

Figure 34-26 When a person in a motor vehicle crash is unrestrained, the brain continues to move forward as the vehicle decelerates suddenly on impact. As the brain strikes the inside of the skull, the anterior portion is compressed and the posterior portion stretched.

© Jones & Bartlett Learning.

▶ Intracranial Pressure

To function properly, the brain must receive a constant supply of oxygen and nutrients, such as glucose. The brain receives about 15% of the cardiac output and consumes about 20% of the body's oxygen. The brain receives its blood supply through the vertebral and internal carotid arteries.

Because the brain is sensitive to decreases in glucose, oxygen, and perfusion, blood flow through the brain (cerebral blood flow) must be maintained at a fairly constant level. If the brain's blood supply is disrupted, then changes in mental status and vital signs may occur. For example, heart rate, respiratory rate, and blood pressure may change.

Remember, the skull houses the brain, its blood vessels, and CSF. In adults, the skull is a rigid, unyielding globe that allows little, if any, expansion of the intracranial contents. Also, the skull has a hard and somewhat irregular interior surface against which brain tissue and its blood vessels can be injured when the head sustains trauma.

Normally, the brain occupies about 80% of the space within the cranium. The remaining space is taken up by blood (12%) and CSF (8%). Accumulations of blood within the skull or swelling of the brain can rapidly lead to an increase in ICP. This increased ICP squeezes the brain against bony prominences within the cranium.

Cerebral perfusion pressure (CPP) is the difference between the **mean arterial pressure (MAP)**, which is the average (or mean) pressure against the arterial wall during a cardiac cycle, and ICP. It is calculated as CPP = MAP − ICP. The MAP is the diastolic blood pressure plus one-third of the pulse pressure (MAP = DBP + 1/3 PP). (Recall from Chapter 8, *Anatomy and Physiology*, that pulse pressure is the systolic blood pressure minus the diastolic pressure.)

MAP is an indicator of how well the brain is being supplied with nutrients. Obviously, decreasing cerebral blood flow (CBF) is a potential catastrophe because the brain depends on a constant supply of blood to furnish the oxygen and glucose it needs to survive.

The normal ICP is 5 to 15 mm Hg, and the normal MAP is 85 to 95 mm Hg. These pressures produce a normal CPP of 70 to 90 mm Hg. At these pressures, the brain receives blood flow, with its oxygen and glucose, sufficient to meet its metabolic needs. Any increase in ICP above 20 mm Hg (such as from cerebral edema or intracranial hemorrhage) decreases CPP and cerebral blood flow.

The diameter of the vessels in the brain affects cerebral blood flow, and therefore CPP. A mechanism called **autoregulation** is the brain's ability to regulate the diameter of the vessels within the brain (and therefore CBF) in response to a wide range of MAPs.

The brain can autoregulate and ensures adequate CBF when the CPP is between 60 and 160 mm Hg. A CPP below the **critical minimum threshold** of 60 mm Hg results in inadequate perfusion of the brain and cerebral ischemia, which can result in permanent neurologic impairment or death. According to the Brain Trauma Foundation, a *single* drop in CPP below 60 mm Hg *doubles* the risk of death in a patient with a brain injury. CPPs of greater than 160 mm Hg produce hypertensive encephalopathy.

Increased ICP disrupts autoregulation by decreasing CPP, as demonstrated using the preceding mathematical formula. As CPP decreases, blood vessels within the brain dilate, increasing the volume of blood in the brain. As a result, ICP increases. This increased ICP further decreases CPP, which leads to further dilation of cerebral vessels, which increases ICP, in a vicious circle.

In an effort to combat increasing ICP, the body uses the Monro-Kellie doctrine, or the Monro-Kellie principle.[34] As we've discussed, the cranial vault is a rigid, nondistensible box—a compartment that cannot expand. This space is 100% filled by the brain, CSF, and blood. In response to an expanding intracranial mass, the body attempts to reduce ICP by expelling CSF and venous blood from the cranial vault. During the early stages, this mechanism is successful in creating more space for the mass and keeping ICP within normal limits **Figure 34-27** .

Without a high index of suspicion, subtle signs and symptoms are easily missed at this stage. As with all compensatory mechanisms, however, this one has physiologic limits. Without intervention, the pressure will eventually

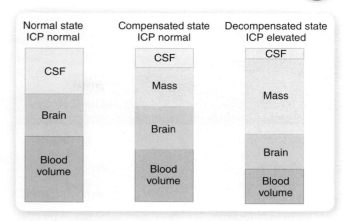

Figure 34-27 The body's attempt to regulate intracranial pressure (ICP). The left represents the normal state. The middle shows the compensated state in which ICP is still normal. The right shows the decompensated state, in which ICP is elevated.

© Jones & Bartlett Learning.

increase to a point at which no more CSF or venous blood can be expelled, and ICP will rise exponentially.

When the ICP begins to rise and the CPP begins to drop, the body attempts to maintain CPP by increasing the MAP. This increase will be indicated not only by an increasing blood pressure (both systolic and diastolic), but also by a widening pulse pressure. To recognize this pattern, you must auscultate a blood pressure, noting both the systolic blood pressure and diastolic blood pressure. You'll miss valuable information by simply palpating the blood pressure.

Other factors also interfere with CPP. For example, excess carbon dioxide in the blood dilates cerebral vessels. This dilation increases cerebral blood volume, which increases ICP, and so on.

Hypotension results in a decreased MAP, which causes a decrease in the CPP. When the MAP drops to 60 mm Hg or less, cerebral blood flow begins to decrease. In response, cerebral vessels become dilated, and the cycle repeats itself. Systolic blood pressure should be maintained at the levels shown in **Table 34-7** .

When swelling or bleeding occurs in the brain, the brain sends signals requesting more oxygen. This triggers a vicious circle. The more blood that enters the brain, the more oxygen it requires, and the more swelling increases. If the ICP gets too high, then the brain tissue has nowhere to go except through the tentorium incisura, the foramen magnum, or both.

Although the exact CPP cannot be calculated in the prehospital setting, you can recognize reduced CPP based on the patient's presentation, vital signs, and trends in the MAP. Many modern monitors will automatically display the MAP, negating the need to perform any mathematical functions during patient care. Prehospital treatment must focus on maintaining CPP (and cerebral blood flow), while mitigating ICP as much as possible—a fine balance to maintain.

Words of Wisdom

It is imperative that you be alert for subtle signs and symptoms when you suspect a TBI. Do not wait for signs of herniation; these signs indicate that the compensatory mechanisms used to keep ICP within normal limits have failed.

Table 34-7	Systolic Blood Pressure Maintenance Levels	
Age Range	**Systolic Blood Pressure Maintenance Level**
Younger than 1 year	Greater than 65 mm Hg
1 to 5 years	Greater than 75 mm Hg
5 to 12 years	Greater than 80 mm Hg
Older than 12 years	Greater than 90 mm Hg[a]

[a]At the time of this printing, there is some evidence that patients age 50 to 69 years should have systolic blood pressure maintained at greater than or equal to 100 mm Hg, and that patients age 15 to 49 years and over age 70 should have systolic blood pressure maintained at greater than or equal to 110 mm Hg.

Data from: Allen BB, Chiu Y, Gerber LM, Ghajar J, Greenfield JP. Age-specific cerebral perfusion pressure thresholds and survival in children and adolescents with severe traumatic brain injury. *Pediatr Crit Care Med.* 2014;15(1):62–70; Haddad SH, Arabi YM. Critical care management of severe traumatic brain injury in adults. *Scand J Trauma Resusc Emerg Med.* 2012;20:12.

▶ Herniation

If increased ICP is not treated promptly in a definitive care setting, then cerebral herniation may occur. In herniation, the brain is forced from the cranial vault, through either the foramen magnum or the tentorium.

Lateral herniation syndrome, also called uncal herniation syndrome, is the most common form of herniation. In this form, a portion of the temporal lobe, called the *uncus*, is displaced laterally before moving downward through the tentorium incisura, compressing the midbrain and posterior cerebral artery.

Because the oculomotor nerve (CN III) also passes through the tentorium incisura, the uncus will compress it. Recall, CN III delivers parasympathetic stimulation to the pupil and therefore is responsible for constriction. The loss of this stimulus results in the pupil dilation that may be seen in TBIs—a strong indicator of herniation.

Because the cranial nerves exert their effects on one side of the body and spinal nerves exert their effect on the opposite side of the body, the patient will exhibit ipsilateral (same-sided) pupil dilation and contralateral (opposite-sided) motor dysfunction. You must evaluate the pupils early in suspected TBI, because a unilateral pupil change may be present for only minutes to hours, depending on the rate of expansion of the intracranial mass.

Herniation shifts the brain tissue downward, ultimately compressing the brainstem from above. This mechanism is called *central herniation syndrome*. Herniation that occurs when part of the cerebellum is forced through the foramen magnum, compressing the brainstem, is called *tonsillar herniation*.

Brainstem compression destroys the respiratory center, induces apnea, decreases perfusion to the rest of the brain, and ultimately causes death. These patients require immediate surgery to place a drain that will allow blood and fluid to escape, alleviating pressure within the cranium. Other areas of the brain may suffer herniation, but such injuries occur less often than either uncal herniation or foramen magnum herniation.

You must closely monitor a patient with head injury for signs and symptoms of increased ICP. The exact clinical signs you encounter depend on the amount of pressure inside the skull and the extent of brainstem involvement. Early signs and symptoms include vomiting (often without nausea), headache, an altered level of consciousness, and seizures.

Later, more ominous signs include hypertension (with a widening pulse pressure), bradycardia, and changes in respirations (**Cushing triad**). The systolic and diastolic blood pressures increase, and the pulse pressure widens, in an attempt to maintain MAP. The baroreceptors respond to this increase in pressure by stimulating the vagus nerve to slow the heart rate in an attempt to reduce the blood pressure. Recall, the baroreceptors are simply pressure receptors and respond only to pressure. They have no way of "knowing" why the pressure is increased.

The changes in respirations can include Cheyne-Stokes respirations or central neurogenic respirations, both of which are efforts to reduce the partial pressure of carbon dioxide, or respiratory patterns that indicate brainstem compression such as apneustic, ataxic, Biot, or agonal respirations. In addition, a unilaterally unequal and nonreactive pupil, coma, and posturing are late signs of increased ICP. **Decorticate (flexor) posturing** is characterized by flexion of the arms and extension of the legs; **decerebrate (extensor) posturing** is characterized by extension of the arms and legs **Figure 34-28**.

▶ Diffuse Brain Injuries

Brain injuries are broadly classified as diffuse or focal. A **diffuse brain injury** is any injury that affects the entire brain. These injuries include cerebral concussion and diffuse (widespread) axonal injury.

Cerebral Concussion

A **cerebral concussion** occurs when the brain is jarred in the skull. This kind of mild, diffuse brain injury is usually caused by rapid acceleration-deceleration. This mechanism produces shearing injuries caused by rotational and angular forces exerted on the brain. These forces damage cell membranes of the neurons, allowing (among other things) potassium to move into the extracellular space, thereby depressing neuronal activity. These injuries may be seen after incidents such as MVCs, falls, and sports injuries. Although most current research on concussions centers on sports-related concussions, the pathophysiology, signs, symptoms, and treatment are the same regardless of the way in which the concussion was sustained.

A concussion injury, caused by a direct or indirect force to the head, results in transient functional dysfunction of the cerebral cortex. The concussion usually resolves spontaneously and rapidly, causing no structural damage

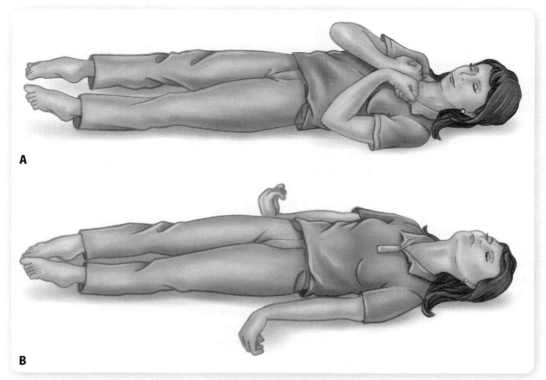

Figure 34-28 Posturing indicates significant intracranial pressure. **A.** Decorticate (flexor) posturing. You can remember this term by thinking of the arms being pulled into the "core" of the body. **B.** Decerebrate (extensor) posturing.

© Jones & Bartlett Learning.

to the brain. Signs of a concussion are nonspecific, with a headache being most common. Additional findings range from transient confusion and disorientation to confusion that may last several minutes. Loss of consciousness is possible, but in most cases, the patient remains conscious. Some report **retrograde amnesia**, a loss of memory relating to events that occurred before the injury, or **anterograde (posttraumatic) amnesia**, a loss of memory relating to events that occurred after the injury.

The exact definition of a concussion has been the subject of much debate over the years. Although the medical community had reached a consensus, the definition continues to evolve as we learn more about this injury. The 5th International Conference on Concussion in Sport in 2016 defined concussion as a traumatic brain injury induced by biomechanical forces. Common features that may be used in clinically defining a concussion include the following four items when the signs and symptoms cannot be explained by drug, alcohol, or medication use, or other injuries or comorbidities [35]:

- Concussion may be caused by either a direct blow to the head or a blow to the face, neck, or elsewhere on the body with an "impulsive" force transmitted to the head.
- Concussion typically results in the rapid onset of short-lived impairment of neurologic function that resolves spontaneously. However, in some cases, signs and symptoms may evolve over a number of minutes to hours.

- Concussion may result in neuropathologic changes, but the acute clinical symptoms largely reflect a functional disturbance rather than a structural injury, and, as such, no abnormality is seen on standard structural neuroimaging studies.
- Concussion results in a range of clinical signs and symptoms that may or may not involve a loss of consciousness. Resolution of the clinical and cognitive features typically follows a sequential course. However, in some cases symptoms may be prolonged.

Words of Wisdom

Medicine is a dynamic and ever-evolving field. As a medical professional, you must keep up with current medical research and literature. For example, the 5th International Conference on Concussion in Sport took place in October 2016. Some of the recommendations and consensus statements about concussions may change before the next such conference. You should review current data and studies while you are reading this section of the text and note any updates or new clinical practice guidelines that occur before the next conference.

As a paramedic, you probably will treat patients who have experienced a concussion. This injury causes more than 1 million visits to EDs annually.[36] Moreover, it is estimated that there are 1.6 to 3.8 million sports-related concussions annually, and many of these patients do not seek immediate medical treatment.[37] As a result, you may very well encounter patients days after their concussive event.

A great deal has been learned about concussions over the last several years. Researchers have exposed the damaging effects of repetitive concussions and the risk of second impact syndrome and postconcussion syndrome. You must not discount a patient with a possible concussion regardless of whether you see him or her at the time of the injury or days to weeks after the concussive event. Do not let helmet use decrease your suspicion of a concussion. While studies have shown that helmets reduce head and facial injury and absorb energy that would otherwise act on the brain, they have not been shown to reduce the incidence of concussions.

Athletic venues are a common site of concussions. You may be on standby for the event or be called to the event after the injury. Most youth coaches are required to take concussion training to be allowed on the field. Upper levels of play usually include athletic trainers who have had extensive concussion training and have likely conducted a prescreening of the injured athlete that they can use for comparison.

At times, you may be the only medical professional on scene. One of the biggest questions in these situations is whether the athlete can return to play. Currently there is no diagnostic test that can reliably be used to for an immediate determination of the presence of a concussion. Therefore it is impossible to rule out a concussion in the setting of a head injury with transient neurologic symptoms. Any time there is a suspicion of a concussion, the player must be removed from play and assessed by a physician.[35] Authorizing an athlete to return to play after a potential concussion is outside the paramedic's scope of practice. If you are faced with this decision, then consult medical control.

If you face a situation in which a coach or parent wants to return the athlete to the game, but you think the player should not return, then explain your concerns to the coach and/or athletic trainer. Point out the signs and symptoms you observe and remind him or her of the steps in the concussion action plans developed by the National Federation of State High School Associations (NFHS) in association with the CDC's "Heads Up" program **Figure 34-29** .[38,39] Both organizations offer free concussion training on their websites.

Assessment and Management. As with any patient, you first complete the primary survey and address any life-threatening conditions you find. If indicated, place the patient in spinal immobilization. The patient with an isolated concussion generally does not face life threats, and your secondary assessment is directed at evaluating for the presence of a concussion.

Always remember, a loss of consciousness or various forms of amnesia do not accurately reflect the severity of a concussion. A patient may experience a severe concussion without losing consciousness. Therefore, if you suspect a concussion, you must complete a thorough evaluation.

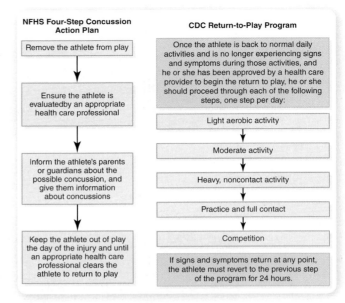

Figure 34-29 Key points of the NFHS and CDC concussion programs.

Data from: National Federation of State High School Associations (NFHS) Sports Medicine Advisory Committee (SMAC). Suggested guidelines for management of concussion in sports. NFHS website. https://www.nfhs.org/sports-resource-content/suggested-guidelines-for-management-of-concussion-in-sports/. Published February 16, 2017. Accessed March 24, 2017; and Centers for Disease Control and Prevention, National Center for Injury Prevention and Control, Division of Unintentional Injuries Prevention. Heads up. Managing return to activities. CDC website. http://www.cdc.gov/headsup/providers/return_to_activities.html. Updated February 8, 2016. Accessed March 24, 2017.

Symptoms may appear immediately or may be delayed, and they generally resolve within 72 hours. Complete recovery occurs 7 to 10 days after the concussive event, but recovery may take longer in children or in any patient with previous concussions.

Your assessment of the concussed patient focuses primarily on cognition, and the findings may be subtle. The patient history is the key component of the assessment of a patient with a concussion. Ask your patient questions to assess his or her memory and awareness of person, place, time, and situation. Questions such as the following can yield valuable information for your assessment:

- "What is your name?"
- "Where are you?"
- "Where were you going?"
- "What were you doing at the time of the incident?"
- "How did it happen?"
- "What is the score?" or "Who are you playing?" (if applicable)

When possible, and with the patient's consent, include people who know the patient during the assessment to verify the answers the patient gives. Ask athletic trainers to compare the current findings to their findings during any preseason screening. To further assess memory, you can ask the patient to remember a series of words or numbers and then repeat them to you later in the call. You can also repeat questions to compare the new answers to the original answers and to evaluate for any change in the patient's mental status and speed of responses. As a paramedic you must realize that in the setting of a concussion, standard orientation questions, such as person, place, time, and situation, are insufficient when compared to a memory assessment.[35]

Findings of a concussion may include the following:[40]

- Headache, the most common finding
- Fatigue or fogginess
- Confusion or altered mental status
- Inability to recognize people or places
- Disorientation
- Dizziness
- Difficulty concentrating
- Memory deficits
- Difficulty maintaining balance
- Visual disturbances
- Delayed responses to questions
- Irritability
- Changes in behavior
- Sleep disturbances
- Sensitivity to light and noise
- Loss of consciousness (about 10% of patients)
- Nausea
- Vomiting

Several assessment tools and scales can help identify a possible concussion:

- The Acute Concussion Evaluation (ACE) tool from the CDC
- The Sport Concussion Assessment Tool (SCAT), for patients 13 years and older
- The child SCAT for patients 12 and younger

Although such assessment tools historically have not been used in EMS, the information they provide can help you evaluate the patient. They also produce excellent standardized baseline information for the receiving physician. Many of these tools are available as software applications, making them quick and easy to use in the field.

The emergency treatment of a patient with an isolated concussion is primarily supportive and consists of patient education, monitoring, and transport to an appropriate facility for further evaluation. The main treatment for concussion is physical and mental rest, because any type of activity, even watching television or reading a book, can increase symptoms and delay the patient's recovery.

The patient, or the parent of a minor whom you suspect of having a concussion, might refuse treatment or transport. As with all refusals, you must obtain an informed refusal, which requires that you explain the benefits of treatment and transport and the risks of refusing. In addition to the standard refusal risks, you must give the patient with a suspected concussion specific information recommended by the CDC. Your system may also require you to consult with medical control in these situations. Patients should be instructed to do the following:

- Call 9-1-1 or go to the ED if they experience any of the signs and symptoms of a concussion.
- Avoid driving, because reaction time, attention, and processing speed may be affected.
- Get adequate sleep at night and avoid fatigue by taking breaks and naps as needed.

- Limit activities that require a lot of thinking or concentration until the patient is free of symptoms.
- Avoid demanding physical activity.
- Avoid a return to athletic activity until the patient has been evaluated by a health care provider and has completed the CDC's recommended five-step program for returning to play (see Figure 34-29). This program does not begin until the patient has been symptom-free for a minimum of 24 hours.

Second Impact Syndrome

When you assess the patient, ask about recent concussions. Ask the patient in particular whether he or she was still experiencing signs and symptoms from the previous concussion at the time of the current incident.

The exact definition and incidence of *second impact syndrome* are controversial, but it is understood to be a rare but often fatal result of receiving a second concussion while still recovering from an earlier concussion.[41,42] Although the exact cause of second impact syndrome is also controversial, it is thought that the brain is vulnerable and autoregulation is disrupted during recovery; therefore even minimal force can result in increased cerebral blood flow, brain herniation, and death.[43,44]

Death can occur as quickly as 2 to 5 minutes after the injury, and children and young adults are the most likely to develop this condition.[41,43] Prompt recognition is crucial. Unfortunately, the MOI may be easily missed. The brain can strike the skull even if the patient does not sustain a blow to the head, as may happen when the head changes direction quickly. This kind of injury can occur, for example, in a MVC or while playing a sport. In most cases, the patient initially appears stunned and may be ambulatory for up to a minute after the injury before suddenly collapsing.[41] Signs and symptoms of second impact syndrome may include the following:

- Sudden loss of consciousness after suffering a blow to the head
- A stunned appearance
- Loss of eye movements
- Dilated pupils (mydriasis)
- Coma
- Respiratory failure
- Cardiac arrest

The emergency treatment of second impact syndrome is supportive. It consists primarily of cardiorespiratory support, assessment and treatment of increased ICP, and perhaps treatment for cardiac arrest. Because of its rapid onset and high rate of mortality, a second concussion that occurs within 7 to 10 days of a previous concussion necessitates immediate transport to the closest facility with neurosurgic capability.

Postconcussion Syndrome

Postconcussion syndrome is another condition you may encounter in the patient with a history of a concussion. In this case, the patient may experience signs and symptoms for 3 to 6 months after the initial concussion. This condition differs from second impact syndrome in that it results from the original concussion, not a second impact. While it does not carry the mortality rate of second impact syndrome, postconcussion syndrome requires that the patient be transported for evaluation by a physician. Postconcussion syndrome should be suspected when the patient has at least three of the following signs and symptoms for at least 3 months after a concussion:

- Headache
- Dizziness
- Fatigue
- Irritability
- Insomnia
- Difficulty concentrating
- Memory difficulty
- Intolerance of stress or emotion

Diffuse Axonal Injury

Diffuse axonal injury (DAI) is one of the most common diffuse brain injuries. It accounts for about 70% of all TBI cases.[45] This injury has a high mortality rate and is one of the leading causes of death from brain injury in patients age 15 to 40 years.[45,46] Survivors have significant morbidity and often experience a rapid onset of coma. It is the most common cause of posttraumatic unconsciousness and the most common cause of a persistent vegetative state after a TBI.[47] DAI is caused by stretching, shearing, or tearing of nerve fibers, with consequent axonal damage.[48] An **axon** is a long, slender extension of a neuron (nerve cell) that conducts electrical impulses away from the **neuronal soma** (cell body) in the brain.

Rotational and angular forces secondary to rapid acceleration and deceleration of the brain, even without impact, lead to shearing of the axons and tensile strain forces on the axons. These forces produce axonal swelling and an interruption of axonal impulses. The white matter is especially vulnerable, but this injury also commonly occurs at the white-gray matter junction because these two tissues differ in their tensile strength.[45,47]

Axonal degeneration can continue for years after the injury, leading to a progressive neurodegeneration. This injury can result from a single incident or from multiple incidents, such as those found in professional boxers or American football players.[48]

DAI most often results from high-speed, rapid acceleration-deceleration forces, such as those produced in MVCs and significant falls. The severity and, thus, the prognosis of DAI depend on the degree of axonal damage (ie, stretching versus shearing or tearing). DAI is classified as being mild, moderate, or severe Table 34-8.

Assessment and Management. The primary findings in DAIs are related to the patient's level of consciousness, with the primary finding being unresponsiveness, often lasting more than 6 hours. As such, treatment is primarily supportive. Be especially wary of airway compromise in the unconscious patient. Perform a primary survey and address any life threats found. If time and resources allow, perform a secondary assessment and treat any injuries appropriately. Patients suspected of having a DAI should be transported to the closest appropriate facility, ideally one with in-house neurologists.

Pathophysiology, Assessment, and Management of Focal Brain Injuries

A **focal brain injury** is a specific, grossly observable brain injury (ie, it can be seen on a computed tomography [CT] scan). Such injuries include cerebral contusions and intracranial hemorrhage.

▶ Cerebral Contusion

In a **cerebral contusion**, brain tissue is bruised and damaged in a local area. Because cerebral contusion is associated with physical damage to the brain, greater neurologic deficits (eg, prolonged confusion, loss of consciousness) are observed with cerebral contusion than with concussion. The same MOIs that cause concussion—acceleration-deceleration forces and direct blunt head trauma—also cause cerebral contusion.

The area of the brain affected most often by cerebral contusion is the frontal lobe. Multiple areas can be damaged by contusion, especially in coup-contrecoup injuries. As with any bruise, the injured tissue reacts by swelling. This swelling inevitably leads to increased ICP and its accompanying negative consequences.

Words of Wisdom

In the prehospital setting, it is generally not possible or necessary to distinguish between cerebral contusion and intracranial hemorrhage. Instead, you should recognize the signs of increasing ICP and appreciate that those signs represent a critically injured patient who needs immediate treatment and prompt transport to an appropriate facility.

▶ Intracranial Hemorrhage

The closed box of the skull has no extra room for accumulation of blood, so bleeding inside the skull also increases ICP. Bleeding can occur between the skull and the dura mater, beneath the dura mater but outside the brain, within the parenchyma (tissue) of the brain itself (intracerebral space), or into the CSF (subarachnoid space).

An **epidural hematoma** is an accumulation of blood between the skull and dura mater; it occurs in about 0.5% to 1% of all head injuries Figure 34-30. An epidural

Table 34-8	**Diffuse Axonal Injury**			
Type of DAI	**Pathophysiology**	**Incidence**	**Signs and Symptoms**	**Prognosis**
Mild DAI	Temporary neuronal dysfunction; minimal axonal damage	Most common result of blunt head trauma; concussion is an example	Loss of consciousness (brief, if present); confusion, disorientation, amnesia (retrograde and/or anterograde)	Minimal or no permanent neurologic impairment
Moderate DAI	Axonal damage and minute petechial bruising of brain tissue; often associated with a basilar skull fracture	20% of all severe head injuries; 45% of all diffuse axonal injuries	Immediate loss of consciousness: secondary to involvement of the cerebral cortex or the reticular activating system of the brainstem. Residual effects: persistent confusion and disorientation; cognitive impairment (eg, inability to concentrate); frequent periods of anxiety; uncharacteristic mood swings; sensory/motor deficits (such as altered sense of taste or smell)	Survival likely, but permanent neurologic impairment common
Severe DAI	Severe mechanical disruption of many axons in both cerebral hemispheres with extension into the brainstem; formerly called "brainstem injury"	16% of all severe head injuries; 36% of all diffuse axonal injuries	Immediate and prolonged loss of consciousness; posturing and other signs of increased ICP	Survival unlikely; most patients who survive never regain consciousness but remain in a persistent vegetative state

Abbreviations: DAI, diffuse axonal injury; ICP, intracranial pressure

© Jones & Bartlett Learning.

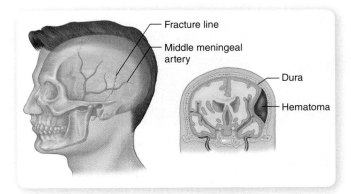

Figure 34-30 An epidural hematoma is usually the result of a blow to the head that produces a linear fracture of the temporal bone and damages the middle meningeal artery. Blood accumulates between the dura mater and the skull.

© Jones & Bartlett Learning.

hematoma is nearly always the result of a blow to the head (eg, low-force impacts such as a fist or a beer bottle) that produces a linear fracture of the thin temporal bone. The middle meningeal artery courses along a groove in that bone, so it is prone to disruption when the temporal bone is fractured.[49] In such a case, brisk arterial bleeding into the epidural space will result in rapidly progressing symptoms.

Signs and symptoms of an epidural hematoma can be deceptive. The classic presentation is a patient who loses consciousness immediately after the injury occurs. The patient then regains consciousness and is coherent during a brief period known as the "lucid interval." Because of the increased ICP resulting from the hemorrhage, the patient ultimately lapses back into unconsciousness.[50] The lucid interval can last from minutes to 24 hours and is generally associated with a headache or other signs that are similar to those associated with a concussion. Remember the lucid interval occurs in only 20% to 30% of epidural hematomas.[51] In the remaining 70% to 80% of cases, the patient exhibits one of the following two behaviors:

- Remains conscious initially and does not lose consciousness until the ICP increases (again, this could be minutes to 24 hours)
- Loses consciousness initially, and the ICP increases before the patient regains consciousness

Thus, you cannot rely solely on the presence or absence of a lucid interval to suspect an epidural hematoma in the setting of a temporal blow and other signs and symptoms.

The greatest risk is a patient who refuses care during the lucid interval or did not lose consciousness immediately after the blow to the head. The following case is a classic example of this risk; a patient suffered a seemingly minor blow to the head while skiing, did not lose consciousness, and despite the efforts of the ski patrol, refused care. She returned to her hotel room, where she lost consciousness an hour later and eventually died from an epidural hematoma.[52]

If you encounter a patient you suspect has an epidural hematoma who refuses transport, then you must inform the patient of that risk. As part of your informed refusal, and in an attempt to change the patient's mind, you will likely have to explain the pathophysiology of epidural hematoma and the fact that the patient can be experiencing such bleeding and still have no symptoms.

With early treatment and surgery, this injury has a high survivability. If the patient loses consciousness because of increased ICP, however, the likelihood of mortality increases significantly.[53]

In the conscious patient, the signs and symptoms of an epidural hematoma typically are limited to those of an associated concussion and any soft-tissue damage or crepitus to the area of impact. As ICP increases, the patient may exhibit signs and symptoms such as ipsilateral pupil dilation, contralateral motor dysfunction, nausea and vomiting, seizures, urinary incontinence, visual disturbances, posturing, and Cushing triad (late).[53]

A **subdural hematoma** is an accumulation of blood beneath the dura mater but outside the brain **Figure 34-31** that usually occurs after falls or injuries involving strong deceleration forces. Although the exact incidence varies among studies, subdural hemorrhages are the most

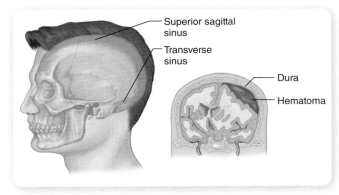

Figure 34-31 In a subdural hematoma, venous bleeding occurs beneath the dura mater but outside the brain.
© Jones & Bartlett Learning.

YOU are the Paramedic PART 3

Within minutes, the engine company arrives for additional assistance. While you manage the airway, the engine crew places a cervical collar and places the patient on the backboard, and your partner completes a rapid head-to-toe exam. He tells you the patient has no apparent movement or sensation of his extremities, and he has lost control of his bowel and bladder.

Recording Time: 5 Minutes	
Respirations	Shallow and labored, assisting with bag-mask ventilation
Pulse	50 beats/min
Skin	Wet and flushed
Blood pressure	80/54 mm Hg
Oxygen saturation (Spo$_2$)	86%
Pupils	PERRLA, but sluggish

5. Why is the patient bradycardic and hypotensive?
6. How would you manage these vital signs?

common intracranial hemorrhage and may or may not be associated with a skull fracture. Bleeding within the subdural space typically results from rupture of the veins that bridge the cerebral cortex and dura.

A subdural hematoma is associated with venous bleeding, so this type of hematoma and the associated signs of increased ICP typically develop more gradually than is seen with an epidural hematoma. The patient with a subdural hematoma often experiences a fluctuating level of consciousness, focal neurologic signs (such as unilateral hemiparesis), or slurred speech.

Subdural hematomas are classified as acute (clinical signs developing within 48 hours after injury), subacute (signs developing between 2 and 14 days after the injury), or chronic (symptoms appearing 14 days to several months after the injury). Acute subdural hematomas have a mortality rate of up to 90% and often are associated with diffuse injuries such as DAIs.[54] The signs and symptoms are directly related to the ICP and the severity of the associated diffuse injury. These patients are often unresponsive when you arrive on scene or may lose consciousness soon after your arrival.

Your role with this patient is primarily recognizing and treating life threats found during the primary survey. Studies have shown a decreased mortality rate when patients are rapidly identified and quickly transported to a facility with immediate neurosurgic capability.[55]

Subacute subdural hematomas have a much lower mortality rate than either acute or chronic subdural hematomas have. The medical community believes that this lower mortality is due to a lower extent of injury to the brain than in an acute subdural injury, and less brain tissue involved than in a chronic subdural injury that has become symptomatic. These types of subdural hematomas appear to be rare, but research is limited, as most studies focus on acute and chronic subdural hematomas.[56]

Patients who have a history of brain atrophy, such as older adults or alcoholics, have a high risk of chronic subdural hematomas. This risk is especially pronounced if the patient takes anticoagulants.[57,58] During the next 14 years, as the population ages, the incidence of chronic subdural hematomas is expected to increase dramatically.[59] This increase is significant because this condition has a mortality rate of 26% at 6 months and 32% one year after it develops.[60]

The risks associated with chronic subdural hematoma are of particular concern because these injuries may be difficult to identify. Patients may have experienced minor trauma weeks to months earlier that they did not consider serious and did not have examined. When you interview the patient or family, do not simply ask about "recent head trauma" because this wording allows them to define *recent*. Instead, ask about any head trauma, no matter how insignificant it may seem, within the past 6 months.

A subacute or chronic subdural hematoma should be considered in any patient with a past history of head trauma associated with a headache, dysphasia, hemiparesis, personality changes, visual disturbances, difficulty

Words of Wisdom

Chronic subdural hematomas are more common among older adults and alcoholics. Because the patient usually presents with an altered mental status, obtaining a good history and performing a thorough assessment are important. You may find that the patient sustained a head injury days, weeks, or months before the present call for EMS assistance.

concentrating, nausea and vomiting, a unilateral dilated pupil, posturing, new-onset seizures, and vital sign changes consistent with Cushing triad.

An **intracerebral hematoma** is bleeding within the brain tissue itself **Figure 34-32** . This type of injury can result from a penetrating injury to the head or from rapid deceleration forces.

Many small, deep intracerebral hemorrhages are associated with other brain injuries, such as DAI. The progression of increased ICP and neurologic deficit depends on several factors. The presence of other brain injuries, the brain region affected (frontal and temporal lobes are the most common), and the size of the hemorrhage, for example, are all important variables. Once symptoms appear, the patient's condition often deteriorates quickly. Intracerebral hematomas are associated with a high mortality rate even if the hematoma is surgically evacuated.

In a **subarachnoid hemorrhage**, bleeding occurs into the subarachnoid space, where the CSF circulates. It results in bloody CSF and signs of meningeal irritation (eg, nuchal rigidity, headache). Common causes of a subarachnoid hemorrhage include trauma or rupture of an aneurysm or arteriovenous malformation.

Many, but not all, patients with a subarachnoid hemorrhage typically present with a sudden, severe headache.[61] This headache is often localized initially but later becomes diffuse secondary to increased meningeal irritation. As bleeding into the subarachnoid space increases, the patient experiences the signs and symptoms of increased

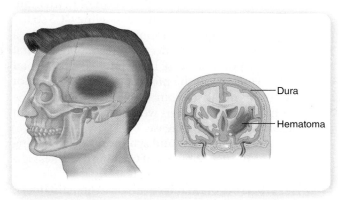

Figure 34-32 An intracerebral hematoma is bleeding within the brain tissue itself.

© Jones & Bartlett Learning.

ICP: decreased level of consciousness, pupillary changes, posturing, vomiting, and seizures. A sudden, severe subarachnoid hemorrhage usually results in death.[62] About 15% of patients die before they reach a medical facility, 40% die within a week, and 50% die within 6 months. People who survive often have permanent neurologic impairment, as rebleeding is common: 15% of survivors experience rebleeding on the first day after the injury, and 40% of survivors experience rebleeding within the first 4 weeks after the injury.[62]

Finally, bleeding between the periosteum of the skull and the galea aponeurosis is called a **subgaleal hemorrhage**. It can occur in conjunction with injuries to the skull and scalp. It is difficult to identify because a large amount of blood may be spread out over the entire surface of the skull. In the newborn and infant population, it can produce enough blood loss to precipitate hypovolemia. In this age group, the accumulation of blood may make the fontanelles and suture lines of the skull difficult or impossible to identify. It is often described as a boggy mass that is moveable and compressible on palpation.

In contrast, a **supragaleal hematoma** often is defined as a firmer, nodular mass, with the idiom "goose egg" occasionally used to describe it.

General Management of Head Trauma

Prehospital assessment and management of a patient with head trauma should be guided by factors such as the severity of the injury and the patient's level of consciousness. As with any patient, your treatment priorities must be based on the conditions that will kill the patient *first*.

A patient with brain injury may have an abnormal rate and pattern of breathing. First, determine whether the patient has an abnormal breathing pattern and note whether it changes while the patient is in your care. Determine a GCS score as early as possible and reassess it often. This baseline will help you detect changes in the patient's condition. Recall from earlier in the chapter that a decrease in the GCS by 2 or more points in a patient with an initial GCS of less than 9 is a sign of herniation.

You must determine an accurate baseline GCS so the patient's progression can be monitored. For example, a patient may have a 1-point decrease in the prehospital setting and a 1-point decrease later in the ED, for a total of 2 points. However, if the prehospital change was not noted and the initial score in the ED was used as the baseline, health care providers would assume the patient had had only a 1-point decrease.

Watch closely for signs and symptoms of increasing ICP, including the development of Cushing triad. Reassess the patient for signs of increasing ICP.

When you care for a patient with head or brain injury, the patient's time on the scene generally should not exceed 10 minutes. The patient requires definitive care at a medical facility staffed and equipped to handle this type

of injury. Continue manual stabilization of the cervical spine until the patient has been completely secured to a backboard if indicated.

Maintain an open airway and ensure the patient's breathing is adequate. Administer oxygen and provide suction as necessary. Refer to the discussions earlier in this chapter about the importance of avoiding hypoxia, hypocapnia, and hypercapnia in the patient with a TBI, as well as strategies for airway management and ventilatory support. Recall, oxygen saturation must never be allowed to drop below 90%, and the ETCO$_2$ should be maintained between 35 and 40 mm Hg unless signs of herniation are present, in which case it should be maintained between 30 and 35 mm Hg. Never allow the ETCO$_2$ to drop below 25 mm Hg as this is associated with increased mortality.

When you are en route, establish vascular access by starting an IV of normal saline or lactated Ringer solution, and infuse the fluid at a rate that will prevent hypotension (systolic blood pressure less than 90 mm Hg) and preserve CPP. Assess the patient's serum glucose level, and administer glucose or glucagon if it is indicated. If the patient is hypotensive (systolic blood pressure less than 90 mm Hg), then look for internal bleeding, because an isolated TBI will almost never present with hypotension. Elevate the head of the stretcher or backboard about a 15° to 30° angle if possible to facilitate the drainage of CSF and venous blood from the cranial vault. Treat seizures if present. Combativeness, agitation, and struggling against immobilization will increase ICP and may worsen existing injuries. Consider sedation or chemical restraint in such situations. Always weigh the risks and benefits of these procedures before performing them.

▶ Thermal Management

Do not allow the patient to become overheated. Patients with a head injury, unlike those with shock, can develop a high body temperature (**hyperpyrexia**), which in turn may worsen the condition of the brain. Do not cover the patient with blankets if the ambient temperature is 70°F (21°C) or higher.

Controversies

There has been some thought that localized hypothermia may benefit patients with acute head injuries because hypothermia increases ICP. However, multiple studies and trials of patients with head injuries have shown that hypothermic therapy did not improve outcomes and that rewarming patients can create additional complications.[63]

▶ Pharmacologic Therapy

Pharmacologic therapy, other than that used to facilitate intubation or treat seizures, is usually not indicated in the prehospital setting for patients with brain injury.

If transport will be prolonged, however, medical control may order the administration of certain medications, such as mannitol (Osmitrol) and/or furosemide (Lasix) to reduce cerebral edema and decrease ICP.[15]

Seizures in a patient with brain injury must be stopped as soon as possible because they provoke further increases in ICP or body temperature. Benzodiazepines, such as diazepam (Valium) or lorazepam (Ativan), should be used to control seizure activity in patients with brain injury.[15] Follow local protocol or contact medical control regarding the doses of these drugs.

When you arrive at the medical facility, neuroprotective agents can be administered to a patient with brain injury. These agents currently are not administered in the prehospital setting, but that could change.

Pathophysiology, Assessment, and Management of Spinal Injuries

Spinal cord injury (SCI) is one of the most devastating injuries that prehospital providers encounter. Unfortunately, treatment options for SCIs are currently limited, with therapy relying heavily on rehabilitation over acute intervention. Preventive measures aimed at reducing the incidence of primary and secondary SCIs are the health care provider's best option for reducing the morbidity and mortality of SCI.

For example, campaigns involving local media, law enforcement, and EMS to encourage and develop habitual use of seat belts by all passengers in an automobile reduce the likelihood of injury during an MVC, especially a rollover incident. Awareness and education about the safe and appropriate use of firearms, anger management education and intervention, and positive conflict resolution programs have the potential to affect rates of SCI that results from violence. Safety education programs for coaches and parents involved in sports and campaigns that encourage the use of adequate protective equipment are attempts to prevent spinal injury on the playing field. As a paramedic, you may very well play a role in these activities.

According to 2016 data from the National Spinal Cord Injury Statistical Center (NSCISC), in the United States an estimated 17,000 new cases of SCI occur each year, which does not include patients who die at the scene of an accident. Cervical spine injuries account for 2% to 3% of trauma admissions to hospitals. Of SCIs, 29% occur in the cervical spine, 24% in the thoracic spine, 37% in the lumbar spine, and 10% in the sacral spine.[64–66]

The NSCISC data show that the current cases of SCI in the United States are 243,000 to 347,000 people.[67] The average age at the time of injury has increased from 29 years during the 1970s to 42 years in 2016. The center's database classifies causes of injury into six major categories: MVCs (38%); falls, especially among older adults (30.5%); acts of violence (13.5%); sports-related activities (9%); medical and surgical causes (5%); and other causes (4%).

Mortality rates for patients with SCIs are highest in the first year after the injury. The leading causes of deaths for SCI patients discharged from a medical facility are pneumonia, pulmonary embolism, and septicemia. About 18% of these injuries result in quadriplegia—paralysis of all four extremities—requiring complete care of the patient for the remainder of his or her life.[68]

Words of Wisdom

Patients with SCI face dramatic changes in lifestyle. A simple walk in the park, a trip to the shopping mall, or a commute to work becomes much more difficult. Care for the patient with SCI also brings significant financial costs.

▶ Mechanism of Injury of Spinal Injury

Any sudden force or change in direction or speed can cause the head and body to move in opposite directions or force the torso to twist, flex, or extend in a way that may cause spinal fracture or SCI. Blunt or penetrating trauma directly to the spinal column can cause vertebral fracture, SCI, or both. When assessing the MOI, you must determine whether force was sufficient to cause injury to the spinal column or cord. Earlier in the chapter, we discussed common mechanisms suggesting that acute SCI should be suspected. Anytime you suspect spinal injury, you should assess whether spinal immobilization is necessary.

Acute spinal injuries are classified according to the associated mechanism, location, and stability of the injury. Vertebral fractures can occur with or without associated SCI. Stable fractures pose less threat to the spinal cord. Unstable injuries involve multiple areas of the spine and are often associated with damage to portions of the vertebrae and ligaments that directly protect the spinal cord and nerve roots. Without appropriate treatment, unstable injuries carry a higher risk of complicating SCI and progression of injury.

When determining whether the patient's MOI is significant enough to cause a spinal injury, consider medical history. Many medical conditions can significantly increase the potential for spinal column and cord injury. You should also consider the patient's age. A newborn or neonate has not developed the muscle tone to control head movement during an incident, has an underdeveloped spinal column and a disproportionately large head, and is unable to communicate pain level.

An older adult may have osteoporosis or osteoarthritis, making him or her more vulnerable to vertebral fracture during a fall. A patient with decreased bone density is also at a higher risk of spinal column injury with or without associated SCI. A variety of factors are associated with decreased bone density:

- Alcohol abuse
- Asian or Caucasian race
- Cigarette smoking
- Diabetes, liver disease, kidney disease
- Family history of osteoporosis
- History of fractures
- Inactive lifestyle
- Use of steroids, barbiturates, anticonvulsants, or thyroid replacement hormones

Most SCIs occur in the area of the cervical spine, with the next most common area being the lumbar region. This is logical considering the anatomy of the human body. The cervical vertebrae support the bowling ball–like head, are the smallest vertebrae, and have no additional protection. The lumbar region, although it includes the largest vertebrae, has no additional support or protection. The thoracic region, which has the fewest injuries, has additional support from the ribs.

Flexion Injuries

Flexion injuries result from forward movement of the head, typically as the result of rapid deceleration (eg, in a MVC) or from a direct blow to the occiput **Figure 34-33** . At the level of C1 to C2, these forces can produce an unstable dislocation with or without an associated fracture. A dislocation can be complete or partial; when partial, it is termed a **subluxation**.

Farther down the spinal column, flexion forces are transmitted anteriorly through the vertebral bodies and can result in an anterior wedge fracture. Depending on

their severity, anterior wedge fractures can be stable or unstable. Loss of more than half the original size of the vertebral body or multiple levels of injury suggest relatively increased instability.

Hyperflexion injuries of greater force can produce teardrop fractures—avulsion fractures of the anterior-inferior border of the vertebral body. The injuries to ligaments associated with teardrop fractures raise concern for possible SCI and qualify teardrop fractures as unstable fractures. Severe flexion can also result in a potentially unstable dislocation of vertebral joints. This condition does not include fracture but can severely injure the ligaments. Strong forces can result in the anterior displacement of **facet joints**. A bilateral facet dislocation is an extremely unstable injury.

Patients can also experience lateral bending, which is similar to a flexion-extension injury. In flexion-extension, the patient's head moves from front to back and is overstretched on one side while being overcompressed on the opposite side. With lateral bending, the patient experiences the same type of injury, but from left to right rather than from front to back.

Rotation With Flexion

The only area of the spine that allows for significant rotation is C1 to C2. Injuries to this area are considered unstable because of the high cervical location and scant bony and soft-tissue support. **Rotation-flexion injuries** often result from high acceleration forces. Rotation with abrupt flexion can produce a stable dislocation in the cervical spine **Figure 34-34** . In the thoracolumbar spine, rotation-flexion forces typically cause fracture rather than dislocation.

Vertical Compression

Vertical compression forces, also called axial loading, are transmitted through vertebral bodies and directed either

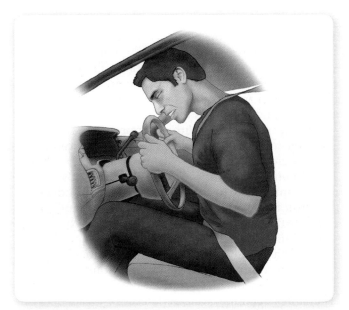

Figure 34-33 A flexion injury.
© Jones & Bartlett Learning.

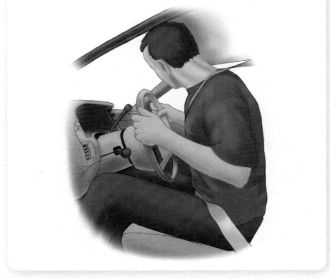

Figure 34-34 A rotation with flexion injury.
© Jones & Bartlett Learning.

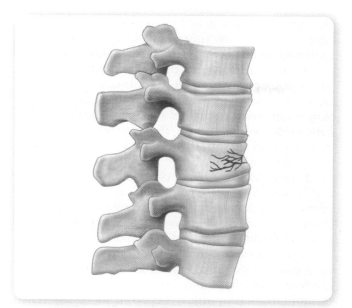

Figure 34-35 A compression fracture.
© Jones & Bartlett Learning.

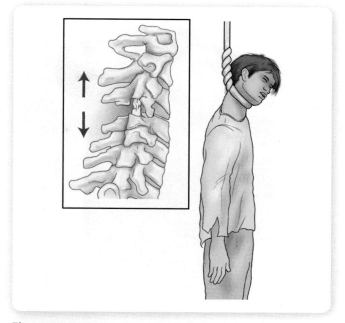

Figure 34-36 Distraction spinal injury.
© Jones & Bartlett Learning.

inferiorly through the skull or superiorly through the pelvis or feet. They typically result from a direct blow to the crown (parietal region) of the skull, commonly affecting the cervical spine, or from rapid deceleration from a fall transmitting impact through the feet, legs, and pelvis, commonly affecting T12 to L2.

These injuries also can occur if the patient falls headfirst, such as in a diving injury, when the head suddenly stops and the weight of the body keeps moving, compressing the cervical spine. Forces transmitted through the vertebral body cause fractures, ultimately shattering and producing a "burst" or compression fracture without associated SCI **Figure 34-35** . Compression forces can cause the herniation of disks, subsequent compression on the spinal cord and nerve roots, and fragmentation into the canal.

Although most fractures resulting from these injuries are stable, primary SCI can result when the vertebral body is shattered and fragments of bone become embedded in the cord. Some compression injuries may be associated with significant retropharyngeal edema, and serious airway compromise is a possibility.

Distraction

Distraction forces are the opposite of compression (axial) forces. Distraction results when parts of the body are pulled in opposite directions **Figure 34-36** . Consider someone who has been hanged. The individual is moving and is jerked to a stop at one point while gravity pulls the rest of the body away from the fixed end. The result is stretching and separation of the spinal column, its ligaments, and its supporting muscles; and tearing of the spinal cord. Although the type of distraction force determines the MOI, the cervical region is most vulnerable to distraction forces because it has the least support and protection.

> ### Words of Wisdom
>
> A distrac*ting* injury is not the same as a distrac*tion* injury. A distrac*ting* injury is an injury to another body part or system (such as a femur fracture) that causes such significant pain and discomfort that it sufficiently distracts the patient's attention, rendering him or her unreliable. In such a case, the patient is unable to report whether there are any signs or symptoms of an occult spinal column injury. Such injury could cause secondary neurologic deficit if not stabilized.
>
> A distrac*tion* injury is one in which there is a physical distraction mechanism that causes separation of spinal column elements and potential SCI. It is very important to clearly recognize the difference between these two terms in evaluating patients with possible spinal column or cord injuries and when determining patients who may be safely managed without spinal immobilization.

The most classic distraction injury is a **hangman's fracture**, which, as its name implies, occurs during a hanging. In addition to distraction forces caused as the rope pulls tight, the rope causes a severe lateral force, snapping the head sideways as the spine stretches. The lateral force causes bending and fractures at the C1 to C2 region, which quickly tears the spinal cord.

Rarely do distraction or compression mechanisms occur alone. Mixed mechanisms with some sort of rotational, flexion, or extension forces usually occur together. Carefully examine the incident and identify the forces that may have been involved. This information will enable

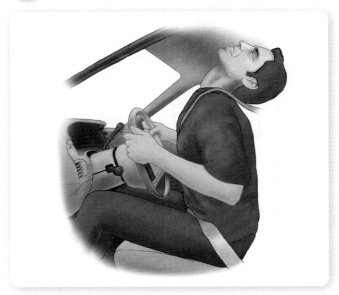

Figure 34-37 A hyperextension injury.
© Jones & Bartlett Learning.

you to better understand the type of injuries the patient may have sustained.

Hyperextension

Hyperextension of the head and neck can produce fractures and ligamentous injury with variable stability Figure 34-37 . Hyperextension injuries can be caused by situations such as a rear-end MVCs in which the body is suddenly pushed out from under the stationary head. This sudden backwards movement of the head can create avulsion fractures of the anterior arch of C1, a vertical fracture through the posterior arch of C1, or fractures of C2.

Hyperextension creates a teardrop fracture of the anterior-inferior edge of the vertebral body, resulting in rupture or tear of the anterior longitudinal ligament. The injury is stable with the head and neck in flexion, but unstable in extension because of loss of structural support.

▶ Categories of Spinal Cord Injuries

Primary Spinal Cord Injury

Primary spinal cord injury is injury that occurs at the moment of impact. Penetrating trauma typically produces transection of neural elements that are incapable of regeneration. These injuries are complete. (The terms *complete* and *incomplete* are discussed in the following section, *Effects of Spinal Cord Injuries*.)

Blunt trauma may displace ligaments and bone fragments, producing compression of portions of the spinal cord or an incomplete dislocation of the vertebral body.

Hypoperfusion and ischemia also may result from this type of injury to the spinal vasculature. Necrosis from prolonged ischemia leads to permanent loss of function.

Spinal cord concussion is characterized by a dysfunction that lasts from 24 to 48 hours, is considered an incomplete injury, and may present in patients with simple compression fractures and in those without radiologic evidence of a fracture. The temporary dysfunction may be due to a short-duration shock or a pressure wave within the cord.

Fracture, dislocation, or direct trauma causes spinal cord contusions. These contusions are associated with edema, tissue damage, and vascular leakage. Hemorrhagic disruption may cause temporary to permanent loss of function despite normal radiographs.

A cord laceration usually results from a projectile or bone entering the spinal canal. Such an injury is likely to produce hemorrhage into the cord tissue, swelling, and disruption of some portion of the cord and its associated communication pathways.

Secondary Spinal Cord Injury

Secondary spinal cord injury results from multiple factors creating a progression of the primary SCI. The ensuing cascade of inflammatory responses may produce further deterioration. Bleeding, swelling, and ischemia can impair the function of the spinal cord.

If a blood vessel is affected or damaged, the swelling may increase, leading to further ischemia and further cord dysfunction. Exposing neural elements to further hypoxemia, hypoglycemia, and hypothermia can exacerbate these effects. Although some SCI may be unavoidable, you should minimize further injury through stabilization, including manual stabilization, neutral alignment, and spinal immobilization. In addition, you must minimize heat loss and maintain oxygenation and perfusion in the care of a patient with a possible SCI.

Effects of Spinal Cord Injuries

Spinal cord compression can result from outside pressure on the spinal cord, or internal pressure exerted on the cord as it swells within the rigid spinal column. Primary cord compression can appear with a crushed vertebra or intervertebral disk. Secondary cord compression occurs when soft tissues around the cord swell after an injury and compress the cord within the spinal column. Both mechanisms can cause ischemia in the compressed portion of the cord. If not corrected, this ischemia can lead to permanent damage.

Regardless of the MOI, all SCIs are classified as complete or incomplete, depending on the degree of damage. **Complete spinal cord injury** means complete disruption of all tracts of the spinal cord, with permanent loss of all cord-mediated functions below the level of injury. The patient will have no sensation, pain, or movement below the site of injury.

When the injury occurs high in the cervical spine, quadriplegia results. A similar injury in the high thoracic area would result in paraplegia.

In an **incomplete spinal cord injury**, the patient retains some degree of cord-mediated function. Recall that various ascending and descending tracts make up the spinal cord. In an incomplete SCI, only some tracts are injured at a specific location, while the rest of the tracts function normally. As a result, the patient loses some cord functions while retaining others. The degree of SCI often cannot be determined for several days after the initial injury; the initial dysfunction may be temporary, and the patient has some potential for recovery.

Anterior cord syndrome results from the displacement of bony fragments into the anterior portion of the spinal cord, often caused by flexion injuries or fractures. The anterior spinal artery provides blood to the anterior two-thirds of the spinal cord. Disruption of this flow will present as an anterior cord syndrome. Physical findings include paralysis below the level of the insult, with loss of sensation to pain and temperature. However, the sense of touch, ability to sense vibrations, and proprioception (the ability to perceive the position and movement of one's body) continue to function normally.[69]

Central cord syndrome, the most common incomplete SCI, accounts for 70% of all incomplete injuries and makes up 20% of all acute SCIs.[70] The most common mechanism is hyperextension injuries to the cervical area causing hemorrhage or edema to the dorsal column of the spinal cord.[70]

This type of damage is rarely associated with fractures or bone disruption but more often accompanies tears to the anterior longitudinal ligament. Central cord syndrome often is seen in older adult patients, who may already have a significant degree of cervical spondylosis and stenosis caused by arthritic changes.[70]

A brief episode of hyperextension can exert pressure on the spinal cord within the relatively constricted spinal canal.[71] Within the central cord, motor (efferent) fibers are uniquely distributed, with more cervical and thoracic motor and sensory tracts than in the periphery of the cord. The patient with central cord syndrome will present with greater loss of function in the upper extremities than in the lower extremities, with variable loss of sensation to pain and temperature. The patient also may have some bowel and bladder dysfunction.[68] The prognosis for central cord syndrome is typically good; many patients regain all motor function or have only some residual weakness in the hands.

Posterior cord syndrome often accompanies extension injuries. This relatively rare syndrome produces dysfunction of the dorsal columns, presenting as decreased sensation to light touch, reduced proprioception, and reduced vibration perception. Most other motor and sensory functions are unaffected. Patients with posterior cord syndrome are less likely to recover function than are patients with central cord syndrome. With therapy and rehabilitation, however, their prognosis is good.

Cauda equina syndrome is defined as a compression of the bundle of nerve roots that resemble a horse's tail, or *cauda equina* in Latin, located at the end of the spinal cord. This region is in the lower back, inferior to the spinal cord, which terminates at L1 as the conus medullaris. Causes of cauda equina syndrome include trauma, swelling after impact, penetrating objects, bone fragments, and an expanding hematoma within the spinal column in the lumbar region. Nontraumatic causes of this syndrome include cord compression caused by a tumor, a herniated disk, infection, or a hematoma.

Cauda equina syndrome can produce the following symptoms:

- Severe low back pain
- Myalgia, paresthesia, or myasthenia in one or both legs
- Loss of sensation, or altered sensation that is severe or worsening, in the legs, buttocks, inner thighs, backs of the legs, or feet. Your patient may report trouble feeling anything in the areas of the body that would sit in a saddle (called saddle anesthesia).
- Acute bladder or bowel dysfunction, such as retention or incontinence, which indicates perineal anesthesia, is clinically diagnostic for cauda equina syndrome. In the trauma center setting, digital rectal tone is evaluated to determine innervation of the entire length of the spinal cord. The absence of rectal tone on this exam is suggestive of SCI or cauda equina syndrome.

Any patient presenting with back pain and bowel or bladder symptoms of any type requires urgent transport to an ED and consultation with a spine surgeon.

Brown-Séquard syndrome occurs typically after penetrating trauma and appears with functional hemisection of the cord and complete damage to all spinal tracts on the involved side. Nontraumatic causes include disk herniation, spinal cord tumors, and spinal epidural hematomas. Injury to the corticospinal motor tracts causes motor loss on the same side as the injury, but below the lesion. Damage to the dorsal column causes loss of motor function, sensation to light touch, proprioception, and vibration on the same side (ipsilateral) as the injury and below the injury. Disruption of the spinothalamic tracts causes loss of sensation to pain and temperature on the opposite side (contralateral) of injury, below the lesion.

Spinal shock is the temporary local neurologic condition that occurs immediately after spinal trauma. Swelling and edema of the cord begin within 30 minutes of the initial insult and can produce a physiologic transection, mechanically disrupting all nerve conduction distal to the injury. The patient may present with a variable degree of acute spinal injury, potentially with flaccid paralysis, flaccid sphincters, and absent reflexes. Sensory function below the level of injury will be impaired, as will thermoregulation and visceral sensation below the lesion, resulting in bowel distention from a loss of peristalsis. Spinal shock usually subsides in hours to weeks, depending on the severity of injury.[17]

Neurogenic shock results from the temporary loss of autonomic function, which controls cardiovascular function, at the level of injury. Marked hemodynamic and systemic effects appear: hypotension results from absent or impaired peripheral vascular tone with the loss of alpha receptor stimulation; blood pools in the enlarged vascular space, causing a relative hypovolemia and making the patient extremely sensitive to sudden position changes; and cardiac preload decreases, resulting in decreased stroke volume and cardiac output. Bradycardia results as well.

In neurogenic shock, the adrenal gland loses its sympathetic stimulation and does not produce epinephrine or norepinephrine. The loss of sympathetic stimulation can lead to hypothermia and an absence of sweating.

The classic case of neurogenic shock is a hypotensive, bradycardic patient whose skin is warm, flushed, and dry below the level of the spinal lesion. The patient also may have loss of bladder control, priapism, and/or paralytic ileus, which is paralysis of the small bowel.

In the case of paralysis of the small bowel, the patient will have hypoactive (slow) bowel sounds. If you note this finding, include it in your report to the receiving facility and in your documentation. Refer to the discussion of treatment of neurogenic shock earlier in this chapter.

Special Populations

General considerations for pediatric, geriatric, and bariatric patients are discussed in Chapter 43, *Pediatric Emergencies*, Chapter 44, *Geriatric Emergencies*, and Chapter 45, *Patients With Special Challenges*, respectively. For example, patients with obesity have special needs related to airway management and transport, and geriatric patients can experience devastating trauma injuries that would be relatively minor for an adult patient. In all three groups, determining the exact location of pain can be difficult: geriatric patients have decreased pain sensation, pediatric patients cannot necessarily verbalize the exact location of their pain, and bariatric patients may be more difficult to palpate in areas of greater tissue.

Special Populations

Spinal cord injury without radiographic abnormalities (SCIWORA) can occur in children because their vertebrae lie flatter on top of each other, which results in the facet joints being more horizontal; in adults, the vertebrae are more curved Figure 34-38 . The child's increased elasticity of the spinal ligaments, weakness of the neck muscles, and disproportionately increased weight of the head also increase the risk of SCIWORA.[72]

A child's vertebrae can easily dislocate and quickly return to their normal positions. The radiograph of a child who has experienced SCIWORA may show no evidence of fracture and show a perfectly aligned vertebral column, while the cord itself has been compressed or transected. You cannot diagnose SCIWORA in the prehospital setting. Sophisticated studies such as magnetic resonance imaging (MRI) may be required even in the hospital.

Patients with Down syndrome are more prone to SCIWORA because they are predisposed to atlantoaxial instability (AAI). The National Down Syndrome Society reports that 15% of people with Down syndrome have asymptomatic AAI, and 1% to 2% have symptomatic AAI.[73] AAI is excessive mobility of the articulation of the atlas (C1) and the axis (C2). This may lead to subluxation of the cervical spine. Radiographs are required for a diagnosis.

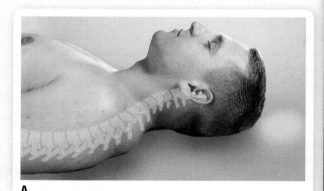

A

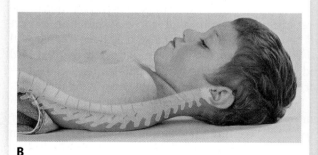

B

Figure 34-38 Comparison of an adult's **(A)** and a child's **(B)** vertebrae.

► The Evolution of Spinal Care

Spinal immobilization is a controversial topic in prehospital medicine. Immobilization has been one of the most common procedures used in EMS for decades because injury to the spinal cord, especially high-level injury, is life threatening and can devastate the patient and his or her quality of life.[74]

Because immobilization has been considered a harmless procedure, and because SCI is potentially devastating, preventive immobilization of all trauma patients became routine. This practice was reinforced in a 1989 paper that stated, "A high index of suspicion and increased vigilance for spinal stabilization prior to evacuation of a patient from a trauma scene is one factor that has contributed to the decline in the percentage of complete spinal cord injury lesions"; this paper recommended that no trauma patient be extricated or transported without spinal immobilization.[75]

As with all treatments, we must evaluate the indications, benefits, and risks of immobilization for each patient. The practice of selective immobilization was first implemented more than 20 years ago in an effort to reduce the number of patients immobilized unnecessarily. According to this concept, only patients with clinical indications of spinal injury are immobilized.

Debate continues regarding potential negative consequences of using cervical collars and backboards. Like any treatment intervention, the tools used in various aspects of patient care can be overused or misused. Therefore, it is imperative that all prehospital providers conduct proper assessments of the scene and the patient to determine what tools are necessary for proper patient care as defined by local protocol.

Studies

Multiple studies have shown that providers can use certain criteria to identify patients who do not need immobilization based on their clinical presentations.[24,25,76-82] Investigators have recently concluded that clinical criteria and the patient's presentation should be considered in the decision to immobilize a patient.

Ambulatory trauma patients have a low risk of spinal injury and an even lower risk of SCI; nevertheless, such patients must be assessed.[83,84] If you find indications of spinal injury, the patient may need some degree of immobilization based on your protocols.

Patients with penetrating trauma but no evidence of neurologic deficit do not require immobilization unless some other factor is present (eg, fell three stories out of a window after being shot). Studies have shown an increased mortality rate for immobilized patients with penetrating trauma compared with those who are not immobilized, potentially due to the increased time on scene necessary to complete the immobilization process. One study reported that the mortality rate of immobilized patients was double that of patients who were not immobilized. SCI is exceedingly rare in penetrating trauma, occurring in less than 1% of patients.[85] In cases in which SCI does occur, a large majority of patients have a complete SCI in which immobilization would have no benefit because the cord already has been damaged.[86]

Complications associated with immobilizing patients with penetrating trauma include the following:

- Immobilization takes time, often causing delays on scene.
- Immobilization takes multiple people, increasing the likelihood that other procedures may be ignored.
- Immobilization can complicate and thereby delay airway management and other procedures within the primary survey.

Potential Negatives of Backboarding

It is important to remember that actions or inactions in the prehospital setting have direct consequences for the patient and the receiving facility. One study found that when immobilization procedures are used, patients spend an average total time of 54 minutes on the backboard with 33 of those minutes, on average, spent in EMS care and 21 minutes spent in the ED.[87]

Hyperextension of the cervical spine that can occur during immobilization procedures can result in neurologic deficit. Therefore, you must immobilize the patient in a neutral position. The adult patient requires 0.5 to 2 inches (1.25 to 5 cm) of padding behind the occiput to achieve a neutral position.[88] Immobilizing the patient's head directly on the backboard produces hyperextension of the cervical spine, thereby increasing the risk of neurologic deficit.

Patients immobilized for a prolonged time also often develop pain in the occipital, sacral, and lumbar areas that they did not have before being immobilized. This can result in potentially unnecessary radiographic studies being taken, and even longer times on the backboard.[89] Padding in the lumbar region and under the patient's knees, to keep the legs slightly flexed, can reduce pain in the lumbar and sacral areas. A vacuum mattress, used either alone or with a rigid backboard, has been shown to reduce pain and neurologic deficit.

Other complications include ulcers and pressure sores, increased risk of aspiration, and respiratory compromise. Cervical collars that are applied too tightly and not reassessed for proper fit can raise ICP, which presents another risk.[90] Head injury is common in trauma, and increased ICP is associated with worse neurologic outcomes. Head injury is far more common in trauma than is cervical injury. Finally, airway management is more difficult with a cervical collar than without.

Guidelines and Position Statements

The approach and recommendation to spinal immobilization has changed significantly over the years. For example, in 2002 the American Association of Neurological Surgeons and the Congress of Neurological Surgeons published their *Guidelines for the Management of Acute Cervical Spine and Spinal Cord Injuries*, in which they found insufficient evidence to support current treatment standards or treatment guidelines.[91] As a result, they recommended that all patients with either cervical spine injury or a mechanism suggesting the possibility of cervical spine injury be fully immobilized. In 2013, they revised their position and recommended the use of selective immobilization criteria.

The National Association of EMS Physicians has also published position statements about spinal immobilization and in 2013 issued a new statement that affected the immobilization of patients in the prehospital setting.[26,92] Its specific recommendations are as follows:

- Appropriate patients for backboard use may include those with any of the following:
  - Blunt trauma and altered level of consciousness

Evidence-Based Medicine

Prior practice was to immobilize everyone.[93,94] Recent publications and position statements have advocated for avoiding immobilization in a subset of patients for whom there is little potential benefit and for whom the discomfort of immobilization, the time to achieve immobilization, and the potential complications of immobilization exceed any potential advantage—in short, those for whom the risk of immobilization outweighs any potential benefits.[95]

Much of the impetus for change has revolved around three concerns: (1) discomfort and risk of skin breakdown associated with immobilization on a hard backboard, (2) decreased ability for a patient to protect his or her own airway when thoroughly immobilized, and (3) increased scene time associated with the immobilization process.[96–99]

An argument against immobilization has also been that it is relatively ineffective. The semantics of the discussion, including the promulgation of new terms (such as *spinal motion restriction*), reflects this argument. It is very true that spinal immobilization results in incomplete immobilization of the spine. It's also true that immobilization of a femur in a traction splint or immobilization of a tibia in a leg splint results in incomplete immobilization. That doesn't make it ineffective or otherwise useless. The purpose of spinal immobilization is to prevent secondary damage to the spinal cord, not to completely immobilize the spine and prevent micromotion at the site of any injury.

The published protocols (including those of the American College of Surgeons Committee on Trauma, National Association of EMS Physicians, and others) make good common sense. Patients with low likelihood of injury based on either low-risk mechanism (eg, gunshot wounds) or reliable physical exam don't need to be immobilized. Unfortunately, trends toward decreasing the frequency of immobilization tend to flow past logic and evidence. In some cases, aggressive and potentially dangerous practices are being implemented, in which immobilization of the spine is effectively eliminated from EMS protocols and cervical collars are applied with no further immobilization of the spine instituted or even attempted. In some cases, careful processes and procedures are employed in the process of transferring patients in lieu of the traditional backboard and collar packaging. Some agencies have gone so far as to remove the backboard (or any equivalent device, such as an air mattress, Kendrick extrication device, or scoop stretcher) from their armamentaria.

It's important to remember that the reason spinal immobilization emerged initially as a tool in EMS was that there were reported cases of patients developing a progression of neurologic deficits during the course of medical care and transport, in the absence of immobilization and recognition of the potential for unstable spinal column injury.[100] We will likely never be able to know if any of those patients' neurologic injuries could have been prevented with better immobilization. The protocols and practices that followed involving the boarding and collaring of all patients with a suspicious MOI, regardless of other signs or symptoms, likely represented unnecessary treatment and may have actually resulted in some degree of harm to a few patients and some degree of discomfort to many. Although the risk of causing an unstable spinal injury in a neurologically uninjured or only partially injured patient to progress to a devastating neurologic consequence is clearly low, it remains the reason we employ spinal immobilization and other precautionary techniques in this patient population. A backboard and collar remind everyone who comes into contact with the patient that there is an unresolved question as to the presence of injury and stability of the spinal column and therefore a potential ongoing risk to the integrity of the patient's spinal cord. Failing to immobilize with a backboard and collar removes that reminder from the view of those who are not necessarily familiar with the history, MOI, or specific symptoms.

It's definitely possible to move a patient safely without use of a backboard, but it's also possible that someone will not think about the need to employ spinal precautions during a transfer and move the patient in a way that will result in permanent devastating neurologic injury. Use of a backboard and collar decreases that risk by increasing the awareness of everyone who comes into contact with the patient. It's also important to consider that between the time a patient is extricated from a vehicle and the time he or she arrives in the ED, the number of times he or she is passively moved, and the forces associated with those moves, are much greater than after arrival at the hospital. Compared to the response scene or even the back of the ambulance, the hospital is a much more controlled environment. Simply put, it's safe to remove the backboard and collar in the ED, but it's not safe to avoid applying it altogether in high-risk patients.

Remember—"first do no harm." You certainly don't want to cause injury or even unnecessary discomfort to someone when immobilization isn't necessary. But you really don't want to cause or even contribute to a permanent paraplegia or quadriplegia in someone who sustained a fracture or dislocation and had intact neurologic function prior to your involvement in his or her treatment.

- Spinal pain or tenderness
- Neurologic complaint (eg, numbness or motor weakness)
- Anatomic deformity of the spine
- High-energy MOI and any of the following:
  - Drug or alcohol intoxication
  - Inability to communicate
  - Distracting injury
- Patients for whom immobilization on a backboard is not necessary include those with all of the following:
  - Normal level of consciousness (GCS of 15)
  - No spine tenderness or anatomic abnormality
  - No neurologic findings or complaints
  - No distracting injury
  - No intoxication
- You can maintain a degree of spinal immobilization by applying a rigid cervical collar and securing the patient to the EMS stretcher without a backboard. These measures are most appropriate for:
  - Patients who are ambulatory at the scene
  - Patients who must be transported for a long time, particularly before interfacility transfer
  - Patients for whom a backboard is not otherwise indicated
- Patients with penetrating trauma to the head, neck, or torso and no evidence of spinal injury should not be immobilized to a backboard.

Application to Current Paramedic Practice

During your EMS education and career, you will encounter many opinions on spinal immobilization. These views may be based on historical approaches to treatment, opinion, interpretation of data, or myriad other factors. For example, a 2013 study of provider attitudes toward immobilization found that most respondents believed immobilization is appropriate with penetrating trauma to the chest or abdomen, but this is not considered appropriate care for such an injury.[101]

Always follow your local protocols when providing any treatment, and this also applies to immobilization. Any changes in protocol and treatment must be developed with your medical director based on current evidence. The three common approaches to immobilization are listed here. You will likely encounter each of them at some time in your career.

1. All trauma patients are immobilized based on mechanism.
2. Patients with an identified mechanism are evaluated for the presence of spinal injury and either fully immobilized or not immobilized, based on selective immobilization criteria.
3. Patients with a mechanism are evaluated for the presence of spinal injury based on selective criteria and are either fully immobilized, placed in a cervical collar only and secured to the stretcher without a backboard, or not immobilized.

▶ Assessment and Management of Spinal Injury

The 2002 *Guidelines for the Management of Acute Cervical Spinal Cord Injuries* stated that 25% of SCIs were believed to be worsened by poor immobilization techniques; however, scientific data have never supported this belief.[91] Medical providers now believe that the deterioration seen in the prehospital setting is due to the progression of secondary cord injuries such as cord swelling. Therefore, limiting the progression of secondary SCI is a major goal of prehospital management of SCI. You should be familiar with the circumstances that often produce SCI and try to determine, through history taking and examination at the scene, whether the patient has any of these conditions.

As with any trauma patient, the primary survey includes the ABCDEs (Airway, Breathing, Circulation, Disability, Exposure) and the formulation of a treatment plan. In the patient with a potential spinal injury, you should manually stabilize the patient at first contact.

Assess the airway, breathing, and circulation, and perform appropriate treatments, as described earlier in this chapter. During the disability phase, perform a neurologic exam and a complete assessment of the spinal column for deformity, crepitus, step-offs, and point tenderness. At this time, you will have gained enough information to develop your approach to immobilization as allowed within your protocols.

Next, place a cervical collar, if indicated, and immobilize the patient by placing the patient on either a backboard, a scoop stretcher, or an air mattress.

If your protocols allow selective immobilization, and immobilization is not indicated, then you generally release manual stabilization at this point and continue the assessment based on the patient's condition.

The amount of time on scene is a concern with every trauma patient. The goal of all EMS providers, regardless of their level, should be to spend no more than 10 minutes on the scene with a critical trauma patient before the patient is transported to the most appropriate facility, unless time is required to extricate the patient or the team is awaiting air evacuation **Figure 34-39**.

Immobilization takes the bulk of your time on scene; however, you must not ignore life threats to the airway, breathing, and circulation by focusing on immobilization and packaging. Recall the effect of hypoxia on head injuries, which are commonly associated with spinal injuries. If you are responding to a patient with a compromised airway or ineffective breathing and you choose to delay treatment of that condition until you have the patient in the ambulance in an attempt to limit your scene time, you must ask yourself whether you gave your patient the best chance of positive outcome. If the patient were to become hypoxic during your time on scene, even if the scene time were 4 minutes, the answer would be no. With practice, you will find that you can easily address life threats, and immobilize and package the patient, within 6 to 10 minutes in most cases.

In the critical trauma patient, we accept the fact that we will likely compromise the spine during rapid extrication, but the benefit of rapid treatment of life threats and transport to definitive care outweighs the risk of spine

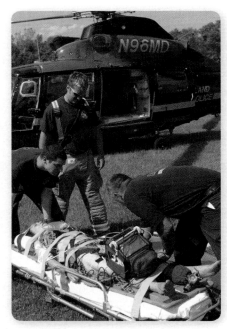

Figure 34-39 Spend no more than 10 minutes on scene with a critical trauma patient unless extrication is underway or you are waiting for air evacuation.
© Mark C. Ide.

Words of Wisdom

Do not ignore life threats to the airway, breathing, and circulation in an attempt to shorten scene time; doing so may worsen patient outcome. With practice you will find that you can easily address life threats, and immobilize and package the patient, within 6 to 10 minutes. Conversely, a 4-minute scene time in which the patient develops hypoxia may lead to a worse outcome than a 10-minute scene time in which the patient did not develop hypoxia because you treated an airway and/or breathing compromise on the scene.

compromise. Fortunately, most trauma patients you see will not be critical, and you will be able to treat patients who have an isolated spinal injury without any life threats. In this case, the greatest threat is their spinal injury, and the benefits of rapid extrication do not outweigh its risks. In such cases, patients may be better served with a slower approach to the treatment of their spinal injuries to produce the least amount of movement possible. This treatment may include a vest-type immobilization device. In this case, your scene time probably will exceed 10 minutes, so you must remember that this approach is appropriate only in the patient with an isolated spinal injury and no critical life threats.

Spinal Splinting Best Practices

For splinting purposes, the spine should be considered one long bone articulating with the head at one end and the pelvis at the other end. Therefore, traditional spinal immobilization uses a cervical collar, a cervical immobilization device, and a long spine board (backboard or scoop).

The following sections of this chapter will focus on the traditional methods of spinal immobilization. You should remember a few caveats about these techniques:

- There is no optimal device for spinal immobilization.
- Vacuum mattresses have been shown to provide effective immobilization with increased patient comfort.
- Padding behind the occiput, lumbar area, and knees reduces pain and pressure.
- Adult patients require 0.5 to 2 inches (1.25 to 5 cm) of padding behind the occiput to maintain neutral position of the cervical spine and avoid hyperextension.
- Because of their large occiput, pediatric patients require padding under the torso to maintain neutral position and avoid hyperflexion. Backboards specifically designed for pediatric patients take this anatomic difference into account, but you must nevertheless evaluate for neutral position.

- Blanket rolls between the legs and along both sides of the body fill voids under the straps, help restrict motion, and increase patient comfort.
- Cloth tape is ineffective at immobilizing the head or the body.
- A rigid cervical collar and rigid cervical immobilization device provide the best immobilization of the head.
- The head, shoulders, and pelvis must be immobilized because these are the weight centers of the body and are subject to the most movement, especially if the patient has to be turned on the backboard.
- Axial movements provide better spinal alignment than do lateral movements.

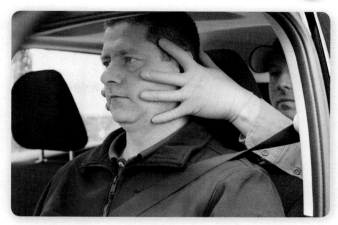

Figure 34-40 Manual in-line stabilization from behind the patient requires thumb placement behind the ears with the fingers spread across the cheeks and jaw.

© Jones & Bartlett Learning.

Words of Wisdom

Think of the spine as a chain. Dragging the chain sideways (lateral movements) will cause the chain to curve—as when the spine moves laterally. However, dragging the chain toward an end (axial movement) keeps all the chain links in line, thus, keeping the spine in line.

Manual Stabilization

You apply manual stabilization during the primary survey when you grasp the patient's head firmly between your hands with the fingers and thumbs extended to avoid extension, flexion, lateral bending, or rotation of the head. You should perform this stabilizing move without exerting traction on the patient's head.

You can maintain manual stabilization from the patient's front, rear, or side. The only difference is how you position your hands. Stabilization from the rear requires thumb placement behind the ears with the fingers spread across the cheeks and jaw **Figure 34-40**. Manual stabilization from the front generally causes less patient anxiety because the patient can see who is touching him or her.

Neutral positioning allows the most space for the spinal cord and may reduce cord hypoxia and excess pressure on the tissues. In some cases, you cannot move the patient's head into a neutral in-line position. You should not move the patient's head and neck if the patient has muscle spasms in the neck; increased pain with movement (ie, interlocked facets); numbness, tingling, or weakness; or a compromised airway or ventilation. In these situations, immobilize the patient in the position in which you found him or her. The risks associated with moving these patients exceed the risks of transporting the patient immobilized on a backboard in the position found.

Cervical collars cannot be adjusted to immobilize these patients, so you should not attempt to apply one. When this situation occurs, stabilize the head and neck with bulky padding and document thoroughly.

Application of the Cervical Collar

A cervical collar is not designed to immobilize the patient's head. Rather, it is intended to reduce flexion and extension of the neck and to place the weight of the head on the shoulders, thus, eliminating the axial load of the head on a compromised cervical spine. A properly applied cervical collar allows the head to remain in a neutral in-line position. It does not prevent the patient from turning his or her head sideways. This is just one reason you must maintain manual stabilization until the patient is fully immobilized.

You must appropriately size the collar. A cervical collar that is too large will cause the patient's neck to hyperextend. Conversely, a cervical collar that is too small will neither eliminate neck flexion nor relieve the axial load. A properly sized collar supports the head in the neutral position by resting on the chest, shoulders, and jaw without applying pressure on the jaw. When the collar is in place, ensure the patient can still speak easily. If the patient pulls down on the collar to speak, then it likely is too large.

Follow the manufacturer's instructions for sizing the cervical collar. Most collars used today are adjustable and have a sizing line used to select the height of the collar. Ensure your hand is parallel to the jaw and measure the distance from the lower jaw to the top of the shoulder by determining the number of fingers needed to completely fill the space **Figure 34-41**. Transfer that measurement to the adjustable or fixed collar to determine the size of collar you need. If you do not have the correct size of collar, then use a rolled towel, tape it to the backboard around the patient's head, and provide continuous manual support. While you are maintaining manual in-line stabilization,

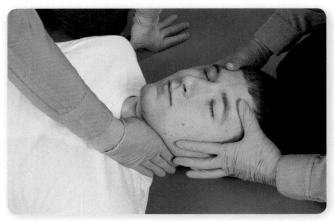

Figure 34-41 To determine the proper cervical collar size, use your fingers to measure the distance from the patient's lower jaw to the top of the shoulder.

© Jones & Bartlett Learning.

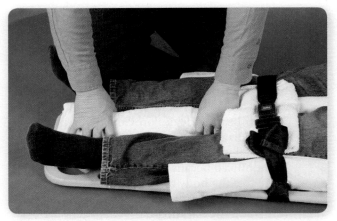

Figure 34-42 Place blanket rolls on each side of the patient's legs to prevent lateral movement and prevent the straps from digging in to the patient.

© Jones & Bartlett Learning.

wrap the collar around the neck and secure the collar to the far side of the chin support. Recheck that the patient is in a neutral in-line position.

Words of Wisdom

When you have been in EMS a while, you will hear the statement, "Everyone is a no-neck." In other words, there is a belief that most patients best fit into the no-neck collar size. In reality, most people require a regular collar size, as found in the manufacturers' studies when they developed the collars. Think about it: if most people were the no-neck size, then why wasn't that size called regular?

Special Populations

Do not automatically accept the labeled sizes of "pediatric" or "infant" for cervical collars. Measure each patient individually. Never place tape across the neck; it may obstruct the airway. Remember to add padding around the outside edges of the pediatric patient so that the padding becomes as wide as the backboard.

Supine Patients

You can immobilize a supine patient by securing him or her to a long backboard. The preferred procedure for moving a patient from the ground to a backboard is the four-person log roll. You should use this procedure whenever you suspect a spinal injury.

In other cases, you may choose to slide the patient onto a backboard or use a scoop stretcher. The patient's condition, the scene, and the available resources will dictate the method you choose. Ideally, the patient should be log rolled onto the uninjured side. Another technique that limits movement of the spine is to use a scoop stretcher to lift the patient a few inches off the floor or ground while crew members slide a long backboard under the patient.

When you immobilize a patient, you must provide the greatest possible stabilization. Multiple studies have shown that prehospital providers often immobilize patients incorrectly. One study found that 30% of patients had at least one point with a head strap unattached, 12% had two points with unattached head straps, and 88% of patients had at least 0.75 inches (2 cm) of slack in the body straps, with an average of 3.4 loose straps per patient.[102]

Even when you tighten the straps as much as possible without compromising chest wall movement, most patients will still have voids between their bodies and the straps that allow movement. These gaps usually appear on the patient's side where the straps come from the backboard and do not make contact with the body. The term "terrible triangle" has been coined to describe them.

Another location that often allows lateral movement is the legs. There is a natural void between the legs because of their attachment to the pelvis. Forcing them together for a prolonged period not only causes pain, but allows voids on the side of the backboard. Allowing the legs to maintain their natural position is preferable; however, this position still allows lateral movement. The easiest solution is to place premade blanket rolls on each side of the patient and between the legs **Figure 34-42**. This step takes only a few seconds and not only fills the voids, but also increases patient comfort, as the straps put pressure on the blankets, which in turn secure the patient. Without such padding, the straps could dig in to the patient and still allow lateral movement.

Therefore, correct strapping is essential for securing the patient to the backboard and most effectively immobilizing the patient. You can choose from many options for securing the patient to the backboard, such as 9-foot (3-m) straps, quick clip straps, and the Spider Strap and its derivatives.

If you are using individual straps to secure the patient to the backboard, you must use at least five straps. In this method, start by bringing one strap over the top of each shoulder, and cross these two straps over the sternum in an X shape. Attach each strap to the side of the backboard opposite the shoulder it crossed several inches below the iliac crest. This process will secure the shoulders and chest.

Next, bring one strap over the top of each iliac crest, cross these two straps over the pelvis, and secure them near the opposite hip, creating an X shape over the hips. Because the shoulder straps were secured below the iliac crest, this second X shape over the hips creates an additional X shape beside the pelvis, creating greater prevention of lateral movement. You can secure the legs with straight straps over the thigh and lower legs Figure 34-43. As discussed, be sure to fill the gaps created between the patient's sides and the backboard straps.

Your job is to ensure that the head, torso, and pelvis move as a unit, with your teammates controlling the movement of the body. You may recruit bystanders to the team if necessary, but instruct them fully before moving the patient.

To immobilize a patient on a backboard, follow the steps in Skill Drill 34-1.

When you find a patient in a prone position or on his or her side, you should log roll the patient into the supine position. Manually stabilize the head and neck in the position in which you found the patient, and then immobilize the patient as described earlier. One rescuer should take control of the cervical spine, using a crossed-hand

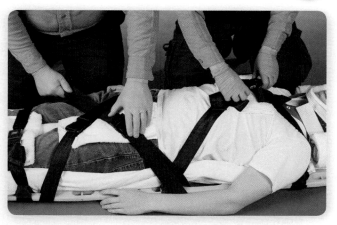

Figure 34-43 Proper strapping of a patient to a backboard.
© Jones & Bartlett Learning.

Special Populations

When you immobilize pregnant patients, tilt the backboard 15 to 20 inches (38 to 50 cm) using a pillow or blankets to avoid supine hypotensive syndrome. This syndrome occurs when the gravid uterus compresses the inferior vena cava and reduces blood return to the right atrium. From a medical perspective, it does not matter if the backboard is tilted to the right or left, but the left is most commonly recommended simply so the patient will be facing you rather than the cabinets in the ambulance, thereby limiting your ability to perform an assessment.

Skill Drill 34-1 · Performing Spinal Immobilization of a Supine Adult Patient

NR Skill

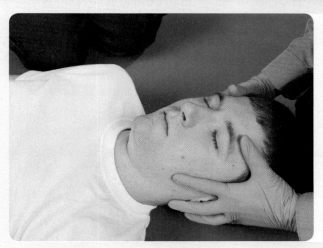

Step 1 Take standard precautions and then begin manual in-line stabilization from a kneeling position at the patient's head: Hold the head firmly with both hands. The provider at the head directs all patient movement. Support the lower jaw with your index and middle fingers, and support the head with your palms. If the patient's head is not facing forward, then gently move it until the patient's eyes are looking straight ahead and the head and torso are in alignment (neutral alignment). Never twist, flex, or extend the head or neck excessively. Do not remove your hands from the patient's head until the patient is properly secured to a backboard and the head is immobilized. Evaluate the patient's reliability in giving a history.

(continued)

Skill Drill 34-1 Performing Spinal Immobilization of a Supine Adult Patient *(continued)*

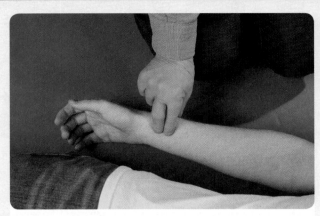

Step 2 Assess distal pulses and motor and sensory function in each extremity.

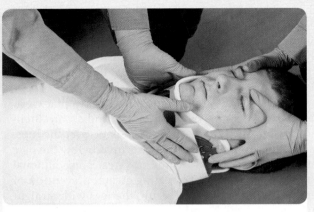

Step 3 Apply a well-fitting cervical collar as previously discussed.

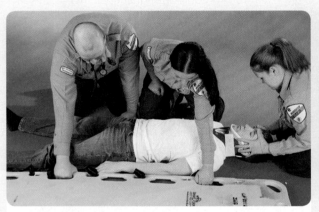

Step 4 The other team members should position the immobilization device (backboard) beside the patient and place their hands on the patient's far side to increase their leverage while kneeling. Instruct them to use their body weight, shoulders, and back muscles to ensure a smooth, coordinated pull. The pull should concentrate on the heavier portions of the body.

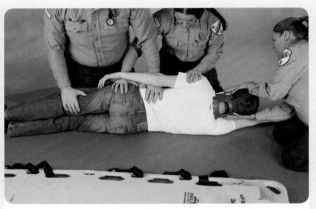

Step 5 On count/command from the paramedic at the patient's head, the rescuers should *roll the patient* toward themselves until the patient is balanced on his or her side. This rolling technique prevents the patient from twisting as he or she is pulled down by gravity and up by the provider. One rescuer should quickly examine the back while the patient is rolled onto the side and then slide the backboard behind and under the patient. The team should then roll the patient back onto the backboard, avoiding rotation of the head, shoulders, and pelvis.

Skill Drill 34-1 Performing Spinal Immobilization of a Supine Adult Patient *(continued)*

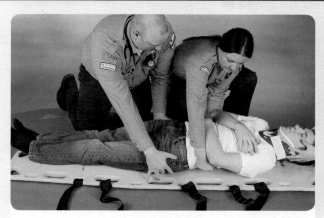

Step 6 Ensure the patient is centered on the backboard. Alternatively, the patient may be moved onto the backboard as follows: The backboard is placed beside the patient with the foot end at the level of the patient's hips. The patient is log rolled, then the patient is pulled onto the backboard along the axis of the spine to a centered position. This alternative method results in only moving the patient twice (one roll and one slide).

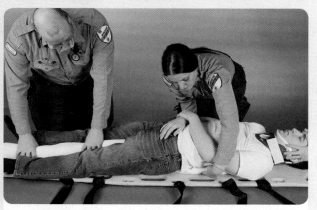

Step 7 Apply padding as necessary to fill the voids between the patient and the device. When possible, prepare blanket rolls ahead of time and have them ready to go. When you have the blankets prepared, you need only seconds to place them. Use of blanket rolls has been shown to dramatically improve the effectiveness of immobilization.

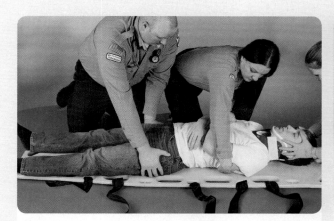

Step 8 Center the patient on the backboard.

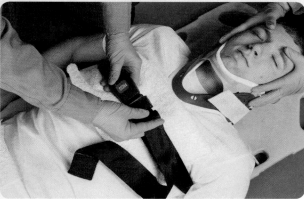

Step 9 Secure the upper torso to the backboard after the patient has been centered on the backboard.

(continued)

Skill Drill 34-1 Performing Spinal Immobilization of a Supine Adult Patient *(continued)*

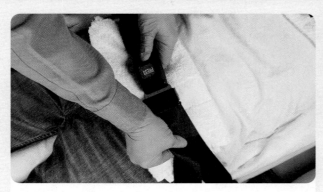

Step 10 Secure the pelvis and upper legs, using padding as needed. For the pelvis, use straps over the iliac crests and/or groin loops (leg straps).

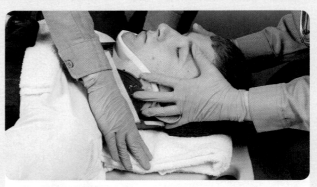

Step 11 Pad behind the patient's neck and head area as needed to maintain a neutral in-line position.

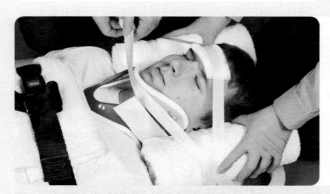

Step 12 Immobilize the head to the backboard with a commercial immobilization device per the manufacturer's instructions. Secure the head to the backboard only after the entire torso has been secured. If the head is secured first and the body shifts, the spine may be compromised. Securing most of the body weight first creates better protection.

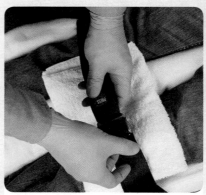

Step 13 Secure the patient's lower legs to the backboard.

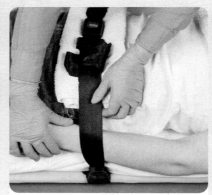

Step 14 Secure the patient's arms with a single strap.

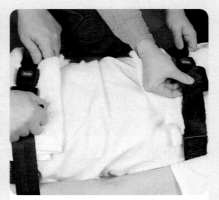

Step 15 Check and readjust straps as needed to ensure the entire body is snugly secured and will not slide during movement of the backboard or during patient transport. Reassess distal pulse, motor, and sensation function in each extremity and repeat periodically.

Special Populations

In some cases, you can immobilize a toddler in an undamaged child seat. If the child and seat must be placed in a supine position, the child must be extricated from the car seat to avoid placing extra pressure on the abdomen and reducing the lung expansion.

Words of Wisdom

When you immobilize the torso, remember you must also immobilize the pelvis. If you immobilize only the shoulders and chest, the body can move laterally if you need to turn the backboard. In most cases, providers simply immobilize the entire body and then the head, and then secure the arms to the device. This approach is acceptable in both the field and National Registry testing, as it meets the critical criteria of the torso being immobilized before the head.

position to roll the patient. The second rescuer should be positioned at the torso, and any other rescuers should be positioned at the pelvis and legs. The rescuer at the head does the count, and the team as a unit rolls the patient into a supine position. You should then continue to assess and immobilize as usual.

As mentioned earlier, patients may be immobilized on other devices, such as a scoop stretcher or a vacuum mattress, rather than a backboard. Skill Drill 34-2 summarizes how to immobilize a patient using a scoop stretcher.

Seated Patients

Patients found in a sitting position (eg, after a MVC) may or may not have spinal injuries. The indications of spinal injury and the severity of associated injuries will dictate your approach to the seated patient. If any of the following criteria are met, then your team should lower the patient directly onto a backboard using the rapid extrication technique discussed later in this chapter:

- You or the patient is in danger.
- You must gain immediate access to other patients.
- The patient has life-threatening injuries that justify rapid extrication.

Place a cervical collar and manually stabilize the entire spine as you move the patient to the backboard.

As with supine patients, seated patients may have no indication for spinal immobilization. In this case, your system may allow you to ask or assist the patient to step out of the vehicle (or otherwise stand up) and sit on a stretcher that has been placed beside him or her. If the patient is unable to do so under his or her own power (due to the presence of non–life-threatening injury or an underlying medical condition), then a backboard can be used for extrication to transfer the patient to the stretcher.

YOU are the Paramedic PART 4

While en route to the medical facility, you intubate the patient while your partner establishes two 18-gauge IV lines and begins fluid resuscitation. In the ambulance, you can better see that the patient's skin is flushed, and he also has an abrasion to his right forehead at the hairline. No other apparent injuries are found. Sinus bradycardia is noted on the monitor.

Recording Time: 15 Minutes	
Respirations	Assisted via bag-mask ventilation and ET tube
Pulse	42 beats/min
Skin	Flushed
Blood pressure	70/42
Oxygen saturation (Spo2)	Unable to obtain
Pupils	PERRLA, but sluggish

7. What other immediate treatments are required?
8. Based on these events, what other factors could complicate the patient's outcome?

Skill Drill 34-2 Using a Scoop Stretcher

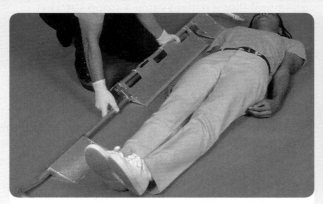

Step 1 With the scoop stretcher separated, measure the length of the scoop and adjust to the proper length.

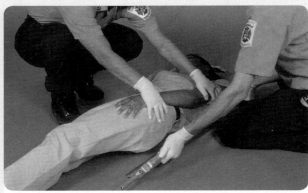

Step 2 Position the stretcher, one side at a time. Lift the patient's side slightly by pulling on the far hip and upper arm, while your partner slides the stretcher into place.

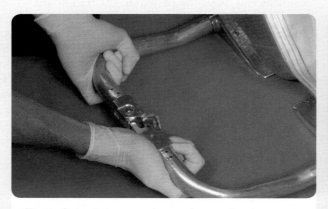

Step 3 Lock the stretcher ends together by engaging their locking mechanisms one at a time, and continue to lift the patient slightly as needed to avoid pinching the patient or your fingers.

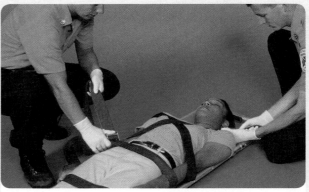

Step 4 Apply and tighten straps to secure the patient to the scoop stretcher before transferring to the stretcher.

© Jones & Bartlett Learning. Courtesy of MIEMSS.

Once the patient is on the stretcher, the backboard can be removed.

If a patient is in cardiac arrest, chest compressions take priority over immobilization. Patients who have no cardiorespiratory function or no hemodynamic compromise but who require spine immobilization have traditionally been extricated using manual stabilization of the head and neck, the placement of an appropriately sized cervical collar, and the use of a vest-type extrication device, followed by placement and securing on a backboard, as described later in this section. However, there are growing questions regarding the effectiveness of the vest-type extrication device and its ability to reduce spinal movement during extrication from a vehicle. Using 16 healthy volunteers and biomechanical markers, one study found there was the least spinal movement when a patient self-extricated from a vehicle without a cervical collar in place. These findings supported the findings of the researchers' earlier proof-of-concept study, which used one healthy paramedic as a patient, as well as the findings of two other studies.[103,104]

While these studies raise interesting questions and indicate the need for further research, the fact that they used such a small sample size of healthy patients, as opposed to those with spinal injury, has not provided enough evidence to recommend a change in the practice of using the vest-type extrication device for seated patients suspected of having a spinal injury.

There is wide variation in the procedures for removing a seated patient without the use of a vest-type extrication device, and it is beyond the scope of this text to address them all. If you work for a system that employs such procedures, you will have to rely on system-specific training to gain the knowledge and skills necessary to implement these protocols.

Once the patient has been removed from the vehicle by self-extrication, vest-type extrication device, or any other locally approved method, the manner in which the patient is immobilized may also vary based on the locality in which you are working. The patient may be secured to a backboard on the stretcher with a cervical collar in place, or he or she may be secured to a backboard with a vest-type extrication device and cervical collar in place.

In the absence of a local protocol that directs you otherwise, follow the steps in **Skill Drill 34-3** to immobilize a seated patient.

Words of Wisdom

As with all factors related to spinal immobilization, there is great variety in the approach to the seated patient. You must apply the principles and concepts you learn during your education to your local protocols and system-specific training when treating a seated patient with a suspected SCI.

Words of Wisdom

After moving the patient to the backboard, be sure to reevaluate any padding you placed between the vest-type immobilization device and the patient's head to ensure the cervical spine is not hyperflexed.

Skill Drill 34-3 Performing Spinal Immobilization of a Seated Adult Patient

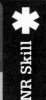

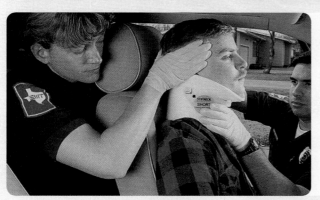

Step 1 Take standard precautions and direct your assistant to place and maintain the head in a neutral in-line position. Stabilize the head and neck with manual in-line stabilization until the patient is secured to the long backboard. Evaluate the patient's reliability as a historian. Assess distal pulse and motor and sensory function in each extremity.

Apply a properly sized cervical collar. Because the cervical collar does not completely stabilize the cervical spine, continue manual stabilization of the head and neck until the patient is fully immobilized on a backboard.

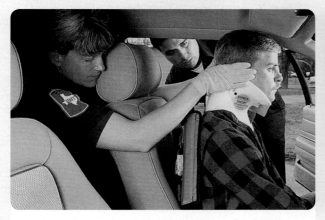

Step 2 Insert the immobilization device between the patient's upper back and the seat back.

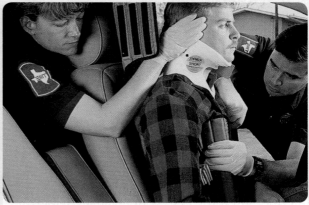

Step 3 Open the backboard's side flaps (if present) and position them around the patient's torso, snug to the armpits.

(continued)

Skill Drill 34-3 Performing Spinal Immobilization of a Seated Adult Patient *(continued)*

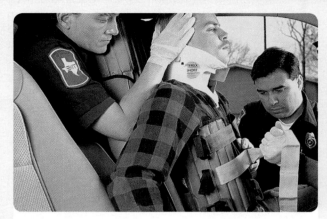

Step 4 When the device is properly positioned, secure the upper torso straps.

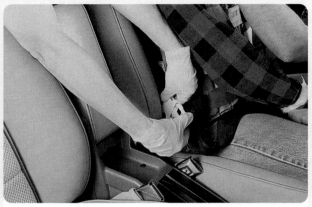

Step 5 Position and fasten both groin loops (leg straps). Pad the groin as needed. Check all torso straps and make sure they are secure. Make any necessary adjustments without excessively moving the patient.

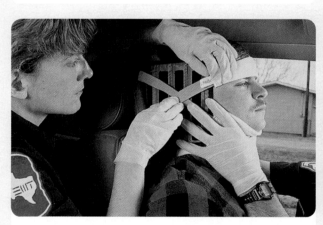

Step 6 Pad any space between the patient's head and the device. Secure the forehead strap or tape the head securely and then fasten the lower head strap around the rigid cervical collar. Reevaluate the patient to ensure that he or she is adequately immobilized. Reassess distal pulses and motor and sensory function in each extremity.

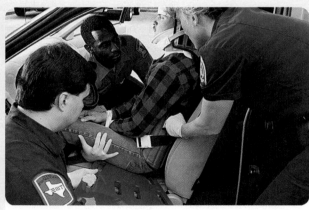

Step 7 Place the long backboard next to the patient's buttocks, perpendicular to the trunk.

© Jones & Bartlett Learning. Courtesy of MIEMSS.

Rapid Extrication

Rapid extrication is the process of manually stabilizing and moving a patient from a sitting position onto an immobilization device without the use of a vest-type immobilization device. With the rapid extrication technique, you can move the patient from sitting in a vehicle to lying supine on a backboard in about 2 minutes. However, as discussed earlier, you cannot ignore immediate life threats and focus only on the extrication.

You should use the rapid extrication technique in the following situations:

- The vehicle or scene is unsafe.
- You cannot properly assess the patient before removing the patient from the vehicle.

Skill Drill 34-3 Performing Spinal Immobilization of a Seated Adult Patient (continued)

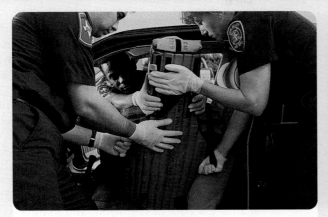

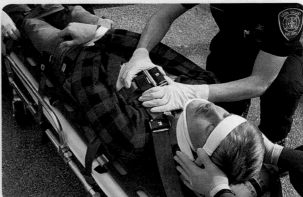

Step 8 Turn the patient parallel to the long backboard and slowly lower him or her onto it. Lift the patient and the vest-type board together as a unit (without rotating the patient), and slip the long backboard under the patient and device. Slide the patient onto the backboard as a unit using any handles that may be built into the device. Release the leg straps and loosen the chest strap to allow the legs to straighten and give the chest room to fully expand.

Step 9 Secure the short backboard and long backboard together. Do not remove the vest-type board from the patient. Reassess distal pulse and motor and sensory function in all four extremities. Note your findings on the patient care report and prepare for transport.

© Jones & Bartlett Learning. Courtesy of MIEMSS.

Special Populations

Osteoporosis in the thoracic and lumbar spine contributes to a high rate of injury in older adult patients. Three types of fractures are usually encountered in these patients:

- *Compression fractures* are stable injuries that often result from minimal trauma (eg, simply bending over, rising from a chair, or sitting down forcefully).
- *Burst fractures* are unstable fractures that typically result from a high-energy MOI such as a MVC or a fall from a substantial height. They may lead to neurologic injury secondary to shifting of the vertebrae with damage to the spinal cord.
- *Seat-belt–type fractures* involve flexion and cause a fracture through the entire vertebral body and bony arch. These injuries typically occur in people who are ejected and in those wearing a lap belt without a shoulder harness.

- The patient needs immediate intervention that requires a supine position.
- The patient's condition requires immediate transport to a medical facility.
- The patient blocks your access to another seriously injured patient.

In such cases, the delay that results from applying a vest-type immobilization device is contraindicated and unacceptable. Unfortunately, the manual support and immobilization that you use with the rapid extrication technique carry a greater risk of spine movement. You should not use the rapid extrication technique if the injuries are not urgent.

The rapid extrication technique requires a team of three providers who know and have practiced the procedure. Follow these steps:

1. The first rescuer manually stabilizes the patient's head and cervical spine in-line from behind. You may apply support from the side, if necessary, by reaching through the driver's door.
2. The second rescuer serves as a team leader and gives the commands to coordinate the

team's moves until the patient is supine on the backboard. Because the second rescuer lifts and turns the patient's torso, he or she must be physically strong enough to move the patient. The second rescuer works from the driver's doorway. If the first rescuer is also working from that doorway, the second rescuer should stand closer to the door hinges toward the front of the vehicle. The second rescuer applies a rigid cervical collar and performs the primary survey.

3. The second rescuer continuously supports the patient's torso until the patient is supine on the backboard. When the second rescuer takes control of the torso, he or she should not let go for any reason. Some type of cross-chest shoulder hug usually works well, but you must choose the method that will work best for the particular patient. You can't simply reach into the vehicle and grab the patient, because doing so will twist his or her torso. You must rotate the body as a unit.

4. The third rescuer works from the front passenger seat and rotates the patient's legs and feet as the torso is turned, ensuring that the feet are free of the pedals and other obstructions. To do this, the third rescuer first should carefully move the patient's nearer leg laterally, without rotating the patient's pelvis and lower spine. The pelvis and lower spine rotate only as the third rescuer moves the second leg during the next step. Moving the nearer leg first makes it much easier to move the second leg in concert with the rest of the body. When the third rescuer moves the legs together, the legs should be moved as a unit Figure 34-44A .

5. The patient is rotated 90°, so the patient's back faces out the driver's door and the feet are on the front passenger's seat. This coordinated movement is done in three or four short, quick, one-eighth to one-quarter turns. The second rescuer coordinates the sequence of moves, and the first rescuer directs each quick turn by saying, "Ready, turn" or "Ready, move." Hand position changes should be made between moves.

6. During the rotation, the first rescuer will work from the backseat in most cases. At some point, either because the doorpost is in the way or because the rescuer cannot reach farther from the backseat, the first rescuer will be unable to follow the torso rotation. At that time, the third rescuer should assume temporary manual in-line stabilization of the head and neck until the first rescuer can regain control of the head from outside the

vehicle. If a fourth rescuer is present, the fourth rescuer stands next to the second rescuer. The fourth rescuer takes control of the head and neck from outside the vehicle without involving the third rescuer. As soon as the change has been made, the rotation can continue Figure 34-44B .

7. When the patient has been fully rotated, place the backboard against the patient's buttocks on the seat. Do not try to wedge the backboard under the patient. If only three rescuers are present, then place the backboard within arm's reach of the driver's door before the move so that you can pull the backboard into place when needed. You can leave the far end of the backboard on the ground. When a fourth rescuer is available, the first rescuer exits the rear seat of the vehicle, places the backboard against the patient's buttocks, and maintains pressure toward the vehicle from the far end of the backboard. When the door opening allows, some rescuers prefer to insert the backboard onto the car seat before they rotate the patient.

8. As soon as the patient has been rotated and the backboard is in place, the second and third rescuers lower the patient onto the backboard while supporting the head and torso so that the neutral alignment is maintained. The first rescuer holds the backboard until the patient is secured Figure 34-44C .

9. The third rescuer moves across the front seat to a position at the patient's hips. If the third rescuer stays at the patient's knees or feet, he or she will be ineffective in helping to move the body's weight. The knees and feet follow the hips.

10. The fourth rescuer maintains in-line support of the head and takes over the giving of commands. If a fourth rescuer is not available, you can direct a volunteer to assist you. The second rescuer maintains the direction of the extrication; this rescuer stands with his or her back to the door, facing the rear of the vehicle. The backboard should be immediately in front of the third rescuer. The second rescuer grasps the patient's shoulders or armpits. On command, the second and third rescuers slide the patient 8 to 12 inches (20 to 30 cm) along the backboard, repeating this slide until the patient's hips are firmly on the backboard.

11. The third rescuer gets out of the vehicle and moves to the opposite side of the backboard, across from the second rescuer. The third rescuer takes control at the shoulders, and the second rescuer moves back to take control of the hips. On command, these

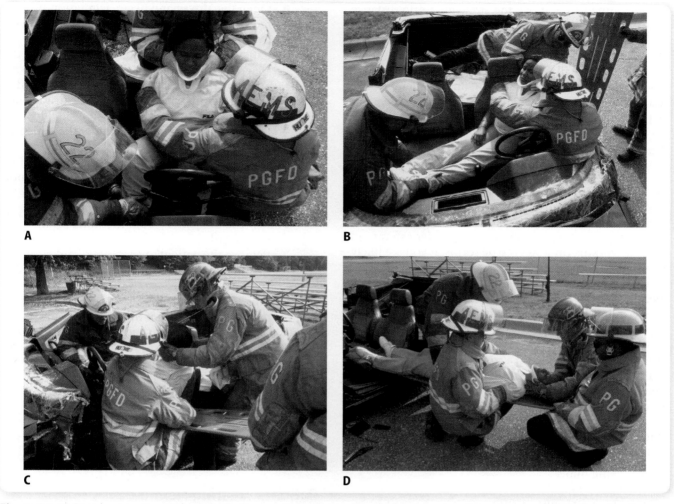

Figure 34-44 Rapid extrication technique. **A.** Moving the patient's legs without moving the pelvis or spine. **B.** Rotating the patient as a unit. **C.** Placing the backboard on the seat. **D.** Sliding the patient onto the backboard.

© Jones & Bartlett Learning. Courtesy of MIEMSS.

two rescuers move the patient along the backboard in 8- to 12-inch (20- to 30-cm) slides until the patient is completely on the backboard **Figure 34-44D** .

12. The first (or fourth) rescuer continues to maintain manual in-line support of the patient's head. The second and third rescuers grasp their sides of the backboard and then carry it and the patient away from the vehicle and onto the nearby prepared stretcher.

Special Populations

To immobilize kyphotic patients, you may need several blankets and pillows or vacuum splints to support the head and upper back. Ensure the empty spaces under the patient's knees and lumbar spine are padded as well.

In some cases, you will be able to place the backboard on the stretcher during rapid extrication. This technique has several advantages. First, the stretcher can be placed out of the way and rolled into place at the vehicle door after the patient has been rotated 90°. This allows more working room when rotating the patient, as the backboard does not take up space. After you rotate the patient, roll the stretcher, which should be at the level of the vehicle seat, into place and slide the foot of the backboard up to, or onto, the seat of the vehicle. Most of the backboard will be on the stretcher, and you simply lower the patient to the backboard and then slide the patient onto it. The other major advantages of this technique are that it can be done with only three providers, it reduces the possibility of the backboard or patient being dropped, and it reduces the risk of injury to a provider who is trying to support the backboard at the head end.

When the backboard and patient have been placed on the stretcher, you should begin lifesaving treatment immediately. If you used the rapid extrication technique because the scene was dangerous, you and your team should immediately move the stretcher a safe distance away from the vehicle before you assess or treat the patient.

The steps of the rapid extrication technique must be considered a general procedure to be adjusted as needed. Every situation will be different—a different vehicle, a different size or priority of patient, and a different crew. Your resourcefulness and ability to adapt are vital elements of a successful rapid extrication.

Packaging and Removing Injured Patients From the Water

Immobilization in water should be performed only by rescuers specifically trained in the procedure. These professionals include swift water rescue specialists, life-guards, rescuers trained in wilderness water safety, and rescuers working on water rescue teams. If you are likely to be called on to treat patients with suspected spinal injuries who are in water, be sure to obtain appropriate specific training.

Even though the patient is in the water, the principles of packaging and removal are the same: keep the head, neck, and trunk in alignment. When the patient may have sustained a spinal injury in a confirmed diving accident, you must begin spinal immobilization even before you remove the patient from the water. The following incidents have the potential to cause spinal injury. As a result, you must appropriately assess for spinal injury, and you must immobilize the patient if indicated by the clinical findings and your local protocols.

- Diving injury
- Boating injury
- Watercraft injury
- Falls from heights such as cliffs or bridges

If you suspect respiratory arrest, you can ventilate while the patient is still in the water. In case of cardiac arrest, however, the rescuer should quickly evaluate the MOI. If a spinal injury is not obvious, immediately remove the patient from the water and begin CPR. However, if the patient shows any indication of a spinal injury, follow these steps to stabilize the patient in the water:

1. If the patient is prone in the water, then approach the patient from the top of the head and place your arm under the body so that the head is supported on your arm and the chest on your hand. Place your other arm across the head and back to splint the head and neck between your arms. Continue to support the patient's head and neck in this fashion, take a step backward and smoothly turn the patient to the supine position **Figure 34-45A** .

2. Two rescuers are usually needed to turn the patient safely, but in some cases one rescuer is enough. Always rotate the entire upper half of the body as a unit. Twisting only the head, for example, may aggravate any injury to the cervical spine.

3. Open the airway and begin ventilation if required. Immediate ventilation is the primary treatment of all drowning and submersion patients. As soon as the patient is faceup in the water, use a pocket mask if one is available. Have the other rescuer support the head and trunk as a unit while you open the airway and begin artificial ventilation **Figure 34-45B** .

4. Float a buoyant backboard under the patient as you continue ventilation.

5. Secure the head and trunk to the backboard to eliminate motion of the cervical spine. Do not remove the patient from the water until this step is complete **Figure 34-45C** .

6. Remove the patient from the water on the backboard.

7. Remove the patient's wet clothes, and cover the patient with a blanket. Administer supplementary oxygen if the patient is breathing adequately; administer positive-pressure ventilation if the patient is apneic or breathing inadequately. Begin CPR if the patient has no pulse. You cannot perform effective chest compressions when the patient is still in the water **Figure 34-45D** .

8. Consider using an advanced airway device to maintain the airway if needed. Place the patient on a cardiac monitor and treat dysrhythmias according to the ACLS algorithms (discussed in other chapters).

Patients Wearing Helmets

Helmets are a relatively common finding in motorcycle and sports-related injuries. The use of helmets has been shown to reduce both the incidence and the severity of brain injuries associated with trauma, and their use is widely encouraged. Most helmets consist of an inner foam layer surrounded by a durable plastic shell.

Helmets can prevent full exposure of the patient and can hinder your efforts to manage the airway and stabilize the spine. Still, there are virtues to leaving a helmet in place. First, removing most types of helmets can cause some spinal motion even under the best circumstances; if the airway and breathing are not compromised, the risk of introducing spinal motion will outweigh the benefit

Controversies

Researchers differ over whether to remove helmets in the field. The key considerations boil down to the urgency of airway management, the fit of the helmet, the presence of well-trained hands to take it off, and the effect the helmet has on immobilizing the patient in a neutral position.

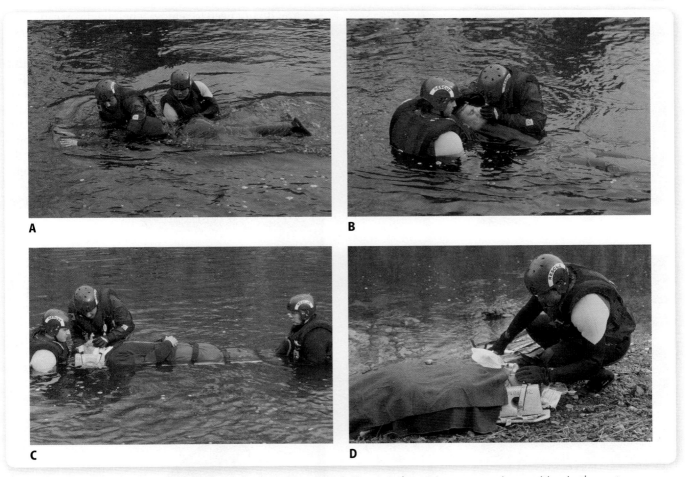

Figure 34-45 Stabilizing a suspected spinal injury in the water. **A.** Turning the patient to a supine position in the water. **B.** Providing artificial ventilation. **C.** Securing the patient to a backboard. **D.** Providing care to the patient out of the water.

© Jones & Bartlett Learning. Courtesy of MIEMSS.

of removing the helmet. Second, a secure-fitting helmet can maintain a degree of stabilization and in some circumstances actually can help maintain the spine in a neutral position.

Only providers familiar with the procedure should attempt helmet removal. A single rescuer should not attempt helmet removal, because the maneuver requires two providers:

1. Kneel at the patient's head. Leave enough room between your knees and the helmet so that you can remove the helmet. Your partner should kneel on one side of the patient, at the shoulder area.
2. Stabilize the helmet by placing your hands on either side of it, with your fingers on the patient's lower jaw to prevent movement of the head. When your hands are in position, your partner can loosen the chin strap.
3. Your partner should open the face shield, if present, and assess the patient's airway and breathing. Remove eyeglasses if present.

4. When the strap has been unfastened, your partner should place one hand on the patient's lower jaw at the angle of the jaw and the other hand behind the head at the back of the helmet. You may then pull the sides of the helmet away from the patient's head Figure 34-46A .
5. Gently slip the helmet partly off the patient's head, stopping when the helmet reaches the halfway point.
6. Your partner then slides his or her hand from the back of the helmet to the occiput, preventing the head from falling back when the helmet is completely removed Figure 34-46B .
7. When your partner's hand is in place, remove the helmet and provide manual in-line cervical spine stabilization Figure 34-46C .
8. Apply a rigid cervical collar and secure the patient to the backboard.
9. With large helmets or small patients, you may need to add padding under the shoulders

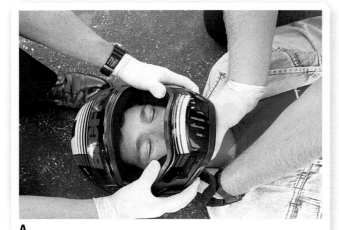

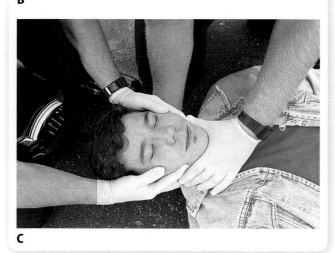

Figure 34-46 Removing a helmet. **A.** Spread the helmet to clear the ears while the other rescuer stabilizes the neck. **B.** Remove the helmet carefully, clearing the nose. **C.** Take over manual in-line cervical spine stabilization.

© Jones & Bartlett Learning. Courtesy of MIEMSS.

to prevent flexion of the neck. If the patient is wearing shoulder pads or a heavy jacket, then you may need to pad behind the head to prevent extension of the neck.

You do not need to remove a helmet if you can access the patient's airway, the head is snug inside the helmet, and the helmet can be secured to an immobilization device. If the patient is wearing padding, remember that the padding and the helmet may work together to align the spine. Removing one without removing the other may cause inadvertent misalignment. If you can remove the face mask of the helmet to access the airway, and if the posterior padding does not prevent treatment, you should leave both of these protection devices in place until the spine has been cleared through radiographic assessment.

Words of Wisdom

When you encounter a patient with a helmet, note whether he or she is wearing a special removal device in the helmet, such as the Eject Helmet Removal System by Simpson Performance Products **Figure 34-47**. This device contains a small air bladder inside the top of the helmet. An air tube descends from the bladder down one side of the helmet. If an emergency provider must remove the helmet, he or she must first cut the helmet's chin strap and remove the patient's goggles or eyeglasses. The provider attaches the inflator bulb to the Eject tube connector, inflating the bladder to gently lift the helmet off the patient's head.

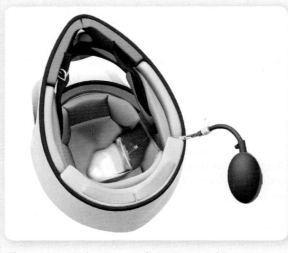

Figure 34-47 The Eject Helmet Removal System from Simpson (simpsonraceproducts.com).
© Simpson Performance Products.

▶ Pharmacotherapy of Spinal Cord Injury

Short-acting, reversible sedatives are recommended for the acute agitated patient after a correctable cause of agitation (eg, hypoxia) has been excluded. The risk of secondary injury caused by movements from acute agitation must be balanced with potential airway and ventilatory compromise as well as a reliable neurologic exam. Pain medication also may be necessary.

Corticosteroids, such as methylprednisolone, are anti-inflammatory agents historically used in the acute phase of SCI, primarily on the basis of three studies. However, the methodology used in these studies came under intense scrutiny after publication, and the findings have never been replicated. Class I, II, and III evidence shows that these medications are associated with harmful side effects and may even result in death.[105] Therefore, the National Association of EMS Physicians, the American Association of Neurological Surgeons, and the Congress of Neurological Surgeons recommend that steroids not be administered in the management of an acute spinal injury.[91,105,106]

▶ Complications of Spinal Cord Injury

The complications of SCI are a consistent cause of the high morbidity and mortality rates and the high financial costs associated with this type of injury. Many of the acute-phase complications of SCI already have been addressed in this chapter, such as the potential for aspiration or respiratory arrest, especially with high cervical injuries. Lower cervical lesions may preserve the diaphragm, but the loss of intercostal muscles ultimately impairs coughing and deep breathing, predisposing the patient to atelectasis and pneumonia. Deep vein thrombosis and pulmonary embolism are late complications that may result from immobility and may become life threatening.

Autonomic dysreflexia, also called autonomic hyperreflexia, is typically a late complication of SCI but can occur acutely. This potentially life-threatening emergency most often occurs with injuries above T4 to T6 and results from the loss of parasympathetic stimulation.[107] About 85% of patients with an SCI above T6 will develop autonomic dysreflexia syndrome, especially when the patient developed spinal shock at the time of injury.[108]

Patients present clinically with evidence of a massive, uninhibited, uncompensated cardiovascular response caused by some stimulation of the sympathetic nervous system below the level of injury Table 34-9 . The irritated area sends a signal that cannot reach the brain, and unabated sympathetic nervous system stimulation results in vasoconstriction, as evidenced by cool, pale extremities, systolic blood pressures of greater than 200 mm Hg, and diastolic blood pressures of 130 mm Hg or greater.

Although a patient can develop severe hypertension, a rise of 20 mm Hg above the patient's normal resting blood pressure along with a history of SCI and associated signs and symptoms indicate the patient is experiencing autonomic dysreflexia. Hypertension activates the vasomotor center in the medulla, leading to parasympathetic stimulation. Vagal compensation causes bradycardia and dilation of peripheral and visceral vessels above the level of the lesion, although vessels below the SCI remain constricted. Selective vasodilation

Table 34-9	Signs and Symptoms of Autonomic Dysreflexia
Hypertension	
Headache	
Nasal congestion	
Dilation of the pupils and blurred vision	
Anxiety	
Bradycardia	
Rebound hypotension	
Flushing and sweating above SCI	
Erect hairs above SCI	
Chills without fever	
Bronchospasm	
Seizures, stroke, and death	
Cardiac dysrhythmias	

Abbreviation: SCI, spinal cord injury
© Jones & Bartlett Learning.

results in flushed skin, sweating, and congestion of nasopharyngeal vessels.[107]

Any noxious stimuli below the level of a cervical or high thoracic SCI can cause autonomic dysreflexia. Common causes include skin lesions such as insect bites, constrictive clothing, or sharp objects compressing the skin. Remove sharp objects from pockets and seat cushions.

Localized wounds such as lacerations, abrasions, decubitus ulcerations, and ingrown toenails are common causes of stimulation.[107] Minimize irritation from skin lesions with cold packs. With bladder distention resulting from obstructed urine outflow, you must suspect spasm or kinked indwelling catheters as well as bladder infection, constipation, or bowel impaction. Catheters should be irrigated, and obstructions should be removed. In men, tight condom catheters can pinch genitalia and should be checked and removed if necessary. In women, menstrual cramps or pregnancy can be a source of the stimulation.

Prehospital management focuses on supporting the vital systems. Inserting a Foley catheter, if authorized, can be lifesaving as it will relieve bladder distention, a common cause of autonomic dysreflexia. If you cannot find the source of the dysreflexia or reduce it effectively, you may need to reduce blood pressure with vasodilators.

Nontraumatic Spinal Conditions

Back pain eventually affects many people and is a common presenting complaint for patients who call for EMS. Most of these patients will have no definite physical or historical cause for their complaint. Back pain is classified into three categories: acute (less than 6 weeks in duration), subacute (from 6 to 12 weeks), and chronic (more than 12 weeks). Most back pain resolves within 4 weeks. Pain lasting longer than that warrants additional examination. Patients younger than 18 years who have chronic conditions have a higher incidence of congenital abnormalities. In those older than 50 years, the pain could be caused by a tumor or could have an intra-abdominal or vascular cause.

Expenses related to back pain can mount quickly. Therapy is expensive, and missed work days mean lost wages. Upright posture places a significant amount of weight on the lumbar spine—specifically at the vertebral level of L4 to L5, where the natural bend in the spine's curvature changes. Thus, many people are susceptible to injury or degenerative disease in this portion of the spine. Spinal tumors can also cause pain and debilitation. People whose occupations require repetitive lifting are at risk of developing low back pain. Those whose work exposes them to vibrations from vehicles or industrial machinery are at risk as well. Such people may also have comorbid diseases, such as osteoporosis. Most low back pain is idiopathic; there is no known cause. As a result, making a precise diagnosis can be difficult.

Controversies

Classic education holds that intervertebral disks have no sensory nerve fibers. In reality, sensory nerves extend into the disk over at least one-third the radius of the outer rim, the annulus fibrosus. In the clinical setting, one cannot tell whether low back pain is coming solely from the irritation of these nerves. However, this etiology is always a possibility, even if MRI and CT scans show no damage. These nerves can be injured at a microscopic level that is undetectable on standard tests.

When evaluating nontraumatic back pain, consider disease processes, including SCI, which can produce severely debilitating lesions (Table 34-10). In the absence of trauma, assess the patient's report of low back pain with the anatomy and neurophysiology of the spine and spinal cord in mind. Pay particular attention to the patient's medications; patients with chronic back pain or tumors may require high dosages of narcotic agents to control their intense pain.

Pain may result from **strain** or **sprain** of paravertebral muscles and supporting ligamentous structures without

Table 34-10	Common Causes of Low Back Pain
Muscle or ligament strains	
Fractures	
Osteomyelitis—bone infection	
Degenerative joint/disk disease	
Spondylolysis	
Bursitis/synovitis	
Disk herniation	
Tumor	

© Jones & Bartlett Learning.

significant injury to nerve elements. Older adult patients (especially women) with a history of osteoporosis are at high risk for spontaneous compression fractures of the spine. These typically stable fractures are not associated with SCI. Tumors in the spine from a variety of metastatic carcinomas can cause pathologic spine fractures, with extension of bone fragments or the tumor itself into the spinal canal causing SCI.

Your assessment of the patient with low back pain should consist of examination of the ABCDEs; obtaining a history, including a SAMPLE history; and evaluation of pain levels. A typical finding with a spinal disorder is that pain diminishes with decreased movement. A patient who is writhing in pain suggests a more severe underlying process, such as abdominal aortic aneurysm or epidural abscess.

Your physical exam of the back should include a search for contusions or abrasions consistent with trauma, warmth or drainage suggesting infection, and point tenderness with percussion along the spine, indicating possible bacterial infection. Pain increasing with leg straightening while supine may indicate a low back herniated disk, particularly if the pain radiates to below knee level.

Any patient with a suspected nontraumatic spinal disorder should undergo a neurologic and function examination before movement. When transporting patients with scoliosis or kyphosis, you may need to adapt your transport modalities.

Words of Wisdom

Spondylolysis is a structural defect of the spine involving the lamina or vertebral arch. It usually occurs between the superior and inferior articulating facets. In most people, it is congenital and therefore chronic. A radiograph is necessary to confirm spondylolysis.

Degenerative disk disease is common in patients older than 50 years. Over time, biomechanical alteration of the intervertebral disk will result in loss of height and reduction of the shock-absorbing property of the disk. Significant narrowing may result in variable segment stability.

Disk herniation may be caused by some degree of trauma in patients with preexisting disk degeneration. It typically affects men between ages 30 and 50 years and may result from poor lifting technique. Herniation most often occurs at L4 to L5 and L5 to S1 but also may occur in C5 to C6 and C6 to C7. Patients will present with pain, usually with straining; they may have spinal tenderness and often have limited range of motion. Patients may have alterations in sensation and motor functions as well. Cervical herniations may present with upper extremity pain or paresthesias that worsen with neck motion. Motor weakness may also result from spinal cord compression.

Words of Wisdom

Some patients with acute low back spasm are literally paralyzed with pain. To move them, use a scoop stretcher that fits under the patient. IV administration of diazepam may be extremely helpful in relieving severe muscle spasm.

Definitive diagnosis of back pain may require multiple types of radiographic imaging. Prehospital management of low back pain in the absence of trauma is primarily palliative, directed at decreasing pain or discomfort with movement.

▶ Spinal Stenosis

Spinal stenosis is a narrowing of the spinal canal that can occur at single or multiple levels, causing compression of exiting nerve roots. Patients with spinal stenosis will report pain radiating from the back into the legs or arms, usually aggravated by prolonged standing and extension and relieved by rest and spinal flexion. These patients should be placed in a comfortable position if transport is required.

■ Injury Prevention

Prevention of head and spine trauma includes general safety measures that can decrease overall risk of injury. Driving safely and always wearing seat belts can reduce the risk of spinal injury, a multitude of other injuries, and death. Motorcycles and all-terrain vehicles are not safe for multiple riders; the operator should be the only rider. Finally, adhering to posted safety alerts, such as those about safe diving at swimming pools, can also help reduce injuries.

YOU are the Paramedic · SUMMARY

1. What should you consider doing?

If you have not already done so, it would be appropriate to request additional resources because this patient's condition is critical and he will require spinal immobilization.

2. What safety concerns do you have?

Dim lighting, slick surfaces, and the swimming pool all are causes for concern. The presence of an emotional crowd should increase your situational awareness. Although the police might have deemed the scene safe, you and your partner must remain aware of your surroundings.

3. What injuries do you suspect?

Given the nature of the scene and the primary survey of your patient, it is highly likely that he has a high cervical spine fracture.

4. What interventions are required?

Airway stabilization and manual stabilization are immediately indicated. If the patient cannot oxygenate well, then you should use a bag-mask device with high-flow oxygen and airway adjuncts. As with any call, start with the basics.

5. Why is the patient bradycardic and hypotensive?

The patient has neurogenic shock. An insult to the cervical spine has disrupted communication between the brain and the body. The sympathetic nervous system has been blocked, resulting in vasodilation and bradycardia.

6. How would you manage these vital signs?

Establish IV access with two 18-gauge catheters. Administer a 20 mL/kg bolus of crystalloids, such as normal saline or lactated Ringer. Don't be surprised if this fails to improve the patient's blood pressure; these patients usually require vasopressors, such as dopamine or norepinephrine. To improve cardiac effects, consider administering atropine or performing transcutaneous pacing. The routine use of IV glucocorticoids, such as methylprednisolone (Solu-Medrol), is controversial. As with all interventions, follow local protocols.

YOU are the Paramedic SUMMARY (continued)

7. What other immediate treatments are required?

The patient is at high risk for hypothermia, not only because of the blood vessel dilation associated with the lack of sympathetic tone, but also because he is wet and naked. Dry the patient, cover him with blankets, and ensure the ambulance is warm. Hypothermia prevents hemoglobin from off-loading oxygen, worsening the patient's condition.

8. Based on these events, what other factors could complicate the patient's outcome?

The presence of alcohol and possibly drugs not only clouds the patient's judgment, but can also reduce the patient's awareness of all injuries. Therefore, the information you obtain from the patient history is most likely unreliable. In addition, with all shallow-water diving incidents, you must consider head injuries as well as spinal trauma.

EMS Patient Care Report (PCR)

Date: 06-01-18	**Incident No.:** 7728		**Nature of Call:** Diving injury	**Location:** Clarke County Swimming Pool	
Dispatched: 0130	**En Route:** 0133	**At Scene:** 0135	**Transport:** 0147	**At Hospital:** 0203	**In Service:** 0218

Patient Information

Age: 19 **Sex:** M **Weight (in kg [lb]):** 75 kg (165 lb)	**Allergies:** No known drug allergies **Medications:** None **Past Medical History:** None **Chief Complaint:** Unresponsive

Vital Signs

Time: 0136	**BP:** Not yet obtained	**Pulse:** Slow, weak, radial	**Respirations:** Snoring, rapid, shallow	**Spo₂:** Not yet obtained
Time: 0140	**BP:** 80/54	**Pulse:** 50	**Respirations:** Shallow, labored	**Spo₂:** 86%
Time: 0150	**BP:** 70/42	**Pulse:** 42	**Respirations:** Assisted	**Spo₂:** None
Time: 0155	**BP:** 70/46	**Pulse:** 42	**Respirations:** Assisted	**Spo₂:** None
Time: 0200	**BP:** 70/42	**Pulse:** 42	**Respirations:** Assisted	**Spo₂:** None

EMS Treatment (circle all that apply)

Oxygen @ _15_ L/min via (circle one): NC NRM (**Bag-mask device** With high-flow oxygen)	(**Assisted Ventilation**)	(**Airway Adjunct:** OPA followed by ET tube)	**CPR**
Defibrillation	(**Bleeding Control:** No external hemorrhage noted)	(**Bandaging:** 4 × 4 to head abrasion)	(**Splinting:** Long backboard) **Other:**

Narrative
Dispatched to an unknown incident at Clarke County Swimming Pool. Arrived to find 19-year-old man lying faceup next to the pool in obvious respiratory distress. According to witnesses, pt dove headfirst into the shallow end of the pool; under water for about 30 seconds; pt was pulled from the water by witnesses; according to witnesses, pt consumed "a couple beers" at about 2400 hours; no known drug allergies, no known PMH. Pt unresponsive; skin, wet/flushed. Addressed ABCDEs with cervical spine precautions. Suspect possible head injury/c-spine injury with neurogenic shock. Called for additional assistance. HEENT—quarter-sized abrasion to right forehead, no major bleeding, otherwise atraumatic. PERRLA (sluggish) 4 mm. No tracheal deviation or JVD. Chest accessory muscle use present. Breath sounds diminished bilaterally, equal excursion, no apparent trauma. Abdomen soft with no distention/rigidity. Pelvis stable. Loss of bowel and bladder. No motor function or reflexes present in upper or lower extremities. Weak, slow pulses present in upper extremities only. Back—no obvious injuries noted. Immobilized on LSB with PMS assessed before and after with no changes. Moved to ambulance. Vital signs as noted above. ETI with 8.0-mm ET tube depth of 21 at the teeth. Two 18-gauge IVs with 250-mL NS bolus administered. Released to trauma center staff.**End of report**

Prep Kit

▶ Ready for Review

- The two primary divisions of insult are head trauma and spinal cord injury.
- *Head trauma* refers to both head injuries and traumatic brain injuries.
- *Head injury* refers to traumatic insult to the head that may result in injury to the soft tissues of the scalp or bony structures of the head and skull, not including the face.
- *Traumatic brain injury* (TBI) refers to impairment of brain function caused by an external force that may involve physical, intellectual, emotional, social, and vocational changes.
- Important anatomic and physiologic structures related to the head and spine include the scalp, the skull, the cranial vault, the brain, the meninges, the spine, the spinal cord, and the spinal nerves.
- The cranial vault creates a nondistensible container for the brain, cerebrospinal fluid, and blood. With an expanding mass, such as a hematoma, the skull cannot expand, and intracranial pressure increases.
- Remember, the patient may have a head injury, spine injury, or both.

- Identifying the type of brain injury in the prehospital setting is almost impossible. Recognizing the presence of brain injury and beginning immediate care is more important than identifying the type.
- A patient with a TBI is presumed to have a cervical spine injury until proven otherwise.
- Certain mechanisms of injury suggest possible spinal injury. Memorize this list and use it to help determine whether the patient should be placed in full spinal immobilization.
- When assessing a patient with a head or spine injury, someone must manually stabilize the cervical spine in a neutral, in-line position as you conduct your assessment. You may apply a cervical collar during assessment if your findings require it. Proper sizing of the cervical collar is crucial. Application of the cervical collar is considered a treatment intervention. Failure to assess pulse, motor, and sensory function prior to application of this medical device could potentially alter your baseline assessment.
- You must maintain manual stabilization during all airway management procedures, including advanced airway management.
- When a patient's ventilations are inadequate, ventilate the patient to maintain an ETCO$_2$ of 35 to 40 mm Hg. In a patient with brain injury, avoid

Prep Kit (continued)

routine hyperventilation; hyperventilation could result in reduced oxygen delivery to the brain and cause cerebral edema. The Brain Trauma Foundation recommends hyperventilation only if signs of cerebral herniation are present.

- Control major bleeding without placing pressure on a potential underlying fracture. Provide fluid resuscitation, but restrict IV fluids in patients with severe closed head injuries to minimize cerebral edema; however, avoid hypotension.

- Placement of the patient on a backboard may be required depending on your findings and your local protocol. If indicated, apply the backboard to a critical patient at the end of your primary survey to enable rapid transport; complete the rest of the assessment en route. In the noncritical patient, apply the backboard after your secondary assessment.

- Time on the backboard should be kept to a minimum; skin breakdown can be a complication of treatment of spinal cord injury. It is crucial to properly pad the backboarded patient and for the emergency department to promptly remove the patient from the backboard. Failure to take these measures will increase the patient's pain and the probability that the patient will develop pressure sores. If your service has alternative devices that can offer improved comfort, such as a vacuum mattress, then you should learn how and when to use them.

- When taking the history of a patient with a head or spine injury, it is important to assess the reliability of the patient as a historian. Perform a physical exam, including a neurologic exam, as part of your secondary assessment.

- You can estimate the severity of intracranial pressure (ICP) based on the patient's clinical presentation. Learn these clinical indicators, and use serial Glasgow Coma Scale scores and pupillary assessments to monitor the progression of ICP.

- Head injuries include scalp injuries, skull fractures (linear, depressed, basilar, and open), TBI and diffuse brain injuries (cerebral concussion and diffuse axonal injury), and focal brain injuries (cerebral contusion and intracranial hemorrhage).

- Do not become distracted by scalp lacerations. Once life threats are managed, evaluate the wound for continued bleeding. With isolated fractures not involving suspected skull fracture, apply direct pressure and use a pressure dressing or hemostatic agent if required.

- Normal intracranial pressure (ICP) is 5 to 15 mm Hg in adults. Increased ICP can squeeze the brain against the interior of the skull and/or press it into sharp edges within the cranium. If severely increased ICP is not promptly treated, cerebral herniation will occur.

- Cerebral perfusion pressure is the pressure of blood flowing through the brain; it is the difference between the mean arterial pressure and the ICP.

- A *single* drop in cerebral perfusion pressure below 60 mm Hg *doubles* the risk of death in an adult patient with a brain injury. You must have a high index of suspicion and watch for subtle signs and symptoms.

- Concussion recommendations continue to evolve, and you will certainly encounter patients with concussions during your practice as a paramedic. As with all patients, address life-threatening conditions, and place the patient in spinal immobilization if indicated. In a sports setting, if you do not believe a patient should return to play, express your concerns and thoroughly explain the risks.

- Second impact syndrome is a rare but sometimes fatal result of receiving a second concussion while still recovering from an earlier one. Postconcussion syndrome is another condition that may occur. Though its mortality rate is not as high, it requires evaluation by a physician. These conditions underscore the importance of obtaining a thorough patient history and maintaining a high index of suspicion.

- Seizures may occur in a patient with brain injury and can aggravate ICP and cause or worsen cerebral ischemia. Treat seizures with a benzodiazepine (such as diazepam or lorazepam).

- Spinal cord injuries (SCIs) are among the most devastating injuries encountered by prehospital providers. To decipher the often subtle findings associated with SCI, you need to understand the form and function of spinal anatomy.

- Acute injuries of the spine are classified according to the associated mechanism, location, and stability of injury.

- Vertebral fractures can occur with or without associated SCI.

- Stable fractures typically involve only a single column and pose a lower risk to the spinal cord.

- A distracting injury is not the same as a distraction injury. A distracting injury is an injury to another body part or system (such as a femur fracture) that causes such significant pain and discomfort that it sufficiently distracts the patient's attention, rendering him or her unreliable. A distraction injury is one in which there is a physical distraction mechanism that causes separation of spinal column elements and potential SCI.

- Primary spinal cord injury occurs at the moment of impact. Secondary spinal cord injury occurs

Prep Kit (continued)

when multiple factors permit a progression of the primary spinal cord injury. The ensuing cascade of inflammatory responses may result in further deterioration.

- Limiting the progression of secondary spinal cord injury is a major goal of prehospital management of spinal cord injury.
- Spinal immobilization is a controversial topic in prehospital medicine. Historically, preventive immobilization of all trauma patients with certain mechanisms of injury was routine. As scientific studies began to show potential negative effects of backboards and cervical collars, selective immobilization—the practice of immobilizing only patients with clinical indications of spinal injury—began to be implemented. Debate continues regarding potential negative consequences of these treatments. The purpose of spinal immobilization is to prevent secondary damage to the spinal cord—not to completely immobilize the spine and prevent micromotion at the site of any injury. Remember, your actions or inactions have direct consequences for the patient and the receiving facility. Your protocols may require you to evaluate the patient's clinical indicators to decide whether to implement spinal immobilization.
- When you perform full spinal immobilization, it is important to use best practices. How you immobilize the patient matters. Hyperextension of the cervical spine that can occur during immobilization procedures can result in neurologic deficit; you must immobilize the patient in a neutral position. Correct cervical collar size is crucial; you must measure each patient for collar size. Pad behind the occiput, lumbar area, and knees to reduce pain and pressure. Use blanket rolls between the legs and along both sides of the patient's body to fill voids under the straps, help restrict motion, and increase patient comfort. There should be no gaps between the patient and the backboard, or beneath the straps. Strapping method is also important; the patient must be strapped so that he or she does not move laterally.
- Pharmacotherapy for SCI includes short-acting, reversible sedatives for the acute patient after a correctible cause of agitation has been excluded.
- Back pain is a common presenting complaint for patients who call for EMS. Obtain the patient's history and perform a physical exam. Any patient with a suspected nontraumatic spinal disorder should undergo a neurologic evaluation.

▶ Vital Vocabulary

anterior cord syndrome A condition that occurs with flexion injuries or fractures, resulting in the displacement of bony fragments into the anterior portion of the spinal cord. Findings include paralysis below the level of the insult and loss of pain, temperature, and touch perception.

anterograde (posttraumatic) amnesia Loss of memory of events that occurred after the injury.

arachnoid The middle membrane of the three meninges that enclose the brain and spinal cord.

autonomic dysreflexia A late, life-threatening complication of spinal cord injury in which stimulation of the sympathetic nervous system below the level of injury generates a massive, uninhibited, uncompensated cardiovascular response; also known as autonomic hyperreflexia.

autoregulation An increase in mean arterial pressure to compensate for decreased cerebral perfusion pressure; compensatory physiologic response that occurs in an effort to shunt blood to the brain; manifests clinically as hypertension.

axon A long, slender extension of a neuron (nerve cell) that conducts electrical impulses away from the neuronal soma.

Babinski reflex Upward movement of the toe(s) in response to stimulation to the sole of the foot. Under normal circumstances, the toe(s) move downward.

basilar skull fracture Fracture generally resulting from the extension of a linear fracture into the base of the skull; usually occurs after a diffuse impact to the head (as in a fall or motor vehicle crash) and can be difficult to diagnose, even with radiography.

Battle sign Bruising over the mastoid bone behind the ear often seen after a basilar skull fracture; also called retroauricular ecchymosis.

Biot (ataxic) respirations Irregular pattern, rate, and depth of respirations with intermittent periods of apnea; result from increased intracranial pressure.

brainstem The midbrain, pons, and medulla, collectively.

Brown-Séquard syndrome A condition associated with penetrating trauma and characterized by hemisection of the spinal cord and complete damage to all spinal tracts on the involved side.

cauda equina The location where the spinal cord separates; composed of nerve roots.

cauda equina syndrome A neurologic condition caused by compression of the bundle of nerve roots located at the end of the spinal cord.

Prep Kit (continued)

central cord syndrome A condition resulting from hyperextension injuries to the cervical area that damage the dorsal column of the spinal cord; characterized by hemorrhage or edema. Findings include greater loss of function in the upper extremities, with variable sensory loss of pain and temperature.

central neurogenic hyperventilation Deep, rapid respirations; similar to Kussmaul, but without an acetone breath odor; commonly seen after brainstem injury.

cerebellum The brain region essential in coordinating muscle movements in the body; also called the athlete's brain.

cerebral concussion Injury that occurs when the brain is jarred around in the skull; a mild diffuse brain injury that does not result in structural damage or permanent neurologic impairment.

cerebral contusion A focal brain injury in which brain tissue is bruised and damaged in a defined area.

cerebral cortex The largest portion of the cerebrum; regulates voluntary skeletal movement and a person's level of awareness—a part of consciousness.

cerebral edema Excessive fluid in the brain; swelling of the brain.

cerebral perfusion pressure (CPP) The pressure of blood flow through the brain; the difference between the mean arterial pressure and intracranial pressure.

cerebrospinal fluid (CSF) Fluid produced in the ventricles of the brain that flows in the subarachnoid space and bathes the meninges.

cerebrum The largest portion of the brain; responsible for higher functions, such as reasoning; divided into right and left hemispheres, or halves.

Cheyne-Stokes respirations A gradually increasing rate and depth of respirations followed by a gradual decrease with intermittent periods of apnea; associated with brainstem insult.

complete spinal cord injury Total disruption of all spinal cord tracts, with permanent loss of all cord-mediated functions below the level of injury.

coup-contrecoup injury Dual impacting of the brain into the skull. Coup injury occurs at the point of impact; contrecoup injury occurs on the opposite side of impact, as the brain rebounds.

cranial vault The bones that encase and protect the brain: the parietal, temporal, frontal, occipital, sphenoid, and ethmoid bones; also called the cranium or skull.

critical minimum threshold Minimum cerebral perfusion pressure required to adequately perfuse the brain; 60 mm Hg in the adult.

Cushing triad Hypertension (with a widening pulse pressure), bradycardia, and irregular respirations; classic trio of findings associated with increased intracranial pressure.

decerebrate (extensor) posturing Abnormal posture characterized by extension of the arms and legs; indicates pressure on the brainstem.

decorticate (flexor) posturing Abnormal posture characterized by flexion of the arms and extension of the legs; indicates pressure on the brainstem.

depressed skull fracture Fracture caused by high-energy direct trauma applied to a small surface area of the skull with a blunt object (such as a baseball bat striking the head); commonly accompanied by bony fragments driven into the brain, causing further injury.

dermatome An area of the body innervated by sensor components of spinal nerves.

diffuse axonal injury (DAI) Diffuse brain injury that is caused by stretching, shearing, or tearing of nerve fibers with consequent axonal damage.

diffuse brain injury Any injury that affects the entire brain.

dura mater The outermost layer of the three meninges that enclose the brain and spinal cord; the toughest meningeal layer.

epidural hematoma An accumulation of blood between the skull and dura.

facet joint The joint on which each vertebra articulates with adjacent vertebrae.

flexion injury A type of injury that results from forward movement of the head, typically as the result of rapid deceleration, such as in a vehicle crash, or with a direct blow to the occiput.

focal brain injury A specific, grossly observable brain injury.

frontal lobe The portion of the brain that is important in voluntary motor actions and personality traits.

hangman's fracture The most classic distraction injury, which occurs when a person is hanged by the neck. Bending and fractures occur at the C1 to C2 region, which quickly tear the spinal cord.

head injury A traumatic insult to the head that may result in injury to soft tissue of the scalp and bony structures of the head and skull, not including the face.

head trauma A general term that includes both head injuries and traumatic brain injuries.

herniation A process in which tissue is forced out of its normal position, such as when the brain is forced from the cranial vault, either through the foramen magnum or over the tentorium.

hyperesthesia Hyperacute pain to touch.

hyperextension Extension of a limb or other body part beyond its usual range of motion.

Prep Kit (continued)

hyperpyrexia A high body temperature.

incomplete spinal cord injury Spinal cord injury in which there is some degree of cord-mediated function. Initial dysfunction may be temporary and there may be potential for recovery.

intracerebral hematoma Bleeding within the brain tissue (parenchyma) itself; also called an intraparenchymal hematoma.

intracranial pressure (ICP) The pressure within the cranial vault; normally 0 to 15 mm Hg in adults.

lamina Posterior arch of the vertebral bone; arises from the posterior pedicles and fuses to form the posterior spinous processes.

limbic system Structures within the cerebrum and diencephalon that influence emotions, motivation, mood, and sensations of pain and pleasure.

linear skull fracture A fracture that usually occurs in the temporal-parietal region of the skull; not associated with skull deformity; accounts for 80% of skull fractures; also called nondisplaced skull fracture.

mean arterial pressure (MAP) The average (or mean) pressure against the arterial wall during a cardiac cycle.

meninges A set of three tough membranes—the dura mater, arachnoid, and pia mater—that encloses the entire brain and spinal cord.

myotome A region of the body innervated by the motor components of spinal nerves.

nerve root injury Injury to a nerve at the level of the spinal cord.

neurogenic shock Shock caused by massive blood vessel dilation and pooling of blood in the peripheral vessels, so that adequate perfusion cannot be maintained.

neuronal soma The body of a neuron (nerve cell).

occipital lobe The portion of the brain responsible for processing visual information.

parasympathetic nervous system Subdivision of the autonomic nervous system; involved in control of involuntary, vegetative functions; mediated largely by the vagus nerve through the chemical acetylcholine.

parietal lobe The portion of the brain that receives and evaluates most sensory information, except smell, hearing, and vision.

pedicles Thick lateral bony struts that connect the vertebral body with the spinous and transverse processes and make up the lateral and posterior portions of the spinal foramen.

periorbital ecchymosis Bruising under or around the orbits that is commonly seen after a basilar skull fracture; also called raccoon eyes.

peripheral nerve injury Injury to a nerve anywhere in the body outside the spinal cord.

petechial hemorrhage A pinpoint red dot in the sclera of the eye.

pia mater The innermost and thinnest of the three meninges that enclose the brain and spinal cord; rests directly on the brain and spinal cord.

plexus A cluster of nerve roots that permits peripheral nerve roots to rejoin and function as a group.

posterior cord syndrome A condition associated with extension injuries in which there is isolated injury to the dorsal portion of the spinal cord. The condition is characterized by decreased sensation to light touch, proprioception, and vibration. Most other motor and sensory functions are unaffected.

primary brain injury Injury to the brain and its associated structures that is a direct result of impact to the head.

primary spinal cord injury Injury to the spinal cord that is a direct result of trauma (eg, spinal cord transection from penetrating trauma or displacement of ligaments and bone fragments, resulting in cord compression).

proprioception The ability to perceive the position and movement of one's body or limbs.

raccoon eyes Bruising under or around the orbits that is commonly seen after a basilar skull fracture; also called periorbital ecchymosis.

reticular activating system (RAS) Located in the upper brainstem; responsible for maintenance of consciousness, specifically one's level of arousal.

retrograde amnesia Loss of memory of events that occurred before the injury.

rotation-flexion injury A type of injury typically resulting from high acceleration forces; can result in a stable unilateral facet dislocation in the cervical spine.

secondary brain injury The aftereffects of the primary injury; includes abnormal processes such as cerebral edema, increased intracranial pressure, cerebral ischemia and hypoxia, and infection. Onset is often delayed after the primary brain injury.

secondary spinal cord injury Injury to the spinal cord, thought to be the result of multiple factors that result in a progression of inflammatory responses from primary spinal cord injury.

spinal shock The temporary local neurologic condition that occurs immediately after spinal trauma. Spinal cord swelling and edema begin immediately after injury, causing severe pain and possible paralysis.

spinal stenosis Narrowing of the spinal canal, causing compression of exiting nerve roots and pain radiating into the legs or arms.

Prep Kit (continued)

sprain Stretching or tearing of ligaments.

strain Stretching or tearing of muscle or tendon.

subarachnoid hemorrhage Bleeding into the subarachnoid space, where the cerebrospinal fluid circulates.

subdural hematoma An accumulation of blood beneath the dura but outside the brain.

subgaleal hemorrhage Bleeding between the periosteum of the skull and the galea aponeurosis.

subluxation A partial dislocation.

supragaleal hematoma Bleeding between the subgaleal area of the skull and the galea aponeurosis.

sympathetic nervous system Subdivision of the autonomic nervous system that governs the body's fight-or-flight reactions by inducing smooth muscle contraction or relaxation of the blood vessels and bronchioles.

temporal lobe The portion of the brain that has an important role in hearing and memory.

tentorium A structure that separates the cerebral hemispheres from the cerebellum and brainstem.

traumatic brain injury (TBI) An impairment of brain function caused by an external force that may involve physical, intellectual, emotional, social, and vocational changes.

trismus Clenched teeth as a result of spasm of the jaw muscles.

vertebral body Anterior weight-bearing structure in the spine made of cancellous bone and surrounded by a layer of hard, compact bone that provides support and stability.

vertical compression A type of injury typically resulting from a direct blow to the crown of the head or rapid deceleration from a fall, with the force moving through the feet, legs, and pelvis, possibly causing a burst fracture or disk herniation.

▶ References

1. Dawodu ST, Yadav RR. Traumatic brain injury (TBI)—definition and pathophysiology. http://emedicine.medscape.com/article/326510. Updated September 22, 2015. Accessed March 27, 2017.
2. Menon DK, Schwab K, Wright DW, Maas AI. Position statement: definition of traumatic brain injury. *Arch Phys Med Rehabil.* 2010;91(11):1637-1640.
3. Prosser JD, Vender JR, Solares CA. Traumatic cerebrospinal fluid leaks. *Otolaryngol Clin N Am.* 2011;44(4):857-873.
4. Centers for Disease Control and Prevention. Guidelines for field triage of injured patients: recommendations of the National Expert Panel on Field Triage, 2011. *Morb Mortal Wkly Rep.* 2012;61(1).
5. Borius PY, Gouader I, Bousquet P, Draper L, Roux FE. Cervical spine injuries resulting from diving accidents in swimming pools: outcome of 34 patients. *Eur Spine J.* 2010;19(4):552-557.
6. Badjatia N, Carney N, Crocco T, et al. Guidelines for prehospital management of traumatic brain injury. 2nd ed. *Prehosp Emerg Care.* 2008;12(suppl 1):S1-S52.
7. Bucher J, Koyfman A. Intubation of the neurologically injured patient. *J Emerg Med.* 2015;49(6):920-927.
8. El-Orbany M, Connolly L. Rapid sequence induction and intubation. *Anesth Analg.* 2010;110(5):1318-1325.
9. Kuzak N, Harrison D, Zed P. Use of lidocaine and fentanyl premedication for neuroprotective rapid sequence intubation in the emergency department. *Can J Emerg Med.* 2006;8(2):80-84.
10. Salhi B, Stettner E. In defense of the use of lidocaine in rapid sequence intubation. *Ann Emerg Med.* 2007;49(1):84-86.
11. Vaillancourt C, Kapur A. Opposition to the use of lidocaine in rapid sequence intubation. *Ann Emerg Med.* 2007;49(1):86-87.
12. Zeiler FA, Sader N, Kazina CJ. The impact of intravenous lidocaine on ICP in neurologic illness: A systematic review. *Crit Care Res Pract.* 2015;15.
13. Arabi YM, Haddad SH. Critical care management of severe traumatic brain injury in adults. *Scand J Trauma Resusc Emerg Med.* 2012;20(12).
14. Carney N, Totten AM, O'Reilly C, et al. Guidelines for the management of severe traumatic brain injury, fourth edition. *Neurosurgery.* 2016;20:1-10.
15. Wood G, Boucher B. *PSAP-VII—Neurology and Psychiatry: Management of Acute Traumatic Brain Injury.* 7th ed. Book 10. Lenexa, KS: American College of Clinical Pharmacy; 2012.
16. Bullock R, Povlishock J. Guidelines for the management of severe traumatic brain injury. 3rd ed. *J Neurotrauma.* 2016;23(suppl 1):S1-S106.
17. Popa C, Popa F, Grigorean V, et al. Vascular dysfunctions following spinal cord injury. *J Med Life.* 2010;3(3):275-285.
18. Alvis-Miranda HR, Castellar-Leones SM, Moscote-Salazar LR. Intravenous fluid therapy in traumatic brain injury and decompressive craniectomy. *Bull Emerg Trauma.* 2014;2(1):3-14.
19. Brain Trauma Foundation. *Guidelines for the Management of Severe Traumatic Brain Injury.* Brain Trauma Foundation website. https://braintrauma .org/uploads/03/12/Guidelines_for_Management _of_Severe_TBI_4th_Edition.pdf. Published September 2016. Accessed March 24, 2017.
20. Kulesza B, Nogalski A, Kulesza T, Prystupa A. Prognostic factors in traumatic brain injury and their association with outcome. *J Pre-Clin Clin Res.* 2015;9(2):163-166.
21. Brenner M, Stein DM, Hu PF, Aarabi B, Sheth K, Scalea TM. Traditional systolic blood pressure

Prep Kit (continued)

targets underestimate hypotension-induced secondary brain injury. *J Trauma Acute Care Surg.* 2012;72(5):1135-1139.

22. King K, Olson D. What you should know about neurogenic shock. *Am Nurse Today.* 2007;2(2):36-38.

23. Lam BL, Thompson HS, Corbett JJ. The prevalence of simple anisocoria. *Am J Opthalmol.* July 1987:104(1);69-73.

24. Domeier R, Frederiksen S, Welch K. Prospective performance assessment of an out-of-hospital protocol for selective spine immobilization using clinical spine clearance criteria. *Ann Emerg Med.* 2005;46(2):123-131.

25. Hoffman J, Wolfson A, Todd K, Mower W. Selective cervical spine radiography in blunt trauma: methodology of the National Emergency X-Radiography Utilization Study (NEXUS). *Ann Emerg Med.* 1998;32(4):461-469.

26. National Association of EMS Physicians Position Statement. EMS spinal precautions and the use of the long backboard. *Prehosp Emerg Care.* 2013;17(3):392-393.

27. Berg G, Nyberg S, Harrison P, Baumchen J, Gurss E, Hennes E. Near-infrared spectroscopy measurement of sacral tissue oxygen saturation in healthy volunteers immobilized on rigid spine boards. *Prehosp Emerg Care.* 2010;14(4):419-424.

28. White CC, Domeier RM, Millin MG. EMS spinal precautions and the use of the long backboard: Resource document to the position statement of the National Association of EMS Physicians and the American College of Surgeons Committee on Trauma. *Prehosp Emerg Care.* 2014;18(2):306-314.

29. Rates of TBI-related emergency department visits, hospitalizations, and deaths—United States, 2001–2010. Centers for Disease Control and Prevention website. https://www.cdc.gov /traumaticbraininjury/data/rates.html. Updated January 22, 2016. Accessed March 21, 2017.

30. Traumatic brain injury and concussion. TBI: get the facts. Centers for Disease Control and Prevention website. http://www.cdc.gov/traumaticbraininjury /get_the_facts.html. Updated March 23, 2017. Accessed March 24, 2017.

31. Chattopadhyay S, Tripathi C. Skull fracture and hemorrhage pattern among fatal and nonfatal head injury assault victims—a critical analysis. *J Inj Violen Res.* 2010;2(2):99-103.

32. Turnage B, Maull K. Scalp laceration: an obvious 'occult' cause of shock. *South Med J.* 2000;93(3):265-266.

33. Qureshi N, Harsh I, Nosko M. Skull fracture: background. Medscape website. http://emedicine. medscape.com/article/248108. Updated May 26, 2016. Accessed May 3, 2016.

34. Levine J, Kumar M. Traumatic brain injury. 2013 Neurocritical Care Society Practice Update. http:// citeseerx.ist.psu.edu/viewdoc/download?doi

=10.1.1.676.6398&rep=rep1&type=pdf. Published 2013. Accessed May 3, 2016.

35. McCrory P, Meeuwisse W, Dvorak J, et al. Consensus statement on concussion in sport—the 5th international conference on concussion in sport held in Berline, October 2016. BMJ Journals website. http://bjsm.bmj.com/content/early/2017/04/26 /bjsports-2017-097699. Accessed May 23, 2017.

36. Scorza K, Raleigh M, O'Connor F. Current concepts in concussion: evaluation and management. *Am Fam Physician.* 2012;85(2):123-132.

37. Giza C, Kutcher J, Ashwal S, et al. Summary of evidence-based guideline update: Evaluation and management of concussion in sports: Report of the Guideline Development Subcommittee of the American Academy of Neurology. *Neurology.* 2013;80(24):2250-2257.

38. HEADS UP: managing return to activities. Centers for Disease Control and Prevention website. http://www.cdc.gov/headsup/providers/return_to _activities.html. Updated February 8, 2016. Accessed March 27, 2017.

39. National Federation of State High School Associations (NFHS) Sports Medicine Advisory Committee (SMAC). *Suggested Guidelines for Management of Concussion in Sports.* NFHS website https://www.nfhs.org/sports-resource-content /suggested-guidelines-for-management-of -concussion-in-sports/. February 16, 2017. Accessed March 27, 2017.

40. Carney N, Ghajar J, Jagoda A, et al. Concussion guidelines step 1. *Neurosurgery.* 2014;75:S3-S15.

41. Bowen A. Second impact syndrome: a rare, catastrophic, preventable complication of concussion in young athletes. *J Emerg Nurs.* 2003;29(3):287-289.

42. Dessy A, Rasouli J, Choudhri T. Second impact syndrome. *Neurosurg Q.* 2015;25(3):423-426.

43. Bey T, Ostick B. Second impact syndrome. *West J Emerg Med.* 2009;10(1):6-10.

44. Wetjen N, Pichelmann M, Atkinson J. Second impact syndrome: concussion and second injury brain complications. *J Am Coll Surg.* 2010;211(4):553-557.

45. Zhang P, Zhu S, Li Y, et al. Quantitative proteomics analysis to identify diffuse axonal injury biomarkers in rats using iTRAQ coupled LC–MS/MS. *J Proteomics.* 2016;133:93-99.

46. Moenninghoff C, Kraff O, Maderwald S, et al. Diffuse axonal injury at ultra-high field MRI. *PLoS One.* 2015;10(3):e0122329.

47. Li X, Feng D. Diffuse axonal injury: novel insights into detection and treatment. *J Clin Neurosci.* 2009;16(5):614-619.

48. Johnson V, Stewart W, Smith D. Axonal pathology in traumatic brain injury. *Exp Neurol.* 2013; 246:35-43.

Prep Kit (continued)

49. Bir S, Maiti T, Ambekar S, Nanda A. Incidence, hospital costs and in-hospital mortality rates of epidural hematoma in the United States. *Clin Neurol Neurosurg.* 2015;138:99-103.

50. Smith S, Clark M, Nelson J, Heegaard W, Lufkin K, Ruiz E. Emergency department skull trephination for epidural hematoma in patients who are awake but deteriorate rapidly. *J Emerg Med.* 2010;39(3):377-383.

51. Ganz J. The lucid interval associated with epidural bleeding: evolving understanding. *J Neurosurg.* 2013;118(4):739-745.

52. Childs D, Marikar S. Was Natasha Richardson's death avoidable? ABC News website. http://abcnews. go.com/Health/MindMoodNews /story?id=7116273&page=1. Published March 19, 2009. Accessed March 27, 2017.

53. National Association of Emergency Medical Technications. Head trauma. In: *PHTLS: Prehospital Trauma Life Support.* 8th ed. Burlington, MA: Jones and Bartlett Learning; 2016.

54. Kamal R. Acute subdural hematoma. In: Mahapatra A, Kumar R, Kamal R, eds. *Textbook of Traumatic Brain Injury.* New Delhi, India: Jaypee Brothers; 2012.

55. Tien HC, Jung V, Pinto R, Mainprize T, Scales DC, Rizolo SB. Reducing time-to-treatment decreases mortality of trauma patients with acute subdural hematoma. *Ann Surg.* 2011;253(6):1178-1183.

56. Takeuchi S, Takasato Y, Otani N, et al. Subacute subdural hematoma. *Brain Edema XV.* 2013; 118:143-146.

57. Ducruet A, Grobelny B, Zacharia B, et al. The surgical management of chronic subdural hematoma. *Neurosurg Rev.* 2011;35(2):155-169.

58. Nayil K, Ramzan A, Sajad A, et al. Subdural hematomas: an analysis of 1181 Kashmiri patients. *World Neurosurg.* 2012;77(1):103-110.

59. Balser D, Farooq S, Mehmood T, Reyes M, Samadani U. Actual and projected incidence rates for chronic subdural hematomas in United States Veterans Administration and civilian populations. *J Neurosurg.* 2015;123(5):1209-1215.

60. Miranda L, Braxton E, Hobbs J, Quigley M. Chronic subdural hematoma in the elderly: not a benign disease. *J Neurosurg.* 2011;114(1):72-76.

61. Agostoni E, Zagaria M, Longoni M. Headache in subarachnoid hemorrhage and headache attributed to intracranial endovascular procedures. *Neurolog Sci.* 2015;36(suppl 1):67-70.

62. Hankey G, Nelson M. Subarachnoid haemorrhage. *Brit Med J.* 2009;339:b2874-b2874.

63. Thompson HJ, Kirkness CJ, Mitchell PH. Hypothermia and rapid rewarming is associated with worse outcome following traumatic brain injury. *J Trauma Nurs.* 2010;17(4):173-177.

64. Abram S, Bulstrode C. Routine spinal immobilization in trauma patients: what are the advantages and disadvantages? *Surgeon.* 2010;8(4):218-222.

65. Bernhard M, Gries A, Kremer P, Böttiger B. Spinal cord injury (SCI)—prehospital management. *Resuscitation.* 2005;66(2):127-139.

66. Domeier RM, Evans RW, Swor RA, Rivera-Rivera EJ, Frederiksen SM. Prehospital clinical findings associated with spinal injury. *Prehosp Emerg Care.* 1997;1:11-15.

67. National Spinal Cord Injury Statistical Center. Spinal cord injury: facts and figures at a glance. Birmingham, AL: University of Alabama at Birmingham. https://www.nscisc.uab.edu/Public /Facts%202016.pdf. Published 2016. Accessed March 27, 2017.

68. Chin L, Dawodu S, Mesfin F. Spinal cord injuries. Medscape website. http://emedicine.medscape.com /article/793582. Updated October 12, 2016. Accessed March 27, 2017.

69. Schneider G. Anterior spinal cord syndrome after initiation of treatment with atenolol. *J Emerg Med.* 2010;38(5):e49-e52.

70. Molliqaj G, Payer M, Schaller K, Tessitore E. Acute traumatic central cord syndrome: a comprehensive review. *Neurochirurgie.* 2014;60(1-2):5-11.

71. Brodell D, Jain A, Elfar J, Mesfin A. National trends in the management of central cord syndrome: an analysis of 16,134 patients. *Spine J.* 2015;15(3):435-442.

72. Brockmeyer D. AANS/CNS section on pediatric neurological surgery. Neurosurgery://on-call website. http://www.neurosurgery.org/sections /section.aspx?Section=PD&%3BPage=ped_spine. asp. Accessed December 21, 2016.

73. Leshin L. Atlantoaxial instability and Down syndrome. National Down Syndrome Society website. http://www.ndss.org/Resources/Health -Care/Associated-Conditions/Atlantoaxial-Instability -Down-Syndrome. Accessed July 24, 2016.

74. De Lorenzo R. A review of spinal immobilization techniques. *J Emerg Med.* 1996;14(5):603-613.

75. Garfin S, Shackford S, Marshall L, Drummond J. Care of the multiply injured patient with cervical spine injury. *Clin Orthopaed Related Res.* 1989;239:19-29.

76. Domeier R, Evans R, Swor R, et al. The reliability of prehospital clinical evaluation for potential spinal injury is not affected by the mechanism of injury. *Prehosp Emerg Care.* 1999;3(4):332-337.

77. Hauswald M. A re-conceptualisation of acute spinal care. *Emerg Med J.* 2012;30(9):720-723.

78. Hauswald M, Braude D. Spinal immobilization in trauma patients: is it really necessary? *Curr Opin Crit Care.* 2002;8(6):566-570.

79. Hauswald M, Ong G, Tandberg D, Omar Z. Out-of-hospital spinal immobilization: its effect on neurologic injury. *Acad Emerg Med.* 1998;5(3):214-219.

Prep Kit (continued)

80. Hoffman J, Mower W, Wolfson A, Todd K, Zucker M. Validity of a set of clinical criteria to rule out injury to the cervical spine in patients with blunt trauma. *N Engl J Med.* 2000;343(2):94-99.

81. Stroh G, Braude D. Can an out-of-hospital cervical spine clearance protocol identify all patients with injuries? An argument for selective immobilization. *Ann Emerg Med.* 2001;37(6):609-615.

82. Theodore N, Hadley M, Aarabi B, et al. Prehospital cervical spinal immobilization after trauma. *Neurosurgery.* 2013;72:22-34.

83. Levy B, Shubert R, Phelan P, et al. Spinal immobilization after motor vehicle collision in patients who are ambulatory at the scene: is it justified? *Ann Emerg Med.* 1999;34(4):S67.

84. Loza A, McCoy E, Puckett J, Penalosa P. Are immobilization backboards and c-collars needed for patients who are ambulatory at the scene of a motor vehicle accident? *Ann Emerg Med.* 2013;62(4):S144.

85. Haut E, Kalish B, Efron D, et al. Spine immobilization in penetrating trauma: more harm than good? *J Trauma.* 2010;68(1):115-121.

86. Brown J, Bankey P, Sangosanya A, Cheng J, Stassen N, Gestring M. Prehospital spinal immobilization does not appear to be beneficial and may complicate care following gunshot injury to the torso. *J Trauma.* 2009;67(4):774-778.

87. Cooney DR, Wallus H, Asaly M, Wojcik S. Backboard time for patients receiving spinal immobilization by emergency medical services. *Int J Emerg Med.* 2013;6:17.

88. De Lorenzo R, Olson J, Boska M. Optimal positioning for cervical immobilization. *Ann Emerg Med.* 1996;28(3):301-308.

89. Kwan I, Bunn F. Effects of prehospital spinal immobilization: a systematic review of randomized trials on healthy subjects. *Prehosp Disast Med.* 2005;20(1):47-53.

90. Sundstrøm T, Asbjørnsen H, Habiba S, Sunde GA, Wester K. Prehospital use of cervical collars in trauma patients: a critical review. *J Neurotrauma.* 2014;31(6):531-540.

91. Hadley M, Walters B. *Guidelines for the management of acute cervical spine and spinal cord injuries.* Section on Disorders of the Spine and Peripheral Nerves of the American Association of Neurological Surgeons and the Congress of Neurological Surgeons. http://www.aans.org/Education%20and%20Meetings/~/media/Files/Education%20and%20Meetingf/Clinical%20Guidelines/TraumaGuidelines.ashx. Accessed March 27, 2017.

92. Domeier R. Indications for prehospital spinal immobilization. *Prehosp Emerg Care.* 1999;3(3):251-253.

93. Blackwell TH. Prehospital care. *Emerg Med Clin North Am.* 1993;11(1):1-14.

94. Hauswald M. A re-conceptualisation of acute spinal care. *Emerg Med J.* 2013;30(9):720–723.

95. White CC 4th, Domeier RM, Millin MG. Standards and Clinical Practice Committee, National Association of EMS Physicians. EMS spinal precautions and the use of the long backboard - resource document to the position statement of the National Association of EMS Physicians and the American College of Surgeons Committee on Trauma. *Prehosp Emerg Care.* 2014;18(2):306-314.

96. Barney RN, Cordell WH, Miller E. Pain associated with immobilization on rigid spine boards. *Ann Emerg Med.* 1989;18:918.

97. Lerner EB, Billittier AJ 4th, Moscati RM. The effects of neutral positioning with and without padding on spinal immobilization of healthy subjects. *Prehosp Emerg Care.* 1998;2:112–116.

98. Sheerin F, de Frein R. The occipital and sacral pressures experienced by healthy volunteers under spinal immobilization: a trial of three surfaces. *J Emerg Nurs.* 2007;33(5):447–450.

99. Jia X, Kowalski RG, Sciubba DM, Geocadin RG. Critical care of traumatic spinal cord injury. *J Intensive Care Med.* 2013;28(1):12-23.

100. Geisler WO, Wynne-Jones M, Jousse AT. Early management of the patient with trauma to the spinal cord. *Med Serv J Can.* 1966;4:512–523.

101. Bouland A, Jenkins J, Levy M. Assessing attitudes toward spinal immobilization. *J Emerg Med.* 2013;45(4):e117-e125.

102. Peery C, Brice J, White W. Prehospital spinal immobilization and the backboard quality assessment study. *Prehosp Emerg Care.* 2007;11(3):293-297.

103. Dixon M, O'Halloran J, Hannigan A, Keenan S, Cummins N. Confirmation of suboptimal protocols in spinal immobilisation? *Emerg Med J.* 2015;32(12):939-945.

104. Bucher J, Dos Santos F, Frazier D, Merlin MA. Rapid extrication versus the Kendrick extrication device (KED): comparison of techniques used after motor vehicle collisions. *West J Emerg Med.* 2015;16(3):453-458.

105. Hurlbert R, Hadley M, Walters B, et al. Pharmacological therapy for acute spinal cord injury. *Neurosurgery.* 2013;72:93-105.

106. Bledsoe B, Wesley K, Salomone J. High-dose steroids for acute spinal cord injury in emergency medical services. *Prehosp Emerg Care.* 2004;8(3):313-316.

107. Bauman C, Milligan J, Lee F, Riva J. Autonomic dysreflexia in spinal cord injury patients: an overview. *J Can Chiropr Assoc.* 2012;56(4):247-250.

108. Leão P, Figueiredo P. Autonomic hyperreflexia after spinal cord injury managed successfully with intravenous lidocaine: a case report. *Patient Saf Surg.* 2016;10(1).

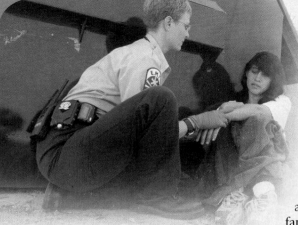

Assessment
in Action

At 0845 hours, you are dispatched for a LifeLine activation at 310 Summit Point Avenue. You arrive to a secured residence with no evidence that it is occupied. You've been here several times for false activations, and after knocking on the door and looking in all of the windows, you see no one and believe this is another false alarm. Just as you are notifying dispatch, a concerned family member runs up to you saying, "I know she's in there! She calls me at 8 o'clock every morning, and I haven't heard from her today."

Because you cannot gain entry to the house, you place a call for law enforcement assistance. The police arrive and break a locked window. As you and your partner enter the home, you hear cries for help. You find an older woman in the upstairs bathroom with a hematoma to her forehead and no other obvious injuries. She tells you she slipped and struck her forehead on the bathtub. Now she's having trouble "making her arms work."

1. Which syndrome is your patient exhibiting?

   A. Anterior cord syndrome
   B. Central cord syndrome
   C. Posterior cord syndrome
   D. Brown-Séquard syndrome

2. What signs and symptoms are unlikely in this patient?

   A. Loss of bowel and bladder functions
   B. Loss of sensation to pain
   C. Loss of sensation to temperature
   D. Loss of proprioception

3. What history may this patient have that could exacerbate her injury?

   A. Acute myocardial infarction
   B. Type 1 diabetes
   C. Type 2 diabetes
   D. Spondylosis

4. The patient's complaint about her arms can be attributed to what kind of disturbance?

   A. Motor fibers
   B. Efferent fibers
   C. Both A and B
   D. Neither A nor B

5. The prognosis for the patient's injury pattern includes:

   A. complete paralysis.
   B. death.
   C. weakness in the hands.
   D. weakness in the feet.

6. This type of injury is typically seen in:

   A. cervical or thoracic fractures.
   B. subluxations.
   C. tears to the supporting ligaments.
   D. pediatric patients.

7. What mechanism of injury is most often associated with this condition?

   A. Hyperflexion
   B. Hyperextension
   C. Axial loading
   D. Lateral displacement

8. How can routine calls place providers and patients at risk?

9. What are the legal implications of forced entry into a home?

10. When you apply spinal precautions to an older adult patient, what considerations should be made?

Chest Trauma

National EMS Education Standard Competencies

Trauma

Integrates assessment findings with principles of epidemiology and pathophysiology to formulate a field impression to implement a comprehensive treatment/disposition plan for an acutely injured patient.

Chest Trauma

Recognition and management of
> Blunt vs. penetrating mechanisms (pp 1789-1790, 1793-1794)
> Open chest wound (pp 1793, 1798-1799)
> Impaled object (pp 1791, 1798)

Pathophysiology, assessment, and management of
> Blunt vs. penetrating mechanisms (pp 1789-1793)
> Hemothorax (pp 1804-1805)
> Pneumothorax (pp 1797-1805)
  • Open (pp 1798-1799, 1804)
  • Simple (pp 1797-1798, 1804)
  • Tension (pp 1800-1804)
> Cardiac tamponade (pp 1806-1808)
> Rib fractures (p 1796)
> Flail chest (pp 1794-1796)
> Commotio cordis (p 1809)
> Traumatic aortic disruption (pp 1809-1810)
> Pulmonary contusion (pp 1805-1806)
> Blunt cardiac injury (p 1808)
> Tracheobronchial disruption (p 1812)
> Diaphragmatic rupture (pp 1811-1812)
> Traumatic asphyxia (pp 1812-1813)

Knowledge Objectives

1. Review the anatomy and physiology of the chest. (pp 1788-1789)
2. Understand the mechanics of ventilation in relation to chest trauma. (p 1790)
3. Describe the assessment process for patients with chest trauma. (pp 1790-1793)
4. Discuss the significance of various signs and symptoms of chest trauma, including changes in pulse rate, dyspnea, jugular venous distention, muffled heart sounds, circulatory changes, and changes in mental status. (pp 1790-1792)
5. Discuss the emergency medical care of a patient with chest trauma. (pp 1793-1794)
6. Discuss the pathophysiology, assessment, and management of chest wall injuries, including flail chest, rib fractures, sternal fractures, and clavicle fractures. (pp 1794-1797)
7. Discuss the pathophysiology, assessment, and management of lung injuries, including simple pneumothorax, open pneumothorax, tension pneumothorax, hemothorax, and pulmonary contusion. (pp 1797-1806)
8. Discuss the pathophysiology, assessment, and management of myocardial injuries, including cardiac tamponade, myocardial contusion, myocardial rupture, and commotio cordis. (pp 1806-1809)
9. Discuss the pathophysiology, assessment, and management of vascular injuries, including traumatic aortic disruption and penetrating wounds of the great vessels. (pp 1809-1811)
10. Discuss the pathophysiology, assessment, and management of other chest injuries, including diaphragmatic injury, esophageal injury, tracheobronchial injuries, and traumatic asphyxia. (pp 1811-1813)

Skills Objectives

1. Describe the steps to take in the assessment of a patient with suspected chest trauma. (pp 1790-1793)
2. Demonstrate the management of a patient with a tension pneumothorax using needle decompression. (pp 1801-1804, Skill Drill 35-1)

▪ Introduction

Trauma accounts for 41 million reported emergency department cases and 2.3 million admissions to the hospital. These types of injuries cost the United States an estimated $671 billion per year in cost of health care and loss of productivity.[1] According to the Centers for Disease Control and Prevention Figure 35-1 , thoracic trauma causes more than 700,000 emergency department visits and more than 18,000 deaths in the United States annually. The National Trauma Data Bank reported 183,813 traumatic incidents involving the thoracic region in 2015, representing 21.36% of all reported traumatic cases.[2] Only traumatic brain injuries account for more deaths among trauma victims. An estimated one in four trauma deaths is directly due to thoracic injuries, and thoracic trauma is a contributing factor in another 25% of trauma patients who die of their injuries.[2]

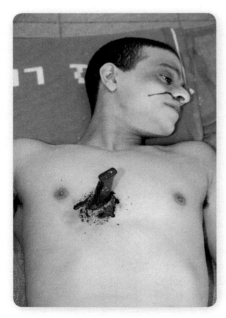

Figure 35-1 Thoracic trauma accounts for a significant number of serious injuries and fatalities.
© PhotoStock-Israel/Alamy.

Given the organs that are housed within the thoracic cavity, it is not surprising that these injuries can be deadly. In addition, the mechanism producing these injuries often involves a great deal of force transmitted to the body.

▪ Anatomy and Physiology Review

The thorax consists of a bony cage overlying some of the most vital organs in the human body. The dimensions of the thorax are defined posteriorly by the thoracic vertebrae and ribs, inferiorly by the diaphragm, anteriorly and laterally by the ribs, and superiorly by the **thoracic inlet** Figure 35-2 .

The dimensions of this area of the body are of great importance in the physical assessment of the patient. Although the thoracic cavity extends to the twelfth rib posteriorly, the diaphragm inserts into the anterior thoracic cage just below the fourth or fifth rib. With the movement of the diaphragm during the ventilation process the size and dimensions of the thoracic cavity will vary, which could in turn affect the organs or cavities (thoracic versus abdominal) in case of blunt or penetrating injury.

Special Populations

Pediatric and older adult patients have anatomic and physiologic differences. For example, the incidence of rib fractures varies with age. The ribs of children are pliable, so they may injure underlying structures without being fractured. In older patients, the brittle nature of the bones makes the ribs more likely to fracture.

YOU ▸ are the Paramedic   PART 1

Your unit is dispatched to meet with law enforcement personnel on the scene of a stabbing. When you arrive, an officer meets you and directs you to the patient. As you approach the patient, you see a man who appears to be about 40 years old. He is sitting upright, with his back against a wall and is responsive. The officer tells you that the patient is extremely intoxicated. A knife is protruding from his left anterior chest, just below the middle of the clavicle. The patient is actively trying to pull the knife out, with little success.

1. What is your primary concern for this patient?
2. What anatomic structures could be damaged in relation to the position of the knife?

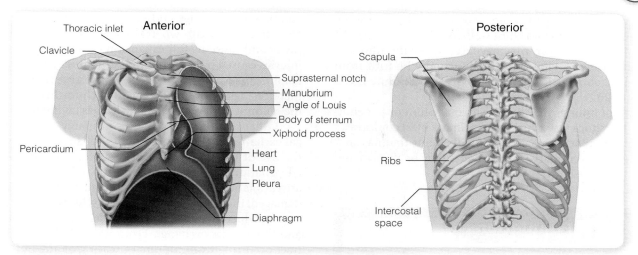

Figure 35-2 The thorax, front and back views.
© Jones & Bartlett Learning.

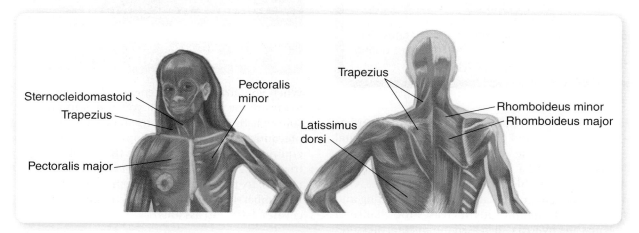

Figure 35-3 The muscles of the thoracic cavity include the trapezius, latissimus dorsi, rhomboids, pectoralis, and sternocleidomastoid muscles.
© Jones & Bartlett Learning.

The thoracic region is not only protected by the skeletal structure of the rib cage and the spine, it also is covered by dense muscle tissues. These muscles assist with the mechanical functioning of the respiratory process and provide movement in this region. They include the trapezius, latissimus dorsi, rhomboids, pectoralis, and sternocleidomastoid **Figure 35-3**.

The primary physiologic functions of the thorax and its contents are to maintain oxygenation and ventilation (via the respiratory system) and to maintain circulation (via the cardiovascular system). These systems require an environment free from disruptions and complications; for this reason, any traumatic injury to the chest is potentially life threatening. If the patient has an underlying medical condition, such as chronic obstructive pulmonary disease or heart failure, even minimal interruptions in the body's normal processes through injury can cripple an already compromised system.

■ Pathophysiology

Traumatic injury to the chest presents the possibility of compromise of ventilation, oxygenation, or circulation. These injuries, if missed or inappropriately treated, could contribute significantly to the patient's morbidity or even cause death.

As in the rest of the body, several injury mechanisms are possible. Conducting a scene size-up will help you determine the forces involved. In a penetrating chest injury, an object, such as a knife, a bullet, or a piece of metal, penetrates the chest wall. Penetrating injuries distribute the forces of injury over a smaller area; however, the trajectory of a bullet is often unpredictable and all thoracic structures are at risk.

In blunt trauma, a blow to the chest may fracture the ribs, the sternum, or whole areas of the chest wall;

bruise the lungs and the heart; and even damage the aorta. Although the skin and chest wall are not penetrated in a closed injury, broken ribs may lacerate the intrathoracic organs. Indeed, vital organs can actually be torn from their attachment in the chest cavity without any break in the skin.

Blast injuries may be classified as blunt or penetrating. The shock wave during the primary blast compresses organs similar to what occurs with blunt trauma, and, during the secondary phase, objects may be thrown and penetrate the body.

Special Populations

Pediatric and older adult patients have differences that you must consider during the assessment process. For example, pediatric signs of pneumothorax or hemothorax are often subtle, and you may not see signs of jugular venous distention as you would in an adult. An older patient experiencing blunt trauma would have considerably higher mortality and morbidity rates than other populations. Consider such differences during the assessment of various populations.

In all age groups, thoracic trauma may impair cardiac output, decreasing blood pressure and perfusion to vital organs. Considering the contents of the thoracic cavity, any injury to the chest has the potential to be lethal. Trauma may result in blood loss, pressure changes, vital organ damage, or any combination of these. Bleeding into the thoracic cavity significantly increases the chance of hypovolemia and hypoxia. Increased intrapleural pressures not only decrease lung volume and oxygenation, but also impair the heart's ability to pump effectively. Blood in the pericardial sac compresses the heart, potentially stopping it altogether. Myocardial valve damage from trauma to the heart can disrupt ventricular filling, allowing for backflow into the atria and further decreasing cardiac output. Vascular disruption may also occur as the result of trauma. A rupture of a major vessel can lead to fatal blood loss, and even a small tear or blockage can cause lack of oxygenation and tissue ischemia. You should have a good understanding of the underlying structures because it increases your assessment abilities and it may increase the patient's chance of survival.

Aside from massive blood loss, impairments in ventilatory efficiency may also be rapidly fatal. Any injury that compromises the chest bellows action decreases air exchange and subsequent oxygenation. A patient experiencing severe chest pain tends to breathe shallowly in an attempt to decrease the discomfort created by movement. This further reduces minute volume, the volume of air exchanged between the lungs and environment in 1 minute. Air entering the pleural space as the result of an open or closed pneumothorax, a tracheal tear, or other damage

compresses the lungs and decreases tidal volume. This condition also occurs when blood collects in the thoracic cavity and prevents full expansion of the lungs. Various injuries caused by chest trauma, such as rib fractures and diaphragmatic injury, result in fewer pressure changes and, therefore, less movement of air, which further decreases the amount of oxygen available for gas exchange.

Other complications are also capable of impairing gas exchange. **Atelectasis** is alveolar collapse that prevents the use of that portion of the lung for ventilation and oxygenation. Atelectasis significantly reduces the surface area available for gas exchange. The more alveoli that are damaged, the less gas exchange occurs. Bruised lung tissue may produce marked hypoxemia as fluid accumulates and impairs gas exchange. Disruption of the respiratory tract occurring from rupture or tearing of any of the respiratory structures prevents oxygen from reaching the alveoli, further impairing gas exchange.

Patient Assessment

Scene Size-up

When you arrive on the scene, your first responsibility is to ensure the safety of both you and your partner. Make sure that the scene is safe to enter and follow standard precautions, using the appropriate personal protective equipment. After you identify the number of patients, triage those patients, and request any additional resources needed, try to determine the mechanism of injury (MOI). Remember that chest injuries are common in motor vehicle crashes, falls, and assaults.

Primary Survey

As you approach the patient, you will form a general impression of the patient's condition. It is important to assess the patient's level of consciousness using AVPU (Awake and alert, responsive to Verbal stimuli, responsive to Pain, Unresponsive). Responsive patients may be able to tell you their chief complaint. Note not only what they say, but also how they say it (ie, three-word sentences), which might require immediate ventilatory assessment.

Difficulty speaking may indicate several conditions, and chest injury is an important one. Assess the patient's entire body for obvious injuries, the appearance of blood, and difficulty breathing. Look for cyanosis, irregular breathing, and chest rise and fall on only one side. Observe the neck, looking for accessory muscle use while breathing; also look for distended or engorged external jugular veins. If no obvious problems are seen, begin looking for them by focusing on the ABCs (Airway, Breathing, Circulation); if the patient is in arrest, then the sequence is CAB (Circulation, Airway, Breathing). The general impression will help you develop an index of suspicion for serious injuries and determine your sense of urgency for medical intervention. A good question to ask yourself is "How sick is this patient?" Patients with significant chest injuries will "look" sick and are often frightened or anxious. Keep in mind that you are rapidly searching for life threats and you will repeat the physical exam in a more detailed manner later in the assessment if time and patient condition allow.

Next, check airway and breathing. Assess the patient's airway status while providing manual in-line stabilization of the cervical spine. Assess for injuries that may result in either obstruction or impairment of the airway. The thoracic injury itself can cause respiratory compromise, which will need to be addressed hand-in-hand with the thoracic injury.

To adequately assess the patient's breathing, the patient's clothing must be removed to expose the thoracic cavity. You should maintain the patient's modesty, but if you do not fully expose the area for visual, palpation, and auscultation assessments, the overall assessment will be incomplete. Taking a systematic approach to assessment will then help you to identify both obvious and subtle injuries or impairments.

Moving from the patient's airway to the chest, be sure to palpate the patient's neck for tracheal deviation and inspect the jugular veins, noting if they are distended or flat. Then begin with an inspection of the patient's thorax. Consider the contour, appearance, and symmetry of the chest wall. Signs of soft-tissue injury (contusions, abrasions, lacerations, or deformity) suggest the possibility of an underlying injury. Paradoxical motion of a section of the chest wall, retractions, subcutaneous air or edema, impaled objects, or penetrating injuries also suggest an underlying injury with the potential to compromise the patient's breathing. If you determine the patient has paradoxical movement of the chest wall or penetrating trauma, address this life threat at once. When further dressings can be applied, apply an occlusive dressing to all penetrating injuries to the chest. Continued treatments of these types of injuries will often depend on local protocols.

Consider the adequacy of both ventilation and oxygenation. To assess ventilation, examine the patient's respiratory rate, depth, and effort. Reliance on accessory muscles or findings such as nasal flaring suggests ventilatory compromise. Inadequate oxygenation may be inferred from findings such as cyanosis or altered mental status.

Administer oxygen with a nonrebreathing mask at 15 L/min. Provide positive pressure ventilations with 100% oxygen if breathing is inadequate based on the patient's level of consciousness and breathing rate and quality. As a note of caution, remember that when you are providing positive pressure ventilation, you are overcoming the normal physiologic functions, and, if your patient has a pneumothorax (collapsed lung), you can quickly exacerbate the injury. Be diligent with auscultation of breath sounds, and evaluate the effectiveness of your ventilatory support with signs of circulation to the skin. Be aware of decreasing oxygen saturation (SpO_2) values because they may indicate the development of hypoxia.

Watch for signs of an impending tension pneumothorax, such as increasingly poor compliance during ventilation.

The final steps in the assessment of the patient's breathing entail the palpation, percussion, and auscultation of the chest. While you are palpating the chest, assess for any evidence of point tenderness, bony instability, **crepitus**, **subcutaneous emphysema**, or edema. Percussion can help to identify either hyperresonance (suggesting increased air within the cavity) or dullness (suggesting blood within the cavity). Auscultation includes the usual assessment for adventitious lung sounds (ie, wheezing, crackles [rales], rhonchi) plus confirmation that lung sounds are present in all lung fields, helping to identify the need for needle decompression.

Assessing the quality of a pulse in a thoracic trauma patient should help you determine the hemodynamic stability of the patient, but can also clue you into clinical findings of a cardiac tamponade (loss of radial pulse on inspiration is a clinical sign of a potential cardiac tamponade). Although an electrocardiogram (ECG) monitor may be applied to evaluate the rhythm at this time, this step is recommended only if it does not cause any delay in completing the primary survey (eg, your partner could perform this task while you continue the primary survey).

Jugular venous distention (JVD) suggests increased central venous pressure—perhaps resulting from a tension pneumothorax, volume overload, right-sided heart failure, or cardiac tamponade **Figure 35-4**. Because true JVD is measured with the patient in a 45° semi-Fowler position, it may be difficult to assess when spine precautions have been implemented. Nevertheless, a lack of JVD in the supine position in combination with other physical findings (eg, tachycardia, altered mental status, thready pulses, poor skin perfusion) may suggest a hypovolemic state.

Auscultation of the heart sounds is another important part of the circulatory assessment. For patients with potential intrathoracic injuries, note whether their heart sounds are easily heard or whether they are muffled. Performing such an assessment may prove difficult in the back

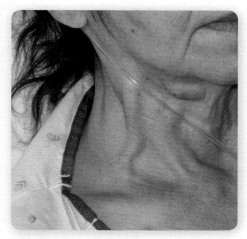

Figure 35-4 Jugular venous distention.
© Ferencga/Wikimedia Commons.

of a moving or running ambulance or because of other noise on the scene. Even so, the presence of muffled heart tones is an important diagnostic clue to the presence of either a tension pneumothorax (because of its resultant mediastinal shift) or a cardiac tamponade.

Even if the assessment of the patient's circulatory status suggests hypovolemic shock, you should recognize that the cause of that state may not lie within the thorax. For this reason, after completing the primary survey, managing any immediate life-threatening conditions, and prioritizing the patient, you must obtain the patient's history and perform a complete physical exam to identify other significant injuries.

When making your transport decision, priority patients are considered patients who have impaired airway, breathing, and/or circulation. Sometimes the priority is obvious, and the decision to transport quickly is easy to make, given the circumstances. At other times, what is happening outside the body may not provide obvious clues to the seriousness of what is happening inside the body. Pay attention to subtle clues such as the appearance of the skin, level of consciousness, or a sense of impending doom in the patient. These symptoms are not as dramatic as a large gash across the chest or air being sucked into the chest; however, they can be equally important indicators of a life-threatening condition. When you find signs of poor perfusion or inadequate breathing, transport quickly and perform the remainder of the assessment en route to the emergency department. A delay on the scene to perform a lengthy assessment will reduce the chances of survival for your patient. With chest injuries, when in doubt, transport rapidly to a hospital. **Table 35-1** lists the "deadly dozen" chest injuries.

Table 35-1	Life-Threatening Chest Injuries

Immediately life-threatening chest injuries that must be detected and managed during the primary survey:

1. Airway obstruction
2. Bronchial disruption
3. Diaphragmatic tear
4. Esophageal injury
5. Open pneumothorax
6. Tension pneumothorax
7. Hemothorax
8. Flail chest
9. Cardiac tamponade

Potentially lethal chest injuries that may be identified during the secondary assessment:

10. Traumatic aortic disruption
11. Myocardial contusion
12. Pulmonary contusion

History Taking

Depending on the severity of the injuries identified up to this point, history taking may need to be done en route to the emergency department.

A relevant patient history should be obtained, including a SAMPLE (Signs and symptoms, Allergies, Medications, Pertinent past history, Last oral intake, Events leading to injury or illness) history. Ask the usual questions related to the patient's symptoms, allergies, medications, past medical history, and last oral intake. Questions about the events surrounding the incident should focus on the MOI: the speed of the vehicle or height of the fall, the use of safety equipment (helmet, air bag, seat belt, life jacket), the type of weapon used, the number of penetrating wounds, and so on.

Words of Wisdom

Any injury below the level of the nipples should be presumed to be an abdominal injury as well as a chest injury.

Secondary Assessment

The secondary assessment, which may be performed en route to the hospital for patients with a significant MOI, should include a complete head-to-toe assessment of the patient. This exam allows you to identify any physical injuries as well as reassess injuries identified in the primary survey. For the chest trauma patient, pay particular attention to the patient's cervical spine, back, and abdomen, as well as the neurologic and circulatory function in the patient's extremities.

Assess for injuries with the potential to compromise the ABCs—namely, aortic transections, great vessel injuries, bronchial disruptions, myocardial contusions, pulmonary contusions, simple pneumothoraces, rib fractures, and sternal fractures. If you have not already done so, obtain a full set of vital signs—including pulse rate, blood pressure, respirations, oxygen saturation, and mental status. The use of monitoring equipment such as capnography and pulse oximetry can aid in the assessment. It is advisable to use the pulse oximeter on any patient with a chest injury to establish a baseline measurement and to help you recognize any downward trends that indicate the patient's condition is worsening.

In a patient who has an isolated injury to the chest with a limited MOI, such as in a stabbing, focus your assessment on the isolated injury, the patient's complaint, and the body region affected. However, it is important in patients with a chest injury not to focus only on a chest wound. With significant trauma, quickly assess the entire patient from head to toe. While you are assessing the skin, look for ecchymosis and other evidence of trauma. Ensure that wounds are identified and control of the bleeding has been established. Note the location and extent of the injury. Assess all underlying systems. Examine the anterior and posterior aspects of the chest wall, and be alert to changes in the patient's ability to maintain adequate respirations.

If there is significant trauma (such as blunt trauma or a gunshot wound) likely affecting multiple systems, perform a full-body scan to determine the nature and extent of thoracic injury. This exam will help you to determine all of the injuries and the extent of the injuries. Inspection or visualization of the region looking for deformities, such as asymmetry of the left and right sides of the chest or shoulder girdle, may reveal the presence of multiple rib fractures, crush injuries, or significant chest wall injury. Identification of discrete areas of contusion or abrasion may pinpoint a specific point of impact. The presence of puncture wounds or other penetrating injuries indicates a possible open chest injury that should be managed accordingly. Be alert for associated burns, which may alter respiratory mechanics. Palpate for tenderness to localize the injury and the presence of fractures. Look for lacerations and local swelling. Application of this systematic approach to patient assessment minimizes the chance of missing significant injury.

Reassessment

When you are reassessing the chest trauma patient, obtain repeated assessments of the patient's vital signs, oxygenation, circulatory status, and breath sounds. Because the progression from pneumothorax to tension pneumothorax

can occur quite rapidly, all patients with a presumptive diagnosis of a pneumothorax should be considered to be in unstable condition and reassessed at least every 5 minutes for worsening dyspnea, tachycardia, and the development of JVD. Similarly, other chest injuries may suggest the presence of more serious underlying pathologic conditions. Because these injuries may have been overlooked during the primary survey, you need to maintain a high degree of clinical suspicion during the on-scene treatment and transport of these patients.

■ Emergency Medical Care

As with any trauma patient, your management of patients with identifiable chest injuries must focus on maintaining the airway, ensuring oxygenation and ventilation, supporting the circulatory status, and expeditiously transporting the patient to an appropriate facility.

With one exception, airway management of the patient with chest trauma should proceed the same as with any other trauma patient. If the status of a potential cervical injury is unknown, the jaw-thrust maneuver should be used rather than the head tilt–chin lift maneuver, because the former technique better limits cervical spine motion. Nasal airways should be avoided in patients with signs of facial injury. Instead, endotracheal intubation should be performed while maintaining manual in-line stabilization of the cervical spine. When a patient with chest trauma has a possible tracheal injury, however, endotracheal intubation should be reconsidered. With a partial tracheal tear, you run the risk of completing the tracheal tear when you are passing the endotracheal tube, a complication that can result in an unmanageable airway. Consequently, when

YOU ▶ are the Paramedic — PART 2

You observe that the patient has labored, shallow breathing. You ask the law enforcement officer to help control the patient's hands while you and your partner conduct a primary survey. Your partner feels for a radial pulse and reports that it is rapid and weak. There is no blood coming from the wound.

Recording Time: 1 Minute	
Appearance	Awake
Level of consciousness	Disoriented
Airway	Open
Breathing	Labored and shallow
Circulation	Poor

3. What immediate treatment do you need to provide to this patient?
4. What steps will you take in your further assessment of this patient?

you suspect your patient has a partial tracheal tear, use the least invasive airway management technique possible.

As part of airway management, you must ensure that the patient maintains adequate oxygenation and ventilation. Oxygenation is accomplished by providing patients with high-flow oxygen via a nonrebreathing mask or, if necessary, with bag-mask ventilation. Ventilation is a more delicate issue in light of the potential complications that can arise from underlying thoracic injuries; therefore, you must provide ventilatory assistance in a highly vigilant fashion. Delivery of positive pressure could potentially hasten the expansion of a pneumothorax, convert a pneumothorax into a tension pneumothorax, or increase the dissection of air through a tracheobronchial injury. Positive pressure ventilation should not be withheld, however; rather, it should be delivered in a manner that minimizes the degree of pressure used. Watch your patient's chest closely—you are looking for visible chest rise without excessive overinflation of the lungs, which would lead to air entering the stomach!

Assessment of the ability of the circulatory system to provide oxygenation and ventilation to the body tissues is the next step in the management of any trauma patient. The patient whose circulatory status is compromised (as evidenced by tachycardia, hypotension, or end-organ dysfunction) requires supportive measures until definitive care can be delivered. Placing the patient in a supine position will deliver blood otherwise held in the venous system of the lower extremities to the central circulation. The provision of judicious intravenous (IV) fluids may also help to expand the intravascular volume while maintaining the oxygen-carrying capacity of the blood.

In general, pharmacologic agents have a limited role in the management of a trauma patient. With the exception of those medications necessary to ensure appropriate airway management, the only drugs currently used are agents for pain management. Narcotic and nonnarcotic analgesics are essential components of the appropriate and compassionate treatment of any trauma patient. As a responsible paramedic, you will take the proper steps to minimize the pain of your patients, although you may often be limited by local protocols, short transport times in more urban settings, and the clinical status of the patient (including appropriate concern about narcotic suppression of the respiratory drive in thoracic trauma patients). Nonpharmaceutical approaches may include appropriate splinting, application of cold packs, and careful handling.

> ## Words of Wisdom
>
> Treatment of pain and anxiety can help with packaging and transport of the patient, thus minimizing secondary injury.

Finally, the global assessment and management of patients with chest trauma includes deciding the appropriate facility to which the patient should be transported. Trauma centers designated to provide multisystem evaluation and management of trauma patients would be the first choice for most patients with chest trauma, particularly those with potentially life-threatening injuries. Sometimes, however, such facilities may not be readily available or may be physically too distant to allow for timely transport (eg, in a rural environment).

The principle of the Golden Period (or Golden Hour) is the time during which treatment of shock or traumatic injuries is most critical and the potential for survival is best.

> ## Words of Wisdom
>
> There are a select few injuries that you must be able to quickly identify and treat during your assessment of the patient's breathing—namely, open pneumothorax and tension pneumothorax. These injuries, if missed, may claim the patient's life.

■ Pathophysiology, Assessment, and Management of Chest Wall Injuries

▶ Flail Chest

Flail chest, a major injury to the chest wall, may result from a variety of blunt force mechanisms such as falls, motor vehicle crashes, and assaults **Figure 35-5**. The associated mortality rates range from 50% to even higher rates in patients older than age 60 years.[3] Mortality rates are directly related to the underlying and associated injuries. Patients are more likely to sustain a mortal injury if they are older, have seven or more rib fractures or three or more associated injuries, present with shock, or have associated head trauma.

A flail segment is defined as two or more adjacent ribs that are fractured in two or more places. The segment between those fracture sites becomes separated from the surrounding chest wall, leaving it free to succumb to the underlying pressures—hence the name *free-floating segment*. Both the location and the size of the segment can affect the degree to which the flail segment impairs chest wall motion and subsequent air movement. In a flail sternum (the most extreme case), the sternum is completely separated from the ribs because of fractures or ruptured costal cartilage. This type of injury results in mechanical dysfunction of both sides of the chest and more severe respiratory impairment.

Once a flail segment has occurred, the underlying physiologic pressures cause paradoxical movement of the segment when compared with the rest of the chest wall. Expansion of the chest wall on inspiration results in

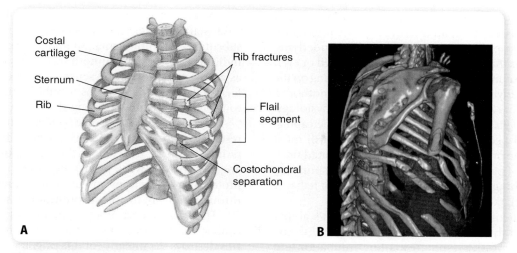

Costal cartilage

Rib fractures

Sternum

Rib

Flail segment

Costochondral separation

A

B

Figure 35-5 A. In flail chest injuries, two or more adjacent ribs are fractured in two or more places. A flail segment will move paradoxically when the patient breathes. **B.** Photo showing flail chest.

A: © Jones & Bartlett Learning; **B:** "Flail Chest in Polytraumatized Patients: Surgical Fixation Using Stracos Reduces Ventilator Time and Hospital Stay", © 2015 Christophe P.M. Jayle et al. BioMed Research International. doi: 10.1155/2015/624723.

negative pressure within the thoracic cavity, which in turn draws the flail segment in toward the center of the chest. As the chest relaxes or is actively contracted (depending on the degree of dyspnea), the resulting positive pressure forces air from the lungs and also forces the flail segment out away from the thoracic cavity. Because of these movements, the lung tissue beneath the flail segment, in addition to being likely contused or otherwise injured, is not adequately ventilated. A flail segment can quickly become life threatening, which explains why it is managed during the primary survey of the patient when significant ventilatory insufficiency is noted. The flailed section might not be immediately apparent due to the intercostal muscle "splinting" the area, thus making paradoxical movement a late sign of flailed segments. Proper assessment of this area includes palpation of the injury site for fractures of the rib cage and the presence of crepitus (bone ends grating together). Typical management involves the use of positive pressure ventilation as well as positive end-expiratory pressure when you are assisting ventilations for the patient.

The blunt force trauma that causes the flail segment can also produce a **pulmonary contusion**, an injury to the underlying lung tissue that inhibits the normal diffusion of oxygen and carbon dioxide **Figure 35-6** . Three physical mechanisms contribute to the formation of a pulmonary contusion: implosion, inertial effects, and the Spalding effect. In the implosion effect, positive pressure created by the trauma compresses the gases within the lung, which quickly reexpand. If this reexpansion is too great, the lung tissue will sustain an implosion injury. Inertial effects are created by tissue density differences between the alveoli and the larger bronchioles. These tissues accelerate and decelerate at different rates, causing them to tear and hemorrhage. With the Spalding effect, the pressure waves generated by either penetrating or blunt trauma disrupt the capillary-alveolar membrane, resulting in hemorrhage.

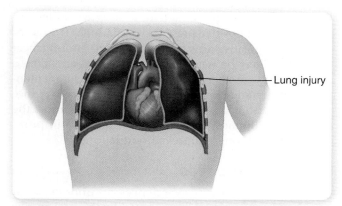

Lung injury

Figure 35-6 A pulmonary contusion is an injury to underlying lung tissue that inhibits diffusion.

© Jones & Bartlett Learning.

If the blunt force that fractures the ribs drives those bone fragments farther into the body, a pneumothorax or hemothorax may result. In addition, the pain associated with the fractures may prevent the patient from taking in adequate tidal volume because he or she is consciously trying to minimize the movement of that segment of the chest. This "self-splinting" action uses the intercostal muscles and purposefully limits chest wall movement to minimize pain. Unfortunately, this action further limits the pulmonary system's ability to compensate for the injury.

Assessment and Management

Physical assessment is the key to identifying a patient with a flail segment. Beginning with general inspection of the chest, you will note evidence of soft-tissue injury to the chest. On further examination, you may observe paradoxical chest wall movement, although the patient's efforts to splint the injury may prevent its visibility.

On palpation, crepitus and tenderness may be noted at the site, and dissection of air into the tissues should raise your clinical suspicion for this injury and an underlying pneumothorax. Auscultation will reveal decreased or even absent breath sounds on the affected side, depending on the degree of underlying injury, splinting, and pneumothorax.

As the injury begins to affect the patient's physiology, the expected signs and symptoms of hypoxia, hypercapnia, and pain will become apparent. The patient will most likely have one or more of the following associated findings: reports of pain, tenderness on palpation, splinting, shallow breathing, agitation/anxiety (hypoxia) or lethargy (hypercapnia), tachycardia, and cyanosis.

Flail segments pose a threat to the patient's ability to breathe and should be treated immediately. When the patient has progressive respiratory failure, intubation and positive pressure ventilation are indicated. Intubating the patient uses positive pressure ventilation as a means of expanding the collapsed alveoli. That portion of the lung parenchyma is then able to contribute to the oxygenation and ventilation of the patient.

The goal is an SpO_2 of at least 95% with supplemental oxygen and positive pressure ventilations. The use of continuous positive airway pressure up to endotracheal intubation may be needed for patients experiencing a reduced SpO_2 with bag-mask ventilation and supplemental oxygen. In addition, the use of medications to reduce the pain associated with chest trauma will promote the patient's willingness to take full breaths and improve oxygenation through improved ventilations.

▶ Rib Fractures

Even when the patient experiences no underlying or associated injury, the pain produced by the broken ribs can result in significant morbidity because it contributes to inadequate ventilation, self-splinting, atelectasis, and the possibility of infection (pneumonia) due to inadequate respiration **Figure 35-7** .

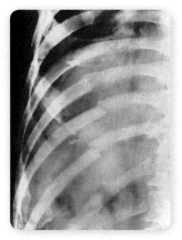

Figure 35-7 Rib fractures.
© BSIP/Science Source.

When you are examining the chest of a patient who has sustained either blunt or penetrating injury, palpate for subcutaneous emphysema (air under the skin), which can indicate a potential pneumothorax. It has been described as a "snap, crackle, pop" sensation under the skin or a feeling like popping the plastic bubbles in the wrap used to protect fragile items during shipping.

In blunt trauma, the force applied to the thoracic cage results in a fracture of the rib in one of three areas: the point of impact, the edge of the object, or the posterior angle of the rib (weak point). Because they are less well protected by other bony and muscular structures, ribs four through nine are the most commonly fractured.

The ribs are part of a ring that helps to expand and contract the thoracic cavity. Because a fracture of one or more ribs destroys the integrity of this ring, the patient's ability to adequately breathe is diminished. Just as importantly, the patient will attempt to limit the pain caused by these injuries by using shallow breathing. This tendency results in atelectasis and may lead to hypoxia or pneumonia.

The presence of rib fractures should also make you suspicious for other associated injuries. When the clinical exam suggests a fracture of ribs four through nine, you should be concerned about associated aortic injury, tracheobronchial injury, pneumothorax, vascular injury, or other more serious injuries. Similarly, fractures of the lower ribs (9 through 11) should raise your concern for an associated intra-abdominal injury.

> ### Words of Wisdom
>
> The sternum is a thick bone. If the thorax receives enough force to fracture the sternum, you must assume that the same force was transmitted to the heart, great vessels, lungs, and diaphragm.

Assessment and Management

Patients with rib fractures typically report pleuritic chest wall pain and mild dyspnea. The physical exam may reveal chest wall tenderness and overlying soft-tissue injury. Crepitus and subcutaneous emphysema may also be noted. When you are assessing the adequacy of the patient's respiratory effort, watch for shallow ventilations as the patient attempts to limit the movement of the affected area of the thoracic cage. The patient may also lean toward the injury site to reduce muscular tension on the fracture or fractures.

The management of rib fractures focuses on the ABCs and evaluating the patient for other, more lethal injuries. Administer supplemental oxygen if indicated and gently splint the patient's chest wall by having the patient hold a pillow or blanket against the area; this measure may allow the patient to take deeper breaths, something that should be encouraged despite the pain. IV analgesics may also assist in this regard.

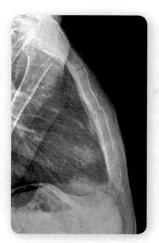

Figure 35-8 Sternal fracture.
© SOVEREIGN, ISM/SCIENCE PHOTO LIBRARY.

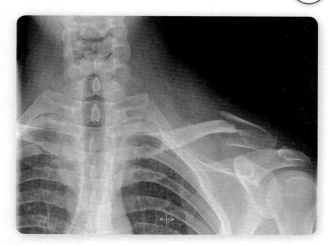

Figure 35-9 Clavicle fracture.
© kalewa/Shutterstock.

► Sternal Fractures

Any suspected fracture of the sternum should increase your index of suspicion for injuries to the underlying organs **Figure 35-8**. There may be involvement of the lungs, great vessels, and the heart itself.

Assessment and Management

On examination, the patient with a sternal fracture will report pain over the anterior part of the chest. Palpation of the area may reveal tenderness, deformity, crepitus, overlying soft-tissue injury, and the possibility of a flail segment. Given the risk of an underlying myocardial contusion, ECG rhythm analysis should be performed.

The treatment of sternal fractures is supportive. Assess the patient's ABCs, and manage associated injuries accordingly. Analgesics in doses sufficient to provide pain relief without suppressing the respiratory drive may aid the patient's ventilatory efforts.

Words of Wisdom

Be alert for the development of a pneumothorax in a patient with a sternal fracture.

► Clavicle Fractures

The **clavicle**, or collarbone, is one of the most commonly fractured bones in the body **Figure 35-9**. Fractures of the clavicle occur most often in children when they fall on an outstretched hand. They are common in cycling crashes and snowboarding. They can also occur with crushing injuries of the chest.

Assessment and Management

A patient with a fracture of the clavicle will report pain in the shoulder and will usually hold the arm across the front of his or her body. A young child often reports pain throughout the entire arm and is unwilling to use any part of that limb. Because the clavicle is subcutaneous, the skin will occasionally "tent" over the fracture fragment. The clavicle lies directly over major arteries, veins, and nerves; therefore, fracture of the clavicle may lead to neurovascular compromise, although this is rare.

Fractures of the clavicle and scapula and acromio-clavicular separations can be splinted effectively with a sling and swathe. A sling is any bandage or material that helps support the weight of an injured upper extremity, relieving the downward pull of gravity on the injured site. To be effective, a sling must apply gentle upward support to the olecranon process of the ulna (at the elbow). The knot of the sling should be tied to one side of the neck so that it does not press uncomfortably on the cervical spine. Note that that this is effective only in the patient who can sit upright; it is not as effective in the supine position.

■ Pathophysiology, Assessment, and Management of Lung Injuries

► Simple Pneumothorax

Small pneumothoraces that are not under tension are a frequent occurrence in the blunt trauma patient. Patients with penetrating trauma to the chest may have a **pneumothorax**—that is, the accumulation of air or gas in the pleural cavity **Figure 35-10**. In this condition, air enters through a hole in the chest wall (that seals itself after air has entered the pleural space) or the surface of the lung as the patient attempts to breathe, causing the lung on that side to collapse as pressure continues to build in the pleural cavity.

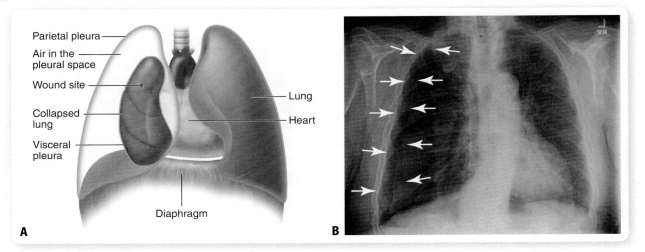

Figure 35-10 A. Pneumothorax occurs when air leaks into the space between the pleural surfaces from an opening in the chest or the surface of the lung. The lung collapses as air fills the pleural space. **B.** Radiograph showing simple pneumothorax. The arrows outline the edges of the pneumothorax.

A: © Jones & Bartlett Learning; **B:** © Steven Needell/Science Source.

Assessment and Management

The presentation and physical findings in a patient with a simple pneumothorax depend on the size of the pneumothorax and the degree of resulting pulmonary compromise. With a small pneumothorax, the patient may report only mild dyspnea and pleuritic chest pain on the affected side. Diminished or unequal breath sounds may be heard on auscultation, a finding that is best heard anteriorly if the patient is in the supine position or in the apices if the patient is upright. (Air will accumulate at the highest point and diminish lung sounds in that area.) Hyperresonance may also be found on the affected side.

As the pneumothorax increases in size, the degree of compromise likewise increases. Patients with larger pneumothoraces will report increasing dyspnea and demonstrate signs of more serious respiratory compromise and hypoxia: agitation, altered mental status, tachypnea, tachycardia, cyanosis, lowered pulse oximetry readings, **pulsus paradoxus** (a drop in blood pressure), and absent breath sounds on the affected side.

The management of the patient with a simple pneumothorax focuses on maintaining the ABCs and provide high-concentration oxygen. Supplemental oxygen aids the patient in overcoming any degree of hypoxia that may exist. Positive pressure ventilation (PPV) can potentially aggravate the condition, possibly resulting in tension pneumothorax, yet PPV should never be withheld from a patient whose presentation calls for such measures. The most critical intervention for these patients is for you to conduct repeated assessments to ensure that the injury has not progressed to a tension pneumothorax. Most pneumothoraces result from a small pulmonary injury that seals itself off, preventing further air loss. For those that do progress, however, rapid recognition and management of this condition can be lifesaving.

▶ Open Pneumothorax

An **open pneumothorax** occurs when a defect in the chest wall allows air to enter the thoracic space. It results from penetrating chest trauma—for example, gunshot wounds, knife wounds, or other impaled objects. The penetrating injury creates a link between the external environment and the pleural space. With each inspiration, the negative pressure created within the thoracic cavity draws more air into the pleural space, resulting in a pneumothorax. As the pneumothorax increases in size, the lung on the involved side loses its ability to expand. In addition, if the "hole" is larger than the glottic opening, the air is more likely to enter the chest wall rather than entering via the trachea. Consequently, the respiratory effort moves air in through the chest wound rather than through the lung, creating the "sucking chest wound" **Figure 35-11**.

The collapse of the involved lung creates a mismatch between ventilation and perfusion. If you assume that the pulmonary vasculature on the involved side remains intact, the heart will continue to perfuse the involved lung while the pneumothorax prevents adequate ventilation. The result is an inability to deliver oxygen to the involved lung (hypoxia) and an inability to eliminate carbon dioxide (hypercapnia).

Assessment and Management

On physical assessment of a patient with an open pneumothorax, exposure of the chest will reveal a chest wall defect or impaled object. If air is being drawn into the chest by the negative inspiratory pressure, a "sucking chest wound" may be noted. If air is being forced out of the chest with the positive pressure of expiration, the result may be a bubbling wound. The movement of air in and out of the open wound may also lead to dissection of that air within the subcutaneous tissue, resulting in subcutaneous emphysema.

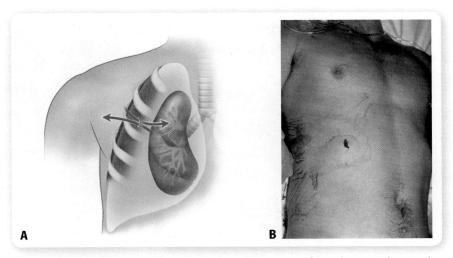

Figure 35-11 A. With a sucking chest wound, air passes from the outside into the pleural space and back out with each breath, creating a sucking sound. The size of the defect does not need to be large to compromise ventilation. **B.** Open pneumothorax.

A: © Jones & Bartlett Learning; B: © Mediscan/Alamy.

With any injury that has the potential to violate the integrity of the thoracic cavity, your assessment should focus on evaluating the patient for the presence of a pneumothorax. Due to the decreased ability to oxygenate and ventilate, the patient will experience tachycardia, tachypnea, and restlessness. These symptoms may be simply a manifestation of the pain from the injury, but other findings may confirm an underlying pneumothorax.

As the air between the pleural membranes increases, the breath sounds diminish on the affected side. Because this expanding volume consists of air, percussion of the chest will aid in the assessment by demonstrating a hyper-resonant sound. These physical findings should confirm your suspicion of an open pneumothorax.

Sucking chest wounds must be treated immediately. The injury should first be converted to a closed injury to prevent further expansion of the pneumothorax. To do so, immediately place your gloved hand over the injury and then replace that hand with an occlusive dressing or a commercial chest seal **Figure 35-12**. Because of the possibility that an underlying lung injury may continue to contribute to the pneumothorax, this dressing should be secured on three sides to facilitate the release of increased pressure, should it develop.

All patients with open pneumothoraces, regardless of their oxygenation status as determined by pulse oximetry, should be placed on high-flow supplemental oxygen via a nonrebreathing mask. If oxygenation or ventilation remains inadequate, endotracheal intubation may be required. You may use sedation or neuromuscular blockade to facilitate this process, depending on your local protocols.

An open pneumothorax usually doesn't progress to a tension pneumothorax, but be aware that it may, and if it does, you must act promptly.

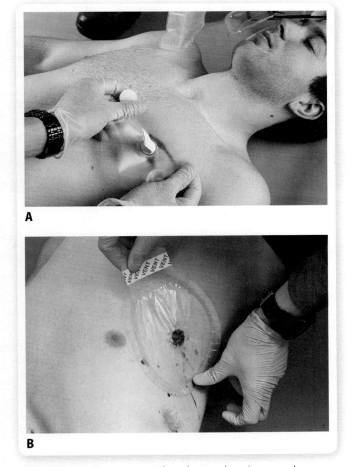

Figure 35-12 A commercial occlusive dressing may be used to seal all four sides of a sucking chest wound. **A.** An Asherman Chest Seal, which is vented. **B.** A HALO Chest Seal, which is unvented.

© Jones & Bartlett Learning.

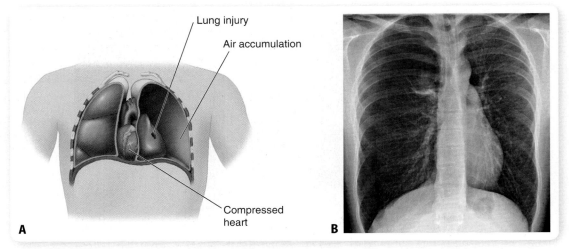

Figure 35-13 A. In a tension pneumothorax, air accumulates in the pleural space, eventually causing compression of the heart and great vessels. **B.** Tension pneumothorax.

A: © Jones & Bartlett Learning; B: © Du Cane Medical Imaging Ltd/Science Source.

► Tension Pneumothorax

A **tension pneumothorax** is a life-threatening condition that results from continued air accumulation within the interpleural space **Figure 35-13**. A tension pneumothorax may result from an open or closed injury. Air may enter the pleural space from an open thoracic injury, an injury to the lung parenchyma due to blunt trauma (the most common cause of tension pneumothorax), barotrauma due to positive pressure ventilation, or tracheobronchial injuries due to shearing forces. Although the exact incidence of this injury is unknown, many trauma patients in cardiac arrest receive emergent treatment for this condition secondary to blunt trauma.

An injury to the lung can cause a one-way valve to develop, allowing air to move into the pleural space but not to exit from it. As it continues to accumulate, the air exerts increasing pressure against the surrounding tissues. This growing pressure compresses the involved lung, diminishing its ability to oxygenate blood or eliminate carbon dioxide from the blood. Eventually, the pressure increase causes the lung to collapse on the affected side

YOU ▷ are the Paramedic   PART 3

Your partner begins to assist the patient's breathing using a bag-mask device at 15 L/min. You listen to lung sounds and find them absent on the left upper lobe with crackles in the left base. The right lung sounds are within normal limits. You request additional assistance to report to the scene.

Recording Time: 5 Minutes	
Respirations	24 breaths/min
Pulse	120 beats/min, weak
Skin	Cool, pale, moist
Blood pressure	92/70 mm Hg
Oxygen saturation (Spo$_2$)	95% at 15 L/min via bag-mask
Pupils	PERRLA

5. Do you remove the knife or bandage it in place?

6. What additional findings would you be looking for in a focused assessment of the chest?

and the mediastinum to shift to the contralateral side. The lung collapse leads to right-to-left intrapulmonary shunting and hypoxia. A reduction in cardiac output occurs as the increased intrathoracic pressure causes compression of the heart and vena cava, reducing preload by decreasing venous return to the heart.

This pressure increase may even exceed the pressure within the major venous structures, decreasing venous return to the heart, diminishing preload, and eventually resulting in a shock state. As venous return decreases, the patient's body attempts to compensate by increasing the heart rate in an attempt to maintain cardiac output.

Assessment and Management

The classic signs of a tension pneumothorax are an absence of breath sounds on the affected side, unequal chest rise, pulsus paradoxus, tachycardia and dysrhythmias such as progression to ventricular tachycardia and ventricular fibrillation, JVD, narrow pulse pressure, and tracheal deviation. Whereas tachycardia may not be a unique finding in the trauma patient, tension pneumothorax induces this change—not because of a hypovolemic state, but rather because of the inability of blood to easily return to the heart from the venous system. The increasing pressure within the thoracic cavity leads to the accumulation of blood within the great vessels just outside the thoracic cavity. As the pressure is translated into the most superficial of these veins—the jugular veins—they become distended with blood. Such JVD is usually a late sign of tension pneumothorax.

During normal inspiration, the negative pressure within the chest decreases blood return, particularly from the legs if the patient is standing, to the heart, thus decreasing preload and slightly decreasing systolic blood pressure (typically less than 10 mm Hg). In pathologic conditions such as tension pneumothorax or pericardial tamponade where the right ventricle is functionally being compressed, the effect on preload of inspiration is magnified, and a drop in blood pressure associated with creating negative intrathoracic pressure is more pronounced. This condition is known as pulsus paradoxus. In many cases, the radial pulse will actually be palpable with expiration and nonpalpable on inspiration, despite irrefutable evidence of cardiac contraction by stethoscope or ECG.

The jugular veins, which exit the thoracic cavity from beneath the clavicles and cross over the sternocleidomastoid muscles as they move superiorly, are considered to be distended when they are engorged to a level one-half to three-quarter inches (1-2 cm) above the clavicle. This assessment is properly done with the patient in a 45° Fowler position; however, this is something that cannot be accomplished during the primary survey of the trauma patient in the field.

Because of the mediastinal shift caused by the increasing pressure, palpation of the trachea may manifest in a deviation of the trachea away from the affected side. However, this late finding in a tension pneumothorax may not be present despite the rapid decompensation of the patient's clinical status. For this reason, you must be vigilant in watching for the cardiopulmonary findings associated with a tension pneumothorax and not rely on the presence of all the classic physical findings in making the diagnosis.

The accumulation of air within the pleural space decreases the lung volume and diminishes the breath sounds on the affected side when you auscultate the chest. Because air causes the loss of breath sounds on that side, the chest will be resonant (like a bell) when percussed, as opposed to the dull sensation expected with fluid or blood.

Due to the injury and the collapsing lung, a patient with a tension pneumothorax often reports pleuritic chest pain and dyspnea. The resulting hypoxia may cause the patient to become anxious, tachycardic, tachypneic, and even cyanotic.

Hypotension, as a late finding of tension pneumothorax, should not be used to either confirm or exclude the possibility of a tension pneumothorax. Its presence may suggest that the pneumothorax has produced such significant pressure as to severely impede preload, or it may represent a simultaneous shock state due to other injuries. Normal blood pressure suggests that, when other signs of a tension pneumothorax are present, the heart is adequately compensating for the diminished venous return.

Words of Wisdom

Shock (a late sign), decreased breath sounds, and hyperresonance to percussion on the same side of the chest mean a tension pneumothorax is present until proven otherwise.

All patients presenting with signs of a tension pneumothorax should immediately be placed on high-flow supplemental oxygen (12 to 15 L/min) via a NRB mask and should be closely evaluated for the need for ventilatory support (if ventilations are too fast/slow or depressed or inadequate volume). Inspect the chest and cover open wounds with a nonporous or occlusive dressing as local protocols require. If signs of tension are present, lift one corner of the dressing to allow air to escape.

In a patient who has a tension pneumothorax and clinical findings that suggest immediate relief of the elevated pressures is needed, you must accomplish this through a **needle decompression**, also referred to as a needle thoracentesis or pleural decompression. Needle decompression is traditionally performed through the second or third intercostal space in the midclavicular line of the affected side; however, some evidence supports placing the catheter at the fifth interspace, slightly anterior to the midaxillary line.[4]

The steps for performing a needle decompression are described in Skill Drill 35-1.

Skill Drill 35-1 Needle Decompression (Thoracentesis) of a Tension Pneumothorax

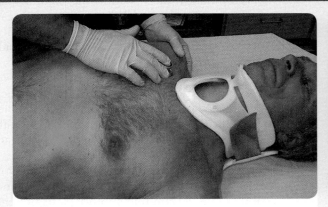

Step 1 Assess the patient to ensure that the presentation matches that of a tension pneumothorax. Look for difficult ventilation despite an open airway, JVD (may not be present with associated hemorrhage), absent or decreased breath sounds on the affected side, hyperresonance to percussion on the affected side, tracheal deviation away from the affected side (late sign, not always present), pulsus paradoxus, and tachycardia.

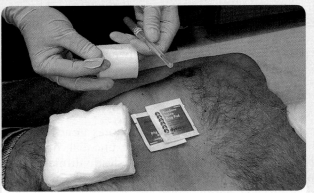

Step 2 Prepare and assemble all necessary equipment, including: a large-bore IV catheter, preferably 14- to 16-gauge and at least 2 inches (5 cm) long (this ensures the ability of the needle to reach the intended depth to relieve pressure); alcohol or povidone iodine (Betadine) preps; a flutter valve (cut off one finger of a glove to use as a substitute if you do not have a commercial device available); and adhesive tape. A two-way or three-way stopcock can also be used to seal or relieve pressure should it begin to build within the thoracic cavity. Obtain medical control order if required by regional protocols.

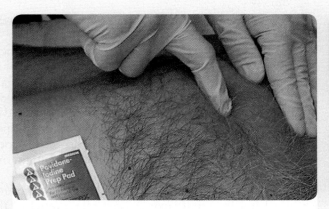

Step 3 Locate the appropriate site Figure 35-14 . Find the second or third rib. Insert the needle just above the third rib into the intercostal space at the midclavicular line on the affected side. If there is significant trauma to the anterior portion of the chest or the chest wall is too deep, use the intercostal space between the fourth and fifth ribs at the midaxillary line on the affected side.

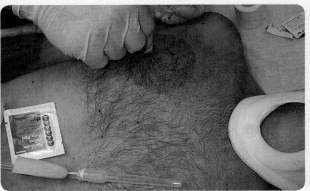

Step 4 Cleanse the appropriate area using aseptic technique.

Skill Drill 35-1 Needle Decompression (Thoracentesis) of a Tension Pneumothorax *(continued)*

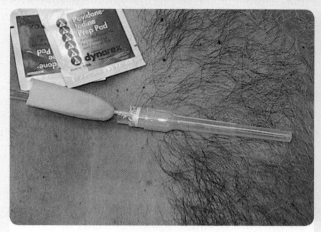

Step 5 Make a one-way valve, or flutter valve, by inserting the catheter through the end of the finger of a medical glove, cut off from the glove. Alternatively, use a commercially prepared device.

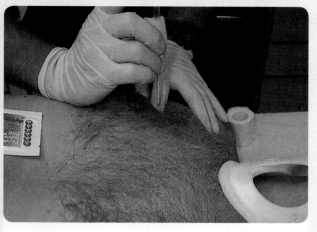

Step 6 Insert the needle at a 90° angle, and listen for the release of air. Insert the needle just superior to the third rib, midclavicular line, or just above the sixth rib, midaxillary line* (to avoid the nerves, arteries, and veins running along the inferior borders of each rib).

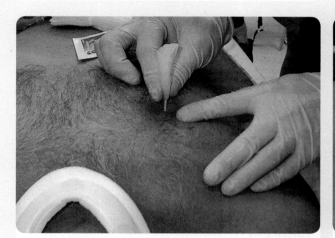

Step 7 Remove the needle, and properly dispose of the needle in the sharps container.

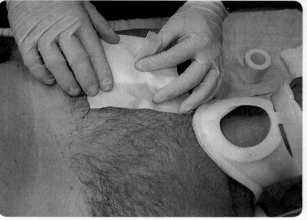

Step 8 Secure the catheter in place in the same manner you would use to secure an impaled object. Monitor the patient closely for recurrence of the tension pneumothorax. This procedure may need to be repeated before arrival at the emergency department.

*Anterior approach is shown here. Some EMS systems are using the lateral approach for this procedure.

© Jones & Bartlett Learning.

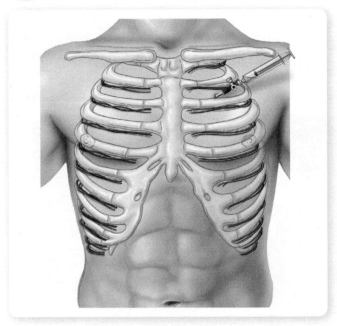

Figure 35-14 Correct placement of the needle for anterior approach to decompression if placing between the second and third rib at the midclavicular line. The positions of nerves, arteries, and veins are shown in relation to the ribs.

© Jones & Bartlett Learning.

Performing a needle decompression is not without risk. If the needle is improperly placed (not inserted over the top of the rib), injury to the intercostal vessels may result in significant hemorrhage. Similarly, passing the needle into the chest may injure the lung parenchyma or even the liver or spleen depending on the position of the diaphragm and the accuracy of the needle position. However, failure to treat tension pneumothorax will cause the patient to progress to cardiopulmonary arrest.

▶ Hemothorax

A **hemothorax** occurs when the potential space between the parietal and visceral pleura is violated and blood begins to accumulate within this space Figure 35-16 . Although it is most commonly caused by tears of lung parenchyma, it may also result from penetrating wounds that puncture the heart or major vessels within the mediastinum or from blunt trauma with deceleration shearing of major vessels. Rib fractures and injuries to the lung parenchyma are the most common sources of injury in the case of a hemothorax. Other causes include injury to the liver, spleen, aorta, internal mammary arteries, intercostal arteries (which can lose up to 50 mL of blood per minute), and other intrathoracic vessels. Due to the location of these

Words of Wisdom

Patients with a pneumothorax, tension pneumothorax, hemothorax, or hemopneumothorax may need a chest tube inserted. A chest tube is a flexible plastic tube that is inserted through the side of the chest into the pleural cavity to remove air, fluid, or pus from the pleural cavity Figure 35-15 . It was traditionally attached to an underwater seal to create a one-way system allowing for air or fluid to drain from the chest with each exhalation, reestablishing the interpleural negative pressure and reinflating the lung. Modern systems no longer use a water chamber, but they have the same effect.

Whereas insertion of a chest tube is not commonly within a paramedic scope of practice, the monitoring and transport of a patient with an existing chest tube is within the National Standards.

When monitoring and transporting a patient with a chest tube in place:

- Make sure all connections are taped or banded with wire to prevent accidental separation.
- Ensure that the dressing over the insertion site is securely taped and occlusive. Use a felt-tip marker to mark the depth of the tube; if there are markings, note the depth of the tube on the transfer chart. Make sure the tube is sutured, wired, or taped so it cannot be accidently pulled out.
- Maintain the drainage unit below the level of the chest at all times during transport. Many units have bed hangers so that the unit can be hung on the stretcher. If there is water in the unit, keep it upright at all times. If attached to a suction device, find out

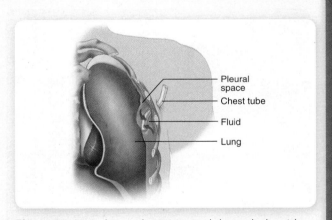

Figure 35-15 A chest tube is inserted through the side of the chest into the pleural space.

© Jones & Bartlett Learning.

if the suction can be discontinued for transport; if not, attach it to portable suction.
- Tubing should be kept coiled to prevent kinks or dependent loops.
- Assess and document bubbling in the water seal (does not have to be continuous), any output in the collection chamber, and its type (eg, blood).
- Do not clamp tubes for transport. This could cause a tension pneumothorax.
- Continuous bubbling may be a sign of tracheobronchial laceration. Large amounts of bloody drainage need to be balanced by transfusion.

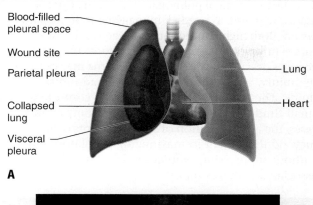

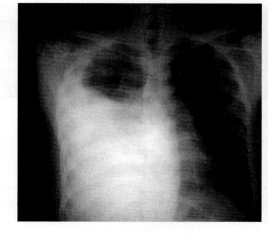

Figure 35-16 A. A hemothorax is a collection of blood in the pleural space produced by bleeding within the chest. **B.** Radiograph of a hemothorax.

A: © Jones & Bartlett Learning; B: © Medicimage/Science Source.

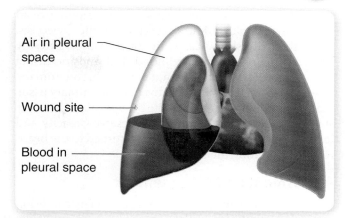

Figure 35-17 In a hemopneumothorax, both blood and air are present.
© Jones & Bartlett Learning.

from other injuries include the lack of tracheal deviation, possible bloody sputum (hemoptysis), and dullness that may be noted on percussion of the affected side of the chest. Neck veins will be flat with associated hypovolemia and distended if there is increased intrathoracic pressure.

The prehospital management of a suspected hemothorax is supportive with rapid transport to the appropriate facility. If the airway does not require intervention, place the patient on high-flow supplemental oxygen via a nonrebreathing mask. Initiate two 18-gauge peripheral IV lines, with fluid resuscitation being guided by local protocols and directed at limiting the duration of hypotension.

> **Words of Wisdom**
>
> The major problem following the occurrence of a massive hemothorax is the development of hypovolemic shock and respiratory compromise.

▶ Pulmonary Contusion

The position of the lungs just beneath the thoracic cage places them at increased risk for injury with thoracic trauma. As the lung tissue is compressed against the chest wall by force or by the positive pressure within the chest during a thoracic injury, alveolar and capillary damage results (see Figure 35-6). This trauma may affect the lungs in a localized area such as a patient with a penetrating injury, or a diffuse area, as in the case of a patient who sustained blunt force trauma to the chest. It leads immediately to a loss of fluid and blood into the involved tissues, followed by white blood cell migration into the area, and, eventually, local tissue edema.

This local tissue injury and edema dilute the local surfactant in the alveoli, diminishing their compliance and causing alveolar collapse (atelectasis). The edema also reduces the delivery of oxygen across the capillary-alveolar interface, resulting in hypoxia. The hypoxia then worsens the situation by thickening the mucus produced, which may

injuries, control of bleeding will be impossible with the usual practices and the amount of circulating blood can be greatly reduced, causing hypovolemic shock.

The collection of blood within the pleural space compresses and displaces the surrounding lung, limiting the patient's ability to adequately oxygenate and ventilate. Unlike a pneumothorax, this injury has the added potential of causing hypovolemia. A **hemopneumothorax** occurs when both blood and air are present in the pleural space **Figure 35-17**.

A massive hemothorax is defined as accumulation of more than 1,500 mL of blood within the pleural space. For the average adult, this amount represents a nearly 25% to 30% blood volume loss, meaning that the patient's condition will have progressed to decompensated (hypotensive) shock. Because each lung can hold up to 3,000 mL, it is possible for a patient to completely bleed out into the thoracic cavity.

Assessment and Management

Physical assessment of a massive hemothorax may reveal signs of both ventilatory insufficiency (hypoxia, agitation, anxiety, tachypnea, dyspnea) and hypovolemic shock (tachycardia, hypotension, pale and clammy skin). The physical findings that help to differentiate this hemothorax

in turn lead to bronchiolar obstruction, air trapping, or an increase in physiologic dead air space and further atelectasis.

If the contusion is large, the body compensates by vasoconstricting pulmonary blood flow and increasing cardiac output. This is an attempt to shunt blood from the injured area and increase its delivery to pulmonary tissue that may be able to oxygenate the blood. This pulmonary shunting decreases the functional reserve capacity and leads to mixed venous blood being returned to the heart, further worsening the hypoxemia.

Assessment and Management

The assessment of the patient with a pulmonary contusion may not initially reveal the presence or severity of the injury because it may take 24 hours before the severity of the injury becomes clinically evident. Because not every trauma patient presents immediately for medical treatment (eg, cases involving domestic violence, assaults, injuries that occur while intoxicated, patients in remote areas who are not immediately located, or search and rescue operations), it is important to be familiar with the clinical presentation of this injury.

Hypoxia and carbon dioxide retention lead to respiratory distress, dyspnea, tachypnea, agitation, and restlessness. Due to the capillary injury and the hemorrhage into the pulmonary parenchyma, the patient may present with hemoptysis (coughing up blood). Evidence of overlying injury may include contusions, tenderness, crepitus, or paradoxical motion. Auscultation may reveal wheezes, rhonchi, crackles, or diminished lung sounds in the affected area. In severe cases, cyanosis and low oxygen saturations may be found.

The treatment of pulmonary contusion begins with the assessment and, as needed, management of the patient's airway. Both high-concentration oxygen and positive pressure ventilation may be used to overcome the pathologic changes described earlier. Because edema may exacerbate the injury, use caution when you are administering IV fluids. The use of IV fluids should be controlled with small fluid boluses to improve cardiac output. In some cases, the administration of small amounts of analgesics may aid the patient in maximizing ventilatory function without suppressing ventilatory drive by reducing pain associated with this injury.

■ Pathophysiology, Assessment, and Management of Myocardial Injuries

▶ Cardiac Tamponade

Cardiac tamponade is defined as excessive fluid in the **pericardial sac**, causing compression of the heart and decreased cardiac output **Figure 35-18** . Cardiac tamponade may also be referred to as pericardial tamponade. The size of the perforation in the pericardium determines the hemodynamic effects of cardiac tamponade, the rate of hemorrhage from the cardiac wound (dependent on the type of vessel—artery vs. vein), and the chamber of the heart involved (the right ventricle is most often penetrated due to its anatomic position). The injury is more commonly caused by a penetrating mechanism, but is also

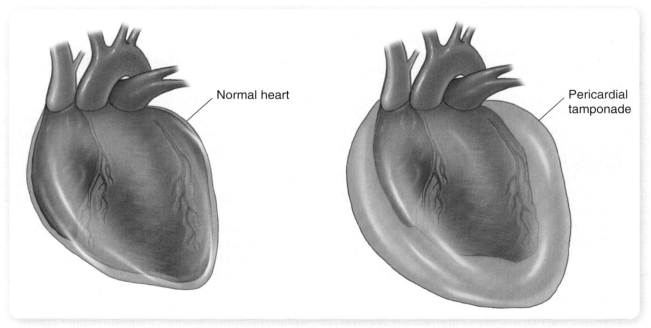

Figure 35-18 Cardiac tamponade is a potentially fatal condition in which fluid builds up within the pericardial sac, compressing the heart's chambers and dramatically impairing its ability to pump blood.

caused by blunt injuries to the chest. Few patients with blunt thoracic trauma experience cardiac tamponade, whereas many patients with cardiac stab wounds develop this condition.

Cardiac tamponade can occur in both medical and trauma patients. In the medical setting, inflammatory processes (ie, pericarditis, uremia, myocardial infarction) lead to the slow collection of fluid within the pericardial sac and the gradual distention of the parietal pericardium. Through this process, 1,000 to 1,500 mL of fluid may accumulate in the pericardial sac. Conversely, the bleeding in the trauma patient is rapid, with blood loss from the coronary vasculature or the myocardium itself quickly collecting between the visceral and parietal pericardium. Because the parietal pericardium is not able to rapidly stretch due to its fibrous tissue, an accumulation of as little as 50 mL of blood can cause a reduction in cardiac output.

As the pericardium fills, the continued bleeding increases the pressure within the pericardium. The more pliable structures within the pericardium—namely, the atria and the vena cavae—become compressed, which drastically reduces preload and thereby diminishes stroke volume. The heart initially attempts to compensate for this reduction in preload by increasing the heart rate. This attempt to maintain cardiac output is only temporary because the continued bleeding will further restrict preload and diastolic filling. The pressure within the pericardial sac will also reduce the perfusion in the myocardium, resulting in global myocardial dysfunction. The combination of these two processes leads to the development of hypotension.

Assessment and Management

The Beck triad is the classic combination of physical findings found in 10% to 40% of patients diagnosed with cardiac tamponade.[5] It includes muffled heart tones, hypotension, and JVD.

Another classic finding in cardiac tamponade (albeit one that is not always present) is the ECG finding of electrical alternans. As fluid accumulates within the pericardial sac, the heart begins to oscillate with each beat. As the heart swings back and forth within the pericardium, its electrical axis changes. Electrical alternans is not commonly seen in acute cardiac tamponade and must be differentiated from bigeminal ectopy, but it is a classic sign of cardiac tamponade. Cardiac output is affected due to an increase in diastolic pressure, and as the condition progresses, a narrowing of pulse pressures will result.

Words of Wisdom

Hypotension and distended neck veins in the presence of normal lung sounds (which rules out pneumothorax), combined with an appropriate history, suggest cardiac tamponade.

Table 35-2	Physical Findings of Cardiac Tamponade Versus Tension Pneumothorax	
Physical Finding	**Cardiac Tamponade**	**Tension Pneumothorax**
Presenting sign/symptom	Shock	Respiratory distress
Neck veins	Distended	Distended
Trachea	Midline	Deviated
Breath sounds	Equal on both sides	Decreased or absent on side of injury
Chest percussion	Normal	Hyperresonant on side of injury
Heart sounds	Muffled	Typically normal

© Jones & Bartlett Learning.

The reduced cardiac output, hypoperfusion, and hypotension observed in cardiac tamponade produce the findings typical of a patient in shock: weak or absent peripheral pulses, diaphoresis, dyspnea, cyanosis, altered mental status, tachycardia, tachypnea, and agitation. Although these symptoms by themselves do not suggest or exclude the presence of cardiac tamponade, identifying them can flesh out the physical assessment.

Physical findings in a patient with cardiac tamponade are not significantly different from those of a tension pneumothorax—namely, hypotension, JVD, tachycardia, altered mental status, and signs of tissue hypoperfusion. One way to differentiate between the two is to remember that in cardiac tamponade, the breath sounds will be equal and the trachea will be midline because the lungs are not affected. **Table 35-2** compares the physical findings of these two emergencies.

The treatment of the patient with cardiac tamponade begins by assessing and managing the ABCs, ensuring adequate oxygen delivery, and establishing IV access. Provide a rapid fluid bolus to maintain cardiac output. Administering IV fluids may slow the patient's deterioration by momentarily increasing preload. The ultimate treatment for cardiac tamponade is **pericardiocentesis**, which involves inserting a needle attached to a syringe into the chest far enough to penetrate the pericardium to withdraw fluid **Figure 35-19**. The patient with a cardiac tamponade should be transported rapidly to a trauma center for pericardiocentesis. Definitive management occurs in the operating room.

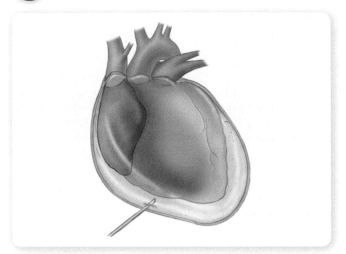

Figure 35-19 Needle aspiration in cardiac tamponade, shown here, is performed in the hospital.

© Jones & Bartlett Learning.

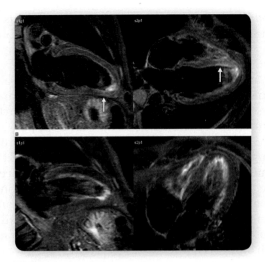

Figure 35-20 Myocardial contusion.

"Cardiac Contusion in a Professional Soccer Player", Vago et al. *Circulation*, June 8, 2010. © American Heart Association.

▶ Myocardial Contusion

The heart's anterior and unprotected position just behind the sternum puts it in a potentially precarious position during a blunt force mechanism. At speeds of greater than 20 to 35 miles per hour, the sudden deceleration of the chest wall may cause the heart to move forward until it collides with the posterior aspect of the sternum, leading to the blunt cardiac injury known as **myocardial contusion** **Figure 35-20**. This type of injury is characterized by local tissue contusion and hemorrhage, edema, and cellular damage within the involved myocardium. Direct damage to the epicardial vessels (coronary arteries and veins) may compromise the blood flow to the heart. Damage to the myocardium tissue at a cellular level may result in ectopic activity, reentry pathways, and dysrhythmias.

Complications of myocardial contusions are similar to the complications seen in patients who experience a myocardial infarction. With this in mind, obtain a 12- or 15-lead ECG to determine the degree of cardiac dysfunction while en route to the hospital. Do not delay transport to obtain the ECG. Dysrhythmias may occur (although they are uncommon in children) due to cellular membrane injury and changes in the myocardial action potential. Structural changes from myocardial blunt injury are rare and often immediately fatal.

Assessment and Management

Sharp, retrosternal chest pain is a common complaint among patients with myocardial contusion. Inspection of the area may reveal soft-tissue or bony injury in the area. Crackles (due to pulmonary edema from left ventricular dysfunction) may be heard on auscultation.

The ECG in a patient with a myocardial contusion is often abnormal. ECG changes may include sinus tachycardia, atrial fibrillation or flutter, premature atrial complexes (PACs) or premature ventricular complexes

(PVCs), a new right bundle branch block, atrioventricular (AV) blocks, nonspecific ST-segment and T-wave changes, and ventricular tachycardia or fibrillation. In the event of a coronary artery injury (likely the right coronary artery), ischemic changes consistent with those seen in myocardial infarction may also occur.

The treatment of patients with possible myocardial contusion begins with supportive care, including oxygen administration, frequent assessment of vital signs, cardiac monitoring, and establishing IV access. Fluid resuscitation should be instituted as needed to maintain the patient's blood pressure with careful monitoring to ensure a fluid overload doesn't occur. Be sure to follow your local protocols regarding fluid boluses and fluid monitoring. Unless allowed by local protocols, consultation with on-line medical control should precede the administration of antidysrhythmic agents to trauma patients.

▶ Myocardial Rupture

Myocardial rupture is an acute perforation of the ventricles, atria, intraventricular septum, intra-atrial septum, chordae tendineae, papillary muscles, or valves. The application of severe blunt force to the chest compresses the heart between the sternum and the vertebrae, which can rupture the myocardium. In penetrating trauma, a foreign object or bony fragment may be propelled into the heart, resulting in a laceration of the myocardial wall. Whether it occurs from a penetrating injury or blunt trauma, a ruptured myocardium is a life-threatening condition.

Assessment and Management

Remember that myocardial rupture is life threatening. Patients may present with acute pulmonary edema or signs of cardiac tamponade. Unless the latter is present and a pericardiocentesis can be done, patients with myocardial rupture should receive supportive care and be rapidly transported to a designated trauma center per local trauma protocols.

Commotio Cordis

If the thorax receives a direct blow during the critical portion of the heart's repolarization period, the result may be immediate cardiac arrest. **Commotio cordis** is ultimately the result of the chest wall impact directly over the heart, especially directly over the left ventricle. Impacts to the chest that are not directly over the heart will not cause commotio cordis.

This phenomenon has been documented to occur following blunt or nonpenetrating chest trauma to the anterior aspect of the chest. Commotio cordis may occur during sports where contact with high-speed objects occurs, including softball, baseball, lacrosse, polo, rugby, boxing, football, or hockey or from items such as bats, snowballs, fists, and even from kicks and punches during kickboxing, boxing, or karate.

Assessment and Management

Patients who are unresponsive, apneic, and pulseless may be experiencing commotio cordis. Many of these patients are cyanotic, and tonic-clonic (grand mal) seizures have been evident in some. Chest wall contusions and localized bruising that correspond to the site of chest impact are also indicators.

Pathophysiology, Assessment, and Management of Vascular Injuries

Traumatic Aortic Disruption

Dissection or rupture of the aorta, also called **traumatic aortic disruption** or aortic dissection, occurs most often in blunt trauma as a result of motor vehicle crashes and falls. One in every five deaths due to blunt trauma includes a transection of the aorta; the most common causes are high-speed motor vehicle crashes and falls from a height.[6] Each year, 5,000 to 8,000 people in the United States die as a result of aortic or great vessel rupture.[7] Given that the body's entire blood volume passes through this vessel, the high mortality associated with such an injury comes as no surprise. Those with transection of the aorta can die quickly from massive hemorrhage, and therefore require immediate transport. Those with less severe injuries can survive until emergency medical services (EMS) units arrive, and with prompt management including surgical intervention at the hospital.

The most widely accepted theory of how this injury evolves holds that the aorta is injured at its fixed points due to shearing forces. The high-velocity, high-energy impacts that result in these injuries cause the aortic arch to swing forward. The resulting tension, along with rotation and torque on the area, causes the descending aorta to rupture at its point of attachment to the posterior thoracic wall **Figure 35-21**.

The aorta includes three layers—the intima, the media, and the adventitia. If the injury tears the intima, the high pressure within the aorta allows the blood to dissect along the media. More severe injuries damage all three layers of the aorta, allowing blood to leak from the aorta into the surrounding tissues. If these tissues cannot stop the bleeding, the patient can survive only with prompt intervention. Otherwise, the injury will be fatal.

Assessment and Management

Depending on the exact nature of the injury, the symptoms and physical exam findings in cases of traumatic aortic disruption or transection will vary from a patient in unstable condition to one with no physical complaints. However, most patients will report tearing pain behind the sternum or in the scapula. Other findings may include signs of hypovolemic shock, dyspnea, and altered mental

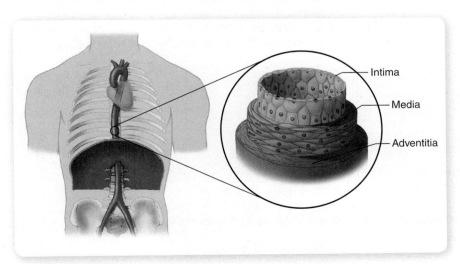

Figure 35-21 The aortic arch, descending aorta, and layers of the aorta.
© Jones & Bartlett Learning.

status. If a hematoma forms in the area of the esophagus, trachea, or larynx, the patient may present with dysphagia, stridor, and hoarseness, respectively. The patient may also have difficulty swallowing. A harsh murmur may be noted due to the turbulence created as the blood passes the site of the injury to the intima in the aorta.

Recognition of traumatic aortic disruption often comes from a high index of suspicion based on the MOI because a high percentage of patients have no signs of external chest trauma. Assessment of the patient's pulses in all extremities is an important key to the identification of these injuries. As the disruption compresses the aorta and progresses along its branch vessels, blood flow to the extremities may be compromised. This phenomenon results in diminished pulses compared with those closer to the site of the injury. On exam, you will note a stronger pulse (and higher blood pressure) in the right arm than in the left arm or the lower extremities. Hypotension and signs of shock may be present.

Because of the high energy involved with aortic injuries, associated injuries are to be expected. They may include multiple rib fractures, flail segment, sternal or scapular fracture, pericardial tamponade, hemothorax or pneumothorax, and clavicle fracture.

The prehospital management of potential aortic injuries is symptomatic. After assessment and management of the ABCs, the patient should receive gradual IV hydration for the treatment of hypotension. Aggressive fluid administration may result in sudden changes in the intra-aortic pressure that could worsen the injury. Do not use vasoactive or vasopressor agents. Expedited transport to a trauma center is essential.

▶ Great Vessel Injury

With the exception of the aorta, the great vessels are located in areas that offer protection from adjacent bony structures and other tissues. Consequently, injury to these vessels is much more likely with penetrating trauma. In rare instances, blunt trauma may damage the overlying structures or produce a severe rotational injury (such as that caused by machinery).

Some great vessel injuries may result in occlusion or spasm of the involved artery. These injuries will present with ischemic changes (pain, pallor, paresthesias, pulselessness, paralysis) in areas in which the blood supply is coming from the involved artery.

Assessment and Management

If bleeding is not prevented, the patient with a great vessel injury will present with signs and symptoms of hypovolemic shock, hemothorax, or cardiac tamponade. If the bleeding results in formation of a hematoma, the compression of adjacent structures (ie, esophagus, trachea) may produce additional signs and symptoms.

> **Words of Wisdom**
>
> Suspect aortic rupture in any accident involving powerful deceleration forces.

The management of potential injuries to the great vessels is no different from the management of any other

YOU are the Paramedic — PART 4

An additional unit arrives on scene to assist. You place the patient in full spinal precautions, to further stabilize the knife and prevent dislodgement or motion with additional injury during transport. You bandage the knife in place, and move the patient to the back of your ambulance for further assessment. Further assessment of the chest reveals no signs of subcutaneous emphysema, muffled heart tones, or rib fractures. You apply the cardiac monitor and find a sinus tachycardia with no ectopy at a rate of 120 beats/min.

Recording Time: 10 Minutes	
Respirations	24 breaths/min
Pulse	120 beats/min, weak
Skin	Cool, pale, moist
Blood pressure	90/72 mm Hg
Oxygen saturation (Spo₂)	96% at 15 L/min via bag-mask device
Pupils	PERRLA

7. What is the next treatment you should consider for this patient?
8. How often should you reassess this patient?

form of acute blood loss. Establish an IV line to provide hydration en route to the trauma center, and treat pericardial tamponade immediately if it is found.

Pathophysiology, Assessment, and Management of Other Thoracic Injuries

▶ Diaphragmatic Injuries

Diaphragmatic injury occurs in a relatively small percentage of all trauma patients, yet the potential for this injury has prompted a change in the management of penetrating trauma in recent years. For example, some surgeons manage penetrating trauma between the midaxillary lines, below the clavicle, and above the iliac crests by undertaking surgical exploration to ensure that the diaphragm is intact. This conservative approach reflects the possibility that a missed diaphragmatic injury may result in significant complications in the years following the injury.

Words of Wisdom

Blunt disruptions of the diaphragm are usually associated with herniation of all or part of the liver into the right side of the chest and the stomach into the left side of the chest. The hiatus is the weakest point and hiatal hernias are common.

Injury to the diaphragm may result from direct penetrating injury or blunt force trauma leading to diaphragmatic rupture. Because the liver protects the diaphragm on the right side, most diaphragmatic injuries (particularly those due to blunt trauma) occur on the left side. Once the diaphragm has been injured, the healing process is inhibited by the natural pressure differences between the abdominal and thoracic cavities.

Injury to the diaphragm and the associated physical findings have been separated into three phases: acute, latent, and obstructive. The acute phase begins at the time of injury and ends with recovery from other injuries (which may overshadow the diaphragmatic injury and serves to explain why less than one-fourth of these injuries are identified during the acute phase). In the latent phase, the patient experiences intermittent abdominal pain due to the periodic herniation or entrapment of abdominal contents in the defect. The obstructive phase occurs when any abdominal contents herniate through the defect, cutting off their blood supply (infarct) in the process.

A rare but ultimate complication of a diaphragmatic injury is the herniation of sufficient abdominal contents into the thoracic cavity. The resulting increased intrathoracic pressure both compresses the lung on the affected

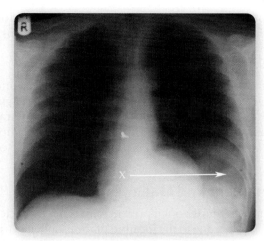

Figure 35-22 Radiograph of a diaphragmatic rupture. The shadow, indicated by the arrow, shows the stomach herniated through the diaphragmatic rupture.
© Hariharan et al; licensee BioMed Central Ltd. 2006.

side and compromises circulatory function; this finding is called a tension gastrothorax.[8]

Assessment and Management

Although diaphragmatic injuries are not likely to be identified in the prehospital setting, you should still maintain clinical suspicion for such injuries **Figure 35-22**. You are most likely to care for the patient during the acute phase, but delayed presentations in the obstructive phase are also possible.

In the acute phase, the patient may present with hypotension, tachypnea, bowel sounds in the chest, chest pain, or absence of breath sounds on the affected side. These signs indicate a large diaphragmatic injury that may be followed by herniation of the abdominal contents into the thoracic cavity.

In the obstructive phase, as the blood supply to the herniated organs becomes compromised, symptoms will include nausea, vomiting, abdominal pain, constipation, dyspnea, and abdominal distention. In many cases, these symptoms are severe and unrelenting. The most severe findings may be consistent with a tension gastrothorax.

In both the acute and obstructive phases, management of diaphragmatic injury focuses on maintaining adequate oxygenation and providing rapid transport to the hospital. Elevate the head of the backboard to keep the abdominal contents in the abdominal cavity, and provide positive pressure ventilation for hypoventilation. In prehospital systems that allow for such procedures, nasogastric

Words of Wisdom

Use of nitrous oxide should be avoided in patients with a possible diaphragmatic injury because it can greatly increase the volume of gas within entrapped viscera.

tube placement may improve the patient's condition by decompressing the involved gastrointestinal organs.

▶ Esophageal Injuries

Esophageal injuries are one of the most rapidly fatal injuries to the gastrointestinal tract, particularly if the diagnosis is not made early. Fortunately, even with penetrating trauma, such injuries are rare. Because of the location of the esophagus, however, it is often associated with other significant injuries.

Assessment and Management

Esophageal injuries often present with other thoracic and spinal injuries due to the location of the esophagus within the thorax. The patient may experience pleuritic chest pain, and particularly pain that is made worse by swallowing or flexion of the neck. Subcutaneous emphysema may occur, but more than half of esophageal injury patients with this finding have an associated tracheal injury.

No specific therapy for esophageal injuries is possible in the prehospital setting. Definitive care occurs once the patient is evaluated in the hospital and an appropriate surgical consultation is achieved. In the meantime, as with every trauma patient, ensure that the patient is given nothing orally to help minimize complications related to this injury.

▶ Tracheobronchial Injuries

Injuries to the major airways are rare. In most instances, they are caused by penetrating injuries, but they may occasionally be seen in severe deceleration injuries. Tracheobronchial injuries have a high mortality rate due to the associated airway disruption **Figure 35-23** .

As with aortic injuries, the site of a tracheobronchial injury is often close to a point of attachment—namely, the carina. The injury to the trachea or mainstem bronchi allows for rapid movement of air into the pleural space or the mediastinum, resulting in a pneumothorax or pneumomediastinum. As this injury progresses to a tension pneumothorax, a needle thoracentesis is often insufficient because the rate of air entry into the pleural space exceeds the rate at which the air can escape from the inserted angiocath.

Assessment and Management

The clinical presentation of tracheobronchial injuries may vary from mildly symptomatic to severe respiratory compromise. Expected physical findings include hoarseness, dyspnea and tachypnea, respiratory distress, and hemoptysis. Look for findings of a pneumothorax or tension pneumothorax.

The treatment of a patient with a suspected tracheobronchial injury centers on adequate assessment and management of the patient's ABCs. The patient with a tenuous airway who can be managed with bag-mask ventilation should not be intubated, because introducing an endotracheal tube may complete a partial tracheal injury and result in complete airway obstruction. Similarly, because of the rapid loss of air into the pleural space, high ventilatory pressures should be avoided when you are providing positive pressure ventilation (bag the patient gently and slowly).

▶ Traumatic Asphyxia

Traumatic injuries that suddenly and forcefully compress the thoracic cavity may induce **traumatic asphyxia** **Figure 35-24** . Traumatic asphyxia may result from an unrestrained driver hitting a steering wheel or a pedestrian who is compressed between a vehicle and a wall. The sudden compression of the chest causes pressure to be translated into the major veins of the head, neck, and kidneys. This massive increase in pressure then passes into the capillary beds, resulting in their rupture.

Assessment and Management

Traumatic asphyxia is characterized by a series of dramatic physical findings. Patients will have cyanosis of

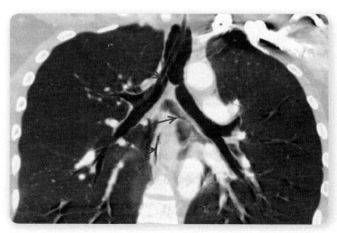

Figure 35-23 Tracheobronchial injury.

Reprinted from Erratum to the August 2014 issue of the Journal of Cardiothoracic and Vascular Anesthesia *J Cardiothorac Vasc Anesth* 28(4), 2015, with permission from Elsevier.

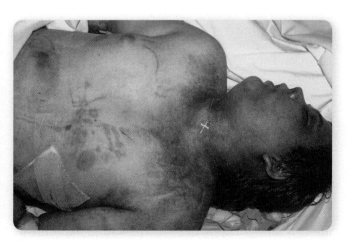

Figure 35-24 Traumatic asphyxia.

the head, the upper extremities, and the torso above the level of the compression. Ocular hemorrhage may be mild, such as bleeding into the anterior surface of the eye (**subconjunctival hematoma**), or extremely dramatic, causing the eyes to protrude from their normal position (**exophthalmos**). Other facial structures, including the tongue and lips, may also become dramatically swollen and cyanotic.

Although the term *asphyxia* implies a uniformly fatal outcome for patients, this is not always the case. Given the significant force required to produce traumatic asphyxia,

however, your suspicion for associated injuries should be quite high. Do not let the dramatic physical findings in the head and neck distract you from those injuries that are immediately life threatening.

After other life-threatening injuries are managed, the treatment of patients exhibiting traumatic asphyxia is relatively brief. In the absence of intubation, provide high-flow supplemental oxygen via a nonrebreathing mask. Take cervical spine precautions, including spinal immobilization. Obtain IV access with two large-bore IV lines. Transport to the nearest appropriate trauma center.

YOU are the Paramedic   SUMMARY

1. What is your primary concern for this patient?

Your immediate concern is the overall presentation of the patient. Does your rapid scan reveal any obvious life threats? Is he responsive? Does he have obvious breathing difficulty or evidence of injury? Does he appear pale, cyanotic, red, or gray? Is he alert and oriented or confused? You already know the cause of injury and that the patient is intoxicated. What you do not know is what damage has been done and how it is affecting the patient.

2. What anatomic structures could be damaged in relation to the position of the knife?

The structures located in the vicinity of the knife blade are the left lung, heart, aorta, and the pleural layers. Do not assume the length of the knife blade as being long or short. Do not assume any single structure in the vicinity of the wound is not damaged.

3. What immediate treatment do you need to provide to this patient?

Immediate treatment is centered on maintaining the patient's airway and providing oxygen. You can be reasonably confident there is damage to the respiratory system due to the location of the knife. You will need to conduct a focused assessment to determine the extent of the damage.

4. What steps will you take in your further assessment of this patient?

The breathing assessment begins with an inspection of the patient's thorax. Consider the appearance of the chest wall and look for signs of soft-tissue injury that suggest the possibility of an underlying injury. Paradoxical motion of a section of the chest wall, retractions, subcutaneous air or edema, impaled objects, or penetrating injuries also suggest an underlying injury with the potential

to compromise the patient's breathing. Next, consider the adequacy of both ventilation and oxygenation. To assess ventilation, examine the patient's respiratory rate, depth, and effort. The final assessment steps entail the palpation, percussion, and auscultation of the chest. Finally, auscultation of the heart sounds is an important part of the circulatory assessment. The presence of muffled heart tones is an important diagnostic clue to the presence of either a tension pneumothorax or a pericardial tamponade.

5. Do you remove the knife or bandage it in place?

The best course of treatment is to leave the knife in the chest and bandage it in place. You have no idea what structures could be damaged by pulling the knife out of the chest.

6. What additional findings would you be looking for in a focused assessment of the chest?

The final steps in the assessment of the patient's breathing entail the palpation, percussion, and auscultation of the chest. While palpating the chest, assess for any evidence of point tenderness, bony instability, crepitus, subcutaneous emphysema, edema, and tracheal position. Percussion can help to identify either hyperresonance (suggesting increased air within the cavity) or dullness (suggesting blood within the cavity).

7. What is the next treatment you should consider for this patient?

The patient whose circulatory status is compromised (as evidenced by tachycardia, hypotension, or end-organ dysfunction) requires supportive measures until definitive care can be delivered. Placing the patient in a supine position will deliver blood otherwise held in the venous system of the lower extremities to the central circulation.

YOU are the Paramedic SUMMARY (continued)

The judicious provision of IV fluids may also help to expand the intravascular volume while maintaining the oxygen-carrying capacity of the blood.

8. How often should you reassess this patient?

In your reassessment of the thoracic trauma patient, obtain repeated assessments of the patient's vital signs, oxygenation, circulatory status, and breath sounds. Because the progression from pneumothorax to tension pneumothorax can occur quite rapidly, all patients with a presumptive diagnosis of a pneumothorax should be considered to be in unstable condition and reassessed at least every 5 minutes for worsening dyspnea, tachycardia, and the development of JVD.

EMS Patient Care Report (PCR)

Date: 05-22-18	**Incident No.:** 73577	**Nature of Call:** Stabbing		**Location:** 1040 Main Street	
Dispatched: 0115	**En Route:** 0116	**At Scene:** 0121	**Transport:** 0129	**At Hospital:** 0142	**In Service:** 0200

Patient Information

Age: 40 **Sex:** M **Weight (in kg [lb]):** 91 kg (200 lb)	**Allergies:** Unknown **Medications:** Unknown **Past Medical History:** Unknown **Chief Complaint:** Stabbing to left upper chest

Vital Signs

Time: 0126	**BP:** 92/70	**Pulse:** 120	**Respirations:** 24	**Spo$_2$:** 95%
Time: 0131	**BP:** 90/72	**Pulse:** 120	**Respirations:** 24	**Spo$_2$:** 96%
Time:	**BP:**	**Pulse:**	**Respirations:**	**Spo$_2$:**

EMS Treatment (circle all that apply)

Oxygen @ ___15___ **L/min via (circle one):** NC NRM (Bag-mask device)	**Assisted Ventilation**	**Airway Adjunct**	**CPR**
Defibrillation	**Bleeding Control**	(Bandaging)	**Splinting**	(**Other:** IV line with saline)

Narrative

Arrived to find approx. 40-year-old male with a knife protruding from his left upper chest ½ inch below mid clavicle. Only the handle of the knife is visible. Law enforcement is present and reports the pt is intoxicated. Pt is responsive and disoriented, actively trying to remove the knife. Officer assisted with restraining pt hands until assessment could be made. Oxygen via bag-mask @ 15 L/min applied. Pt's chest wall is intact with no bleeding from the wound noted. Lung sounds absent in the left upper lobe and crackles in all left lower fields. Right lung sounds are within normal limits. Spinal precautions taken to help stabilize knife and prevent additional injury during transport. Knife secured in place with a bulky dressing. IV normal saline established with 18-gauge in left antecubital vein. Pt is transported to the trauma center with no change in condition. Reported to Dr Morrison on arrival.**End of report**

Prep Kit

▶ Ready for Review

- The thorax contains the ribs, thoracic vertebrae, clavicle, scapula, sternum, heart, lungs, diaphragm, great vessels (including the aorta), esophagus, lymphatic channels, trachea, mainstem bronchi, and nerves.
- Oxygenation and ventilation (delivery of oxygen and removal of carbon dioxide) take place within the thorax, as well as some aspects of circulation.
- Injuries to the thorax can cause air or blood to enter the lungs, or may prevent the organs from being able to move properly, inhibiting oxygenation and ventilation.
- Begin the assessment of a thoracic trauma patient as you would any other patient—with a scene size-up and assessment of the ABCs.
- When you are assessing breathing, note any signs of injury to the thorax, which could indicate additional underlying injuries. Look for paradoxical motion, retractions, subcutaneous emphysema, impaled objects, or penetrating injuries.
- Consider the adequacy of ventilation and oxygenation. Watch for signs of hypoxia, an irregular pulse, changes in blood pressure, and jugular venous distention.
- Because the mechanism of injury that caused the thoracic condition may have been traumatic, always consider cervical spine immobilization in such cases.
- Several types of chest injuries may have similar signs and symptoms, such as hypoxia, pain, tachycardia, cyanosis, and shock. Managing the various chest injuries involves several common steps: maintaining the airway, ensuring oxygenation and ventilation, supporting circulatory status, and transporting quickly. Learning the subtle differences between various chest injuries will help you manage them more specifically.
- Chest wall injuries include flail chest, rib fractures, sternal fractures, and clavicle fractures.
- In flail chest, two or more ribs are broken in two or more places. It can result in a free-floating segment of rib that moves paradoxically when compared with the rest of the chest wall. As a result, the lung tissue beneath the flail segment is not adequately ventilated.
- Management of flail chest includes airway management and possibly positive pressure ventilation, if the patient experiences respiratory failure. Intubation may also be necessary.
- Rib fractures produce significant pain and can prevent adequate ventilation. Sternal and clavicle fractures are also problematic because they are usually associated with other serious injuries.
- Management of rib fractures should focus on the ABCs.
- Lung injuries include simple pneumothorax, open pneumothorax, tension pneumothorax, hemothorax, and pulmonary contusion.
- A pneumothorax occurs when air leaks into the space between the pleural surfaces from an opening in the chest or the surface of the lung. The lung collapses as air fills the pleural space. The result is a mismatch between ventilation and perfusion.
- Management of a pneumothorax begins with the ABCs and administration of high-concentration oxygen. Cover a sucking chest wound with a nonporous dressing.
- A tension pneumothorax is a life-threatening condition and results from collection of air in the pleural space. The air exerts increasing pressure on surrounding tissues as it accumulates, compromising ventilation, oxygenation, and circulation.
- Patients with a tension pneumothorax should be placed on high-flow supplemental oxygen via a nonrebreathing mask. Cover open wounds with a nonporous or occlusive dressing. If signs of tension are present, lift one corner of the dressing to allow air to escape.
- A hemothorax is the accumulation of blood between the parietal and visceral pleura. It results in compression of structures around the collection of blood and compromises ventilation, oxygenation, and circulation.
- If the airway of a patient with a hemothorax does not require intervention, place the patient on high-flow supplemental oxygen via a nonrebreathing mask. Initiate two large-bore peripheral IV lines, with fluid resuscitation being guided by local protocols and directed at limiting the duration of hypotension.
- A hemopneumothorax is the collection of both blood and air in the pleural space.
- A pulmonary contusion occurs from compression of the lung. It results in alveolar and capillary damage, edema, and hypoxia.
- For patients with a pulmonary contusion or cardiac tamponade, assess and manage the ABCs and consider administering IV fluids.
- Myocardial injuries include cardiac tamponade, myocardial contusion, myocardial rupture, and commotio cordis.
- Cardiac tamponade occurs when excessive fluid builds up in the pericardial sac around the heart. The heart becomes compressed and stroke volume is compromised.

Prep Kit (continued)

- The treatment of the patient with cardiac tamponade begins by managing the ABCs, ensuring adequate oxygen delivery, and establishing IV access. Provide a rapid fluid bolus to maintain cardiac output. Pericardiocentesis is the ultimate treatment option for this condition, a risky technique that is rarely performed by paramedics.
- Myocardial contusion is essentially blunt trauma to the heart. Hemorrhage, edema, and cellular damage result, and dysrhythmias may occur.
- Management of patients with a myocardial contusion should be supportive, but also includes cardiac monitoring and establishing IV access. Fluid resuscitation should be instituted as needed to maintain the patient's blood pressure. Consultation with online medical control may precede the administration of antidysrhythmic agents.
- Myocardial rupture is perforation of one or more elements of the anatomy of the heart, such as the ventricles, atria, or valves. It can occur from blunt or penetrating trauma.
- Patients with myocardial rupture should receive supportive care and be rapidly transported to a trauma center where a thoracotomy can be performed.
- Commotio cordis occurs from a direct blow to the chest during a critical portion of the heart's repolarization period, resulting in possible cardiac arrest.
- Vascular injuries include traumatic aortic disruption and great vessel injury.
- Traumatic aortic disruption is literally ripping of the aorta. Injuries to other great vessels may cause similar conditions of potentially fatal bleeding.
- Care for patients with traumatic aortic disruption focuses on symptom control. After assessment and management of the ABCs, the patient should receive gradual IV hydration for the treatment of hypotension. Management of patients with great vessel injuries is no different from those with acute blood loss.
- Other thoracic injuries include diaphragmatic injuries (abdominal contents may herniate through the injury and cut off the blood supply); esophageal injuries, which can be rapidly fatal; tracheobronchial injuries (injury to the airways); and traumatic asphyxia (sudden compression of the chest leading to pressure on the head, neck, and kidneys, causing capillary beds to rupture).

▶ Vital Vocabulary

atelectasis Alveolar collapse that prevents use of that portion of the lungs for ventilation and oxygenation.

cardiac tamponade A condition in which the atria and right ventricle are collapsed by a collection of blood or other fluid within the pericardial sac, resulting in a diminished cardiac output.

clavicle An S-shaped bone, also called the collarbone, that articulates medially with the sternum and laterally with the shoulder.

commotio cordis An event in which an often-fatal cardiac dysrhythmia is produced by a sudden blow to the thoracic cavity.

crepitus A grating sensation made when two pieces of broken bone rub together or subcutaneous emphysema is palpated.

exophthalmos Protrusion of the eyes from the normal position within the socket.

flail chest An injury that involves two or more adjacent ribs fractured in two or more places, allowing the segment between the fractures to move independently of the rest of the thoracic cage.

hemopneumothorax A collection of blood and air in the pleural cavity.

hemothorax The collection of blood within the normally closed pleural space.

jugular venous distention (JVD) A prominence of the jugular veins due to increased volume or increased pressure within the central venous system or the thoracic cavity.

myocardial contusion Blunt force injury to the heart that results in capillary damage, interstitial bleeding, and cellular damage in the area.

myocardial rupture An acute traumatic perforation of the ventricles, atria, intraventricular septum, intra-atrial septum, chordae, papillary muscles, or valves.

needle decompression Also referred to as a needle thoracentesis, this procedure introduces a needle or angiocath into the pleural space in an attempt to relieve a tension pneumothorax.

open pneumothorax The result of a defect in the chest wall that allows air to enter the thoracic space.

pericardial sac The potential space between the layers of the pericardium.

Prep Kit (continued)

pericardiocentesis A procedure in which a needle or angiocath is introduced into the pericardial sac to relieve cardiac tamponade.

pneumothorax The collection of air within the normally closed pleural space.

pulmonary contusion Injury to the lung parenchyma that results in capillary hemorrhage into the tissue.

pulsus paradoxus A drop in the systolic blood pressure of 10 mm Hg more than during inspiration; commonly seen in patients with cardiac tamponade or severe asthma.

subconjunctival hematoma The collection of blood within the sclera of the eye, presenting as a bright red patch of blood over the sclera but not involving the cornea.

subcutaneous emphysema A physical finding of air within the subcutaneous tissue.

tension pneumothorax A life-threatening collection of air within the pleural space; the volume and pressure have both collapsed the involved lung and caused a shift of the mediastinal structures to the opposite side.

thoracic inlet The superior aspect of the thoracic cavity, this ring like opening is created by the first vertebral vertebra, the first rib, the clavicles, and the manubrium.

traumatic aortic disruption Dissection or rupture of the aorta.

traumatic asphyxia A pattern of injuries seen after a severe force is applied to the thorax, forcing blood from the great vessels and back into the head and neck.

▶ References

1. Trauma statistics. National Trauma Institute website. http://nationaltraumainstitute.org/home/trauma_statistics.html. Updated February, 2014. Accessed April 3, 2017.

2. American College of Surgeons, National Trauma Data Bank. National Trauma Data Bank 2015 annual report. https://www.facs.org/~/media/files/quality%20programs/trauma/ntdb/ntdb%20annual%20report%202015.ashx. Accessed April 3, 2017.

3. Aggarwal S, Qamar A, Sharma V, Sharma A. Abdominal aortic aneurysm: a comprehensive review. *Exp & Clin Cardiol.* 2011;6(1):11-15.

4. Inaba K, Branco BC, Eckstein M, et al. Optimal positioning for emergent needle thoracostomy: a cadaver-based study. *J Trauma.* 2011;71(5):1099-103.

5. Ariyarajah V, Spodick DH. Cardiac tamponade revisited: a postmortem look at a cautionary case. *Tex Heart Inst J.* 2007;34(3):347-351.

6. Naude GP, Back M, Perry MO, Bongard FS. Blunt disruption of the abdominal aorta: report of a case and review of the literature. *J Vasc Surg.* 1997;25(5):931-935.

7. Blunt trauma to the great vessels of the chest. Barnard Health Care Emergency Medicine website. https://www.barnardhealth.us/emergency-medicine/blunt-trauma-to-the-great-vessels-of-the-chest.html. Published January 17, 2017. Accessed April 3, 2017.

8. Naess PA, Wiborg J, Kjellevold K, Gaarder C. Tension gastrothorax: acute life-threatening manifestation of late onset congenital diaphragmatic hernia (CDH) in children. *Scand J Trauma Resusc Emerg Med.* 2015;23:49.

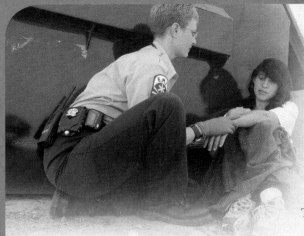

Assessment in Action

Your unit is dispatched to a local soccer field for a player down. When you arrive on scene, a man in his 20s appears to be in a great deal of pain. The patient is responsive and lying supine on the ground holding his chest. The coach states the patient was hit in the chest by an opposing player's head. The patient fell to the ground but did not lose consciousness.

1. Given the mechanism of injury described and the presentation of the patient, what is the most common thoracic injury that he would be experiencing?

    A. Pulmonary contusion
    B. Rib fractures
    C. Flail chest
    D. Penetrating trauma

2. When you assess this patient, you find his respiratory rate and quality is rapid and shallow. You suspect the patient is limiting his chest expansion due to pain. If the patient continues this respiratory pattern, what condition may develop?

    A. Pulmonary contusion
    B. Subcutaneous emphysema
    C. Atelectasis
    D. Cardiac contusion

3. When you are assessing the patient's chest, you find extensive bruising and instability over the right lower ribs. What other type of injury may you want to consider?

    A. Abdominal injuries
    B. Cardiac contusion
    C. Pelvic injuries
    D. Flail segment

4. When the patient has a thoracic injury as described and free air is in the pleural cavity, this condition is known as a:

    A. hemothorax.
    B. cardiac contusion.
    C. pulmonary contusion.
    D. pneumothorax.

5. When the thoracic trauma patient presents with air bubbles trapped below the skin, the patient is presenting with which sign?

    A. Pulmonary contusion
    B. Subcutaneous emphysema
    C. Atelectasis
    D. Cardiac contusion

6. What treatments might help the patient the most with his respiratory effort?

    A. Place the patient on a long spine board and protect his cervical spine
    B. IV access and fluid bolus
    C. Supplemental oxygen via nasal cannula at 2 L/min
    D. IV access and administration of pain medications

7. If this patient had gone into sudden cardiac arrest following the traumatic experience, which of the following would have been the most common cause of the arrest?

    A. Hemothorax
    B. Tension pneumothorax
    C. Commotio cordis
    D. Cardia tamponade

8. Describe the mechanism in which barotrauma causes a pneumothorax.

9. Describe the steps in assessing JVD.

10. Describe the steps in performing a detailed assessment of the chest.

Abdominal and Genitourinary Trauma

National EMS Education Standard Competencies

Trauma

Integrates assessment findings with principles of epidemiology and pathophysiology to formulate a field impression to implement a comprehensive treatment/ disposition plan for an acutely injured patient.

Abdominal and Genitourinary Trauma

Recognition and management of
> Blunt versus penetrating mechanisms (pp 1824-1826, 1831-1832, 1836)
> Evisceration (p 1832)
> Impaled object (p 1832)

Pathophysiology, assessment, and management of
> Solid and hollow organ injuries (pp 1824-1825, 1833-1834)
> Blunt versus penetrating mechanisms (pp 1824-1826, 1831-1832, 1836)
> Evisceration (p 1832)
> Injuries to the external genitalia (pp 1836-1838)
> Vaginal bleeding due to trauma (pp 1837-1838, and see Chapter 22, *Gynecologic Emergencies*)
> Sexual assault (pp 1837-1838, and see Chapter 22, *Gynecologic Emergencies*)
> Vascular injury (pp 1834-1835)
> Retroperitoneal injuries (pp 1834-1835)

Knowledge Objectives

1. Describe the anatomy and physiology of the abdomen, including an explanation of abdominal quadrants and boundaries. (pp 1821-1822)
2. List the vascular structures contained in the abdomen. (pp 1821-1822)
3. Discuss the solid and hollow organs of the abdomen. (p 1822)
4. Describe the anatomy and physiology of the female and male genitourinary systems, and distinguish between hollow and solid organs. (pp 1823-1824)
5. Discuss closed abdominal injuries, providing examples of the mechanisms of injury that are

likely to cause this type of trauma in a patient. (pp 1824-1825)
6. Discuss open abdominal injuries and provide examples of the mechanisms of injury that would cause these. (p 1826)
7. Discuss the assessment of a patient who has experienced an abdominal or genitourinary injury. (pp 1828-1831)
8. Discuss special considerations related to patient privacy when assessing a patient with a genitourinary injury. (p 1830)
9. Describe the different ways solid organs of the abdomen, including the liver, spleen, pancreas, and diaphragm, can be injured, and list the signs and symptoms a patient might exhibit depending on the organ or organs involved. (pp 1833-1834)
10. Describe the different ways hollow organs of the abdomen, including the small intestine, large intestine, and stomach, can be injured, and list the signs and symptoms a patient might exhibit depending on the organ involved. (p 1834)
11. Discuss the emergency medical care of a patient who has sustained a closed abdominal injury. (pp 1833-1836)
12. Discuss the emergency medical care of a patient who has sustained an open abdominal injury, including penetrating injuries and abdominal evisceration. (pp 1833-1836)
13. Describe how retroperitoneal injuries can occur and the signs and symptoms associated with these. (p 1834)
14. Discuss abdominal vascular injuries and the signs and symptoms associated with these. (pp 1834-1835)
15. Describe duodenal injury and the signs and symptoms associated with it. (p 1835)
16. Discuss the assessment and emergency medical care of a patient who has sustained a genitourinary injury related to the kidneys, ureters, urinary bladder, and urethra. (pp 1835-1836)
17. Discuss the assessment and emergency medical care of a patient who has sustained trauma to the internal or external genitalia. (pp 1836-1838)

Skills Objectives

1. Demonstrate proper emergency medical care of a patient who has experienced a blunt abdominal injury. (pp 1831-1832, 1836)

2. Demonstrate how to apply a dressing to an abdominal evisceration wound. (p 1832)

3. Demonstrate proper emergency medical care of a patient who has a penetrating abdominal injury with an impaled object. (p 1832)

Introduction

The abdominal cavity is the largest cavity in the body. Because this cavity extends from the diaphragm to the pelvis, the evaluation and management of patients with abdominal trauma can be challenging. There is great variability in the presentation of conditions, which are rarely resolved in the prehospital setting. Abdominal injuries may be life threatening; therefore, patient assessment should be rapid so management and transport to an appropriate facility can be started.

The abdominal cavity contains several vital organ systems such as the digestive, urinary, and genitourinary systems. These organ systems are vulnerable to trauma partly because of their location, but they also lack some of the protective structures afforded by the skeletal system. Abdominal trauma may be caused by a blunt or penetrating force and ranges from minor single-system injuries to the more complicated and potentially devastating multisystem injuries. Abdominal injuries are difficult to prevent because the risk of people being involved in crashes and sustaining other forms of trauma cannot be eliminated. Factors such as an empty bladder and toned abdominal muscles can help decrease potential damage should trauma occur to the abdomen.

Because of the broad spectrum of abdominal injuries, assessment and interventions should be performed quickly and cautiously. Delays in the recognition and management of abdominal injuries can have fatal consequences.

YOU ▶ are the Paramedic   PART 1

You are the second unit dispatched to the scene of a motor vehicle crash. On arrival, you find the vehicle has sustained front-end damage from striking a utility pole. There are approximately 20 inches (51 cm) of frontal intrusion. The driver and the passenger in the backseat behind the driver are still in the vehicle. You notice that the driver's side airbag deployed. The first crew arrived on scene seconds before your crew and is caring for the passenger. Your crew is assigned the care of the driver.

Your patient is a 45-year-old male who was not wearing a seat belt. As you access the patient, you find him slouched down in the front seat. He is alert and answers your questions, but appears pale and diaphoretic as you approach. You notice the lower portion of the steering wheel is bent inward.

Recording Time: 1 Minute	
Appearance	Eyes open; slouched down
Level of consciousness	Alert and oriented
Airway	Patent
Breathing	Rapid and shallow
Circulation	Rapid radial pulse

1. What are your immediate concerns?
2. What are your immediate treatment priorities?

Assessments in the field can be difficult because of other system injuries that may lead to changes in a patient's mental status and sensation. For example, an unresponsive patient or a patient who does not feel pain after spinal trauma may not be able to communicate, leaving the determination of existing injuries to be based solely on presenting signs and the mechanism of injury (MOI). Sometimes it is difficult to perform a proper assessment on a patient who is intoxicated, has used illicit drugs, has injury to the brain or spinal cord, or has sustained injury to adjacent structures such as the pelvis or ribs.

In recent years, there has been a concerted effort to reduce morbidity and mortality resulting from abdominal trauma. This process has taken shape at several different levels. The education of prehospital providers in recognizing the need for rapid transport has significantly reduced the time from injury to definitive care. Advances in hospital care, such as improved diagnostic equipment (eg, ultrasonography), surgical techniques, and postoperative care, have also improved patient outcomes. Furthermore, trauma system development has played a large role in providing advanced interventions and detection of traumatic injuries.

Trauma to the genitourinary system—ie, the kidneys, ureters, bladder, and male and female reproductive organs—may result from either blunt or penetrating trauma. Most injuries to the genitourinary system involve the kidneys. You should consider trauma to the genitourinary system whenever a patient has sustained injuries to the lower rib cage, abdomen, pelvis, or upper legs.

Words of Wisdom

Unrecognized abdominal injury remains a cause of preventable death after trauma to the trunk of the body.

The purpose of this chapter is to supply the information necessary for you to assess and begin managing the trauma patient as quickly and with as much confidence as possible. This chapter provides the concepts and vocabulary for the effective understanding and communication of key data that will improve the assessment of the trauma mechanism. Your field account from the scene is the only source of information for physicians and surgeons to help them understand the events and mechanism that led to any given trauma presentation. This information is crucial in visualizing and searching for injuries that may not be obvious on physical examination, as is often seen with abdominal trauma.

Anatomy and Physiology Review

The oval-shaped abdominal cavity extends from the diaphragm, the large muscle that separates the thoracic cavity from the abdomen, to the pelvic brim. The pelvic

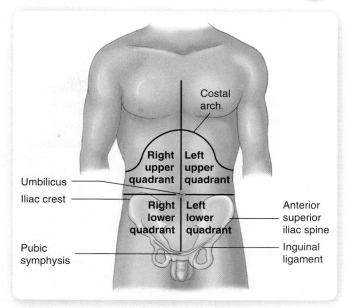

Figure 36-1 The abdomen is often referred to by quadrants.
© Jones & Bartlett Learning.

brim stretches at an angle from the intervertebral disk between L5 and S1 to the pubic symphysis. For a complete discussion of the abdominal and genitourinary systems, see Chapter 8, *Anatomy and Physiology*.

▶ Anatomic Regions

Knowledge of the anatomic boundaries of the abdomen is important when you are looking for potential injury patterns, such as hollow organ injury, vascular injury, solid organ injury, or injuries to the retroperitoneal area. To describe a location in the abdomen, or a source of pain found when you are conducting your assessment, the quadrant system is generally used **Figure 36-1**. The area around the umbilicus is referred to as the **periumbilical** area.

▶ Abdominal Organs and Vital Vessels

The abdomen contains many organs, primarily those of the digestive system. **Figure 36-2** shows the abdominal organs and the regions in which they are located: the peritoneal cavity, the retroperitoneal space, and the pelvis. The **peritoneal cavity** is the area in the abdomen encased in the peritoneum. The upper peritoneal cavity (the thoracoabdominal component of the abdomen) contains the diaphragm, liver, spleen, stomach, gallbladder, and transverse colon. The lower peritoneal cavity contains the small bowel, sigmoid colon, parts of the descending and ascending colon, and, in women, the internal reproductive organs. The **retroperitoneal space** is the area posterior to the peritoneal lining of the abdomen. The abdomen also contains many vital vessels, shown in **Figure 36-3**.

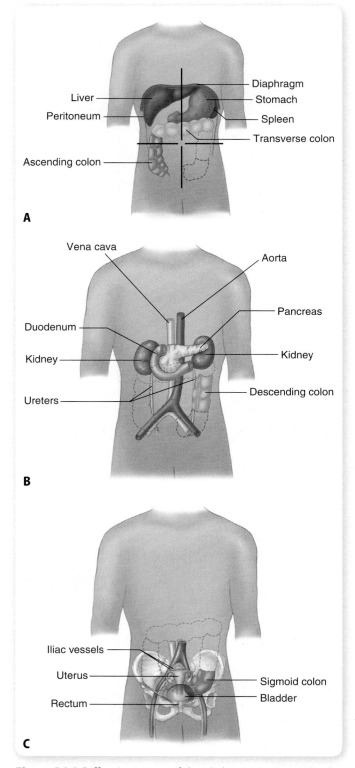

A

B

C

Figure 36-2 Different organs of the abdomen are contained in the peritoneal cavity **(A)**, the retroperitoneal space **(B)**, and the pelvis **(C)**.

© Jones & Bartlett Learning.

Solid Organs

The liver lies in the right upper quadrant (extending to the epigastrium), superior and anterior to the gallbladder and the hepatic and cystic ducts, and superior to the stomach.

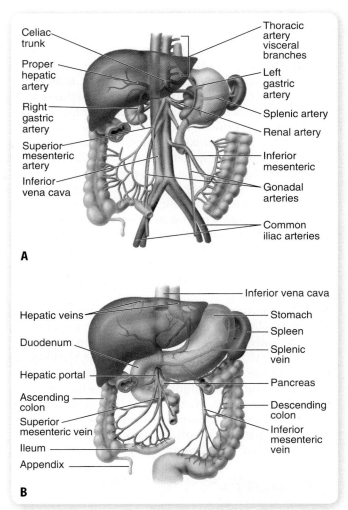

A

B

Figure 36-3 A. Arteries of the abdomen. **B.** Veins of the abdomen.

© Jones & Bartlett Learning.

It has a significant blood supply provided by the hepatic artery and the hepatic-portal vein. Like the liver, the spleen is a solid organ in the peritoneum and is highly vascular. Its shape resembles a baseball catcher's mitt.[1] The pancreas is a solid organ located in the retroperitoneal space under the liver and behind the stomach. It produces and secretes digestive enzymes and the hormone insulin. The spleen, liver, and vascular system of the abdomen are the primary sources of exsanguination during abdominal trauma.[2]

Hollow Organs

The stomach is an intraperitoneal hollow organ that lies in the left upper quadrant and epigastric region. It serves primarily as the storage area for ingested food and liquid.

The gallbladder is a saclike organ located on the lower surface of the liver that acts as a reservoir for bile, one of the digestive enzymes produced by the liver.

The small and large intestines run from the end of the stomach to the anus. The majority of the intestines are in the intraperitoneal area. They digest and absorb water and nutrients.

► Organs of the Genitourinary System

The abdomen also contains organs of the urinary system. Located in the retroperitoneal space, the kidneys filter blood and excrete body wastes in the form of urine. The kidneys are discussed in greater detail in Chapter 21, *Genitourinary and Renal Emergencies*. The urinary bladder, a hollow organ, stores urine until it is excreted. The ureters carry urine from the kidneys to the urinary bladder.

The abdomen also contains organs of the reproductive system. The female reproductive system contains the uterus and the ovaries **Figure 36-4** . These organs can be injured from crushing and compression forces as well as shearing injuries that may result when a restraint device, such as a lap belt or shoulder belt, are worn improperly.

The male reproductive system **Figure 36-5** contains the penis, which is the male external reproductive organ, and the testes, also known as the testicles. The testes produce sperm and secrete male hormones such as testosterone.

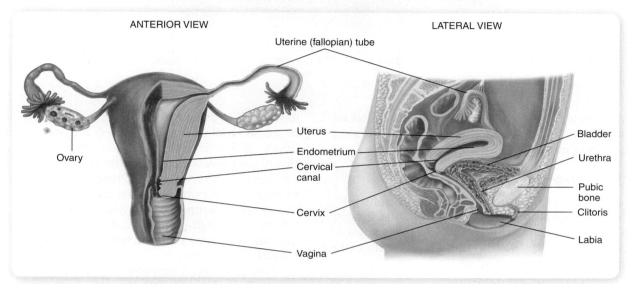

ANTERIOR VIEW
LATERAL VIEW

Uterine (fallopian) tube
Uterus
Endometrium
Cervical canal
Cervix
Vagina
Ovary
Bladder
Urethra
Pubic bone
Clitoris
Labia

Figure 36-4 The female genitals and reproductive system.

© Jones & Bartlett Learning.

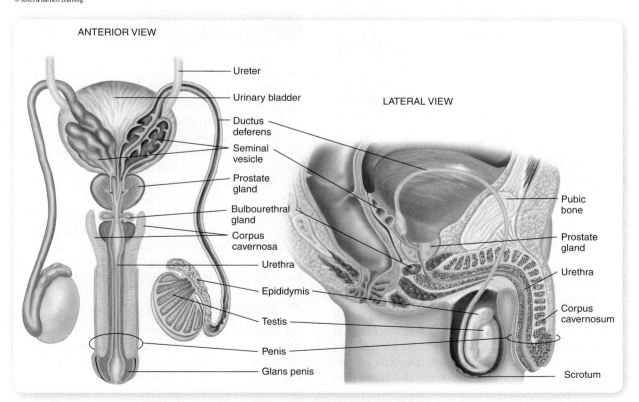

ANTERIOR VIEW
LATERAL VIEW

Ureter
Urinary bladder
Ductus deferens
Seminal vesicle
Prostate gland
Bulbourethral gland
Corpus cavernosa
Urethra
Epididymis
Testis
Penis
Glans penis
Pubic bone
Prostate gland
Urethra
Corpus cavernosum
Scrotum

Figure 36-5 The male genitals and reproductive system include the testicles, vas deferens, seminal vesicles, urethra, and penis.

© Jones & Bartlett Learning.

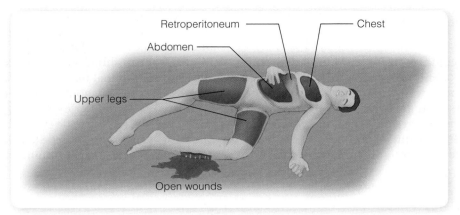

Figure 36-6 The places where enough blood can be lost to cause shock.
© Jones & Bartlett Learning.

The testicles are held outside the body in the scrotal sac and can be retracted into a more protected position by the cremaster muscles.

▶ The Diaphragm

One additional structure in the abdomen is the diaphragm—the dome-shaped muscle that separates the thoracic cavity from the abdominal cavity. It curves from its point of attachment in the flanks at the 12th rib and peaks in the center at the 4th intercostal space.

▶ Pathophysiology of the Injury

The abdomen, retroperitoneal space, and muscle compartments of the proximal lower extremities are areas of the body that can house significant amounts of blood following a blunt or penetrating injury **Figure 36-6**. Because the abdomen and retroperitoneum can accommodate large amounts of blood, the bleeding may produce few signs and symptoms of the trauma. Even the patient's vital signs and physical exam may not indicate the extent of the bleeding.

Solid organs, such as the liver and spleen, can easily be crushed by blunt trauma to the abdomen. The spleen is the most commonly injured organ in blunt abdominal trauma; the liver is second.[2] With penetrating trauma, the liver is most frequently injured. If a trauma patient has unexplained symptoms of shock, you should suspect abdominal trauma.

Hollow organs are more resilient to blunt trauma and less likely to be injured by trauma—unless they are full. When a hollow organ is full, it is likely to be injured and can burst in the same way a chemical cold pack breaks when you apply pressure to the outer bag. The danger of bursting hollow organs is that they hold substances (such as urine, feces, bile, or stomach acids) that can spill out into the abdominal cavity. This spillage can cause **peritonitis**, an inflammation of the lining of the abdomen (the **peritoneum**). Peritonitis is a life-threatening infection. There are two types of peritonitis: chemical and bacterial. Chemical peritonitis—caused, for example, by the release

of stomach acids into the abdomen—may have a sudden onset. Bacterial peritonitis—caused, for example, by the release of feces into the abdomen—may develop more slowly, over several hours. Peritonitis can also be classified as primary or secondary. Primary peritonitis occurs when infection travels from the blood or lymph nodes into the peritoneum. Secondary peritonitis occurs when infection travels from the gastrointestinal or biliary tract into the peritoneum. Of the two, secondary peritonitis is much more common.

You must have a high index of suspicion and a clear understanding of the MOI to which your trauma patient was exposed.

■ Mechanism of Injury

Blunt abdominal trauma may occur as the result of falls, motor vehicle crashes, bicycle and motorcycle crashes, or vehicle-pedestrian crash, or because of any force striking the abdomen, as in assaults, sporting activities, and explosions. Penetrating abdominal trauma most often results from stab wounds and gunshot wounds. A combination of blunt and penetrating trauma also can occur. More detailed information with regard to MOI and blunt versus penetrating trauma can be found in Chapter 29, *Trauma Systems and Mechanism of Injury*.

The likelihood of significant intra-abdominal injury is high when a patient has hypotension in the field, a major chest injury, or pelvic fracture.[2] Unrecognized abdominal trauma is a leading cause of death in trauma patients because of delays in surgical intervention.

▶ Blunt Trauma

An abdominal injury is most often the result of blunt trauma and is associated with mortality rates of 10% to 30%.[3] A direct blow to the abdomen, such as contact with the lower rim of a steering wheel or a door intruding into the passenger space from a motor vehicle crash, can cause compression and crushing injuries. These forces can deform solid organs and can cause hollow organs to rupture, spilling their contents into the abdomen and increasing the risk of infection.

Blunt trauma to the abdomen can often lead to a closed abdominal injury—one in which soft-tissue damage occurs inside the body, but the skin remains intact Figure 36-7. When you are assessing the abdominal region in a patient who has received blunt trauma, consider three common MOIs: shearing, crushing, and compression. In the rapid deceleration of a patient during a motor vehicle crash or fall from a height, a shearing force can be created as the internal organs continue their forward motion. This MOI

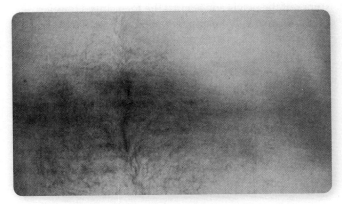

Figure 36-7 Blunt abdominal trauma typically leads to closed abdominal injury—the internal organs are injured, but the skin remains intact.

© American Academy of Orthopaedic Surgeons.

causes hollow, solid, and visceral organs and vascular structures to tear, especially at their points of attachment to the abdominal wall. Organs that shear or tear include the liver, kidneys, small and large intestines, and spleen. In motor vehicle crashes, this MOI has been described as the third collision (such as the car into the wall, the patient into the steering column, and the internal organs into the patient's inner rib cage).

Crush injuries are the result of external factors at the time of impact; they differ from decelerating injuries occurring before impact. When abdominal contents are crushed between the anterior abdominal wall and the spinal column (or other structures in the rear), crushing occurs. Solid organs like the kidneys, liver, and spleen are at the greatest risk of injury from this mechanism. Direct application of crushing forces to the abdomen would come from objects such as the dashboard, the front hood of a car (in a vehicle-pedestrian crash), or falling objects. Additionally, these injuries can be caused by a restraining device that has not been properly attached or worn or by the steering wheel striking the abdominal cavity of an unrestrained driver as the person is propelled forward.

The last MOI to consider is compression injury resulting from a direct blow or external compression from a fixed object (such as a lap belt or airbag). These compression forces will deform hollow organs, increasing the pressure within the abdominal cavity. This dramatic change in abdominal pressure can cause a rupture of the small intestine or diaphragm. Rupture of organs can lead to uncontrollable hemorrhage and peritonitis.

YOU are the Paramedic PART 2

The patient is alert and complains of significant abdominal pain. He tells you that he is becoming nauseated. His skin is cool, pale, and diaphoretic.

Before moving your patient, you perform a primary survey and a rapid trauma assessment and find that he is guarding his abdomen with significant bruising noted on the right side. He yells out as you push down over his right upper quadrant.

Recording Time: 5 Minutes	
Level of consciousness	Alert and oriented to person, place, time, and event.
Skin	Cool, pale, and diaphoretic
Pulse	140 beats/min; weak and regular
Blood pressure	100/64 mm Hg
Respirations	20 breaths/min
Oxygen saturation (Spo₂)	92% on room air

3. What do you recall about solid versus hollow organs in regard to blunt trauma?
4. What do these signs indicate to you?
5. What can you conclude from the patient's vital signs?

► Penetrating Trauma

Penetrating trauma results in tissue damage by lacerating or cutting, resulting in an open abdominal injury—one in which a break in the surface of the skin or mucous membrane exposes deeper tissue to potential contamination. In general, gunshot wounds cause more injury than stab wounds cause because bullets travel deep into the body and have more kinetic energy, increasing the damage lateral to the track of the missile due to temporary cavitation. Gunshot wounds to the abdomen most commonly involve injury to the small bowel, colon, liver, and vascular structures; the extent of injury is less predictable than is the injury caused by stab wounds because gunshot wounds depend mostly on the characteristics of the weapon and the characteristics of the bullet. In penetrating trauma from stab wounds, the liver, small bowel, diaphragm, and colon are the organs most frequently injured.

Words of Wisdom

Always remember the concept of associated injuries. On the basis of the MOI, some of the following syndromes are common:

- Fractures of the lower rib cage: suspect spleen and/or liver injuries
- Upper abdominal injuries: suspect chest trauma
- Pelvic fractures: suspect intra-abdominal trauma (bladder laceration)
- Penetrating wounds at or below the nipple line: suspect intra-abdominal injury

► Motor Vehicle Crashes

In motor vehicle crashes, there are five typical patterns of impact—frontal, lateral, rear, rotational, and rollover—which are discussed in Chapter 29, *Trauma Systems and Mechanism of Injury*. In a head-on or other frontal impact, the patient, especially an unbelted driver or front-seat passenger, often is pushed down and under the dashboard. These types of impacts can also result in patients being thrown forward through the windshield and up and over the hood of the car. Traumatic aortic disruptions, liver and spleen injuries, and many nonabdominal injuries can result.

In a lateral, side-impact, or "T-bone" collision, the diaphragm, liver or spleen (depending on which side of the patient was hit), and pelvis often are injured. In some circumstances, a vehicle may spin out of control, exposing the passengers to rotational forces. These forces often result in cervical spine and abdominal visceral injuries. In a rear-impact collision, intra-abdominal injuries can occur from compression and deceleration forces. The patient is less likely to have an injury to his or her abdomen if he or she has been restrained properly. However, if restraints are improperly worn or not used at all, the potential for injury is great.

Rollover impacts present the greatest potential to inflict lethal injuries. Unrestrained occupants may change direction several times, with an increased risk of ejection or partial ejection from the vehicle. The occupants involved in a rollover may collide with each other as well as with the vehicle interior, producing a wide range of probable injuries. The criteria for referral to a trauma center are discussed in Chapter 29, *Trauma Systems and Mechanism of Injury*.

Seat belts have prevented thousands of injuries and saved many lives, including those of people who would have otherwise been ejected from the vehicle. When worn properly, a seat belt lies below the anterior superior iliac spines of the pelvis and against the hip joints. However, seat belt use, especially improper seat belt use, can occasionally cause compression injuries to the pancreas, liver, spleen, small bowel, or kidneys when the car suddenly decelerates or stops Figure 36-8 . Occasionally, fractures of the lumbar spine have been reported.

► Motorcycle Falls or Crashes

With the popularity of motorcycles and the production of high-performance racing bikes that are most attractive to younger and inexperienced riders, the number of motorcycle crashes continues to increase. In a motorcycle

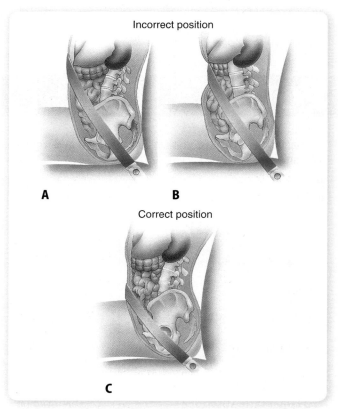

Incorrect position

A   **B**

Correct position

C

Figure 36-8 (A) and **(B)** show improper positioning of seat belts. The proper position for a seat belt is below the anterior superior iliac spines of the pelvis and against the hip joints, as shown in **(C)**.
© Jones & Bartlett Learning.

crash, any structural protection from a steel cage, as is provided in an automobile, does not exist. The motorcyclist's only protection is that which he or she wears, such as the helmet and abrasion-resistant or leather pants, gloves, jacket, and boots. Although helmets are designed to protect against impact to the head, they transmit any impact to the cervical spine, so they do not protect against severe cervical injury. You should consider transport to a trauma center with crashes occurring at speeds of greater than 20 mph or with separation of the rider from the motorcycle.

▶ Falls From Heights

When an adult falls from a height, the fall usually occurs in the context of criminal activity, attempted suicide, or intoxication. The position or orientation of the body at the moment of impact will help determine the type of injuries sustained and their survivability. The surface onto which the person has fallen and the degree to which that surface can deform (plasticity) under the force of the falling body can help in dissipating the forces of sudden deceleration. For adults, consider immediate transport to a trauma center with falls of greater than 20 ft (6 m). For a child, falls more than 10 ft (3 m) or two or three times

the height of the child warrant consideration for transport to a trauma center.

▶ Blast Injuries

Although most commonly associated with military conflict, blast injuries are also seen in civilian practice in mines, shipyards, and chemical plants; they are also increasingly associated with terrorist activities. Blast injuries, particularly those from weapons designed specifically for antipersonnel effects (such as mines or grenades), can generate fragments traveling at velocities of 4,500 feet per second (1,372 m/s). This is nearly double the velocity of a projectile from a high-speed rifle. Any energy transmitted from a blast fragment will cause extensive and disruptive damage to tissue.

■ General Pathophysiology

Hemorrhage is a major concern in patients with abdominal trauma. It can occur when there is external or internal blood loss. When you are caring for patients with abdominal trauma, especially blunt abdominal trauma, the estimation of the volume of blood lost is difficult.

YOU ▶ are the Paramedic   PART 3

As a precaution, you initiate spinal immobilization. Oxygenation is supported by the placement of a nonrebreathing mask at 15 L/min. Based on the MOI and the stability of the patient, you have decided to transport the patient to a Level 1 trauma center.

En route, you establish two 18-gauge intravenous (IV) lines. You initiate fluid resuscitation in 250-mL boluses with reassessment after each bolus. You complete your secondary assessment, remaining suspicious about his right upper quadrant pain and guarding. You observe a 6-inch by 1-inch (15-cm by 2.5-cm) contusion on the right side of his abdomen, likely from impact with the lower portion of the steering wheel. No other injuries are noted during your secondary assessment.

Recording Time: 10 Minutes	
Level of consciousness	Alert and oriented × 4
Skin	Cool, pale, and diaphoretic
Pulse	152 beats/min; weak and regular
Blood pressure	86/43 mm Hg
Respirations	24 breaths/min
Oxygen saturation (Spo$_2$)	98% while receiving 15 L/min via nonrebreathing mask
Pupils	PERRLA 4 mm

6. What does right upper quadrant pain suggest?
7. What may the right shoulder pain indicate?
8. What are some possible causes for the patient's hypotension?

Signs and symptoms will vary greatly depending on the volume of blood lost and the rate at which the body is losing blood. Key indicators of hemorrhagic shock will become apparent with the assessment of the neurologic and cardiovascular systems.

As hypovolemia increases, the patient will have initial agitation and confusion. The heart compensates early for this loss by an increase in heart rate (tachycardia) and stroke volume. As hypoperfusion continues, the coronary arteries can no longer meet the increased demands of the myocardium, which leads to ischemia and heart failure. The symptoms of cardiac dysfunction are demonstrated by the presence of chest pain, tachypnea with adventitious (abnormal) lung sounds, and dysrhythmias. If left untreated, hypoperfusion will result in anaerobic metabolism and acidosis.

Injuries to hollow or solid organs can result in the spillage of their contents into the abdominal cavity. When the enzymes, acids, or bacteria leak from hollow organs into the peritoneal or retroperitoneal space, they cause irritation of the nerve endings. These nerve endings are found in the fascia of the surrounding tissues. As the inflammation affects deeper nerve endings (such as the endings of the afferent nerves), localized pain will result. Pain is localized if the extent of the contamination is confined; pain becomes generalized if the entire peritoneal cavity is involved.

Patient Assessment

Scene Size-up

As with all other aspects of prehospital care, scene safety remains the priority before providing any patient care. It is always important to remember that if a patient has penetrating or blunt trauma, some external force caused this injury (such as a gun, a knife, or the baseball bat in the corner of the room). These situations could also potentially be dangerous to the paramedic.

Primary Survey

Because most significant abdominal injuries require definitive care in the hospital, your main goal in assessing victims of abdominal trauma is determining which patients need rapid transport to the hospital, perhaps to a trauma center. Failure to make this determination rapidly and effectively can lead to increased morbidity and mortality rates from unrecognized abdominal injury.

Approach the patient using the ABCDE approach (Airway, Breathing, Circulation, Disability, and Exposure), as discussed in Chapter 11, *Patient Assessment*. Recognize that if there is life-threatening bleeding or cardiac arrest, the order of your assessment will be CABDE. Form a general impression, noting the manner in which the patient is lying. Movement of the body or the abdominal organs irritates the inflamed peritoneum, causing additional pain. To minimize this pain, patients may lie still, usually with the knees drawn up, and breathe using rapid and shallow breaths. For the same reason, they may contract abdominal muscles (guarding). Therefore, a quiet, still patient may have severe injuries, whereas a patient who is moving around is less likely to have peritonitis.

Quickly determine if the patient has an altered mental status or signs of airway compromise. If the patient has an altered mental status, keep the airway clear of vomitus so that it is not aspirated into the lungs. Turn the patient to one side, using spinal precautions if necessary, and try to clear any material from the throat and mouth. Note the nature of the vomitus: undigested food, blood, mucus, or bile.

Quickly assess the patient for adequate breathing. A distended abdomen or pain may prevent adequate inhalation. When these guarded respirations decrease the effectiveness of the patient's breathing, providing supplemental oxygen with a nonrebreathing mask will help improve oxygenation. If the patient's level of consciousness is decreased and respirations are shallow, consider supplementing respirations with a bag-mask device. Use airway adjuncts as necessary to ensure a patent airway.

As you check circulation, remember that superficial abdominal injuries usually do not produce significant external bleeding. Internal bleeding from open or closed abdominal injuries, however, can be profound. Trauma to the kidneys, liver, and spleen can cause significant internal bleeding. Significant bleeding is an immediate life threat and must be controlled quickly using appropriate methods. In dark environments, bleeding can be difficult to see. Thick clothing may also hide bleeding. Wounds should be covered and bleeding controlled as quickly as possible. If you suspect shock, treat the patient for shock according to your protocols.

When you are caring for a potential genitourinary emergency, remember that the genitourinary system can be a significant source of bleeding. Quickly assess the patient's pulse rate and quality; determine the skin condition, color, and temperature; and check the capillary refill time. These assessments will help you determine the presence of circulatory problems or shock. Closed injuries do not have visible signs of bleeding. Because the bleeding is occurring inside the body, shock may be present. Your assessment of the pulse and skin will give you an indication as to how aggressively you need to treat your patient for shock.

When you are removing the patient's clothing, note whether there is the presence of blood from the vagina or rectum. If blood is noted, be sure to inspect those areas more closely during your physical exam.

Next, you need to make a transport decision. Because of the nature of abdominal injuries, a short on-scene time and quick transport to the hospital are generally indicated. Abdominal pain together with an MOI that suggests injury to the abdomen or flank is a good indication for rapid transport. Because it is not possible to diagnose organ rupture in the field, do not delay transport when internal injuries are possible. The condition of a patient with visible significant bleeding or signs of significant internal bleeding may quickly become unstable. Treatment should be directed at quickly addressing life threats and providing rapid transport to the closest appropriate hospital.

Patients with abdominal injuries should be evaluated at the highest level of trauma center available because of the hidden or occult nature of most abdominal injuries. Transport to a trauma center is indicated for any patient who has an MOI that produces a high index of suspicion and who has any visible significant trauma, whether blunt or penetrating. Follow local protocols when you are considering a lower level of care such as acute care sites and clinics.

A patient with a genitourinary system injury should be taken to a trauma center for evaluation and treatment. Any injury to this system can prove to be life altering and often requires a medical specialist to provide specialized care. When possible and protocols allow, transport the patient to a facility capable of treating this subset of injuries.

Words of Wisdom

Delay in recognizing intra-abdominal or pelvic injury leads to early death from hemorrhage or delayed death from visceral injury. Pelvic injury can include fractures, but torn ligaments can also be associated with life-threatening bleeding.

History Taking

Try to obtain as many details about an injury as possible, keeping in mind that trauma patients should be transported to the hospital quickly. In other words, in addition to getting information about the patient, such as the SAMPLE history (Signs and symptoms, Allergies, Medications, Pertinent past history, Last oral intake, Events leading to injury or illness), it is important to obtain details on how the injury occurred, whether from the patient, witnesses, police, or other emergency medical services (EMS) providers.

When a patient receives blunt trauma caused by a motor vehicle crash, determine the types of vehicles involved, the speed at which they were traveling, and how the vehicles collided. You should also try to find out other information about the event, such as the use of seat belts, the deployment of airbags, and the patient's position in the vehicle.

When a patient has sustained penetrating trauma, it is helpful to identify the type of weapon used; however, this is often impossible because assailants usually leave with their weapon. In a gunshot case, determine the type of gun and the number of shots, if possible. Also, try to ascertain an estimated distance between the victim and the assailant whenever possible. In patients with stab wounds, determine the type of knife, the possible angle of the entrance wound, and the number of stab wounds. Patient care, however, always remains the priority.

Secondary Assessment

Although this chapter primarily concerns victims of abdominal trauma, you must remember that patients may sustain more than one injury, the true nature of the injury may not be immediately apparent, and injuries may change over time. Therefore, you still must perform an overall assessment of the patient with an apparent abdominal injury. Of note, head injury or the presence of intoxicants such as drugs or alcohol can mask the signs and symptoms of shock from abdominal trauma. Likewise, **hemoperitoneum** (a collection of blood in the abdominal cavity) from either a solid organ or vascular injury may not immediately be apparent on abdominal examination alone. In fact, this condition often is associated with an initially normal abdominal examination and is then identified by the presence of unexplained shock or shock out of proportion to the known injuries. Clearly, you can make this determination only after a thorough examination that includes all other areas, not simply the abdomen.

Visible wounds and/or the MOI may suggest intra-abdominal injury; however, a focused but complete abdominal examination for the victim of abdominal injury still is warranted. For example, peritonitis from a hollow organ injury may be present with a subjective complaint of abdominal pain as well as the objective finding of tenderness on palpation or percussion of the abdomen. You also may note the presence of guarding, rigidity, or distention, although the latter is a late finding and should not be relied on to determine the absence of peritonitis or significant abdominal pathology. In fact, subtler clues such as ecchymosis or abrasions may be the only clues to significant intra-abdominal injury, particularly when the MOI or the presence of unexplained shock also suggests that intra-abdominal injury may have occurred.

Words of Wisdom

An injury to the chest anywhere below the nipples should also be considered an injury to the abdomen.

Examine the patient's neck and chest, paying particular attention to the trachea (tracheal deviation due to mediastinal shift), symmetry of the chest during expansion, and absence of breath sounds. Remember that the diaphragm plays a large role in the mechanical process of breathing. Signs and symptoms of a diaphragmatic

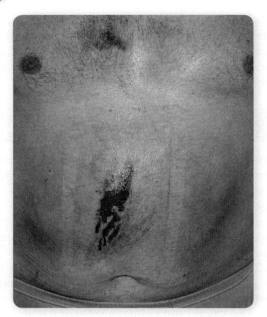

Figure 36-9 Examine the abdomen closely for bruising, road rash, localized swelling, lacerations, distention, and pain.
© Dr. P. Marazzi/Photo Researchers, Inc.

rupture can include abdominal pain, acute respiratory distress, decreased breath sounds, abdominal sounds in the chest, subcutaneous emphysema, and a sunken abdomen or an abdomen that appears empty.

The secondary assessment should include inspection for abrasions, bruising, distention, obvious external blood loss, wounds, an **evisceration** (displacement of an organ outside the body), and the presence of impaled objects, although you probably already took a quick look for these findings during the primary survey **Figure 36-9** . You may not have noticed a seat belt sign or other specific injury pattern during the primary survey because of your search for life-threatening injuries. A complete inspection of the abdomen also includes inspecting the back.

Words of Wisdom

Always examine the back of the patient as carefully as you examine the front. Gunshot wounds or stab wounds can easily be missed within creases of the body, especially if the patient is obese or has large quantities of body hair.

An abdominal wall contusion is not usually difficult to recognize, even with a brief inspection of the abdomen. Alone, an abdominal wall contusion may be impressive, but it is not a critical finding; however, it can indicate that significant blunt force trauma has been applied to the underlying structures. Therefore, especially in the presence of otherwise unexplained shock, consider an abdominal wall contusion a valuable clue to possible hemorrhagic shock. When present, abdominal wall contusions and hematomas may be clues to underlying injuries. However, as with all such bruises, the appearance, including the distinct color, of these abdominal wall injuries is from the presence of blood visible under the skin. This blood can result from a variety of sources, ranging from the rupture of capillaries to lacerations of solid organs, such as the liver or spleen. A ruptured spleen may lead to intra-abdominal hemorrhage that eventually becomes visible as ecchymosis around the umbilicus (Cullen sign). Depending on the briskness and severity of hemorrhage, visible ecchymosis may be delayed for several hours from the time of initial injury. Therefore, the absence of a visible bruise does not indicate a lack of intra-abdominal injury.

Palpation can elicit signs of tenderness associated with any abdominal injury as well as the guarding or rebound tenderness associated with peritoneal irritation. Palpation also includes assessing extra-abdominal structures, such as checking for pelvic stability and tenderness and checking for tenderness in the back that may indicate retroperitoneal injury. Carefully palpate the entire abdomen, beginning with the quadrant that is farthest from the injury, while assessing the patient's response and noting abdominal masses and deformities. Retroperitoneal hemorrhage may be present because of damaged muscle, lacerated or avulsed kidneys, and injuries to the vessels of the supporting **mesentery** (membranous double fold of tissue in the abdomen that attaches various organs to the body wall). All abdominal organs have a generous blood supply, making them susceptible to significant bleeding as a result of blunt forces causing a shearing-type injury. The injury can be slow to develop, and may be subtle and difficult to locate and assess.

Controversies

In a hospital setting, auscultation for the presence or absence and character of bowel sounds is part of the standard medical assessment of patients with abdominal trauma. To properly auscultate bowel sounds, it is necessary to listen for several minutes. This is not practical in the field, and the ambient noise is often too great to determine the presence or absence of bowel sounds.

When you are assessing a genitourinary injury, there is a potential for embarrassing the patient. Maintain a professional presence at all times when assessing and treating these injuries. Remember to provide privacy for the patient during the assessment process. Look for blood first on the patient's undergarments, and inspect the external genitalia only when the patient reports pain or there are external signs of injury. During your physical exam, also note whether the patient has **hematuria** (blood in the urine). This is a cardinal sign of renal and urinary tract injury, which can occur when renal or urinary vessels rupture, or when blood is able to enter the urine during glomerular filtration. Note the color of the urine—a darker brown suggests bleeding in the upper urinary tract, whereas a brighter red is most likely due to bleeding in the lower portion of the tract.

The presence of pregnancy should also be determined. Traumatic injuries to pregnant patients can be further complicated by the physiologic changes experienced by the patient. Some changes can mimic shock. For example, the pregnant patient's heart rate can increase by as much as 20 beats/min, blood volume increases by 50% during midpregnancy, and a pregnant woman can experience relative anemia from hemodilution. Because of the increase in blood flow to the uterus, the risk for massive blood loss is greatly increased with trauma to the bony pelvis.

Management of pregnant patients should always start with the ABCDEs. There is a higher risk of aspiration and increase in gastric acidity. All pregnant patients should receive maximum oxygenation because of increased oxygen consumption and reduced reserve. Also, remember that if the pregnant patient is more than 20 weeks' gestation, she should be tilted at least 15° to her left to relieve uterine pressure on the inferior cava and prevent supine hypotensive syndrome. If the patient is secured to a long backboard or scoop stretcher, towel rolls can be placed underneath it to accomplish the tilting.

Finally, several newer technologies are useful when assessing abdominal trauma in the prehospital environment. Focused Assessment with Sonography for Trauma (FAST) is an ultrasonographic scan performed using a portable machine. A FAST exam can be used early in the patient's evaluation and has been shown to decrease the time to surgery, treatment costs, and the length of hospital stays.[4] Another technology entering the arena of prehospital care is telemedicine, which allows physicians from remote areas (such as base medical centers) to receive and review images and diagnostic data from rural EMS providers on scene or en route.

Assess the patient's pain using the OPQRST (Onset, Provocation/palliation, Quality, Region/radiation, Severity, Timing) mnemonic and quantify the severity on a pain scale. Recall that **somatic pain** is often described as sharp and localized to the area of injury. It comes from skin and muscle, as well as joints, ligaments, and tendons. Bleeding, swelling, and cramping may exist with somatic pain. This pain usually responds well to medications such as opioids and nonsteroidal anti-inflammatory drugs. **Visceral pain** comes from organs inside the body with injury or illness and is often described as a deep ache with cramping. There are three main areas where visceral pain is felt: the thorax, abdomen, and pelvis. Pain receptors in these cavities respond to stretching, oxygen deprivation, and swelling. Visceral pain can radiate to other locations such as the back and chest. Opioids are the most effective for this type of pain.

Words of Wisdom

Cullen sign is a black-and-blue discoloration (ecchymosis) in the umbilical region caused by peritoneal bleeding. Grey Turner sign includes ecchymosis present in the lower abdominal and flank regions. They are both caused by intra-abdominal bleeding found 12 to 24 hours after the initial injury. The presence of these signs is helpful, but their absence does not rule out life-threatening abdominal hemorrhage.

Reassessment

Reassessment includes repeating the primary survey, as well as retaking vital signs and checking interventions on the patient.

Pertinent field documentation of the abdominal trauma assessment should include the following: whether or not seat belts were worn, which type, and their position on the patient; the location, intensity, and quality of pain; whether or not nausea or vomiting is present; the contour of the abdomen; any ecchymosis or open areas present on inspection; the presence or absence of rebound tenderness, guarding, rigidity, spasm, or localized pain; any changes in the level of consciousness and serial vital signs; other injuries found; the presence or absence of alcohol, narcotics, or any type of analgesic; and the results of your reassessment.

■ Emergency Medical Care

Not all victims of abdominal trauma have *serious* abdominal injuries. However, critical findings during the primary survey, such as unexplained shock, and physical signs of significant abdominal injury necessitate rapid transport to a facility with immediate surgical capability. However, some patients may be appropriately transported to other facilities or even not transported at all. Your local protocols should address this and identify the closest appropriate facility for victims of abdominal injury.

You should pay careful attention to the patient's ABCDEs in all cases of trauma—and abdominal trauma is no exception. Airway and breathing are seldom affected by isolated abdominal injury. But many patients have more than one injury; therefore, you must address the ABCDEs in all cases to avoid missing potentially life-threatening injuries. Ensure an open airway while taking spinal precautions and administer supplemental oxygen.

Because the major cause of morbidity and mortality in abdominal trauma is hemorrhagic shock, begin shock resuscitation immediately and continue it during transport.

Resuscitation usually consists of administering IV fluids, usually normal saline or lactated Ringer solution (follow your local protocol), through two 18-gauge peripheral IV lines. In the absence of a traumatic brain injury, the goal of fluid replacement is to maintain a systolic blood pressure of 80 to 90 mm Hg.[3] Do not delay transport to initiate IV therapy; establish IV lines whenever possible during transport. Minimize external hemorrhage by applying pressure dressings. Apply a cardiac monitor and pulse oximetry as well as capnography, if possible. Transport the patient to the appropriate hospital or regional trauma center, depending on your local transport protocols. Note that the assessment should also not delay patient care and transport. Repeated abdominal examinations are the key to discovering a patient's worsening condition before vital signs change.

> ## Words of Wisdom
>
> A distended, tender abdomen after injury means internal bleeding and significant blood loss. Treat for shock and transport immediately.

Administering pain medication is somewhat controversial because it may mask symptoms and often is contraindicated because of the patient's hypotension. In most instances, it may be appropriate to consult with medical direction en route to the hospital to discuss analgesia. While historically it was thought best not to mask the pain until the patient was diagnosed in the emergency department (ED), today many medical directors feel that pain management is a more humane approach and will order an analgesic such as fentanyl.

▶ Evisceration

An evisceration is externalization of abdominal organs through a wound in the abdominal wall **Figure 36-10**. The protrusion may be small or large. Generally, little pain is associated with this type of injury; do not apply any material that will adhere to the abdominal structures. Do not attempt to place the organ back into the body. Apply a normal saline-soaked sterile dressing over the top of the evisceration. Cover the injured area to keep it warm. Transport the patient immediately to the closest appropriate hospital. Strangulation of the bowel by the abdominal wall causes decreased blood flow to the protruding part and can cause death to that part of the bowel. Early symptoms are localized pain, nausea, and vomiting. Also, the patient can experience peritonitis if the bowel is leaking fluids into the abdominal cavity. Patients may feel more comfortable with their knees bent because flexing the knees relieves abdominal muscle tension. Encourage the patient not to cough or bear down, and consider providing pain relief.

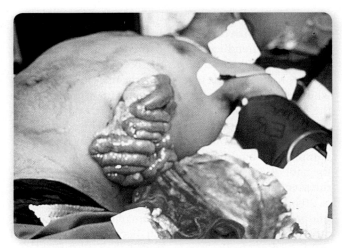

Figure 36-10 An abdominal evisceration is an open abdominal wound from which internal organs or fat protrude.

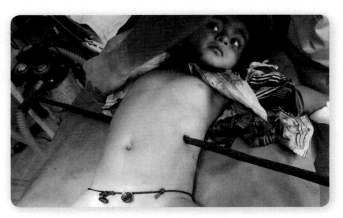

Figure 36-11 An object impaled in the abdomen.
© STRDEL/AFP/Getty.

▶ Impaled Objects

You may encounter a patient who has an impaled object **Figure 36-11**. Stabilize the impaled object in place and transport the patient. Do not attempt to remove or manipulate the object; doing so may cause further injury or increase bleeding. In unusual situations, it may be necessary to shorten a portion of the object while it is still within the abdominal cavity to enable transport. To minimize tissue damage, make every attempt to move the object as little as possible in these situations.

■ Pathophysiology, Assessment, and Management of Specific Injuries

▶ Pathophysiology

Abdominal trauma can be life threatening. Injuries of the abdominal organs, especially those in the retroperitoneal area, can bleed profusely and can hold a large amount of blood. Solid organs such as the kidneys and liver can bleed profusely when torn or cut, as do the major blood vessels that run through the abdominal cavity.

Injuries to hollow organs such as the stomach, although not likely to result in shock, produce a serious risk of infection. The bowel can spill its contents into the abdominal cavity, causing peritonitis and systemic infection. The main causes of death that result from abdominal trauma are hemorrhage and systemic infection.

Diaphragm Injuries

The diaphragm plays the primary role in a patient's ventilatory process. An injury to the diaphragm can cause signs and symptoms of ventilatory compromise. The degree of diaphragmatic injury and associated herniation of abdominal contents upward into the chest cavity is frequently small at first and extends over time; therefore, this injury often is subtle and not appreciated on initial field examination.

Diaphragmatic injuries or ruptures are not isolated incidents; patients often have associated thoracic, abdominal, head, and extremity injuries. A patient who has a right-sided diaphragmatic tear most likely also has a liver injury; a patient who has a left-sided tear most likely also has a spleen injury.

Injuries to the diaphragm are rare, resulting both from blunt trauma (typically high-speed motor vehicle crashes) and from penetrating trauma. A lateral impact during a motor vehicle crash is most likely to cause a diaphragmatic rupture because of the twisting or distortion of the chest wall that may shear or tear the diaphragm. In frontal motor vehicle crashes, the patient may strike the steering wheel or column. This impact may cause a significant change in abdominal pressure, which may also tear the diaphragm.

Injuries to Solid Abdominal Organs

The solid organs in the abdomen include the liver, spleen, kidneys, and pancreas. When a solid organ in the abdomen is injured during blunt or penetrating trauma, the organ releases blood into the peritoneal cavity. This bleeding can cause nonspecific signs such as tachycardia

and hypotension. Findings relate to the size of the injury and the time since the injury occurred.

Liver Injuries. The liver is the largest organ in the abdominal cavity and the most vascular. Because of its size and location, it is the most vulnerable organ in the abdomen. The superior border of the liver can be as high as the patient's nipples, so a liver injury must be suspected in all patients who have right-sided chest trauma as well as abdominal trauma. Also, the ligament in front of the liver (ligamentum teres) can slice the liver in situations involving sudden deceleration. The liver can be contused or lacerated, and a hematoma can develop. The patient may present with a history of an injury to the right upper or central abdomen or right lower chest, fractures of the lower right ribs, right upper quadrant ecchymosis and tenderness, abdominal wall spasm and rigidity, involuntary guarding and rebound tenderness, and hypotension or signs of hypovolemic shock.

Spleen Injuries. Falls and motor vehicle crashes can injure the spleen. However, less obvious injury patterns in activities such as sports (for instance, tackling in football or checking in lacrosse) can also cause injury to the spleen. There are case reports of patients who sustained a ruptured spleen even though the contact was relatively minor. This is especially true if the spleen is enlarged from mononucleosis or other underlying disease. Approximately 5% of circulating blood filters through the spleen every minute. It gets direct vascular supply from the aorta, and its drainage goes directly into the inferior vena cava. When the spleen ruptures, blood spills into the peritoneum, which can ultimately cause shock and death. Because the spleen can bleed profusely, a ruptured spleen can be life threatening. Unlike the liver, penetrating trauma does not present as much of an immediate threat of shock unless a major blood vessel supplying the organ is lacerated. Suspect a spleen laceration when fractures of the 9th through 10th ribs on the left side are present. The patient may present with left upper quadrant tenderness, signs of peritoneal irritation (rebound tenderness and guarding), referred pain to the left shoulder (**Kehr sign**), and hypotension or signs of hypovolemic shock.

YOU ▶ are the Paramedic   PART 4

On arrival at the hospital, the patient's condition is immediately evaluated by the trauma team, and a computed tomography (CT) scan of the abdomen, head, neck, chest, and spine is completed. According to the attending physician, there is no injury to the head, chest, neck, or spine, but the abdominal CT scan reveals hemorrhage from the liver. The patient is evaluated by the trauma team and taken emergently to the operating room for packing of his liver to control the hemorrhage.

9. Why is it important to transport trauma patients (especially those with abdominal trauma) to trauma centers?

10. Why would you be cautious about the amount of IV fluid that you give this patient?

Injuries to Hollow Abdominal Organs

The hollow organs of the abdomen include the small and large intestines, stomach, and bladder. Hollow visceral injuries produce most of their symptoms from peritoneal contamination. When a hollow organ such as the stomach or bowel is injured, it releases its contents into the abdomen. These contents may irritate the abdomen, producing symptoms. A patient who has the seat belt sign—a contusion or abrasion across the lower abdomen—usually also has intraperitoneal injuries.

> ### Words of Wisdom
>
> During a crash, lap belts cause compression, potentially resulting in the rupture of the small or large intestine.

Injuries to the Small and Large Intestines. The intestines are most commonly injured from penetrating trauma, although they can be injured from severe blunt trauma as well. When ruptured, the intestines spill their contents (which contain fecal matter and a large amount of bacteria) into the peritoneal or retroperitoneal cavities, resulting in peritonitis. Blunt trauma to the abdominal wall most commonly causes injury to the duodenum because of its location and ligamentous attachment. It can present as back pain. Penetrating trauma will cause injury to the small bowel, then the stomach and large intestine. The most common cause is the seat belt, because the lap belt lies along the lower quadrant of the abdominal cavity. Symptoms will be caused by the contents rather than the blood loss. Small-bowel and colon injury may present with only generalized pain.

Stomach Injuries. Most injuries to the stomach result from penetrating trauma; the stomach is rarely injured from blunt trauma. When rupture of the stomach does occur after blunt trauma, it is usually associated with a recent meal or inappropriate use of a seat belt. Trauma to the stomach frequently results in the spillage of acidic material into the peritoneal cavity, creating a chemical irritation that produces abdominal pain and peritoneal signs relatively quickly, although patients taking antacid medications may have delayed symptoms.

> ### Words of Wisdom
>
> Every injured patient should be assumed to have a full stomach and bladder.

Retroperitoneal Injuries

Structures contained within the retroperitoneal cavity are the pancreas, vascular structures, part of the small intestine, and kidneys. Injuries confined to the retroperitoneum can be very difficult to diagnose. In general, they are in an area that is remote from physical examination, and an injury initially does not present with signs and symptoms of peritonitis.

Because the blood or other contaminants are held in the retroperitoneal space, they do not frequently cause abdominal pain, peritoneal signs, or abdominal distention. Occasionally, retroperitoneal bleeding can lead to ecchymosis of the flanks (Grey Turner sign) or around the umbilicus (Cullen sign).

> ### Words of Wisdom
>
> Use this mnemonic to recall how to distinguish between Grey Turner sign and Cullen sign: Grey TURNer sign is located when you TURN toward your flank. CUllen sign is located around the Umbilicus.

Pancreatic Injuries. Because of the anatomic position of the pancreas in the retroperitoneum, it is relatively well protected. It typically takes a high-energy force to damage the pancreas. These high-energy forces are most commonly produced by penetrating trauma. With blunt trauma, an unrestrained driver who hits the steering column or a bicyclist who hits the handlebars is at risk of pancreatic injury. When the pancreas is injured from either blunt or penetrating trauma, the enzymes it normally produces to aid digestion are released into the peritoneum instead. These chemicals have an irritating effect on the peritoneum and intra-abdominal structures. Because these are digestive enzymes, they start to break down the internal organs and tissue with which they have come in contact. This process often is described as autodigestion because the pancreatic enzymes literally start to digest the patient's own tissues. Although this enzymatic breakdown leads to chemical peritonitis, the assessment of patients with potential retroperitoneal injuries such as pancreatic trauma can be difficult. As previously stated, peritonitis from this irritation and autodigestion may be readily recognized on physical examination by findings such as abdominal rigidity, guarding, and rebound tenderness. However, because the posterior peritoneum separates the pancreas from the true abdomen, these findings may be significantly delayed.

Vascular Injuries. Intra-abdominal vascular injuries are associated with extremely rapid rates of blood loss, and injury to these structures are often masked by other injuries.[5] The significance of the injury depends on how many vessels were injured and the length of time that has passed since the injury occurred. Besides the kidneys, the vascular structures found in the retroperitoneal space include the descending aorta (and its branches), the superior phrenic artery, the inferior phrenic artery, the inferior vena cava, and the mesenteric vessels. Injuries to these structures occur with both blunt and penetrating trauma, but penetrating trauma is the major cause. Patients with gunshot wounds to the abdomen will have major vessel injury in 20% to 25% of cases.[5] Penetrating trauma that causes injury to the great vessels of the abdomen will also be associated with injuries to multiple intra-abdominal organs. Blunt trauma can cause injuries to vascular structures in the peritoneal cavity because they are sheared from their points of attachment. Compression or deceleration forces applied to the abdomen can result in avulsion of small vessels from the larger vessels from which they branch, resulting in exsanguination. Intimal tears within the vessel itself can occur, resulting in thrombosis formation.[2]

Words of Wisdom

Blunt abdominal injury may be much more serious than it looks. Do not dawdle at the scene!

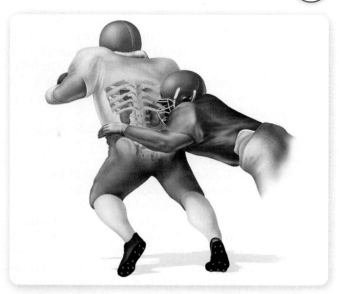

Figure 36-12 A football tackle that results in blunt trauma to the lower rib cage or flank can cause renal injury.
© Jones & Bartlett Learning.

Duodenal Injuries. In abdominal trauma, the duodenum (the first part of the small intestine) can rupture, spilling its contents into the retroperitoneum, usually because of high-speed deceleration injuries. Contamination of the retroperitoneum with duodenal contents may ultimately produce abdominal pain or fever, although symptoms will not likely develop for hours to days. Abdominal pain, nausea, and vomiting may develop, although belatedly. Because of the delayed presentation and variable symptoms, a high degree of suspicion for duodenal injury must be maintained in any abdominal trauma, but especially in high-speed deceleration crashes. As a result of the duodenum's close proximity to multiple organs, it is unlikely that it will be injured by itself. A duodenum injury should be suspected in children who are thrown from a bicycle and strike their abdomen on the handlebars.

Kidney and Ureter Injuries

The kidneys and ureters can be injured in association with abdominal trauma, often as a result of direct trauma (blunt or penetrating) to the back or flank. Such injuries can result in contusions, hematomas, and disruptions of the collecting system (ureters). Injuries to the kidneys generally involve significant forces, such as those sustained in falls from height, high-speed motor vehicle crashes, or sports-related injuries. Suspect injury with fractures of the 11th and 12th ribs or flank tenderness.

Blunt renal trauma results when the kidney becomes compressed against the lower ribs or lumbar spine (as is seen in sports injuries, also known as kidney punch) or when the upper abdomen becomes compressed just below the rib cage (such as when a child is run over by a car). Contact sports such as football, soccer, hockey, boxing, and rugby are some of the more common culprits in renal injury **Figure 36-12**. A ruptured kidney will usually present with pain on inspiration in the abdomen and flank areas. Gross hematuria will almost always be present.

Penetrating renal trauma can occur with gunshot or stab wounds in the abdomen or lower chest. A high suspicion for significant injury must be maintained regardless of the site of the entry wound. Penetrating renal trauma is more likely to be associated with injury to the liver, lung, and spleen. For instance, the upward motion of stabbing may cause a renal laceration as well as a pneumothorax. A gunshot wound may result in direct injury to the kidney, but produce greater surrounding tissue destruction due to the expanding cavity created by the traveling bullet.

Ureteral injuries are difficult, if not impossible, to identify in the prehospital setting. However, they rarely lead to an immediate life-threatening condition. A high index of suspicion should remain, just the same.

Words of Wisdom

Prehospital care of renal injuries relies on the basics of abdominal trauma. Any obvious external abdominal hemorrhage must be addressed. If hemorrhage is not readily apparent but the patient has a large abdominal bruise in the region of the kidneys or is hypotensive, you should assume that the patient has significant internal hemorrhage and begin IV fluid resuscitation in the field per protocol.

Bladder and Urethra Injuries

Trauma to the bladder or urethra is often associated with other significant injuries. A blunt or penetrating injury to the bladder may result in bladder rupture or laceration, usually as a result of blunt trauma. The likelihood of a bladder injury varies by the severity of the mechanism, but also by the degree of the bladder distention. The fuller the bladder, the greater the opportunity for injury. A seat belt that causes contusions to the lower abdomen may also cause blunt trauma to the bladder.

Bladder injuries are usually associated with pelvic injuries from motor vehicle crashes, falls from heights, and physical assaults to the lower abdomen. These MOIs may cause a pelvic fracture to perforate the bladder.

Bladder rupture is associated with a high mortality rate because the trauma required to pierce the bladder frequently damages other organs or vascular structures. If a bladder rupture results from sudden deceleration forces, such as those occurring in motor vehicle crashes, urine may be spilled into either part of the abdominal cavity, leading to intraperitoneal, extraperitoneal, or retroperitoneal rupture.

The signs and symptoms of bladder injuries are generally nonspecific but may present as gross hematuria, suprapubic pain and tenderness, difficulty voiding, and abdominal distention, guarding, or rebound tenderness. The presence of signs of peritoneal irritation may also indicate the possibility of an intraperitoneal bladder rupture.

▶ Assessment

Because signs such as tachycardia and hypotension may not develop until a patient has lost a significant volume of blood, normal vital signs do not rule out the possibility that there has been a significant intra-abdominal injury. Bleeding into the peritoneal cavity from solid organ injuries can also produce abdominal tenderness or distention even though the distention may not be evident until the patient has lost nearly all the blood in the abdomen. Palpation of the abdomen may reveal localized or generalized tenderness, rigidity, or rebound tenderness, all of which suggest a peritoneal injury.

Injuries to the pancreas have subtle or absent signs and symptoms initially and should be suspected in any rapid deceleration injury. Injury should be suspected after a localized blow to the midabdomen. These patients usually experience a vague upper and midabdominal pain that radiates to the back. Peritoneal signs may develop several hours after the injury.

Assessment findings in a patient with vascular injuries depend on whether the bleeding is contained (a hematoma) or there is active hemorrhage. In active hemorrhage, the patient will present with significant hypotension, tachycardia, and shock.

The most frequent presentation of blunt renal trauma is flank pain and hematuria, which usually goes undetected until evaluation in the ED. Suspicion for renal injuries should be high whenever a patient has obvious hematomas or ecchymoses over the upper abdomen, lateral aspects of the middle back, or lower rib cage. Fractures of the lower rib cage should also raise the suspicion for renal trauma.

Bladder injury should be suspected in any patient with trauma to the lower abdomen or pelvis. Bladder injury may also be suspected in the prehospital setting if a patient reports an inability to urinate, blood is noted at the penile opening during history taking and secondary assessment, or the patient has tenderness on palpation of the suprapubic region.

Finally, ultrasonography is being used with increasing frequency in some areas.

▶ Management

As mentioned previously, it is crucial for you to have a high index of suspicion when the MOI suggests possible internal abdominal damage. As with other abdominal injuries, management includes support of the ABCDEs, spinal immobilization (if indicated), rapid patient evaluation, and transport to an appropriate receiving facility with close monitoring for changes in vital signs and patient condition.

■ Pathophysiology, Assessment, and Management of Injuries to the Male Genitalia

▶ Pathophysiology

Injuries to the Testicle or Scrotal Sac

Severe injuries to the testicles are rare because of their mobility and natural position. Although loss of fertility is the major concern when a patient sustains a testicular injury, the exact outcome depends on whether the testicle can be preserved via definitive treatment in the hospital setting.

Blunt trauma to the testicles or scrotal sac can result from motor vehicle crashes, physical assaults, or sports injuries. Blunt testicular trauma can result in simple contusions, rupture of the testicle, and, in rare cases, torsion (twisting) of the testicle. Testicular injuries frequently present following trauma to the thighs, buttocks, penis, lower abdomen, and pelvis.

Penetrating trauma to the testicles or scrotal sac may result from stab wounds, gunshot wounds, blast wounds, or animal bites. You should have a high suspicion for other associated injuries in cases of obvious penetrating trauma.

Penis Injuries

The penis is a vital organ for both proper urination and sexual function. Injuries to the penis may result from blunt or penetrating trauma but also may arise from sexual behavior or self-mutilation. Physiologically, the penis becomes erect when blood fills the corpus cavernosa. Priapism—a painful, tender, persistent erection—can have nontraumatic causes, such as sickle cell disease or adverse medication reaction.

A fractured penis may occur when an erect penis is accidentally impacted against the partner's pubic symphysis or bent too far via self-manipulation.

Penetrating trauma to the penis most often results from gunshot wounds. Also, reports in the medical literature describe self-mutilation or amputation of the penis. Typically, this type of injury occurs in patients with significant psychiatric disorders.

▶ Assessment

Contusions of the testicles or scrotal sac result in painful hematomas that may respond to application of ice packs. Rupture of the testicle is difficult to identify in the prehospital setting, although tender scrotal swelling should be a presenting complaint. Similarly, you will not be able to determine if a particular blunt trauma has resulted in a testicular torsion. Although serious injury to the testicles is rare, it does not require much force to cause intrascrotal bleeding. If enough bleeding or concomitant swelling occurs, pressure necrosis (tissue death) may result. For this reason, you should not ignore testicular complaints even in the face of other trauma, and should communicate this concern to the ED staff.

In the case of a penile fracture, the wall of the corpora cavernosa is torn; pain and a large hematoma are the presenting signs and symptoms.

When there is penetrating trauma to the penis, attention should be paid to controlling hemorrhage and assessing the patient for other injuries associated with the trauma.

Special Populations

In the pediatric population, penile contusions have been reported to occur when a toilet seat falls unexpectedly and compresses the child's penis. Ice packs can help decrease swelling. Note that penile trauma in a child may be a sign of abuse, and an evaluation for other injuries may be warranted.

▶ Management

Scrotal lacerations or avulsions should be treated with proper attention to any hemorrhage or testicular evisceration. Gentle compression and the application of ice packs may help decrease bleeding, swelling, and pain. Provide pain relief and emotional support.

A scrotal laceration may serve as a portal through which bacteria can enter the scrotum or perineum. The resulting infection, called Fournier gangrene, causes necrosis of the muscle and other subcutaneous tissue within the scrotum. The scrotum may feel spongy, and the accumulation of gas in the scrotal sac may produce the distinctive sounds of crepitus. The scrotal tissues will become gray-black, drainage will occur at the wound site, and fever and scrotal pain will be present. A scrotal laceration is a true emergency, and prompt transport to the hospital is indicated. If left untreated, the infection can enter the bloodstream, causing systemic sepsis.

In the case of an amputation, attempts should be made to recover the amputated penis because surgical repair is often possible.

A number of reports have described people who have placed objects around the penis, testicles, or both. Inability to remove the object can result in incarceration of the organ, with tissue death being the most feared consequence. No attempt to remove the object should be made in the field. Instead, the patient should be transported to the hospital for proper evaluation and treatment, which may necessitate the use of cutting devices or aspiration of the distal edema.

■ Pathophysiology, Assessment, and Management of Injuries to the Female Genitalia

▶ Pathophysiology

Vaginal trauma may be the result of blunt or penetrating trauma or may be self-inflicted. Blunt trauma may result from motor vehicle crashes in which high-energy impacts cause significant abdominal and pelvic trauma or from saddle-type injuries, such as falling on the handlebars of a bicycle. Lacerations to the vaginal wall can occur, as well as uterine rupture or ovarian contusion. Trauma to the external genitalia may produce contusions to the vulva or labia.

Penetrating trauma to the reproductive organs may result from stabbings to the lower pelvis or gunshot wounds. Because the path of a bullet cannot be predicted from the entry wound alone, any injuries to the abdomen or upper legs may have also damaged the reproductive organs.

Self-inflicted trauma has been reported in female children and in psychiatric patients who insert foreign bodies into their genitalia.

▶ Assessment

Signs of trauma may include hematomas and ecchymoses in the lower pelvic area and on the external female genitalia, bleeding from the vagina, and tenderness on palpation of the lower pelvis. The assessment may reveal clues of sexual assault; this topic is covered in Chapter 22, *Gynecologic Emergencies*.

▶ Management

Use compression to stem any external hemorrhage, and administer replacement fluids to treat the hypotensive patient. Use any pain medication with extreme caution in the hypotensive patient.

Occasionally, women of reproductive age can cause vaginal lacerations by using devices or tools to remove tampons, pads, and other products that they could not digitally remove from the vaginal canal. Do not attempt to remove any objects; immediately transport the patient for treatment at the hospital. Finally, remember emotional considerations and be familiar with your reporting requirements for assault.

Words of Wisdom

Pelvic fractures may result from blunt trauma from motor vehicle crashes, motorcycle crashes, or vehicle-pedestrian crashes. Pelvic fractures are commonly associated with internal abdominal injuries; signs and symptoms such as pain in the pelvis, groin, or hips; hematomas or contusions to the pelvic region; obvious external bleeding; or hypotension without obvious external bleeding. Pelvic fractures are covered in Chapter 37, *Orthopaedic Trauma.*

YOU are the Paramedic — SUMMARY

1. What are your immediate concerns?

Immediate concerns may include spinal cord injuries, occult abdominal trauma, and injuries to the airway. The patient possibly struck the steering wheel, potentially causing blunt force trauma to his abdomen and trauma to his chest and neck.

2. What are your immediate treatment priorities?

Immediate treatment priorities include spinal precautions and supporting airway and breathing.

3. What do you recall about solid versus hollow organs in regard to blunt trauma?

Solid organs, such as the liver and spleen, can easily be crushed by blunt trauma to the abdomen, resulting in blood loss. Hollow organs are more resilient to blunt trauma and less likely to be injured by trauma—unless they are full. When a hollow organ is full, it is likely to be injured and can burst.

4. What do these signs indicate to you?

His cool, pale, and moist skin could be a result of peripheral-vascular shunting, as seen in the early stages of shock. When the sympathetic nervous system stimulates the release of epinephrine and norepinephrine from the adrenal glands, peripheral vasoconstriction occurs and the sweat glands are opened.

5. What can you conclude from the patient's vital signs?

The patient's blood pressure is in the low normal range and the pulse rate is rapid. The patient's tachycardia could be caused by the body's attempt to compensate. Considering his abdominal exam findings, the tachycardia could be a sign of shock in this patient.

6. What does right upper quadrant tenderness suggest?

Right upper quadrant tenderness may indicate injury to the liver.

7. What may the right shoulder pain indicate?

The right shoulder pain (from diaphragmatic irritation) may indicate referred pain indicative of a liver injury; however, it may also indicate musculoskeletal injury such as a sprain or strain.

8. What are some of the possible causes for the patient's hypotension?

With the presentation of the patient and the MOI evidence presented, you would suspect that the patient is in a hemorrhagic shock state from internal bleeding as a result of the blunt trauma.

9. Why is it important to transport trauma patients (especially those with abdominal trauma) to trauma centers?

Trauma centers have the specialized staff, equipment (eg, imaging devices), and resources to provide the best care for trauma patients. The closest hospital may not have the appropriate imaging devices and staff ready to diagnose and treat this patient.

10. Why would you be cautious about the amount of IV fluid that you give this patient?

Although maintaining perfusion is imperative to a positive patient outcome, you must be cautious with the amount of IV fluid you give to a patient who has uncontrolled bleeding. With excessive IV fluid, you could raise pressure sufficiently to disrupt clots and in turn, increase the internal bleeding.

YOU are the Paramedic   **SUMMARY** *(continued)*

EMS Patient Care Report (PCR)

Date: 10-20-18	Incident No.: 126		Nature of Call: MVC		Location: Pine & Chestnut
Dispatched: 1304	**En Route:** 1305	**At Scene:** 1311	**Transport:** 1321	**At Hospital:** 1336	**In Service:** 1406

Patient Information

Age: 45 **Sex:** M **Weight (in kg [lb]):** 100 kg (220lb)	**Allergies:** No known drug allergies **Medications:** None **Past Medical History:** None **Chief Complaint:** Right upper quadrant abdominal pain

Vital Signs

Time: 1316	BP: 100/64	Pulse: 140	Respirations: 20	Spo$_2$: 92%
Time: 1321	BP: 86/43	Pulse: 152	Respirations: 24	Spo$_2$: 98%
Time: 1335	BP: 96/72	Pulse: 124	Respirations: 20	Spo$_2$: 98%

EMS Treatment (circle all that apply)

Oxygen @ __15__ L/min via (circle one): NC (NRM) Bag-mask device	Assisted Ventilation	Airway Adjunct	CPR
Defibrillation	**Bleeding Control**	**Bandaging**	**Splinting**	**Other:** Spinal immobilization, IV NS in R and L AC with 16g, Zofran

Narrative

Called to a single vehicle MVC. Upon arrival found a 45-year-old A/Ox4 male sitting in the front seat. Pt was an unrestrained driver with heavy damage noted to the vehicle. Steer wheel deformity was noted to the lower ring of the wheel. Pts C/C was of abdominal pain and right shoulder pain. Pt denies LOC and is able to recall all events. C-spine was controlled with negative step off noted; good PMS before and after immobilization. Trauma exam showed bruising across the right side of the abdomen and an increase in pain with palpation to the right upper quadrant, pt rated pain at a "10" when palpated. Pt also complained of a dull pain in his right shoulder, no findings found upon exam to shoulder. Rest of trauma exam was unremarkable. V/S noted, lungs CTA, skin pale/warm/diaphoretic, PERRLA 4mm, GCS 15. Secured patient for transport to Level 1 trauma center. Right and left AC IVs were established with 18g @ a 250-mL bolus. Pt complained of nausea. Pt was given 4 mg of Zofran IVP @ 1322 with relief of the nausea. Secondary exam was unremarkable. Contacted medical control with negative orders. Transported and left in care of ED staff.**End of report**

Prep Kit

▶ Ready for Review

- Unrecognized abdominal trauma is the leading cause of unexpected death in trauma patients. Recognizing abdominal injuries and providing rapid transport are key contributions you can make to a patient who has these injuries.
- The abdomen contains many vital organs and structures, including the kidneys, liver, spleen, pancreas, diaphragm, small and large intestines, stomach, bladder, and several great vessels.
- The quadrant system is generally used to describe a location in the abdomen. The four quadrants consist of the right upper quadrant, the right lower quadrant, the left lower quadrant, and the left upper quadrant.
- The peritoneum is a membrane that lines the abdominal cavity. Abdominal trauma can lead to peritonitis, an inflammation of the peritoneum that results from either blood or hollow organ contents spilling into the abdominal cavity. This is a life-threatening infection.
- The retroperitoneal space is the area behind the peritoneum and contains the aorta, vena cava, pancreas, kidneys, ureters, and portions of the duodenum and large intestine.
- When a patient has experienced trauma to the chest or abdomen, you should suspect that he or she also has additional internal abdominal injuries. Also, suspect abdominal trauma in patients who have unexplained symptoms of shock.
- Injury to the abdomen may be slow to develop and can be fatal. An injury may be subtle and difficult to locate and assess.
- Solid organs such as the liver and spleen have a large blood supply and can easily be crushed by blunt trauma. The abdomen and retroperitoneum can accommodate large amounts of blood but produce few signs and symptoms.
- Injury to hollow organs can cause the release of toxins such as urine, bile, or stomach acid into the abdominal cavity, causing major peritonitis.
- Penetrating trauma results in tissue damage by lacerating or cutting, causing open abdominal injury.
- During patient assessment, note the manner in which the patient is lying; patients who are quiet or still should increase your index of suspicion of injuries. Prioritize the ABCDEs, remembering that a distended abdomen can prevent adequate inhalation, and internal unseen injuries can lead to shock. Assessment findings of the pulse and skin will give you an indication as to how aggressively you need to treat for shock.

- Assessment should never delay patient care and transport! Short on-scene time and quick transport to a trauma center are generally indicated. Evaluate subtler signs and symptoms during history taking and the secondary assessment.
- Try to obtain as many details about an injury as possible. Also, note the use of seat belts, deployment of airbags, and the patient's position in the vehicle. If a weapon was involved, note the type of weapon if this information is available.
- Peritonitis can take hours to days to develop. Shock, tachycardia, and confusion may not develop until the patient has lost a significant amount of blood. Maintain a high index of suspicion for a patient who has a mechanism of injury consistent with abdominal trauma, regardless of vital signs and other findings.
- Kidney trauma can cause flank pain and hematuria. Management is the same as for other types of abdominal trauma.
- Suspect a bladder injury in any patient who has trauma to the lower abdomen or pelvis. Symptoms include inability to urinate, blood at the urethral opening, and tenderness of the suprapubic region. Management follows basic trauma principles.
- Blunt trauma to the testicles can cause painful hematomas, testicular rupture, or testicular torsion. The scrotum may be tender and swollen. Lacerations or avulsions should be treated with gentle compression and ice packs.
- Blunt trauma to the penis can cause a large hematoma and pain. Management follows basic trauma principles.
- Vaginal trauma can cause hematomas and ecchymoses in the lower pelvic area and on the external female genitalia, bleeding from the vagina, and tenderness on palpation of the lower pelvis.

▶ Vital Vocabulary

evisceration Displacement of an organ outside the body.

hematuria The presence of blood in the urine.

hemoperitoneum The presence of extravasated blood in the peritoneal cavity.

Kehr sign Left shoulder pain that may indicate a ruptured spleen.

mesentery A membranous double fold of tissue in the abdomen that attaches various organs to the body wall.

peritoneal cavity The area in the abdomen encased in the peritoneum. It consists of an upper and a lower part. The upper portion contains the diaphragm, liver, spleen, stomach, gallbladder, and transverse colon. The lower portion contains the small bowel, sigmoid colon, parts of the descending

Prep Kit *(continued)*

and ascending colon, and, in women, the internal reproductive organs.

peritoneum A membrane in the abdomen encasing the liver, spleen, diaphragm, stomach, and transverse colon.

peritonitis Inflammation of the peritoneum, the protective membrane that lines the abdominal and pelvic cavities.

periumbilical Pertaining to the area around the umbilicus.

retroperitoneal space The area in the abdomen containing the aorta, vena cava, pancreas, kidneys, ureters, and portions of the duodenum and large intestine.

somatic pain Localized pain, usually felt deeply, that represents irritation or injury to tissue, causing activation of peripheral nerve tracts.

visceral pain Crampy, aching pain deep within the body, the source of which is usually difficult to pinpoint; common with genitourinary problems.

▶ References

1. Olthof DC, van der Vlies CH, Goslings JC. Evidence-based management and controversies in blunt splenic trauma. *Curr Trauma Rep.* 2017;3(1):32-37.
2. Holleran RS. Abdominal trauma. In Holleran RS, ed. *ASTNA Patient Transport: Principles and Practice.* 4th ed. St. Louis, MO: Mosby; 2010:340-354.
3. Bloom I, White M, Yancey AH II. Abdominal trauma. In Campbell JR, Alson RL, eds. *International Trauma Life Support for Emergency Care Providers.* 8th ed. Boston, MA: Pearson Education; 2016:255-264.
4. Nelson BP, Chason K. Use of ultrasound by emergency medical services: a review. *Int J Emerg Med.* 2008;1(4):253-259.
5. Tonks SA. Abdominal vascular injuries. Medscape website. http://emedicine.medscape.com/article/1984639-overview. Updated October 6, 2016. Accessed March 31, 2017.

Assessment in Action

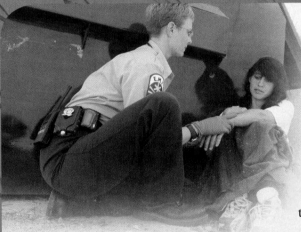

You are dispatched to the scene of a 19-year-old man who has been assaulted. When you arrive, you find the patient sitting on the sidewalk. A police officer at the scene is holding pressure to the patient's right upper abdomen with a blood-soaked gym towel. You observe no other obvious trauma injuries.

Your partner takes over control of applying pressure to the patient's abdomen with a sterile trauma dressing. As the bloody towel is replaced, you note a 2-inch (5-cm) deep laceration to the right upper quadrant with constant slow bleeding. The patient is alert and oriented and states, "I got stabbed!" He is reporting only right upper abdominal pain and denies associated trauma injuries. The patient is pale and diaphoretic and asks to lie down. His vital signs are as follows: respirations, 24 breaths/min; pulse, 136 beats/min; blood pressure, 100/66 mm Hg; and pulse oximetry, 93% on room air. The patient is placed on the stretcher in a supine position as requested.

1. On the basis of the information provided, is this patient a priority patient?

    A. Maybe. Serial vital signs and reassessment will be needed before making this decision.

    B. No. The patient is alert and oriented and his vital signs appear relatively stable at this time.

    C. Yes. The patient's skin color, diaphoresis, and tachycardia indicate the need for limited scene time and rapid transport.

    D. No. Based on the patient's age, he is able to compensate longer and will remain stable for a longer period of time.

Assessment *in Action* (continued)

2. On the basis of the location of the patient's wound, you should suspect injury to which of the following?

    A. Liver and possibly the gallbladder
    B. Stomach and possibly the spleen
    C. Urinary bladder
    D. Appendix

3. On-scene care of this patient should include which of the following?

    A. Comprehensive physical exam
    B. Initiation of IV fluid therapy
    C. Endotracheal intubation
    D. Oxygen administration

4. An open abdominal injury is one in which:

    A. organs are crushed or rupture.
    B. there is soft-tissue damage inside the body but the skin remains intact.
    C. there is a break in the surface of the skin, exposing deeper tissue to potential contamination.
    D. the inner lining of the abdomen is inflamed, resulting in tensing of the abdominal muscles.

5. En route, you note that the patient's abdomen is distended and rigid. The patient reports tenderness at the site of injury. A repeat set of vital signs reveals the following: respirations, 26 breaths/min; pulse, 148 beats/min; blood pressure, 86/56 mm Hg; and pulse oximetry, 97% (with nonrebreathing mask). On the basis of these findings, you suspect:

    A. septic shock.
    B. tension pneumothorax.
    C. compensated shock.
    D. decompensated (hypotensive) shock.

6. Which of the following signs are consistent with abdominal hemorrhage?

    A. Tender abdomen, hypertension, and bradycardia
    B. Distention, hypotension, tachycardia, and shock
    C. Tachycardia, hypertension, and distention
    D. Periumbilical ecchymosis, distention, bradycardia, and shock

7. You have established two 18-gauge IVs. Although all vital signs are important, which of the following should be most closely monitored en route to the nearest trauma center?

    A. Mental status, heart rate, blood pressure, and skin color and temperature
    B. Respiratory rate and blood pressure
    C. Mental status, oxygen saturation, and skin color and temperature
    D. Respiratory rate and mental status

8. Discuss the value of performing percussion of the abdomen as part of the prehospital abdominal exam.

9. Is auscultation of bowel sounds useful in assessing for abdominal trauma?

10. What are the primary sources of exsanguination during abdominal trauma?

Orthopaedic Trauma

National EMS Education Standard Competencies

Trauma

Integrates assessment findings with principles of epidemiology and pathophysiology to formulate a field impression to implement a comprehensive treatment/disposition plan for an acutely injured patient.

Orthopaedic Trauma

Recognition and management of
> Open fractures (pp 1848-1851, 1857-1863, 1866-1874)
> Closed fractures (pp 1848-1851, 1857-1863, 1866-1874)
> Dislocations (pp 1851, 1874-1877)
> Amputations (see Chapter 31, *Soft-Tissue Trauma*)

Pathophysiology, assessment, and management of
> Upper and lower extremity orthopaedic trauma (pp 1848-1863, 1866-1868, 1872-1877)
> Open fractures (pp 1848-1863, 1866-1874)
> Closed fractures (pp 1848-1863, 1866-1874)
> Dislocations (pp 1851-1857, 1874-1877)
> Sprains/strains (pp 1851-1857)
> Pelvic fractures (pp 1868-1871)
> Amputations/replantation (see Chapter 31, *Soft-Tissue Trauma*)
> Compartment syndrome (p 1864)
> Pediatric fractures (see Chapter 43, *Pediatric Emergencies*)
> Tendon laceration/transection/rupture (Achilles and patellar) (pp 1852, 1877)

Medicine

Integrates assessment findings with principles of epidemiology and pathophysiology to formulate a field impression and implement a comprehensive treatment/disposition plan for a patient with a medical complaint.

Nontraumatic Musculoskeletal Disorders

Anatomy, physiology, pathophysiology, assessment, and management of
> Nontraumatic fractures (pp 1878-1880)

Anatomy, physiology, epidemiology, pathophysiology, psychosocial impact, presentations, prognosis, and management of common or major nontraumatic musculoskeletal disorders, including
> Disorders of the spine (see Chapter 34, *Head and Spine Trauma*)
> Joint abnormalities (pp 1878-1879)
> Muscle abnormalities (p 1879)
> Overuse syndromes (pp 1879-1880)

Knowledge Objectives

1. Describe the incidence, morbidity, and mortality of musculoskeletal injuries. (p 1844)
2. Review the anatomy and physiology of the musculoskeletal system. (pp 1844-1846)
3. Describe age-associated changes in the bones. (p 1846)
4. Predict injuries based on the mechanism of injury, including:
   a. Pathologic (p 1846)
   b. Direct (p 1846)
   c. Indirect (pp 1846-1847)
5. Discuss the general pathophysiology of musculoskeletal injuries, including fractures, ligament injuries, dislocations, muscle injuries, tendon injuries, and injuries that may signify fractures. (pp 1847-1852)
6. Discuss fracture classifications, including linear, transverse, oblique, spiral, impacted, comminuted, segmental, complete, incomplete, nondisplaced, and displaced. (pp 1848-1850)
7. Discuss the pathophysiology of open versus closed fractures. (p 1848)
8. Discuss the signs and symptoms of a fracture. (pp 1848, 1850-1851)
9. Discuss the need for assessment of pulses, motor, and sensation before and after splinting. (p 1851)
10. Explain the process of assessing a patient with a musculoskeletal injury. (pp 1852-1857)
11. Discuss the assessment findings associated with musculoskeletal injuries. (pp 1852-1855)
12. Identify the need for rapid intervention and transport when dealing with musculoskeletal injuries. (p 1853)

13. List the primary signs and symptoms that can indicate less obvious extremity injury. (p 1854)
14. List the 6 Ps of musculoskeletal injury assessment. (p 1854)
15. List the other signs and symptoms that can indicate less obvious extremity injury. (p 1854)
16. Discuss the general emergency care principles used in managing musculoskeletal injuries. (pp 1857-1863)
17. Discuss the relationship between volume of hemorrhage and open or closed fractures. (p 1858)
18. Discuss methods of pain control for a patient with a musculoskeletal injury. (p 1858)
19. Discuss the general guidelines of splinting. (p 1859)
20. Describe the special considerations involved in femur fracture management. (pp 1862-1863, 1872)
21. Discuss the pathophysiology, assessment, and management of complications of musculoskeletal injuries, including peripheral nerve injuries, compartment syndrome, crush injuries, and thromboembolic disease. (pp 1863-1866)
22. Discuss the pathophysiology, assessment, and management of specific fractures, including shoulder girdle fractures, midshaft humerus fractures, elbow fractures, forearm fractures, wrist and hand fractures, pelvic fractures, hip fractures, femoral shaft fractures, knee fractures, tibia and fibula fractures, ankle fractures, and calcaneus fractures. (pp 1866-1874)

23. Describe the procedure for reduction of an ankle, finger, or knee dislocation or fracture. (pp 1873-1874, 1876-1877)
24. Discuss the pathophysiology, assessment, and management of specific joint injuries and dislocations, including those to the shoulder girdle, elbow, wrist and hand, finger, hip, and knee. (pp 1874-1877)
25. Explain the importance of manipulating a knee dislocation or fracture with an absent distal pulse. (p 1877)
26. Discuss the pathophysiology, assessment, and management of bony abnormalities, including osteomyelitis and tumors. (p 1878)
27. Discuss the pathophysiology, assessment, and management of joint abnormalities, including arthritis, osteoarthritis, rheumatoid arthritis, gout, and septic arthritis. (pp 1878-1879)
28. Discuss the pathophysiology, assessment, andmanagement of muscle abnormalities, such as myalgia. (p 1879)
29. Discuss the pathophysiology, assessment, and management of overuse injuries, including tendinitis, bursitis, carpal tunnel syndrome, and polyneuropathy. (pp 1879-1880)

Skills Objectives

1. Demonstrate how to perform a motor function and sensory exam. (pp 1855-1857, Skill Drill 37-1)
2. Demonstrate how to properly splint an injured extremity. (pp 1859-1863)

■ Introduction

Musculoskeletal injuries are one of the most common reasons that patients seek medical attention. From 2009 to 2011, an estimated 102.5 million persons reported a musculoskeletal disease.[1] This number represents nearly one-third of the US population. These injuries may result in musculoskeletal impairment. The direct and indirect costs (eg, missed workdays) to the US economy approached 5.7% of the gross domestic product in 2011 ($873 billion).[1] Some areas of public policy, legislative changes, and public education have been effective in reducing the number of work-related injuries and other preventable injuries.[2] For example, efforts made to increase seat belt use in motor vehicles and to reduce falls in older people have had positive effects.[3,4]

Injuries related to the musculoskeletal system are usually easily identifiable because of the associated pain, swelling, and deformity. Although these injuries are rarely fatal, they often result in short- or long-term disability. By providing prompt temporary measures, such as splinting and analgesia, paramedics may help reduce the period during which patients are disabled. However, despite the sometimes dramatic appearance of these injuries, you should not focus on the musculoskeletal injury without first determining that no life-threatening injury exists. *Never forget the ABCDEs!*

■ Anatomy and Physiology Review

The musculoskeletal system gives the body its shape and allows for its movement. It is essential that you understand its basic anatomy and physiology. Chapter 8, *Anatomy and Physiology*, provides complete anatomic descriptions of the musculoskeletal system.

► Functions of the Musculoskeletal System

The musculoskeletal system performs many important functions, such as providing support to the soft tissues. It enables erect posture and body movement. The musculoskeletal system also provides protection to critical underlying organs and structures. Remember, damage to the musculoskeletal structure may be a surrogate marker for deeper and more significant injuries, so it is important to understand its basic anatomy and physiology.

► The Body's Scaffolding: The Skeleton

The integrated structure formed by the 206 bones of the body is called the skeleton. It may be divided into two distinct portions: the **axial skeleton** and the **appendicular skeleton**. The axial skeleton is composed of the bones of the central part, or axis, of the body; its divisions include the vertebral column, skull, ribs, and sternum. It is reviewed in detail in Chapter 34, *Head and Spine Trauma*. The appendicular skeleton is divided into the **pectoral girdle**, the **pelvic girdle**, and the bones of the upper and lower extremities.

Shoulder and Upper Extremities

The shoulder girdle is the base of the upper arm. It consists of a scapula and clavicle. The scapula and clavicle work together to keep the glenohumeral joint stable and in a position of function. They also serve as important sites of muscle attachment, which allow for upper arm flexion and extension, abduction and adduction, and internal and external rotation.

The upper extremity consists of the shoulder, elbow, wrist, and hand joints as well as the bones of the upper arm, forearm, and hand. The upper arm allows us to reach above and away from our body core. It serves as an important anchor point for muscles of the shoulder girdle and for muscles that permit flexion and extension and supination through the elbow. Upper extremity injuries occur frequently because of the tendency to extend the arm outward to stop a fall. This type of injury is referred to as a fall on outstretched hand, or FOOSH.

Attached to the forearm are important muscles that affect wrist, hand and finger flexion and extension, and supination and pronation. Many small muscles, tendons, nerves, and blood vessels run independently through the forearm to the hand. The majority of hand function comes from muscles in the forearm that have long tendons that extend to the hand and fingers. There are only a few

> **Words of Wisdom**
>
> To remember the difference between supination and pronation, think of soup. The SUPinated hand can hold a cup of SOUP.

YOU ► are the Paramedic   PART 1

You are dispatched to the scene of a private residence for a 24-year-old male roofer who fell off a ladder while carrying shingles up to the roof. Coworkers witnessed the fall and tell you that he fell about 15 to 20 feet, landing feet first on the lawn.

When you arrive, you find the patient lying supine on the grass next to the ladder. He is alert and is slow to answer all questions. He recalls the event and describes feeling light-headed when he was climbing up the ladder before he fell. He reports feeling sleepy and weak and has low back pain, bilateral lower extremity pain.

Recording Time: 1 Minute	
Appearance	Lying supine, complaining of pain
Level of consciousness	Alert; slow to answer questions
Airway	Patent with clear speech
Breathing	Nonlabored and shallow
Circulation	Rapid radial pulse, no obvious external bleeding

1. What are your initial assessment and treatment priorities?
2. What other information would you obtain about the patient and the incident?
3. What are your early communication and transport plans?

small muscles located within the hand itself. Because humans work primarily with their hands, the hands are often in harm's way and are common sites of injury. Even lacerations to the hand and wrist area that appear minor should be closely evaluated for tendon, blood vessel, and nerve injury.

Pelvis and Lower Extremities

The pelvic girdle forms the base of the torso and connects it with the lower extremities. The pelvic bones form a ring, which is extremely strong and allows multiple sites for muscle attachment. Because of humans' upright posture, the muscles spanning this area are large and numerous. These muscles allow for flexion and extension, abduction and adduction, and rotation of the hip.

The lower extremity consists of the hip, knee, and ankle joints, as well as the bones of the thigh, leg, and foot. The thigh functions to allow the foot to be positioned away from the body to facilitate balance and strength. Muscles of the hip and thigh also direct flexion and extension of the knee joint. Below the knee joint, the tibia runs down the front of the leg. The tibia is vulnerable to direct blows. It can be felt precariously close to the skin. The tibia supports 90% of the weight of the upper body while the fibula serves as more of a strut. The function of the leg is to facilitate walking by allowing the foot and ankle to be propelled forward of the body. The ankle and foot allow for balance adjustment on uneven terrain.

Patterns and Mechanisms of Musculoskeletal Injury

Skeletal injury results when skeletal tissues are impacted by forces that exceed the tissues' physiologic limitations. In some cases, a force that might not generally cause harm to healthy bone produces a fracture. Such a pathologic fracture occurs when a medical condition causes the bone to become abnormally weak. In adults and children, motor vehicle crashes (MVCs), falls, and athletic activities are common causes of injury. Among children, intentional trauma or abuse is a common cause of fractures and musculoskeletal injuries. Sports activities account for a significant number of musculoskeletal injuries.

Bone ages just like any other tissue of the body, decreasing in density after age 35 years, eventually leading to a loss of height. In women, this decrease in density is accelerated once menopause is reached. A significant decrease in bone density, called osteoporosis, is associated with a higher risk of fracture. People with osteoporosis are at risk for incurring a fracture, especially in the hip, spine, and wrist. Other changes associated with aging of bone include aging of muscles, cartilage, and other connective tissues that may also lead to degradation of joints and disk herniation.

Special Populations

In the older adult patient, fractures and dislocations may be associated with osteoarthritis or the normal atrophy and weakening processes associated with aging. A high degree of suspicion is necessary in the older adult population for low-energy fracture due to age-related changes. Signs of abuse are most likely to be detected by conducting a thorough patient history and looking for environmental clues.

▶ Injury Forces and Motions

Direct Force

An object that strikes a person will transfer its energy to its point of impact. If the force of the object exceeds the strength of the bone, a fracture occurs. If the point of impact is close to a joint, then there can be a dislocation, which may or may not be associated with a fracture. Soft tissues local to the injury are often contused and occasionally rupture.

Penetrating injuries, in addition to soft-tissue damage, may lead to a fracture or other musculoskeletal injury. A high-velocity injury, such as that caused by a high-power rifle, typically severely shatters bone and causes extensive soft-tissue damage. Remember, the speed of the penetrating object has more effect than the size of that object.

An impalement injury commonly causes a soft-tissue injury similar to that seen in a low-velocity penetrating injury. If the impaled object happens to strike a bone, then it may cause a fracture. In any case of impalement, it is essential to stabilize the object to protect the soft tissues from further injury.

Indirect Force

An indirect injury occurs when a force is applied to one region of the body but causes an injury in another region of the body. In this type of injury, the force is transmitted through the skeleton until, at some point, it reaches an area that is structurally weak in comparison with the other parts of the musculoskeletal system through which the force has traveled.

For example, a hip fracture may occur when a person's knee strikes the dashboard during an MVC. In this case, the force is applied to the knee and travels proximally along the femur. When this force reaches the femoral neck, it causes the femoral neck to fracture.

Forces may be transmitted along the entire length of a bone or through several bones in series and may cause an injury anywhere along the way. Thus, a person falling on an outstretched hand may have one or more injuries as the result of forces transmitted proximally from the point of impact: (1) fracture of the scaphoid bone of the hand

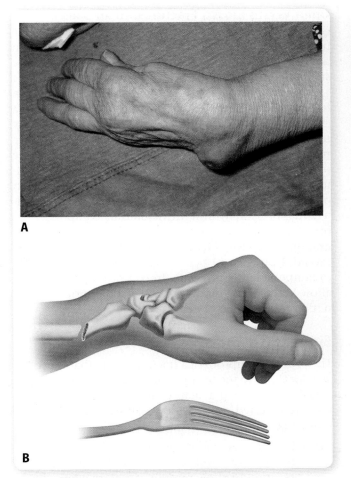

Figure 37-1 A. Exceeding the range of motion of an extremity can cause a fracture. **B.** Fractures of the distal radius can be caused by hyperextension of the wrist secondary to falling on an outstretched hand. This mechanism of injury produces a characteristic "silver fork" deformity.

A: © Dr. M.A. Ansary/Science Source; **B:** © Jones & Bartlett Learning.

Table 37-1	Musculoskeletal Injuries That Commonly Occur Together
If You Find	**Look For**
Scapular fracture	Rib fracture, pulmonary contusions, pneumothorax
Scaphoid fracture	Wrist, elbow, or shoulder fracture
Pelvic fracture	Lumbosacral spine and other long bone fractures, intra-abdominal or genitourinary injury
Hip dislocation	Fracture of the acetabulum or femoral head
Femoral fracture	Dislocation of ipsilateral hip
Patellar fracture	Fracture-dislocation of ipsilateral hip
Knee dislocation	Tibial fracture; distal pulse may be absent
Calcaneal fracture	Fracture of the ankle, leg, hip, pelvis, lumbar spine, and the other calcaneus

© Jones & Bartlett Learning.

(direct blow), (2) fracture of the distal ulna and radius (Colles fracture) **Figure 37-1**, (3) fracture-dislocation of the elbow, (4) fracture-dislocation of the shoulder, or (5) fracture of the clavicle.

Twisting injuries, such as those that commonly occur in football or skiing, result in fractures, sprains, and dislocations. Typically, the distal part of the limb remains fixed, as when cleats or a ski holds the foot to the ground, while torsional force increases in the proximal section of the limb; the resulting force causes tearing of tendons and ligaments and spiral fractures of bone.

Stress fractures, also called **fatigue fractures**, are caused by repetitive stress. Stress fractures typically occur in segments of poor vascularity. A repetitive submaximal load causes microcracks in the cortical bone, resulting in an imbalance of bone resorption and formation. In the case of pathologically weakened bone, stress fractures may occur by simple activities of daily living. Endocrine dysfunction is a risk factor for developing a stress fracture. Symptoms of pain at the site are often reported long before the fracture is visible by radiograph.

Some injuries are commonly encountered together because of the way the causative forces are transmitted; fractures that occur in this manner are called **associated fractures**. If you find one of these fractures, then look for the others **Table 37-1**. Pain and swelling over the scaphoid (navicular) bone of the wrist, for example, means that the patient fell hard against an outstretched hand, so he or she may have other injuries anywhere along the axis from the hand to the shoulder.

■ Pathophysiology

▶ Fractures

A **fracture** is a break in the continuity of a bone. Fractures occur when the magnitude of the force applied to a bone (a single application or an accumulation of repetitive applications) overcomes the strength of the bone. The strength of a bone is affected by age, osteoporosis, nutritional status, and disease processes.

Fracture Classification

Fracture Type. A fracture may be classified based on the direction that the fracture line travels through a bone, number of fractures on the bone, or number of cortices (layers) involved **Figure 37-2** and **Table 37-2**.

Fracture Classification Based on Displacement. Fractures may be classified based on the type of displacement **Table 37-3**. The visual appearance of the limb can characterize the fracture. Deformities of the limb can be angulated, rotated, or shortened.

Angulation of a fracture means that each end of the fracture is not aligned in a straight line and that an angle has formed between them. Angulation may occur in the frontal plane, sagittal plane, or both.

Open Versus Closed Fractures. In an **open fracture** **Figure 37-3**, a break in the overlying skin allows the fracture to communicate with the outside environment. In a **closed fracture** **Figure 37-4**, the skin over the fracture site remains intact.

In addition to having a higher risk of infection, open fractures have the potential for more blood loss than a closed fracture for two reasons. First, open fractures usually result from high-energy injuries, so they typically involve more soft-tissue damage. Second, in most fractures, the periosteal vessels and the vessels supplying the surrounding soft tissues are disrupted, leading to the formation of a hematoma. In a closed fracture, the increased interstitial pressure within the hematoma compresses the blood vessels, limiting the size of the hematoma. For example, in a closed femur fracture, the blood loss may exceed 2 pints (1 L) before enough pressure develops to tamponade the bleeding. In contrast, open fractures allow much of the blood to escape, so tamponade does not occur as readily or at all.

Signs and Symptoms of a Fracture

The primary symptom of a fracture is *pain* that is usually well localized to the fracture site. In addition, the patient may report hearing a snap or feeling a break. Signs of fracture detected on physical examination include the following:

- *Deformity* is one of the most reliable signs of a fracture. The limb may be found in an unnatural position or show motion at a place where there

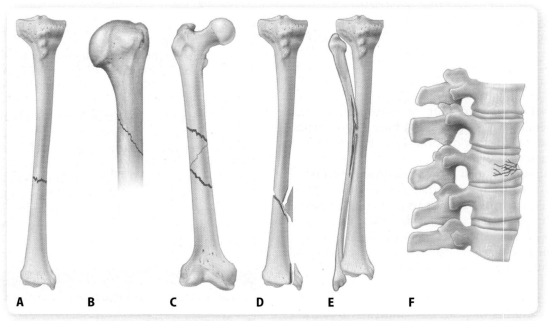

Figure 37-2 Types of fractures. **A.** Transverse fracture of the tibia. **B.** Oblique fracture of the humerus. **C.** Spiral fracture of the femur. **D.** Comminuted fracture of the tibia. **E.** Greenstick fracture of the fibula. **F.** Compression fracture of a vertebral body.

Table 37-2	Fracture Classification Based on Fracture Type		
Category	**Type of Fracture**	**Description**	**Common Causes**
Direction the fracture line travels through a bone	**Linear fracture**	Parallel to the long axis of the bone	Low-energy stress injuries
	Transverse fracture	Straight across a bone at right angles to each cortex	Direct, low-energy blow
	Oblique fracture	At an angle across the bone	Direct or twisting force
	Spiral fracture	Encircles the bone	Twisting injury
	Impacted fracture	End of one bone becomes wedged into another bone	Fall from a significant height
	Pathologic fracture	Can present as either a localized erosive destruction of the cortical bone or as an abnormal overgrowth of bone	Primary or metastatic cancer
Number of fractures on one bone	**Comminuted fracture**	More than two fracture fragments located in one area of the bone	High-energy injury (such as crush injury)
	Segmental fracture	More than two fracture fragments, but breaks occur in different parts of the bone	High-energy injury
Number of cortices injured	**Complete fracture**	Break through both cortices	High-energy injury
	Incomplete fracture	Break through one cortex	Low-energy injury
	■ **Greenstick fracture**	Typically occurs in the proximal metaphysis or diaphysis of the tibia or radius; when this fracture occurs in the shaft, the cortex on the convex side of the deformity is broken, but the cortex on the concave side remains intact	Occurs exclusively in children
	■ **Buckle fracture** (**torus fracture**)	Occurs in the metaphysis of long bones in response to excessive compression loading on one side of the bone; the compressed cortex buckles and the opposite cortex is pulled away from the physis	Unique to children; most commonly seen in the distal radius, usually resulting from a fall on an outstretched hand
	■ Plastic deformation	When a compression force is applied to a bone, numerous small fractures on the compressed side of the bone cause it to bend, resulting in plastic deformation of the bone	Often occurs in children and young adults; most commonly affects the radius, ulna, tibia, fibula, or clavicle
	■ Fatigue fracture (**stress fracture**)	Occurs when the muscle develops faster than the bone and places exaggerated stress on the less-developed bone; may also be due to repetitive small injuries that eventually lead to bone failure	Usually occurs in the legs or feet of people who engage in strenuous, repetitive activities (such as dancers, joggers, military recruits)

Table 37-3	**Fracture Classification Based on Displacement**	
Type of Fracture	**Description**	**Common Causes**
Nondisplaced fracture	Bone remains aligned in its normal position, despite the fracture.	Low-energy injury
Displaced fracture	Ends of the fracture move from their normal positions.	High-energy injury
▪ **Overriding**	Muscles pull the distal fracture fragment alongside the proximal one, leading them to overlap; the limb becomes shortened.	Occurs only when a fracture is fully displaced and there is no bone contact
▪ **Distraction injury**	A powerful tensile force is rapidly applied to a bone, causing it to fracture; the bone ends are pulled apart.	Industrial equipment, machinery
▪ Impacted fracture (impaction injury)	A massive compressive force is applied to a bone, causing it to become wedged into another bone.	More likely to happen in **cancellous bone**
▪ **Avulsion fracture**	A powerful muscle contraction causes the insertion site of the muscle to be fractured off of the bone.	Sudden "jerking" of a body part
▪ **Depression fracture**	Blunt trauma to a flat bone (such as the skull) causes the bone to be pushed inward.	Blunt injury

© Jones & Bartlett Learning.

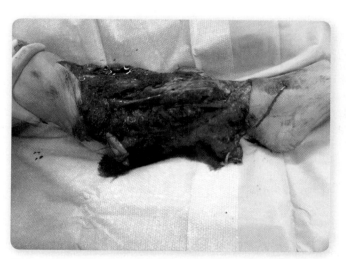

Figure 37-3 An open fracture.

© Andrew Pollak, MD. Used with permission.

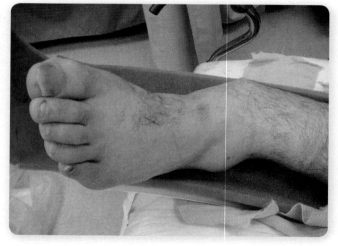

Figure 37-4 A closed fracture.

Courtesy of Rhonda Hunt.

is no joint. Compare the deformed limb with the extremity on the other side **Figure 37-5**.
- *Shortening* occurs in fractures when the broken ends of a bone override one another. It is characteristic of femur fractures, for example, because the broken femur can no longer serve as a strut to oppose spasm in the powerful thigh muscles.

- Visual inspection will usually reveal *swelling* at the fracture site due to bleeding from the broken bone and the accumulation of fluid. As blood infiltrates the tissues around the broken bone ends, *ecchymosis* will become apparent.
- *Guarding* and *loss of use* characterize most fractures. The patient will try to keep a fractured

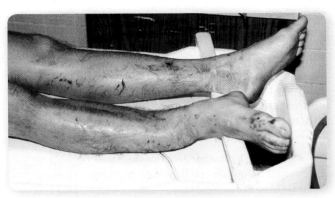

Figure 37-5 Obvious deformity is a sign of bone fracture.
© Charles Stewart, MD, EMDM, MPH.

bone still and will avoid putting any stress on it. Sometimes the measures a patient takes to protect a fractured bone from movement are so characteristic that one can almost diagnose the fracture without examining the extremity. A patient who walks to the ambulance holding the dorsum of one wrist in the other hand, for example, likely has a Colles fracture. A patient standing with the head cocked toward a "knocked-down shoulder" probably has a fracture of the clavicle on the side to which the head is leaning.

- A fractured bone is almost invariably *tender to palpation* over the fracture site.
- Palpation may reveal **crepitus**, a grating sound or sensation caused by bone ends touching, over the broken bone ends. Crepitus may be noted as an incidental finding during splinting attempts. Avoid excessive manipulation of the injured extremity, as this will cause unnecessary pain.
- In an open fracture, *exposed bone ends* may be visible in the wound. Any break in the skin near a fracture should raise suspicion of an open fracture even if you do not see bone. Often, the fracture end ruptures the skin and then retracts back into the soft tissue.

▶ Ligament Injuries and Dislocations

The shapes of the bones that form a joint and the tightness of the ligaments that hold them in place are key factors in determining a joint's **range of motion (ROM)**. When forced beyond their normal limit, the bones that form a joint may break or become displaced, and the supporting ligaments and joint capsule may tear.

Dislocations, Subluxations, and Diastases

In a **dislocation**, a bone is totally displaced from the joint. Typically, at least part of the supporting joint capsule and some of the joint's ligaments are disrupted. Dislocations occur when a body part moves beyond its normal ROM and the articular surfaces are no longer intact. The dislocated bones are then held in position by muscle spasms. Evaluation of the patient usually reveals an obvious and significant deformity, a significant decrease in the joint's ROM, and severe pain. In all cases of a dislocation, a fracture should be suspected until ruled out by radiographs.

The partial dislocation of a joint is a **subluxation**. In this type of injury, the articular surfaces of the bones that form the joint are no longer completely in contact. In some cases, part of the joint capsule and supporting ligaments may be damaged. Despite the subluxation, the patient may be able to move the joint to some degree. Failure to recognize and treat a subluxation may lead to persistent joint instability and pain. A **luxation** is a complete dislocation.

When the ligaments that hold two bones in a fixed position with respect to one another are disrupted and the space between them increases, a situation known as a **diastasis** occurs. An example of this would be an injury to the ligaments that hold the pubic symphysis together, causing the width of the joint to increase (diastasis of the pubic symphysis).

The principal symptom of a dislocation is pain or a feeling of pressure over the involved joint, plus loss of motion of the joint. A patient with a posterior dislocation of the shoulder, for example, is unable to raise the arm but holds it against the side instead. Sometimes the joint will seem "frozen." The principal sign of dislocation is deformity.

A dislocation is considered an urgent injury because of its potential to cause **neurovascular compromise** distal to the site of injury. If the dislocated bone presses on a nerve, then there may be numbness or weakness distally; if an artery is compressed, there may be absent distal pulses (such as in a knee dislocation occluding the popliteal artery). For these reasons, you should always assess the patient's neurovascular status distal to the site of dislocation (check pulse, motor function, and sensation [PMS]) prior to and after splinting.

Sprains

Sprains are injuries in which ligaments are stretched or torn. They usually result from a sudden twisting of a joint beyond its normal ROM that also causes a temporary subluxation. The majority of sprains involve the ankle or the knee because most occur after a person misjudges a step or landing. Evasive moves, like those done during a sporting event, commonly cause sprains in athletes.

Sprains are typically characterized by pain, swelling, and discoloration over the injured joint and unwillingness to use the limb. In contrast with fractures and dislocations, sprains usually do not involve deformity and joint mobility is usually limited by pain, not by joint incongruity **Figure 37-6** .

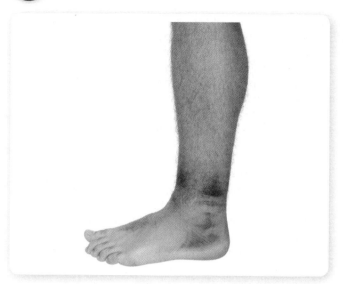

Figure 37-6 Swelling around an ankle from an injury. It is often not possible without radiographic imaging to determine whether a patient has a fracture.

© iStockphoto/Thinkstock/Getty.

Words of Wisdom

It may be difficult to differentiate among the various types of injuries in the field. Diagnosing a severe sprain versus a fracture is one such challenge. Certain clinical tools (eg, Ottawa ankle rules) have been developed to assist in making these decisions. Injuries associated with a high-force mechanism of injury should elicit a high degree of suspicion for fracture when evaluating joint injuries. General treatment of sprains and strains is similar to that of fractures and includes immobilization of the extremity by splinting.

▶ Muscle and Tendon Injuries

Muscle and tendon injuries include strains, Achilles tendon rupture, and injuries related to inflammatory processes, such as bursitis and tendinitis, discussed later in this chapter.

A **strain** (pulled muscle or tendon) is an injury to a muscle and/or tendon that results from a violent muscle contraction or from excessive stretching. Often no deformity is present and only minor swelling is noted at the site of injury. Some patients may report increased pain with passive movement of the injured extremity.

Words of Wisdom

To help remember that a strain involves a tendon, note that the word *strain* includes a *T* (for tendon). The word *sprain* does not include a *T*; sprains do not involve tendons, but rather ligaments.

■ Patient Assessment

When you are assessing an injured patient, *do not be distracted by visually impressive injuries!* It is essential to complete the primary survey of the patient before focusing on the extremities. In cases of musculoskeletal injuries, patients may be classified based on the presence or absence of associated injuries:

- Life- or limb-threatening injury or condition, including life- or limb-threatening musculoskeletal trauma
- Life-threatening injuries and only simple musculoskeletal trauma
- Life- or limb-threatening musculoskeletal trauma and no other life-threatening injuries
- Isolated non–life- or non–limb-threatening injuries

Scene Size-up

As with all patients, you should conduct a scene size-up, focusing on safety and standard precautions. Consider the mechanism of injury (MOI), the need for spinal stabilization, and the potential hazards that may be present at such a scene. Once on scene, observe for hazards and don personal protective equipment (PPE) appropriate for the MOI. A mask, gown, and eye protection may be needed for severe MOIs or when there is the possibility of hidden bleeding. Finally, request additional resources as needed.

Documentation & Communication

Some services take pictures at MVC scenes to include in reports to the receiving hospital. These images allow emergency department staff to better understand the forces involved. Standards relating to the Health Insurance Portability and Accountability Act (HIPAA) and patient privacy should be carefully observed when images are obtained. Some agencies issue company cameras to emergency medical services (EMS) personnel, to be returned at the end of the shift, to help minimize violations of HIPAA.

Primary Survey

Perform a primary survey focusing on the patient's mental status, ABCDEs, and priority. The primary survey usually follows an ABCDE sequence (Airway, Breathing, Circulation, Disability, and Exposure), but if the patient appears lifeless or has severe external bleeding, use a CABDE sequence (Circulation, Airway, Breathing, Disability, and Exposure). The injuries in this region often are some of the first you see when you arrive at the side of the patient. You should use caution to prevent yourself from focusing solely on these distracting injuries at the risk of missing other life threats.

The patient's emergency will often be simple and non–life threatening; however, some situations will include multiple problems, only one of which involves musculoskeletal injuries. If there was significant trauma and multiple body systems are affected, then the musculoskeletal injuries may be a lower priority. Do not waste scene time on prolonged musculoskeletal assessment or splinting. Use a scoop or long backboard as a "full-body" splint and complete additional assessment of musculoskeletal injuries during transport. This is an acceptable splinting option when time precludes specific splinting of individual fractures or when patient condition precludes taking the time to splint individual fractures.

If a spinal injury is suspected, then take the appropriate precautions and prepare for stabilization.

If musculoskeletal injuries in the extremities are suspected, then they must be at least initially stabilized, if not splinted, prior to moving. Assess for pulses distal to the injury and note any circulatory changes before and after any manipulation as well as frequently during transport.

Open fractures can cause significant external bleeding (usually slow and steady). It is often possible to observe fatty droplets in the blood, which come from the bone marrow. Bleeding from the fractured bone ends and medullary canal is difficult to control. After limb alignment and splinting, a sterile dressing and compressive wrap can be effective. The bandage should be secure enough to control bleeding without restricting circulation distal to the injury. Monitor bandage tightness by assessing the circulation, sensation, and movement distal to the bandage. Swelling from fractures and internal bleeding may cause bandages to become too tight. If bleeding cannot be controlled, then you should quickly proceed to apply a tourniquet.

After assessing ABCDEs, you need to make a transport decision. If the patient you are treating has an airway or breathing problem or significant bleeding, then provide rapid transport to the hospital for treatment and apply individual splints en route. A patient who has a significant MOI but whose condition appears otherwise stable also should be transported promptly to the closest appropriate hospital. Patients with bilateral fractures of the long bones (humerus, femur, or tibia) have been subjected to a high amount of kinetic energy, which should dramatically increase your index of suspicion for serious unseen injuries.

Patients with a simple MOI, such as twisting of an ankle or dislocation of a shoulder, may be further assessed

YOU are the Paramedic — PART 2

The patient remains slow to respond, but alert and oriented to person, place, time, and event. Both of the patient's lower extremities are obviously deformed. Bilateral femur deformity is observed. His skin is pale, cool, and slightly moist.

Before moving your patient, you splint his legs, fit him with a cervical collar, and initiate spinal precautions. His back reveals deformity and pain at L4 and L5. The patient tells you that he has type 1 diabetes and has been feeling light-headed intermittently over the past few days. You obtain his blood glucose level, which is 46 mg/dL.

Recording Time: 5 Minutes	
Level of consciousness	Alert (oriented to person, place, time, and event)
Skin	Cool, pale, and slightly moist
Pulse	116 beats/min; weak and regular
Blood pressure	104/60 mm Hg
Respirations	24 breaths/min
Oxygen saturation (Spo$_2$)	98% on room air
Blood glucose level	46 mg/dL

4. What do these physical findings indicate to you?
5. Why is a history of type 1 diabetes significant?
6. What can you conclude from the patient's vital signs?
7. Why is a blood glucose reading of 46 mg/dL significant?

and their condition stabilized on scene prior to transport if no other problems exist. Handle fractures carefully while preparing for transport. Careful handling is necessary to limit pain and prevent sharp bone ends from breaking through the skin or damaging nerves and blood vessels in the extremity.

History Taking

Obtain the patient's medical history using the standard SAMPLE (Signs and symptoms, Allergies, Medications, Pertinent past history, Last oral intake, Events leading to injury or illness) format. This history should also identify any preexisting musculoskeletal disorders and attempt to learn more about the injury. Some information obtained will be relevant to the injury, such as the patient having osteoporosis or taking anticoagulant medications.

Obtain information about the incident that led to the injury from the patient and any bystanders who witnessed it. In particular, determine the condition and position of the patient immediately before the incident, the details of the incident, and the patient's position after the incident. Also, ask the patient for a subjective description of the injury: How did this happen? Did you hear a pop? Do you have pain? What functional limitations do you now have?

Special Populations

Children with fractures may not want you to see, touch, or splint the injured extremity. You should always be honest with children about what you are doing and whether it will hurt. In particular, splinting is a necessary and sometimes painful intervention for a child with a fracture. Once the splint is in place, cold packs are applied, and analgesia is considered, the child will likely have less pain because the fracture is stabilized. Pediatric fractures are covered in Chapter 43, *Pediatric Emergencies*.

Secondary Assessment

When examining the patient, obtain a baseline set of vital signs. The focus can then shift to evaluating the injured extremity. One of the simplest ways to assess an extremity is to compare one side with the other, noting any discrepancy in length, position, or skin color. Next, complete an exam, noting swelling, deformity, discoloration, tenderness, abrasions, lacerations, punctures, or burns as you observe and palpate the soft tissue from head to toe and assess the patient for limitations, such as inability to move a joint. While performing the exam, be sure to cover the **6 Ps of musculoskeletal assessment**: Pain, Paralysis, **Paresthesias** (numbness or tingling),

Pulselessness, Pallor (pale or delayed capillary refill in children), and Pressure.

During the secondary assessment is the time to consider distracting injuries; that is, the injuries that are immediately obvious. In the case of an obvious open fracture of the femur, a patient might direct you only to the site of greatest pain. Distal extremity injuries (fractures and dislocations of the feet and hands) are classically overlooked due to a distracting injury.[5]

Pain

When assessing a patient's pain, remember the OPQRST mnemonic: Onset of the pain; Provoking or Palliating factors; Quality of the pain (such as sharp, pressure, crampy); Region of the pain, including its primary location and areas where pain radiates or refers; Severity of the pain; and the Time (duration) that the patient has been experiencing pain. It is also useful to have the patient quantify the severity of the pain by using a scale of 1 to 10 or with visual images, such as faces that appear to be happy or in pain (see Chapter 43, *Pediatric Emergencies*).

Inspection

When you are inspecting an injured extremity, always evaluate the joint above and the joint below the site of injury because the injuring force may have affected these sites as well. In particular, compare the injured side with the uninjured side. While inspecting a patient's injuries, look for the following signs:

- Deformity, including asymmetry, angulation, shortening, and rotation
- Skin changes, including contusions, abrasions, avulsions, punctures, burns, lacerations, and bone ends
- Swelling
- Muscle spasms
- Abnormal limb positioning
- Increased or decreased ROM
- Color changes, including pallor and cyanosis
- Bleeding, including estimating the amount of blood loss

Words of Wisdom

The ends of a fractured bone are sharp. Use caution whenever bone ends are exposed to prevent a puncture injury to yourself, your crew, or the splint.

Palpation

Palpation of an injured extremity should include the injury site and the regions above and below it. Regions of **point tenderness** (those that the patient identifies as painful) should be identified. Reassess any tender areas frequently to determine whether there are changes in the location or severity of the pain or tenderness. Note that while point tenderness is one of the best indicators of an injury, it may be absent in patients who are intoxicated or who have an injury to the spinal cord.

When you are palpating an injured site, attempt to identify instability, deformity, abnormal joint or bone continuity, and displaced bones. Feel for crepitus, which is commonly found at the site of a fracture. Palpate distal pulses on all extremities, with special attention to comparing the strength of the pulses in the injured extremity with those in a normal one.

On occasion, an arterial injury may be identified while palpating an extremity. Signs of an arterial injury include a pulsatile expanding hematoma, diminished distal pulses, a palpable thrill (vibration) over the site of injury that correlates with the patient's heartbeat, and difficult-to-control bleeding.

The purpose of palpating the pelvis is to identify instability and point tenderness. Apply pressure over the pubic symphysis to evaluate for tenderness and crepitus. Next, press the iliac wings toward the midline and then posteriorly. Any gross instability found during this examination should be reported to hospital personnel because it may indicate a severe pelvic injury. Do not repeatedly examine the pelvis if instability is found because the manipulation may disrupt blood clots and cause further bleeding.

The upper and lower extremity exam should include palpation of the entire length of each arm and leg to identify any sites of injury. The most efficient way to palpate these body parts is to place your hands around the extremity and squeeze. Repeat this procedure every few centimeters until you reach the end of the extremity. When evaluating the upper extremities, always examine the cervical spine and shoulder because complaints relating to the arm may be caused by a more proximal disorder. Likewise, with the lower extremities, always conduct an exam of the pelvis and hip if the patient reports pain in the leg.

Motor Function and Sensory Exam

In the case of a musculoskeletal injury, it is essential to assess a patient's distal pulse as well as motor and sensory function. A motor function exam should be performed whenever a patient has an injury to an extremity, provided the patient does not also have a life-threatening injury. When you are assessing motor function, consider the preinjury level of function. In some cases, weakness or motor deficits may be due to prior injuries or medical problems. For this reason, you should perform a careful review of the patient's history whenever a patient reports being weak or unable to move an extremity.

Also, perform the test on both sides of the body simultaneously so that each extremity can be compared. See Chapter 11, *Patient Assessment*, for more detail about performing a motor function and sensory exam. If you are evaluating a patient with a specific extremity or joint complaint, conduct the portion of the motor function and sensory exam that relates to the specific injured extremity or joint. Skill Drill 37-1 demonstrates how to perform an entire motor and sensory exam.

Skill Drill 37-1 Performing a Motor Function and Sensory Exam

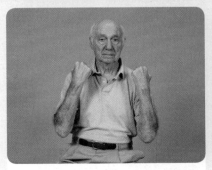

Step 1 Have the patient flex his or her arms at the elbow to test musculocutaneous nerve motor function.

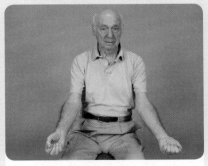

Step 2 Have the patient extend the arms at the elbow to test radial nerve motor function.

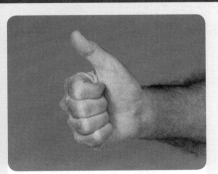

Step 3 Have the patient extend the thumbs (thumbs up) to test radial nerve motor function.

(continued)

Skill Drill 37-1 Performing a Motor Function and Sensory Exam *(continued)*

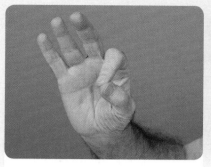

Step 4 Have the patient make an "okay" sign to test median nerve motor function.

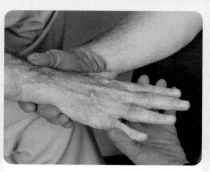

Step 5 Have the patient spread his or her fingers apart to test ulnar nerve motor function.

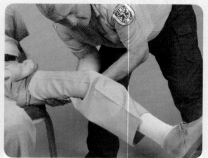

Step 6 Instruct the patient to extend his or her legs at the knee to test femoral nerve motor function.

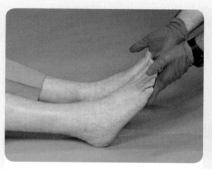

Step 7 Have the patient flex his or her feet and ankles downward (**plantarflex**) to test tibial nerve motor function.

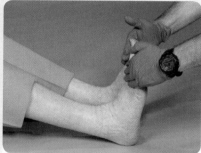

Step 8 Instruct the patient to flex the feet and ankles upward (**dorsiflex**) to test deep peroneal nerve motor function.

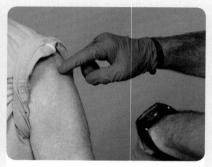

Step 9 Lightly touch the lateral surface of the shoulder (over the deltoid) to test axillary nerve sensory function using the corner of a bandage or tissue to make contact with the skin.

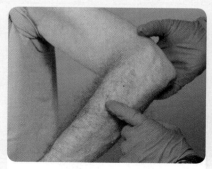

Step 10 Lightly touch the anterolateral surface of the forearm to test musculocutaneous nerve sensory function.

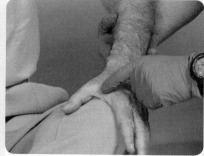

Step 11 Lightly touch the dorsal surface of the web space of the thumb to test radial nerve sensory function.

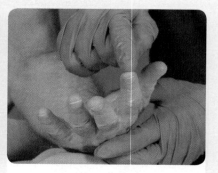

Step 12 Lightly touch the **volar** surface of the distal thumb, index, and middle fingers to test median nerve sensory function.

Skill Drill 37-1 Performing a Motor Function and Sensory Exam (continued)

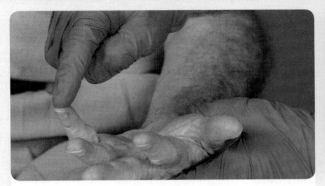

Step 13 Lightly touch the distal volar surface of the small finger to test ulnar nerve sensory function.

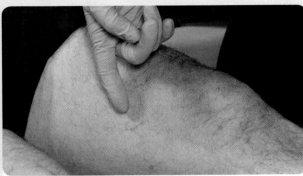

Step 14 Lightly touch the anteromedial surface of the thigh to test femoral nerve sensory function.

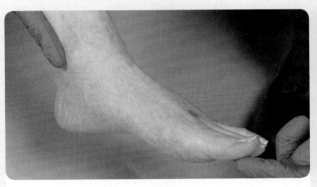

Step 15 Lightly touch the plantar surface of the toes to test tibial nerve sensory function.

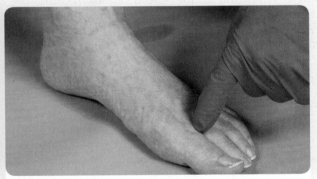

Step 16 Lightly touch the web space between the great toe and the second toe to test peroneal nerve sensory function.

© Jones & Bartlett Learning. Courtesy of MIEMSS.

Reassessment

The condition of the injured extremities requires regular reassessment after the initial exam and stabilization of the injuries. Repeating the neurovascular exam periodically will allow for the recognition of developing neurologic deficits or compartment syndrome.

Documentation & Communication

Always document the findings of a musculoskeletal exam, even if they are normal. When an abnormality is identified, document the specific deficit—for example, "the patient was unable to extend the thumb or the wrist."

Emergency Medical Care

General treatment of fractures includes controlling external bleeding and preventing infection in open fractures, managing internal bleeding (shock considerations), and immobilizing the limb.

General treatment of sprains and strains is similar to that of fractures and includes RICES (Rest, Ice, Compression, Elevation, and Splinting). Treat a closed soft-tissue injury by applying the mnemonic RICES:

- **Rest.** Keep the patient as quiet and comfortable as possible.
- **Ice.** Use ice or cold packs to slow bleeding by causing blood vessels to constrict and also to reduce pain.

- **Compression.** Apply pressure over the injury site to slow bleeding by compressing the blood vessels.
- **Elevation.** Raise the injured part just above the level of the patient's heart to decrease swelling.
- **Splinting.** Immobilize a soft-tissue injury or an injured extremity to decrease bleeding and reduce pain.

▶ Volume Deficit Due to Musculoskeletal Injuries

Fractures may lead to significant blood loss from damage to vessels within the bone and musculature around the bone and, in some cases, from damage to large blood vessels in the region of the fracture. When you are caring for patients with fractures, perform interventions such as applying direct pressure, splinting, and administering intravenous (IV) fluids to prevent hypotension and unstable condition of the patient. **Table 37-4** lists the potential blood loss in the first 2 hours from various fracture sites and may serve as a guideline for estimating the amount of resuscitation required. The goal of prehospital management should be to keep the patient's volume, vital signs, and mental status normal. This management is especially important for a patient with multiple injured extremities, because total blood loss can be significant.

▶ Pain Control

Orthopaedic injuries are associated with pain that may be caused by continued movement of an unstable fracture, muscle spasm, soft-tissue injury, nerve injury, or muscle ischemia. These injuries are often extremely painful, so the goal of prehospital pain control should be to diminish the patient's pain to a tolerable level.

A number of interventions may be performed in the field to control pain from a musculoskeletal injury.

Table 37-4	Potential Blood Loss From Fracture Sites
Fracture Site	**Potential Blood Loss (mL)**
Pelvis	1,500–3,000
Femur	1,000–1,500
Humerus	250–500
Tibia or fibula	250–500
Ankle	250–500
Elbow	250–500
Radius or ulna	150–250

The first step is to assess the level of pain. Establishing a baseline level of pain and reassessing it after each intervention allow you to determine the effectiveness of the treatment being provided. Simple methods for controlling pain include splinting in an anatomic position, resting and elevating the injured part, and applying ice or heat packs.

When simple procedures do not effectively control a patient's pain, consider the administration of medications. Medications for this purpose in the field include ketamine, a dissociative anesthetic; narcotics, such as fentanyl, morphine, and nitrous oxide; or antispasmodic agents, such as diazepam and lorazepam. These agents should be reserved for patients in hemodynamically stable condition who have an isolated musculoskeletal injury. Medications are discussed in detail in Chapter 13, *Principles of Pharmacology*. Obtain vital signs before and after administering any medication for pain and spasm. Further, when these medications are used, you must be prepared to support the airway. Continuous monitoring of the patient's oxygen saturation and end-tidal carbon dioxide level are essential. After pain medication is administered, reassess the patient's pain to ensure that pain relief is adequate.

Administering pain medication before splinting may allow the extremity to be stabilized more effectively. Remember, *it hurts* to have an injured extremity held in the proper position for splinting. Pain medication may make it possible for the patient to tolerate that position longer and allow the splint to be applied properly.

▶ Cold and Heat Application

Cold packs or ice are useful for treating patients during the initial 48 hours following an injury and are effective at decreasing pain and swelling. Cooling the injured area causes vasoconstriction of the blood vessels in the region and decreases the release of inflammatory mediators. As a result, swelling and inflammation are reduced when cold packs are used during the acute stage of an injury.

Conversely, heat therapy should generally be avoided during the initial 48 to 72 hours following an injury because it may actually increase pain and swelling during this period. Once the acute phase of the injury ends and the damaged blood vessels become clotted, heat packs are useful for increasing blood flow to the region to decrease stiffness and to promote healing. As a consequence, heat packs may be beneficial for patients who report an injury that occurred several days before contacting paramedics.

▶ Splinting

Splinting is intended to provide support to and prevent motion of the broken bone ends and two adjacent joints **Figure 37-7**. Correctly splinting an injured extremity not only decreases the pain a patient experiences, but also reduces the risk of further damage to muscles, nerves, blood vessels, and skin. In addition, splinting helps to control bleeding by allowing clots to form where vessels were damaged. When a patient with multiple orthopaedic injuries must be transported immediately, you will not

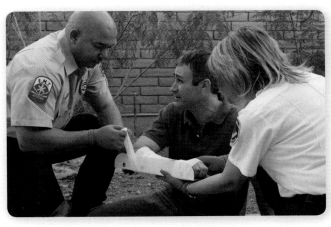

Figure 37-7 Splinting reduces pain and helps prevent additional damage to the extremity.

© Jones & Bartlett Learning. Courtesy of MIEMSS.

have time to splint each fracture one by one. One way to stabilize multiple fractures when the patient's overall condition is critical is to use a vacuum mattress and a scoop stretcher. This method will serve three purposes: (1) it will protect against a spinal injury, (2) it will reduce the movement of injured extremities by securing them to the board, and (3) it will save time at the scene.

Whenever there is time, apply a traction splint for a femur fracture. For a physiologically unstable patient, do not spend time applying traction splints; rather, use something faster, such as a vacuum mattress, long board, or scoop stretcher.

Principles of Splinting

Splinting is one of the most crucial skills to learn when caring for patients with musculoskeletal injuries. Failure to properly splint an injured extremity leads to unnecessary discomfort and the possibility of further injury or harm. Keep the following points in mind when applying a splint:

1. The injured area must be adequately visualized before splinting. Remove clothing as necessary so that you can inspect the area thoroughly.
2. Assess and *record* distal PMS functions before and after splinting.
3. Cover all wounds with a sterile dressing before applying the splint. To prevent infection following an open fracture, you should brush away any obvious debris on the skin surrounding an open fracture before applying a dressing. Do not enter or probe the open fracture site in an attempt to retrieve debris, because doing so may lead to further contamination. Do not attempt to push exposed bone ends back under the skin.
4. Do not move the patient before splinting unless an immediate hazard exists.
5. *For fractures*, the splint must immobilize the bone ends and the two adjacent joints.

For dislocations, the splint must extend along the entire length of the bone above and the entire length of the bone below the dislocated joint.
6. Pad the splint well to prevent local pressure and to provide optimal motion restriction.
7. Support the injured site manually with one hand above and one hand below the injury, and minimize movement until the splint is applied and secured.
8. If a long bone fracture is severely angulated, then gently apply longitudinal traction (tension) to attempt to realign the bone into a more natural position and improve circulation. Use a smooth, firm grip to apply manual traction, and take care to avoid any sudden, jerky movements of the limb. *Do not attempt to straighten fractures involving joints without first obtaining medical direction.* The pain associated with straightening an unstable joint injury generally outweighs the benefits of doing so in the field, unless there is a loss of distal circulation, in which case it makes sense to attempt repositioning of the injured joint.
9. If the patient can tolerate it, then splint the knee straight if not directly injured and angulated; splint the elbow at a right angle.
10. If the patient reports severe pain or is resistant to movement, then discontinue applying traction, splint in the position of deformity, and carefully monitor the distal neurovascular status (PMS).
11. Splint firmly, but not so tightly as to occlude the distal circulation.
12. If possible, to allow for monitoring of skin color, temperature, and condition, do not cover fingers and toes with the splint.
13. If possible, apply cold packs and elevate the splinted limb to minimize swelling.
14. When the patient has a life-threatening injury, individual splint application for possible fractures must not delay transport and might not be accomplished.

Words of Wisdom

Always check the pulses, strength, motor function, and sensation distal to a musculoskeletal injury.

Types of Splints

Any device used to immobilize a fracture or dislocation is considered a splint. Commercially available splints include board splints, inflatable or vacuum splints, and traction splints. Lack of a commercially made splint should never prevent proper immobilization of an injured patient; multiple casualties may tax the resources of even the best-equipped ambulance, requiring improvisation.

Rigid Splints. A rigid splint is any inflexible device that may be attached to a limb to maintain stability—a padded board, a piece of heavy cardboard, or an aluminum "ladder" or SAM (structural aluminum malleable) splint molded to fit the extremity. More elaborate rigid splints are designed to quickly fit around two or three sides of an extremity and be secured with self-adhesive (Velcro) straps or cravats. Some rigid splints are made of a radiolucent material that allows radiographs to be obtained without removal of the splint. Whatever its construction, the splint must be generously padded to ensure even pressure along the extremity and long enough to be secured well above and below the fracture site (beyond the proximal and distal joints).

Documentation & Communication

Document the neurovascular exam and distal PMS functions before and after splinting.

When you are applying a rigid splint, grasp the extremity above and below the fracture site, and apply gentle traction. Another provider should then place the splint alongside the limb. While one provider maintains traction, the other wraps the limb and splint in self-adhering bandages that are tight enough to hold the splint firmly to the extremity but not so tight as to occlude circulation **Figure 37-8**. (If the splint has its own straps that are used to secure it to the extremity, then this step is not required.) Leave the fingers or toes out of the bandage so that distal circulation can be monitored.

Sling and Swathe. An arm sling may be fashioned from a triangular bandage and is useful to stabilize injuries

that involve the shoulder or as an adjunct to a rigid splint of the upper extremity. The sling holds the injured part against the chest wall and takes some of the weight off the injured area.

To apply a sling, place the splinted extremity in a comfortable position across the chest and lay the long edge of a triangular bandage along the patient's side opposite the injury. Bring the bottom edge of the bandage up and over the forearm and tie it *at the side* of the neck to the other end. Tie or pin the pointed end of the sling, at the elbow, to form a cradle. Secure the sling so that the hand is carried higher than the elbow and the fingers are visible for checking peripheral circulation **Figure 37-9**. If the patient is large, then tie two cravats together using a square knot, to give you more material. Cushion the sling with gauze pads to secure the splint and increase patient comfort.

An arm that is splinted with a sling can be further stabilized by adding a swathe. Create a swathe by using one or more triangular bandages to secure the arm firmly to the chest wall. This technique is particularly useful for injuries to the clavicle and for anterior dislocations of the shoulder. Do not use a sling if the patient has a neck injury. Be careful not to secure the swathe so tight as to reduce chest expansion during respirations.

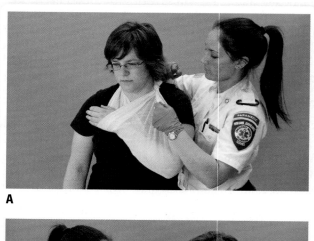

A

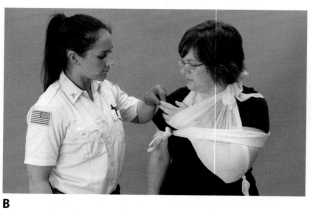

B

Figure 37-9 A. Apply the sling so that the knot is tied at one side of the neck. **B.** Secure the sling. Leave the fingers exposed to allow for circulation checks.

© Jones & Bartlett Learning. Photographed by Glen E. Ellman.

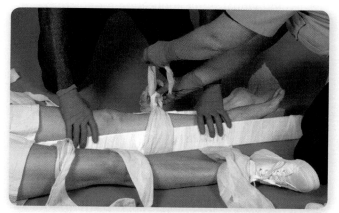

Figure 37-8 In applying a rigid splint, wrap the limb and splint so that the splint is firmly in place but does not cut off circulation.

© Jones & Bartlett Learning.

Pneumatic Splints. Pneumatic splints (also known as air splints or inflatable splints) are useful for stabilizing fractures involving the lower leg or forearm. They are not effective for angulated fractures or for fractures that involve a joint because they will forcefully attempt to straighten the fracture or joint. Likewise, air splints should not be used on open fractures in which the bone ends are exposed.

Air splints offer two distinct advantages: they can help slow bleeding, and they can minimize swelling by applying pressure over fracture sites to decrease small-vessel bleeding.

The method of application for an air splint depends on whether it is equipped with a zipper. If it is not, then gather the splint on your own arm so that its proximal edge is just above your wrist. Grasp the patient's hand or foot while an assistant maintains proximal countertraction, then slide the air splint over your hand and onto the patient's extremity. Position the air splint so that it is free of wrinkles. Then, while you continue to maintain traction, instruct your assistant to inflate the splint with a commercially available device that is compatible with the splint system. Do *not* use a compressed air tank to inflate an air splint. If the air splint has a zipper, then apply it to the injured area while an assistant maintains traction proximally and distally; then zip it up and inflate **Figure 37-10** . In either case, inflate the splint just to the point at which finger pressure will make a slight dent in the splint's surface.

You must watch air splints carefully to ensure they do not lose pressure or become overinflated. Overinflation is particularly likely when the splint is applied in a cold area and the patient is subsequently moved to a warmer area because the air inside the splint will expand as it gets warmer, possibly increasing pressure and causing pulses to cease. Air splints will also expand when going to a higher altitude if the patient compartment is unpressurized, a factor that must be considered when patients are transported by air ambulance.

Vacuum Splints. A vacuum splint consists of a sealed plastic container that is filled with air and thousands of small plastic beads **Figure 37-11** . The device is wrapped around or otherwise formed to the limb being treated. A suction pump attached to the splint is then used to evacuate the air from inside. The resulting evacuation of air from inside the device compresses the beads in such a way that the whole splint becomes rigid, much like a plaster cast that has been molded to conform to the contours of the patient's limb.

A smaller vacuum splint is available to splint individual limbs. This type of splint is applied by positioning the injured limb on the splint and then evacuating the air from inside of it. The result is a splint that is molded to the extremity **Figure 37-12** . This type of vacuum splint requires less space than a mattress-style vacuum splint but is still relatively expensive compared with standard rigid splints.

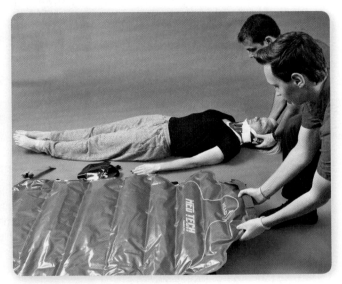

Figure 37-11 A vacuum splint.
© Jones & Bartlett Learning.

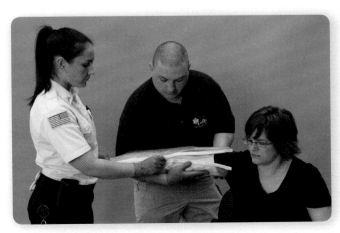

Figure 37-10 Positioning an air splint that features a zipper.
© Jones & Bartlett Learning. Photographed by Glen E. Ellman.

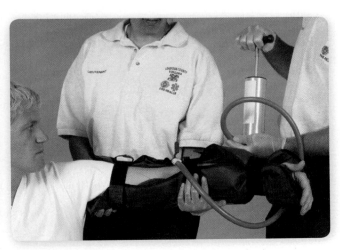

Figure 37-12 Applying a vacuum splint to a limb.
© Jones & Bartlett Learning.

Vacuum Mattress. The vacuum mattress is an excellent immobilization device, but there are a few factors that may limit its broad appeal. A vacuum mattress is simply a vacuum splint applied as a mattress underneath the patient. After vacuum air evacuation, the mattress provides excellent stabilization of the patient's spine and any included extremities. The mattress is quite bulky however, so it not only takes up a lot of storage room in the vehicle, but can also be difficult to work with in cramped quarters. Furthermore, like all vacuum splints, it requires a mechanical suction pump, yet another piece of equipment to grab.

Special Populations

Because vacuum mattresses conform to the body, they may be useful for older adult patients who have abnormal curvatures of the spine and are suspected of having spinal column injuries.

Traction Splints. Following a femur fracture, the strong muscles of the thigh go into spasm, which often leads to significant pain and deformity. Traction splints provide constant pull on a fractured femur, thereby preventing the broken bone ends from overlapping as a result of unopposed muscle contraction. In addition, these splints help maintain alignment of the fracture pieces and provide effective stabilization of the fracture site. As a result, patients are likely to experience less pain.

Traction splints also reduce blood loss. By pulling the femur nearer to its anatomic length, the muscles of the thigh are placed back under physiologic tension. This tension applies compression to injured blood vessels. The combination of this compression and the immobilization provided by the splint allow for a stable hematoma formation.

Traction splints are indicated for the treatment of most isolated femur fractures. They should not be used when the patient has an additional fracture below the knee on the same extremity. The most commonly used traction splints are the Sager and the Hare traction splints **Figure 37-13**. The basic principles of application are

YOU are the Paramedic   PART 3

Before moving your patient into the ambulance, you reassess his most distal pulses as well as sensation and motor function.

En route to a trauma center, an IV line is established. You administer IV dextrose and begin fluid resuscitation per protocol. You complete your secondary assessment, remaining suspicious about continued hemorrhage from multiple long bone fractures and impending shock. The patient's abdomen remains unremarkable. The patient responds more rapidly to questions and states he feels less "sleepy" after the glucose administration. He now reports pain to his legs.

Recording Time: 15 Minutes	
Level of consciousness	Alert, still oriented to person and place, time, and event; able to respond quickly to questions
Skin	Cool, pale, and slightly moist
Pulse	128 beats/min; weak and regular
Blood pressure	84/44 mm Hg
Respirations	24 breaths/min
Oxygen saturation (Spo$_2$)	98% on room air
Pupils	PERRLA
Pain scale	Visual analog scale; pain is an "8" on "0 to 10" scale.
Blood glucose level	126 mg/dL (after glucose administration)

8. Why should this patient be transported to a trauma center?
9. What do his vital signs indicate?

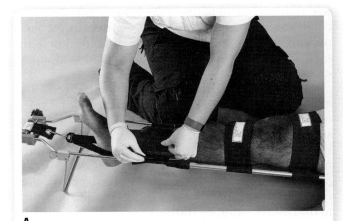

A

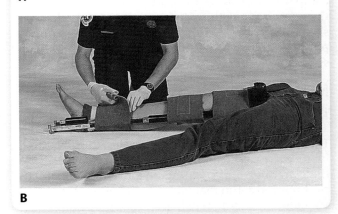

B

Figure 37-13 Applying a Hare traction splint **(A)** and a Sager traction splint **(B)**. With both devices, one rescuer connects the straps and another checks distal pulse, motor function, and sensation.

A: © Jones & Bartlett Learning; B: © Jones & Bartlett Learning. Courtesy of MIEMSS.

the same for both splints. After assessing the injured extremity for distal PMS functions, place the splint next to the uninjured leg to determine the proper length. The traction splint should extend 6 to 10 inches (15 to 25 cm) beyond the foot.

After applying the proximal securing device (ischial strap), support and stabilize the leg to minimize movement while another rescuer applies the ankle hitch. When the hitch is secure, the second rescuer will apply gentle longitudinal traction using enough force to realign the extremity. Then secure the Velcro straps. With prolonged transport (greater than 2 hours), caution should be exercised when using traction splints, as overtensioning can result in nerve injury and/or pressure sores. After applying the splint, reassess PMS functions, then secure the patient to a long backboard or scoop stretcher to prevent movement during transport.

Buddy Splinting. Buddy splinting is used to splint injuries that involve the fingers or toes. With this technique, an adjacent uninjured finger or toe serves as a splint to the injured one. To buddy splint, tape the injured digit to an uninjured one. Place a gauze pad between the digits

that are taped together, and ensure that the tape does not pass over joints. Ensure the tape is not so tight as to cut off circulation.

▪ Pathophysiology, Assessment, and Management of Complications of Musculoskeletal Injuries

Musculoskeletal injuries can lead to numerous complications—not just those involving the musculoskeletal system, but also systemic changes or illness. It is essential to not focus all of your attention on the musculoskeletal injury: keep in mind that there is a patient attached to the injured extremity!

The likelihood of having a complication is often related to the strength of the force that caused the injury, the injury's location, and the patient's overall health. Any injury to a bone, muscle, or other musculoskeletal structure is likely to be accompanied by bleeding. In general, the greater the force that caused the injury, the greater the hemorrhage that will be associated with it.

Following a fracture, the sharp ends of the bone may damage muscles, blood vessels, arteries, and nerves, or the ends may penetrate the skin and produce an open fracture. A significant loss of tissue may occur at the fracture site if the muscle is severely damaged or if the bone's penetration of the skin causes a large defect.

Long-term disability is one of the most devastating consequences of a musculoskeletal injury. In many cases, a severely injured limb can be repaired and made to look almost normal. Unfortunately, many patients cannot return to work for long periods because of the extensive rehabilitation required and because of chronic pain. Paramedics have a critical role in mitigating the risk of long-term disability. By preventing further injury, reducing the risk of wound infection, minimizing pain by the use of cold packs and analgesia, and transporting patients with musculoskeletal injuries to an appropriate medical facility, they help reduce the risk or duration of long-term disability.

▶ Peripheral Nerve Injury

When blood vessels are damaged following a musculoskeletal injury, loss of blood flow can occur in the body part supplied by that vessel. This is called **devascularization**. Additionally, neurovascular injuries can occur. The skeletal system normally protects the peripheral nerves within the limbs from injury. These critical structures typically lie deep within the limb and close to the skeleton. For example, the brachial plexus is situated within the axilla and the inner aspect of the arm, shielded from injury by the shoulder girdle. When the shoulder girdle or proximal humerus is fractured, displaced fracture fragments may lacerate or impale the nerves of the plexus, leading to a neurologic deficit. Peripheral nerve injuries are also likely to occur following a joint dislocation because the nerves and vessels in the region of a joint tend to be more securely tethered to the soft tissues and are less likely to escape injury. This outcome is particularly common following knee joint dislocations.

Assessment and Management

A thorough neurologic exam should be performed to identify the affected nerve and where along its course it has been affected. Splinting the injury in an anatomic position can help relieve pressure on the damaged nerve.

▶ Compartment Syndrome

Within a limb, groups of muscles are surrounded by an inelastic membrane called **fascia**. Thus, the muscles are confined to an enclosed space, or compartment, that can accommodate only a limited amount of swelling. When bleeding (hematoma) or swelling occurs within a compartment for any reason but typically because of a fracture or severe soft-tissue injury, the pressure within it rises. Pressure that is too high may prevent blood flow in vessels supplying the muscles within the same fascial compartment. This reduced blood flow leads to muscle ischemia and then possible subsequent muscle death with symptoms including severe pain, tenderness and sensory changes. This condition, known as **compartment syndrome**, is one of the most devastating consequences of a musculoskeletal injury.

External and internal factors can lead to the development of compartment syndrome. External factors include bandages, splints, and casts that are applied too tightly and restrict circulation. A number of internal factors can also increase the amount of swelling within a compartment. For example, bleeding within a compartment may occur because of a fracture, dislocation, crush injury, vascular injury, soft-tissue injury, bleeding disorder, or snakebite (though this is unusual). Alternatively, fluid leakage or edema may occur secondary to ischemia, excessive exercise, trauma, burns, or any condition associated with the leakage of proteins and fluid from vessels into the interstitial space. Circulatory problems, including compartment syndrome, can result from a cast that is too tight around a swollen limb. A common misconception is that open fractures are safe from compartment syndrome—this is not true.

Assessment

Signs and symptoms of compartment syndrome include early and late findings. Typically, the first complaint is a searing or burning *pain* that is localized to the involved compartment and out of proportion to the injury. This pain is often severe and typically not relieved with pain medication, including narcotics. When you examine the patient, passive stretching of an ischemic muscle will result in *severe* pain. In the lower leg, test for this condition through flexion and extension of the great toe and through dorsiflexion and plantar flexion of the foot. In the forearm, use finger and hand flexion and extension.

During examination of the patient, the affected area may feel very firm and there may be skin pallor. Typical neurologic changes include paresthesias, such as a burning sensation, numbness, or tingling, and paralysis of the involved muscles, which occurs late in the condition. A very late consequence of compartment syndrome is pulselessness. If a plaster cast has been applied, then check pulses and check sensory and motor function distal to the cast terminus. By the time the pressure within the compartment reaches the point that it totally occludes the artery passing through it, significant muscle necrosis has probably occurred. The presence of peripheral pulses does not exclude the possibility of compartment syndrome.

Management

The goal of prehospital care is to deliver the patient to an emergency facility before the extremity is pulseless. Thus, management should include elevating the extremity to heart level (not above!), placing cold packs over the extremity, and opening or loosening constrictive clothing and splint material. Give a bolus of an isotonic crystalloid solution to help the kidneys flush out toxins from resulting rhabdomyolysis, which is discussed in the next section.

> ### Words of Wisdom
>
> A patient who shows evidence of compartment syndrome must be transported on an emergency basis to the hospital. There is no treatment for this syndrome other than surgery. Do not delay transport.

▶ Crush Syndrome

Crush syndrome occurs because of a prolonged compressive force that impairs muscle metabolism and circulation and presents following the extrication or release of an entrapped limb. When limbs are crushed, muscle tissue becomes ischemic and dies and necrosis develops resulting in release of harmful products, a process known as **rhabdomyolysis**. Rhabdomyolysis is an emergency that occurs not only in trauma patients, but also in patients who have been lying on an extremity, on their back, or in the same position for an extended period (4 to 6 hours of compression)—for example, when a person who has experienced a drug overdose or stroke is not found for an extended period. It can also present in the setting of excessive exertion, genetic defects, infection, hyperthermia, hypothermia, metabolic disorders, or use of certain drugs/medications.

After a muscle is compressed for 4 to 6 hours, the muscle cells begin to die and release their contents into the localized vasculature. When the force compressing the region is released, blood flow is reestablished and the necrotic tissue is released into the systemic vasculature. The primary substances that are of concern are lactate, potassium and myoglobin. The release of these substances into the circulation can result in decreased blood pH (a condition known as acidosis).

Renal failure is another serious complication that may develop after release of the crushing force. **Glomerular filtration** is the process by which toxins and waste products are removed from circulating blood. A typical clinical finding is tea-colored urine. The exact mechanism that leads to glomerular filtration impairment remains unclear, although injury from circulating myoglobin resulting in renal vasoconstriction, ischemic tubule injury, and tubular obstruction are likely to contribute.[6] The release of large quantities of myoglobin into the central circulation can clog the distal tubules of the glomerulus, causing cytotoxicity in the proximal tubules. Cytotoxicity is caused by the development of oxygen free radicals. These products travel throughout the affected area, scavenging oxygen molecules and damaging and destroying tubule cells.[7]

Renal dysfunction that results from rhabdomyolysis can lead to significant electrolyte abnormalities that can cause significant problems. Increased blood potassium (**hyperkalemia**) can occur very quickly. Hyperkalemia can lead to cardiac dysrhythmias and electrocardiogram (ECG) changes affecting the appearance of waveforms and interval measurements. **Hyperphosphatemia** can lead to calcifications that can interfere with normal blood flow and normal nervous tissue function. Increased levels of uric acid, lactic acid, and potassium may also cause metabolic acidosis.

Assessment and Management

Treatment of crush syndrome, which aims to prevent complications due to toxin release, should always be performed with medical direction. A number of steps must be taken *before* releasing the compressing force. As with all patients, assess ABCDEs in case of suspected crush syndrome. Ensure that the patient is being given high-flow supplemental oxygen, and then administer a bolus of crystalloid solution to increase the intravascular volume and to protect the kidneys from the forthcoming myoglobin load. Volume replacement is a keystone of treatment for rhabdomyolysis. Upon removal of the crushing item, you can expect the damaged muscles to release potassium and lactate into the circulation. Establish cardiac monitoring to evaluate for ECG changes related to hyperkalemia. To protect against the surge of potassium, a nebulizer treatment with albuterol may be given during extrication

(beta-2 agonists promote the movement of potassium into cells). Once the patient is freed, if the ECG shows changes consistent with hyperkalemia, administer calcium to stabilize the myocardium. Sodium bicarbonate can be given to promote alkalization. Insulin may also be given intravenously with dextrose to facilitate the intracellular movement of potassium. In the hospital intensive care units, hemodialysis can be employed to clear the excess potassium and other products of rhabdomyolosis from the circulation. Rapid transport is indicated. En route, you should complete a rapid full-body scan and care for injuries not treated on scene. Open injuries can be handled with dressings and bandaging, and fractures can be splinted, if time permits. Be prepared to administer additional fluids as indicated by patient condition or via online medical direction. Obtain vital signs and ECG every 5 minutes at a minimum.

▶ Thromboembolic Disease

Thromboembolic disease, including **deep vein thrombosis (DVT)** and **pulmonary embolism**, is a significant cause of death following musculoskeletal injuries, especially when injuries to the pelvis and lower extremities lead to prolonged immobilization.

Assessment and Management

Signs and symptoms of DVT include disproportionate swelling of an extremity, discomfort in an extremity that worsens with use, and warmth and erythema of the extremity. When a DVT dislodges, it may cause a pulmonary embolism—a blood clot that occludes a portion or all of the pulmonary arteries **Figure 37-14**. Signs and symptoms of a pulmonary embolism include a sudden onset of dyspnea, pleuritic chest pain (either side), tachypnea, tachycardia, low-grade fever, right-sided heart failure, shock, and, in some cases, cardiac arrest.

A history of recent orthopaedic surgery or prolonged immobilization due to orthopaedic injury should raise suspicion when performing the history. Treatment for thromboembolic disease in the field is limited to maintaining the airway, adequate oxygenation, and intravascular volume and providing rapid transport to an emergency department.

Fat Embolism

Patients with long bone fractures are at risk for developing a fat embolism. In this condition, fat droplets become lodged in the vasculature of the lungs. Affected patients have inflammation of the vasculature of the lungs and other blood vessels where fat is deposited. Generally, symptoms begin within 12 to 72 hours of injury; they include tachycardia, dyspnea, tachypnea, pulmonary congestion, fever, petechiae, change in mental status, and organ dysfunction.

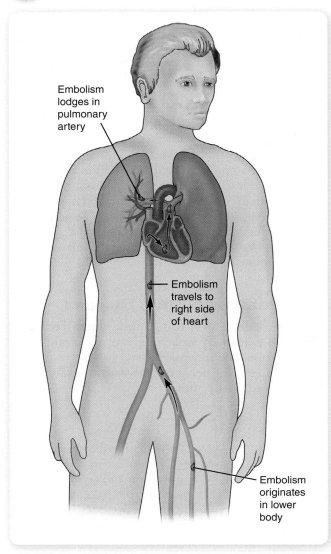

Embolism lodges in pulmonary artery

Embolism travels to right side of heart

Embolism originates in lower body

Figure 37-14 When a portion of a deep vein thrombosis dislodges, it may travel to the pulmonary arteries and inhibit blood flow from the heart to the lungs.

© Jones & Bartlett Learning.

Pathophysiology, Assessment, and Management of Specific Fractures

▶ Shoulder Girdle Fracture

The shoulder girdle consists of the clavicle, shoulder, and scapula.

Clavicle Fracture

Clavicle fractures are very common and often occur in children. In most cases, the clavicle fractures in the middle third of the bone, typically from a fall onto an outstretched hand or from direct lateral trauma to the shoulder (as in contact sports, snowboarding, and cycling).

Shoulder Fracture

Fractures of the shoulder include those that involve the **glenoid fossa** of the scapula, the humeral head, and the humeral neck. Most shoulder fractures are caused by a fall onto an outstretched hand and usually occur in older patients (younger patients tend to dislocate the shoulder because they have stronger bones).

Scapula Fracture

Injuries to the scapula usually result from violent, direct trauma. Therefore, when a scapular injury is suspected, it is essential to look for associated injuries—particularly intrathoracic injuries, such as pneumothorax, hemothorax, and fractured ribs.

Assessment

Patients with a clavicle fracture have pain in the region of the shoulder, swelling, unwillingness to raise the arm, and tilting of the head toward the injured side.

Patients with a shoulder fracture rarely have evidence of a significant deformity, but instead have considerable swelling, ecchymosis, and pain with movement of the arm. In some cases, an associated injury to the brachial plexus may be identified during the neurologic examination.

Signs and symptoms of a scapular fracture include pain that increases with arm abduction and swelling in the region of the scapula. Potential complications include axillary artery or nerve injury, brachial plexus injury, pulmonary contusion, and clavicle fractures.

Management

Fractures in the shoulder region may usually be treated by using a sling and swathe. These bindings should be applied to maintain the extremity in the position of comfort, often keeping the arm against the chest wall to allow the body to act as a splint. In cases of suspected scapula fractures, full spinal immobilization will often be warranted given the amount of force required to cause a fracture.

▶ Midshaft Humerus Fractures

Fractures of the shaft of the humerus usually occur in younger patients secondary to high-energy injuries, such as MVCs. Unlike fractures that occur more proximally, these injuries typically involve substantial deformity.

Assessment

Examination of the extremity usually reveals a significant amount of swelling, ecchymosis, gross instability of the region, and crepitus. If the force that caused the injury is severe enough, then the nerves and blood vessels in the upper arm may be damaged. Of particular concern is the radial nerve, which may be injured by the force itself or could become entrapped within the fracture site. The classic sign of a radial nerve injury is wrist drop.

Management

If the fracture is angulated, then longitudinal traction may be applied to correct the deformity, but efforts should be halted if the patient's pain is too severe or if neurovascular status worsens. Once the extremity is in the desired position, apply a rigid splint that extends from the axilla to the elbow. Next, apply a sling and swathe to stabilize the arm to the chest wall, and place cold packs over the fracture site to decrease the patient's pain and swelling.

▶ Elbow Fractures

Distal Humerus

Supracondylar fractures of the humerus occur often in children. The typical mechanism is a fall onto an outstretched hand with the elbow in extension, thereby breaking the distal humerus; as a result, the distal fragment of the humerus is pushed posteriorly and the humeral shaft is pulled anteriorly, where it compresses the brachial artery and the radial and median nerves. If the brachial artery is compromised, then the patient could develop compartment syndrome in the forearm. When this complication occurs, the patient is at risk for a **Volkmann ischemic contracture**, a condition in which muscles of the forearm degenerate from prolonged ischemia. The patient's muscles that allow for movement of the fingers become contracted and nonfunctional, and the patient loses the ability to use the hand.

Proximal Radius and Ulna

Radial head fractures may result from a fall onto an outstretched hand or from a direct blow to the bone. Similar to distal humerus fractures, these injuries may lead to an injury of the nerves or blood vessels in proximity to the fracture site. Therefore, a careful neurovascular examination should be performed.

Assessment and Management

Patients with a distal humerus fracture will report pain in the area of the elbow and typically have a significant degree of swelling and ecchymosis. Radial head fractures cause significant pain when the patient attempts supination or pronation. In either case, the patient is likely to have pain and ecchymosis in the region of the injury.

Treatment of injuries in the region of the elbow is the same regardless of the exact location of the injury. The injured extremity must be repeatedly assessed for evidence of compartment syndrome. Before splinting the extremity, it is mandatory to document a neurovascular exam. The injured extremity should be splinted in the position in which it is found if the patient has a strong distal pulse, and cold packs should be used only if there is no evidence of compartment syndrome. If the patient has an absent distal pulse or neurologic deficits, then consult with the appropriate medical facility to determine whether you should attempt fracture reduction. In any event, the patient must be transported urgently to the closest appropriate medical facility for definitive treatment.

▶ Forearm Fractures

Fractures of the forearm may involve the radius, the ulna, or, more commonly, both. Injury may result from a direct blow to the bone, the classic example of which is the nightstick fracture of the ulna. In other cases, injury occurs because of a fall onto an outstretched hand, as in a Colles fracture, also called a silver fork fracture. This fracture typically occurs in older patients with osteoporosis who have fallen, but it may be found in younger patients as well. Forearm fractures and other upper extremity fractures have also been associated with airbag deployment during MVCs.[8]

Assessment and Management

A patient with a Colles fracture usually has a dorsally angulated deformity of the distal forearm (the "**silver fork deformity**") and pain and swelling near the injured site.

A variety of splints may be used to secure a forearm fracture. Regardless of the type, the splint should provide stabilization of the entire forearm and, in cases of more proximal fractures, the elbow. Apply cold packs to the injury site to decrease pain and swelling. Frequent neurovascular exams are warranted to monitor for evidence of compartment syndrome and acute carpal tunnel syndrome.

▶ Wrist and Hand Fractures

Injuries to the wrist and hand may lead to significant long-term disability, especially in people who rely on the use of their hands to earn a living. Sometimes these injuries occur while working at the job or at home; in other cases, they result from a fall or during a sporting event. Careful splinting of the injured site is essential to help reduce the risk of long-term disability.

Scaphoid

The **scaphoid**, also called the carpal navicular, is located just distal to the radius. It may be injured from a fall onto an outstretched hand. The major complication of a scaphoid fracture is **avascular necrosis** of the bone, or poor fracture healing because of the limited blood supply to this bone.

Boxer's Fracture

A **boxer's fracture** is a fracture of the neck of the fifth metacarpal (small finger). It commonly occurs after punching a hard object, such as a wall or a door.

Metacarpal Shaft

Fractures of the metacarpals may result from a crush injury or from direct trauma.

Mallet Finger (Baseball Fracture)

A **mallet finger** occurs when a finger is jammed into an object, such as a baseball or basketball, resulting in an avulsion fracture of the extensor tendon.

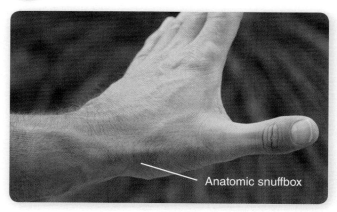

Figure 37-15 The region between the two tendons shown is the anatomic snuffbox.

© Jones & Bartlett Learning.

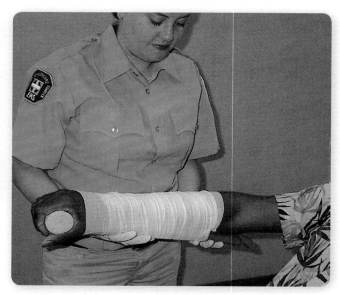

Figure 37-16 Splinting the hand and wrist.

© American Academy of Orthopaedic Surgeons.

Assessment

The classic finding for a scaphoid fracture is pain and tenderness in the anatomic snuffbox. To identify the anatomic snuffbox on yourself, extend your thumb. Two tendons will be visible at the base of the thumb on the radial aspect of the wrist. The region between these two tendons is the **anatomic snuffbox** Figure 37-15 .

The patient with a boxer's fracture typically has pain over the ulnar aspect of the hand and may have noticeable swelling.

Assessment of the injured hand with metacarpal fractures may reveal abnormal rotation or alignment of the fingers, swelling of the palm, and pain and tenderness in the region of injury. You should assess the neurovascular function of the hand and fingers following a crush injury because development of compartment syndrome is possible within the hand.

The patient with mallet finger will not be able to extend the distal phalanx of the finger and will maintain it in a flexed position.

Management

If possible, then splint the injured hand in the position of function by placing the wrist in about 30° of extension, with fingers slightly flexed (a roll of gauze approximately 2 to 3 inches [5 to 8 cm] in diameter accomplishes this nicely). Next, secure the extremity to an armboard or other rigid splint that extends proximally to the elbow and is slightly elevated to help reduce swelling Figure 37-16 . For injuries that are isolated to the digits, use a foam-padded flexible aluminum splint to splint the injured digit, if available. In the case of penetrating injuries, regardless of whether a fracture is present, apply bulky dressings to the site of injury and splint the injured hand in the position of function.

▶ Pelvis Fractures

Pelvic fractures are relatively uncommon injuries, accounting for fewer than 3% of all fractures. Despite their low incidence, these injuries are responsible for a significant number of deaths in blunt trauma patients. The risk of death following a pelvic fracture can range as high as 55%, depending on the severity of the injury.[9] Death after a pelvic fracture commonly results from massive hemorrhage caused by damage to the arteries and veins of the pelvis. The mortality rate due to pelvic fracture with hemorrhage ranges 25% to 40%.[9]

Disruptions of the pelvic ring occur secondary to high-energy trauma. The majority of pelvic fractures are a result of blunt trauma from MVCs, motorcycle crashes, or vehicles striking pedestrians. Pelvic fractures may also result from crush injuries and falls from a significant height. Because of the forces required to break the pelvis, suspect multisystem trauma until disproven, including abdominal trauma and head injury Figure 37-17 .

A number of structures within the pelvis are at risk for injury when it is fractured—the bladder, urethra, rectum, vagina, and sacral nerve plexus. The blood vessels that are most prone to damage are the veins within the pelvis, but there may be damage to the internal or external iliac vessels and to arteries in the lumbar region. The nerves at greatest risk of injury are those in the lumbar and sacral regions and the sciatic and femoral nerves.

There are four main types of pelvic fractures, listed in Table 37-5 . Specific types of fractures are discussed in the next sections.

Lateral Compression Pelvic Ring Disruptions

Lateral compression injuries result from an impact on the side of the body (such as being struck by a car from the side or falling from a significant height and landing on one side of the body). The side of the pelvis that sustains the impact becomes internally rotated around the

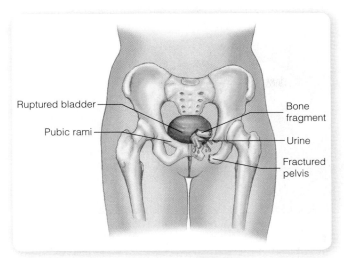

Figure 37-17 Pelvic fractures occasionally cause laceration of the bladder as a result of penetration by bony fragments. Externally, pelvic fractures can cause severe bruising and swelling.

© Jones & Bartlett Learning.

Table 37-5	**Types of Pelvic Fractures**
Type	**Fractures in Category**
Type I	Avulsion fractures Fracture of pubis or ischium Fracture of iliac wing Fracture of sacrum Fracture of coccyx
Type II	Single fracture of pelvic ring (including unilateral fractures of both pelvic rami) Subluxation of the pubic symphysis Fracture near the sacroiliac joint
Type III	Multiple breaks of pelvic ring
Type IV	Fracture involving acetabulum

© Jones & Bartlett Learning.

sacrum, and the actual volume within the pelvis decreases **Figure 37-18** . This MOI does not usually result in an unstable pelvis. Because the volume in the pelvis is reduced, not increased, life-threatening hemorrhage is less common in such cases. However, lateral compression is often associated with injuries in other regions of the body.

Anterior-Posterior Compression Pelvic Ring Disruptions

These injuries may occur following a head-on MVC, motorcycle crash, or fall or in a pedestrian who is struck head-on by a vehicle. The force of the impact compresses the pelvis in the anterior-to-posterior direction, causing the pubic symphysis and posterior supporting ligaments to be disrupted and tear apart. The pelvis then spreads apart and opens like a book—hence the name **open-book pelvic fracture**. Such an injury has the potential for massive blood loss because the volume of the pelvis is greatly increased.

Vertical Shear

Vertical shear injuries occur when a major force is applied to the pelvis from above or below, such as when a person falls from a significant height and lands on the feet. On landing, the force is transmitted through the legs to the pelvis, leading to the complete displacement of one or both sides of the pelvis toward the head, with disruption of the bony or ligamentous structures. Thus, this kind of injury has anterior and posterior components. The anterior component involves a fracture of the rami or disruption of the pubic symphysis. The posterior component involves a fracture of the ilium or sacrum or a disruption of the sacroiliac joint. This unstable fracture results in an increase in pelvic volume.

Straddle Fracture

A **straddle fracture** occurs when a person falls and sustains an impact in the region of the perineum, producing bilateral fractures of the inferior and superior rami. This injury does not interfere with weight bearing, but it does carry a risk owing to its associated complications, particularly those of the lower genitourinary system.

Open Pelvic Fractures

Although penetrating trauma to the pelvis may result in bony fractures, the more worrisome injury is to the major vascular structures, which can cause life-threatening hemorrhage. Such an injury is defined by the presence of a laceration of the skin in the pelvic region, vagina, or rectum. Open fractures (not to be confused with open-book fractures) are uncommon and may result from either penetrating or blunt trauma caused by a high-velocity mechanism. This MOI causes subsequent massive hemorrhage and has a mortality rate ranging from 5% to 16%.[10] When the patient does survive, the frequent result is chronic pain and permanent disability.

Assessment

Patients with pelvic ring disruptions who have a stable injury, such as a minimal lateral compression injury, may report pain in the pelvis and difficulty bearing weight. Patients with a more severe injury may show evidence of profound shock, gross pelvic instability, and diffuse pelvic and lower abdominal pain. There may also be bruising or lacerations in the perineum, scrotum, groin, suprapubic region, and flank and hematuria (blood in the urine) or blood coming from the meatus of the penis, vagina, or rectum.

The patient with a vertical shear is likely to have significant shortening of the limb on the affected side and is at risk for massive hemorrhage into the pelvis.

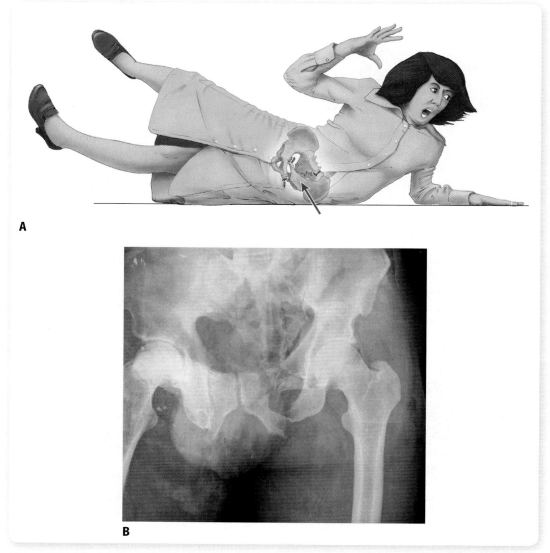

Figure 37-18 A. A lateral compression injury to the pelvis. **B.** A radiograph of a lateral compression injury.

A: © Jones & Bartlett Learning; B: Courtesy of Andrew N. Pollak, MD, FAAOS.

When there is an MOI for pelvic fracture, any bleeding seen in the area of the rectum or vagina should increase your suspicion of a pelvic fracture. However, properly evaluating and treating a patient is more important than is identifying the specific type of pelvic fracture which is almost impossible without a complete radiographic evaluation. Assessment of the patient with a possible pelvic fracture should begin as in any other trauma patient—with a primary survey of the mental status and ABCDEs, taking spinal precautions. During the rapid full-body scan of the patient, you should search for injuries typically associated with pelvic fractures. Assess the pelvis for bleeding, lacerations, bruising, and instability. To assess for instability, apply pressure over the iliac wings in a medial direction and in a posterior direction. Once instability of the pelvis

is identified, the pelvis should not be reassessed for instability to avoid causing increased bleeding.

A search for entry and exit wounds for a penetrating trauma is helpful, but an extended search should never delay quick transport and treatment of hypotension.

Management

Treatment should include careful monitoring of the ABCs, spinal stabilization, and IV access. Patients with open-book pelvic fractures will require IV fluids with lactated Ringer solution or normal saline but may still remain hypotensive in the field. Management of the pelvic injury is aimed at reducing the amount of bleeding. Large-volume bleeding into the pelvic cavity can amount to more than 6 pints (3 L) of blood loss. Methods used to accomplish stabilization may include application of a pelvic binder or simply tying a sheet around the pelvis. Applying lateral pressure to the greater trochanters of the hip forces the unstable pelvis to internally rotate and reduces the potential space within the pelvis, which may allow for tamponade of the bleeding vessels.

Follow these steps to apply a pelvic binder **Figure 37-19** :

1. Log roll the patient onto a backboard to get the binder into position behind the pelvis. Alternatively, the binder can be placed onto the board prior to moving the patient onto the backboard.
2. Ensure the binder is centered over the greater trochanters and not over the iliac wings. If the binder is over the abdomen or impinging the rib cage, then it has been positioned too proximally. This positioning can cause obstruction of the diaphragm and chest wall expansion during respiration.
3. Connect the two sides of the binder together anteriorly using the Velcro straps.
4. Apply gentle but firm pressure from either side of the patient to close down the pelvic volume by pushing the two sides of the unstable disrupted pelvis together.
5. Perform definitive tightening of the binder to hold the reduced position of the pelvic ring.
6. Ensure the patient can still breathe easily and that the binder is not impeding chest excursion with ventilation. If it is, then open the binder immediately and reposition it lower.

Once immobilized, the patient should be rapidly transported to a trauma center, and IV fluid should be administered to maintain adequate tissue perfusion, but hypertension should be avoided because too much fluid can exacerbate bleeding and disrupt the natural hemostasis.

▶ Hip

A hip fracture involves a fracture of the femoral head, femoral neck, intertrochanteric region, or proximal femoral shaft. Fractures of the femoral head are uncommon injuries that are usually associated with a hip dislocation. Femoral neck and **intertrochanteric fractures** typically occur in older patients with osteoporosis who have fallen and sustained direct trauma to the hip. They may occur in younger patients with healthy bone, typically as the result of a high-energy mechanism. Proximal femoral shaft fractures can occur in patients of any age and result from a high-energy mechanism.

Assessment

Patients with a hip fracture will report pain in the affected hip, especially with attempts at movement, and will report an inability to bear weight. They may also report hearing or feeling something snap. If the fracture is displaced, then the patient almost always has an externally rotated and shortened leg. If there is no displacement, then the leg may appear normal. Examination of the injury site usually finds tenderness to palpation, and there may be noticeable swelling, deformity, or ecchymosis.

Management

The treatment of hip fractures depends on the MOI. Hip fractures in older patients who sustained a low-energy injury, such as a fall from a standing position, do not require traction splints. Treat these injuries by supporting the injured extremity in the position in which it is found. This may be accomplished by placing pillows or blankets under the affected extremity and securing them in place **Figure 37-20** .

Treat young patients and patients who have sustained high-energy injuries as you would any other trauma patient: fully immobilize the patient, establish vascular access, monitor for shock, and transport to a trauma center.

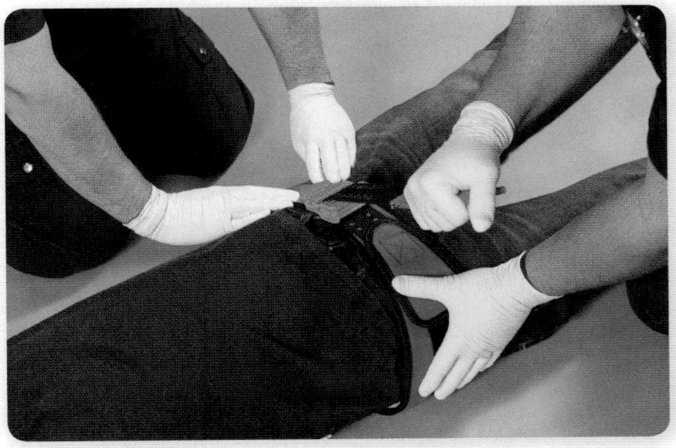

Figure 37-19 Application of a pelvic binder is one of the best ways to stabilize the pelvis and control hemorrhage.
© Jones & Bartlett Learning.

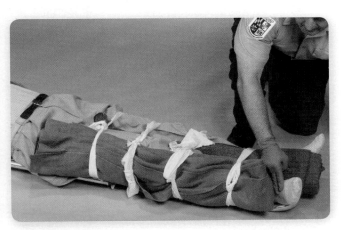

Figure 37-20 An acceptable method for splinting a hip fracture.
© Jones & Bartlett Learning. Courtesy of MIEMSS.

Definitive treatment of a hip fracture almost always requires surgery. If possible, the bone is repaired with plates, rods, or screws. Sometimes, however, the hip must be replaced.

Patient Safety

A hip fracture in an older patient can be a debilitating and life-altering injury. In many cases, these injuries occur in the home after slipping on a throw rug, tripping over an object that extends into the walkway, or stumbling because of poor lighting. To help prevent this injury and other fall-related problems, you should point out any safety hazards in the home to the patient or a family member. Doing so takes only a minute, and most patients and families appreciate the advice.

▶ Femoral Shaft

Femoral shaft fractures occur following high-energy impacts. Thus, the presence of a fracture of the femoral shaft should alert you to the risk of other injuries.

Assessment and Management

Patients with femoral shaft fractures will report severe pain. The fracture may be severely angulated or lead to significant limb shortening, or it may be open. Examination may identify significant thigh edema, bruising, crepitus, and muscle spasm.

There is often significant blood loss (perhaps 1 to 3 pints [0.5 to 1.5 L]) at the fracture site. In addition, damage to the neurovascular structures of the thigh is possible. Femoral shaft fractures also place the patient at risk for fat emboli.

Management of femoral shaft fractures includes monitoring for evidence of shock and establishing vascular access. Place the injured extremity in a traction splint to achieve stability and hemorrhage control. Because these injuries may be extremely painful, consider the administration of pain medication.

▶ Knee

Fractures of the knee may involve the distal femur, proximal tibia, or patella. An injury to this region may result from a direct blow to the knee, an axial load of the leg, or powerful contractions of the quadriceps.

YOU ▶ are the Paramedic   PART 4

En route, you reassess the patient's splints and distal pulses, motor function, and sensation to his lower extremities. His pedal pulses are absent bilaterally, and he is unable to move his toes and cannot feel you touch them. You administer a 500-mL normal saline bolus and reassess his condition. You receive an order to administer 50 mcg of fentanyl IV push every 15 minutes as necessary and as vital signs permit. His pain improves, and he thanks you for your care. Blankets are placed to keep him warm. His blood glucose level is now 122 mg/dL. On arrival at the hospital, the patient's pedal pulses and sensation to his toes return.

Recording Time: 20 Minutes	
Level of consciousness	Remains alert and oriented to person, place, time, and event
Skin	Cool, pale, and dry
Pulse	110 beats/min; weak and regular (after fluid bolus)
Blood pressure	95/56 mm Hg
Respirations	20 breaths/min
ECG	Sinus tachycardia
Oxygen saturation (Spo$_2$)	98% on room air
Pupils	PERRLA
Pain scale	Visual analog scale; pain is a "3" on "0 to 10" scale
Blood glucose level	122 mg/dL

10. What do absent pedal pulses, absent motor function, and lack of sensation in the toes indicate?

11. Why is it important to treat the patient's pain?

Assessment and Management

Assessment of the patient generally reveals significant pain in the knee, decreased ROM, pain with movement and weight bearing, ecchymosis, swelling, and, in the case of displaced fractures, deformity.

Management of knee fractures depends on the position of the leg and the status of distal pulses. If the patient has intact distal circulation, then splint the extremity in the position that it is found. If there is no distal pulse, then seek medical consultation to determine whether you should attempt manipulation before transport. When possible, elevate the leg to the heart level and apply cold packs. Frequent neurovascular checks are mandatory, given the high incidence of compartment syndrome and neurovascular injury in cases of knee fracture.

Words of Wisdom

When you find a knee injury in the victim of a MVC, look for posterior dislocation of the hip.

▶ Tibia and Fibula

Fractures of the tibia and/or fibula may result from direct trauma to the lower leg or from application of rotational or compressive forces.

Assessment and Management

These injuries often present with significant deformity and soft-tissue injury. Complications may include compartment syndrome, neurovascular injury, infection, poor healing, and chronic pain.

Apply a rigid, long leg splint, and administer pain medication as necessary. If there is gross angulation, then attempt to align the leg after administering pain medication, documenting the premanipulation and postmanipulation neurovascular status. Monitor the patient for evidence of compartment syndrome, elevate the extremity to heart level, and apply cold packs.

Words of Wisdom

Whenever an open fracture is reduced, there is a risk that blood will be splashed. Always wear safety glasses and a gown, in addition to gloves, when splinting or manipulating an open fracture.

▶ Ankle

Fractures of the ankle usually result from sudden, forceful movements of the foot that damage the malleoli and sometimes produce dislocation (called a fracture-dislocation) Figure 37-21 . In other cases, an axial load is transmitted through the foot and causes the **talus** (the bone of the foot that articulates with the tibia) to impact the distal tibia, leading to a fracture.

Assessment and Management

Signs and symptoms of an ankle fracture include pain, deformity, and swelling. Ankle fractures may lead to damage of the nerves and blood vessels that supply the foot, the development of compartment syndrome, and chronic ankle pain and arthritis.

Ankle fractures should be stabilized using a commercially available splint or a pillow splint. The toes should be exposed to allow for frequent checks of distal neurovascular function. Elevate the extremity to the heart level, and apply cold packs to reduce swelling.

If an ankle fracture-dislocation is associated with a pulseless foot, then medical direction may recommend that you attempt reduction. To reduce a fracture-dislocation of the ankle, first relax the calf muscles to allow the foot

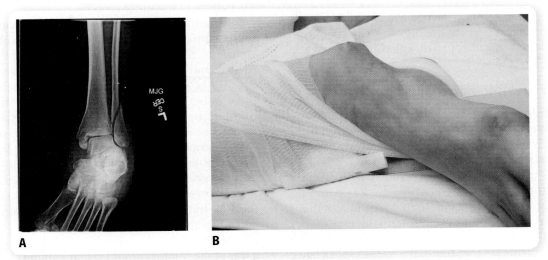

A   **B**

Figure 37-21 A radiographic image **(A)** and a clinical image **(B)** demonstrating severe fractures of the ankle.

Courtesy of Andrew N. Pollak, MD, FAAOS.

to move more freely by flexing the patient's leg at the knee. With the leg flexed, grasp the heel and the foot just proximal to the toes and apply gentle traction. Next, rotate the foot back into its normal position without forcing it. If this procedure is successful, then reassess the distal neurovascular status and splint the extremity in the reduced position, using care not to allow the ankle to dislocate again. If the fracture-dislocation cannot be reduced, then notify medical control and expedite transport after splinting the ankle in the position in which it was found.

► Calcaneus

The calcaneus may be fractured when a patient jumps from a height and lands on his or her feet or when a powerful axial force is otherwise applied directly to the heel.

Assessment and Management

These injuries present with foot pain, swelling, and ecchymosis and should alert providers to the possibility of injuries in the knee, pelvis, and spine.

When a calcaneus fracture is suspected, splint the injured extremity with a pillow and apply ice packs to help decrease swelling. Any patient with a suspected calcaneus fracture requires spinal stabilization, given the high risk of an associated spinal injury, particularly bilateral fracture.

■ Pathophysiology, Assessment, and Management of Ligament Injuries and Dislocations

► Shoulder Girdle Injuries and Dislocations

Acromioclavicular Joint Separation

Separation of the acromioclavicular (AC) joint usually occurs from a direct blow to the superior aspect or point of the shoulder, as may happen during contact sports and falls Figure 37-22 .

Posterior Sternoclavicular Joint Dislocation

Posterior dislocation of the clavicle at its junction with the sternum most often occurs as a result of a direct blow to the clavicle but is sometimes seen after strong pressure is applied to the posterior shoulder (as when a football player ends up at the bottom of a pileup). This injury is rarely difficult to identify because there is pain and swelling at the sternoclavicular joint. What makes this a potentially dangerous and even potentially fatal injury is not the dislocation itself, but the possible damage to underlying structures—specifically, the trachea, esophagus, jugular vein, subclavian vein and artery, carotid artery, and other vascular structures.

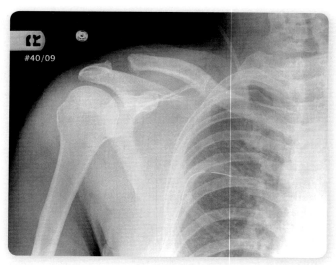

Figure 37-22 Separation of the acromioclavicular joint. This space is wider than it should normally be.
Courtesy of Anand M. Murthi, MD.

Shoulder Dislocation

Most shoulder dislocations are anterior dislocations.[11] Anterior shoulder dislocations are often caused by a fall onto an outstretched arm that is abducted and externally rotated.

Assessment

Patients with AC joint separation generally report pain and tenderness in the region of the AC joint, and the prominence of the distal clavicle may lead to a noticeable protrusion.

Any symptoms of a posterior dislocation of the clavicle that suggest an underlying injury—such as dyspnea, pain on swallowing, a sensation of choking, loss of pulses, or a sensory deficit in the upper extremity on the same side—are danger signals and should prompt rapid transport of the patient to a trauma center.

Patients experiencing shoulder dislocation report severe pain and have significantly decreased ROM at the shoulder. The arm is usually abducted and externally rotated, and any efforts at moving it result in extreme pain Figure 37-23 . A prominent bulge from the acromion is often noted on the anterior surface of the shoulder, the humeral head may be palpable, and the patient may experience frequent and painful muscle spasms.

Posterior shoulder dislocations are much less common and are often caused by massive muscle contractions such as those seen with electrical shocks and seizures. These injuries present with the same reports of pain and limited motion, but the arm is maintained in internal rotation and adduction.

In some patients, a shoulder dislocation will produce a tear of the rotator cuff or a fracture of the glenoid. Some patients may have a concomitant injury to the brachial plexus, axillary artery, or axillary vein. The axillary nerve

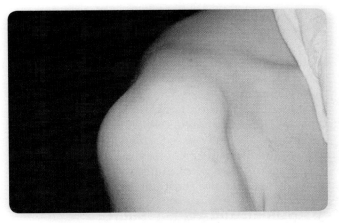

Figure 37-23 The typical appearance of an anterior shoulder dislocation.
© American Academy of Orthopaedic Surgeons.

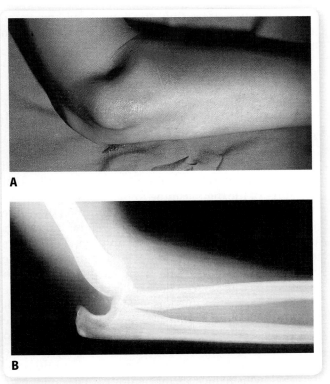

Figure 37-24 A posteriorly dislocated elbow. **A.** The clinical appearance of an elbow dislocation. **B.** Radiographic appearance of the same elbow.

is also prone to injury during a shoulder dislocation; assess sensation over the deltoid muscle to determine whether there is a sensory deficit in the distribution of this nerve. Patients with a shoulder dislocation are also at risk for future dislocations, especially during the first 2 years following the injury and if the patient is young.

Management

In cases of an AC joint separation, a sling and swathe will often provide significant pain relief. Consider administration of medication to relieve the pain as well.

For a dislocated shoulder, splint the injured extremity in the position in which it was found by using blankets, pillows, and, when possible, a sling and swathe. When applying the swathe, it may be necessary to connect two cravats together so as to encircle the patient's body, extremity, and pillows or blankets. Given the likelihood of muscle spasm and pain, use of pain medication may be necessary. Perform neurovascular assessments frequently to monitor for changes in function.

▶ Elbow Dislocation

Elbow dislocations are medical emergencies because of the high risk of neurovascular injury. The vast majority of elbow dislocations are posterior injuries that result from a fall onto an outstretched hand or from hyperextension of the elbow joint.

Subluxation of the radial head is also referred to as **nursemaid's elbow**. It commonly occurs in children younger than 6 years and is caused by a sudden pull on the child's arm.

Assessment and Management

Patients usually report significant pain in the region of the elbow and may have a large degree of swelling and ecchymosis. A palpable deformity may be present at the elbow from the prominence of the **olecranon** process **Figure 37-24**, and there is typically locking or resistance

to movement of the joint. Major complications of an elbow dislocation include an associated fracture in the region of the joint, brachial artery injury, median nerve injury, and injury to the ulnar nerve.

Clinically, for patients with radial head subluxation, the injured arm is held in flexion and the child will often refuse to move the hand or elbow on the injured side. In general, there is only mild swelling in the region of the elbow.

When you suspect a dislocation or subluxation in the elbow, splint the injured extremity in the position in which it was found. A sling and swathe may be applied to provide additional stabilization to the injured elbow.

▶ Wrist and Hand Dislocation

The wrist can become dislocated when it is hyperextended beyond its normal ROM.

Assessment and Management

A patient with a wrist or hand dislocation will have pain, swelling, and deformity, much like that seen with fractures. Treatment for fractures and dislocations, sprains, and strains of the wrist or hand is essentially the same.

Use a padded board or pillow splint with a sling and swathe to stabilize a dislocated hand or wrist. As always, use cold packs and elevation, and consider administering pain medication. If possible, the hand should be placed in the position of function and a roll of gauze placed in the curled palm.

► Finger Dislocation

Finger dislocations are caused by a sudden "jamming" force or from extension of the fingers beyond the normal ROM.

Assessment and Management

There is generally pain and deformity at the affected joint, and there may be compromise of the neurovascular structures of the digit, leading to paresthesias.

Manage the dislocated finger by splinting the entire hand in the position of function and using soft dressings as needed to support the digit, or simply tape the fingers together (buddy system). Do not attempt to relocate the injured digit in the field unless you are directed to do so by medical control. To reduce a dislocated digit, if the digit is dislocated to the dorsal side, extend the digit; if it is dislocated to the volar side, flex the digit. Next, use gentle longitudinal traction to bring the digit back into its normal position. It may be helpful to apply pressure at the dislocated joint to push the distal part into position. Following reduction, the neurovascular status of the digit should be reassessed and the digit should be fully immobilized to prevent it from dislocating again.

► Hip Dislocation

More than 90% of all hip dislocations involve posterior dislocation.[12] The majority of these dislocations occur due to deceleration injuries, in which a flexed knee strikes an immobile object with a great degree of force **Figure 37-25** .

When a patient has a posterior hip dislocation, the leg of the affected side is typically found in flexion, adduction, and internal rotation, and it is noticeably shorter. Patients report severe pain and inability to move the leg, and significant soft-tissue swelling may be evident. Complications arising from such injuries include sciatic nerve injury, avascular necrosis of the hip, and associated fractures of the acetabulum.

Anterior hip dislocations usually follow a forceful spreading injury that occurs while the hip is flexed. The affected leg is usually flexed, abducted, and externally rotated, and the patient reports severe pain. Major complications of this type of injury include injury to the femoral artery or nerve and avascular necrosis of the hip.

Assessment and Management

Because the majority of hip dislocations are associated with a high-energy mechanism, a secondary assessment of the entire body should be conducted and the patient fully stabilized. Splint the injured extremity in the position in which it is found by using blankets and pillows. Perform and document frequent neurovascular checks on your patient care report. Once at the hospital, the patient generally requires general anesthesia to allow the hip to be reduced within the socket.

► Knee Dislocation

Dislocations of the knee are true emergencies that may threaten the limb. When the knee is dislocated, the ligaments that provide support to it may be damaged or torn. The knee may be dislocated by high-energy trauma (as in MVCs), or it may dislocate secondary to powerful twisting forces (as when athletes attempt to avoid another player). In most cases, the knee will spontaneously relocate itself following the injury and there may be no obvious evidence of injury.

The direction of dislocation refers to the position of the tibia with respect to the femur. Anterior knee dislocations, which result from extreme hyperextension of the knee, are the most common, occurring in almost one-half of all cases. Commonly, the posterior cruciate ligament is torn. There is a relatively low risk of injury to the popliteal artery in the form of intimal tear. In posterior dislocations, a direct blow to the knee forces the tibia to shift posteriorly. There is a high risk of damage to the anterior cruciate ligament and the popliteal artery.

Medial dislocations result from a direct blow to the lateral part of the leg. Because the deforming force causes the medial aspect of the knee to stretch apart, there is a high likelihood of injury to the medial collateral and cruciate ligaments. When the force is applied from the medial direction, a lateral dislocation occurs and the lateral part of the knee is stretched apart, injuring the lateral collateral ligament. Lateral and medial dislocations happen less commonly and have a lesser risk of injuring the popliteal artery.

Assessment and Management

Patients with a knee dislocation will typically report pain in the knee and report that the knee "gave out." If the knee

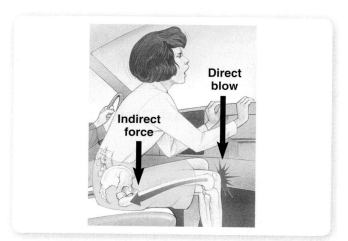

Figure 37-25 When a flexed knee strikes a dashboard, the force may be transmitted to the femur, causing it to be driven posteriorly. The hip may dislocate, and the acetabulum may fracture.

did not spontaneously replace itself, then there may be evidence of significant deformity and decreased ROM. Complications may include limb-threatening popliteal artery disruption; injuries to the popliteal, peroneal, and tibial nerves; and joint instability. Do not confuse this injury with a relatively minor patella dislocation.

In all cases of knee dislocation, distal neurovascular function must be assessed frequently and will often guide the management. If a pulse is palpable in the foot, then splint the knee in the position in which it is found. If there is no palpable pulse, then you may need to reduce the knee to restore circulation. A number of factors, including time to the hospital and duration of dislocation, will affect this decision, so you should always seek medical direction before reducing a dislocated knee.

To reduce a dislocated knee, apply longitudinal traction to the tibia in the direction of the foot. While the first rescuer is applying traction, a second provider should apply pressure to the distal femur and proximal tibia. If the knee is dislocated anteriorly, then apply pressure to the femur in the anterior direction and to the tibia in the opposite direction. In the case of a posterior dislocation, apply pressure in the opposite manner, with the tibia pressed anteriorly and the femur pressed posteriorly. Once the reduction has been accomplished, check the patient's neurovascular status and splint the leg securely. If the attempt at reduction fails, then splint the knee in the position in which it is found and undertake rapid transport to an appropriate facility.

▶ Tendon/Ligament Lacerations, Transections, and Ruptures

Knee Injury

The knee can be twisted during sports, resulting in potential laceration, transection, or rupture of the anterior cruciate ligament, the posterior cruciate ligament, the lateral collateral ligament, or the medial collateral ligament. The meniscus is another structure that is commonly injured in both sporting and nonsporting activities. This structure can be damaged during twisting (noncontact injury) or as a result of a direct blow (contact injury). Direct blows to the knee can result in an "unhappy triad" of injuries, which include tears of the anterior cruciate ligament, medial collateral ligament, and meniscus.

In addition, the knee can be hyperextended (stretched beyond its usual ROM) or can experience a torsion injury when the foot is fixed but the body pulls in another direction.

Shoulder Injury

Sternoclavicular sprain can occur from a direct blow, or from twisting of a posteriorly extended arm. Also, rotator cuff injury can occur from a violent pull on the arm, an abnormal rotation, or a fall on an outstretched arm. Rotator cuff injuries are often associated with chronic degenerative changes on the undersurface of the acromion.

Assessment and Management

Special assessment findings include muscle weakness, pain, edema, and loss of ROM. You should treat these as joint injuries and splint in place.

Principles of treating tendon injuries are the same as those used in treating other musculoskeletal injuries. Compare the symmetry of the injured limb with the opposite limb. Determine the extremity's ROM. Use cold packs, elevate the extremity, assess PMS distal to the injury site, and stabilize if needed. As always, provide psychological support to the patient, and adjust your approach when working with a pediatric patient. If an athletic trainer is on site, then he or she may have specialized knowledge of sports injuries and may be able to provide additional assistance.

▶ Achilles Tendon Rupture

A rupture of the Achilles tendon usually occurs in athletes older than 30 years who are involved in start-and-stop sports such as basketball or football.

Assessment and Management

The most immediate indications are pain from the heel to the calf and a sudden inability for plantar flexion of the foot. As time passes, the calf muscles begin to contract proximally and a deformity within the calf may develop. Additionally, there is often ecchymosis of the skin in the posterior calf, and there can be a palpable defect along the length of the tendon. The **Thompson test** can be performed in the field to identify an Achilles tendon rupture. To perform this test, have the patient assume a prone position and then squeeze the calf muscles of the injured leg **Figure 37-26**. If the foot plantarflexes while squeezing, then the tendon is at least partially intact. If there is no movement of the foot, then the Achilles tendon has likely been torn.

Management of an Achilles tendon injury includes RICES and pain control. These injuries are treated with surgery or multiple casts and can require up to 6 months for recovery.

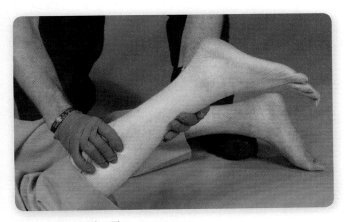

Figure 37-26 The Thompson test.
© Jones & Bartlett Learning. Courtesy of MIEMSS.

Pathophysiology, Assessment, and Management of Nontraumatic Musculoskeletal Disorders

Musculoskeletal complaints range from those requiring minimal treatment and evaluation to those necessitating extensive systematic testing, examination, and treatment. Both a systematic physical examination and a thorough history are necessary to appropriately evaluate and treat patients with musculoskeletal problems.

Patients presenting with nontraumatic musculoskeletal disorders generally do not have an acute life-threating condition, although there is frequently concern for the neurovascular status of an affected limb. Nontraumatic musculoskeletal disorders can be complex medical issues encompassing aspects of rheumatology, neurology, oncology, hematology, and infectious diseases. Generally, these patients have a history of musculoskeletal disorders and are already under a physician's care. It is important to ask whether the patient is following the advice given— that is, is the patient compliant with medications and physical therapy?

► Bony Abnormalities

Osteomyelitis

Osteomyelitis is a bacterial infection of the bone. It can be caused by systemic or local infections, and can develop in people with weakened immune systems, such as those with diabetes, older adults, or drug addicts. Any open wound over a bone or decubitus ulcer can lead to an infection, resulting in osteomyelitis.

The signs and symptoms of osteomyelitis are the same as in any infection. They can include fever, chills, erythema over the site, swelling, and pain. Onset can be slow or rapid.

EMS treatment is recognition, splinting, and transport. The patient will need antibiotics and often surgery to treat the disease.

Tumors

A tumor is a growth of abnormal tissue. Bone tumors can cause pathologic fractures in the bone as they increase in size. These tumors can be benign or malignant. The most common primary tumors of the bone are multiple myelomas, Ewing sarcoma (primarily found in children and adolescents), osteosarcoma, and chondrosarcoma.

Usually there will be pain in the affected area. There may be signs of infection such as night sweats or difficulty in using the affected extremity, but there may be no pain or discomfort at all. Swelling or a mass of tissue at the bone site is possible. You should compare the extremities for asymmetry. Splint the area of concern and transport for further evaluation.

► Joint Abnormalities: Arthritis

Arthritis means inflammation of a joint. Arthritis can have multiple etiologies and presentations and can lead to joint destruction, sepsis, and death in the worst cases. The three most common types of arthritis are osteoarthritis, rheumatoid arthritis, and gouty arthritis.

Osteoarthritis (OA) is a disease of the joints that occurs as they age and begin to wear. In general, the risk of developing OA increases with age, but other factors also increase the risk, such as obesity and prior joint injury.

Rheumatoid arthritis (RA) is a systemic inflammatory disease that affects joints and other body systems. RA can be a mild, nonprogressive disease or can be a full-blown, fatal illness. In RA, significant bone erosion at the affected joints makes them more susceptible to fractures and dislocations. Of particular concern is the cervical spine, which is at high risk of subluxating following trauma or during intubation.

Gout, or crystal-induced arthritis, is a condition in which the body has difficulty eliminating uric acid (**hyperuricemia**), and the result is buildup of the salts of uric acid. When the concentration of uric acid in the blood becomes too great, the uric acid may crystallize within the synovial fluids of a joint.

Septic arthritis typically involves the knee, shoulder, hip, ankle, elbow, or wrist. This condition is caused by a bacterial infection such as *Streptococcus* or *Staphylococcus*.

OA is characterized by pain and stiffness, which typically get worse with use, and "cracking" or "crunching" of the affected joints. The spine, hands, knees, and hips are the most commonly affected sites.

For the patient with RA, inflammation of almost any joint combination is possible; however, symmetric involvement of the hands, feet, or wrists are most common. Onset can be either insidious or acute.

The patient with gout will have a hot, red, swollen joint with decreased ROM. Most cases involve the big toe, although the ailment can present in multiple other locations, such as fingers and elbow joints, or as kidney stones.

Patients with septic arthritis may have a history of IV drug use and a fulminant presentation of a marked toxicity, fever, and altered level of consciousness. In older patients, septic arthritis can have a more insidious onset with malaise, anorexia, and lack of fever.

Treatment of OA involves low-impact physical therapy, pain control, anti-inflammatory medications, joint injections, and, in severe cases, joint replacement surgery.

Give extra attention to the cervical spine of a patient with RA to prevent further injury. Primary medical treatment typically includes use of various nonsteroidal anti-inflammatory drugs (NSAIDs).

Prehospital treatment of gout involves stabilization, pain relief (NSAIDs and corticosteroids), and transport to an emergency department, where the fluid in the joint can be aspirated to search for the characteristic crystals of gouty arthritis. Primary treatment then relies on dietary and lifestyle changes to reduce uric acid levels.

▶ Muscle Disorders

Muscle disorders can present in a wide variety of ways, from simple overuse syndromes to serious viral illnesses. The term **myalgia** refers to muscle pain that is a symptom of some other underlying issue. The most common cause is simple stress or straining of the muscle, but myalgia may involve viral infections, nutritional deficiencies, or metabolic myopathy. Medication-induced myalgia can be caused by vaccinations, angiotensin-converting enzyme inhibitors, cholesterol-lowering medication, and cocaine use. Diseases resulting in a symptom of myalgia can range from the common flu, Lyme disease, malaria, roundworm (trichinosis), lupus, and muscle abscesses.

As mentioned, the most common cause of myalgia is a repetitive strain injury or muscle overuse. Strain and overuse can result from ergonomic conditions such as repetitive motion for extended periods or prolonged use of a body part in a less than optimal position. A common symptom is short periods of intense pain in a diffuse area of the body. The pain typically gets worse with activity and can subside with rest. Treatment primarily relies on cessation of activity and NSAID treatment for inflammation and pain.

▶ Overuse Syndromes

Tendinitis and Bursitis

When a muscle is subjected to frequent, repetitive use, its tendon or nearby bursa is at risk for becoming inflamed. When inflammation of the tendon causes pain, the patient is said to have **tendinitis**. When it is the bursa that becomes inflamed and painful, the patient has **bursitis**.

With tendinitis, there will typically be point tenderness on the inflamed tendon, with pain often increasing if the person performs the movement that led to the inflammation. Patients with bursitis often complain of pain in the region of the inflamed bursa, especially with motions that cause the space where the bursa sits to become smaller.

Examination of the site may reveal tenderness, swelling, erythema, and warmth.

Tendinitis and bursitis are treated with RICES and pain relievers. In many cases, in-hospital treatment includes corticosteroid injections.

Carpal and Cubital Tunnel Syndromes

In contrast with the diffuse, nonanatomically specific form of most myalgias, syndromes such as **carpal tunnel syndrome** or **cubital tunnel syndrome** present with specific anatomic symptoms that are more readily identifiable. The symptoms of carpal tunnel syndrome are caused by compression of the median nerve at the wrist where it passes through the carpal canal. This compression can be caused by inflammation and swelling of tissue around the canal, by narrowing of the canal, or by pressure from outside the canal. Similarly, in cubital tunnel syndrome, also known as ulnar nerve entrapment, the ulnar nerve is compressed at the cubital tunnel along the outer edge of the elbow.

Patients with carpal tunnel syndrome have numbness and tingling in the hands, in particular to the index, thumb, and middle fingers that are innervated by the median nerve. Cubital tunnel syndrome exhibits burning, numbness, tingling, and possible partial loss of function of the little finger, and in the medial aspect of the ring finger.

Prehospital management of both cubital and carpal tunnel syndromes includes recognition, splinting, and transport. Definitive treatment of both syndromes includes rest of the affected extremity, removal of the underlying cause (typically occupational or positional), and possibly physical therapy. In the worst cases, surgical decompression of the canal may be required.

Polyneuropathy

In contrast to the nerve compression of tunnel syndromes, peripheral neuropathy, or peripheral nerve syndrome, stems from actual nerve damage of the peripheral nervous system. Causes are potentially numerous, and in a majority of cases the pathophysiology is not well understood. In the prehospital environment, it is important for you to obtain a comprehensive history to help determine onset, duration, patterns, and symmetry of symptoms; this information ultimately helps a physician begin to make a diagnosis of the patient with peripheral neuropathy.

Polyneuropathy occurs when there is simultaneous dysfunction of multiple peripheral nerves. Symptoms can present as motor, sensory, or both. Polyneuropathies can develop over days to weeks and are considered to be an acute condition. The most significant polyneuropathy is Guillain-Barré syndrome. This syndrome has an unclear etiology but results in inflammation and demyelination of peripheral nerves. Typically, the patient has a recent history of illness such as an upper respiratory tract infection, surgery, or vaccination. Motor weakness begins proximally and progresses during a period of days to weeks in an ascending fashion to full motor paralysis. The illness typically peaks in 10 to 14 days; however, recovery can take months, and full recovery is sometimes not possible.

Poliomyelitis is a polyneuropathy affecting the musculoskeletal system in a less organized and more centralized pattern than is seen in Guillain-Barré syndrome. It produces asymmetric paralysis primarily of the lower extremities and by definition does not include sensory loss. The greatest risk in poliomyelitis is of respiratory muscle paralysis.

Progression of paralysis stops when the patient becomes afebrile. Thanks to effective vaccination programs, poliomyelitis is exceedingly rare in the United States today.

Most cases of polyneuropathy that you will see will be acute cases. Because the causes are often unknown, PPE is essential. Assessment of ABCDEs, current history, and transport are mandated so that a definitive diagnosis can be reached at the hospital. Pain management should be considered.

YOU are the Paramedic   SUMMARY

1. What are your initial assessment and treatment priorities?

Initial assessment priorities include ABCDEs and assessing for head and spinal cord injuries, occult abdominal trauma, and bleeding from multiple fractures. The patient is feeling sleepy and weak and has a rapid radial pulse. Therefore, treatment priorities will focus on treatment for possible shock. In addition, treatment priorities include spinal precautions and supporting airway and breathing.

2. What other information would you obtain about the patient and the incident?

It is important to attempt to understand why the patient fell. What does the patient recall regarding the event? Are alcohol or drugs involved? Or, can any information be revealed from the patient's medical history or recent health complaints?

3. What are your early communication and transport plans?

Effective early communication with the receiving facility and transport to a trauma center will improve this patient's outcome. Depending on your location, you may consider transport by air.

4. What do these physical findings indicate to you?

His pale, cool, moist skin could be a result of peripheral-vascular shunting as seen in early stages of shock. When the sympathetic nervous system stimulates the release of epinephrine and norepinephrine from the adrenal glands, peripheral vasoconstriction occurs and the sweat glands are opened. Deformity to his bilateral femurs and lower extremities are most likely due to fractures.

5. Why is a history of type 1 diabetes significant?

The history of type 1 diabetes may explain the report of feeling light-headed during the past few days and may have contributed to the same complaint experienced before he fell. His blood glucose level should be checked.

6. What can you conclude from the patient's vital signs?

The patient's blood pressure is normal, but his pulse rate is rapid. The patient's tachycardia could be caused by the body's attempt to compensate for blood loss. Considering his physical exam findings, the tachycardia could be a sign of shock.

7. Why is a blood glucose reading of 46 mg/dL significant?

A normal glucose level should be between 60 and 120 mg/dL. Therefore, his blood glucose level is too low. This would explain his feeling of light-headedness and could be the cause of his falling off the ladder. The finding that his mental status improved after the IV administration of glucose also supports this thinking.

8. Why should this patient be transported to a trauma center?

Trauma patients in all age groups benefit from treatment at trauma centers. Transport of this patient to a trauma center may improve this patient's outcome. Depending on your location and regional resources, you may consider transport by air.

9. What do his vital signs indicate?

The level of tachycardia has increased, indicating that the body is compensating for shock. The patient is now hypotensive, indicating that internal bleeding from multiple long bone fractures is significant.

10. What do absent pedal pulses, absent motor function, and lack of sensation in the toes indicate?

Absent pedal pulses, absent motor function, and lack of sensation in his toes may indicate neurovascular damage to his extremities. These findings may also be a result of poor peripheral circulation secondary to his hypotension.

YOU are the Paramedic   SUMMARY *(continued)*

11. Why is it important to treat the patient's pain?

It is very important to make the patient comfortable and treat his pain because pain causes unfavorable physiologic changes in perception and vital signs. However, careful monitoring is required when narcotic analgesics are given to trauma patients with probable internal hemorrhage. Remember, the side effects of narcotic analgesics include respiratory depression, bradycardia, and hypotension.

EMS Patient Care Report (PCR)

Date: 10-15-18	Incident No.: 128		Nature of Call: Fall		Location: 12301 Matthews Lane
Dispatched: 1304	**En Route:** 1305	**At Scene:** 1311	**Transport:** 1327	**At Hospital:** 1342	**In Service:** 1412

Patient Information

Age: 24 **Sex:** M **Weight (in kg [lb]):** 75 kg (150 lb)	**Allergies:** No known drug allergies **Medications:** Humulin and Novolog **Past Medical History:** Type 1 diabetes **Chief Complaint:** Bilateral thigh and lower extremity pain

Vital Signs

Time: 1316	BP: 104/60	Pulse: 116	Respirations: 24	Spo₂: 98%
Time: 1321	**BP:** 94/53	**Pulse:** 122	**Respirations:** 24	**Spo₂:** 98%
Time: 1326	**BP:** 84/44	**Pulse:** 128	**Respirations:** 24	**Spo₂:** 98%
Time: 1331	**BP:** 95/56	**Pulse:** 110	**Respirations:** 20	**Spo₂:** 98%

EMS Treatment (circle all that apply)

Oxygen @ _____ L/min via (circle one): NC NRM Bag-mask device	Assisted Ventilation	Airway Adjunct	CPR
Defibrillation	**Bleeding Control**	**Bandaging**	(**Splinting:** Femurs and lower extremities)	(**Other:** IV NS lock #16 GA left AC, cervical stabilization, 50 mcg fentanyl IVP, blankets)

Narrative

Pt 24-year-old male roofer who fell about 20 feet, landing on his feet, impacting the lawn. On arrival found pt lying supine on ground alert and oriented × 3 but slow to answer questions. Skin is pale, cool, and moist. Obvious deformity observed to bilateral femurs and bilateral lower extremities. Pt recalls entire event and denies LOC, neck pain, numbness/tingling in extremities, headache, nausea/vomiting, abdominal pain, chest pain, or dyspnea, but states he was "light-headed" while climbing the ladder before he fell. Complains of bilateral femur pain, low back pain, and bilateral lower extremity pain. Pain an "8" on "0 to 10" scale. Fitted pt with c-collar and immobilized to long backboard. After splinting, pedal pulses are absent, sensation to toes is absent, and the pt is unable to move his toes upon command. Blood glucose 46 mg/dL. D₅₀ 25 g IVP given per protocol. Improved to 126 mg/dL. En route, called medical direction and spoke to Dr. Hartmann, who advised a 500-mL NS IV bolus and gave orders for fentanyl 50 mcg IVP PRN and as vital signs permit. Fentanyl 50 mcg IVP given and 500-mL NS IV bolus given. Pain now a "3" on "0 to 10" scale and blood glucose is 122 mg/dL. Transported pt to St. Anthony's Hospital room #14 and report given to Julia, RN. No pt belongings transported.**End of report**

Prep Kit

▶ Ready for Review

- Injuries and complaints related to the musculoskeletal system are one of the most common reasons that patients seek medical attention.
- Musculoskeletal injuries are sometimes very dramatic, but attention should not be focused on them until life-threatening conditions have been addressed.
- You have a vital role in reducing the complications associated with musculoskeletal injuries by promptly and effectively splinting injured extremities.
- Assume the existence of a fracture whenever a patient who reports a musculoskeletal injury has deformity, bruising, decreased ROM, or swelling.
- Always perform and record an accurate neurovascular examination before and after splinting an injured extremity.
- Check penetrating injuries for underlying fractures or other musculoskeletal injury.
- Musculoskeletal injuries are likely to be accompanied by hemorrhage.
- When a dislocation is associated with absent distal pulses, obtain medical direction to determine whether the injury should be reduced.
- Look for injuries to the chest and abdomen, and fully stabilize the spine when patients have evidence of a high-energy injury, such as a femoral shaft or scapular fracture.
- Because fractures may be associated with significant blood loss, resuscitation with IV fluid may be necessary.
- Pelvic fractures are potentially lethal injuries owing to the massive potential for blood loss.
- Posterior sternoclavicular joint dislocations are potentially fatal due to possible damage to underlying structures.
- *Never forget the ABCDEs!* Do not become distracted; the fracture can wait if airway, breathing, or circulation problems are noted.
- Musculoskeletal injuries can lead to numerous complications, including vascular injuries, neurovascular injuries, compartment syndrome, crush syndrome, and thromboembolic disease.
- Blood vessels can be damaged following a musculoskeletal injury. Loss of blood flow to the area of the musculoskeletal injury is called devascularization.
- Neurovascular injuries include impalement or laceration of nerves of a plexus, leading to a neurologic deficit. Neurovascular injuries can also occur following a joint dislocation.

- Compartment syndrome occurs when bleeding or swelling increases within a compartment to the point that the pressure within that compartment impairs circulation. This pressure and decreased blood flow can cause pain, sensory changes, and muscle death.
- Crush syndrome occurs when a prolonged compressive force impairs muscle metabolism and circulation. When the compressive force is released, toxins enter the patient's circulation.
- Nontraumatic musculoskeletal disorders can be highly complex medical issues encompassing aspects of rheumatology, neurology, oncology, hematology, and infectious diseases. Nontraumatic musculoskeletal disorders include bony abnormalities, such as osteomyelitis and tumors; disorders of the spine, including low back pain and disc disorders; joint abnormalities; muscle abnormalities; and overuse syndromes.
- Types of arthritis include osteoarthritis, rheumatoid arthritis, gout, and septic arthritis. Gout can be treated with immobilization, pain relief, and transport.
- Muscle disorders include myalgia, muscle pain that is a symptom of some other underlying issue. Treatment will be based on the patient's complaint and history. Transport for definitive diagnosis.
- Tendinitis and bursitis are overuse syndromes, which occur from frequent and repetitive use that results in inflammation. Tendinitis and bursitis are treated with RICES, pain relievers, and steroid injections.
- Paramedics may encounter patients with numbness, tingling, or pain in their wrist or hand. This can be from carpal tunnel syndrome or cubital tunnel syndrome. Prehospital treatment includes recognition, splinting, and transport.
- Polyneuropathy, or peripheral nerve syndrome, stems from actual nerve damage of the peripheral nervous system. Good history taking is important to provide a basis for a physician to begin diagnosis and treatment. Also, prehospital pain management should be considered.

▶ Vital Vocabulary

6 Ps of musculoskeletal assessment Pain, Paralysis, Parasthesias, Pulselessness, Pallor, and Pressure.

anatomic snuffbox The region at the base of the thumb where the scaphoid may be palpated.

angulation The presence of an abnormal angle or bend in an extremity.

appendicular skeleton The part of the skeleton comprising the upper and lower extremities.

arthritis Inflammation of the joints.

Prep Kit (continued)

associated fractures Musculoskeletal injuries that commonly occur together.

avascular necrosis Tissue death resulting from the loss of blood supply.

avulsion fracture A fracture that occurs when a piece of bone is torn free at the site of attachment of a tendon or ligament.

axial skeleton The part of the skeleton comprising the skull, spinal column, and rib cage.

boxer's fracture A fracture of the head of the fifth metacarpal that usually results from striking an object with a clenched fist.

buckle fracture A common incomplete fracture in children in which the cortex of the bone fractures from an excessive compression force; also called a torus fracture.

buddy splinting Securing an injured digit to an adjacent uninjured one to allow the intact digit to act as a splint.

bursitis Inflammation of a bursa.

cancellous bone Trabecular or spongy bone.

carpal tunnel syndrome Compression of the median nerve at the wrist where it passes through the carpal canal, causing numbness and tingling in the hand, and possibly pain.

closed fracture A fracture in which the skin is not broken.

comminuted fracture A fracture in which the bone is broken into three or more pieces.

compartment syndrome An increase in tissue pressure in a closed fascial space or compartment that compromises the circulation to the nerves and muscles within the involved compartment.

complete fracture A fracture in which the bone is broken into two or more completely separate pieces.

crepitus A grating sensation felt when moving the ends of a broken bone.

crush syndrome A condition that arises after a body part that has been compressed for a significant period is released, leading to the entry of potassium and other metabolic toxins into the systemic circulation.

cubital tunnel syndrome Compression of the ulnar nerve at the tunnel along the outer edge of the elbow, causing numbness, tingling, and possible partial loss of function of the little finger and medial aspect of the ring finger.

deep vein thrombosis (DVT) The formation of a blood clot within the larger veins of an extremity, typically following a period of prolonged stabilization.

depression fracture A fracture in which the broken region of the bone is pushed deeper into the body than the remaining intact bone.

devascularization The loss of blood to a part of the body.

diastasis An increase in the distance between the two sides of a joint.

dislocation The displacement of a bone from its normal position within a joint.

displaced fracture A break in which the ends of the fractured bone move out of their normal positions.

distraction injury An injury that results from a force that tries to increase the length of a body part or separate one body part from another.

dorsiflex To bend the foot or hand backward.

fascia A strong, fibrous membrane that covers, supports, and separates muscles.

fatigue fracture A fracture that results from multiple compressive loads.

femoral shaft fracture A break in the diaphysis of the femur.

fracture A break or rupture in the bone.

glenoid fossa The socket in the scapula in which the head of the humerus rotates.

glomerular filtration The process by which the kidneys filter the blood, removing excess wastes and fluids.

gout A painful disorder characterized by the crystallization of uric acid within a joint.

greenstick fracture A type of fracture occurring most frequently in children in which there is incomplete breakage of the bone.

hyperkalemia An abnormally elevated level of potassium in the blood.

hyperphosphatemia An abnormally elevated serum phosphate; often associated with decreased calcium. Normal phosphate levels are between 0.81 and 1.45 mmol/L.

hyperuricemia High levels of uric acid in the blood.

impacted fracture A broken bone in which the cortices of one bone become wedged into another bone, as could be the case in a fall from a significant height.

incomplete fracture A fracture in which the bone does not fully break.

indirect injury An injury that results from a force that is applied to one region of the body but leads to an injury in another area.

intertrochanteric fracture A fracture that occurs in the region between the lesser and greater trochanters.

Prep Kit (continued)

lateral compression A force that is directed from the side toward the midline of the body.

linear fracture A fracture that runs parallel to the long axis of a bone.

luxation A complete dislocation.

mallet finger An avulsion fracture of the extensor tendon of the distal phalynx caused by jamming a finger into an object.

myalgia Muscle pain.

neurovascular compromise The loss of the nerve supply, blood supply, or both to a region of the body, typically distal to a site of injury; characterized by alterations in sensation.

nondisplaced fracture A break in which the bone remains aligned in its normal position.

nursemaid's elbow The subluxation of the radial head that often results from pulling on an outstretched arm.

oblique fracture A fracture that travels diagonally from one side of the bone to the other.

olecranon The proximal bony projection of the *ulna* at the elbow; the part of the ulna that constitutes the "funny bone."

open-book pelvic fracture A life-threatening fracture of the pelvis caused by a force that displaces one or both sides of the pelvis laterally and posteriorly.

open fracture Any break in a bone in which the overlying skin has been damaged.

osteoarthritis (OA) The degeneration of a joint surface caused by wear and tear that lead to pain and stiffness.

osteoporosis A condition characterized by decreased bone density and increased susceptibility to fractures.

overriding The overlap of a bone that occurs from the muscle spasm that follows a fracture, leading to a decrease in the length of the bone.

paresthesia An abnormal sensation such as burning, numbness, or tingling.

pathologic fracture A fracture that occurs in an area of abnormally weakened bone.

pectoral girdle The shoulder girdle.

pelvic girdle The large bone that arises in the area of the last nine vertebrae and sweeps around to form a complete ring.

plantarflex To bend the foot toward the ground.

point tenderness The tenderness that is sharply localized at the site of the injury, found by gently palpating along the bone with the tip of one finger.

polyneuropathy A type of disorder in which multiple nerves become dysfunctional.

pulmonary embolism Obstruction of a pulmonary artery or arteries by solid, liquid, or gaseous material swept through the right side of the heart into the lungs.

range of motion (ROM) The arc of movement of an extremity at a joint in a particular direction.

rhabdomyolysis The destruction of muscle tissue leading to a release of potassium and myoglobin.

rheumatoid arthritis (RA) An inflammatory disorder that affects the entire body and leads to degeneration and deformation of joints.

scaphoid The wrist bone that is found just beyond the most distal portion of the radius.

segmental fracture A bone that is broken in more than one place.

septic arthritis Inflammation of a joint based on a bacterial or fungal infection.

silver fork deformity The dorsal deformity of the forearm that results from a Colles fracture.

spiral fracture A break in a bone that appears like a spring on a radiograph.

sprain An injury, including a stretch or a tear, to the ligaments of a joint that commonly leads to pain and swelling.

straddle fracture A fracture of the pelvis that results from landing on the peroneal region.

strain Stretching or tearing of a muscle or tendon by excessive stretching or overuse.

stress fracture A fracture that results from exaggerated stress on the bone caused by unusually rapid muscle development.

subluxation A partial or incomplete dislocation.

supracondylar fracture A fracture of the distal humerus that occurs just proximal to the elbow.

talus The bone of the foot that articulates with the tibia.

tendinitis Inflammation of a tendon that most commonly results from overuse.

Thompson test Squeezing of the calf muscle to evaluate for plantar flexion of the foot to determine whether the Achilles tendon is intact.

thromboembolic disease The condition in which a patient has a deep vein thrombosis or pulmonary embolism.

torus fracture *See* buckle fracture.

transverse fracture A fracture that runs in a straight line from one edge of the bone to the other and that is perpendicular to each edge.

Prep Kit *(continued)*

twisting injury An injury that commonly occurs during athletic activities in which an extremity rotates around a planted foot or hand.

vertical shear The type of pelvic fracture that occurs when a massive force displaces the pelvis superiorly.

volar Pertaining to the palm or sole; referring to the flexor surfaces of the forearm, wrist, or hand.

Volkmann ischemic contracture Contraction of the fingers and sometimes the wrist following severe injury around the elbow joint; characterized by loss of muscular power and rapid onset of death and resultant contracture of the forearm musculature.

▶ References

1. MEPS: Medical Expenditures Panel Survey. Agency for Healthcare Research and Quality, US Department of Health and Human Services, website. https://meps.ahrq.gov/mepsweb/. Accessed March 17, 2017.
2. US Department of Labor, Bureau of Labor Statistics. Occupational Injuries and Illnesses (Annual) News Release. https://www.bls.gov/news.release/archives/osh_10272016.htm. Accessed March 31, 2017.
3. Beck LF, West BA. Vital signs: nonfatal motor vehicle-occupant injuries (2009) and seat belt use (2008) among adults—United States. *MMWR.* 2011; 59(51):1681-1686.
4. Lee R, Parker E, Bergen G, et al. Older adult fall prevention—getting to outcome measures in the clinical setting. *Inj Prev.* 2016;22:A35.
5. Stawicki SP, Lindsey DE. Trauma corner—missed traumatic injuries: a synopsis. *OPUS 12 Sci.* 2009; 3(2):35-13.
6. Zager RA, Gamelin LM. Pathogenetic mechanisms in experimental hemoglobinuric acute renal failure. *Am J Physiol.* 1989;256:F446-F455.
7. Bosch X, Poch E, Grau JM. Rhabdomyolysis and acute kidney injury. *N Engl J Med.* 2009; 361(1):62-72.
8. Jernigan MV, Duma SM. The effects of airbag deployment on severe upper extremity injuries in frontal automobile crashes. *Am J Emerg Med.* 2003; 21(2):100-105.
9. Raafat A, Wright MJ. Current management of pelvic fractures. *South Med J.* 2000;93(8). http://www.medscape.com/viewarticle/410597_3. Accessed March 31, 2017.
10. Fiechtl J. Pelvic trauma: initial evaluation and management. UpToDate website. http://www.uptodate.com/contents/pelvic-trauma-initial-evaluation-and-management. Updated January 19, 2017. Accessed May 4, 2017.
11. Cothran VE. Shoulder Dislocation. Medscape website. http://emedicine.medscape.com/article/93323-overview. Updated December 21, 2016. Accessed April 18, 2017.
12. McMillan SR. Hip dislocation in emergency medicine. Medscape website. http://emedicine.medscape.com/article/823471-overview#a6. Updated April 11, 2016. Accessed May 8, 2017.

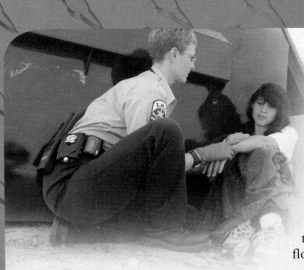

Assessment in Action

You are dispatched to the scene of a 69-year-old woman who fell while dancing at her granddaughter's wedding reception. When you arrive, you find the patient lying supine on the dance floor holding her right hip and grimacing in pain. According to the patient, she was dancing when she tripped on a rug, hitting her right leg on the wooden dance floor. She states she has a history of osteoporosis.

Assessment *in Action* (continued)

You observe that the right leg is abnormally externally rotated and shortened in contrast to the left leg. Pedal pulses are strong and regular bilaterally, and she has normal sensation to her toes and moves them upon command. The patient is alert and oriented and states, "My hip really hurts." She is reporting only intense right hip pain and denies associated injuries. The patient's skin is pink, warm, and dry. Her vital signs are as follows: respirations, 24 breaths/min; pulse, 112 beats/min; and blood pressure, 126/68 mm Hg. A pulse oximetry reading is 98% on room air. The patient is placed on the stretcher in a supine position as requested with her right leg and hip supported with pillows and blankets. Her right femur and hip reveal swelling and ecchymosis. En route, a full-body exam is performed and found to be unremarkable except for her right hip deformity. A large-bore IV line is initiated and oxygen is applied. Medical direction is contacted and a narcotic analgesic is administered for pain. The patient is transported to the closest trauma center.

1. Unopposed pull of which muscles leads to the observed deformity in the right lower extremity?

   A. Quadriceps muscles
   B. Gastrocnemius/soleus muscle
   C. Gluteus muscles
   D. Hamstring muscles

2. By what mechanism does osteoporosis increase the risk for fractures?

   A. Pathologic thickening of bone
   B. Thinning of the bone by excessive resorption
   C. Excessive calcium supplementation
   D. Genetic mutation

3. In this patient, pain at the fracture site is likely associated with:

   A. rupture of the sciatic nerve.
   B. fat embolism.
   C. ischemia of the limb.
   D. shortening of the hip girdle muscles.

4. Based on the deformity observed in this patient, you conclude that the fracture is a(n):

   A. complete fracture.
   B. incomplete fracture.
   C. comminuted fracture.
   D. stress fracture.

5. A fracture of the hip would be definitively treated with:

   A. a cast.
   B. traction.
   C. a splint.
   D. surgery.

6. Placing a fractured extremity in anatomic position typically:

   A. decreases blood pressure.
   B. decreases transport time.
   C. improves pain.
   D. impairs circulation to the distal limb.

7. Faced with a high-force MOI combined with lower pelvis instability, lower extremity deformity, and hemodynamic instability, you should:

   A. place a pelvic binder/sheet over the iliac crests.
   B. place a pelvic binder/sheet over the greater trochanters.
   C. administer morphine analgesia.
   D. call for medical direction.

8. How should paramedics manage musculoskeletal injuries in the field when they cannot be differentiated as sprains, strains, or fractures?

9. What are the principles of fracture splinting?

10. Why are elbow dislocations medical emergencies?

CHAPTER 38

Environmental Emergencies

National EMS Education Standard Competencies

Trauma

Integrates assessment findings with principles of epidemiology and pathophysiology to formulate a field impression to implement a comprehensive treatment/disposition plan for an acutely injured patient.

Environmental Emergencies

Recognition and management of
> Submersion incidents (pp 1907-1911)
> Temperature-related illness (pp 1892-1907)

Pathophysiology, assessment, and management of
> Near drowning (pp 1907-1911)
> Temperature-related illness (pp 1892-1907)
> Bites and envenomations (pp 1923-1929)
> Dysbarism
  • High-altitude (pp 1918-1921)
  • Diving injuries (pp 1911-1918)
> Electrical injury (pp 1921-1922)
> Radiation exposure (see Chapter 32, *Burns*)
> High-altitude illness (pp 1918-1921)

Knowledge Objectives

1. Describe four factors that affect how a person deals with exposure to a cold or hot environment and how each one relates to emergency medical care. (p 1889)
2. Explain the four different ways a body can lose heat and ways the rate and amount of heat loss or gain can be modified in an emergency situation. (pp 1891-1892)
3. Describe the various forms of illnesses caused by heat exposure, the signs and symptoms, and the people who are at the greatest risk of developing one of them. (pp 1892-1894)
4. Explain emergency medical care of a patient who has sustained a heat injury, including assessment of the patient, review of signs and symptoms, and management of care. (pp 1893-1899)
5. Explain local cold injuries and the underlying causes. (pp 1899-1900)

6. Describe the process of providing emergency medical care of a patient who has sustained a local cold injury, including assessment of the patient, review of signs and symptoms, and management of care. (pp 1901-1902)
7. Discuss hypothermia, including its definition, the signs and symptoms of its four different stages, the risk factors for developing it, and its management and treatment. (pp 1902-1907)
8. Explain the importance of following protocols in wilderness EMS operations. (p 1907)
9. Discuss drowning, including its definition, incidence, risk factors, assessment, treatment, and prevention. (pp 1907-1911)
10. Describe the various types of diving emergencies and the process of providing emergency medical care to a patient who has been involved in a diving emergency, including assessment of the patient, review of signs and symptoms, and management of care. (pp 1911-1918)
11. Discuss the types of dysbarism injuries that may be caused by high altitudes, including the signs and symptoms and emergency medical treatment in the field. (pp 1918-1921)
12. Discuss lightning injuries, including the incidence, risk factors, assessment, and emergency medical treatment. (pp 1921-1922)
13. Discuss the emergency medical care of patients who have been stung by hymenoptera, including steps the paramedic should follow if a patient develops a severe reaction to the sting or bite. (pp 1923-1924)
14. Identify the species of arachnids (spiders, scorpions, and ticks) found in the United States that may cause life-threatening injuries, and the emergency medical care of patients who have been bitten by each type. (pp 1926-1929)

Skills Objectives

1. Demonstrate how to treat a patient with heat cramps. (pp 1894-1895)
2. Demonstrate how to treat a patient with heat exhaustion. (p 1896)
3. Demonstrate how to treat a patient with heatstroke. (pp 1898-1899)

4. Demonstrate the emergency medical treatment of local cold injuries in the field. (pp 1901-1902)
5. Demonstrate using a warm-water bath to rewarm the limb of a patient who has sustained a local cold injury. (pp 1901-1902)
6. Demonstrate how to care for a patient who is suspected of having an air embolism or decompression sickness following a diving emergency. (pp 1916-1917)
7. Demonstrate how to care for a patient who is experiencing altitude illness. (pp 1920-1921)

8. Demonstrate how to care for a patient who has been struck by lightning. (p 1922)
9. Demonstrate how to care for a patient who has been bitten by a crotalin or elapid and is showing signs of envenomation. (pp 1925-1927)
10. Demonstrate how to care for a patient who has been bitten by a black widow or brown recluse spider. (p 1928)
11. Demonstrate how to care for a patient who has been bitten by a tick. (p 1929)

■ Introduction

According to the Centers for Disease Control and Prevention (CDC), more than 13,400 people in the United States died of hypothermia-related causes from 2003 to 2013—a rate of 0.5 per 100,000 people. In addition, the incidence of this type of environmentally induced death is increasing.[1] Similarly, deaths from heat-related issues between 2005 and 2009 rose to higher rates than have been observed during any other 5-year period in the past 35 years.[2] Ambient temperatures on Earth continue to rise: March 2016 was the hottest month on record, 2016 was the warmest year on record, and since the late 19th century,

YOU are the Paramedic   PART 1

You are dispatched to the scene of a private residence for a 20-year-old man who came stumbling home after falling through the ice while out riding his snowmobile. His mother tells you he walked home, approximately half a mile (0.8 km). She states she had him remove his clothes; she then wrapped him in a warm blanket and gave him some hot coffee. She went to prepare a warm bath when she heard a "thud" in the kitchen. When she entered the kitchen, she found him sitting on the floor and he "wasn't acting right," so she called EMS. The current ambient temperature outside is 36°F (2°C).

When you arrive, you find the patient sitting on the kitchen floor alert and shivering. He responds to your voice but has difficulty answering questions. His face is pink, but his lips are dusky. He recalls the event and denies any injuries, but reports "aching all over" and "feeling weak and sleepy."

Recording Time: 1 Minute	
Appearance	Eyes open and shivering
Level of consciousness	Alert
Airway	Patent with clear speech
Breathing	Nonlabored, slow, and shallow
Circulation	Rapid radial pulse; no obvious external bleeding

1. What are your assessment and treatment priorities?
2. What other information would you obtain about the patient and the incident?
3. What are your early communication and transport plans?

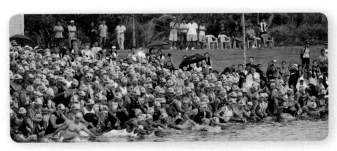

Figure 38-1 Environmental emergencies can occur in a variety of settings, including endurance sports events.
© patrimonio designs ltd/Shutterstock.

the hottest years on record have all been from 1997 to the present.[3] From 1999 through 2009, extreme heat exposure caused or contributed to more than 7,800 deaths in the United States.[4] The heat wave that afflicted Europe in the summer of 2003 was estimated to have caused as many as 70,000 deaths.[5] **Environmental emergencies** are medical conditions caused or worsened by the weather, terrain, fauna, or unique atmospheric conditions present at high altitude or underwater. Most emergency medical services (EMS) providers would recognize the obvious problem of a child who has fallen into an icy lake. The challenge lies in recognizing patients with environmental emergencies in the unusual settings of endurance sports events or at mass gatherings, and even acutely confused older adult patients **Figure 38-1**.

Unique to environmental emergencies are the conditions that directly cause harm or complicate treatment and transport considerations. Wind, rain, snow, temperature extremes, and humidity may all affect the body's ability to adapt to its environment. The locations of these outings can also have a huge impact on the ability to know about, respond to, and rescue people in remote settings **Figure 38-2**.

Certain common risk factors predispose people to environmental emergencies. Conditions such as diabetes, cardiac disease (for example, coronary artery disease, heart failure), restrictive lung disease, thyroid disease, and psychiatric illnesses can alter the body's ability to compensate for environmental extremes. In addition, young and older people have unique disadvantages when it comes to thermoregulation. A patient who is dehydrated can be at risk. Finally, the patient's overall health and fitness status and ability to acclimatize (that is, physiologically adjust to the new environment) can mean the difference between life and death.

This chapter first describes the techniques that the healthy body uses to respond to changes in temperature. It then assesses factors that can interfere with the body's ability to shed or gain heat, thereby increasing a person's risk of experiencing an environmental emergency. Next, it examines the pathophysiology, assessment, and management of environmental illnesses.

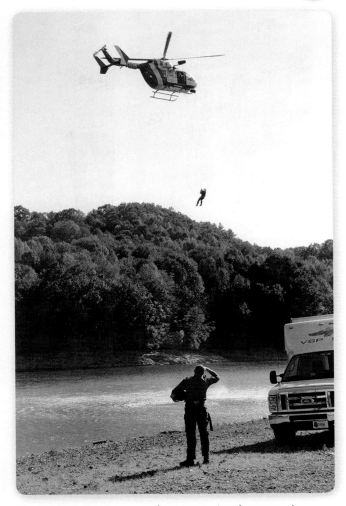

Figure 38-2 Environmental emergencies that occur in remote settings can make rescue particularly challenging.
© Earl Neikirk/AP Photo.

■ Anatomy and Physiology Review

▶ Homeostasis and Body Temperature

Homeostasis refers to body processes that balance the supply and demand of the body's needs. Ensuring the balance between heat production and heat dissipation (**thermoregulation**) is the job of thermosensitive neurons in the anterior **hypothalamus**. The hypothalamus acts similar to a thermostat in activating the mechanisms for increasing or decreasing body temperature. A rise in core body temperature (CBT) elicits responses that increase heat loss and shut off normal heat production pathways (thermogenesis); a fall in the CBT prompts heat production and conservation and turns off normal heat-liberating pathways (thermolysis) **Figure 38-3**.

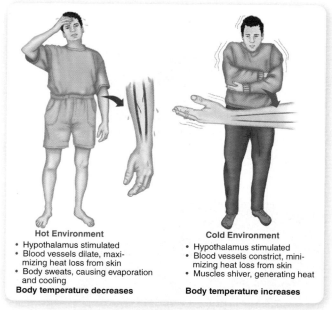

Hot Environment
- Hypothalamus stimulated
- Blood vessels dilate, maximizing heat loss from skin
- Body sweats, causing evaporation and cooling

Body temperature decreases

Cold Environment
- Hypothalamus stimulated
- Blood vessels constrict, minimizing heat loss from skin
- Muscles shiver, generating heat

Body temperature increases

Figure 38-3 Like a thermostat, the hypothalamus notes a rise or fall in core body temperature and elicits responses to regulate it.
© Jones & Bartlett Learning.

> **Words of Wisdom**
>
> Do not become a victim yourself. Stay hydrated, dress for the weather, and store oral fluids in a cooler in your rig.

The human body maintains a constant core temperature of approximately 98.6°F (37°C) that represents a balance between the heat produced or absorbed by the body and the heat released to the outside. At this temperature, the body's metabolism functions normally. Temperatures in the core (the brain and thoracoabdominal organs) remain relatively constant. The temperature of the periphery (the skin and extremities) can fluctuate, so this part of the body has a major role in thermoregulation. **Hypothermia** is commonly defined as a decreased **core body temperature (CBT)** starting at 95°F (35°C). **Hyperthermia** is generally defined as elevated CBT starting at 100.4°F (38°C). CBT is defined as the temperature in the trunk of the body comprising the heart, lungs, brain, and abdominal viscera.

In the field, the oral temperature is commonly used, although it may not be sufficiently accurate. It can vary dramatically from the CBT if the patient has been mouth breathing or drinking hot or cold liquids, and can vary by nearly 1°F (0.6°C) from the CBT even in a patient at rest and not drinking liquids.[6] Axillary temperatures are discouraged due to high inaccuracy.[7] The most accurate means of determining CBT is to use a rectal thermometer capable of measuring extremes of temperatures. This can be done with a mercury or electronic thermometer.

Tympanic temperatures, which are taken with a device that measures the heat reflected off the eardrum, as well as various commercial devices for measuring skin temperatures, may be increasingly accurate and may be more appropriate for some field operations than rectal temperature.

▶ Thermoregulatory Mechanisms

The body's main thermoregulatory center is located in specialized tissue found in the hypothalamus. The thermogenic (heat-generating) function of the hypothalamus is mediated by the sympathetic nervous system; the thermolytic (heat-liberating) tissues are mediated by the parasympathetic nervous system. Peripheral and central thermoreceptors are integrated with the central nervous system (CNS), enabling a balance of heat loss and heat production while maintaining the CBT within relatively normal limits. Peripheral thermoreceptors that are present on the surface of the body relay information to the hypothalamus about ambient temperature.

At rest, the body produces heat chiefly by the metabolism of nutrients (carbohydrates, fats, and rarely proteins). The liver and skeletal muscles are the major contributors to the **basal metabolic rate (BMR)**, the heat energy produced at rest from normal body metabolic reactions. The BMR of the average 154-pound (70-kg) adult is in the range of 60 to 70 kilocalories per hour. Many factors affect this rate, including age, gender, stress, and hormones. The most important factor, however, is body surface area. As the ratio of body surface area to body volume increases, heat loss to the environment increases. Thus, when two people have the same weight, the shorter person will have a higher BMR.

Exertion also affects the metabolic rate. For example, a brisk walk can produce heat totaling 300 kcal/h. The recommended daily caloric intake is around 2,000 to 2,500 kcal (a food "calorie" is actually a kilocalorie). Men's bodies require slightly higher calorie intake than women's (for example, a moderately active woman between ages 19 and 30 requires 2,000 to 2,200 calories per day, while a man in the same category requires 2,600 to 2,800 calories).

Some of the heat generated by metabolism and glycogen breakdown during muscle activity is used to warm the body; the excess is dissipated, ordinarily by taking advantage of the temperature gradient between the body and the outside environment. If the environmental temperature is higher than the body temperature, then heat can be absorbed from the environment. For example, standing in bright sunshine on a hot, breezeless day can add up to 150 kcal/h to the internal heat load.

Lastly, the skin plays a vital role in body temperature regulation. Although the mechanisms are quite complicated, the body has the ability to both conserve and liberate large amounts of heat energy through the skin. In an effort to liberate heat, blood flow to the skin can involve up to 8 liters per minute and 60% of cardiac output.

▶ Physiologic Responses to Heat and Cold

Thermolysis

The body reacts to its daily production of heat energy and to hot environmental conditions in much the same way—**thermolysis**, the release of stored heat and energy from the body. An increase in the CBT causes the hypothalamus to send signals via efferent pathways in the autonomic nervous system, causing vasodilation and sweating.

Because of cutaneous vasodilation, the effective volume of the vascular system is increased (when the diameter of a vessel, such as an artery, is increased, its volume increases); the heart must increase its output to compensate for this effect. The pulse rate and stroke volume increase, and the work of the heart is markedly increased. If vasodilation increases dramatically, the person may have a complete loss of vasomotor control (that is, the ability of the arteries to constrict in response to sympathetic stimulation). In that case, blood pools in the periphery, and the patient could experience neurogenic shock.

When warmed blood from the core and overheated muscles heads for the peripherally dilated cutaneous vessels, it may be cooled in four ways (in addition to behavioral changes, such as slowing down or seeking shade):

- **Radiation**, the transfer of heat away from the body, accounts for more than 65% of heat loss.[8] Heat loss through the head is especially notable. If the ambient temperature is high (68°F [20.0°C] or greater), body heat will be gained.
- **Conduction** is the transfer of heat from a hotter object to a cooler object by direct physical contact.

Air is a poor conductor of heat (only 2% of body heat is lost to it), whereas the ground is a good conductor. Water is the best conductor. A person who falls into a cold lake will lose heat 25 times faster than a dry person exposed to air of the same temperature. Clothing soaked with rain, snow, or perspiration can be just as dangerous.

- **Convection** refers to the transfer of energy that takes place when moving air (or liquids) disturbs molecules next to an object. It can be thought of as a property that aids in conduction. A person instinctively uses this principle when blowing on hot food to cool it. Likewise, air moving across the body surface can pick up heat and carry it away. The faster the air is moving, the faster it can remove heat from the body. The **wind-chill factor** measures the chilling effect of a given temperature at a given wind speed. For example, the chilling effect of a 30°F (−1.1°C) ambient temperature with a 35 mph wind is −4°F (−20.0°C) **Figure 38-4** .
- **Evaporation**, the conversion of a liquid to a gas, liberates 1 kcal per 1.7 mL of sweat. Sweating and heat dissipation by evaporation normally account for about 30% of cooling. Evaporation is the primary method of cooling in higher temperatures until a high humidity level slows the evaporative rate. It has a minor role via respiration. This phenomenon is also behind the evaporative method of cooling for heatstroke patients. In cold conditions, wet clothes can cause heat loss by conduction and, as they dry, further heat loss by evaporation.

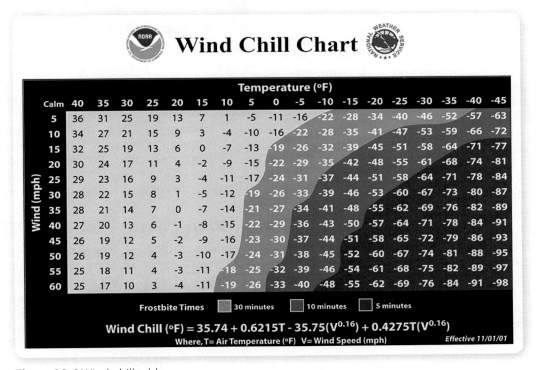

Figure 38-4 Wind-chill table.
Courtesy of the National Weather Service/NOAA.

Temperature (°F)

Relative Humidity (%)	80	82	84	86	88	90	92	94	96	98	100	102	104	106	108	110
40	80	81	83	85	88	91	94	97	101	105	109	114	119	124	130	136
45	80	82	84	87	89	93	96	100	104	109	114	119	124	130	137	
50	81	83	85	88	91	95	99	103	108	113	118	124	131	137		
55	81	84	86	89	93	97	101	106	112	117	124	130	137			
60	82	84	88	91	95	100	105	110	116	123	129	137				
65	82	85	89	93	98	103	108	114	121	128	136					
70	83	86	90	95	100	105	112	119	126	134						
75	84	88	92	97	103	109	116	124	132							
80	84	89	94	100	106	113	121	129								
85	85	90	96	102	110	117	126	135								
90	86	91	98	105	113	122	131									
95	86	93	100	108	117	127										
100	87	95	103	112	121	132										

Likelihood of Heat Disorders with Prolonged Exposure or Strenuous Activity

Caution | Extreme Caution | Danger | Extreme Danger

Figure 38-5 Heat index.

Courtesy of NOAA.

These four mechanisms require a thermal gradient between the body and its surroundings; that is, the mechanisms work only as long as the temperature of the skin surface is higher than that of the outside environment (and metabolism does not produce an overwhelming heat load) **Figure 38-5**. When the environmental temperature exceeds the skin temperature, the body absorbs heat. In those circumstances, the increase in blood flow to the skin becomes counterproductive because it promotes increased heat absorption.

The only way the body can dissipate heat when the ambient temperature approaches body temperature is by the evaporation of sweat, up to a point. A healthy adult can sweat a maximum of about 1 L/h. Furthermore, for effective evaporation of sweat, the ambient air must be relatively unsaturated with water. As the relative humidity increases, the rate of evaporation decreases; effective sweat evaporation ceases when the relative humidity reaches about 75%.

Thermogenesis

In a cold environment, the skin serves as the body's thermostat. If your skin is cold, your body will shiver even if your CBT is not lowered. **Thermogenesis**, the production of heat and energy for the body, is the primary method of dealing with cold stressors. In addition to normal heat production from the BMR and physical exertion, the hypothalamic center and sympathetic nervous system can increase muscle tone and initiate shivering in the short term and increase thyroid levels in the long term. The hypothalamus also stimulates peripheral vasoconstriction, thereby shunting blood to the core. The eccrine sweat glands receive cholinergic stimuli to decrease sweating. The thicker the outer shell, the better the insulation. All other factors being equal, heavier people are more effectively insulated from the cold.

Pathophysiology, Assessment, and Management of Heat Illness

Heat illness is an increase in CBT due to inadequate thermolysis. The fundamental problem is the inability to get rid of the heat buildup in the body, often because of hot and humid conditions. A person's general state of health, clothing, mobility, age, comorbidities, and certain medications **Table 38-1** can add to the problem. When the thermoregulatory system is taxed beyond its limits or fails for any reason, the CBT soars, sometimes rising from normal to about 106°F (41°C) in less than 15 minutes. That is the situation in heatstroke, for example.

▶ Risk Factors for Heat Illness

Certain factors increase a person's risk for ill effects from any given heat stress; the factors are summarized in **Table 38-2**. Older adults are at particular risk because they do not adjust as well to the heat: they perspire less; they acclimatize more slowly; they feel thirst less readily in response to dehydration; and their decreased mobility can affect the ability to obtain fluids. Older adults are also more likely to have chronic conditions, such as diabetes and cardiovascular disease, which can dramatically interfere with normal heat regulation. In addition, they are more apt to be taking medications that disrupt the body's mechanisms for dissipating heat.

Numerous medications can affect the body's ability to regulate its temperature. Diuretics may result in dehydration and electrolyte disturbances. These conditions

Table 38-1	Substances Contributing to Heat Illness

Alcohol
Alpha agonists
Anticholinergics
Antihistamines
Antiparkinsonian agents
Antipsychotics
Beta-blockers
Calcium channel blockers
Diuretics
Heroin
Laxatives
Lithium
Monoamine oxidase inhibitors
Hallucinogens
Sympathomimetic medicines
Thyroid agonists
Tricyclic antidepressants

© Jones & Bartlett Learning.

may then interfere with peripheral vasodilation needed for heat transfer. Beta-blockers can lessen a tachycardic response to heat stress, as can normal age-related decreases in maximum pulse rate. Acclimatization has numerous adaptive physiologic effects. It can decrease the likelihood of heat illness, but it takes days of a person performing controlled, progressive exertion in a hot environment to be effective.

Among young and healthy people, infants and young children are most vulnerable to heat stress when exposed to a hot environment. Children, compared with adults, have proportionally higher metabolic heat production, have a CBT that rises faster during dehydration, and do not dissipate heat as well owing to their smaller organ and vascular systems. Athletes and military recruits engaging in heavy exertion in hot conditions are also at increased risk.

The following subsections discuss the major types of heat illness Table 38-3 .

▶ Heat Cramps
Pathophysiology

Heat cramps are acute, involuntary, painful muscle spasms, usually in the lower extremities, the abdomen, or both, that occur because of profuse sweating and subsequent sodium losses in sweat. Three factors contribute to heat cramps: salt depletion, dehydration, and muscle fatigue. Heat cramps most often afflict people in good physical condition—for example, athletes, military personnel, and physical laborers. A recent study of US

Table 38-2	Factors That Predispose to Heat Illness

Factors That Increase Internal Heat Production	Factors That Interfere With Heat Dissipation
<ul><li>Physical exertion</li><li>Response to infection (fever)</li><li>Hyperthyroidism</li><li>Agitated and tremulous states (Parkinson, psychosis, mania, drug withdrawal—opiate and alcohol)</li><li>Drug overdoses (such as cocaine, caffeine, LSD, phencyclidine hydrochloride, methamphetamine, ecstasy)</li></ul>	<ul><li>High ambient temperature</li><li>High humidity</li><li>Obesity (insulation effect, less efficient dissipation)</li><li>Impaired vasodilation</li><li>Diabetes</li><li>Alcoholism</li><li>Drugs: diuretics, tranquilizers, beta-blockers, antihistamines, phenothiazines, antidepressants</li><li>Impaired ability to sweat (cystic fibrosis, skin diseases, healed burns)</li><li>Heavy or tight clothing (especially PPE)</li></ul>
Factors That Increase Heat Absorption	**Factors That Impair the Body's Response to Heat Stress**
<ul><li>Confined, unventilated, hot living quarters</li><li>Working in hot conditions</li><li>Being in non–air conditioned parked automobiles in high temperatures</li></ul>	<ul><li>Dehydration (including recent GI or respiratory infections)</li><li>Prior episode of heatstroke</li><li>Hypokalemia</li><li>Cardiovascular disease</li><li>Previous stroke or other central nervous system lesion</li></ul>

Abbreviations: GI, gastrointestinal; LSD, lysergic acid diethylamide; PPE, personal protective equipment
© Jones & Bartlett Learning.

Table 38-3	Comparing Conditions Resulting From Heat Stress		
Variable	**Heat Cramps**	**Heat Exhaustion**	**Heatstroke**
Pathophysiology	Sodium and water loss	Sodium and water loss, hypovolemia	Failure of heat-regulating mechanisms
Mental and neurologic status	Normal	Normal or mild confusion	Altered, delirium, seizures
Temperature	May be mildly elevated	Usually mildly elevated	Usually >104°F (40.0°C)
Skin	Cool, moist	Pale, cool, moist	Dry, hot, but sweating may persist, especially with exertional heatstroke
Muscle cramping	Severe	May or may not be present	Absent

© Jones & Bartlett Learning.

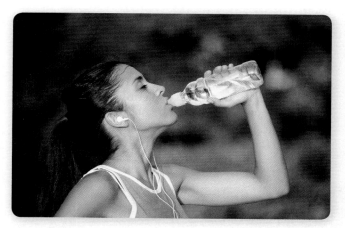

Figure 38-6 If you drink plain water, you will not replace sweat sodium losses.

© Peter Bernik/Shutterstock.

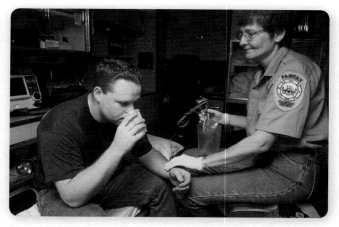

Figure 38-7 Give the patient with heat cramps one or two glasses of a salt-containing solution if he or she is not nauseated.

© Jones & Bartlett Learning.

college football players showed a twofold increase in sweat sodium losses in athletes prone to heat cramps.[9] Usually a person exerting himself or herself in a hot environment will become thirsty and will increase fluid intake. But if the person is sweating heavily, he or she is losing fluids and salt through the skin. If the person drinks plain water, then he or she will not replace sweat sodium losses **Figure 38-6** . Note that this principle is equally important for EMS support services, such as the rehabilitation sector for a wildland fire operation, which should have approved electrolyte solutions available instead of just plain water.

Assessment

Heat cramps usually start suddenly during strenuous and/ or prolonged physical activity. They may be mild, characterized by only slight abdominal cramping and tingling in the extremities. More often, however, the patient presents

with severe pain in the extremities and abdomen and may have nausea. Patients with heat cramps remain alert. The pulse is generally rapid, the skin pale and moist, and the temperature normal.

Management

Treatment of heat cramps aims to eliminate the exposure and restore lost salt and water to the body:

- Move the patient to a cool environment. Have the patient lie down if he or she feels faint.
- If the patient is not nauseated, give one or two glasses of a balanced electrolyte liquid. **Figure 38-7** . Instruct the patient to drink the solution slowly. Have the patient munch on salty chips or pretzels. Salt tablets can irritate the stomach lining and may precipitate or worsen nausea.

- If the patient is too nauseated to take liquids by mouth, then insert an intravenous (IV) catheter and infuse normal saline (NS).
- Do not massage the cramping muscles; this may actually aggravate the pain.
- As the patient's salt balance is restored, the symptoms will abate and the patient may want to resume activity. In the field, this decision is best made with medical control.

▶ Heat Syncope

Pathophysiology

Heat syncope is an orthostatic syncopal, or near-syncopal, episode that typically occurs in nonacclimated people who may be under heat stress. Whereas older adults are certainly at higher risk, they are also at higher risk for cardiac syncope and atypical acute coronary syndromes, and due caution is advisable. Heat syncope can occur with prolonged standing, as in mass outdoor gatherings, or when standing suddenly from a sitting or lying position. One of the body's thermoregulatory functions is peripheral vasodilation. The causes are thought to be an upright posture in which gravity causes dependent pooling of blood, which can also possibly be exacerbated by some degree of dehydration and/or hypokalemia.

Assessment and Management

Treatment involves placing the patient in a supine position and replacing fluid deficits. If the patient does not recover quickly in the supine position, then consider other differentials, which may include heatstroke, cardiac syncope, or atypical acute coronary syndromes.

▶ Heat Exhaustion

Pathophysiology

Heat exhaustion is a clinical syndrome thought to represent a milder form of heat illness on a continuum leading to heatstroke. Its hallmarks are volume depletion and heat stress. Classically, two forms are described: water-depleted and sodium-depleted. Water-depleted heat exhaustion occurs primarily in geriatric patients owing to immobility, medications that contribute to dehydration, and decreased thirst sensitivity and in active younger workers or athletes who do not adequately replace fluids in a hot environment. Sodium-depleted heat exhaustion results from huge sodium losses from sweating but replacing only free water, not sodium.

A concept closely related to sodium-depleted heat exhaustion is **exercise-associated hyponatremia (EAH)**. Studies from the Boston Marathon, the Grand Canyon National Park, and the military point to a common thread: prolonged exertion usually in a hot environment coupled with excessive fluid intake.[10-12] Most victims have too much water in their bodies in relationship to total sodium. Sodium is depleted with excessive sweating and/or excessive free water intake. This results in an imbalance of the sodium levels in the body's serum. The body tries to compensate by fluid shifting and moving fluids into the interstitial and intracellular spaces. Recent evidence also points to arginine vasopressin (AVP) as a contributing factor (AVP is a hormone that increases water absorption in the kidneys). The first symptoms are often nonspecific and include nausea, vomiting, weight gain, and headache. As the severity worsens, mental status changes (confusion, agitation, disorientation) become common. Cerebral edema, pulmonary edema, respiratory distress, seizures, coma, and death may ensue if the condition goes untreated or unrecognized. This situation and the increasing prevalence of EAH are partly a result of a recommendation that prevailed over the past decades—to drink before becoming thirsty. It was commonly taught that the threshold where thirst appears signifies that the person has already passed into early dehydration. Outdoorspeople and athletes were encouraged to drink prescribed amounts of liquids to prevent this. It is now known that no single recommendation fits all people under all conditions in terms of fluid, salt, and electrolyte consumption. The current, evidence-based consensus recommendation from the Wilderness Medical Society (WMS) is ad libitum fluid intake—allowing thirst to drive the extent of drinking—to avoid excessive fluid intake *or* serious dehydration.[13]

Evidence-Based Medicine

The WMS now teaches ad libitum fluid intake—allowing thirst to drive the extent of drinking—to avoid excessive fluid intake *or* serious dehydration.[13] This replaces the teaching that thirst was a sign that occurred too late to be used to dictate hydration.

Remain alert for older, debilitated adult patients (who may simply be hyponatremic without the exercise-induced component) and patients who participate in endurance sports of more than three hours' duration, such as marathons and Ironman competitions. The Third International Exercise-Associated Hyponatremia Consensus Development Conference, held in 2015, recommended that patients with exercise-associated hyponatremia and signs or symptoms of encephalopathy should be treated immediately with a bolus infusion of 3% sodium chloride (NaCl) to acutely reduce brain edema. Additional 3% NaCl bolus infusions should be administered if there is no clinical improvement.[14] If local protocols do not permit you to administer 3% NaCl, then confirmed EAH is a contraindication to administration of hypotonic fluids (such as ½NS), isotonic fluids (such as NS), or lactated Ringer solution, all of which can worsen the patient's condition. To aid in confirmation of EAH, these experts also state that a mechanism for measuring serum sodium on site of athletic events or responses is optimal, but acknowledge that capability is not always practical or possible.[14]

Be aware that rapid transport to the ED may be mandated based on the patient's presenting symptoms and history.

Assessment

Symptoms of heat exhaustion can be nonspecific and may include headache, fatigue, weakness, dizziness, nausea, vomiting, and, sometimes, abdominal cramping. The patient is usually sweating profusely, and the skin is pale and clammy. The core temperature may be normal or slightly elevated (less than 104°F [40°C]). Tachycardia is present, although this response may be blunted if the patient is taking a beta-blocker or other heart rate-limiting medication. Respirations are fast and shallow. Tachypnea may produce symptoms of hyperventilation: carpopedal spasm, perioral numbness, and a low end-tidal carbon dioxide level (ETCO$_2$). Blood pressure may be decreased due to peripheral pooling of blood or volume depletion; if not decreased at rest, blood pressure will almost certainly drop when the patient tries to sit or stand from a recumbent position (**orthostatic hypotension**). If the patient reports brown urine, then you should suspect rhabdomyolysis (the destruction of muscle tissue leading to a release of potassium and myoglobin).

Heat exhaustion is sometimes mistaken for "summer flu," and the condition may be misdiagnosed. If left untreated, then heat exhaustion may progress to heatstroke. Older adult patients with primary gastrointestinal (GI) infections (nausea/vomiting and diarrhea) may be mistaken for experiencing heat exhaustion especially if they are found in a hot environment. However, be cautious because GI symptoms can also occur with heatstroke.

Management

The treatment of heat exhaustion is aimed at removing the patient from exposure to heat and repairing the derangement in fluid and electrolyte balance:

- Move the patient to a cool environment; remove excess clothing, and place supine.
- If the patient's temperature is elevated, then sponge, spray, or drip the patient with tepid water and fan gently to make him or her more comfortable—but do not overdo it. Heroic measures to rapidly lower body temperature are unnecessary, and chilling the patient can cause shivering and thermogenesis.
- Consider specially designed cooling chairs for hand and forearm immersion in cold water for rehabilitation at fire scenes, mass gatherings, and endurance sports.
- Most commercial sports drinks have excessive carbohydrates—oral hydration solutions should not be more than 6% carbohydrate. You can make an oral rehydration solution by mixing 1 teaspoon of salt and 2 tablespoons of sugar with 1 quart (1 liter) of water. If nausea and vomiting are present, then start a normal saline IV line and

draw blood for electrolyte determinations. Use the pulse rate and blood pressure to guide the fluid amounts administered.
- If exercise-associated hyponatremia is suspected, then do not give fluids by mouth. Instead, draw blood for checking the blood sodium level and administer IV normal saline or hypertonic saline following local protocols.
- Monitor cardiac rhythm, vital signs, and temperature.
- If you cannot determine whether the patient has heat exhaustion or heatstroke, then use a thermometer, and if elevated CBT, treat for heatstroke. You may also want to consider administration of an antiemetic (eg, ondansetron [Zofran]).

Controversies

The actual diagnosis of heat exhaustion versus heatstroke can be challenging, and there is a great deal of overlap in signs and symptoms. This determination is further complicated if the patient already has a preexisting altered mental status and the fact that the patient may continue to sweat. The safest and easiest way to differentiate between the two conditions is to remember heatstroke involves an elevated temperature and an altered mental status.

▶ Heatstroke

Pathophysiology

Of all heat illnesses, **heatstroke** is the least common but the deadliest. It is caused by a severe disturbance in the body's thermoregulation and is a profound emergency, with mortality rates as high as 10% in treated patients and 30% to 80% in untreated patients.[15] Emergency diagnosis typically depends on two findings: elevated core temperature and altered mental status.

As would be expected, the pathophysiologic consequences are related to the effects of elevated temperatures on the body's cells. This is evidenced by disruption of cell membranes, adenosine triphosphate transport channels, enzymes, breakdown of muscle cells (as evidenced by the presence of elevated serum creatine phosphokinase and presence of the muscle protein myoglobin in the urine), and electrolyte disturbances. Heat-labile proteins break down and lead to edema and hemorrhage. This increased vascular permeability leads to decreased cardiac output, hypotension, and shock. Loss of sweating is a consequence, not a cause of heatstroke.

Two heatstroke syndromes are distinguished: classic and exertional Table 38-4 . **Classic heatstroke** (passive heatstroke), which usually occurs during heat waves, is most likely to strike very old, very young, or people with reduced mobility. Patients with chronic illnesses, such as diabetes or heart disease, are particularly susceptible, as

Table 38-4	Classic Versus Exertional Heatstroke	
Characteristic	**Classic Heatstroke**	**Exertional Heatstroke**
Age	Older	Younger
General health	Chronic diseases, schizophrenia	Healthy person
Medications	Beta-blockers, diuretics, anticholinergics	Often none, consider stimulant abuse
Activity	Very little to bedridden	Strenuous
Sweating	May be absent	Present
Skin	Hot, red, dry	Moist, pale
Blood glucose level	Normal or high	Hypoglycemic
Rhabdomyolysis	Rare	Common
Acute renal failure	Rare	Common

© Jones & Bartlett Learning.

are people with alcoholism and patients taking certain medications (diuretics, sedatives, anticholinergics). In this syndrome, high environmental temperatures initially elicit thermolysis, but heat dissipation strategies begin to fail. The CBT rises as dehydration worsens and the body can no longer sweat as it seeks to retain fluids to ensure adequate perfusion. This leads to the typical signs and symptoms of heatstroke. Some research has shown that being confined to a bed, not leaving home daily, and not being able to care for oneself are the greatest risk factors of death during heat waves. Preexisting psychiatric illness tripled the risk of death followed by cardiovascular and pulmonary diseases.[16]

Exertional heatstroke is typically an illness of young people exercising in hot and humid conditions. When the ambient temperature approaches body temperature, radiation and convection are no longer effective means of shedding excess heat. If the relative humidity rises above 75%, then evaporative cooling becomes ineffective. People who continue exercising in such conditions will continue generating heat without any means of releasing that heat. They often sweat profusely. Heat will then build up within the body, causing the CBT to rise rapidly. This is a common scenario with high school or college athletes, military recruits, and others participating in intense, prolonged activity in hot and/or humid conditions.

Assessment

Both types of heatstroke present with similar signs and symptoms, which may or may not be recognized as the consequence of heat exposure. Patients most likely will not be able to give a coherent history because they will be confused, delirious, or comatose. Often the earliest signs of heatstroke are changes in behavior—irritability, combativeness, signs the patient is hallucinating—which may mislead bystanders and EMS workers into thinking the patient is having a behavioral or substance-related emergency. Older adult patients with heatstroke may present with signs resembling those of a suspected stroke, including trouble walking, talking, or using an arm or leg. Other CNS disturbances that commonly occur are seizures and constricted pupils.

> **Words of Wisdom**
>
> Suspect heatstroke and check CBT in any person behaving strangely in a hot environment.

The diagnostic vital sign is, of course, a markedly elevated body temperature, usually of greater than 104°F (40.0°C). However, it may be lower and, thus, misleading if any cooling techniques have been undertaken by bystanders. Never assume that a temperature of 104°F (40.0°C) is required for the diagnosis of heatstroke. Signs of a hyperdynamic state are usually present: tachycardia, hyperventilation with a lowered ETCO$_2$, and lowered peripheral vascular resistance from efforts of the body to cool itself with vasodilation. Heatstroke is characterized by some degree of dehydration that worsens the problem by decreasing the body's ability to get the hotter core blood to the periphery for thermolysis. Blood pressure can be normal or decreased depending on the level of dehydration. The skin can be dry, red, and hot in classic heatstroke or pale and sweaty in exertional heatstroke. However, the presence or absence of sweating is not important! If the patient's temperature is markedly elevated and he or she has an altered mental status, assume heatstroke regardless of whether the patient is sweating or not.

The diagnosis of heatstroke is easy to miss. It may develop rapidly in a patient whose heat exhaustion was mistaken for the flu, or it may present as coma of unknown origin. Unless you keep the possibility of heatstroke in mind during the hot months of the year or in conditions of extreme temperatures and assess the patient's temperature as part of the vital signs, you may waste precious time searching for some other cause of the patient's symptoms.

Fever and Conditions That Mimic Heatstroke. New paramedics may face a perplexing challenge: Why is this nursing home patient's temperature elevated? Is it heatstroke, a febrile illness, or sepsis? Neurologic changes can be present in all three situations. The history, however, may suggest infectious causes. For example, is there a change in the urine color in a catheter bag, a recent complaint of cough and dyspnea, or an obvious skin infection? Complaints of a fever, rash, photophobia, and stiff neck may point to meningitis. An intermittent shaking chill also favors infectious causes of increased temperature.

A fever can signal that the body is fighting an infection by inhibiting reproduction of harmful toxins. Pyrogens (proteins secreted by infective organisms and the body's immune system) act on the hypothalamus by increasing the thermal set point, which results in a fever. The body then uses its thermoregulatory tools to maintain the new temperature setting. The patient with a reset temperature may adapt to this change by wearing more clothes, and sometimes the body creates more heat via shivering. Although aspirin and nonsteroidal anti-inflammatory drugs can lower a fever (by blocking prostaglandins), they are dangerous to use when you are treating heat illnesses and are not recommended.[17]

Anticholinergic poisoning presents with an elevated temperature; dry, red skin; mental status changes; and tachycardia. Anticholinergic poisonings usually cause dilated pupils, whereas patients with heatstroke usually have constricted pupils.

Two rare syndromes also cause hyperthermia. **Neuroleptic malignant syndrome (NMS)** is caused by antipsychotic and some antiemetic medications, and patients present with hyperthermia, muscular rigidity, altered mental status, and a hyperdynamic state. **Malignant hyperthermia** can occur as a result of common anesthesia medications (notably succinylcholine) and presents similarly to NMS. Fever is a very late finding and ETCO$_2$ may be an earlier and more effective diagnostic tool to recognizing malignant hyperthermia. Researchers are exploring a common genetic contributor to malignant hyperthermia and heatstroke.

Management

If you are unsure about what exactly is causing the patient's elevated temperature, the prudent step is for you to treat for heatstroke because of the deadly consequences of missing the diagnosis. Online medical control may also help you with treatment plans.

Heatstroke treatment requires two things: removing the patient from the offending environment and rapid cooling. The main methods used for rapid cooling are total immersion of the body in cold or ice water and evaporative cooling by spraying cold or cool water over the patient accompanied by the use of fans to promote convection. Further, dousing patients with water or spraying them with a mist and fanning them was found to be acceptable. Ineffective methods included ice packs alone or in combination with fanning, fanning without use of water, and cooling blankets. Evidence-based guidelines

YOU are the Paramedic   PART 2

The patient remains slow to respond, but is alert and oriented to person, place, time, and event. He continues to shiver as you dry him off, examine him, and cover him with dry blankets. His skin is pale, cold, and slightly moist.

His head, neck, and back are unremarkable. Besides his report that he is "aching all over," he reports pain to his hands, fingers, feet, and toes. He has absent distal pulses, is unable to move his toes on command, and cannot feel you touch his toes. His fingers and toes are soft to the touch. He moves his lower extremities on command, but they are weak and uncoordinated. The patient reveals no health history.

Recording Time: 10 Minutes	
Level of consciousness	Alert (oriented to person, place, time, and event), but slow to respond
Respirations	10 breaths/min; slow and shallow
Pulse	104 beats/min; weak and irregular
Skin	Cold, pale, and slightly moist
Blood pressure	80/40 mm Hg
Oxygen saturation (Spo$_2$)	95% on room air

4. What do these physical findings indicate to you?
5. Why is his shivering significant?
6. What can you conclude from the patient's vital signs?

from the American College of Sports Medicine reiterate the importance of rapid cooling first, then providing transport.[18] Obvious limitations include the need for ice and responsive patients not tolerating this measure well. A summary of treatment for heatstroke is as follows:

- Evaluate the ABCDEs (Airway, Breathing, Circulation, Disability, Exposure) as needed, administer supplemental oxygen, consider sedation if the patient is agitated or combative, and be prepared to intubate.
- Move the patient to a cool environment, and remove the patient's clothes. Cooling efforts should continue until the rectal temperature reaches about 102°F (38.9°C). Further aggressive cooling can overshoot or cause shivering.
- Cool as rapidly as possible by the most expeditious means available:
  - Consider ice water immersion as a rapid cooling method, especially when circulating the water to pull heat away from the patient. Cooling with ice water–soaked blankets and fanning is nearly as effective as immersion. Pay close attention to airway status and watch for seizures.
  - Spray the patient with cold or cool water while fanning constantly to promote rapid evaporation. The ambulance should carry a portable fan during the summer months for this purpose or use a fire department ventilation fan.
- Start an IV line, administer normal saline, and check the blood glucose level. Be careful with fluids—pulmonary edema is a known complication of heatstroke. Remember that cooling promotes peripheral vasoconstriction that can raise the blood pressure.
- Monitor cardiac rhythm, and remember rhabdomyolysis can occur with resultant hyperkalemia.
- Be prepared to treat seizures with common antiseizure medicines (lorazepam, midazolam, or diazepam).

Evidence-Based Medicine

Recent research conducted at the University of Arkansas found the "TACO (tarp-assisted cooling with oscillation) method" an effective alternative to traditional immersion methods. In the study, rescuers had participants who had exerted themselves to a temperature of 102°F (39°C) lie down on a tarp. The rescuers then lifted the edges of the tarp and poured ice water over the participants. On average, body temperatures declined 0.25°F (about 0.14°C); this was a marked difference from the results of a second group of participants, who lay down on the tarp without the addition of ice water.[19]

Prevention of Heat Illness. Military organizations have understood the effects of heat illness for decades. They were one of the first groups to understand the importance of acclimatization. More modern contributions have included standards for conducting training in hot environments. Heat stress indices are a variety of scientific measurements that allow for an estimation of the effect of variables such as temperature, humidity, and wind speed on the ability to work in hot environments. These indices have applications not just for the military but are regulated for numerous industries and even scholastic sports.

The following measures can help protect you, your colleagues, and the communities you serve from heat illness:

1. Acclimatize whenever possible. Maintain personal fitness.
2. Limit time spent in heavy activity in PPE (eg, wildland duties in bunker gear), especially during the hottest parts of the day or season. Paramedics working in hot climates should have appropriate summer uniforms.
3. Maintain hydration, eat appropriately, and rest. Avoid beverages with a high sugar and caffeine content. Some ambulances are equipped with an on-board refrigerator for hot weather. Otherwise, carry a portable cooler, fill it about half full with crushed ice, and stock it with sports drinks or other salt-containing drinks for patients and the crew.
4. Develop or research standards on activities in hot weather from professional organizations (eg, National Fire Protection Association, Occupational Safety and Health Administration, American College of Sports Medicine, Wilderness Medical Society).
5. Improve your own physical fitness, both in terms of cardiovascular endurance and muscular strength.
6. Conduct community-based programs aimed at high-risk populations—for example, nursing home risk assessments and prevention programs.

Be alert for early symptoms of heat illness, such as headache, nausea, cramps, and dizziness. If you experience any of those symptoms, then immediately get out of the hot environment and get medical attention.

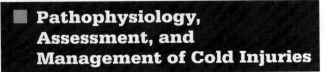

■ Pathophysiology, Assessment, and Management of Cold Injuries

▶ Local Cold Injury/Frostbite

Pathophysiology

Most injuries from the cold are localized to the extremities or exposed parts of the body, such as the tips of the

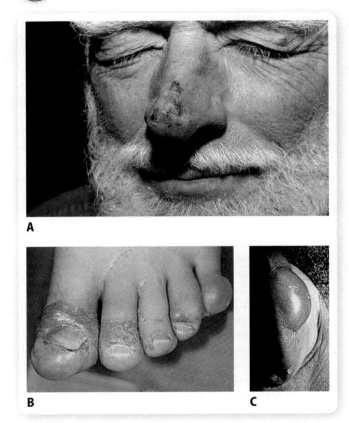

A

B   **C**

Figure 38-8 The tip of the nose **(A)**, the extremities **(B)**, and the ears **(C)** are particularly susceptible to frostbite.

A: © Dr. P. Marazzi/Science Source; **B and C:** © American Academy of Orthopaedic Surgeons.

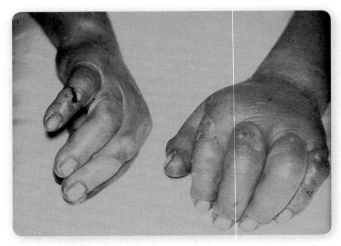

Figure 38-9 Frostbitten skin is hard and usually waxy to the touch.

© American Academy of Orthopaedic Surgeons.

ears, nose, upper cheek, and tips of the fingers or toes **Figure 38-8**. Local freezing injuries fall under the general heading of frostbite. **Frostbite** is an ischemic injury that is classified as superficial, partial thickness, or full thickness.

A mild form of frostbite, sometimes called **frostnip**, develops slowly and generally is not painful; however, the patient may report numbness. It is common among people who participate in winter sports. This problem is easily treated by firmly placing a warm hand over the chilled nose or ear. If the fingers have frostnip, they can be warmed by placing them into the armpit. The return of warmth to a frostnipped area is usually signaled by some redness and tingling. A warming technique called windmilling involves rapidly making a large circle with your arm and hand, starting with your hand next to your side, raising it backward and up until you are reaching straight up, and moving it rapidly down frontward. This technique forces blood into the cold hand.

Deeper degrees of frostbite involve freezing of tissues and can occur in ambient temperatures that are well below the freezing point. This freezing injury cascade starts with initial freezing of tissues with microvasoconstriction and local fluid shifting. Cells are composed chiefly of water, so when they are subjected to low enough temperatures, the water within them turns into ice crystals, causing cellular shrinkage and a hyperosmolar state. This problem is further complicated by increased viscosity accompanied by "sludging," poor flow, capillary leakage due to osmotic imbalance, and resultant thrombus and ischemic injury.

Risk Factors for Frostbite. Several factors predispose a person to frostbite:

- Cold exposure without adequate clothing
- Impeding the circulation to the extremities:
  - Wearing restrictive or tight clothing
  - Smoking, which constricts arteries
  - Drinking alcohol, which helps peripherally dilate blood vessels and causes diuresis
- Fatigue, dehydration, or hunger
- Coming in direct contact with cold objects (conduction)
- Hypothermia (experiencing generalized hypothermia is the most likely way to sustain a local cold injury)

Assessment

Superficial Frostbite. The most common symptom of **superficial frostbite** is an altered sensation: numbness, tingling, or burning. The skin typically appears white and waxy and has been compared with frozen halibut **Figure 38-9**. Because it is frozen, the skin is firm to palpation, but the underlying tissues remain soft. Once thawing occurs, the injured area turns cyanotic, and the patient experiences a burning, stinging sensation. Capillary leakage produces edema in the frostbitten area, though development of blisters (blebs) is more characteristic of deep frostbite. Dull or throbbing pain may persist for days or weeks after the injury.

Deep Frostbite. **Deep frostbite** usually involves the hands or the feet. A frozen extremity looks white, yellow-white, or mottled blue-white, and it is hard, cold, and without sensation. The major tissue damage occurs not from the

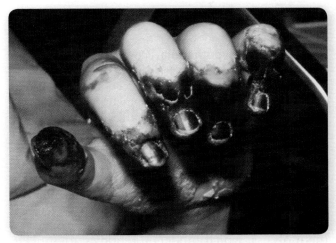

Figure 38-10 Gangrene can occur when tissue is frozen and chemical changes occur in the cells.

Courtesy of Dr. Jack Poland/CDC.

freezing of the tissues, but rather when the tissues thaw out. When tissues thaw slowly, partial refreezing of melted water may occur. Because these new ice crystals tend to be much larger than those formed during the original freeze, they cause even greater tissue damage. As thawing occurs, the injured area turns purple and becomes excruciatingly painful. **Gangrene** (permanent cell death) may set in within a few days, requiring amputation of all or part of the injured limb **Figure 38-10**.

Management

The prehospital treatment of superficial frostbite does not differ significantly from that of deep frostbite. Usually, it is difficult to determine the depth of the injury when you first see it. As the affected area is rewarmed, what was moderate or mild pain can become severe as the second phase of frostbite damage occurs: reperfusion injury. The most important factors at this time are distance to the hospital and whether the injured area has been partially or completely thawed before your arrival at the scene. If the area is still frozen when you reach the patient, you may opt to leave it frozen until the patient arrives at the hospital because rapid rewarming is difficult to carry out properly in the field. Contact medical control to discuss various options.

General principles include the following:

- Get the patient out of the cold. Take the patient indoors or into a heated ambulance depending on circumstances. Remove wet clothing.
- Do not rub or massage the frostbitten area; massage will cause further damage to injured tissues.
- Transport the patient to the hospital with the injured area elevated.
- Administer analgesia as needed.
- Cover blisters with a dry, sterile dressing.
- Consider rewarming only if the potential to refreeze does not exist.

Principles of rewarming are as follows:

1. If rewarming is agreed to by medical control, then rewarm the injured extremity (if hand or foot) before transport. To do so, you will need a water bath—a large, clean container in which the extremity can be immersed without touching the container's side or bottom. Water should be heated in a second container and then stirred into the water bath until the temperature of the bath is between 98°F and 100°F (about 37°C and 38°C). While you are heating the water, administer IV analgesia such as fentanyl or hydromorphone. The patient will experience severe pain as the limb thaws out, and you want to mitigate that pain as much as possible.

2. When the water bath has reached the appropriate temperature, gently immerse the injured extremity. Keep a thermometer in the water. When the water temperature falls below 98°F (37°C), temporarily remove the injured extremity from the bath while you add more hot water to the container. Stir the water around and keep adding more hot water until the bath is again in the appropriate temperature range; then reimmerse the injured extremity.

   The rewarming procedure typically takes 10 to 30 minutes. It is complete when the frozen area is warm to the touch and is deep red or blue (and remains red when you remove the limb from the water bath). While rewarming is in progress, keep the patient warm, preferably indoors, with insulated clothing and blankets. Do not permit the patient to smoke because nicotine causes vasoconstriction and, therefore, interferes with blood flow to the injured area. Do not allow the patient to ingest anything by mouth.

3. Once rewarming is complete, dry the extremity and gently apply sterile dressings. Use sterile gauze to separate frostbitten fingers and toes.

> **Words of Wisdom**
>
> Do not attempt rewarming in the field if there is any possibility of refreezing or if the patient must walk on the frostbitten foot.

▶ Trench Foot and Chilblains

Trench foot involves a process similar to frostbite but can occur at ambient temperatures as high as 60°F (16°C). It is caused by prolonged exposure to cool, wet conditions. The mechanism of injury can be explained by conduction: Wet feet lose heat 25 times faster than dry feet. Vasoconstriction and an ischemic cascade similar to that seen with frostbite then set in. Prevention—keeping the feet dry and warm—is the best treatment.

Chilblains describe itchy red or purple lesions usually on the face or extremities. These are believed to represent longer exposure to temperatures just above freezing.

Treatment is removal from environmental extremes and room temperature rewarming.

▶ Hypothermia

Pathophysiology

Hypothermia is defined as a decrease in CBT generally starting at 95°F (35°C), owing to inadequate thermogenesis and/or excess environmental cold stress. This definition is somewhat arbitrary because pathophysiologic mechanisms start at a higher temperature than 95°F (35°C). Extreme cold weather does not need to be present for a person to become hypothermic. For example, a geriatric patient with alcoholism who has had a stroke and is now living alone can become hypothermic in a home heated to 60°F (15.6°C). Other examples include an unprepared hiker caught in a summer wind and rainstorm or a person who becomes submerged in icy water Figure 38-11 .

Hypothermia is sometimes also called accidental hypothermia to distinguish it from therapeutic or induced hypothermia, which is a key step in the last link in the chain of survival for comatose patients with return of spontaneous circulation.

The body regulates cold stress by increasing thermogenesis, decreasing thermolysis, and pursuing adaptive behavioral changes. Simply put, vasoconstriction produces peripheral tissue ischemia. Continued drops in temperature cause the hypothalamic center to stimulate shivering. If cold continues, vasoconstriction is lost and then vasodilation occurs with loss of core body heat to the periphery.

Risk Factors for Hypothermia. People at risk for hypothermia have increased thermolysis, decreased thermogenesis, impaired thermoregulation, or other contributing factors. Many issues can lead to the development of a hypothermic condition, including cold temperatures, fatigue, improper gear for adverse conditions, wetness, dehydration, malnutrition, and the length of exposure and intensity of weather conditions Table 38-5 .

Alcohol is a common contributor to hypothermia.[20] It predisposes the patient to hypothermia by impairing shivering thermogenesis (decreased thermogenesis) and by promoting cutaneous vasodilation (increased thermolysis), which hinders the body's attempts to create an insulating shell around its warm core. Liver

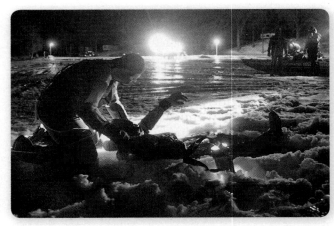

Figure 38-11 Patients who have been submerged in cold water are at high risk for hypothermia.
© Andy Barrand, *The Herald Republican*/AP Photo.

Table 38-5	**Factors That Predispose to Cold Illness**		
Factors That Increase Heat Loss	**Factors That Impair Thermoregulatory Mechanisms**	**Factors That Decrease Heat Production**	**Miscellaneous Causes**
■ Cold water submersion ■ Wet clothes ■ Wind-chill temperature ■ Impaired judgment from drugs or alcohol ■ Vasodilation from: • Alcohol • Acute spinal cord injury ■ Diabetic peripheral neuropathies	■ Dehydration ■ Parkinson disease or dementia ■ Multiple sclerosis ■ Anorexia nervosa ■ Central nervous system bleeding or ischemia, spinal cord injury with neurogenic shock ■ Multisystem trauma ■ Drugs interfering with vasoconstriction: • Alcohol • Benzodiazepines • Phenothiazines • Tricyclic antidepressants	■ Hypothyroidism ■ Age (very young or very old) ■ Hypoglycemia ■ Malnutrition ■ Inability to shiver and immobility	■ Sepsis ■ Meningitis ■ Overzealous heatstroke treatment ■ Overzealous burn cooling

disease, which leads to inadequate glycogen stores, and the subnormal nutritional status of most people with alcoholism further impair metabolic heat generation. Finally, alcohol impairs judgment, which often leads to inappropriate behavior in cold conditions. Impaired thermoregulation can also occur with therapeutic use or overdoses of sedative medications, tricyclic antidepressants, and phenothiazines, primarily by interfering with CNS-mediated vasoconstriction.

Older adults often cannot generate heat effectively because of reduced muscle mass and a diminished shivering response. Atrophy of subcutaneous fat cells also reduces an older adult patient's insulation against heat loss. Medications commonly prescribed to older adults may interfere with vasoconstriction as well. Hypothyroidism and malnutrition may further contribute to an older adult's vulnerability (decreased thermogenesis).

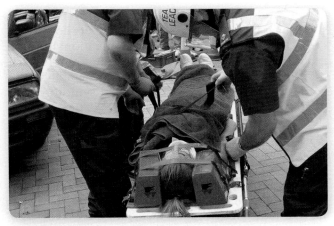

Figure 38-12 Trauma patients need to be moved to the stretcher as soon as is safe and medically appropriate. Place a blanket beneath the patient to conserve body heat.
© Jim Cole/AP Photo.

Words of Wisdom

Simply covering a patient hit by a motor vehicle and lying in the street is not good enough; body heat continues to be conducted away into the cold pavement. Quickly remove the patient from the street onto a patient transport device, such as a scoop stretcher or basket, and move to the ambulance.

The most important of the other factors contributing to hypothermia is trauma. Hypotension and hypovolemia can interfere with normal thermoregulation. Patients with CNS trauma, shock, and burns will not be able to mount a shivering response owing to the nature of their injuries. Last, hypothermia in trauma patients can lead to lethal coagulation problems and acidosis. If you are wearing protective gear in the cold, then ensure your ambulance is preheated, ask the patient if he or she is cold, and do what you can to conserve the patient's body heat **Figure 38-12**.

Special Populations

Older adults living alone should be checked on during cold spells. Education on preventing hypothermia can be done at community and senior centers. Infants and toddlers, who have a large head-to-body surface area, should always have their heads covered during the winter.

Assessment

The National Institutes of Health has initiated a public awareness campaign informing the public to watch for "umbles"—stumbles, mumbles, fumbles, and grumbles.

These behaviors are good indicators of how the cold affects the cerebral and cognitive functioning of patients in the early stages of hypothermia.

The 2014 WMS "Practice Guidelines for Out-of-Hospital Evaluation and Treatment of Hypothermia" defines mild hypothermia as a CBT of 95°F to 90°F (35°C to 32°C), moderate hypothermia as between 90°F and 82°F (32°C and 28°C), and severe hypothermia as below 82°F (28°C).[21] Some experts have proposed an additional level of severe hypothermia, representing CBT of less than 75°F or 68°F (24°C or 20°C). The American Heart Association (AHA) guidelines, most recently updated in 2015, define mild hypothermia as >93°F (34°C), moderate hypothermia as between 93°F and 86°F (34°C and 30°C), and severe hypothermia as <86°F (30°C).[22] These guidelines have been criticized, however, as being inconsistent with more standard classifications and emphasizing response to defibrillation (which is less likely to be successful below 86°F [30°C]), a single criteria, versus more universal and widely relevant physiologic changes present at each stage. It is important to emphasize that in the early, clinical stage of hypothermia, before the technical threshold for hypothermia has been met and when the CBT may still be greater than 95°F (35°C), the patient still may show obvious signs and symptoms of hypothermia. Fortunately, the body may compensate for this condition through thermogenesis until the patient finds a way to increase heat production or the glycogen energy stored in the muscles and liver is exhausted.

Hypothermia may also be classified according to the time to onset. Acute hypothermia occurs rapidly (as in cold water submersion), subacute hypothermia occurs over a short period (as in exposure to cold conditions during a short time), and chronic hypothermia may occur over days (for example, an urban homeless person or a poorly heated home with an older resident). In yet another classification, primary hypothermia is caused by cold exposures, whereas secondary hypothermia is due to problems such as severe sepsis.

In mild hypothermia, the hypothalamic-induced shivering is in full force and the "umbles" are noticeable: the patient develops fumbles (coordination and fine motor control problems), stumbles, mumbles (speech difficulty), and crumbles (incoherence, hemodynamic collapse). Often, however, the initial symptoms are vague. Older people may simply have a flatter affect, be slightly more confused, or develop symptoms suggestive of a possible stroke, including dysarthria and **ataxia**. No strong correlation has been observed between signs or symptoms and a specific CBT.

The net effect of hypothermia is to slow things down, but different body systems react in different ways. The overall slowdown of function is most dramatically apparent in the CNS, where just about everything slows—thinking, feeling, and speaking. A hypothermic patient is typically apathetic and often shows impaired reasoning ability. Speech is slow and may be slurred; coordination is impaired; and the gait is ataxic. These signs and symptoms may closely resemble those associated with stroke, head injury, acute psychiatric disturbance, or alcohol intoxication, which most likely explains why many cases of hypothermia are initially misdiagnosed.

In the cardiovascular system, hypothermia induces several changes. Initially, as peripheral vasoconstriction shunts blood to the body core, the body's volume receptors interpret the increased flow as an increase in volume. The sodium reabsorption mechanism becomes impaired, leading to an increase in urine output (**cold diuresis**). At the same time, cooling of the tissues induces a flow of water from the intravascular to the extravascular spaces. The net effects are to increase the viscosity of the blood, thereby impairing circulation, and to produce a state of hypovolemia. Meanwhile, the heart is being affected by the drop in body temperature. Cold initially speeds up the heart, then slows the rate and disrupts the electric conduction system. At a CBT of approximately 90°F (32°C), the body experiences cardiac dysrhythmias, including atrial fibrillation. A unique Osborn wave may be observed if shivering does not obscure the tracing **Figure 38-13** . Of special concern is ventricular fibrillation, to which a hypothermic heart becomes susceptible at a CBT of around 82.4°F (28°C). The 2015 AHA CPR, ECC, and

ACLS guidelines suggest attempting defibrillation once.[22] If ventricular fibrillation persists, the advice and evidence is unclear and treatment may include repeated attempts in conjunction with rewarming strategies.

Initially, the respiratory rate speeds up, but later it slows, leading to a decrease in minute volume. Tracheobronchial secretions increase, and bronchospasm may occur. Non-cardiogenic pulmonary edema may occur, especially in older adult patients. At 90°F (32.2°C), hypoventilation is profound, protective airway reflexes decline, and oxygen consumption decreases by about half.

The muscular system also slows down in response to cold. The initial muscular reaction to cold is shivering, one of the most powerful ways to increase body temperature (shivering raises core temperatures about 2°F/h (about 1°C/h). However, shivering can cause challenges because while it generates heat, it also makes skilled movements more difficult, uses large amounts of energy, stresses the cardiovascular system, and may be uncomfortable for the patient. Shivering, in any case, ceases around 91°F (32.8°C). Thereafter, cold muscles become progressively weaker and stiffer, impairing the exposed person's ability to save himself or herself.

Finally, cold affects the body's metabolism. Shivering can deplete the body of glucose, leading to hypoglycemia. Meanwhile, insulin levels fall, making further glucose metabolism impossible, so the body switches to the metabolism of fat. The liver's metabolism of drugs is also affected by the cold. Because medications are metabolized more slowly than normal, the effects of those drugs last much longer. A traditional treatment for hypothermia is to provide warm, sugar-containing drinks. The reason for this is not that the warmth of the drink will increase CBT. In fact, warm drinks do not significantly increase CBT (although they may provide psychological benefit). The primary benefit of this intervention is in the provision of carbohydrates to provide caloric support of shivering.

Management

This section first discusses general care and then explains how to manage cardiac arrest in a hypothermic patient. General care is aimed at preserving further heat loss and rewarming. The patient should be stripped of wet clothes and insulated from further heat loss. **Figure 38-14** illustrates recommendations for prehospital care.

Breathing Patients With a Pulse

Mild Hypothermia Cases (95°F [35°C]). The treatment is passive rewarming that involves removing wet clothing and drying the patient's skin. Depending on the patient's location and the relative ease of transport, you may have to promote heat generation by feeding the patient, giving warm, oral fluids with simple sugars (not containing caffeine or alcohol), and getting the patient to move about. Warm the ambulance for the patient and apply blankets. During transport, physiologically, the ideal patient compartment temperature is 82°F (28°C), the

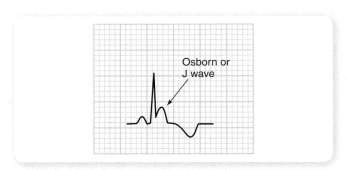

Figure 38-13 Osborn or J wave.
Reproduced from *12-Lead ECG: The Art of Interpretation*, courtesy of Tomas B. Garcia, MD.

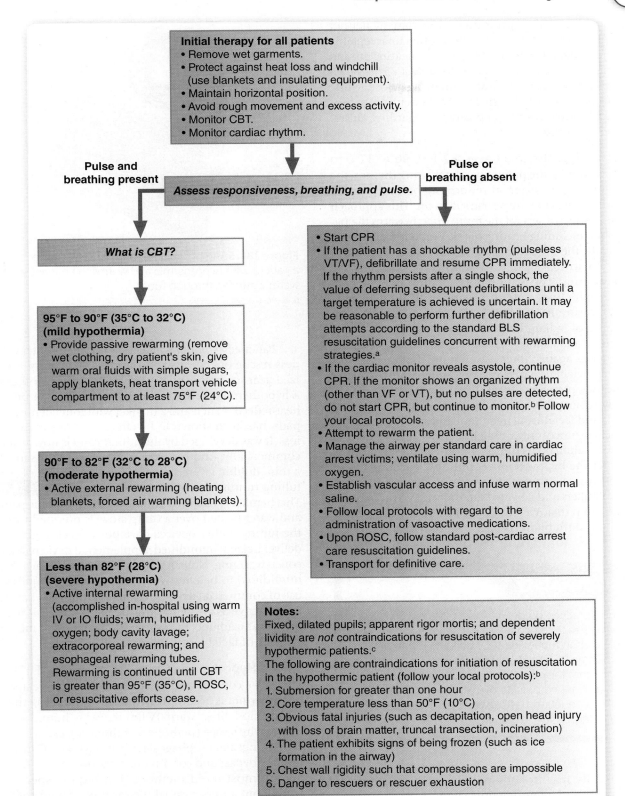

Initial therapy for all patients
- Remove wet garments.
- Protect against heat loss and windchill (use blankets and insulating equipment).
- Maintain horizontal position.
- Avoid rough movement and excess activity.
- Monitor CBT.
- Monitor cardiac rhythm.

Assess responsiveness, breathing, and pulse.

Pulse and breathing present

Pulse or breathing absent

What is CBT?

95°F to 90°F (35°C to 32°C) (mild hypothermia)
- Provide passive rewarming (remove wet clothing, dry patient's skin, give warm oral fluids with simple sugars, apply blankets, heat transport vehicle compartment to at least 75°F (24°C).

90°F to 82°F (32°C to 28°C) (moderate hypothermia)
- Active external rewarming (heating blankets, forced air warming blankets).

Less than 82°F (28°C) (severe hypothermia)
- Active internal rewarming (accomplished in-hospital using warm IV or IO fluids; warm, humidified oxygen; body cavity lavage; extracorporeal rewarming; and esophageal rewarming tubes. Rewarming is continued until CBT is greater than 95°F (35°C), ROSC, or resuscitative efforts cease.

- Start CPR
- If the patient has a shockable rhythm (pulseless VT/VF), defibrillate and resume CPR immediately. If the rhythm persists after a single shock, the value of deferring subsequent defibrillations until a target temperature is achieved is uncertain. It may be reasonable to perform further defibrillation attempts according to the standard BLS resuscitation guidelines concurrent with rewarming strategies.[a]
- If the cardiac monitor reveals asystole, continue CPR. If the monitor shows an organized rhythm (other than VF or VT), but no pulses are detected, do not start CPR, but continue to monitor.[b] Follow your local protocols.
- Attempt to rewarm the patient.
- Manage the airway per standard care in cardiac arrest victims; ventilate using warm, humidified oxygen.
- Establish vascular access and infuse warm normal saline.
- Follow local protocols with regard to the administration of vasoactive medications.
- Upon ROSC, follow standard post-cardiac arrest care resuscitation guidelines.
- Transport for definitive care.

Notes:
Fixed, dilated pupils; apparent rigor mortis; and dependent lividity are *not* contraindications for resuscitation of severely hypothermic patients.[c]
The following are contraindications for initiation of resuscitation in the hypothermic patient (follow your local protocols):[b]
1. Submersion for greater than one hour
2. Core temperature less than 50°F (10°C)
3. Obvious fatal injuries (such as decapitation, open head injury with loss of brain matter, truncal transection, incineration)
4. The patient exhibits signs of being frozen (such as ice formation in the airway)
5. Chest wall rigidity such that compressions are impossible
6. Danger to rescuers or rescuer exhaustion

Abbreviations: BLS, basic life support; CBT, core body temperature; CPR, cardiopulmonary resuscitation; IO, intraosseous; IV, intravenous; ROSC, return of spontaneous circulation; VF, ventricular fibrillation; VT, ventricular tachycardia

Figure 38-14 Prehospital hypothermia treatment algorithm.

Data from: [a]Web-based Integrated 2010 & 2015 American Heart Association Guidelines for Cardiopulmonary Resuscitation and Emergency Cardiovascular Care. Part 10: special circumstances of resuscitation. © 2015 American Heart Association. https://eccguidelines.heart.org/index.php/circulation/cpr-ecc-guidelines-2/part-10-special-circumstances-of-resuscitation/. Accessed May 4, 2017.
[b]Hypothermia. In: National Model EMS Clinical Guidelines. National Association of State EMS Officials. V.08-16. https://www.nasemso.org/Projects/ModelEMSClinicalGuidelines/index.asp. Accessed May 4, 2017.
[c]Zafren K, Giesbrecht GG, Danzl DF, et al. Wilderness Medical Society practice guidelines for the out-of-hospital evaluation and treatment of accidental hypothermia: 2014 update. *Wilderness Environ Med.* 2014;25(suppl 4):S66-S85.

temperature at which a normothermic patient neither gains nor loses heat.[21] However, this is often unacceptably hot for providers. The WMS recommends heating ground and air ambulance compartments to at least 75°F (24°C) in hypothermia cases to limit patient heat loss, while maintaining a reasonable operational environment for providers. Follow your local protocols regarding ambulance temperature.

Moderate Hypothermia Cases (82°F to 90°F [32°C to 28°C]). Assuming the patient has a perfusing rhythm, the treatment is active external rewarming because passive rewarming will generally not be sufficient. This approach involves the use of several means to directly warm the patient's skin, including heating blankets and forced hot air. Technically, the use of warmed IV fluids at temperatures from 102°F to 105°F (39°C to 41°C) is considered active core rewarming. The National Association of State EMS Officials guidelines state that warmed IV fluids ideally should measure 107°F (42°C). The 2015 AHA guidelines suggest use of radiant heat from hot packs placed in the groin, neck, and axillae.[22] However, the WMS specifically recommends against their use, arguing that they do not provide sufficient heat to affect core temperature to counter the risk they present of local thermal burns.[21] The WMS does advise hot packs be used to prevent local cold injury to hands and feet during treatment and transport. Follow your local protocols regarding hot packs. It is prudent to administer a fluid bolus (unless otherwise contraindicated) to counter the hypovolemia commonly encountered in hypothermia. Commercial warming devices that use special blankets and a heated fan unit can warm patients at a rate of up to 4.3°F (2.9°C) per hour, which is much faster than warm blankets (2.2°F [1.2°C]).

Patient Safety

In their practice guidelines, the WMS reminds EMS providers that charcoal HeatPac warming units can cause carbon monoxide (CO) buildup within patient compartments and should not be used in aircraft. In ground units they should be used only after the device has been ignited outside the vehicle and after initial smoke production has subsided, with ongoing CO monitoring.[21]

Carefully monitor the patient for direct thermal tissue injury and hemodynamic changes because active external rewarming measures can cause **afterdrop**. Afterdrop is the continued lowering of the CBT even after the patient is removed from the cold. In theory, it is caused by rewarming peripheral blood before the core is warmed, leading to peripheral vasodilation (rewarming shock), although inadequate fluid resuscitation may also play a role.

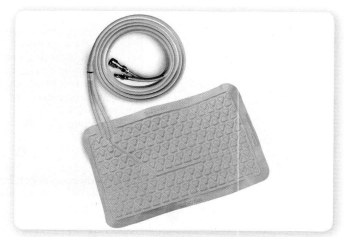

Figure 38-15 The hydraulic sarong can be wrapped around a patient with hypothermia and warms the patient via warm water fed through tubes.

Courtesy of Cincinnati Sub-Zero Products, Inc.

Paramedics working in regions in which winter wilderness rescue operations are routine should carry specialized gear for prehospital management of hypothermia. A hypothermia prevention management kit, comprising a heat-reflective shell and a blanket with four chemical heat pads, has been shown to be effective at preventing heat loss. It was developed by the military and is now available commercially. Another example, the hydraulic sarong, is a thin, double-layered blanket with a network of plastic tubing running between the two layers **Figure 38-15**. This blanket is wrapped around the hypothermic patient, and water heated over a camp stove is pumped through the tubing. Other devices have been developed to help deliver heated, humidified supplemental oxygen to aid in core rewarming. Note that the oxygen must be heated *and* humidified to be effective, which generally requires the use of commercial devices. Heated, humidified oxygen is not effective as a sole rewarming method, but it may be useful as an adjunct in combination with other methods. The risk of facial burns must be mitigated.

Severe Hypothermia Cases (Less Than 82°F [28°C]). The active core rewarming sequence used to treat severe hypothermia is accomplished in-hospital using the following modalities: warm IV fluids; warm, humid oxygen; body cavity lavage (peritoneal or thoracic); extracorporeal rewarming; and esophageal rewarming tubes. Cardiopulmonary bypass and continuous arteriovenous rewarming are the most rapid methods, but require specialized equipment and personnel. Rewarming should continue until the CBT is greater than 95°F (35°C).

Patients With No Pulse or Not Breathing

The 2015 AHA guidelines for basic life support (BLS) recommend CPR if no signs of life are present.[22] Rhythm identification should be rapidly accomplished. As mentioned previously, one attempt at defibrillation seems prudent. Other authorities argue that if there is an organized rhythm on the electrocardiogram (ECG), then CPR should be withheld because it represents a viable rhythm; follow your local guidelines. Establish IV access. Infuse warm normal saline. Attempt to insert an advanced airway, and ventilate with warm, humid oxygen. Commercial devices are available for both IV fluids and oxygen delivery. The 2015 AHA ACLS guidelines suggest "it may be reasonable to consider administration of a vasopressor during cardiac arrest according to the standard ACLS algorithm concurrent with rewarming strategies."[22] However, the 2014 WMS practice guidelines recommend that providers "not administer any vasoactive drug until the patient has been rewarmed to 86°F (30°C)."[21] Follow your local protocols regarding administration of vasoactive drugs.

Withholding and Cessation of Resuscitative Efforts

In the field, patients with obvious lethal traumatic injuries or those so solidly frozen as to block the airway or chest compression efforts generally are dead. If submersion preceded the arrest, then successful resuscitation is unlikely, with the possible exception of people who have been submersed in icy waters. Trauma, alcohol overdose, and drug overdose could have led to hypothermia in the first place and can hamper resuscitation efforts. Try to factor these conditions into your treatment decisions and seek medical control input. For example, a heroin user who was found outdoors and quickly recovers after naloxone administration requires a full set of vital signs, including body temperature.

Some providers believe that patients who appear dead after prolonged exposure to cold temperatures are not dead until "warm and dead." The effects of hypothermia may essentially protect the brain and organs if hypothermia develops quickly, a fact that is being used to successfully treat some cardiac arrest patients. Sometimes it may be impossible to know which came first—a cardiac arrest and then hypothermia or vice versa. In those situations, it is prudent to attempt resuscitation. Although a cutoff of 50°F (10°C) for possible survival of accidental hypothermia has been proposed, there is no compelling evidence or consensus that there is any single reasonable temperature below which a human cannot survive. However, there are clearly physiologic signs that indicate a patient is "cold and dead" with no chance of resuscitation. The WMS includes in such criteria obvious fatal injuries (such as decapitation, open head injuries with loss of brain matter, truncal transection, incineration), or a chest wall that is so stiff that compressions are not possible. It is worth noting that, according to the 2014 WMS practice guidelines, fixed, dilated pupils, apparent rigor mortis, and dependent lividity are *not* contraindications for resuscitation of severely hypothermic patients. Follow your local protocols regarding resuscitation.

Controversies

There is a widespread belief that rough handling of a hypothermic patient may cause the heart rhythm to change to ventricular fibrillation. Although people in severe hypothermia are prone to a ventricular fibrillatory arrest, it has not been clearly demonstrated that intubation or roughly handling the patient causes ventricular fibrillation. In fact, Danzl's multicenter hypothermia survey showed no case of ventricular fibrillation in 117 hypothermic patients who were intubated, although case reports exist of ventricular fibrillation occurring during endotracheal intubation of hypothermic patients.[23] Do not let concern for possible ventricular fibrillation prevent you from inserting an advanced airway or moving the patient if this is necessary in the course of care.

■ Pathophysiology, Assessment, and Management of Drowning

▶ Pathophysiology

According to the CDC, 46,419 drowning deaths were recorded between 1999 and 2010 in the United States, yielding an average of 3,868 deaths per year, or an average of about 10 deaths per day.[24] In the United States, drowning is the second leading cause of injury-related death among children younger than age 15 years, and is the leading cause of death in the group age 1 to 4 years, with 388 deaths in 2014 alone. In many countries it is the leading cause of accidental death in many age groups. The high rates of drowning in the United States and worldwide, coupled with the degree to which such deaths are highly preventable, make this a critically important topic for EMS injury prevention.[25,26]

The first task in understanding drowning is to define it. In 2002, the First World Congress on Drowning adopted a consensus definition,[27] which was subsequently endorsed by the World Health Organization (WHO), the International Liaison Committee on Resuscitation (ILCOR), and numerous other American and international organizations.[25] Their definition is currently the standard in medical science and clinical care and will be used here: **Drowning** is the process of experiencing respiratory impairment from submersion or immersion in liquid. Drowning outcomes include death, morbidity, and no morbidity. Terms such as near-drowning, wet, dry, and secondary drowning are confusing and while previously popular have no effect on care and should no longer be used.

People may live or die based on what happens when a liquid-air interface occurs at the airway's entrance. Consequently, the drowning continuum progresses from

Table 38-6	**Risk Factors for Drowning**

- Male sex
- Younger than 20 years (even higher for <5 years)
- Preexisting conditions, such as seizure disorder, mental/physical handicaps
- Alcohol use
- Ineffective safety barriers (gates, locks, or use of a solar cover on a pool)
- Hyperventilation (see diving section on shallow water blackout syndrome)

© Jones & Bartlett Learning.

breath holding, to **laryngospasm**, to the accumulation of carbon dioxide and the inability to oxygenate the lungs, to subsequent respiratory and cardiac arrest from multiple-organ failure due to tissue hypoxia. The patient can be resuscitated at any point along this continuum and generally speaking, the earlier the resuscitation takes place, the better the success rate.

Table 38-6 lists the risk factors for drowning. Note that toddlers typically drown in bathtubs, school-age children in pools, and teens in lakes or rivers. Comorbidities such as a seizure disorder or medical or physical handicaps may also contribute to drowning in an apparently safe environment such as a bathtub.

Drowning generally follows a predictable sequence starting when the victim cannot keep his or her face out of the liquid medium:

1. The length of breath holding depends on the victim's state of health and fitness, his or her level of panic, and the water temperature; duration of breath holding is shorter in colder water.

2. As water enters the mouth and nose, coughing and gasping ensue, and the victim may swallow considerable amounts of water. While some theoretic differences distinguish saltwater and freshwater drownings, this information is not clinically useful while you are resuscitating a patient. Both freshwater and saltwater can lead to pulmonary injuries, but the water composition does not significantly affect electrolytes or blood volume, as was previously thought.

3. After the step of coughing and gasping, one of two pathophysiologic paths is possible: laryngospasm or aspiration.

   a. In the laryngospasm path, water in the pharynx and laryngeal areas leads to spasms of the laryngeal muscles (laryngospasm). Laryngospasm leads to asphyxia—that is, a combination of **hypoxemia** (low oxygen levels in arterial blood) and **hypercapnia** (increased carbon dioxide in the blood)—and the patient may become unresponsive. Hypoxemia stimulates the body to shift from aerobic to anaerobic metabolism, with the ensuing production of lactate and development of metabolic acidosis. Eventually laryngospasm ceases and various amounts of water begin to enter the lungs.

   b. In the aspiration path, water enters the lungs before laryngospasm. Surfactant, a critical agent needed for gas exchange, is washed away, and the patient succumbs to the same effects of asphyxia (hypoxemia and hypercapnia). Historically, these were separated into the terms "wet" (aspiration) and "dry" (laryngospasm) drowning, with wet drowning estimated to occur about 85% of the time. This is a historical distinction of little clinical relevance. Consistent with the philosophy of the 2002 World Congress definition, researchers and clinicians (and EMS personnel) are discouraged from using "wet drowning" or "dry drowning" terminology.

4. It is believed that the initial hypoxic insult occurs from apnea; however, as time progresses, the lungs are injured directly in a process called **acute lung injury**. Here the lung tissue is directly damaged via complex biochemical processes (including dysfunction of basement membranes, and surfactant and cytokine damage leading to problems with the normal alveolar-capillary interface including fluid-filled airspaces and alveolar collapse). The net result is poor lung compliance and difficulty effectively ventilating and oxygenating the patient, leading to hypoxic brain damage. In addition, all of the deleterious effects of hypoxia on the myocardium may occur, including dysrhythmias and cardiac arrest.

▶ Assessment and Initial Treatment

To assess a drowning patient, you must reach him or her. People who have specialized training and experience in water rescue are best able to accomplish this task Figure 38-16 . Many fire departments and law enforcement agencies have water rescue teams, as does the US Coast Guard. The water rescue training should match the environment in question, which can range from swift water, to open water, to surf, all of which have different characteristics and rescue standards and techniques. Rescuers with no formal training should attempt rescue only by avoiding water entry and using other techniques (reaches and throws) to access a responsive patient.

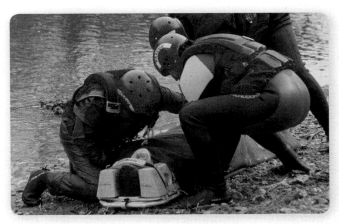

Figure 38-16 Rescuers must wear proper personal protective equipment, including a personal flotation device, when performing a water rescue.

© Jones and Bartlett Learning. Courtesy of Ellis & Associates.

When you reach the victim, the steps of treatment follow the usual sequence of ABCs (Airway, Breathing, Circulation). The first priority is establishing the airway. Cervical spine precautions should then be taken if necessary. The 2015 AHA ACLS guidelines recommend against routine cervical spine immobilization as this may hamper patient transport and care. The exceptions are patients who have a history of diving or using a waterslide, signs of injury, and alcohol intoxication. The 2014 WMS practice guidelines also recommend no routine cervical spine immobilization, and recommend that immobilization be considered only in settings of blunt trauma in association with any of the following:[28]

- Significant mechanism for cervical spine injury
- Altered mental status (Glasgow Coma Scale score <15; evidence of intoxication)
- Focal neurologic deficit
- Significant distracting injury

According to the WMS practice guidelines, patients without a pulse who are still in the water should be brought to a firm surface before CPR is begun in all circumstances. Rescue breathing and in-water resuscitation (IWR) under very specific circumstances may be warranted, and is endorsed by consensus statements from the International Lifesaving Federation, the US Lifesaving Association, the American Red Cross, and the Young Men's Christian Association, as well as the WMS practice guidelines. Requisite circumstances for IWR include extended distance from point of extrication, a patient with a pulse but inadequate breathing, presence of a flotation device (if in deep water), and a rescuer trained in IWR.[28] Always follow your local protocols.

Once a patient is brought to a firm surface, oxygenation and ventilation are the most important priorities. High flow oxygen should be administered to awake and alert patients in distress, and significant respiratory impairment, unresponsiveness, or apnea requires immediate ventilation.

▶ Management

Continue rescue breathing until the patient is on land. Once the patient is on a solid surface, start supplementary oxygen and at the same time quickly determine whether the patient has a pulse. A drowning victim, in accordance with 2015 AHA ACLS guidelines, continues to be treated according to the traditional ABC guidelines, as opposed to the CAB (Circulation, Airway, Breathing) approach used in most resuscitations, because of the paramount importance of establishing the airway and ensuring adequate ventilations in patients drowning due to non-cardiac causes. Once two breaths have been given, chest compressions are then started and continued in accordance with ACLS and Pediatric Advanced Life Support guidelines: establish IV access, administer indicated medications such as epinephrine, perform cardiac monitoring, and defibrillate any shockable rhythms. Note that only the patient's chest needs to be dried prior to automated external defibrillator (AED) placement; the entire body does not need to be dried. Additional drying of the patient can be performed when it will not delay further defibrillation attempts. Because ventricular fibrillation is rare in submersion, the AED should only be used in such a way that it does not interfere with the more critical interventions of oxygenation and ventilation.

Do not perform manual abdominal thrusts (Heimlich maneuver) to remove water from the lungs because they may displace water from the stomach into the lungs, increasing the risk of pneumonitis and subsequent lung infections. Suction may be used to clear the airway. Early advanced airway placement is indicated if BLS airway interventions fail.

Most drowning victims receiving rescue breathing or compressions will vomit; remove vomit from the mouth via suction, finger swipes, or other devices such as towels. Consider placing the patient on his or her side (or log rolling if on a backboard) to avoid aspiration. Most submersion patients have significant amounts of foam in the mouth and airway. The foam is mostly surfactant and debris and does *not* need to be cleared; it can be pushed back into the lungs during ventilation and will be reabsorbed.[29] Do not spend significant amounts of time trying to clear foam from the airway.

During normal, spontaneous breathing, the pressure in the airways at the end of exhalation is effectively zero. As a result, some alveoli normally collapse during the expiratory phase of the respiratory cycle. When there is widespread atelectasis—as in submersion—it is essential to maintain some positive pressure at the end of exhalation to keep the alveoli open and to drive any fluid that may have accumulated in the alveoli back into the interstitium or capillaries. Positive end-expiratory pressure (PEEP) focuses on maintaining some degree of positive pressure at the end of the expiratory phase of respiration. In the field, PEEP may be indicated for intubated patients who must be transported over long distances to the hospital after submersion. Several commercial devices are designed to allow PEEP via an endotracheal (ET) tube. In addition, portable ventilators usually have a PEEP setting.

If an ET tube has been inserted, then insert a nasogastric tube to decompress the stomach (discussed in Chapter 15, *Airway Management*). If a pulse is absent, then implement advanced life support measures similar to those used in any other case of cardiopulmonary arrest: establish IV access, administer epinephrine, and perform cardiac monitoring and defibrillation as indicated.

Patients rescued from submersion incidents are prone to bronchospasm from the irritation to their airways. If you hear wheezes, then administer a beta-2 adrenergic drug, such as albuterol by nebulizer, as you would for a patient having an acute asthmatic attack.[25] However, avoid corticosteroids because they are associated with adverse outcomes in drowning victims.[30]

Some drownings may have unexpectedly good outcomes with prolonged resuscitation, especially if the patient is a child and the incident occurred in very cold water. Successful resuscitation with complete neurologic recovery has been reported even in cases in which the victim had been submerged for more than 1 hour in icy water.[31] This is because hypothermia decreases the body's metabolic demand, likely protecting the body and brain from the effects of prolonged hypoxia. However, because hypothermia is more often dangerous than protective, remember to consider the effects of hypothermia on a drowning patient, including using the hypothermia algorithm. Do not forget to search for comorbidities, including trauma, hypoglycemia, acute coronary syndrome, cerebrovascular accident, or alcohol or drug intoxication.

YOU are the Paramedic   PART 3

Before moving the patient into the ambulance, you reassess distal pulses, sensation, and motor function. Oxygenation is supported by the placement of oxygen via a nasal cannula at 4 L/min.

En route you complete your secondary assessment, remaining suspicious about a possible head injury. Except for his frostbitten upper and lower extremities, his exam is unremarkable. The patient's fingers and toes remain soft, but sensation remains absent. The hands, fingers, toes, and feet are wrapped with bulky dressings to protect them. The patient rates his pain an "8" on a "0 to 10" scale. An 18-gauge IV line is established. The patient's blood glucose level is 48 mg/dL. Medical direction is consulted regarding fluid resuscitation, pain management, and glucose administration. Warm IV fluids are infused and a 500-mL normal saline bolus PRN is ordered. Dextrose 50% 25 grams IV push is administered, and morphine sulfate 2 mg IVP is given every 15 minutes PRN and as vital signs permit, titrated to effect. Heat packs are placed to his groin, neck, and axillae and the heat is turned up in the back of the ambulance. You transport the patient to a trauma center.

Recording Time: 20 Minutes	
Level of consciousness	Alert, still oriented to person, place, time, and event; able to respond quickly to questions
Respirations	12 breaths/min
Pulse	104 beats/min; weak and irregular
Skin	Cold, pale, and slightly moist
Blood pressure	89/54 mm Hg
Temperature	Oral, 87°F (30.6°C); rectal, 91°F (32.8°C)
ECG	Atrial flutter
Oxygen saturation (Spo$_2$)	98% while receiving 4 L/min via nasal cannula
Pupils	PERRLA
Pain scale	Visual analog scale; pain is an "8" on "0 to 10" scale

7. Why is the blood glucose reading of 48 mg/dL significant?
8. Would you support the patient drinking warm fluids?
9. What is the significance of his dysrhythmia?

Table 38-7	**Management of Submersion**

- Rescuers trained and practiced in doing so should perform the water rescue.
- Protect the cervical spine in cases of obvious trauma, diving, waterslides, or alcohol intoxication.
- Ensure basic life support measures are being carried out with an emphasis on airway and oxygenation.
- Anticipate vomiting; have suction immediately available.
- Administer supplemental oxygen and intubate if needed.
- Establish IV access.
- Measure core body temperature; prevent or treat hypothermia.
- Administer a beta-2 adrenergic for wheezing.
- Monitor $ETCO_2$ and pulse oximetry.
- Insert a nasogastric tube in intubated patients.
- Transport every submersion patient to the hospital, including patients who seem to recover at the scene.

Abbreviations: $ETCO_2$, end-tidal carbon dioxide; IV, intravenous

© Jones & Bartlett Learning.

Evidence-based guidelines adopted by ILCOR and the AHA maintain that length of submersion alone predicts survival. Of patients with submersion times less than 5 minutes, 85% have a good outcome, while patients with greater than 10 minutes of submersion have only a 4% chance of good outcome. Times greater than 25 minutes showed nearly universal poor outcomes.[32] This emphasizes the extreme time sensitivity of drowning care and removing the patient from a submerged state.

Paramedics have a unique opportunity to participate in injury prevention activities. This can be as simple as commenting on pool safety practices during a call, to more formal participation in community education and prevention programs. Table 38-7 summarizes the management of submersion.

Postresuscitation Complications

Adult respiratory distress syndrome, hypoxic brain injury, multiorgan failure and sepsis syndromes are common complications that can occur hours to days after a submersion. These factors highlight the importance of an emergency department evaluation of submersion victims. Their symptoms may be subtle (slight cough, mild tachypnea), or they may be asymptomatic. Patients may still die of drowning hours after the incident and after a period of apparent stability.

▶ Submerged Vehicle Incidents

According to the WMS, Project ALIVE, the Wilderness EMS Medical Director Course, and drowning experts, the current best evidence suggests that the safest time to escape from a submerging vehicle is immediately after it enters the water, during the initial floating phase, which usually lasts 60 seconds or less.[28] A sequence of steps has been established to ensure that occupants in a submerging vehicle prioritize egress strategies: seat belts, windows, children, out. These steps indicate that seat belts should be removed (one's own and anyone else unable to do it themselves), followed by opening or breaking windows, releasing children (oldest to youngest), then immediately exiting the vehicle.

Nearly every year, deaths occur while callers are on the phone with emergency medical dispatchers because they are not instructed to immediately exit the vehicle. At least one major prehospital dispatch system has changed its protocols to address this. Many people drown in submerging vehicles without contacting 9-1-1 and without exiting the vehicle. One reason is a prevailing myth that victims in a submerging vehicle should allow the passenger compartment to fill with water before attempting egress. This action is not evidence-based and is extremely dangerous.

When arriving on the scene of an actively submerging vehicle, attempt to remove the passengers from the vehicle as quickly as possible, usually through the rear window after breaking it. Attempt this only if you have adequate training for water entry and the circumstances are reasonable from a scene safety perspective.

■ Pathophysiology, Assessment, and Management of Diving Injuries

There are 3.5 million recreational scuba divers in the United States, not to mention people engaged in diving for commercial and military purposes.[33] Paramedics who work in coastal or lakefront areas in which diving is popular are likely to encounter a diving casualty; therefore, they should become familiar with diving medicine.

Four modes of diving are distinguished:

- **Scuba diving.** The most popular form of diving, scuba diving is named for the **self-contained underwater breathing apparatus** that the diver carries on his or her back.
- **Breath-hold diving.** Also called free diving, it does not require any equipment, except sometimes a snorkel.
- **Surface-tended diving.** Air is piped to the diver through a tube from the surface.
- **Saturation diving.** The diver remains at depth for prolonged periods.

All divers, irrespective of the type of diving they do, are subject to the increased ambient pressures that occur underwater. Injury results from the physical effect of these pressures on the body. To understand these changes, it is important to review how gases act under different physical conditions.

▶ General Pathophysiology: Physical Principles of Pressure Effects

Pressure, which is defined as force per unit area, may be expressed in a number of ways. The weight of air at sea level, for example, can be expressed as 14.7 pounds per square inch (psi), as 760 mm Hg, or as 1 **atmosphere absolute (ATA)**. The latter system—measurement in ATA—is most commonly used in diving medicine. Because water is much denser than air, relatively small changes in depth produce large changes in pressure. For every 33 **feet of seawater (fsw)**, the pressure increases 1 ATA. The depth of the dive can be used to estimate the pressure to which the diver was exposed: At sea level, the pressure is 1 ATA; at a depth of 33 fsw, the pressure is 2 ATA; at 66 fsw, it is 3 ATA; and so forth. The majority of scuba diving is done at depths between 60 and 120 fsw (3 to 5 ATA).

Liquids such as water are not compressible—that is, their volumes do not change with pressure. Because the body and its tissues are composed primarily of water, their volumes are not significantly affected by the pressure changes experienced in descent or ascent through water. Gas-filled organs are another matter, however, because gases *are* compressible and follow several physical laws:

- **Boyle's law** states that at a constant temperature, the volume of a gas is inversely proportional to its pressure (if you double the pressure on a gas, you halve its volume):

$$PV = K$$

where P = pressure, V = volume, and K = a constant. As a diver descends (and the pressure goes up), gas volume is reduced; as the diver ascends (pressure goes down), gas volume increases. As shown in **Figure 38-17**, this effect is most extreme near the water's surface. This law explains the barotrauma that can occur in gas-filled spaces in the body (including lungs, GI tract, sinuses, and parts of the ear).

- **Dalton's law** deals with the pressures exerted by mixtures of different gases. Dalton's law states that each gas in mixture exerts the same **partial pressure** that it would exert if it were alone in the same volume and that the total pressure of a mixture of gases is the sum of the partial pressures of all gases in the mixture. Thus, for fresh air:

$$P_{total} = P_{O_2} + P_{CO_2} + P_{N_2}$$

When total pressure increases, the partial pressure of each gas increases proportionally. This law helps explain **nitrogen narcosis**, oxygen toxicity, and the dangers of contamination in pressurized breathing systems. Because

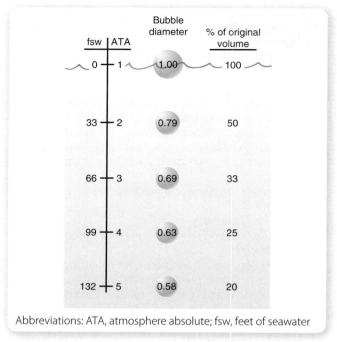

fsw	ATA	Bubble diameter	% of original volume
0	1	1.00	100
33	2	0.79	50
66	3	0.69	33
99	4	0.63	25
132	5	0.58	20

Abbreviations: ATA, atmosphere absolute; fsw, feet of seawater

Figure 38-17 Boyle's law: As a bubble descends through water, its volume changes in inverse proportion to the ambient pressure.
© Jones & Bartlett Learning.

the relative percentage of each gas remains constant at different pressures, it also explains why pulse oximetry readings in divers with nitrogen narcosis remain unaffected.

- **Henry's law** states that the amount (concentration) of gas dissolved in a liquid is directly proportional to the partial pressure of the gas above the liquid:

$$P = kC$$

Where P is partial pressure of the gas above the liquid, k is a constant, and C is concentration of gas in the liquid. A classic example of this law is when a sealed bottle that has dissolved carbon dioxide is opened. The opened bottle allows carbon dioxide to escape, lowering the partial pressure (P) of the gas. This forces the concentration of carbon dioxide in the soda to decrease as well, and the extra carbon dioxide escapes as bubbles. This law explains decompression sickness (the "bends").

Fresh air is composed of about 79% nitrogen and 21% oxygen. Nitrogen is an inert fat-soluble gas (it prefers to dissolve in fatty or lipid-rich tissues including the nervous system). Nitrogen in the body follows the laws described above. Per Boyle's law, the volume of nitrogen decreases as pressure increases (during descent) and its volume increases as pressure decreases (during ascent) leading to barotrauma. Per Dalton's law, the partial pressure of nitrogen increases as total pressure increases. Nitrogen at a high enough partial pressure becomes an anesthetic, leading to nitrogen narcosis at depths of around 100 fsw.

Per Henry's law, as pressure decreases during ascent, nitrogen comes out of solution in the blood and may cause bubbles in tissue, leading to decompression sickness, or the bends. Oxygen also follows these laws, and it can cause oxygen toxicity at depths via the same mechanism as nitrogen narcosis. However, because oxygen is taken up and metabolized by the body, oxygen does not contribute to decompression sickness.

To avoid the problems listed above, commercial divers use a decompression schedule to allow gases time to equilibrate. Recreational divers usually adhere to a "no-decompression" limit (a table outlining safe times at various depths) so they do not have to decompress on surfacing. Use of enriched Nitrox gas, which is a gas with a lower nitrogen and higher oxygen concentration, decreases the risk of nitrogen narcosis and **decompression illness (DCI)** (these illnesses will be discussed later), but it increases the risk of oxygen toxicity. Dive tables and dive computers provide guidelines for divers regarding when to take decompression stops during the dive, but they are not perfect. Even if divers follow recommended tables or use the appropriate gas mixture, they may still be at risk for any type of diving injury.

► General Assessment: Diving History

It is important for you to obtain as many details as you can about the dive and the onset of the patient's symptoms. As you obtain the diving history, it is helpful to use a special form that records the following information:

- When did symptoms start (during ascent or descent)? Decompression sickness will usually manifest within the first hour of surfacing and usually within 24 hours. If the patient flew after diving, then consider decompression sickness up to 72 hours afterwards. Symptoms occurring within 10 minutes of surfacing suggest air embolism, especially when they are accompanied by a loss of consciousness.
- What type of diving was done and what type of equipment was used?
- What type of tank was used (compressed air or a Nitrox system [combination of nitrogen and oxygen] with distinctive yellow and green stripes on the tank or a different mixed gas)?
- Where is the diving site, and what was the water temperature?
- How many dives were made during the past 72 hours, and what were the depth, bottom time, and surface interval for each?
- Was a dive computer used?
- Were safety stops used?
- Were there any attempts at in-water decompression (considered risky)?
- Were there any dive complications?
- What were predive and postdive activities?

► Injuries at Depth
Pathophysiology

Nitrogen narcosis ("rapture of the deep" or "narc'ed") is a state of altered mental status caused by breathing compressed nitrogen-containing air at depth. The human body does not use nitrogen for metabolism; thus, in a breathing gas mixture, nitrogen dilutes the concentration of oxygen. Nitrogen, which makes up 79% of fresh air, will also make up 79% of compressed air according to Dalton's law. When the pressure increases, the partial pressure of nitrogen increases as well. At a partial pressure of about 3.2 ATA, reached at about 100 feet, nitrogen begins to have anesthetic properties and divers may begin to feel the effects of nitrogen narcosis. It becomes more pronounced at 150 fsw, and is why sport divers should not use compressed air for dives of greater than 120 feet.

Assessment

Signs and symptoms include a euphoric feeling; inappropriate behavior at depth, including lack of concern for safety, apparent stupidity or inappropriate laughter; and tingling of the lips, gums, and legs. A diver may suddenly become panicked and spit out the regulator or surface too quickly. Divers report that they are able to better tolerate breathing compressed air as their diving experience increases.

Management

The only effective way to counteract the narcotic effect of nitrogen is to lower the nitrogen partial pressure through controlled ascent or use a mixed gas for diving with a decreased nitrogen percentage.

► Injuries During Descent and Ascent
Barotrauma

Pathophysiology. The major problem divers encounter during descent is **barotrauma** ("squeeze"). This injury results from a pressure imbalance between gas-filled spaces inside the body and the external atmosphere. Barotrauma can result from two different mechanisms: compression of gases within body spaces during descent or expansion of gases within those spaces during ascent (discussed later). Barotrauma can affect any gas-filled space in the body, including the sinuses, the inner and middle ears, and even teeth. Table 38-8 summarizes the types of barotrauma.

A person who is scuba diving is generally protected from barotrauma by breathing compressed air that matches the pressure of the surrounding environment. Thus, as long as the air-filled cavities of the body can equilibrate freely, they will not implode. This no longer holds true if there is an obstruction, such as with a sinus or ear infection.

As the diver ascends and the ambient pressure around him or her decreases, the gases within the body's air-filled spaces expand. As in barotrauma during descent, this

Table 38-8	**Diving Injuries (Types of Barotrauma)**			
Mechanisms and Pathophysiology	**Body Region**	**Condition**	**Clinical Features**	**Treatment**
During *descent:* compression of gas in closed spaces	Ear	External ear squeeze (*barotitis externa*)	Otalgia, bloody otorrhea	Keep ear canal dry; no swimming or diving until healed
		Middle ear squeeze (*barotitis media*)	Severe ear pain, tympanic membrane can rupture; emesis, vertigo, nystagmus; self-limited facial nerve palsy	Decongestants; no diving until healed, may need IV antiemetic
		Inner ear squeeze	Tinnitus, vertigo, hearing loss; emesis, pallor, diaphoresis	May need IV antiemetic medications, decongestants; surgical repair
	Paranasal sinuses	Sinus squeeze	Severe pain over affected sinuses and upper teeth, epistaxis	Topical and oral decongestants
	Face	Face mask squeeze	Ecchymoses and petechiae of skin beneath face mask; scleral/conjunctival hemorrhage	Cold compresses, prevent by forced exhalation through nose
During *ascent:* expansion of gas in closed spaces	Gastrointestinal tract	"Gas in gut" (*aerogastralgia*)	Colicky belly pain, belching, flatulence; rare pneumoperitoneum	Rare reports of rupture; usually, no care needed
	Lungs	Pulmonary barotrauma "burst lung," pulmonary overpressurization syndrome (POPS)	Dyspnea, dysphagia, hoarseness, substernal pain; subcutaneous emphysema around neck; pneumothorax, syncope	100% oxygen; decompress pneumothorax
		Arterial gas embolism (AGE)— complication of POPS	Altered mental status, vertigo, dizziness, seizures, dyspnea, pleuritic chest pain, sudden loss of consciousness on surfacing; sudden death	100% oxygen; transport supine; if air embolism suspected, place in left lateral recumbent position; hyperbaric therapy; consider steroids
Decompression sickness	Skin		Pruritus, subcutaneous emphysema, swelling, rashes	100% oxygen; observe for complications
	Joints and muscles	Bends ("pain-only bends")	Arthralgias, especially in elbows and shoulders, relieved by pressure	100% oxygen, analgesia; observe

Mechanisms and Pathophysiology	Body Region	Condition	Clinical Features	Treatment
	Cerebrum		Multiple sensory and motor disturbances	100% oxygen, hyperbaric therapy; IV fluids
	Cerebellum	The "staggers"	Unsteadiness, incoordination, vertigo	100% oxygen, hyperbaric therapy; IV fluids
	Spinal cord		Paraplegia, paraparesis, bladder dysfunction (inability to void), back pain	100% oxygen, hyperbaric therapy; IV fluids
	Lungs	Venous air embolism (the "chokes")	Chest pain, cough, dyspnea, signs of pulmonary embolism	100% oxygen, hyperbaric therapy; IV fluids
Dissolved nitrogen	Central nervous system	Nitrogen narcosis ("rapture of the deep")	Symptoms like those of alcohol intoxication	Controlled ascent to shallow water
Hyperventilation before dive	Central nervous system	Shallow water blackout (in breath-hold dives)	Loss of consciousness just before reaching surface	100% oxygen; assisted breathing

Abbreviations: AGE, arterial gas embolism; IV, intravenous; POPS, pulmonary overpressurization syndrome
© Jones & Bartlett Learning.

commonly affects the ears and sinuses. In one common scenario in which a diver has used decongestants before a dive, the medication may wear off before ascent. The increased mucosal swelling allows air to become trapped in the sinuses and ears, creating a "reverse squeeze" in which the increasing pressure cannot equalize during ascent. Symptoms are identical to those observed during descent.

Assessment and Management. If there is a blockage in the eustachian tube, which connects the middle ear with the nasopharynx, or if the diver cannot equalize ear pressures with a Valsalva maneuver, then the pressure in the middle ear cannot be equalized with that of the outside water. A characteristic "middle ear squeeze" syndrome then develops with severe ear pain. If the tympanic membrane ruptures, then nausea, vomiting, and vertigo may occur. This effect is especially likely in cold waters. At depths, this reaction may cause panic, rapid ascent, and the problems associated with such an ascent. Treatment involves a loose dressing for ear bleeding; some patients may require IV antiemetics or sedatives. Note that some symptoms, such as hearing loss and vertigo, may be a sign of decompression sickness.

Pulmonary Overpressurization Syndrome (POPS)

Pathophysiology. A more dangerous form of barotrauma can occur when divers fail to exhale during an ascent,

and pressure in the lungs is increased. The lung volume of scuba divers who have inhaled to their total lung capacity at a depth of 33 fsw (1 ATA) doubles by the time divers reach the surface if they hold their breath during ascent. This is likely to occur in an emergency ascent, for example, when divers panic due to difficulty with their equipment and give in to the instinctive impulse to hold their breath under water. The result is one of the worst forms of barotrauma of ascent—**pulmonary overpressurization syndrome (POPS)**, also known as "burst lung." It can cause pneumothorax, mediastinal and subcutaneous emphysema, alveolar hemorrhage, and a lethal **arterial gas embolism (AGE)**, discussed in the next section. Because the relative pressure and volume changes are greatest near the surface of the water, a small overpressurization—that produced by breath holding for the last 6 feet (2 m) of ascent, for example—can suffice to rupture alveoli. For that reason, all diving students are trained to exhale constantly as they are ascending so as to vent air from their lungs. People with chronic obstructive pulmonary disease (COPD) and asthma are at a slightly increased risk owing to their already altered air movement dynamics.

Assessment and Management. When alveoli rupture, the signs and symptoms depend in part on where the escaping air ends up. Most commonly, it leaks into the mediastinum and beneath the skin, causing mediastinal and subcutaneous emphysema. The patient may report a sensation of fullness in the throat, pain on swallowing (**odynophagia**), dyspnea, or substernal chest pain. When the patient speaks, he or she may be hoarse or have a brassy quality to the voice. Physical examination may reveal palpable subcutaneous air above the clavicles. Sometimes a crunching noise that is synchronous with the heartbeat may be audible by auscultation (called Hamman sign). Another less common result of alveolar rupture is pneumothorax; therefore, you should always look for unequal breath sounds, low pulse oximetry values, and hyperresonance on the affected side of the chest.

The prehospital treatment of a patient with pulmonary barotrauma depends—at least in terms of urgency—on whether the patient has an arterial gas embolism (discussed next). A diver with only pneumomediastinum and subcutaneous emphysema will most likely be managed symptomatically in the hospital. A pneumothorax may require needle decompression or a chest tube. In the field, provide 100% oxygen (by nonrebreathing mask; if you must bag the patient be careful—that is, do not give PEEP to a patient with POPS!) because it increases oxygen's partial pressure and may decrease bubble size and speed up "off-gassing."

Arterial Gas Embolism

Pathophysiology. By far the most dangerous possible consequence of POPS is AGE, which is second only to drowning as a cause of death among divers. Air bubbles from ruptured alveoli enter the pulmonary capillaries and coalesce into increasingly larger bubbles as they travel through the pulmonary veins back to the left side of the heart. From the left ventricle, these bubbles may enter the coronary arteries, producing all of the effects of acute myocardial infarction, including cardiac arrest. The vast majority of air emboli, however, rise to the head, generally the highest point in the diver's body, where they cause stroke-like symptoms within the cerebral circulation.

Assessment. The clinical picture of a patient with AGE tends to be dramatic. Symptoms usually appear within seconds or minutes (most commonly within 10 minutes) after surfacing and may involve just about any cerebral function. There is usually a history of panic or an uncontrolled ascent, although it can occur in shallow water. The patient may experience weakness or paralysis of one or more of the extremities, seizure activity, or unresponsiveness. A variety of other neurologic symptoms—including paresthesias, visual disturbances, deafness, and changes in mental status—are also reported.

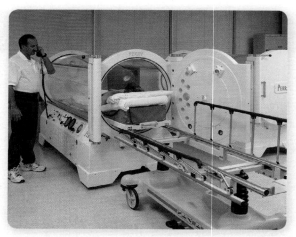

Figure 38-18 A hyperbaric chamber, usually a small room, is pressurized to more than atmospheric pressure and used in the treatment of decompression sickness and air embolism.
Courtesy of Perry Baromedical Corporation.

Management. If you suspect an AGE, then transport the patient to a hyperbaric chamber facility as soon as possible for recompression **Figure 38-18**. Treatment of a suspected AGE is summarized below:

- Ensure an adequate airway. Intubate an unresponsive patient with an advanced airway, but remember to fill air balloons with saline—not air—to allow for hyperbaric therapy.
- Administer 100% supplemental oxygen by nonrebreathing mask.
- Transport in a supine position. If you suspect an air embolism, then place in the left lateral recumbent position. Monitor/treat for hypothermia if appropriate.
- Ground transport is preferred to air owing to cabin pressures, but in general, the most expeditious form of transportation to a center capable of hyperbaric oxygen therapy should be utilized.
- Establish IV access, and administer normal saline solution.
- Monitor cardiac rhythm, and be prepared to treat dysrhythmias.
- Have drugs ready for immediate use if needed:
  - Seizures may require sedatives (lorazepam, midazolam, or diazepam).
  - Dopamine infusion (10 mcg/kg/min) may be needed for hypotension.
- Follow local protocols for direct referral to a hyperbaric chamber facility.
- Lidocaine and steroid administration are controversial—follow local protocols.

Decompression Sickness

Pathophysiology. **Decompression sickness (DCS)** refers to a broad range of signs and symptoms caused by nitrogen bubbles in blood and tissues coming out of solution during

Words of Wisdom

Any diver who experiences loss of consciousness right after a dive has experienced an air embolism until proved otherwise.

ascent. Bubbles do damage in two ways: by interfering mechanically with tissue perfusion and by triggering chemical changes within the body. The ensuing multisystem disorder can potentially affect almost every organ in the body. Because nitrogen is highly lipid-soluble, the CNS and the spinal cord are more susceptible to DCS.

As a diver descends, increasing quantities of nitrogen and oxygen become dissolved in the blood (per Henry's law) and are then carried to the tissues, where oxygen is metabolized but nitrogen remains. As the diver ascends and ambient pressure decreases, the reverse process occurs: Nitrogen begins to diffuse out of the tissues. If the ascent is slow enough, then the amount of nitrogen in the tissues will equilibrate with that in the alveoli and escape harmlessly with each breath. If the ascent takes place more rapidly than nitrogen can be removed, however, then the diver's tissues will literally begin to bubble. This effect can be worsened if the diver undertakes multiple dives in a short time without allowing for nitrogen off-loading after each dive.

Other risk factors for DCS include obesity (more fatty tissues), dehydration, fatigue, and flying (going to higher altitude) within 12 to 14 hours of diving. Note that the activity of diving alone can lead to dehydration because it often involves activity in tropical climates while breathing dry air. Another risk factor for severe neurologic DCS is the presence of a patent foramen ovale, which affects as much as one-third of the general population. This congenital defect arises when the foramen ovale between the atria fails to close at birth; it may allow nitrogen bubbles to travel from the pulmonary circulation directly into the systemic circulation, leading to increased damage of the CNS and proximal spinal cord.

Assessment. Historically, decompression sickness was classified as type I or type II. Type I refers to mild forms of DCS that involve only the skin, lymphatic system, and musculoskeletal system. Joint pain, the most common symptom, causes the patient to "bend" over in pain. The skin may become mottled and pruritic. The patient may be fatigued and weak. Lymph dysfunction is rarely seen and can lead to edema. Type II includes all the other organs, including pulmonary, cardiovascular, and nervous systems, and is more dangerous. A much more informative way to describe DCS is to specify the systems affected and the precise symptoms (see Table 38-8).

Management. You may not always be able to distinguish between DCS and AGE in the field, especially when the patient has neurologic symptoms **Figure 38-19**. The term *DCI* is sometimes used to refer to both DCS and AGE. As a general rule, symptoms produced by air embolism usually reflect cerebral dysfunction, whereas the spinal cord is more likely to be involved in DCS. A loss of consciousness points to AGE. In terms of prehospital treatment, management in either case is basically the same: administer 100% oxygen, manage acute problems such as dysrhythmias and seizures, and transport the

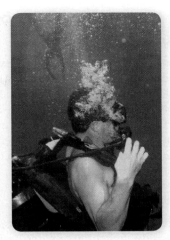

Figure 38-19 Decompression sickness (the "bends") affects divers who ascend to the surface too quickly.
Courtesy of Mass Communication Specialist 2nd Class Rebecca J. Moat/U.S. Navy.

patient to a hyperbaric facility in optimal condition even if symptoms appear to resolve. Treatment of DCS is summarized as follows:

- Ensure an adequate airway.
- Administer 100% supplemental oxygen by nonrebreathing mask.
- Insert an IV line for normal saline, and administer fluids at the rate ordered. (For long-range transport of a catheterized patient, adjust fluids to produce a urine output of 1 to 2 mL/kg per hour.)
- Do not use nitrous oxide/oxygen (Nitronox) for analgesia.
- Arrange for transport per protocol to a hyperbaric facility. If you do not know where the facility is, then contact the Divers Alert Network (DAN) for assistance: (919) 684-9111.

Hyperbaric Oxygen Therapy. Hyperbaric oxygen therapy involves intermittent inhalation of pure oxygen under a pressure of greater than 1 ATA. This treatment mechanically reduces bubble size, reduces nitrogen content, and increases oxygen delivery to ischemic tissues. Treatment pressures and times are dictated by established tables such as the US Navy Treatment Tables. Hyperbaric oxygen is indicated in patients with AGE and DCS as well as carbon monoxide poisoning and some other subacute or chronic medical conditions. It is also used in routine decompression of industrial divers. Hyperbaric oxygen does have some risks: it can convert a pneumothorax into a tension pneumothorax if there is no chest tube. It can cause seizures due to oxygen toxicity, and it can cause barotrauma via the same mechanism as diving. Care is recommended with pregnant patients and those with lung disease such as asthma or COPD, fever, or seizure disorders due to the potential for barotraumas or seizures. However, in the setting of a patient with a possible AGE or DCS, the benefits of hyperbaric oxygen treatment may certainly outweigh the risks.

▶ Other Gas-Related Problems

Pathophysiology

Most recreational divers breathe compressed air. Tanks that hold various mixtures of nitrogen and oxygen allow divers to remain underwater for longer periods. Such divers are less likely to develop DCS because they are breathing less nitrogen. Conversely, these divers are more prone to oxygen toxicity, which constitutes a CNS emergency. Air with an oxygen concentration of 21% can cause toxicity at a depth of about 200 feet.

Assessment

An affected diver may experience dizziness, lack of coordination, confusion, twitching or paresthesia symptoms, and underwater seizures.

Management

Evacuation from the water involves a controlled ascent to the surface by the diver or dive partner while ensuring the diver continues to maintain an airway and has access to air during ascent. Whereas DCS may be a concern after an emergent ascent, the risk of AGE is actually not increased when a seizing or postictal patient is brought to the surface.

On rare occasions, a scuba tank may be filled with contaminated air, especially if the compressor that fills the tank malfunctions. Carbon monoxide and carbon dioxide will affect the diver early in the dive—a characteristic that helps distinguish this condition from DCS. Treatment, once back in the boat or on the shore, involves 100% oxygen and supportive therapy; hyperbaric oxygen therapy in pregnant patients or those with significant exposure has been shown to decrease long-term neurologic consequences of carbon monoxide poisoning.

▶ Shallow Water Blackout

Pathophysiology

Shallow water blackout is a condition that may be seen by paramedics in any part of the country, even in desert states. The blackout is frequently seen in swimmers performing breath-holding exercises (for fun, to see who can remain the longest underwater, or for functionality, such as among military personnel or competitive swimmers). One way of theoretically extending a person's underwater endurance is to hyperventilate just before going beneath the surface. Hyperventilation decreases Pa_{CO_2} and causes cerebral vasoconstriction. Meanwhile, as the swimmer descends, his or her Pa_{O_2} increases. Because the Pa_{CO_2} is relatively low, the swimmer's respiratory drive is suppressed, so he or she has the sensation of being able to remain underwater longer than normal while oxygen continues to be removed from the alveoli. The swimmer remains conscious because cerebral function is maintained by the increased Pa_{O_2} at depth. On surfacing, however, ambient pressure rapidly decreases, the Pa_{O_2} plummets, and hypoxemia combined with cerebral vasoconstriction causes blackout just before reaching the surface. Even without the pressure changes associated with Pa_{O_2}, the Pa_{O_2} drops more quickly than the P_{CO_2} rises. This means that the swimmer may pass out before ever sensing the need to breathe.

Assessment and Management

Treatment is the same as for any other case of drowning. When the patient regains consciousness, however, you need to explain the seriousness of what just happened. Explain to the patient and any other participants that hyperventilation before a breath-hold dive is a dangerous activity that can result in death.

▶ Getting Help for Diving Injuries

A valuable resource for emergency medical personnel dealing with underwater diving accidents is DAN, which provides a 24-hour emergency consultation service at (919) 684-9111. Calls are received at DAN headquarters at Duke University Medical Center, Durham, North Carolina, and the caller is immediately connected with a physician experienced in diving medicine who can assist with diagnosis, provide advice for early management of the accident, and supervise referral to an appropriate recompression chamber when necessary. DAN also produces many excellent training and continuing medical education resources that are available on its website.

Documentation & Communication

In case of a diving emergency, pass along the following information to the emergency department: how long the diver was at the bottom, how many dives were performed, whether the patient was carrying a computer that recorded dive-related data, whether there was a decompression stop before fully ascending, and how deep the diver was.

■ Pathophysiology, Assessment, and Management of Altitude Illness

Altitude is considered to be a terrestrial elevation above 5,000 feet (1,500 m) because this is the level where the body normally begins to have physiologic changes due to the hypobaric hypoxia to which it is exposed. Altitude illness is a problem of hypobaric hypoxia—that is, low partial pressure of oxygen leading to hypoxemia. As per Dalton's law (discussed in the diving section), the amount of a gas that is available for the body to use is determined by the partial pressure driving that gas. As a person ascends in elevation, atmospheric pressure decreases, and therefore the partial pressure of oxygen decreases (hypobaric). This results in a decreasing amount of oxygen available for the body to use. Whereas the partial pressure of oxygen in the atmosphere decreases with increasing altitude, it remains a constant 21% of the makeup of atmospheric gases. For example, the partial pressure of arterial oxygen (Pao$_2$) is 103 mm Hg at sea level but only 81 mm Hg in Denver (elevation 5,280 feet [1,600 m]). Barometric pressure also varies according to how far from the equator you are located (it is lower the farther you are from it) and is typically lower in the winter. Interestingly, local changes in barometric pressures can alter the "relative altitude" by 500 to 2,500 feet (150 to 760 m).

▶ Pathophysiology

Altitude illnesses are illnesses caused by the effects of hypobaric (low atmospheric pressure) hypoxia on the CNS and pulmonary system as a result of unacclimatized people ascending to a higher altitude. It runs the gamut from the common acute mountain sickness (AMS) to the

rare deaths from high-altitude cerebral edema (HACE) and high-altitude pulmonary edema (HAPE).

Altitude illness typically occurs in people who rapidly ascend to heights above 8,000 feet (2,400 m) but can occur at altitudes as low as 6,500 feet (2,000 m). Symptoms usually occur within 6 to 10 hours. The incidence of altitude illness is directly related to both how high people ascend as well as how quickly they arrive at that elevation. If people ascend slowly, then their bodies are more likely to acclimatize to altitude. Altitude illness develops when people ascend higher or faster than their body can acclimatize to the altitude. Studies have shown that among Americans who go from lowland locations to higher elevations and sleep at around 8,200 feet (2,500 m), there is a 22% chance of developing AMS, rising as high as 42% for those sleeping above 9,800 feet (3,000 m).[34] AMS is even more common among climbers of Mt. Rainier (who typically go from sea level to 14,400 feet (4,400 m) in as little as 18 to 24 hours), averaging 70% of all climbers.[35]

In a simplified description, the body adjusts or acclimatizes to altitude by defending the amount of oxygen available for delivery to the tissues. The first response

YOU are the Paramedic | PART 4

En route you reassess the patient's distal pulses, motor function, and sensation to his upper and lower extremities. His pedal pulses are now present bilaterally. He is unable to move his fingers and toes, but they remain cold and he cannot feel you touch them. You administer an additional 500-mL warm normal saline bolus and reassess. The patient's shivering has ceased. His pain has improved and he thanks you for your care. Blankets and heat packs are replaced to keep him warm. On arrival at the hospital, the patient's sensation to his toes returns.

Recording Time: 30 Minutes	
Level of consciousness	Alert, still oriented to person, place, time, and event; able to respond quickly to questions
Respirations	14 breaths/min
Pulse	104 beats/min; strong and regular
Skin	Cool, pale, and dry
Blood pressure	110/64 mm Hg (after 1,000 mL of warm normal saline)
Temperature	Oral, 90°F (32.2°C); rectal; 93°F (33.9°C)
ECG	Normal sinus rhythm
Oxygen saturation (Spo$_2$)	98% while receiving 4 L/min via nasal cannula
Pupils	PERRLA
Pain scale	Visual analog scale; pain is a "4" on "0 to 10" scale

10. What are your reassessment priorities?
11. Why is it important to treat the patient's pain?

to hypobaric hypoxia is hyperventilation; this allows for the blowing off of carbon dioxide in exchange for holding onto oxygen. However, this quickly leads to a respiratory alkalosis, for which the body must compensate in order to continue to hyperventilate. This is done by the kidneys secreting bicarbonate in the urine. This causes a compensatory metabolic acidosis and the body can continue to hyperventilate. Other changes such as the increased production of red cells and changes at the cellular level to improve oxygen transfer also occur, but take several days to a week.

Hypoxemia is the main culprit behind the pathophysiologic responses observed in altitude illness, but the exact mechanism remains poorly understood. The hypoxemia is believed to initiate a complex series of reactions (often sympathetically mediated) that result in overperfusion to the brain and lungs, with resultant increases in capillary pressures, leakage, and then cerebral and pulmonary edema. HAPE, while part of the spectrum of altitude illness, results from marked vasospasm of the pulmonary arteries; this results in a high-pressure driving fluid from the pulmonary vasculature into the lungs and causing pulmonary edema. HAPE does not result from a volume overload state (as can be seen in cardiogenic pulmonary edema). The treatments for HAPE therefore differ markedly from standard pulmonary edema, and nitroglycerin and furosemide (Lasix) are not used to treat HAPE.

Risk Factors for Altitude Illness

Several factors predispose a person to altitude illnesses. The most important risk factor is a prior history of AMS. In cases where people have previously become ill, they should slow their ascent and/or use prophylactic medicines to decrease the likelihood of illness. Normal residence below 3,000 feet (900 m), obesity, and rapid or high ascents also increases the risk of developing altitude illness **Figure 38-20**. Physical fitness is not a factor. Age does not matter, although there is some suggestion that older adults may be less likely to develop such an illness. The susceptibility to altitude illness is individually variable and not predictable other than by a past history of altitude exposure.

▶ Assessment

When people ascend to an elevation higher or faster than their body can acclimatize, altitude illness develops. Altitude illness is a spectrum of illness ranging from mild AMS to life threatening HACE and HAPE. AMS is a clinical diagnosis; there are no specific physical findings that define it. HACE and HAPE have a combination of historic and physical findings that define them. The following definitions of altitude illness have been internationally established:

- **Acute mountain sickness (AMS).** Headache plus at least one of the following: fatigue or weakness, gastrointestinal symptoms (nausea, vomiting, or loss of appetite), dizziness or light-headedness, or difficulty sleeping. The headache is often described as throbbing that is worse over the temporal or occipital areas and is exacerbated by the Valsalva maneuver.
- **High-altitude pulmonary edema (HAPE).** At least two of the following symptoms: dyspnea at rest, cough, weakness or decreased exercise performance, or chest tightness or congestion. Also, at least two of the following signs: central cyanosis, audible crackles (rales) or wheezing in at least one lung field, tachypnea, or tachycardia. Patients may or may not exhibit symptoms if AMS precedes symptoms of HAPE.
- **High-altitude cerebral edema (HACE).** HACE requires the presence of a change in mental status and/or ataxia in a person with AMS or the presence of mental status changes and ataxia in a person without AMS. HACE can progress to coma.

Other conditions can mimic AMS, and the emergence of symptoms 4 or more days after being at higher elevations, a lack of a headache, or the failure of descent to improve signs or symptoms points to other causes.

▶ Management

The mainstay of management of all altitude illness includes oxygen, descent, and evacuation, though the specifics of each illness vary. Prevention is best accomplished via acclimatization, and/or the use of acetazolamide in those persons likely to be susceptible for developing altitude illness given a planned ascent rate. A standard for slow ascent is to ascend sleeping altitude only 1,000 feet (300 m) per day once over 8,000 feet (2,500 m) in elevation. This is, of course, a slow ascent rate. Acetazolamide is a carbonic anhydrase inhibitor, which means it causes the kidneys to secrete bicarbonate. This causes a metabolic acidosis that the body compensates for by hyperventilating to create a respiratory alkalosis. Acetazolamide thus helps the body to acclimatize by causing the needed physiologic

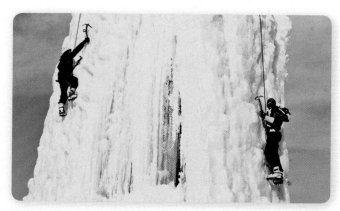

Figure 38-20 Rapid or high ascents increase the risk of developing altitude illness.
© Alan Heartfield/Shutterstock.

changes, though in reverse. Acetazolamide also decreases cerebrospinal fluid production, so it may cause some affect through decreasing minimal cerebral edema. Side effects commonly seen are diffuse and migratory paresthesias, mild diuresis, and because it hydrolyzes carbon dioxide on the tongue, it makes all carbonated beverages taste bad. Acetazolamide is a sulfa-based drug, so traditionally, people who develop anaphylaxis to sulfa-based antibiotics have been discouraged from taking it. However, this should be discussed with a physician on a case-by-case basis, because the evidence supporting this association is weak and acetazolamide may be safe in many patients with sulfa allergies.[36] Acetazolamide is the only drug with a US Food and Drug Administration (FDA) approval for prevention and treatment of altitude illness.

The treatment of AMS can be both symptomatic and physiologic. Acetaminophen or aspirin can be used for headache. Antiemetics such as prochlorperazine (Compazine) or ondansetron (Zofran) can be used for nausea. Acetazolamide both treats AMS and helps the body to acclimatize to altitude. Oxygen, if available, is helpful. A patient with AMS does not mandatorily need to descend (though descent will rapidly improve AMS), but should not ascend further until the symptoms have resolved.

Descent and oxygen are the mainstays of HAPE treatment. A patient with HAPE should descend immediately. The use of medications for HAPE as adjunctive treatment is limited to those patients where descent and oxygen are not readily available or when these are not resulting in a rapid improvement in the patient. The failure of significant descent and oxygen to improve HAPE should also cause you to consider a different cause of the pulmonary symptoms.

Because a primary physiologic change causing HAPE is elevated pulmonary arterial pressure, the medications used to treat and prevent HAPE are predominantly pulmonary artery vasodilators. Nifedipine remains the gold standard for prevention and adjunctive treatment of HAPE. Salmeterol has also been shown to be beneficial in preventing HAPE.[37] The phosphodiesterase inhibitors sildenafil and tadalafil are used for treatment of pulmonary hypertension and are becoming more popular for use in prevention and treatment of HAPE. However, an international medical alpinism commission has recommended caution in their use because of potentially dangerous side effects. Albuterol has not been studied but should be as effective as salmeterol. Dexamethasone has also been shown in a single study to be effective in preventing HAPE, though its use has not become routine because of the lack of further clinical experience and research data.[37] Remember, HAPE is not a fluid overload problem, so nitrates and furosemide (Lasix) should not be used.

HACE treatment involves oxygen, mandatory descent, and use of dexamethasone. Whereas the former two are the most important, it has become standard procedure for dexamethasone to be given as soon as possible. As discussed in the Appendix to Volume 1, *Emergency Medications*, a dose of 8 mg is given by any accessible route followed by 4 mg every 6 hours during descent/evacuation.

Portable Hyperbaric Chambers

Another adjunct useful for prehospital treatment of altitude illness when descent cannot be carried out is the use of the portable hyperbaric chamber. These are available as the Gamow bag, the PAC, and the Certec bag. The patient is placed inside these bags and air is pumped in under pressure by foot pump or electric pump. The increased pressure around the patient provides the equivalent of the patient having descended several hundred to several thousand feet (100 to 1,000 m). These bags are even more effective when the patient is placed on oxygen inside the bag. However, they are cramped, claustrophobic for the patient, and make it difficult to treat a patient once they are locked inside.

Pathophysiology, Assessment, and Management of Lightning Strike

▶ Pathophysiology

In contrast to the proverbial suggestion that lightning strikes are rare, about 20-50 deaths per year in the United States are attributed to lightning, with Florida being the leading state for lightning strikes.[38] Lightning strike morbidity is even higher, with between three to five times more people being struck than are killed, though this number may be higher because the actual number struck remains unknown. Lightning strikes are different from industrial electrical injuries, and should be treated differently. Lightning is neither an alternating current nor direct current; it is a massive unidirectional flow of electrons, with voltages in the millions, up to 30 million volts or more. As opposed to industrial injuries from high voltage, however, the duration of the current is miniscule, on the order of only one thousandth or even ten thousandth of a second; thus, much of this energy is not typically transferred into the victim but rather flows over them.

The most common cause of lightning injury is a side splash injury in which lightning hits an object and then spreads out from that point, though it can also strike a person directly.

The energy from a bolt of lightning may act as a giant depolarizing charge to the entire body. This can cause asystole and respiratory arrest both via diaphragm depolarization as well as a brainstem-induced central apnea. After this depolarization, the heart, due to its automaticity, will usually resume a sinus rhythm spontaneously. However, the body's respiratory effort does not spontaneously restart, and if the patient remains apneic, the heart will then go into a secondary hypoxic arrest. Thus, if CPR is

instituted promptly, most lightning strike victims will survive. However, while correct prehospital treatment results in a low death rate from lightning strike, morbidity is high; as many as 75% of people struck by lightning will have some long-term complication. Clinically significant burns are not usually seen with lightning strikes unless victims have metal objects on them that can heat up and can cause thermal burns (large metal belt buckles for example), or if they are wet and the water is converted to steam causing steam burns. Lightning strike victims may have a "Lichtenberg figure" Figure 38-21 . This is pathognomonic of a lightning strike, though it is not an actual burn, but rather caused by blood cells forced out of contracting capillaries on the skin, similar to a bruise.[39,40] Lightning strike victims may also have been thrown by the strike and should be evaluated for trauma.
Table 38-9 lists prevention techniques to avoid being struck by lightning.

▶ Assessment and Management

Assessment and management of injuries resulting from lightning strikes are covered in Chapter 32, *Burns*. Recall that the initial approach and triage of lightning victims is different than encountered in other situations. It is best summed up as "reverse triage": If patients have any signs of life, then they will likely recover and can be attended to secondarily; those who appear dead are the ones who must be attended to first. A lightning strike induces cardiac and respiratory arrest. As mentioned, the heart will often restart spontaneously; however, respirations will not, and the victim therefore becomes hypoxemic, preventing the heart from recovering. If CPR/rescue breathing is given, then hypoxemia may be prevented and the heart may restart. All victims of lightning strike need to be evaluated at a medical facility.

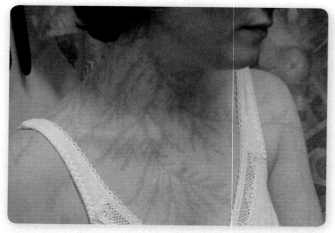

Figure 38-21 A Lichtenberg figure, pathognomonic of a lightning strike. It is caused by the electron shower over the skin and can last for hours to days.
© 2007 British Association of Plastic, Reconstructive and Aesthetic Surgeons.

Table 38-9	**Techniques to Avoid Being Struck by Lightning**

- Avoid open areas in which you are the tallest object.
- Avoid extremes of high or low ground.
- Avoid direct contact with metal or current-carrying objects.
- Avoid seeking shelter under a lone tree or in the middle of an open area.
- Seek shelter amidst trees of uniform size.
- If caught alone in an open area, then keep the feet together and squat close to the ground. If legs are spread apart this theoretically provides the path of least resistance for current to run up one leg, through the body, and down the other leg, which is a path of lower resistance than through the ground.
- If caught with a group in an open area, then spread out to prevent the splash effect of a lightning strike, but remain within eyesight. Each person should keep the feet and knees together and squat close to the ground.
- Being inside of a metal vehicle is extremely safe because electricity flows around the metal vehicle without entering the vehicle itself. The safety has nothing to do with the insulating effect of rubber tires. A metal vehicle would be just as effective if it were sitting on the ground on its rims. In a lightning storm, stay in your rig.
- The 30-30 rule: if the time from lighting until thunder is 30 seconds or less, ensure you are under cover. Do not leave until 30 minutes after the storm has passed. Remember the most dangerous time is just before arrival of the storm and just afterward.
- Many have learned the counting rule to determine distance from a storm, but have misunderstood the calculation. The number of seconds between lightning flash and thunder boom can be counted, but because of the different speeds of light and sound, the number must be divided by 5 to determine the distance in miles of a storm cell (by 3 if using kilometers). So, in other words, if time from lightning to thunder is 30 seconds—as in the 30-30 rule—the lightning is not 30 miles (50 km) away, it is 6 miles (10 km) away! Additionally, lightning has been known to strike as far as 10 to 15 miles (16 to 24 km) away from the storm cell's center. This means that even the 30-30 rule will not eliminate the chance of a lightning strike. Correctly calculating lightning distance is crucial to avoid minimizing storm distance by as much as a factor of 5!

■ Pathophysiology, Assessment, and Management of Envenomation: Bites and Stings

There are thousands of creatures in the continental United States that produce and secrete venom. Fortunately, most of them do not have an effective method of injecting or spreading that venom to humans. The commonly encountered venomous creatures that you need to be aware of are the following:

- Insects of the order Hymenoptera (bees, wasps, hornets, and fire ants)
- Snakes of the Elapidae family and Crotalinae subfamily (elapids like coral snakes and crotalins like rattlesnakes)
- Spiders, specifically *Latrodectus mactans* (black widow), *Loxosceles reclusa* (brown recluse), and *Tegenaria agrestis* (hobo)
- Scorpions of the genus *Centruroides*

The most frequent cause of mortality from all **envenomations** is not the venom itself but an anaphylactic reaction to it. Anaphylaxis can occur with exposure to any venom, but is most commonly seen with hymenopteran envenomation, and, thus, the most deaths related to envenomation result from hymenopteran bites or stings. Anaphylaxis is covered in Chapter 25, *Immunologic Emergencies*. The important point is that treatment of anaphylaxis resulting from envenomations is no different than treatment of anaphylaxis from any other cause.

The mainstay of treatment of all envenomations that do not involve anaphylaxis is the management of the ABCs and transport. No antivenins are commonly used in the prehospital environment in the United States, although some agencies such as Venom One in Florida do provide prehospital antivenin. Vascular access should be obtained for all patients transported following an envenomation. Do not overlook scene safety; the venomous creatures may still be around. It is also not uncommon for the patient or friends to have captured the offending creature and placed it in a bag or container with the intention of bringing it to the hospital for identification. Be careful how you handle the bag or container because some creatures, even when dead, can cause envenomation.

▶ Hymenoptera

Pathophysiology

As mentioned, the most common cause of envenomation-related deaths in the United States is the order Hymenoptera, which includes European (honey) bees (Apidae); yellow jackets, wasps, hornets (Vespidae); and fire ants (Formicidae) `Figure 38-22`. There are estimated to be more than 1 million hymenopteran stings annually in

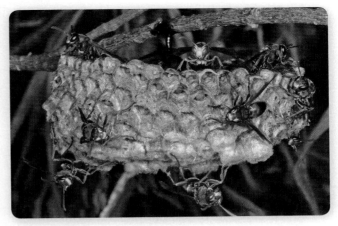

Figure 38-22 Hymenopteran stings include those from bees, wasps, hornets, yellow jackets, and fire ants.
© Stuart Elflett/Shutterstock.

the United States, 3% of which require treatment for anaphylaxis.[41] Among the Hymenoptera there is a degree of cross reaction in the venom of all three of these subfamilies with each other. For example, a person who experiences anaphylaxis after a bee sting could also develop anaphylaxis following a fire ant bite. In the case of stinging by a honeybee, the stinger/venom sac is pulled from the bee's body and remains attached to the skin. This only rarely occurs with any of the other subfamilies.

Assessment

Hymenopteran venom is a complex mixture of proteins that cause a local reaction with symptoms of erythema, swelling, and pruritus. Melittin is a protein in the venom that causes the immediately painful feeling of a sting. It works through a direct effect on skin pain receptors. The more severe hymenopteran sting reactions, when they occur, are immunoglobulin-E mediated. In a quarter of those people stung, a local reaction develops, and can become quite extensive over the day or two following the sting. It is exceedingly rare for an infection to develop after a hymenopteran sting. Erythema and swelling, often with associated pruritus that begins within a day of the sting, is a local reaction and not an infection.

Anaphylaxis after a hymenopteran sting occurs rapidly, typically within 10 minutes.

Management

If the patient has no history of allergy to bee stings and does not have a systemic reaction, then transport to the hospital is usually unnecessary. When this decision is made, advise the patient of the warning signs of anaphylaxis and the urgency of calling 9-1-1 in such an event. Instruct the patient to have the wound checked by a physician if it does not improve markedly within 24 hours. Infection is likely after the stings of fire ants, which roam the southeastern United States throughout the late spring and early summer. Fire ant stings typically produce small pustules at the sting site about 6 hours after the sting. When the pustules are broken open—often when the patient starts to scratch—the affected area is vulnerable to secondary infection.

Treatment of a hymenopteran sting focuses primarily on pain relief and minimization of the risk of infection. First, determine whether the stinger and venom sac are still attached to the skin. If so, remove the stinger as rapidly as possible using the most readily available technique. For many years it has been recommended that you use a scalpel blade to gently scrape the stinger and venom sac from the wound. This was suggested because it was felt that using an improper technique would inadvertently release additional venom into the skin during removal. Subsequently, it has been found that rapid removal is by far more important than how removal is accomplished.

After removing the stinger, clean the wound thoroughly with soap and water or an antiseptic solution such as povidone-iodine. Local reactions are treated with cool compresses and elevation. Antihistamines are also used for symptomatic treatment. Antihistamines can be given orally as well as in the topical form sprayed onto the sting site. In small, localized reactions, topical hydrocortisone can be used.

Specific treatment of fire ant stings includes moving the patient (and crew) away from the site, brushing off ants, and providing supportive care.

▶ Snake Bites
Pathophysiology

There are two families of snakes in the United States that are of concern for envenomation: the Viperidae, (specifically, the subfamily Crotalinae, also known as "pit vipers"), which cause 99% of all bites, and the Elapidae, which cause the remaining 1%.[42,43] Approximately 10,000 snake bites occur in the United States every year, with about 30% being venomous.[44] Whereas morbidity can be significant, fatalities are rare, with fewer than 10 usually seen per year. Bites are most commonly seen in the southeastern United States, although Texas has the greatest number of recorded snake fatalities.[45]

Pit viper venom contains hemolytic and proteolytic enzymes that lead to extensive local tissue damage in addition to systemic effects. This explains the medically important consequences of these bites; namely, the injection of these hemotoxic substances creates soft-tissue swelling and necrosis, local and then systemic bleeding, and coagulopathies. In contrast, coral snakes possess potent neurotoxic venom that leads to paresthesias, fasciculations, weakness, respiratory difficulty, and other stroke-like symptoms, but little in the way of direct local tissue injury.

Crotalins: Pit Vipers. The family Vipiridae, subfamily Crotalinae, are the "pit vipers" and the cause of the greatest number of bites and morbidity. The name *pit viper* is

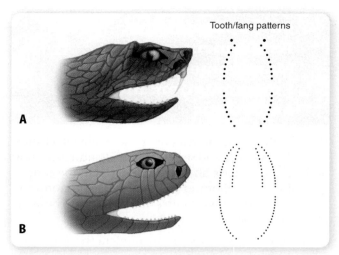

Figure 38-23 Characteristics of pit vipers and nonpoisonous snakes. **A.** Pit vipers have vertical pupils, a pit between the eye and the nostril, a single row of teeth, and two erectile fangs. **B.** Nonpoisonous snakes have round pupils and often a double row of upper teeth; they do not leave fang marks.
© Jones & Bartlett Learning.

derived from the heat-sensing pits that are located between the eye and the nostril Figure 38-23 . Other common findings in all crotalins include elliptical eyes and a single row of subcaudal plates (scales on the underside of the snake near the tail). Commonly encountered pit vipers include rattlesnakes (timber rattler, prairie rattler, and the eastern and western diamondback), cottonmouths (water moccasins), and copperheads. Eastern and western diamondbacks cause the greatest morbidity and mortality from snake bite.

Elapids: Coral Snakes. Coral snakes are members of the venomous snake family Elapidae, the same family that includes mambas, cobras, and sea snakes. There are three main coral snakes of concern in North America: the eastern coral snake, the Texas coral snake, and the Sonoran coral snake. The "new world" coral snakes found in North America have small heads and lack the retractable front fangs exhibited by other crotalins—their front fangs are smaller to fit inside their smaller heads. It is a misconception that coral snakes are rear-fanged, just as it is a misconception that they must chew to deliver their powerful venom. The envenomation causes few local symptoms and it may be several hours before systemic symptoms develop. For this reason, any patient with a possible elapid bite needs to be transported. In the continental United States only, the elapid can be described by its banding pattern and separated from its nontoxic mimic snakes: "Red on yellow, kill a fellow, red on black, venom lack" differentiates the coral snake from its nontoxic mimics such as the king snake Figure 38-24 . However, local variants or albinism within the United States can lead to deviation from the mnemonic.

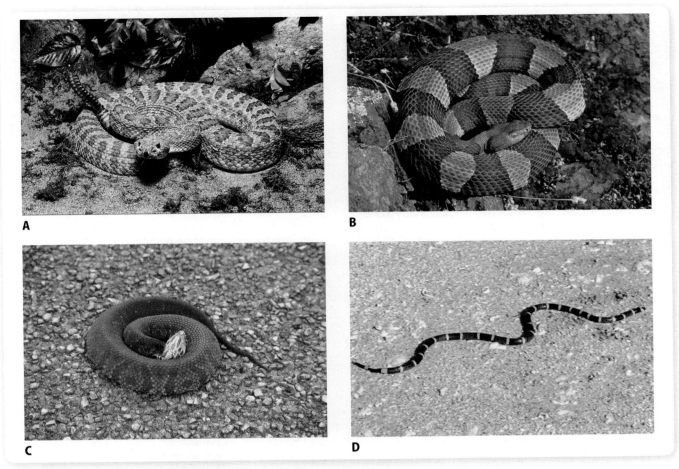

Figure 38-24 A. Rattlesnake. **B.** Copperhead. **C.** Cottonmouth. **D.** Coral snake.

A: © Photos.com/Getty; B: Courtesy of Ray Rauch/U.S. Fish & Wildlife Service; C: © SuperStock/Alamy; D: Courtesy of Luther C. Goldman/U.S. Fish & Wildlife Service.

Assessment

First and foremost, you need to make certain that the scene is safe and is not a threat to the EMS team or the patient. Confirm that the snake is dead, trapped, or gone. Note the time at which the bite occurred. Due to the serious damage that venom can cause, the amount of time that passes from the bite to the time of care is important. Determine the type of snake, if possible. This needs to be done without endangering yourself or others—dead snakes can still bite. Consider taking a picture of the snake instead of killing it, which may be safer and still convey important information to health care providers in the hospital.

Venoms. Crotalin venom is a mixture of enzymes that promote tissue destruction through proteolysis, hemolysis, thrombogenesis, and some degree of neurologic and cardiac toxicity in higher doses. These venom components cause the signs and symptoms of toxicity. Severity is determined by how much venom is injected as well as the location. Upwards of 25% of bites are actually "dry bites," in which no venom was injected.[46, 47] The ultimate severity of a bite is difficult to determine immediately after the bite, and therefore all patients should be transported. Elapid venom is primarily a neurotoxin, the injection of which leads to respiratory failure and death. The Mojave rattlesnake is an exception to the typical separation of crotalins and elapids. It is a crotalin, but it also has a potent neurotoxin in its venom, and thus its bites are a varied combination of crotalin and elapid envenomation. Crotalin bites cause swelling and pain at the bite site ▶ Figure 38-25 .

Bites with envenomation will usually be painful and bleed from the wound site and, as severity increases, swelling progresses up the affected extremity. Systemic symptoms also occur. Initial symptoms include an abnormal taste in the mouth, often described as metallic. Weakness, dizziness, altered mental status, and loss of consciousness can occur. Diaphoresis and tachycardia can occur. Nausea and vomiting are common. As coagulopathies develop, spontaneous bleeding is seen, which may be followed by shock and cardiovascular collapse.

The degree of envenomation of a crotalin bite is determined by the degree of swelling of the affected extremity as well as the presence of any systemic symptoms. Severity of pain and fasciculation are also good ways to monitor progressive envenomation.

- A mild envenomation has minimal local swelling only with no systemic symptoms.

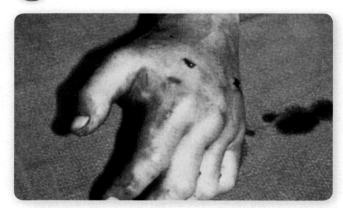

Figure 38-25 A snake bite wound from a poisonous snake has characteristic markings: two small puncture wounds about 0.5 inch (25 mm) apart, discoloration, and swelling.

© American Academy of Orthopaedic Surgeons.

- Moderate envenomation has swelling extending up the extremity and the possible presence of systemic symptoms and fasciculation. Coagulation abnormalities, if they occur, are minimal and no significant bleeding is seen.
- Severe envenomation has extensive soft-tissue swelling and severe systemic effects and bleeding up to and including disseminated intravascular coagulation and shock. Coagulation abnormalities are prominent.

Management

The treatment for any significant snake envenomation is the provision of antivenin. There are no pediatric doses of antivenin—snakes do not differentiate children from adults; the antivenin directly counters the venom. EMS and hospital systems that encounter envenomations should have protocols in place for appropriate triage to facilities with antivenin, or they should have a system in place to retrieve antivenin from other facilities.

Monitor the ABCs. Gain IV access and initiate oxygen therapy if required. Keep the patient calm, supine, and motionless to decrease venom spread and absorption. Quickly clean the wound with available antimicrobial agents. If local protocols allow, then draw blood for hospital use because coagulation studies may be unreliable in blood obtained later in the patient's course of treatment. Immobilize the involved extremity in a neutral position below the level of the heart, avoiding excessive constriction. Swelling occurs rapidly in a crotalin envenomation, so remove rings and any other constricting jewelry from both sides (ie, unaffected as well as affected side). Finally, begin rapid transport to a facility where the patient can receive antivenin. Note that even with appropriate delivery of antivenin, repeat symptoms of severe bites can occur 7 to 10 days later.

Table 38-10 outlines lay treatments for snake bites that are *not* beneficial and may be outright dangerous.

Table 38-10	Snake Bites: Treatments to Avoid

Do not ice bites. Ice has no benefit and can increase tissue damage.

Do not incise and suck. Incision markedly increases tissue damage because a coagulopathy may have developed. The rapidity of absorption of the toxin and angle of the fangs in injecting the venom also precludes incision and suction from being of any benefit other than to increase tissue damage. Commercial suction devices without incision have been shown to be of limited benefit only if used within the first 3 minutes of the bite. If used after this time, then they are of no benefit.

Do not provide electric shock to the bite. Electric shock has been touted as a method of decreasing the toxicity of venom by denaturing the venom proteins. This does not work; the amount of electricity that would be required to actually denature the snake venom would be such that it would cause third-degree burns and massive tissue destruction.

Do not use tourniquets. Tourniquets will localize the venom and in crotalin envenomation will increase the local tissue damage. This is as opposed to a constriction dressing that is designed only to limit lymphatic flow. In elapid bites, which contain a neurotoxin and little-to-no toxin that causes local tissue damage, there is a benefit to the use of constriction dressings. By inhibiting lymphatic flow, the constriction bandage slows the absorption of the neurotoxin. Constriction dressings have been used for years in the treatment of elapid bites outside of the United States. Previously felt to be inappropriate for American species of elapids, constriction dressings are now sometimes recommended for elapid bites in the United States. However, the constriction bandage must be applied correctly or it can be ineffective or even harmful. Hands-on instruction should be obtained in the technique to ensure correct application and pressure, and local protocols should be followed regarding whether this intervention is appropriate. In theory, a constriction bandage is made by wrapping an elastic compressive bandage tightly and proximally up the bitten extremity starting just over the site of the bite. The wrap is extended up above the next major joint and then wrapped back down the extremity to the bite site. The extremity is then immobilized.

© Jones & Bartlett Learning.

▶ Spider Bites

Pathophysiology

There are an estimated 34,000 species of spiders worldwide.[48] Most spiders are carnivores and can bite; they normally use their venom to subdue their prey. There are three important spider species that cause envenomation in the United States. They are the black widow, brown recluse, and the hobo spiders.

Controversies

The use of constriction dressings in the United States is controversial. In elapids, it been shown that envenomation effects from Australian species are decreased with a specific pressure-immobilization (P-I) technique.[49] However, it is unclear whether this technique is applicable to American elapid species. The procedure has drawbacks, including studies that suggest most providers, even physicians, are unable to properly apply it and the subsequent requirement that patients (even those with upper extremity bites) must be immobilized.[50] In a crotalin bite, a constriction dressing (different from a P-I technique) may slow systemic absorption of the toxin if applied correctly; however, it has also been shown that if too much pressure is applied, local tissue destruction will be increased.[51] Adding to the controversy is the changed recommendation from the American Red Cross advocating the use of constriction bands for prehospital care of crotalin (pit viper) bites. Most emergency medicine physicians, toxicologists, and wilderness medicine experts believe constriction will increase the degree of local tissue damage without much benefit to systemic toxicity. Thus the controversy continues. EMS providers are encouraged to follow their local protocols.

Only the female of the black widow species poses a danger to humans. Her name derives from her disagreeable practice of devouring her mate. This spider is glossy black with a 0.5-inch (25-mm) oval body, a leg span of about 1.5 inches (38 mm), and a characteristic red-orange hourglass mark on the abdomen **Figure 38-26**.

The black widow spider is found throughout the United States, but especially in the Southeast. Black widow spider bites occur in the United States most often between the months of April and October.[52] This spider makes its home in sheds, basements, garages, woodpiles, and similar areas. Because it likes to live in outhouses, bites may occur in some rather sensitive

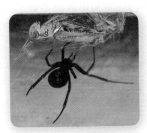

Figure 38-26 Black widow spiders are distinguished by their glossy, black body and bright red-orange hourglass marking on the abdomen.

© Crystal Kirk/Shutterstock.

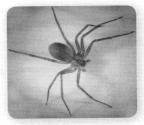

Figure 38-27 Brown recluse spiders are dull brown and have a dark, violin-shaped mark on the back.

Courtesy of Kenneth Cramer, Monmouth College.

areas of the anatomy. However, most wounds involve the hands or forearms.

The brown recluse spider, also known as the fiddleback spider due to its unique violin-like back marking, is found from the southern Midwest of the United States to Texas and across the Southeast **Figure 38-27**. It is not found in the far West unless accidently transported to the region from a native state. There are other species of *Loxosceles* found in every state, but these are not known for causing envenomation. The Northwest, however, is home to the hobo spider—a member of the genus *Tegenaria*—whose bite may be similar clinically to the brown recluse, and thus is grouped with it for clinical approach. The brown recluse is not aggressive and bites only when accidently pressed against the skin—for example, when a person puts on clothes that the spider has crawled into. The hobo spider, while described as an "aggressive house spider," is considered to be only slightly more aggressive than the brown recluse spider.

Assessment

A history of a spider bite is not often confirmed. Instead, the patient may report a sudden, sharp prick followed by a cramping or numbing pain that begins at the bite area and gradually spreads. Extreme restlessness is the classic sign of the reaction to a black widow spider bite.

Special Populations

In children, a black widow spider bite can be fatal.

The black widow is one of the most venomous of North American spiders. Its venom is predominantly a neurotoxin (which triggers multiple neurotransmitters from presynaptic nerves) that causes local pain and swelling followed by muscle spasm and paralysis. The local pain is rapid in onset, occurring within 30 to 60 minutes of the bite. Local muscle spasm and localized diaphoresis can occur. Diffuse and more pronounced muscular spasms may then follow. These typically involve the thigh and shoulder girdle and later the abdomen. The abdominal spasm can cause a "boardlike" appearance and can be confused with an acute abdomen. Systemic symptoms of nausea and vomiting also occur. Respiratory difficulty may develop as the diaphragm becomes affected by the venom.

Brown recluse spider bites are typically painless, and most people go on to have little or no subsequent symptoms, local or systemic. In a small percentage of people bitten, local and/or systemic symptoms may develop. There is a small subset of patients who, for unknown reasons, will have more pronounced symptoms and will develop **loxoscelism** Figure 38-28 . Loxoscelism is a potentially fatal condition resulting from a brown recluse spider bite that begins with a painful, inflamed vesicle that may progress to a gangrenous sloughing of the skin. Most commonly this condition presents cutaneously with pruritus and pain developing 2 to 8 hours after the bite. These symptoms worsen over the next day to day and a half, followed by the development of a necrotic lesion that can take a month or more to heal and may require skin grafting. Systemic symptoms are more rare and include nausea, vomiting, and fever. In rare cases it has been reported that hemolysis and coagulopathies have led to death.

Management

Treatment for a black widow spider bite includes intermittent use of ice and antimicrobial cleansing of the wound, as well as providing pain and muscle spasm relief, and prompt transport. ABCs and monitoring are standard. Obtain IV access and apply oxygen. Narcotics and muscle relaxants/ sedatives are the other prehospital mainstays of therapy. Treat severe muscle spasms with the benzodiazepines diazepam or lorazepam. Use narcotics for pain relief. An antivenin is available for treatment of black widow spider bites, but its use is typically reserved for severe envenomation in extremes of patient age or for immunocompromised patients. This antivenin has a high incidence of allergic reactions inherent in all equine-derived antivenin.

Treatment for both brown recluse and hobo spider bites is supportive. Antivenin is not routinely available.

> ### Words of Wisdom
>
> Calcium gluconate given intravenously was previously recommended for treatment of the muscle spasms and pain associated with black widow spider bites but is no longer recommended because it has been shown to be no better than placebo in symptom relief.[53] Antivenin is available in the United States. Contact your poison control center.

▶ Scorpion Stings

Pathophysiology

There are approximately 90 scorpion species in the continental United States.[54] Only one genus, *Centruroides* (bark scorpion), is of any potential threat to humans Figure 38-29 . The vast majority of the 15,000 scorpion stings seen in the United States are from other species and result only in a painful local reaction.[55] The bark scorpion is found living along the Mexican border of Arizona and California, though its habitat extends up to parts of Nevada, New Mexico, and Utah. It is not aggressive, but is nocturnal and can crawl into places such as shoes or other personal items. The bark scorpion can also climb walls, where it can be accidently encountered.

A scorpion's venom is located in the glands of the stinger with which the scorpion will stab its prey after grasping it with its claws. Scorpion venom is made up of a mixture of many toxins that affect virtually every body system.

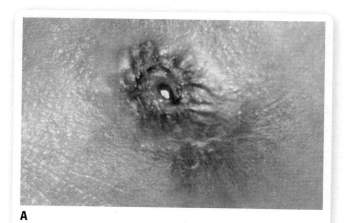

A

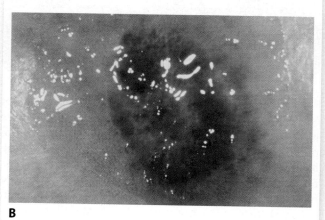

B

Figure 38-28 Brown recluse spider bite in early stage **(A)** and late stage **(B)**.

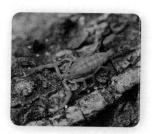

Figure 38-29 The bark scorpion.

Assessment

Local scorpion sting symptoms are similar to hymenopteran stings, with development of erythema, pruritis, urticaria, and a sharp burning pain or paresthesia. The paresthesias have been described as feeling like a strong electric shock. Local effects begin within minutes of a sting, and last for several hours. Local tissue necrosis is not common. These local symptoms are all that occur in the vast majority of scorpion stings. In contrast, a sting from the more neurotoxic bark scorpion causes minimal local symptoms. Systemic symptoms typically begin within minutes and peak by 4 to 6 hours, with resolution in 24 to 72 hours if treated symptomatically only (without the use of antivenin).

The most predominant effect of the bark scorpion venom is a neurotoxic one that causes an autonomic excitation. The toxin causes nerve sodium channels to remain open, allowing continuous activation of nerves of the sympathetic, parasympathetic, and somatic nerve systems. The symptoms seen are due to this diffuse neuronal excitation. These symptoms are myriad and depend to a great extent on which portion of the nervous system is most in overdrive, the sympathetic or parasympathetic. If the sympathetic is predominant, then tachycardia, palpitations, tachypnea, hypertension, dry mouth, and elevated temperature are seen. Sympathetically induced pulmonary edema also may be seen. If the parasympathetic stimulation predominates, then bradycardia, hypotension, lacrimation, salivation, urination, priapism, and defecation are seen. Cranial nerve findings are common and include nystagmus or wandering eye movements as well as tongue fasciculations and dysphagia. Muscle contractions, myoclonic jerking, and fasciculations are signs of somatic nervous system involvement. The typical bark scorpion victim has nystagmus, hypersalivation, dysphagia, mydriasis, and restlessness.

Management

Prehospital treatment primarily involves maintenance of ABCs, monitoring of the patient, and transport to the hospital. Intubate the patient, if required for airway maintenance. Initiate an IV line and give volume as required for the maintenance of blood pressure. Apply ice packs to areas of local pain and swelling. There is no role for suction or extraction devices. Immobilize the extremity. Application of a constricting band just above the wound site (but not tight enough to occlude the pulse) may reduce lymph flow and the subsequent spread of venom; follow your local protocol. In the unlikely event of seizures, treat with benzodiazepines per local protocol and transport the patient to an appropriate facility.

For a bark scorpion sting in which the patient shows signs of severe toxicity, a reasonable treatment is now available. The FDA approved Anascorp, a Mexican-manufactured scorpion antivenin, in 2011. This ovine-derived antivenin can rapidly decrease morbidity in those with more severe toxicity.

In-hospital treatment is protection of the ABCs through supportive care. This may include the use of alpha- and

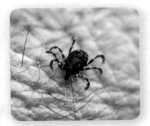

Figure 38-30 Ticks typically attach themselves directly to the skin.
© Joao Estevao A. Freitas (jefras)/Shutterstock.

beta-blockers as well as atropine to control the excessive nervous system symptoms. Vasoactive drugs are used as required to control the neurologic overstimulation. If available, then administer bark scorpion antivenin.

▶ Tick Bites
Pathophysiology

Ticks are blood-sucking arthropods found around the world, often in rural, wooded areas Figure 38-30 . Ordinarily, tick bites are not a medical emergency, but they are of concern because ticks serve as disease vectors. Bacteria, viruses, and protozoa can be transmitted via a tick bite, and they are linked to a variety of serious illnesses, including febrile illness, Lyme disease (associated with a bull's-eye rash around the location of the bite), Rocky Mountain spotted fever, and tularemia.

In rare cases, a tick bite on the back of the head, neck, or spine may produce potentially life-threatening "tick paralysis" that cannot be reversed unless the tick is removed. The clinical presentation mirrors that of Guillain-Barré syndrome. Although this is a rare occurrence, consider this possibility in unexplained weakness or paralysis after a person (especially a child) has recently been out in a wooded area.

Assessment and Management

The principal treatment of a tick bite is careful removal of the tick. Ticks attach themselves tenaciously to their victims using their mouth parts and a cement-like adhesive. If you try to pull the tick away from the skin, then the mouth parts may remain embedded. To remove the tick, after putting on gloves, use a curved forceps to grasp the skin immediately adjacent to the tick's head or the head itself as close to the skin as possible, and pull straight upward using steady, gentle traction. As you pull, use even pressure, and avoid twisting or jerking the tick. Do not squeeze or crush the tick's body. Dispose of the tick in a container of alcohol.

Once you have removed the tick, wash the area around the bite with soap and water. Depending on your local protocol, there may be no reason to transport the patient if he or she remains asymptomatic, but do advise your patient to see a physician. If you suspect tick paralysis or Lyme disease (with its cardiac or neurologic manifestations), then transport the patient.

YOU are the Paramedic

SUMMARY

1. What are your assessment and treatment priorities?

Assessment priorities include assessing for trauma injuries. The patient is feeling sleepy and weak and has a rapid radial pulse. Therefore, treatment priorities will focus on treatment of occult trauma injuries as well as passive rewarming. In addition, treatment priorities include spinal precautions (because he fell through the ice) and supporting airway and breathing. Assessment and treatment for cold-related injuries (frostbite) are also important.

2. What other information would you obtain about the patient and the incident?

It is important to identify any trauma injuries, especially head and spine trauma. What does the patient recall about the event? Were alcohol or drugs involved? Or, can any information be revealed from the patient's medical history or recent health complaints?

3. What are your early communication and transport plans?

Effective early communication with the receiving facility and transport to a trauma center will improve this patient's outcome. Depending on your location, you may consider transport by air.

4. What do these physical findings indicate to you?

His pale, cold, and moist skin could be a result of peripheral vasoconstriction as a result of frostbite. The fact that his peripheral-vascular and motor assessment is abnormal can be attributed to his frostbite. This is also evidenced by his weak and uncoordinated lower extremity movements. His fingers and toes are soft to the touch so they most likely sustained superficial frostbite. If they were firm, then you should suspect deep frostbite.

5. Why is his shivering significant?

The shivering means that his core body temperature (CBT) is still probably above 91°F (32.7°C) because shivering usually ceases when the CBT drops below 91°F (32.7°C). It also means that his body is compensating for the hypothermia and trying to generate heat through movement of skeletal muscle. The implication of this action is that he will burn energy at a faster rate than if he were resting. Therefore, checking his blood glucose level is important.

6. What can you conclude from the patient's vital signs?

The patient's blood pressure and pulse rate are low. His pulse is irregular and indicates some type of dysrhythmia.

He will need a 12-lead electrocardiogram and continuous cardiac monitoring for lethal dysrhythmias. In addition, you should obtain a CBT.

7. Why is the blood glucose reading of 48 mg/dL significant?

Normal blood glucose level ranges from approximately 60 to 120 mg/dL. Therefore, his blood glucose level is too low. This would explain his feeling of being sleepy and weak. It is possible that the hypoglycemia was a contributing factor to the snowmobile accident, but unlikely because he is healthy otherwise and has no history of diabetes.

8. Would you support the patient drinking warm fluids?

Drinking warm fluids would have to be limited in this patient. The patient should not have caffeinated beverages because they have a diuretic effect and hypovolemia is often associated with hypothermia. Because the patient is immobilized and he is still shivering, he may be at risk for aspiration.

9. What is the significance of his dysrhythmia?

The patient is shivering and has a CBT of 91°F (32.7°C). Atrial flutter may be observed in such patients until their CBT increases. The patient remains at risk for lethal dysrhythmias, so continuous cardiac monitoring is important.

10. What are your reassessment priorities?

It is important to reassess his vital signs and CBT for hemodynamic changes because active external rewarming can cause *afterdrop*—the continued lowering of the CBT even after the patient is removed from the cold. Because he is still at risk for dysrhythmias, cardiac monitoring remains important. Continue to reassess his frostbitten extremities for peripheral-vascular, motor, and sensory changes.

11. Why is it important to treat the patient's pain?

It is important to make the patient comfortable and treat his pain because pain causes unfavorable physiologic changes in perception and vital signs. However, careful monitoring is required when narcotic analgesics are given. Remember that side effects of narcotic analgesics include respiratory depression, bradycardia, and hypotension.

YOU ▸ are the Paramedic $\quad$ SUMMARY *(continued)*

EMS Patient Care Report (PCR)

Date: 01-10-18	**Incident No.:** 130		**Nature of Call:** Hypothermia	**Location:** 1090 County Aire Dr	

Dispatched: 1400	**En Route:** 1405	**At Scene:** 1415	**Transport:** 1445	**At Hospital:** 1525	**In Service:** 1555

Patient Information

Age: 20 **Sex:** M **Weight (in kg [lb]):** 100 kg (220 lb)	**Allergies:** No known drug allergies **Medications:** None **Past Medical History:** None **Chief Complaint:** Upper & lower extremity pain/hypothermia

Vital Signs

Time: 1425	**BP:** 80/40	**Pulse:** 104	**Respirations:** 10	**SpO₂:** 95%
Time: 1435	**BP:** 89/54	**Pulse:** 104	**Respirations:** 12	**SpO₂:** 98%
Time: 1445	**BP:** 110/64	**Pulse:** 104	**Respirations:** 14	**SpO₂:** 98%

EMS Treatment (circle all that apply)

Oxygen @ __4__ L/min via (circle one): (**NC**) $\quad$ **NRM** $\quad$ **Bag-mask device**	**Assisted Ventilation**	**Airway Adjunct**	**CPR**
Defibrillation	**Bleeding Control**	**Bandaging**	(**Splinting:** Spinal immobilization)	(**Other:** IV NS Lock #18 GA left AC, heat packs, blankets)

Narrative

Pt 20-year-old male who fell through the ice while riding his snowmobile about 1300 today. Pt then walked about ½ mile home unassisted. Upon arrival found pt sitting on kitchen floor A&O x 4, but slow to answer questions. Skin is pale, cold, and moist. Shivering noted. Extremities cold with absent distal pulses, absent sensation, and unable to move fingers and toes upon command. Wet clothes removed and pt dried and blankets applied. Physical exam otherwise unremarkable. Pt recalls entire event and denies LOC, neck pain, numbness/tingling in extremities, headache, N/V, abdominal pain, chest pain, or dyspnea. Reports bilateral hand, foot, finger/toe pain and "aching all over." Pain an "8" on "0–10" scale. Fitted pt with cervical collar and immobilized to long backboard. Heat packs applied to groin, neck, and axillae. En route fingers and toes remain soft and now pt can move fingers/toes, but sensation remains absent. Bulky dressings applied to hands, feet, fingers, and toes. Blood glucose 48 mg/dL. Medical direction is called and spoke to Dr. Patterson who advised a 500-mL warm NS IV bolus PRN and gave orders for morphine sulfate 2 mg IVP PRN and as vital signs permit titrated to effect and D₅₀ 25 grams IVP. Meds given as ordered and IV bolus X 2 given. Pain now a "4" on "0–10" scale and blood glucose is 149 mg/dL. Transported pt to St. Anthony's Hospital room #14 and report given to Julia, RN. No pt belongings transported. Paramedic Fred #12211.**End of report**

Prep Kit

► Ready for Review

- Environmental emergencies are medical conditions caused or worsened by the weather, terrain, or unique atmospheric conditions such as high altitude or being underwater.
- Risk factors that predispose people to environmental emergencies include being very young, being an older adult, being in a poor state of health, and taking certain medications.
- Thermoregulation is the body's ability to ensure a balance between heat production and release. The hypothalamus is the organ involved in regulating this balance. The skin also has a major role.
- The body produces heat through metabolism. The basal metabolic rate is the heat energy produced at rest from normal metabolic reactions. Metabolism can be increased through exertion, which also creates body heat. Absorption of heat from the environment can also occur.
- Thermolysis is the release of heat and energy from the body. Thermogenesis is the production of heat and energy for the body.
- The body has four main means of cooling itself: radiation—transfer of heat to the environment; conduction—transfer of heat to a cooler object through direct contact; convection—loss of heat to air moving across the skin; and evaporation—conversion of liquid to a gas (sweating).
- Heat illness is the increase in core body temperature due to inadequate thermolysis; the body cannot get rid of a heat buildup.
- Heat cramps are acute, involuntary muscle pains in the abdomen or lower extremities resulting from profuse sweating and sodium loss. The patient's pulse rate is usually rapid, the skin pale and moist, and the temperature normal. Treatment includes moving the patient to a cool environment, providing a salt-containing solution if the patient is not nauseated, or administering IV normal saline.
- Heat syncope can occur when an overheated patient suddenly changes position. Treatment includes placing the patient supine and replacing fluids.
- Heat exhaustion can result from dehydration and heat stress. Symptoms include headache, fatigue, dizziness, nausea, vomiting, and abdominal cramping. Skin is usually pale and clammy, and the pulse rate and respirations are rapid. Treatment consists of removing the patient from heat and providing fluids through sports drinks or an IV line.
- Heatstroke is defined as altered mental status with elevated body temperature. Signs include changes in behavior, nervous system disturbances (such as tremors), elevated temperature, tachycardia, hyperventilation, and skin that is dry and red or pale and sweaty. Treatment is to remove the patient from the heat, perform cooling measures, administer normal saline, and monitor the cardiac rhythm.
- Fever can mimic heatstroke. Obtain a thorough history, and treat for heatstroke if in doubt.
- To prevent heat illness, dress appropriately, stay hydrated, and stay in the shade or air conditioning. Community-based programs aimed at high-risk populations can provide valuable education.
- Frostbite is local freezing of a body part; it is classified as superficial or deep. Frostnip is a mild form of frostbite.
- Superficial frostbite is characterized by numbness, tingling, or burning. The skin is white, waxy, and firm to palpation. When thawed, the skin turns cyanotic and the patient feels a hot, stinging sensation. Treatment consists of getting the patient out of the cold; rewarming the injured part with body heat; covering with a warm, sterile dressing; and transporting the patient.
- In deep frostbite, the injured body part looks white, yellow-white, or mottled blue-white and is hard, cold, and without sensation. Major tissue damage can occur when the part thaws. Gangrene (permanent cell death) can result in the need for amputation. Treatment includes leaving the part frozen if it is found frozen, or rewarming the part if it is partially thawed.
- Trench foot is similar to frostbite but results from prolonged exposure to cool, wet conditions. Prevention is the best treatment.
- Hypothermia is a decrease in core body temperature. It can be mild, moderate, or severe.
- Mild hypothermia is a core body temperature of less than 95°F (35°C). The patient shivers and may be confused, have slurred speech, or have impaired coordination. Treatment is passive rewarming such as removing wet clothing or drying the patient's skin and possibly providing warm fluids. The Wilderness Medical Society (WMS) defines mild hypothermia as 95°F to 90°F (35°C to 32°C).
- Moderate hypothermia is a core body temperature in the range of 82°F to 90°F (28°C to 32°C). Treatment is passive rewarming, active external rewarming

Prep Kit (continued)

of truncal areas, administering warmed IV fluids, and potentially using special rewarming devices.

- Severe hypothermia is a core body temperature of less than 82°F (27.7°C). Treatment is active internal rewarming, such as administering warm IV fluids, and in-hospital measures.

- Hypothermic patients who are not breathing or who do not have a pulse need resuscitation. Patients in cardiac arrest require high-quality CPR and possibly a single shock depending on the heart rhythm; follow local guidelines. Attempt to insert an advanced airway; deliver ventilation with warm, humidified oxygen; and provide IV fluids.

- Hypothermic patients with obvious lethal traumatic injuries, or patients who are so frozen as to block the airway or chest compression efforts, are generally dead. If the patient appears dead after prolonged exposure, then hypothermia may protect the brain and organs. Resuscitation can be attempted in cases of cardiac arrest and hypothermia.

- Drowning is the process of experiencing respiratory impairment from submersion or immersion in liquid.

- Caring for a patient who was submersed starts with reaching the patient, a task that should be undertaken by specially trained rescuers. Treatment includes caring for the ABCs and taking cervical spine precautions. A nasogastric tube may be inserted to decompress the stomach if the patient is intubated. Submersion patients may develop bronchospasm and may require administration of a beta-2 adrenergic drug.

- In diving injuries, obtain as many details as possible about the patient, including the type of diving, type of tank, number of dives in the past 72 hours, and predive and postdive activities.

- Barotrauma can result during dive descent, owing to a pressure imbalance between the inside of the body and the outside atmosphere. It may result in ear pain. Treatment is a loose dressing for ear bleeding, and possibly IV antiemetics or sedatives.

- Nitrogen narcosis is a state of altered mental status caused by breathing compressed air at depth. Signs and symptoms include feeling euphoric; exhibiting inappropriate, foolish behavior; and tingling of the lips, gums, and legs.

- When a diver ascends too quickly, pulmonary overpressurization syndrome (POPS, also known as burst lung) can occur. Signs and symptoms include

mediastinal and subcutaneous emphysema, a sense of fullness in the throat, pain on swallowing, dyspnea, and substernal chest pain.

- Arterial gas embolism is a dangerous consequence of pulmonary overpressurization syndrome. Air bubbles may travel to the coronary arteries, causing cardiac arrest. Symptoms include weakness or paralysis of the extremities, seizure activity, unresponsiveness, and other neurologic symptoms.

- Treatment of barotrauma depends on whether an air embolism is present. A pneumothorax may require needle decompression. With an air embolism, the patient must receive treatment in a hyperbaric chamber.

- Decompression sickness encompasses a broad range of signs and symptoms caused by nitrogen bubbles in blood and tissues coming out of solution on dive ascent. Symptoms include itchy skin, subcutaneous emphysema, swelling, rashes, joint and muscle pain, sensory and motor disturbances, incoordination, paralysis, chest pain, and dyspnea. Treatment is 100% oxygen, IV normal saline, and transport to a hyperbaric facility.

- Shallow water blackout occurs when a person hyperventilates just before swimming underwater and passes out before resurfacing. Treatment is the same as for any other submersion.

- The Divers Alert Network (DAN) is a valuable resource for diving-related injuries. Callers are immediately directed to advice regarding management, and when necessary, to a physician experienced in diving medicine. DAN is particularly helpful in locating hyperbaric chambers.

- Altitude illness occurs when unacclimatized people ascend to altitude. Types of altitude illness include acute mountain sickness, high-altitude cerebral edema, and high-altitude pulmonary edema.

- Symptoms of acute mountain sickness include headache plus fatigue, weakness, gastrointestinal symptoms, dizziness, light-headedness, and difficulty sleeping.

- Symptoms of high-altitude cerebral edema include a change in mental status and/or ataxia in a person with acute mountain sickness or the presence of both in a person without acute mountain sickness.

- Symptoms of high-altitude pulmonary edema include at least two of the following: dyspnea at rest, cough, weakness, or chest tightness or congestion and

Prep Kit *(continued)*

at least two of the following: central cyanosis, audible crackles, wheezing, tachypnea, or tachycardia.

- Treatment of altitude illnesses includes descending or using a portable hyperbaric chamber, providing oxygen, and administering certain IV medications.
- Cardiopulmonary resuscitation should be started promptly for lightning strike victims.
- Lightning strike victims should be evaluated using "reverse triage," meaning that those people who appear to be dead should be treated first.
- Anaphylactic reaction is the most frequent cause of mortality from all insect bites and envenomations.
- Prompt removal of hymenopteran stingers or venom sacs can decrease toxin exposure.
- Fire ant stings often result in infection.
- Pit vipers (crotalins) are responsible for the greatest number of snake bites in the United States.
- With a crotalin bite, if there are visible fang marks with no bleeding, this indicates that a "dry bite" (with no venom) has occurred.
- In terms of scene safety, it is important to ensure the snake is dead, gone, or trapped in cases of envenomation.
- All significant snake envenomations require treatment with antivenin; transport promptly. The time between the occurrence of the bite and the time of treatment is crucial.
- The female black widow, the brown recluse, and the hobo spider produce the most concerning spider bites.
- A small subset of patients with brown recluse spider bites may develop loxoscelism.
- Scorpion stings produce a neurotoxic reaction that causes autonomic excitation.
- Treatment of scorpion stings is largely supportive, with protection of the airway.
- Tick bites can transmit a variety of serious illnesses, and in rare cases, can cause life-threatening paralysis. Principal treatment is careful removal of the tick, and washing the area around the bite. Transport all patients with any neurologic symptoms.

▶ Vital Vocabulary

acute lung injury A condition in which lung tissue is damaged, characterized by hypoxemia, low lung volume, and pulmonary edema.

acute mountain sickness (AMS) An altitude illness characterized by headache plus at least one of the following: fatigue or weakness, gastrointestinal symptoms (nausea, vomiting, or anorexia), dizziness or light-headedness, or difficulty sleeping.

afterdrop Continued fall in core body temperature after a victim of hypothermia has been removed from a cold environment, due at least in part to the return of cold blood from the body surface to the body core.

altitude illnesses Conditions caused by the effects from hypobaric (low atmospheric pressure) hypoxia on the central nervous system and pulmonary systems as a result of unacclimatized people ascending to altitude; range from acute mountain sickness to high-altitude cerebral edema and high-altitude pulmonary edema.

arterial gas embolism (AGE) The resultant gaseous emboli from the forcing of gas into the vasculature from barotrauma.

ataxia Inability to properly coordinate the muscles; often used to describe a staggering gait.

atmosphere absolute (ATA) A measurement of ambient pressure; the weight of air at sea level, equivalent in pressure to 33 feet (10 m) of seawater (fsw).

barotrauma Injury resulting from pressure disequilibrium across body surfaces.

basal metabolic rate (BMR) The heat energy produced at rest from normal body metabolic reactions, determined mostly by the liver and skeletal muscles.

Boyle's law At a constant temperature, the volume of a gas is inversely proportional to its pressure (if you double the pressure on a gas, you halve its volume); written as $PV = K$, where P = pressure, V = volume, and K = a constant.

breath-hold diving Also called free diving, this type of diving does not require any equipment, except sometimes a snorkel.

chilblains Itchy red and purple swollen lesions that occur primarily on the extremities, due to longer exposure to temperatures just above freezing or sudden rewarming after exposure to cold.

classic heatstroke Also called passive heatstroke, this is a serious heat illness that usually occurs during heat waves and is most likely to strike very old, very young, or bedridden people.

cold diuresis Secretion of large amounts of urine in response to cold exposure and the consequent shunting of blood volume to the body core.

conduction Transfer of heat to a solid object or a liquid by direct contact.

Prep Kit (continued)

convection Mechanism by which body heat is picked up and carried away by moving air currents.

core body temperature (CBT) The temperature in the part of the body comprising the heart, lungs, brain, and abdominal viscera.

Dalton's law Each gas in a mixture exerts the same partial pressure that it would exert if it were alone in the same volume, and the total pressure of a mixture of gases is the sum of the partial pressures of all the gases in a mixture.

decompression illness (DCI) A term for decompression sickness (DCS) and air gas embolism (AGE).

decompression sickness (DCS) A broad range of signs and symptoms caused by nitrogen bubbles in blood and tissues coming out of solution on ascent.

deep frostbite A type of frostbite in which the affected part looks white, yellow-white, or mottled blue-white and is hard, cold, and without sensation.

drowning The process of experiencing respiratory impairment from submersion or immersion in liquid.

envenomation The injecting of venom via a bite or sting.

environmental emergencies Medical conditions caused or exacerbated by the weather, terrain, or unique atmospheric conditions such as high altitude or underwater.

evaporation The conversion of a liquid to a gas.

exercise-associated hyponatremia (EAH) A condition due to prolonged exertion in hot environments coupled with excessive hypotonic fluid intake that leads to nausea, vomiting, and, in severe cases, mental status changes and seizures (also known as exertional hyponatremia or exercise-induced hyponatremia).

exertional heatstroke A serious type of heatstroke usually affecting young and fit people exercising in hot and humid conditions.

feet of seawater (fsw) An indirect measure of pressure under water, equal to one atmosphere absolute (ATA).

frostbite Localized damage to tissues resulting from prolonged exposure to extreme cold.

frostnip Early frostbite, characterized by numbness and pallor without significant tissue damage.

gangrene Permanent cell death.

heat cramps Acute and involuntary muscle pains, usually in the lower extremities, the abdomen, or both, that occur because of profuse sweating and subsequent sodium losses in sweat.

heat exhaustion A clinical syndrome characterized by volume depletion and heat stress that is thought to be a milder form of heat illness and on a continuum leading to heatstroke.

heat illness The increase in core body temperature due to inadequate thermolysis.

heatstroke The least common and most deadly heat illness, caused by a severe disturbance in thermoregulation, usually characterized by a core temperature of more than 104°F (40°C) and altered mental status.

heat syncope An orthostatic or near-syncopal episode that typically occurs in nonacclimated people who may be under heat stress.

Henry's law The amount of gas dissolved in a liquid is directly proportional to the partial pressure of the gas above the liquid.

high-altitude cerebral edema (HACE) An altitude illness in which there is a change in mental status and/or ataxia in a person with acute mountain sickness or the presence of mental status changes and ataxia in a person without acute mountain sickness.

high-altitude pulmonary edema (HAPE) An altitude illness characterized by at least two of the following: dyspnea at rest, cough, weakness or decreased exercise performance, or chest tightness or congestion. Also, at least two of the following signs: central cyanosis, audible crackles or wheezing in at least one lung field, tachypnea, or tachycardia.

homeostasis A tendency to constancy or stability in the body's internal environment; processes that balance the supply and demand of the body's needs.

hypercapnia Increased carbon dioxide in the blood.

hyperthermia Unusually elevated body temperature.

hypothalamus Portion of the brain that regulates a multitude of body functions, including core temperature.

hypothermia Condition in which the core body temperature is significantly below normal.

hypoxemia A decrease in arterial oxygen level.

laryngospasm Severe constriction of the larynx in response to allergy, noxious stimuli, or illness.

loxoscelism A potentially fatal condition resulting from a brown recluse spider bite that begins with a painful, inflamed vesicle that may progress to a gangrenous sloughing of the skin.

malignant hyperthermia A condition that can result from common anesthesia medications (notably

Prep Kit *(continued)*

succinylcholine) and present with hyperthermia, muscular rigidity, altered mental status, and a hyperdynamic state.

neuroleptic malignant syndrome (NMS) A condition caused by antipsychotic and even common anti-emetic medications that presents with hyperthermia, muscular rigidity, altered mental status, and a hyperdynamic state.

nitrogen narcosis A state resembling alcohol intoxication produced by nitrogen gas dissolved in the blood at high ambient pressure; also called rapture of the deep.

odynophagia Painful swallowing.

orthostatic hypotension A fall in blood pressure that occurs when moving from a recumbent to a sitting or standing position.

partial pressure The amount of the total pressure contributed by various gases in solution.

pulmonary overpressurization syndrome (POPS) Also called burst lung, this diving emergency can occur during rapid ascent and can cause pneumothorax, mediastinal and subcutaneous emphysema, alveolar hemorrhage, and the lethal arterial gas embolism (AGE).

radiation Emission of heat from an object into surrounding, colder air.

saturation diving A type of diving in which the diver remains at depth for prolonged periods.

self-contained underwater breathing apparatus The expansion of the acronym SCUBA for specialized underwater breathing equipment.

shallow water blackout A diving emergency that occurs when a person hyperventilates just before submerging underwater and becomes unresponsive before resurfacing due to hypoxemia and cerebral vasoconstriction.

superficial frostbite A type of frostbite characterized by altered sensation (numbness, tingling, or burning) and white, waxy skin that is firm to palpation, but the underlying tissues remain soft.

surface-tended diving A type of diving in which air is piped to the diver through a tube from the surface.

thermogenesis The production of heat in the body.

thermolysis The liberation of heat from the body.

thermoregulation The process by which the body compensates for environmental extremes, for example, balancing between heat production and heat release.

trench foot A process similar to frostbite but caused by prolonged exposure to cool, wet conditions.

wind-chill factor A measurement that takes into account the temperature and wind velocity in calculating the effect of a given ambient temperature on living organisms.

▶ References

1. Centers for Disease Control and Prevention. Hypothermia-related deaths: Wisconsin, 2014, and United States, 2003-2013. *Morb Mortal Wkly Rep.* 2015;64(6):141-143.

2. 17 Shocking Heat Exhaustion Statistics. Health Research Funding website. http://healthresearchfunding.org/17-shocking-heat-exhaustion-statistics/. Posted Mar 23, 2015. Accessed March 13, 2017.

3. NASA, NOAA data show 2016 warmest year on record globally. National Aeronautics and Space Administration website. https://www.nasa.gov/press-release/nasa-noaa-data-show-2016-warmest-year-on-record-globally. NASA Media Release 17-006: January 18, 2017. Accessed March 13, 2017.

4. Kochanek KD, Xu J, Murphy SL, Miniño AM, Kung H-C, Division of Vital Statistics. Deaths: preliminary data for 2009. *Natl Vital Stat Rep;* 59(4). Hyattsville, MD: National Center for Health Statistics; 2011.

5. Robine JM, Cheung SL, Le Roy S, et al. Death toll exceeded 70,000 in Europe during the summer of 2003. *C R Biol.* 2008;331(2):171-178.

6. Mazerolle SM, Ganio MS, Casa DJ, Vingren J, Klau J. Is oral temperature an accurate measurement of deep body temperature? A systematic review. *J Athl Train.* 2011;46(5):566-573.

7. Sund-Levander M, Grodzinsky E. Time for a change to assess and evaluate body temperature in clinical practice. *Int J Nurs Pract.* 2009;15(4):241-249.

8. Cold exposure: ways the body loses heat. University of Michigan, Michigan Medicine website. http://www.uofmhealth.org/health-library/tw9037. Updated May 27, 2016. Accessed March 21, 2017.

9. Stofan JR, Zachwieja JJ, Horswill CA, Murray R, Anderson SA, Eichner ER. Sweat and sodium losses in NCAA football players: a precursor to heat cramps? *Int J Sport Nutri Exerc Metab.* 2005;15:641-652.

Prep Kit (continued)

10. Almond CSD, Shin AY, Fortescue EB, et al. Hyponatremia among runners in the Boston Marathon. *N Engl J Med.* 2005;352:1550-1556.

11. Backer HD, Shopes E, Collins SL, Barkan H. Exertional heat illness and hyponatremia in hikers. *Am J Emerg Med.* 1999;17(6):532-539.

12. O'Donnell FL, ed. Army Medical Surveillance Activity. Update: exertional hyponatremia, active component, U.S. Armed Forces, 1999-2011. *MSMR.* 2012;19:20-23.

13. Bennett BL, Hew-Butler T, Hoffman MD, Rogers IR, Rosner MH. Wilderness Medical Society practice guidelines for treatment of exercise-associated hyponatremia. *Wilderness Environ Med.* 2013;24(3):228-240.

14. Hew-Butler T, Rosner MH, Fowkes-Godek S, et al. Statement of the third international exercise-associated hyponatremia consensus development conference, Carlsbad, California, 2015. *Clin J Sport Med.* 2015;25(4):303-320.

15. Brege D. Recognizing and treating heatstroke. *Nurs Made Incredibly Easy!* 2009;7(4):13-18.

16. Mann D. Public health & policy. Residence, medication key factors linked to heatstroke-related deaths. Medpage Today website. http://www.medpagetoday.com/publichealthpolicy/publichealth/6401. Posted August 13, 2007. Accessed March 21, 2017.

17. Lipman G, Eifling K, Ellis M, Gaudio F, Otten E, Grisson C. Wilderness Medical Society practice guidelines for the prevention and treatment of heat-related illness: 2014 update. *Wilderness Environ Med.* 2014;S55-S65.

18. Armstrong LE, Casa DJ, Millard-Stafford M, Moran DS, Pyne SW, Roberts WO. Exertional heat illness during training and competition. *Med Sci Sports Exerc.* 2007;39(3):556-572.

19. Luhring KE, Butts CL, Smith CR, et al. Cooling effectiveness of a modified cold-water immersion method after exercise-induced hyperthermia. *J Athl Train.* 2016 Mar;51(3):252-257. http://natajournals.org/doi/10.4085/1062-6050-51.12.07?code=nata-site. Accessed March 15, 2017.

20. Centers for Disease Control and Prevention: Hypothermia-Related Deaths-United States, 2003, *MMWR Weekly.* 2004;53(08);172-173. https://www.cdc.gov/mmwr/preview/mmwrhtml/mm5308a2.htm. Accessed March 21, 2017.

21. Zafren K, Giesbrecht GG, Danzl DF, et al. Wilderness Medical Society practice guidelines for the out-of-hospital evaluation and treatment of accidental hypothermia: 2014 update. *Wilderness Environ Med.* 2014;25(suppl 4):S66-S85. https://www.ncbi.nlm.nih.gov/pubmed/25498264. Accessed November 15, 2016.

22. CPR and ECC guidelines: cardiac arrest in accidental hypothermia. American Heart Association website. https://eccguidelines.heart.org/index.php/circulation/cpr-ecc-guidelines-2/part-10-special-circumstances-of-resuscitation/cardiac-arrest-in-accidental-hypothermia/. Accessed November 15, 2016.

23. Danzl DF, Pozos RS, Auerbach PS, et al. Multicenter hypothermia survey. *Ann Emerg Med.* 1987;16(9):1042-1055. https://www.ncbi.nlm.nih.gov/pubmed/3631669. Accessed November 15, 2016.

24. Xu JQ. Unintentional drowning deaths in the United States, 1999-2010. National Center for Health Statistics Data Brief, no 149. Hyattsville, MD: National Center for Health Statistics. 2014. http://www.cdc.gov/nchs/data/databriefs/db149.pdf. Accessed November 15, 2016.

25. Sempsrott JS, Schmidt AC, Hawkins SC, Cushing TA. Drowning and submersion injuries. In: Auerbach PS, ed. *Auerbach's Wilderness Medicine.* 7th ed. Philadelphia, PA: Elsevier; 2017.

26. 10 leading causes of injury deaths by age group highlighting unintentional injury deaths, United States-2014. Centers for Disease Control and Prevention website. Available at https://www.cdc.gov/injury/images/lc-charts/leading_causes_of_injury_deaths_unintentional_injury_2014_1040w740h.gif. Accessed March 13, 2017.

27. Bierens JJLM, ed. *Handbook on Drowning: Prevention, Rescue, Treatment.* Germany: Springer; 2006.

28. Schmidt AC, Sempsrott JR, Hawkins SC, Arastu AS, Cushing TA, Auerbach PS. Wilderness Medical Society practice guidelines for the prevention and treatment of drowning. *Wilderness Environ Med.* 2016;27(2):236-251.

29. Schmidt AC. Drownings present as hypoxic events. *J Emerg Med.* 2012;37(7). http://www.jems.com/articles/print/volume-37/issue-7/patient-care/drownings-present-hypoxic-events.html. Accessed March 13, 2017.

30. Foex, BA, Boyd R. Towards evidence based emergency medicine: best BETs from the Manchester Royal Infirmary. Corticosteroids in the management of near-drowning. *Emerg Med J.* 2001;18:465-466.

31. Bolte RG , Black PG, Bowers RS. The use of extracorporeal rewarming in a child submerged for 66 minutes. *JAMA.* 1988;260(3):377-379.

32. Sempsrott J. Drowning: 2015 in review. *Wilderness Medicine Magazine.* January 6, 2016.

33. van Hoesen KB, Lang MA. Diving medicine. In: Auerbach PS, ed. *Auerbach's Wilderness Medicine.* 7th ed. Philadelphia, PA: Elsevier; 2017.

Prep Kit (continued)

34. Zafren K. Management of acute high altitude illnesses. In: Hawkins SC, ed. *Wilderness EMS.* Philadelphia, PA: Wolters Kluwer; 2018.

35. Harris FS, Terrio J, Miser WF, Yetter JF. High-altitude medicine. *Amer Fam Physician.* 1998;57(8):1907-1914.

36. Hawkins SC, Simon RB, Beissinger JP, Simon D. *Vertical Aid: Essential Wilderness Medicine for Climbers, Trekkers, and Mountaineers.* New York, NY: The Countryman Press; 2017.

37. Luks AM, McIntosh SE, Grissom CK, et al. Wilderness Medical Society consensus guidelines for the prevention and treatment of acute altitude illness: 2014 update. *Wilderness Environ Med.* 2014;25(suppl 4):S4-S14.

38. U.S. lightning deaths in 2017: 0. National Oceanic and Atmospheric Administration website. http://www.lightningsafety.noaa.gov/fatalities.shtml. Accessed March 21, 2017.

39. Cooper MA, Andrews CJ, Holle RL, Bliumenthal R, Aldana NN. Lightning-related injuries and safety. In: Auerbach PS, ed. *Auerbach's Wilderness Medicine.* Philadelphia, PA: Elsevier; 2017.

40. Cooper MA, Holle RL, Andrews CJ. Distribution of lightning injury mechanisms. Presented at 20th International Lightning Detection Conference; April, 2008; Tucson, AZ.

41. Park R. Hymenoptera stings. Medscape website. http://emedicine.staging.medscape.com/article/768764-overview#a6. Updated April 27, 2017. Accessed May 9, 2017.

42. Juckett G, Hancox JG. Venomous snakebites in the United States: management review and update. *Am Fam Physician.* 2002;65(7):1367-1375.

43. Ferri FF. Ferri's Clinical Advisor 2013. Philadelphia, PA: Elsevier; 2013:162.

44. Sanders L. Management of venomous snake bites in North America. emDocs website. http://www.emdocs.net/management-of-venomous-snake-bites-in-north-america/. September 11, 2015. Accessed May 9, 2017.

45. Frequently asked questions about venomous snakes. Department of Wildlife Ecology & Conservation, UF Wildlife-Johnson Lab website. http://ufwildlife.ifas.ufl.edu/venomous_snake_faqs.shtml. Updated May 2, 2012. Accessed March 15, 2017.

46. Young, BA, Zahn K. Dry bites are real. Venom flow in rattlesnakes: mechanics and metering. *J Exp Biol.* 2001;204:4345-4351.

47. Kanaan NC, Ray J, Stewart M, et al. Wilderness Medical Society practice guidelines for the treatment of pit viper envenomations in the United States and Canada. *Wilderness Env Med.* 2015;26(4):472-487.

48. Sharma S, Vyas A, Sharma R. Diversity and abundance of spider fauna of narmada river at Rajghat (Barwani) (Madhya Pradesh) India. *Researcher.* 2010;2(11):2.

49. Currie BJ, Canale E, Isbister GK. Effectiveness of pressure-immobilization first aid for snakebite requires further study. *Emerg Med Australasia.* 2008;20(3):267-270.

50. Norris RL, Ngo J, Nolan K, Hooker G. Physicians and lay people are unable to apply pressure immobilization properly in a simulated snakebite scenario. *Wilderness Environ Med.* 2005;16:16-21.

51. Howarth DM, Southee AS, Whytw IM. Lymphatic flow rates and first aid in simulated peripheral snake or spider envenomation. *Med J Australia.* 1994;161:695-700.

52. Black widow spider bite—topic overview. WebMD website. http://www.webmd.com/first-aid/tc/black-widow-spider-bite-topic-overview#1. Accessed May 9, 2017.

53. Clark RF, Wethern-Kestner S, Vanc MV, Gerkin R. Clinical presentation and treatment of black widow spider envenomation: a review of 163 cases. *Ann Emerg Med.* 1992 Jul;21(7):782-787.

54. Forrester MB, Stanley SK. Epidemiology of scorpion envenomations in Texas. *Vet Hum Toxicol.* 2004;46(4):219-221. https://www.ncbi.nlm.nih.gov/labs/articles/15303401/. Accessed May 9, 2017.

55. Mowry JB, Spyker DA, Cantilena LR, Bailey JE, Ford M. The 2014 annual report of the American Association of Poison Control Centers' National Poison Data System (NPDS): 30th annual report. https://aapcc.s3.amazonaws.com/pdfs/annual_reports/2012_NPDS_Annual_Report.pdf. Accessed March 23, 2017.

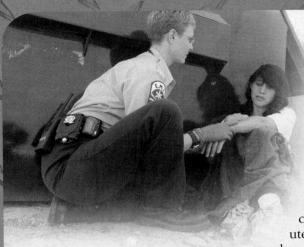

Assessment in Action

It is a hot, humid summer day (98°F [37°C] ambient air temperature/80% humidity) and you are dispatched to the scene of a local grocery store for a 2-year-old girl who is unresponsive. According to law enforcement personnel at the scene, the child was left in the vehicle "with the windows cracked" while her mother went into the store "for just a minute." When you arrive, you find the child with the police who now have her in their air-conditioned patrol vehicle; she is lying supine on some towels in the back seat. A police officer is fanning the child as he sits next to her in the squad vehicle.

The child is extremely flushed and her skin is hot, dry, and red. Her extremities are mottled and her lips are gray. She is unresponsive to voice and pain (no motor response), and without eye opening. Her airway is open with dried secretions around the mouth.

Her vital signs are: respirations, 70 breaths/min with retractions; carotid pulse, 180 beats/min, weak and regular; blood pressure cannot be measured; and pulse oximetry, 88% on room air; rectal thermometer reads 106°F (41.1°C); capillary refill time is 5 seconds. Breath sounds are diminished, but clear and equal bilaterally. Her weight is estimated at 35 pounds (16 kg) using a length-based resuscitation tape. There are no signs of trauma injuries. The patient's clothes are removed as she is placed on the stretcher and bag-mask ventilations are initiated with 100% oxygen. While en route to the closest pediatric specialty center, IV access is attempted twice without success. Intraosseous access in the left tibia is obtained. Cold packs are applied to the patient's neck, groin, and axillae, and the air conditioner in the back of the ambulance is turned to its lowest setting. Medical direction is consulted and a rapid infusion of a 10 mL/kg NS bolus is ordered PRN. Her blood glucose level is 38 mg/dL. D_{25} 12.5 grams IVP is given per protocol. En route a complete trauma assessment is performed and found to be unremarkable.

1. The patient's body reacted to hot environmental conditions by releasing stored heat and energy by a process called:

   A. thermolysis.
   B. hemolysis.
   C. thermogenesis.
   D. shivering.

2. All of the following are ways the patient's body can compensate for an increased core body temperature EXCEPT:

   A. increased cardiac output.
   B. opening of sweat glands.
   C. increased basal metabolic rate.
   D. cutaneous vasoconstriction.

3. The only way the patient's body can dissipate heat when the ambient temperature approaches body temperature is through:

   A. perspiration (sweat).
   B. decreasing respirations.
   C. shivering.
   D. increased basal metabolic rate.

4. A severe heat-related disturbance in the body's thermoregulation system characterized by mental status changes, typically accompanied by a core body temperature more than 104°F (40°C), is called:

   A. heat exhaustion.
   B. heatstroke.
   C. heat syncope.
   D. heat cramps.

Assessment *in Action* (continued)

5. When you treat this patient for heatstroke, cooling should:

   A. occur in such a way as to not allow her core body temperature to drop more than 1 degree per hour.
   B. occur as slowly as possible.
   C. not be considered a priority.
   D. occur as rapidly as possible.

6. Patients with heatstroke, such as in this case, are at risk for the development of:

   A. metabolic alkalosis.
   B. seizures.
   C. hyperglycemia.
   D. exertional hypernatremia.

7. All of the following would be an effective means of cooling the patient EXCEPT:

   A. cold water or ice immersion.
   B. spraying the patient with tepid water while fanning constantly.
   C. administering antipyretics.
   D. applying ice packs to the patient's groin, neck, and axillae.

8. How can you differentiate a patient experiencing heatstroke from a patient with a febrile illness or sepsis?

9. Why are older adults at more risk than younger adults for cold-related emergencies?

10. What is the most frequent cause of mortality from all envenomations?

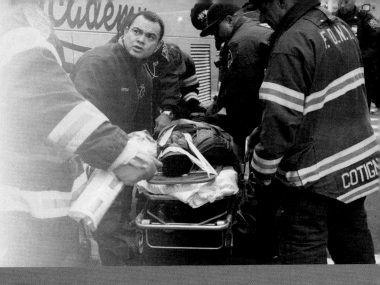

SECTION 8

Shock and Resuscitation

Responding to the Field Code

National EMS Education Standard Competencies

Shock and Resuscitation

> Integrates comprehensive knowledge of causes and pathophysiology into the management of cardiac arrest and pre-arrest states.

Knowledge Objectives

1. Describe how paramedics, the field code team, and the emergency medical services agency can incorporate the latest *Guidelines for Cardiopulmonary Resuscitation and Emergency Cardiac Care* from the American Heart Association and International Liaison Committee on Resuscitation into the management of field codes. (pp 1945, 1947-1957, 1962-1970)
2. Discuss the importance of the five links of the out-of-hospital chain of survival during a successful field code. (p 1945)
3. Describe the management mnemonic SMART, including how communities can apply it to improve the survival rates of patients in out-of-hospital cardiac arrest. (pp 1945-1946)
4. Discuss the use of simulation technology in cardiopulmonary resuscitation (CPR) training. (pp 1946-1947)
5. Describe the resuscitation pyramid and how it relates to high-quality CPR. (p 1947)
6. Discuss some of the theories about blood flow during CPR that have shifted the focus of certain CPR techniques. (p 1948)
7. Summarize the steps of the Basic Life Support Healthcare Provider Adult Cardiac Arrest Algorithm and identify the key to a successful outcome in patients in cardiac arrest. (pp 1948-1950)
8. Explain how two-rescuer CPR can benefit the paramedic and the patient. (p 1951)
9. Explain how to perform two-rescuer adult CPR, including the method for switching positions during the process. (pp 1951-1953)
10. Define the five age groups for the purposes of resuscitation. (pp 1951, 1953)
11. Explain how to perform child and infant CPR, including the method for switching positions during the process. (pp 1954-1957)
12. Discuss guidelines for circumstances that require the use of an automated external defibrillator on both adult and pediatric patients in cardiac arrest. (pp 1957-1958)
13. Describe situations in which manual or automated defibrillation would be appropriate. (p 1957)
14. Describe how to manage a witnessed cardiac arrest versus a nonwitnessed cardiac arrest. (pp 1958-1959)
15. Summarize how to perform manual or automated defibrillation on an adult versus a child or infant. (pp 1959-1960)
16. Explain special situations related to the use of defibrillation. (p 1961)
17. Review the management of a cardiac arrest based on analysis of the electrocardiogram as either a shockable rhythm (ventricular fibrillation [VF] or pulseless ventricular tachycardia [pVT]) or a nonshockable rhythm (pulseless electrical activity [PEA] or asystole). (pp 1964-1967)
18. Describe the possible causes and treatment of cardiac rhythms (the "Hs and Ts"), including how the management of these conditions begins in the field. (p 1966)
19. Discuss the different mechanical adjuncts to circulation that are used to assist in delivering chest compressions during CPR. (pp 1967-1969)
20. Describe the general steps of postresuscitative care and the importance of transporting the patient to the most appropriate facility. (p 1969)
21. Describe the ethical issues related to patient resuscitation, including examples of when not to start CPR on a patient. (pp 1969-1970)
22. Explain the various factors involved in the decision to stop CPR after it has been started on a patient. (pp 1970-1971)
23. Discuss the value of scene choreography and crew resource management during a field code. (pp 1970-1972)
24. Describe the typical roles of the code team leader and code team members during a field code. (p 1972)
25. Describe the importance of debriefing after a field code. (p 1973)

Skills Objectives

1. Demonstrate how to perform one- and two-rescuer adult CPR. (pp 1949-1953, Skill Drill 39-1)
2. Demonstrate how to perform CPR in a child who is between age 1 year and the onset of puberty. (pp 1953-1955, Skill Drill 39-2)
3. Demonstrate how to perform CPR in an infant who is between ages 1 month and 1 year. (pp 1953-1954, 1956-1957, Skill Drill 39-3)
4. Demonstrate how defibrillation is integrated into the field code for the adult or pediatric patient. (pp 1958-1961)
5. Demonstrate how to manage a patient in VF or pVT. (pp 1964-1966)
6. Demonstrate how to manage a patient in asystole or PEA. (pp 1964-1967)
7. Demonstrate the roles of the code team members and code team leader in a resuscitation. (p 1972)

■ Introduction

In the early 1970s, when the first edition of this text was written, the technique of cardiopulmonary resuscitation (CPR) was only in its second decade of existence. A sudden cardiac arrest in the out-of-hospital environment was a terminal event and few people survived. In the mid 1970s, stories began to circulate about the success of programs such as the Medic One CPR training in Seattle and surrounding King County, Washington. These programs brought CPR training to the public through schools, firehouses, and postal mailings. The training programs resulted in a paradigm shift. The expectations of the 1970s that most cardiac arrests would result in death soon gave way to the current expectation for a **return of spontaneous circulation (ROSC)**.

Today, the best emergency medical services (EMS) systems take the time to train the public in CPR and place **automated external defibrillators (AEDs)** in certain public places such as those where there is a relatively high likelihood of witnessed cardiac arrest, such as airports, stadiums, etc. These EMS systems are achieving tremendous success in increasing the number of patients with ROSC. It is not unusual to find communities with a ROSC rate as high as 40%.[1,2] EMS providers are no longer surprised when they get a patient's pulse back; they expect it to come back! It is clear that treating a sudden cardiac arrest is a discipline that requires attention to all the details, as well as involvement of the entire community.

YOU ▶ are the Paramedic   PART 1

At 1415 hours you are dispatched to a golf course located in a gated island community. Local volunteer emergency medical responders (EMRs) have also been dispatched. You are advised that you are responding to a 54-year-old man who has collapsed while golfing. He is reported to be pulseless and apneic, and hands-only CPR is in progress. You have requested that your field supervisor respond to the call with you. On arrival you find CPR being performed on a man lying on the ground. An AED is attached to the patient. You are met by a man who tells you that his friend was reporting "indigestion" after lunch when they began playing. Thanks to a recent community CPR course, he initiated compressions immediately. The bystander is not aware of any medical history or medications taken regularly by his friend. He explains that the patient's wife is being driven to the scene from their home within the community.

The EMRs assist you and your paramedic partner as you begin two-rescuer CPR and ventilating the patient with a bag-mask device. You are told CPR has been in progress for approximately 6 minutes. The AED was retrieved and one shock was delivered prior to your arrival. You connect your cardiac monitor and analyze the electrocardiogram (ECG). The patient's rhythm is ventricular fibrillation. You are aware that this is a lethal but shockable rhythm, and you prepare to defibrillate while the EMRs continue high-quality compressions at a rate of 100 to 120 per minute and your partner provides ventilations using high-concentration oxygen. You assume the role of code team leader.

1. Which links of the out-of-hospital chain of survival are present that would make you optimistic about this patient's potential for ROSC?
2. On the basis of the events occurring prior to your arrival and your own analysis of the ECG, what are your next steps as code team leader?

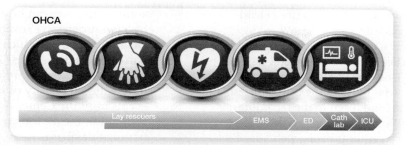

Figure 39-1 The five links of the out-of-hospital chain of survival.
Reprinted with permission. Highlights of the 2015 American Heart Association Guidelines Update for CPR & ECC. © 2015 American Heart Association, Inc.

This chapter explores ways that practice and planning can help increase your success with resuscitation. You will learn about planning for the resuscitation or "field code," and what actions are performed by the **code team leader** and **code team members**. The expression, "Failure to plan is planning to fail," is never more apparent than during the resuscitation of the patient who has experienced sudden cardiac arrest. In the past, the American Heart Association (AHA), in concert with the International Liaison Committee on Resuscitation, came together to revise the *Guidelines for Cardiopulmonary Resuscitation and Emergency Cardiac Care (ECC)* every 5 years. However, it was recognized in the 2015 guidelines that a 5-year cycle is insufficient to keep pace with the rapidly evolving research in resuscitation science, and you should expect to see updates released more frequently in the future. This chapter describes how you, your team, and your agency can incorporate the latest guidelines into the management of field codes in adults, children, and infants. The care of newborn and neonatal patients is discussed in Chapter 42, *Neonatal Care.*

Words of Wisdom

According to the AHA Statistics Committee and Stroke Statistics Subcommittee, each year roughly 359,800 people experience EMS-assessed out-of-hospital cardiac arrest in the United States.[3] For patients of any age, survival to hospital discharge after EMS-treated non-traumatic cardiac arrest with any first recorded rhythm was 10.6%.[3] Of the approximately 20,150 patients with bystander-witnessed out-of-hospital cardiac arrest in 2011, 31.4% (6,327) survived to hospital discharge.[3]

Improving the Response to Cardiac Arrest

▶ The Chain of Survival

To achieve success in the assessment and management of a patient in cardiac arrest in the field, all the links in the out-of-hospital chain of survival must be solidly in place **Figure 39-1** . As determined by the AHA, the five links are as follows:[4]

1. Recognition and activation of the emergency response system
2. Immediate high-quality CPR
3. Rapid defibrillation
4. Basic and advanced EMS care
5. Advanced life support (ALS) and postarrest care (that is, transport to a hospital that can provide state-of-the-art procedures such as **targeted temperature management (TTM)**, continuous electroencephalogram [EEG] or brain wave monitoring, cardiac catheterization, and seizure control)

This process takes a team of skilled providers, beginning with community members who are trained in CPR, to the first EMRs who arrive with an AED, to the emergency medical technicians (EMTs) and paramedics who have been well trained in high-quality CPR and frequently practice simulated codes. The prehospital team should practice so they are able to work together in tandem, with their moves choreographed by a code team leader. A slightly different version of the chain of survival exists for in-hospital providers. The in-hospital chain of survival emphasizes surveillance and prevention of the patient in peri-arrest (a condition that is highly likely to lead to cardiac arrest if left untreated).

▶ Developing Out-of-Hospital Program Objectives: The SMART Way

When you are undertaking a community-based program to improve the survival of patients in out-of-hospital cardiac arrest, consider adopting the management mnemonic **SMART** to describe the objectives of the program: Specific, Measurable, Attainable and Achievable, Realistic and Relevant, and Timely. The following are a few questions that members of progressive communities must ask themselves to improve their responses:

■ Is a universal access number (ie, 9-1-1) available, and do all members of the public know how and when to use it?

- Do all citizens have an address number clearly posted on their residence?
- Are all public safety telecommunicators trained to provide instruction in hands-only CPR-T (telephone CPR) Does the medical director for the dispatch center review 100% of the cardiac arrests to analyze the times and listen to the recordings for compliance with medical dispatch protocols?
- Does your dispatch center utilize a web-based system or mobile app that alerts nearby CPR-trained bystanders in the community of the location of patients in cardiac arrest?
- Is a community CPR training program readily available at all times of the day and days of the week at little to no cost for the citizens? If so, then does the public know such a program is available? Have 25% to 50% of the population been trained? (Part of attaining this objective can be addressed by convincing the public to take the self-help approach to CPR training as provided by the AHA's 20-minute CPR Anytime program.)
- Is CPR training a requirement to graduate high school in your state? (Advocates have proposed such legislation in all 50 states. As of September 2016, 32 states require CPR, and lives are being saved every day as a result.[5])
- Are 100% of the responders to emergencies (police, fire, EMS) currently trained in CPR and use of an AED? Are they required to keep their certification current? Do all emergency response vehicles have an AED?
- Are AEDs and trained personnel available in all locations of public assembly for more than 500 people or in high-risk locations (ie, golf courses, sports arenas, concert venues, nursing homes)?
- Do all schools have AEDs readily available to travel with their athletic teams when competing in all sporting events?
- Do fitness centers in your community have personnel trained in CPR and AEDs readily available?
- How long does it take for the first EMR to arrive on the scene? How long does it take for the paramedics to arrive? Is this data published on a regular basis for all to see? If such data does not get measured and evaluated, then it is difficult to improve the response.
- Is the medical director for the EMS system actively involved in reviewing all cardiac arrests and making quality improvements to the response of the EMS system based on these reviews?
- Are all the cardiac arrests in your community reported using the Recommended Guidelines for Uniform Reporting of Data from Out-of-Hospital Cardiac Arrest, "The Utstein Resuscitation Registry Templates," so data from your community can be compared with the data of other progressive communities?[6]
- Do all hospitals to which you transport patients participate in the AHA's Get With The Guidelines quality improvement suite? This database is the only national registry of in-hospital resuscitation events until the Centers for Disease Control and Prevention moves forward and implements a national database.
- Do the out-of-hospital and in-hospital resuscitation teams practice their response with simulation technology on a regular basis? These code drills should focus on teamwork, following current guidelines, and ensuring a minimal amount of interruptions during high-quality CPR.

If you answered no to some of these questions, then there is more work to be done in your community! If you answered yes to all of the questions, then share your best practices with neighboring communities to help them improve their response to sudden cardiac arrest.

Words of Wisdom

According to the Centers for Disease Control and Prevention, an estimated 70% of all out-of-hospital cardiac arrests occur in the home or residence.[7] The remainder occur in public places. Do your family members or the family members of your coworkers know how to access EMS and begin CPR?

▶ Simulation Training

In the past, simulation or mock code training in medicine typically involved using so-called simulated patients in a classroom setting. The students assessed people who were instructed to mimic having symptoms of different ailments. However, modern technology has helped to streamline this training method by creating simulation modules. Regardless of the type of industry or training, one question always comes up: "How do I train my personnel for the 'low-frequency, high-risk' situation?" As a paramedic, for example, you must be able to recognize and manage a life-threatening condition (eg, lethal dysrhythmia, cardiac arrest, multisystem trauma).

Modern simulation technology allows you to gain knowledge about real-life scenarios by performing in a virtual world where no one is injured if you make a mistake. Using high-fidelity manikins and video recordings to mimic the field code for review and analysis, this type of training is invaluable because your actions and results are tracked and available to critique, to review, and to learn from. High-fidelity manikins integrate with a computer simulator and have the ability to play out preprogrammed scenarios involving alterations in the vital signs, ECG tracing, SpO_2 level, end-tidal carbon dioxide ($ETCO_2$) level, and other parameters.

Many EMS systems spend time in simulation centers to practice their codes and team leadership. This practice helps to compensate for a lack of actual skill performance on actual patients. According to one 2015 report, even the busiest EMS systems only see about 57 to 124 out-of-hospital cardiac arrests per year per 100,000 population.[8]

▶ Ongoing Development of CPR Guidelines

Strong Emphasis on Quality CPR

During the 1990s, the emphasis on performing quality CPR seemed to slip as providers became more focused on traditionally advanced skills such as intubation, drug administration, and other aspects of field code management. Studies in medical journals, which prompted the development of the 2005 ECC guidelines, demonstrated that the quality of CPR was poor in both the in-hospital and out-of-hospital settings for the following reasons: The depth of compressions was inadequate, the rate of compressions was too slow, almost half the time no compressions were being provided, the ventilations were too fast, and the chest was rarely allowed to fully recoil. Studies investigating the value of intubation and the use of resuscitation drugs were inconclusive at best, but it was determined that performing CPR is clearly important both before and immediately after defibrillation. In addition, it was determined that immediate CPR can double or triple the rate of survival in a patient who is experiencing ventricular fibrillation (VF) or sudden cardiac arrest.

All AHA guidelines published since 2005 emphasize the importance of providing high-quality CPR beginning with compressions. The goal is to push hard and fast, and allow full chest recoil. (Never lean on the chest between compressions.) In fact, the so-called resuscitation pyramid is built on a strong base of high-quality CPR beginning with compressions, as illustrated in **Figure 39-2**. On

arrival at the scene of a patient in cardiac arrest, you need to understand that the success of the resuscitation does not rely on an intravenous (IV) line, an endotracheal (ET) tube, a circulatory adjunct, or drugs you have in your drug box. Your best chance of succeeding at resuscitation hinges on providing continuous, uninterrupted, high-quality CPR compressions as promptly as possible. In many EMS systems, the saying is "BLS owns CPR." In other words, patient survival is based on excellent basic life support, and ALS skills performed by the paramedic must not interrupt basic care!

Airway Management

If you were to compare the first edition of this textbook with this current edition on the management of cardiac arrest, then an obvious difference would be the de-emphasis of securing the patient's airway with endotracheal intubation, a technique that was previously considered the gold standard. Clearly, the airway is no less important today than it was four decades ago. However, with research showing that high-quality chest compressions can double—if not triple—the chance of survival if administered promptly, the focus has shifted to interventions that make a measurable difference in survival (ie, defibrillation).[9,10] If you can open the airway and successfully ventilate the patient using basic adjuncts (ie, oropharyngeal airway, nasopharyngeal airway, and bag-mask ventilation), then it is not a priority for you to ensure that an ET tube is inserted. Today, paramedics are taught to consider the use of advanced airways during the field code if a basic airway is inadequate or the airway needs to be better protected (ie, a vomiting patient). You should be trained to place an advanced airway with little to no interruption in chest compressions (less than 10 seconds). If you cannot accomplish this step, then a rescue airway (ie, King LT, Combitube) is an acceptable alternative.

Another consideration with airway maintenance and adjunct placement is control of the volume and rate of ventilation. During a field code, administer each ventilation over 1 second, and only with sufficient volume for you to see visible chest rise. Do not hyperventilate the patient because this can cause gastric distention or regurgitation and induce hypotension during CPR.[11] Excessive gas in the chest has been shown to significantly reduce coronary artery perfusion pressure. Some EMS medical directors have encouraged paramedics to use an impedance threshold device (ITD), which is placed in the ventilation circuit between the mask and the bag-mask device or **automatic transport ventilator (ATV)**. The ITD helps to reduce excessive pressure within the chest and is discussed later in this chapter.

Another consideration to take into account when you are using advanced airways early in the treatment of the field code is whether the five links of the out-of-hospital chain of survival are all in place (see Figure 39-1). Studies have shown that the probability of ROSC in the patient

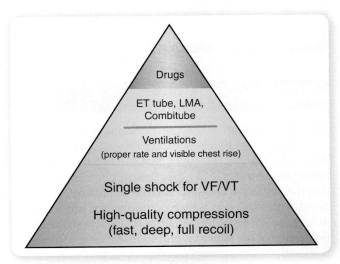

Figure 39-2 The resuscitation pyramid.

after cardiac arrest is about 40%. If the patient wakes up, then it is best to not have an ET tube in place. If the patient does not wake up and is a candidate for TTM, then you may now find it necessary to intubate the patient and provide medication to prevent shivering. Most paramedics sedate patients in need of TTM post ROSC. These examples show that the decision to place an advanced airway during the field code should be based on the patient's situation, rather than performed automatically as it may have been in the past.

Blood Flow During CPR

The theories about blood flow during CPR have evolved over the years. An early thought was the "heart pump theory," in which the heart is directly squeezed by compression between the sternum (breastbone) and the spinal column. The pressure is increased within the chambers of the heart and blood flows from high-pressure chambers to the low-pressure vessels and organs. However, the heart valves need to be properly functioning to keep the blood flowing in the right direction and to prevent retrograde flow of blood.

The next thought on how blood flows during CPR was the "thoracic pump theory," in which compression of the sternum raises the pressure in the entire chest cavity. With the pressure in the extrathoracic spaces remaining low, the pressure gradient is established in which venous collapse prevents the backflow of blood and open arteries allow for the forward flow of blood out of the chest. Administration of vasopressors is thought to be a benefit in helping to keep those essential arteries open. Building on the concepts of both these theories, researchers have found success in promoting the use of harder and faster chest compressions that can increase the pressure to a greater degree. However, all of this blood movement ceases when chest compressions are interrupted; thus, the emphasis is for continuous chest compressions with minimum, if any, interruptions.

Finally, the current theories on blood flow during CPR consider the importance of negative intrathoracic pressure. Because patients in cardiac arrest are not breathing on their own, they do not produce negative inspiratory pressure (provided there is full chest recoil) to assist in circulatory system blood flow, most specifically the coronary arteries. During CPR, some negative pressure develops in the chest as the sternum and ribs rebound to their normal position during the decompression (relaxation) phase. In fact, researchers have noted that in the studies on pigs, using mechanical chest compression devices to deliver the chest compressions, it is essential to ensure that the pad of the compressor releases complete pressure on the chest wall or else there is little to no coronary blood flow. This finding contributed to the current emphasis on full chest recoil. When a greater amount of negative pressure can be achieved in the chest (remember, push hard and fast and allow full chest recoil without leaning on the chest), a

greater amount of blood is returned to the heart. Then on the next compression, a greater amount of blood is forced to circulate to the coronary arteries of the heart and the rest of the vital organs. You can see how the concept of a device, such as the ITD in combination with an **active compression-decompression CPR (ACD-CPR)** device, could be effective in enhancing this negative pressure gradient. (An ACD-CPR device is a manual suction cup-type device that is placed in the center of the chest and then used to pull the chest wall up and down during CPR.) As the theories of how to best resuscitate a patient in cardiac arrest continue to evolve through ongoing research, it is apparent that providing the highest quality of CPR in a timely manner, with little to no interruptions, is the patient's best chance for ROSC.

> ### Words of Wisdom
>
> When the heart stops contracting, the blood stops flowing and blood, oxygen, and essential substrates cannot be delivered or removed from the cells of the body. The body cannot survive when the heart stops because organ damage begins quickly after the blood stops circulating. Of all the organs, the brain is the most sensitive to lack of blood flow and oxygen. Brain damage begins within 4 to 6 minutes after the patient experiences a cardiac arrest. The arrest is considered irreversible within 8 to 10 minutes. Reperfusion of the brain with oxygenated blood is essential to ROSC.
>
> The heart can stop beating for many reasons but the primary reasons are sudden death due to a life-threatening dysrhythmia (ie, VF or ventricular tachycardia [VT]), heart disease, electrolyte imbalances, and severe trauma. Medical emergencies such as asthma, anaphylaxis, opioid overdose, and being struck in the chest at the wrong time in the cardiac cycle (ie, commotio cordis) can also lead to cardiac arrest. The downward spiral from respiratory distress to respiratory failure, respiratory arrest, and finally, cardiac arrest commonly occurs in infants and children.

■ Adult CPR

The initial steps for managing the adult patient in cardiac arrest follow the BLS Healthcare Provider Adult Cardiac Arrest Algorithm **Figure 39-3** . Adult BLS procedures are summarized in **Table 39-1** . Research findings showed that the key to a successful outcome in patients in cardiac arrest is the speed at which compressions are initiated. As per the AHA guidelines, after you verify scene safety, establish that the patient is unresponsive. Shout for nearby help and alert the emergency response system using your mobile device. Assign someone to quickly get the AED.

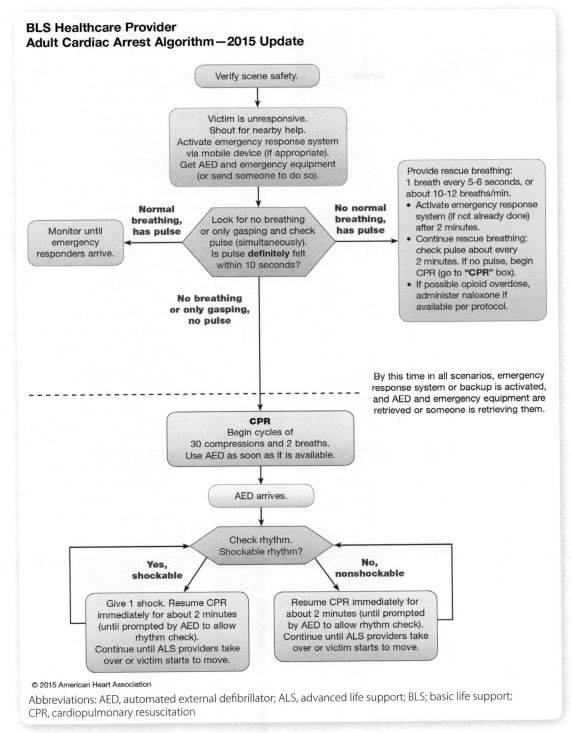

BLS Healthcare Provider
Adult Cardiac Arrest Algorithm—2015 Update

Verify scene safety.

Victim is unresponsive.
Shout for nearby help.
Activate emergency response system
via mobile device (if appropriate).
Get AED and emergency equipment
(or send someone to do so).

Provide rescue breathing:
1 breath every 5-6 seconds, or
about 10-12 breaths/min.
- Activate emergency response
  system (if not already done)
  after 2 minutes.
- Continue rescue breathing;
  check pulse about every
  2 minutes. If no pulse, begin
  CPR (go to "CPR" box).
- If possible opioid overdose,
  administer naloxone if
  available per protocol.

Normal breathing, has pulse

Monitor until emergency responders arrive.

Look for no breathing
or only gasping and check
pulse (simultaneously).
Is pulse **definitely** felt
within 10 seconds?

No normal breathing, has pulse

No breathing or only gasping, no pulse

By this time in all scenarios, emergency
response system or backup is activated,
and AED and emergency equipment are
retrieved or someone is retrieving them.

CPR
Begin cycles of
30 compressions and 2 breaths.
Use AED as soon as it is available.

AED arrives.

Check rhythm.
Shockable rhythm?

Yes, shockable

Give 1 shock. Resume CPR
immediately for about 2 minutes
(until prompted by AED to allow
rhythm check).
Continue until ALS providers take
over or victim starts to move.

No, nonshockable

Resume CPR immediately for
about 2 minutes (until prompted
by AED to allow rhythm check).
Continue until ALS providers take
over or victim starts to move.

© 2015 American Heart Association

Abbreviations: AED, automated external defibrillator; ALS, advanced life support; BLS; basic life support;
CPR, cardiopulmonary resuscitation

Figure 39-3 The BLS Healthcare Provider Adult Cardiac Arrest Algorithm.
Reprinted with permission. Highlights of the 2015 American Heart Association Guidelines Update for CPR & ECC. © 2015 American Heart Association, Inc.

Next, observe for a lack of normal breathing (ie, agonal gasps or absent breathing), and simultaneously check for a pulse. Take no more than 10 seconds to do this. If the patient has no pulse and is either not breathing or only gasping, then begin CPR and continue for 2 minutes or five cycles of 30 compressions and two ventilations. Always bring your AED or defibrillator/monitor to the

patient on any potential cardiac arrest call. In all patients, begin CPR and attach the AED as soon as it is available. In some instances, CPR may have been started prior to your arrival.

To help make CPR easier to learn, remember, and perform, the general public or lay rescuers are taught to provide hands-only CPR. In some cases, bystanders may

Table 39-1	Review of Adult BLS Procedures
Procedure	
Circulation	
Pulse check	Carotid artery
Compression area	In the center of the chest (two hands on lower half of the sternum)
Compression depth	2 in. to 2.4 in. (5 cm to 6 cm)
Compression rate	100 to 120/min
Compression-to-ventilation ratio (until advanced airway is inserted)	30:2
Foreign body obstruction	Responsive: abdominal thrusts (Heimlich maneuver); chest thrusts if patient is pregnant or is obese Unresponsive: CPR
Airway	
Airway positioning	Head tilt-chin lift; jaw-thrust maneuver if spinal injury is suspected
Breathing	
Ventilations	1 breath every 5 to 6 s (10 to 12 breaths/min); about 1 s per breath; visible chest rise
Ventilations with advanced airway placed	1 breath every 6 s (a rate of 10 breaths/min)

Abbreviations: BLS, basic life support; CPR, cardiopulmonary resuscitation

Data from: Kleinman ME, Brennan EE, Goldberger ZD, Swor RA, Terry M, Bobrow BJ, Gazmuri RJ, Travers AH, Rea T. Part 5: adult basic life support and cardiopulmonary resuscitation quality: 2015 American Heart Association Guidelines Update for Cardiopulmonary Resuscitation and Emergency Cardiovascular Care. Circulation. 2015;132(suppl 2):S414–S435.

trained previously in CPR are often reluctant to begin this procedure for the following reasons:

- The steps of CPR may have been too complicated and included too many steps to remember. However, the AHA guidelines reflect a significant effort to simplify the steps taught to the public with the emphasis on hands-only CPR with the focus on compressions.
- Training methods may have been inadequate, and skill retention typically declines rapidly after a course. This issue is being studied to try to determine which methods of training will produce the greatest skill retention. A video-based watch-and-do method, as opposed to watch-then-do, has been incorporated into most courses.
- Some members of the public may be afraid of transmitted diseases and, therefore, may be reluctant to perform mouth-to-mouth resuscitation. Although the AHA guidelines strongly emphasize that the risk of transmission of infection is low, those people who are concerned about disease are encouraged to use barrier devices. Personal protective equipment and specific disease risk levels are discussed in Chapter 26, *Infectious Diseases*. In addition, the technique of hands-only/compression-only CPR is encouraged for those people who are reluctant to perform ventilations and for dispatcher-assisted CPR instruction.
- Finally, many bystanders who are trained in CPR may not help when confronted with a cardiac arrest because they are afraid they might do the wrong thing.

Words of Wisdom

To perform high-quality CPR, remember the following steps:
- Maintain a compression rate between 100 and 120 compressions per minute.
- Maintain a compression depth of at least 2 inches (5 cm). Do not exceed 2.4 inches (6 cm) in adults or one-third the depth of the chest in infants and children.
- Allow full chest recoil (no leaning) after each compression.
- Minimize interruptions in chest compressions.
- Avoid hyperventilation.

Even brief interruptions can significantly diminish the coronary artery perfusion pressure. In resuscitation, the compressions are provided at a rate between 100 and 120 per minute as the code team adds ventilations, IV or intraosseous (IO) medications, and an advanced airway. However, the code stops as soon as the compressions are interrupted!

have taken a traditional CPR course, which taught the compression to ventilation ratio of 30:2. The public is generally not taught to take a pulse, to perform rescue breathing, or to perform two-rescuer CPR. Unfortunately, studies have shown that bystander CPR is performed in only one-third or fewer of witnessed cardiac arrests and is often poorly performed.[7] Bystanders who have been

Two-Rescuer CPR

Two-rescuer CPR is always preferable over one-rescuer CPR because it is less tiring and facilitates effective chest compressions. In fact, a team approach to CPR and AED use is far superior to the one-rescuer approach. Once one-rescuer CPR is in progress, additional rescuers can be added easily. Prior to assisting with CPR, a second rescuer should apply the AED and then set up airway adjuncts including a bag-mask device and suction, and insert an oropharyngeal airway. If CPR is in progress, then the second rescuer should enter the procedure after a cycle of 30 compressions and two ventilations.

When you use two or more rescuers, the compressor and ventilator should rotate every 2 minutes. To do so, position a third rescuer so he or she is kneeling on the other side of the patient's chest across from the compressor. Now, you can have an "active compressor" and an "on-deck compressor" who is ready to take over after the five cycles or 2-minute intervals. Studies of rescuer fatigue show that the compressor tires after only 2 to 5 minutes and that the quality of compressions will decrease if the compressor is not replaced.

To perform adult CPR with two or more rescuers, follow the steps in Skill Drill 39-1 .

Words of Wisdom

During switches, make every effort to minimize the time that no compressions are being administered. This break between compression cycles should last approximately 5 seconds but no more than 10 seconds.

The switch between the two rescuers can be easily accomplished. Rescuer one should finish the cycle of 30 compressions while rescuer two moves to the opposite side of the chest and moves into position to begin compressions. Rescuer one should deliver two rescue breaths and then rescuer two should take over compressions by administering 30 chest compressions. Rescuer one will then deliver two ventilations and the CPR cycles will continue as needed until the next 2-minute mark is reached, at which time the process will be repeated.

CPR for Infants and Children

A question often asked is, "For the purposes of resuscitation, what age defines a child?" Many pediatricians say, "If the patient looks like a child, then he or she is a child; if the

YOU are the Paramedic PART 2

Your field supervisor arrives as you prepare to defibrillate. After the defibrillator has charged, you announce that everyone should "Clear the patient!" After you have confirmed that the patient is clear and the bag-mask device has been removed from the patient, you deliver a 200-J biphasic shock. The volunteer EMRs immediately resume CPR and your field supervisor prepares to gain venous access. After delegating medication preparation, she has 1 mg of epinephrine 0.1 mg/mL (1:10,000) ready to administer via the IV line while the EMRs complete their five cycles of compressions. You check the patient's rhythm and find pVT on the cardiac monitor. You confirm that the patient has no pulse and complete the assessment in less than 10 seconds. The epinephrine has been administered so you prepare to defibrillate again. As the EMRs complete their fifth cycle, you announce that everyone should "Clear the patient" and after verifying that the patient is clear, deliver another shock of 200 J. Your field supervisor has now prepared 300 mg of amiodarone for IV administration. After she administers this medication, she prepares the intubation equipment for your partner, who is continuing to ventilate the patient using a bag-mask device.

Recording Time: 6 Minutes	
Appearance	Pale and mottled
Level of consciousness	Unresponsive
Airway	Patent
Breathing	Apneic; ventilations provided at a rate of 10 breaths/min via bag-mask device
Circulation	Pulseless with CPR in progress; skin is cool

3. What alternative medications are indicated for VF/pVT and at what dosages?

4. If the rhythm had been analyzed as torsades de pointes, then what medication might be beneficial and at what dosage?

Skill Drill 39-1 Performing Two-Rescuer Adult CPR

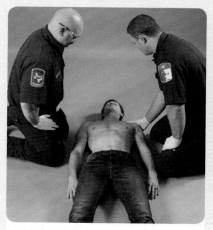

Step 1 Take standard precautions and ensure scene safety. Move to the patient's head and establish unresponsiveness while your partner moves to the patient's side to be ready to deliver chest compressions.

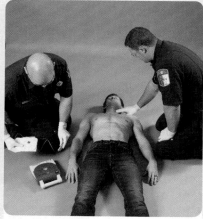

Step 2 If the patient is unresponsive, then simultaneously check for breathing and palpate for a carotid pulse; take no more than 10 seconds to do this. If the patient has no pulse and is either not breathing or only gasping, then apply an AED if available.

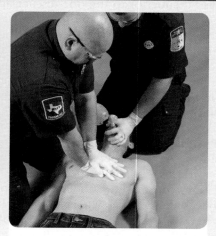

Step 3 If an AED is unavailable, then begin CPR at a ratio of 30 chest compressions to 2 ventilations. After an advanced airway is inserted, rescuers should switch from cycles of CPR to continuously delivered compressions at a rate of 100 to 120/min.

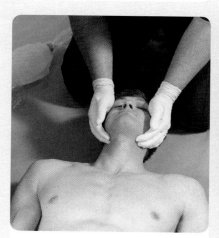

Step 4 If the patient has a pulse, then position the patient to open the airway according to your suspicion of spinal injury. If breathing is adequate, then place the patient in the recovery position and monitor breathing and pulse.

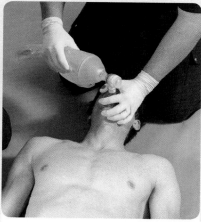

Step 5 If the patient has a pulse but is not breathing adequately, then deliver rescue breaths at a rate of 1 breath every 6 s (10 to 12 breaths/min).

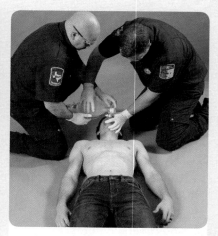

Step 6 If CPR was started, then the compressor and ventilator should switch positions after 2 min. Minimize the time between compression cycles to approximately 5 s but no more than 10 s. If a third rescuer is available, then position him or her at the chest opposite the compressor. If only two rescuers are available, then switch mid-cycle during compressions.

Skill Drill 39-1 Performing Two-Rescuer Adult CPR *(continued)*

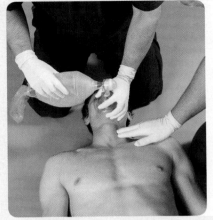

Step 7 Reassess the patient every few minutes. Each assessment should last no more than 10 s. Depending on the patient's condition, continue CPR, continue rescue breathing only, or place the patient in the recovery position and monitor breathing and pulse.

Note: After an advanced airway has been inserted, the compressions and ventilations are no longer performed in cycles. Instead, they are performed individually, are not timed, and do not require waiting for the other rescuer to pause (**asynchronous**). The compressor provides between 100 and 120 compressions/min without pausing for breaths, and the ventilator gives 10 breaths/min (1 breath every 6 s). Because the compressor will inevitably get tired, switch compressors every 2 min, but minimize the break in the compression cycle to approximately 5 s.

© Jones & Bartlett Learning.

patient looks like an adult, then he or she is an adult." The AHA guidelines use the following definitions of age groups for the purposes of resuscitation:[12,13]

- **Newly born.** An infant within the first few hours after birth.
- **Neonate.** An infant within the first month after birth. (Neonatal resuscitation is covered in Chapter 42, *Neonatal Care*.)
- **Infant.** Age 1 month to 1 year.
- **Child.** Age 1 year to adolescence (signs of puberty or secondary sexual characteristic development, such as axillary hair in boys or breast development in girls).
- **Adult.** Adolescent and older.

In most cases, cardiac arrest in infants and children follows respiratory arrest, which triggers hypoxia and ischemia of the heart. Children consume oxygen two to three times as rapidly as adults. Therefore, you must open the airway and provide artificial ventilation. Often, this step will be enough to allow the child to resume spontaneous breathing and, thus, prevent cardiac arrest. Therefore, airway and breathing are a focus of pediatric BLS Table 39-2.

Respiratory conditions leading to cardiopulmonary arrest in children can have a number of different causes, including the following:

- Injury, both blunt and penetrating
- Infections of the respiratory tract or another organ system
- A foreign body in the airway
- Submersion
- Electrocution
- Poisoning or drug overdose
- Sudden infant death syndrome

Pediatric BLS can be divided into the following four steps:

1. Determining responsiveness
2. Circulation
3. Airway
4. Breathing

Evidence-Based Medicine

As mentioned previously, the use of advanced airway devices seems to be deemphasized in the AHA guidelines—particularly the use of endotracheal intubation. When used by skilled providers, a bag-mask device with supplemental oxygen can be as effective as an ET tube in terms of oxygenation, ventilation, and protection from aspiration for short transportation times.

Many EMS medical directors have been reluctant to train their EMTs in the optional endotracheal intubation skill because of the marginal results when the skill is not practiced frequently. In the past, unrecognized, uncorrected esophageal intubations or tube dislodgements occurred with unacceptable frequency. Major complications of emergency tracheal intubation, such as esophageal intubation, have been reported in as little as 1.8% and as many as 17% of pediatric patients in the out-of-hospital setting.[14,15] Another study in a large adult group of cardiac arrests found that 25% of the tubes were incorrectly placed by paramedics.[16] As a consequence, the advanced airway option now favors the use of easier-to-insert rescue airway devices (ie, LMA, Combitube, or King LT).

Table 39-2	Review of Pediatric BLS Procedures	
Procedure	**Infants (between age 1 month and 1 year[a])**	**Children (1 year to onset of puberty[b])**
Circulation		
Pulse check	Brachial artery	Carotid or femoral artery
Compression location	Just below the nipple line	In the center of the chest (lower half of the sternum)
Hand placement	Two-finger technique for single rescuer or two-thumb encircling-hands technique with two rescuers	Heel of one or both hands
Compression depth	At least one-third anterior-posterior diameter (about 1.5 in. [4 cm])	At least one-third anterior-posterior diameter (about 2 in. [5 cm])
Compression rate	100 to 120/min	100 to 120/min
Compression-to-ventilation ratio (until advanced airway is inserted)	30:2 (one rescuer); 15:2 (two rescuers)[c]	30:2 (one rescuer); 15:2 (two rescuers)[c]
Foreign body obstruction	Responsive: Back slaps and chest thrusts Unresponsive: CPR	Responsive: Abdominal thrusts (Heimlich maneuver) Unresponsive: CPR
Airway		
Airway positioning	Head tilt–chin lift; jaw thrust maneuver if spinal injury is suspected	Head tilt–chin lift; jaw thrust maneuver if spinal injury is suspected
Breathing		
Ventilations	1 breath every 3 to 5 s (12 to 20 breaths/min); about 1 s per breath; visible chest rise	1 breath every 3 to 5 s (12 to 20 breaths/min); about 1 s per breath; visible chest rise
Ventilations with advanced airway	1 breath every 6 to 8 s (8-10 breaths/min); with at least 100 chest compressions delivered per minute, continuously, without pauses for ventilation	1 breath every 6 to 8 s (8-10 breaths/min); with at least 100 chest compressions delivered per minute, continuously, without pauses for ventilation

Abbreviations: BLS, basic life support; CPR, cardiopulmonary resuscitation

[a]The AHA defines neonatal patients as birth to age 1 month, and infants as age 1 month to 1 year. Neonatal resuscitation is covered in Chapter 42, *Neonatal Care*.
[b]Onset of puberty is approximately 12 to 14 years of age, as defined by secondary sexual characteristics (eg, breast development in girls and axillary hair in boys).
[c]Pause compressions to deliver ventilations.

Data from: Atkins DL, Berger S, Duff JP, Gonzales JC, Hunt EA, Joyner BL, Meaney PA, Niles DE, Samson RA, Schexnayder SM. Part 11: pediatric basic life support and cardiopulmonary resuscitation quality: 2015 American Heart Association Guidelines Update for Cardiopulmonary Resuscitation and Emergency Cardiovascular Care. *Circulation*. 2015;132(suppl 2):S519–S525.

▶ Technique for Children

The technique of CPR has a few slight variations for children compared to the adult technique. These variations are shown in **Skill Drill 39-2**.

▶ Technique for Infants

The technique of CPR for an infant has a few slight variations from the adult and child technique, as shown in **Skill Drill 39-3**.

Skill Drill 39-2 — Performing CPR on a Child

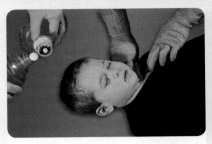

Step 1 Take standard precautions and ensure scene safety. Move the child's head and establish unresponsiveness while your partner moves to the patient's side to be ready to deliver chest compressions. If the patient is unresponsive, then simultaneously check for breathing and palpate for a brachial pulse; take no more than 10 seconds to do this. If the patient has no pulse and is either not breathing or only gasping, then apply an AED if available.

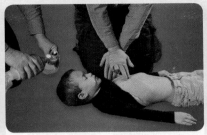

Step 2 Place the child on a firm surface. Place the heel of one or two hands in the center of the chest, on the lower half of the sternum, avoiding the xiphoid process.

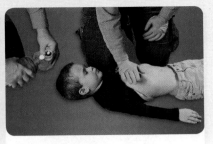

Step 3 Compress the chest one-third the anterior-posterior diameter of the chest (approximately 2 in. [5 cm] in most children) at a rate of 100 to 120/min. In between compressions, allow the chest to fully recoil; do not lean on the chest. Compression and relaxation time should be the same duration. Use smooth movements. Hold your fingers off the child's ribs, and keep the heel of your hand or hands on the sternum.

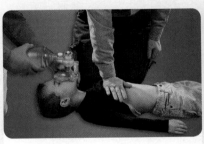

Step 4 Coordinate compressions and ventilations in a 30:2 ratio for one rescuer and 15:2 for two rescuers, making sure the chest rises with each ventilation. At the end of each cycle, pause for two ventilations.

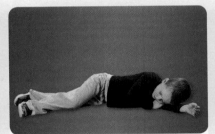

Step 5 Continue cycles of compressions and ventilations until an AED becomes available or the patient shows signs of spontaneous breathing. If the child resumes effective breathing, then place him or her in a position that allows for frequent reassessment of the airway and vital signs during transport.

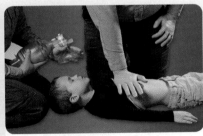

Step 6 If the child remains in cardiac arrest, continue CPR. Rotate compressors every 2 minutes of CPR.

Note: After an advanced airway has been inserted, the compressions and ventilations are no longer performed in cycles. Instead, they are performed continuously at a rate of at least 100 breaths/min, without pauses for ventilation. Ventilations should be delivered at 1 breath every 6 to 8 s (8-10 breaths/min). Because the compressor will inevitably get tired, switch compressors every 2 min but limit the break in compressions to approximately 5 s.

Skill Drill 39-3 Infant CPR

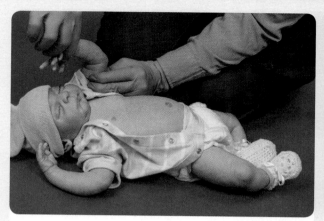

Step 1 Take standard precautions and ensure scene safety. Move the infant's head and establish unresponsiveness while your partner moves to the patient's side to be ready to deliver chest compressions. If the patient is unresponsive, then simultaneously check for breathing and palpate for a brachial pulse; take no more than 10 seconds to do this. If the patient has no pulse and is either not breathing or only gasping, then apply an AED if available.

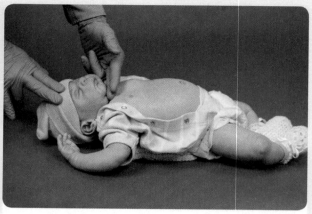

Step 2 Place the infant on a firm surface, using one hand to keep the head in an open airway position. You can also use a pad or wedge under the shoulders and upper body to keep the head from tilting forward.

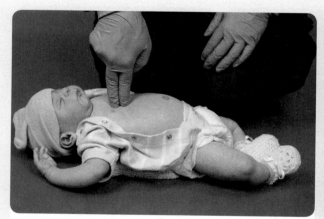

Step 3 Imagine a line drawn between the nipples. Place two fingers in the middle of the sternum, about 0.5 in. (1 cm) below the level of the imaginary line (one finger width). Using two fingers, compress the sternum at least one-third the anterior-posterior diameter of the chest (approximately 1.5 in. [4 cm] in most infants). Compress the chest at a rate of 100 to 120/min. After each compression, allow the sternum to return briefly to its normal position. Allow equal time for compression and relaxation of the chest. Do not remove your fingers from the sternum, and avoid jerky movements.

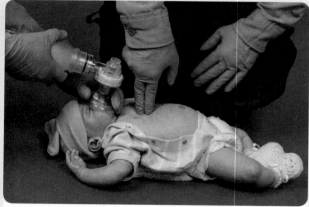

Step 4 Coordinate compressions and ventilations in a 30:2 ratio for one rescuer and 15:2 for two rescuers, making sure the chest rises with each ventilation. At the end of each cycle, pause for two ventilations. Continue cycles of compressions and ventilations until an AED becomes available or the infant shows signs of spontaneous breathing. If the infant resumes effective breathing, place him or her in a position that allows for frequent reassessment of the airway and vital signs during transport.

If two rescuers are available, then compressions can also be performed using the two-thumb encircling-hands technique **Figure 39-4**. If the chest does not rise, or rises only a little, then use a head tilt–chin lift to open the airway. Reassess the infant for signs of spontaneous breathing after five cycles (about 2 minutes) of CPR.

Defibrillation

When an unresponsive patient is receiving CPR, the defibrillator is probably one of the first pieces of equipment you will obtain from the ambulance. As you learned in Chapter 17, *Cardiovascular Emergencies*, **defibrillation** is the process by which a surge of electric energy is delivered to the heart. As a paramedic, you are likely to administer electricity to a patient in one of three different ways: defibrillation, cardioversion, or transcutaneous pacing. In the context of a patient who is in cardiac arrest, defibrillation is needed when the patient is in one of the two shockable rhythms (VF or pVT). Occasionally you may be the first responder to arrive on scene. For example, you may encounter a patient in cardiac arrest in a public place such as a school where you are playing in a community basketball league, or while exercising in a health club. In those situations, you are likely to use an AED rather than the manual defibrillator/monitor you would carry on your paramedic unit. Many communities

YOU are the Paramedic — PART 3

After 2 minutes of compressions, you check the patient's rhythm. The patient continues to be in VT. While the EMRs continue CPR and the field supervisor assists your partner with intubation, you remind them that intubation should delay compressions no longer than 10 seconds. The intubation is completed and while tube placement is confirmed by cord visualization, auscultation, and the use of ETCO$_2$ monitoring, you prepare to administer 1 mg of epinephrine 0.1 mg/mL (1:10,000) to the patient. The supervisor prepares the second dose of amiodarone 150 mg for the patient as you note that the ETCO$_2$ is 37 mm Hg and appropriate waveforms are present. The EMRs complete another five cycles of CPR and you identify that the patient remains in VT. You prepare to deliver the third shock by charging to 200 J. You again announce and verify the patient should be cleared and then defibrillate. Compressions resume as the second dose of amiodarone is administered.

The patient's wife arrives and you take this opportunity to obtain a SAMPLE (Signs and symptoms, Allergies, Medications, Pertinent past medical history, Last oral intake, Events leading up to the illness or injury) history. She advises you her husband has reported occasional indigestion for the last week and finally contacted his physician this morning. He was scheduled for a stress test tomorrow. Current medications are limited to over-the-counter products such as acid-reducers and pain relievers. She is aware of no allergies. She tells you that until now she believed her husband to be healthy because he regularly exercised and watched his diet. She thinks he ate lunch with friends immediately prior to beginning this round of golf. You advise her that her husband's condition is extremely critical but that you are providing him with the best care possible.

Recording Time: 12 Minutes	
Respirations	10 breaths/min via ET tube ventilations
Pulse	Pulseless with CPR in progress at 100 to 120 compressions/min
Skin	Pale and cool
Blood pressure	Not obtainable
Oxygen saturation (Spo$_2$)	Not obtainable
Pupils	Equal, round, and unresponsive to light
End-tidal carbon dioxide (ETCO$_2$)	37 mm Hg

5. Why is intubation not an early intervention consideration in the patient in cardiac arrest?
6. What is the importance of ETCO$_2$ monitoring in the patient in cardiac arrest?
7. If resuscitative efforts are eventually successful, then what is the significance of transporting the patient in cardiac arrest to a facility capable of advanced cardiac care?

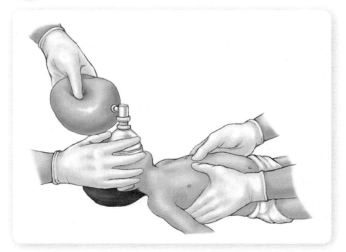

Figure 39-4 The two-thumb encircling hands technique for infant chest compressions can be used when two rescuers are available.

© Jones & Bartlett Learning.

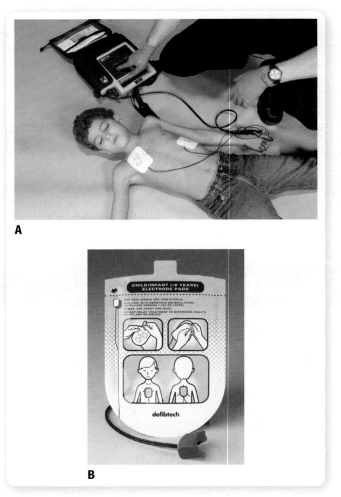

Figure 39-5 The pediatric dose-attenuator system.
A. Attenuator pads in use. **B.** Attenuator pads in packaging.

A: © Jones & Bartlett Learning. Courtesy of MIEMSS; B: Courtesy of Defibtech, LLC.

have placed AEDs in public places such as health clubs, swimming pools, concert venues, sports arenas, airports, schools, and government buildings. These public access defibrillation programs, when properly managed, include regular checks on the units as well as regular training for those who are likely to use them. It is also helpful to package a disposable razor with the AED in case the patient has a hairy chest that makes it difficult for the pad to stick properly.

Aside from CPR, the AED has been shown to be one of the most effective lifesaving treatments for patients found in cardiac arrest. Although you will usually arrive with a manual defibrillator, it is essential that you also know how to use an automated unit as you may encounter one in the field. Remember the following guidelines for AED use:

- **Adults**: Use a standard adult AED unit.
- **Children (age 1 year to the onset of puberty)**: Use an AED with pediatric dose-attenuation and a pediatric-sized pad, if available **Figure 39-5** . If a pediatric dose-attenuator system is unavailable, then use a standard adult AED.
- **Infants (ages 1 month to 1 year)**: Use a manual defibrillator if available. If a manual defibrillator is unavailable, then use a pediatric dose-attenuator. If neither is available, then use a standard adult AED with the pads in the anterior-posterior position.
- **Newborns (birth to age 1 month)**: Focus attention on CPR with emphasis on ventilation. For more information, refer to Chapter 42, *Neonatal Care*.

If the patient is in either VF or pVT, then defibrillation is needed as soon as possible because the likelihood of

its success declines rapidly over time. If you witness a patient's cardiac arrest, then attach the AED as quickly as possible and proceed to analyze. However, if the patient's cardiac arrest was unwitnessed, then first perform five cycles (about 2 minutes) of CPR and quickly apply the AED. The rationale for this sequence is that the heart is more likely to respond to defibrillation within the first few minutes of the onset of VF. If the cardiac arrest interval is prolonged, however, then metabolic waste products accumulate within the heart, energy stores are rapidly depleted, and the chance of successful defibrillation is reduced. Therefore, a 2-minute period of CPR before applying the AED to patients with prolonged cardiac arrest can "prime the pump," thus, restoring oxygen to the heart, removing metabolic waste products, and increasing the chance of successful defibrillation. If two rescuers are available on the scene, then both compressions and AED application can occur simultaneously.

If the cardiac arrest is unwitnessed and CPR is not in progress, then immediately start CPR while preparing the AED to assess for a shockable rhythm. If the patient converts to VF or pVT and the defibrillator is already attached, then perform CPR only long enough to charge the defibrillator and then defibrillate. Defibrillation is not useful in either asystole (flatline) or pulseless electrical activity (PEA). PEA refers to an organized cardiac rhythm (other than pVT) on the cardiac monitor that is not accompanied by any detectable pulse. Defibrillation of asystole is unlikely to be beneficial and is harmful (due to the unnecessary interruption of compressions). Thus, if you are unsure about asystole or PEA after checking more than one ECG lead, then resume CPR and follow the asystole pathway in the cardiac arrest algorithm until the next pulse and rhythm check.[17] To shorten the post-defibrillation interval, many EMS systems practice defibrillation with the compressor hovering over—but not touching!—the patient's chest.

▶ Manual Defibrillation

Some defibrillators are combination units that can perform either manual or automated defibrillation. In **manual defibrillation**, you interpret the cardiac rhythm and determine whether defibrillation is needed. Manual defibrillator units require you to select the appropriate dose. A default setting of 200 J is usually used; however, settings may range from 120 J to 200 J, depending on the specifications of the manufacturer (primarily based on biphasic units, because most monophasic units have been replaced) **Figure 39-6**. For simplicity, this text uses the default setting of 200 J. After delivering a shock, it is important to immediately begin chest compressions for a 2-minute cycle and then reassess the patient for pulse return and rhythm change. If your unit has both manual and AED mode, then it is faster to use the unit in the manual mode because you can notice rhythm changes on the screen and interpret the ECG as a shockable rhythm (VF or pVT) more quickly than the time it takes an AED to do the same.

Evidence Based Medicine

In 2015, the Institute of Medicine of the National Academies* released a report entitled *Strategies to Improve Cardiac Arrest Survival: A Time to Act.*[18] The key recommendations in this report included the following:

- Establish a national cardiac arrest registry.
- Foster a culture of action through public awareness and training.
- Enhance the capabilities and performances of EMS systems.
- Set national accreditation standards related to cardiac arrest for hospitals and health care systems.
- Adopt continuous quality improvement programs for cardiac arrest response in EMS systems, health care systems, and hospitals.
- Accelerate research on pathophysiology, new therapies, and translation of science for cardiac arrest.
- Accelerate research on the evaluation and adoption of cardiac arrest therapies.
- Create a national cardiac arrest collaborative to raise the visibility of cardiac arrest for policy makers and members of the public.[18]

*As of March 2016, the Institute of Medicine of the National Academies was renamed the Health and Medicine Division of the National Academies of Sciences, Engineering, and Medicine.[19]

The six steps for manual defibrillation are as follows:

1. Take standard precautions.
2. Prepare the skin for placement of the adhesive defibrillation pads, if needed. Attach the pads to the patient's chest as instructed on the package.
3. Turn on the main power switch and then set the energy level to 200 J, or follow the defibrillator manufacturer's recommendations regarding the appropriate energy level.

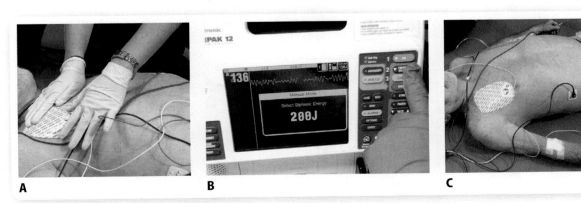

Figure 39-6 The use of a manual defibrillator on an adult patient in cardiac arrest. **A.** Attach the pads to the patient's chest. **B.** Turn on the main power switch. **C.** Clear the area and press the button on the machine to deliver the shock.

4. Charge the defibrillator. Remember not to defibrillate a patient who is lying in pooled water. Ensure that the patient is not touching metal.

5. Clear the area. Ensure the compressor is hovering over, but not touching, the patient's chest. Announce, "All clear!" Then press the button on the machine to deliver the shock.

6. Resume CPR immediately. Continue CPR for 2 minutes or five cycles, and then pause to check for a pulse and reevaluate the rhythm. If at any point you see an organized rhythm on the cardiac monitor, then check for a pulse (maximum of 10 seconds).

   Note: Prehospital agencies use defibrillation pads and have not used paddles in the past decade. If you have to use a unit with paddles, then you will need to use a conductive jelly and exert firm pressure (20 to 25 lb [9 kg to 11 kg]) on each paddle to make good skin contact.

See Chapter 17, *Cardiovascular Emergencies*, for a more complete description of this procedure (Skill Drill 17-4: Performing Manual Defibrillation).

The steps for manual defibrillation of an infant or child are similar to those of an adult, with the following additional points to keep in mind:

- Place one adhesive defibrillation pad on the anterior chest wall to the right of the sternum, inferior to the clavicle. Place the other pad on the left midclavicular line at the level of the xiphoid process **Figure 39-7**.
- For children who are younger than 1 year or who weigh less than 22 pounds (10 kg), you may use anterior-posterior placement **Figure 39-8**.

Pediatric defibrillation pad sizes are listed in **Table 39-3**.

Most EMS systems use pre-gelled defibrillator pads that are often interchangeable with the AED pads that might be used by EMRs. Know your equipment and determine whether it will be necessary to apply new pads or cables to the patient. When you apply the pads, ensure that no air pockets are present in the pad-skin interface because they may result in skin burns and decreased defibrillation effectiveness. The initial energy setting for defibrillation of pediatric patients is 2 J/kg. If this level is unsuccessful, then repeat the defibrillation at 4 J/kg. Further defibrillation should occur at 4 J/kg after cycles of CPR, as needed. With ongoing CPR, remember to search for and manage any underlying reversible causes (discussed later in this chapter). Administer epinephrine only after you have delivered two shocks, doubling the dose of electricity for the second attempt.

Consult with your medical director, medical control physician, or local protocols for the decision on when and where to transport pediatric patients who are in cardiopulmonary arrest. Early ROSC (less than 5 min) and VF or pVT as a presenting rhythm are associated with improved neurologic outcome for survivors of pediatric cardiopulmonary arrest.

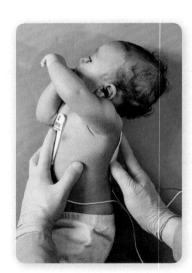

Figure 39-8 Anterior-posterior pad position for children who are younger than 1 year or who weigh less than 22 pounds (10 kg).

© Jones & Bartlett Learning.

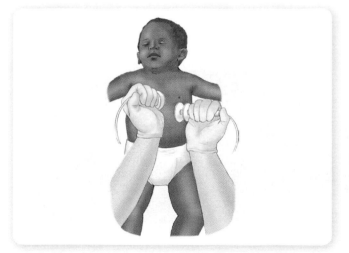

Figure 39-7 Anterior chest wall placement of paddles (shown here) or pads (commonly used in prehospital care) for the infant.

© Jones & Bartlett Learning.

Table 39-3	**Pediatric Defibrillation Pad Size**	
Age/Weight	**Pad Size**
Older than 1 year or weighing >22 lb (10 kg)	3-in. (8-10-cm) pads (adult)
Up to 1 year or weighing <22 lb (10 kg)	2-in. (4.5-cm) pads (pediatric)

Data from: Haskell SE, Atkins DL. Defibrillation in children. J Emerg Trauma Shock. 2010;3(3):261-266.

▶ Shockable ECG Rhythms

The two shockable ECG rhythms are VF and pVT. When a patient is in a shockable rhythm, the heart is quivering but blood is not pumping. As you have learned, defibrillation stuns the heart muscle momentarily and allows the patient's normal conduction system to resume control. If the patient is not defibrillated, then the VF will ultimately deteriorate to asystole.

In the first moments of a cardiac arrest, when the patient is in VF or pVT, the heart is oxygenated and "ready" to receive a shock. This condition explains why the rescuer should begin the steps of CPR and attach the AED as quickly as possible. If a shock is recommended in this circumstance, then administer it immediately—the chances of a successful defibrillation drop 7% to 10% for every minute that passes.

If a patient is in cardiac arrest for an interval of 4 to 5 minutes or longer, even if the initial ECG showed a shockable rhythm, then the success rate of defibrillation may be poor because the heart is not "ready" for a shock. Therefore, a rapid shock is not the best initial treatment. Instead, perfusion and oxygenation are needed first. Begin the steps of CPR, proceeding with five cycles (2 minutes of 30 compressions to two ventilations) and then apply the AED as soon as possible. If the patient is in VF or pVT at this point, then he or she is ready for a dose of electricity.

▶ Effective Shocks and Special Circumstances

When a shock is effective, occasionally the patient wakes up. However, the majority of effective defibrillations take a minute or so to produce ROSC. The defibrillation actually stuns the heart, allowing the pacemaker to begin to beat. This heartbeat may not be enough to generate a pulse just yet. For this reason, as soon as the patient is defibrillated, you should immediately begin compressions. The success rate for a biphasic dose is excellent (better than 95%) if the heart is ready to receive the shock.[20] Do not be surprised if the patient begins to move after a minute or so. After a cycle of 2 minutes of CPR, it is then acceptable to take 10 seconds to check for a pulse and review the rhythm if the patient continues to show signs of life or advanced monitoring show signs of ROSC. If ROSC is present, you can then cease the compressions and check for a pulse, respirations, and blood pressure.

When using a manual defibrillator/monitor, the patient's ECG is monitored and displayed throughout the arrest—not just when you are asking an AED to analyze the rhythm. Thus, it is possible to observe a rhythm change to a shockable rhythm while compressions are being done and then begin to charge the unit. After the AED is fully charged, the operator should clear all rescuers and deliver the shock. With this approach, compressions should be delivered while the AED is charging to minimize the interruption, and the compressor should hover over the patient's chest.

It is also recommended that the ventilation device be removed from the patient or detached from the advanced airway to prevent oxygen from flowing across the patient's chest while a shock is being delivered, because the simultaneous delivery poses a fire hazard.

Controversies

In some settings, the LMA, Combitube, or King LT are thought to be superior to bag-mask ventilation and oxygenation. Surprisingly, research shows that these devices are equivalent to the ET tube in the adult patient. In addition, the Combitube and King LT offer protection from aspiration of the stomach contents into the lungs. The LMA, Combitube, and King LT are similar in the following ways:

- They are advanced airway devices that are inserted blindly.
- They are placed orally and inserted past the hypopharyngeal space.
- They are easy to use and do not require extensive training in laryngoscopy.

By training selected EMS providers on the use of these devices, your service may expand the number of patients who have access to an advanced airway. The specifics on how to use these devices are included in Chapter 15, *Airway Management*.

Review the following special circumstances for defibrillation and understand the solutions or modifications to the procedure should they arise:

- The patient is an infant. Use the appropriate pediatric pads and an attenuator if available.
- The patient has a hairy chest and the electrodes will not stick. Quickly shave the patient just as you would to obtain a 12-lead ECG.
- The patient is submersed in water or is soaking wet. Get out of the rain, quickly moving the patient to your ambulance, or remove the patient from the pool and dry off him or her prior to applying the electrodes or providing a shock.
- The patient has an automatic implantable cardioverter defibrillator or pacemaker. Avoid these devices by a few inches when you are placing the electrodes.
- The patient has a transdermal medication patch on the chest. Quickly remove the patch and wipe the chest dry. Wear disposable gloves while removing the patch to avoid absorbing the nitroglycerin into your skin.

A comparison of the key elements of adult, child, and infant CPR is shown in **Table 39-4**.

Table 39-4	Key Elements of CPR for Adults, Children, and Infants		
Procedure	**Age 9 Years to Adult**	**Age 1 to 8 Years**	**Younger Than 1 Year[a]**
Circulation			
Recognition	Unresponsive with no breathing, or only agonal (gasping) respirations		
Pulse check	Carotid artery	Carotid artery	Brachial artery
Compression location	In the center of the chest (lower half of the sternum)	In the center of the chest (lower half of the sternum)	Just below the nipple line
Hand placement	Heel of both hands	Heel of one or both hands	Two-finger or two-thumb encircling-hands technique
Compression depth	At least 2 in. (5 cm); not to exceed 2.4 in. (6 cm)	At least one-third of anterior-posterior diameter of chest; approximately 2 in. (5 cm)	At least one-third of anterior-posterior diameter of chest; approximately 1.5 in. (4 cm)
Compression rate	100 to 120/min		
Chest wall recoil	Allow full chest recoil in between compressions. No leaning! Rotate rescuers delivering compressions every 2 min		
Interruptions	Limit interruptions in delivery of chest compressions to less than 10 s		
Compression-to-ventilation ratio (until an advanced airway is inserted)	30:2 (one or two rescuers)	30:2 (one rescuer); 15:2 (two professional rescuers)	
Airway			
Airway positioning	Head tilt–chin lift maneuver; jaw-thrust maneuver if spinal injury is suspected		
Breathing			
Untrained rescuer	Compressions only		
Ventilations without advanced airway	2 breaths with a duration of 1 s each, with enough volume to produce chest rise[b]		
Ventilations with advanced airway	1 breath every 6 s (10/min) Asynchronous with chest compressions; duration of 1 s each, with enough volume to produce chest rise	*Age 1 month to the onset of puberty:* 1 breath every 6 to 8 s (8-10 breaths/min) Chest compressions delivered continuously at a rate of at least 100/min with no pauses for ventilations; duration of 1 s each, with enough volume to produce visible chest rise	
Rescue breathing	1 breath every 5–6 s (10–12 breaths/min)	1 breath every 3–5 s (12–20 breaths/min)	1 breath every 3–5 s (12–20 breaths/min)
Defibrillation			
Device	Adult AED	Use pediatric dose-attenuator unit if available; if unavailable, then use adult unit	Use manual defibrillator if available; if unavailable, use unit with pediatric dose-attenuator; if neither is available, then use adult unit

Procedure	Age 9 Years to Adult	Age 1 to 8 Years	Younger Than 1 Year[a]
Procedure	Attach AED as soon as it is available. If two rescuers are available, then one should immediately begin CPR while the second retrieves and applies the AED. Minimize CPR interruptions. Resume CPR immediately after shock, beginning with chest compressions.		
Airway Obstruction			
Foreign body obstruction	Responsive: abdominal thrusts Unresponsive: CPR[c]	Responsive: abdominal thrusts	Responsive: back slaps and chest thrusts

Abbreviations: AED, automated external defibrillator; CPR, cardiopulmonary resuscitation

[a] Excluding newborns, in whom arrest is usually the result of asphyxiation and requires the rescue ventilations.

[b] Pause compressions to deliver ventilations.

[c] Look in the mouth for objects before delivering breaths in a patient with a known airway obstruction.

Data from: Kleinman ME, Brennan EE, Goldberger ZD, Swor RA, Terry M, Bobrow BJ, Gazmuri RJ, Travers AH, Rea T. Part 5: adult basic life support and cardiopulmonary resuscitation quality: 2015 American Heart Association Guidelines Update for Cardiopulmonary Resuscitation and Emergency Cardiovascular Care. Circulation. 2015;132(suppl 2):S414–S435; and Atkins DL, Berger S, Duff JP, Gonzales JC, Hunt EA, Joyner BL, Meaney PA, Niles DE, Samson RA, Schexnayder SM. Part 11: pediatric basic life support and cardiopulmonary resuscitation quality: 2015 American Heart Association Guidelines Update for Cardiopulmonary Resuscitation and Emergency Cardiovascular Care. Circulation. 2015;132(suppl 2):S519–S525.

YOU ▶ are the Paramedic   PART 4

You reassess your patient to find that his skin appears to have more color and you quickly check for a pulse. A carotid pulse rate of 68 beats/min is detected. The compression device has been paused and you analyze the patient's rhythm. You detect clear ST-segment elevation and begin to obtain a 12-lead ECG. You identify the presence of the ST elevation myocardial infarction and your partner transmits the ECG to the hospital. You prepare to call in your report to the receiving facility while your partner obtains vital signs. Although the patient has not shown signs of responsiveness, you are pleased to have achieved a ROSC. After completing your radio report, the hospital advises you they have received your ECG transmission and you should take the patient to the cardiac catheterization laboratory on arrival without stopping in the emergency department (ED).

You and your team move to the back of the ambulance with the patient loaded and secured to a backboard. Your partner has also applied a cervical collar to help secure the ET tube. Your partner continues to deliver ventilations while the field supervisor prepares the ATV. The patient is connected to the ATV and the field supervisor advises she will drive you to the hospital. Transport time is estimated to be approximately 10 minutes.

You obtain another set of vital signs prior to reaching the hospital. On arrival, you unload the patient with the assistance of your partner and field supervisor. Your field supervisor goes to locate your patient's wife to update her on her husband's location in the hospital. While you transfer your patient to the staff in the lab, you provide a bedside report and your updated assessment findings to the receiving nurse and cardiologist. You return to the EMS workroom in the ED to complete your patient care report (PCR). You are aware of the importance of accurate and specific documentation of this field resuscitation for data collection and reporting for cardiac arrests.

Recording Time: 21 Minutes	
Respirations	10 breaths/min via ET tube using an ATV
Pulse	68 beats/min
Skin	Pink, cool, and dry
Blood pressure	88/54 mm Hg
Oxygen saturation (Spo₂)	99% on 100% F$_{IO_2}$
Pupils	Equal, round, and sluggish but reactive to light
End-tidal carbon dioxide (ETCO₂)	38 mm Hg

8. What is the significance of completing ALS care prior to transport?
9. What is the significance of good documentation for improvement of survival in out-of-hospital cardiac arrests?

■ The Advanced Cardiac Life Support Algorithm

The Advanced Cardiac Life Support (ACLS) Algorithm **Figure 39-9** used to manage an adult in cardiac arrest builds on the BLS Healthcare Provider Adult Algorithm discussed earlier in this chapter. After making sure the patient has been placed on supplemental oxygen, the cardiac monitor/defibrillator is used to determine whether the patient is still in a shockable rhythm. The ACLS Algorithm separates the treatment approach into two basic pathways: shockable rhythms (VF or pVT) or nonshockable rhythms (asystole or PEA).

Preplanning is needed so that the medications are drawn up and ready to administer prior to the rhythm checks. The medications are administered during CPR, and compressions should not be interrupted just to administer a medication.

As long as the patient has an effective airway and is being adequately ventilated, placement of an advanced airway (ie, LMA, Combitube, King LT, or ET tube)—although helpful—should never take priority over delivery of high-quality compressions or defibrillation when needed. Practice your intubation techniques so you are able to insert the advanced airway device with no more than a 10-second interruption in chest compressions. With practice, placement of an advanced airway can be done while chest compressions are proceeding in many situations. Refer to in Chapter 15, *Airway Management*, for more information about advanced airway devices.

▶ Managing Patients in VF or pVT

If patients in VF or pVT receive timely and appropriate care, then these patients are the most likely to be resuscitated. Continue to perform high-quality CPR and do a rhythm check at each 2-minute point. If the patient is in a shockable rhythm, then administer a single shock and immediately begin compressions. If three rescuers are performing CPR (ventilator, active compressor, and on-deck compressor) and an advanced airway has been placed, then the compressions and ventilations can be asynchronous. Medications should be prepared and administered while performing CPR. A timekeeper, if available, can remind the code team leader what steps should be coming up in the next 30 seconds, in the next 15 seconds, and so on.

Drug therapy for VF or pVT includes a vasopressor (epinephrine). Epinephrine (0.1 mg/mL [1:10,000]) is given as a 1-mg IV push; this dose should be repeated every 3 to 5 minutes as long as the pulse is absent. Per the AHA guidelines, vasopressin is no longer recommended because research has found it to be neither more nor less effective than epinephrine when measuring survival after ROSC.

After the third shock, you may decide to administer an antidysrhythmic such as amiodarone, which is given as a 300-mg bolus during CPR. Amiodarone may be repeated once at 150 mg in 3 to 5 minutes after the initial dose. If amiodarone is unavailable, then you may administer lidocaine (1 to 1.5 mg/kg IV push, then 0.5 to 0.75 mg/kg, up to a maximum of 3 doses, or 3 mg/kg). Do not combine these two antidysrhythmics and always follow your local protocol.

If the patient has torsades de pointes, then consider administering magnesium (loading dose 1 to 2 g IV or IO).

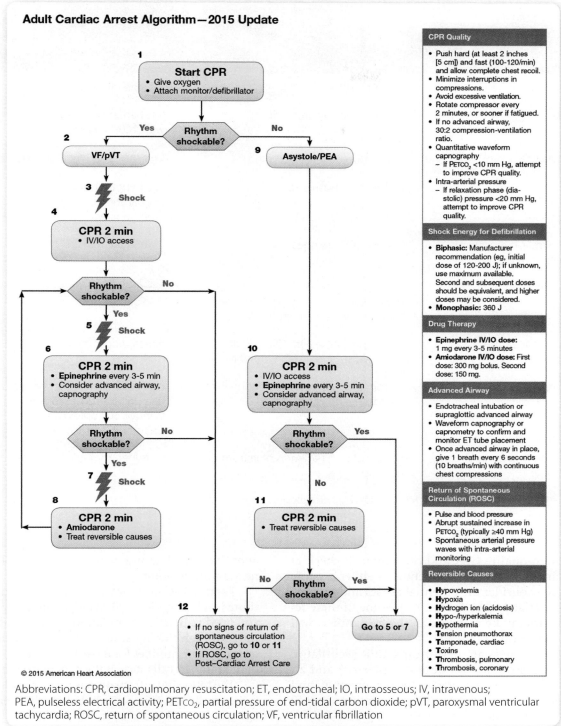

Figure 39-9 Advanced Cardiac Life Support (ACLS) Algorithm for cardiac arrest (adult or pediatric).

Reprinted with permission. Web-based Integrated 2015 American Heart Association Guidelines for CPR & ECC. Part 7: Adult Advanced Cardiovascular Life Support. © 2015 American Heart Association, Inc.

After each drug has been administered, allow it to circulate and then reanalyze the patient at the next 2-minute point. If the patient remains in a shockable rhythm, then administer another shock and consider possible reversible causes of cardiac arrest (the "Hs and Ts") (Table 39-5).

▶ Managing Patients in PEA or Asystole

Recall that PEA refers to an organized cardiac rhythm (other than VT) on the cardiac monitor that is not accompanied by any detectable pulse. Continue to

Table 39-5	Possible Reversible Causes of Cardiac Arrest	
Causes	**Clues**	**Treatment (Beyond Managing the Cardiac Arrest)**
Hypovolemia	Patient history	Volume infusion
Hypoxia	Cyanosis; airway problem	Intubation and ventilation with 100% oxygen
Hypoglycemia	Blood glucose level <60 mg/dL	Dextrose 50% in water, 25 g
Hypothermia	History of exposure to cold	See hypothermia algorithm in Chapter 38, *Environmental Emergencies.*
Hyperkalemia, hypokalemia, Hydrogen ions (acidosis)	History, ECG changes	Immediate transport
Tension pneumothorax	History; no pulse with CPR; unequal breath sounds with hyperresonance to percussion on affected side	Needle decompression of the affected side of the chest
Tamponade (cardiac)	History; no pulse with CPR; jugular venous distention; stab wound to heart	Pericardiocentesis (immediate transport)
Toxins (drug overdose)	History of accidental or intentional overdose	Naloxone (Narcan) for opioid or narcotic overdose; consult with Poison Control. See opioid algorithm in Chapter 27, *Toxicology.*
Thrombosis (pulmonary or coronary)	History of clot; patient is blue from neck up	Consider immediate transport.

Abbreviations: CPR, cardiopulmonary resuscitation; ECG, electrocardiogram

© Jones & Bartlett Learning.

provide high-quality CPR and do a rhythm check at each 2-minute point. If the patient is in either asystole or PEA, then consider the potential causes and manage them appropriately (see Table 39-5). Some of these reversible issues can be managed in the field; others will require intervention in the ED.

If three rescuers are performing CPR (ventilator, active compressor, and on-deck compressor) and an advanced airway has been placed, the compressions and ventilations can be asynchronous. Medications should be prepared and administered while doing CPR. A timekeeper, if available, can remind the code team leader what should be coming up in the next 30 seconds, in the next 15 seconds, and so on.

Drug therapy for PEA or asystole includes a vasopressor (epinephrine). Epinephrine (0.1 mg/mL [1:10,000]) is given as a 1-mg IV push; this dose should be repeated every 3 to 5 minutes as long as the pulse is absent.

If the patient converts to VF or pVT at any point or when the rhythm is checked every five cycles of CPR (approximately 2 minutes), move back to the shockable side of the algorithm. After each drug has been administered,

allow it to circulate and then reanalyze the patient at the next 2-minute point.

Paramedics are trained to follow the current algorithms and use good medical judgment. To be successful, you need to practice. Simulation is very helpful because modern high-fidelity simulators can provide excellent learning opportunities for those low-frequency, high-risk, or high-impact calls such as the patient in cardiac arrest.[22]

The following information is *not* an algorithm; rather, these are the key points to remember when you are managing a patient in cardiac arrest:

- Perform high-quality CPR beginning with compressions; minimize interruptions from start to completion of the field code. Organize the code around 2-minute cycles of 30 compressions and two ventilations, and then switch compressors and analyze the rhythm. If an advanced airway is inserted, then switch to asynchronous compressions at a rate of 100 to 120 per minute and ventilate every 6 seconds (a rate of 10 breaths/min).

- If a shockable rhythm is identified, then continue compressions until the defibrillator is charged to the appropriate dose and then stop, clear, deliver the shock, and immediately begin compressions unless the patient wakes up.
- Without interrupting CPR, obtain IV/IO access and administer epinephrine every 3 to 5 minutes for the duration of the code (provided the patient is not hypothermic). After a cycle of CPR and shock, if necessary, administer an antidysrhythmic drug for VF/pVT (amiodarone 300 mg which may be repeated at 150 mg).
- For asystole or PEA, do not deliver shocks.
- For all cardiac arrests, regardless of the rhythm, consider the possible reversible causes ("Hs and Ts") and manage them appropriately.
- If you decide to insert an advanced airway (supraglottic or ET tube), then confirm and monitor with waveform capnography and switch to asynchronous compressions and ventilations. Never hyperventilate the patient because this can negatively affect coronary perfusion pressure.
- If the patient experiences ROSC, then the capnography readings might show a sustained increase in ETCO$_2$ level (typically greater than or equal to 40 mm Hg). Turn your attention to monitoring vital signs, obtain a 12-lead ECG, and prepare to transport the patient to the most appropriate facility that can perform postresuscitative care (ie, TTM, EEG monitoring, cardiac catheterization).

Mechanical Adjuncts to Circulation

The AHA guidelines maintain manual chest compressions as the standard of care for treatment of cardiac arrest, but recommend use of mechanical adjuncts in certain settings where the delivery of high-quality chest compressions could be difficult or dangerous. For example, mechanical chest compression devices may make it possible to provide high-quality CPR during a prolonged arrest (ie, lengthy ambulance transport to the catheterization lab or a patient with hypothermia).[23] Some EMS systems have had marked success incorporating mechanical adjuncts into their field codes. The use of mechanical adjuncts to circulation is a medical decision and should involve a careful analysis of your agency's operations, transport distances, and available personnel on the field code team, as well as a review of the most recent published studies.

▶ Load-Distributing Band CPR Device

The load-distributing band CPR device (eg, AutoPulse) is designed to deliver consistent, uninterrupted adult chest compressions and therefore improve hemodynamics

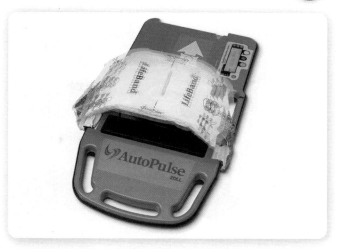

Figure 39-10 The AutoPulse load-distributing band device.
Courtesy of ZOLL.

during cardiac arrest **Figure 39-10** . This automated, portable device offers an easy-to-use, load-distributing band that squeezes the entire chest, thereby improving blood flow to the heart and brain during cardiac arrest. Its use can also free up rescuers to focus on other lifesaving interventions and eliminate fatigue from the performance of chest compressions.

The load-distributing band CPR device can be integrated into a field code as follows:

1. Ensure that CPR is in progress and that effective, high-quality compressions are being provided.
2. Align the patient on the platform of the device.
3. Close the chest band over the patient's chest.
4. Press the start button (device performs the compressions automatically).
5. Provide bag-mask ventilation at a rate of two ventilations for every 30 compressions. Each ventilation should be given over 1 second to provide visible chest rise.
6. If an advanced airway is in place, then the compressions and ventilations become asynchronous.

▶ Mechanical Chest Compression Device

A mechanical chest compression device (eg, the Thumper) is an adjunct to adult CPR that provides both continuous chest compressions (between 100 and 120 per minute) and ventilations **Figure 39-11** . It can be used with a pocket mask or an advanced airway. Because this device is powered by oxygen and delivers oxygen when it ventilates, it requires a large volume of oxygen. If you use a mechanical chest compression device, then plan to carry additional portable oxygen tanks equipped with high-pressure hose adapters to facilitate rapid transfer of the gas. Use these high-pressure adapters in the ambulance and keep them

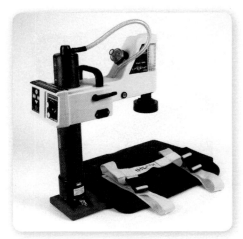

Figure 39-11 The Thumper CPR system.
Courtesy of Michigan Instruments, Inc.

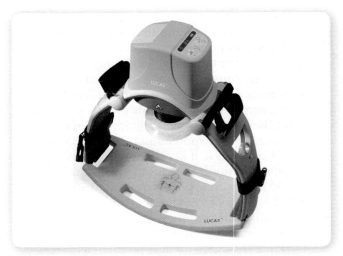

Figure 39-12 The Lucas 2 mechanical piston device.
Courtesy of Physio-Control, Inc.

available for use in the ED if the device is used to transport the patient to the ED. The mechanical chest compression device has been particularly useful in lengthy arrests (eg, hypothermic arrest), because it can produce high-quality CPR compressions for a long time.

In the past, some EMS systems reserved the use of mechanical chest compression devices for transport to the hospital. Given that high-quality compressions are important to the success of the resuscitation, it makes more sense for the code team to practice simulated codes to ensure they can apply the device as early as possible without any interruptions in manual CPR.

▶ Mechanical Piston Device

A mechanical piston device (eg, Lucas 2) is a mechanical chest compression device that depresses the adult sternum via a compressed gas-powered plunger mounted on a backboard **Figure 39-12**. This device is not designed to offer a ventilation component because many EMS systems use an ATV for this purpose. The mechanical piston device is portable and easy to deploy; a small backplate fits behind the patient and allows the piston to snap down directly into the backplate. The device is powered by a small battery at the top of the piston.

When you are using any of the mechanical adjuncts to circulation, it is important that they are easy to deploy without interrupting high-quality, manual chest compressions. If the adjunct is not easy to deploy, then it will not be used early in the field code. If your EMS agency purchases an adjunct to circulation, then practice with the device so all members of your service can deploy it and make sure it arrives on the scene as early as possible in the field code.

▶ Impedance Threshold Device

The ITD (eg, ResQPOD) is designed to enhance chest compressions by creating a vacuum in the chest that allows

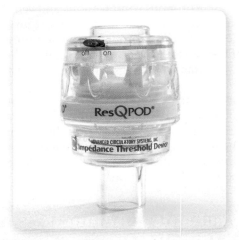

Figure 39-13 The ResQPOD is thought to improve perfusion during compressions when used in combination with an active compression-decompression cardiopulmonary resuscitation device.
Courtesy of Advanced Circulatory.

more blood to flow to the heart and brain **Figure 39-13**. Imagine a bellows fanning a fireplace. As the bellows opens to its full size, it sucks in air. A similar process occurs when the chest wall re-expands—the vacuum that results pulls air into the lungs and blood back into the heart. An ITD selectively prevents that unnecessary air from rushing into the chest, maximizing the vacuum during the recoil phase of the compression. The ITD also has a prompt that helps the ventilator keep track of the rate of ventilations to avoid exceeding the recommended rate. The AHA guidelines do not recommend the use of an ITD as an adjunct during conventional CPR (the ITD is categorized as Class III: No Benefit).[24] However, use of an ITD has been to be shown to enhance the effects of the ACD-CPR device. If your EMS system is still using the ITD, then it should be removed from the ventilation system

Words of Wisdom

The AHA guidelines include recommendations regarding confirmation of ET tube placement and continuous monitoring of the position of the tube to avoid its dislodgement. After you see the ET tube pass through the vocal cords and verify the tube position by chest expansion and auscultation during positive pressure ventilation, obtain additional confirmation of placement using continuous waveform ETCO$_2$ (capnography). No single confirmation technique is completely reliable. Your initial techniques of verification should include the following measures:

- Direct visualization of the tube going through the vocal cords
- Bilateral chest expansion
- Five-point auscultation (epigastrium and two in each lung)
- Initial monitoring of ETCO$_2$ level
- Use of an esophageal detector device

Be sure to provide continuous monitoring of the ETCO$_2$ level throughout the field code and closely note and respond to any changes. Not only will the ETCO$_2$ level tell you if the tube is misplaced, but it will also give you an indication of ROSC.

as the patient's pulse returns because it is designed to be used solely in conjunction with compressions.

Postresuscitative Care

Postresuscitative care is an important component of caring for patients in cardiac arrest. If an effective cardiac rhythm is restored in the field, then provide immediate transport because the patient needs careful monitoring and titrated therapy that can most effectively be provided in an intensive care unit.

The following is a summary of postresuscitative care:

1. Stabilize the cardiac rhythm (ie, administer an antidysrhythmic for post-VF or post-VT), administer atropine or use a transcutaneous pacemaker for symptomatic bradycardia).
2. Normalize the blood pressure (administer a dopamine [Intropin] or norepinephrine infusion to raise the systolic pressure to at least 100 mm Hg).
3. Elevate the patient's head to a 30° angle if the blood pressure levels allow.
4. Obtain a 12-lead ECG, monitor glucose level, assess oxygen needs, and prevent seizure activity.
5. Provide TTM for the patient with ROSC who is in a coma (usually provided in the ED setting).

When to Start and When to Stop CPR

As a paramedic, it is your responsibility to start CPR in all patients who are in cardiac arrest, with only two general exceptions.

First, do not start CPR if the patient has obvious signs of death such as absence of a pulse and breathing, along with any one of the following findings:

- Rigor mortis: stiffening of the body after death
- Dependent lividity (livor mortis): a discoloration of the skin caused by pooling of blood
- Putrefaction: decomposition of the body
- Evidence of nonsurvivable injury, such as decapitation, dismemberment, or burned beyond recognition

Rigor mortis and dependent lividity develop after a patient has been dead for a long period.

Second, do not start CPR if the patient and his or her physician have previously agreed not to resuscitate. This condition may apply only to situations in which the patient is known to be in the terminal stage of an incurable disease. In this situation, CPR serves only to prolong the patient's death. However, this issue can be complicated. Do not resuscitate (DNR) orders, Medical Orders for Life-Sustaining Treatment (MOLST) forms, and advance directives such as living wills may express the patient's wishes; however, these documents may not be readily producible by the patient's family or caregiver. In such cases, the safest course is to assume that an emergency exists, begin CPR under the rule of implied consent, and contact medical control for further guidance. Conversely, if a valid DNR, MOLST form, or living will is produced, then resuscitative efforts may be withheld. Learn your state laws and local protocols as well as the standards in your system for treating terminally ill patients, and refer to Chapter 4, *Medical, Legal, and Ethical Issues*, for further discussion on advance health care directives. Some EMS systems have electronic notes on patients who are preregistered with the system, specifying the amount and extent of treatment desired. Other states have specific DNR forms that allow EMS providers to withhold care when the patient, family, and physician have agreed in advance that such a course is most appropriate. It is crucial that you understand your local protocols and are aware of the specific restrictions these advance directives imply.

In all other cases, begin CPR on anyone who is in cardiac arrest. It is usually impossible to know how long the patient has been without oxygen to the brain and vital organs unless you were there to witness the cardiac arrest. Factors such as air temperature and the basic health of the patient's tissues and organs can affect his or her ability to survive. Therefore, most legal advisors recommend that, when in doubt, always give too much care rather than too little. Always start CPR if any doubt exists.

After you begin CPR in the field, do not stop until one of the following events occurs:

- The patient starts breathing and has a pulse (ROSC).
- The patient is transferred to another health care provider of equal or more advanced training.
- You are completely out of strength and energy and are no longer physically able to perform CPR.
- A physician who is present or providing online medical direction assumes responsibility for the patient and gives direction to terminate the resuscitative efforts.

In short, always continue CPR until the patient's care is transferred to a physician or higher medical authority in the field. In some cases, your medical director or a designated medical control physician may order you to stop CPR on the basis of the patient's condition. Every EMS system should have clear standing orders or protocols that provide guidelines for starting and stopping CPR. Your medical director and the legal adviser of your EMS system should agree on these protocols, which should be closely administered and reviewed by your medical director.

► Terminating Resuscitative Efforts

The AHA guidelines say the following about lengthy resuscitative efforts and transporting patients in cardiac arrest:

- Few instances require transporting a patient in nontraumatic cardiac arrest who has failed a successfully executed prehospital ACLS resuscitation effort to an ED to continue the resuscitation attempt.

- In the absence of mitigating factors, prolonged resuscitative efforts are unlikely to be successful. If ROSC of any duration occurs, however, then it may be appropriate to consider extending the resuscitative effort.
- Rare exceptions may include severe prehospital hypothermia (eg, submersion in icy water) and drug overdose. A successfully executed prehospital resuscitation includes an adequate trial of BLS and ALS.

Transporting a deceased patient who is refractory to proper BLS and ALS care is usually not appropriate. Protocols for pronouncement of death and appropriate transport of the body by non-EMS vehicles should be established.

► Termination Rules

The quality of CPR is compromised during transport and survival is linked to optimizing scene care, rather than simply rushing to the hospital. Specifically, for a patient who is receiving only BLS, the BLS termination of resuscitation rule was established to consider terminating BLS support before ambulance transport if all of the following criteria are met:

1. The arrest was not witnessed by anyone.
2. No ROSC after three full rounds of CPR and AED analysis.
3. No AED shocks were delivered.

For situations where ALS personnel are present to provide care for an adult in out-of-hospital cardiac arrest, the ALS termination of resuscitation rule was established to consider terminating resuscitative efforts before ambulance transport if all of the following criteria are met:

1. The arrest was not witnessed by anyone.
2. Bystander CPR was not provided.
3. No ROSC after complete ALS care in the field.
4. No AED shocks were delivered.

Of course, the local decision on transportation should involve preplanning by the regional and service medical directors.

▉ Scene Choreography and Teamwork

During resuscitation, many tasks need to be performed. This is where teamwork comes in. Teamwork divides the task while multiplying the chances for a successful resuscitation. A role is available for each health care provider who is committed to fulfilling his or her part. Teams who practice together regularly are more successful in their resuscitation attempts.

Consider an analogy from the world of sports, where it is essential that all team members practice to be successful. In 2016, Christopher Froome and his international team of cyclists won the Tour de France **Figure 39-14** . The Tour is a grueling 21-stage bike race that covers roughly 2,000 miles (3,500 km) through the tallest mountains and smallest towns into Paris. Cycling is a team sport, just like baseball, soccer, football, or basketball. Each member of the team had a specific role that helped the team succeed—for example, maintaining the pace, blocking the wind, and collecting water bottles and food bags. All team members must be totally committed to the success of the team rather than to their individual achievements.

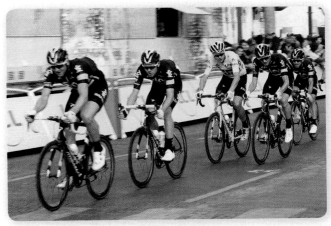

Figure 39-14 Even though Christopher Froome (yellow jersey) is the only member of Great Britain's Team Sky wearing the overall race leader's jersey, his entire team worked hard to get him through the race safely, because cycling is a team sport.
© Jean Catuffe/Getty.

The intense preparation and teamwork that characterize any type of high-level sports team hold a few pertinent lessons for field code team members:

- Athletes do not only excel on their own. They need the support of their team and coach.
- The coach helps the team members understand the rules of the game and prepare for its challenges.
- The coach drills the athletes with routines or "plays" and provides constant feedback and plenty of practice opportunities to measure their progress.
- The team trains with the best equipment, eats nutritious meals, develops a positive mental attitude about winning, and gets plenty of rest after enduring rigorous demanding physical and mental exercise.
- When it is time to compete, team members are well prepared, on time, and ready to go. The coach can support them from the sidelines and may offer signals and guidance or plays in some sports, but he or she cannot compete for the team.

Field code team members who are rested, fit, and well nourished, and who bring a positive attitude to their work, practice their skills, know the plays, and work together as a team, are on top of their game. They are ready to resuscitate patients. To be successful, your team needs to take the following steps:

- Know the plays (ie, the algorithms) expertly and automatically. This knowledge takes much practice. When the team has questions, use posters and pocket cards to ask, explain, and prepare.
- Listen to your "coaches." They have the best interests of the patients in mind—and your best interests, too.
- Have a practice ethic. Pull out the manikins and run simulations frequently. Collect data on the cumulative time of interruptions of compressions so that the team has feedback and can work to improve its performance. How long does it take you to do each procedure? If you measure it and provide feedback, then you can improve performance. Many EMS systems have incorporated a pit crew approach to the management of cardiac arrest.[25] The term originated in motor racing, in which teams of technicians rapidly assess and repair vehicles in a manner of seconds. Following this model, each team member is assigned a specific role before beginning care of the patient. The pit crew model clarifies each team member's role and responsibilities, and minimizes confusion on the scene. Therefore, this model minimizes the time to first compression.

- Remember that success requires practice, a positive mental attitude, well-designed plays, and excellent coaching.
- Utilize CPR feedback devices. Several devices are available to provide immediate feedback to rescuers on the rate and depth of their compressions.
- Recognize that the effectiveness of the team is not about you. It is about succeeding as a group. Patients and their families are counting on you to get this right, so come prepared!

▶ Code Team Member and Code Team Leader Roles

Whether you are a code team member or a code team leader, you should know both your own role and the roles of the other members of your code team during the resuscitation attempt. This knowledge will help you anticipate what steps are coming next and see how your role is an essential part of the resuscitation attempt. Whatever skills you are trained and appropriately authorized to perform, it is essential to the success of the resuscitation that you are prepared, have practiced regularly, have mastered the algorithms, and are committed to success.

Code Team Member Roles

A code team member may be called on to perform all of the following roles (and more):

- **Ventilator.** Responsible for managing the airway. This team member's duties include suctioning the patient, ventilating the patient with a bag-mask device or ATV, and inserting an advanced airway device (ie, LMA, Combitube, King LT, or ET tube).
- **Active compressor.** Responsible for providing high-quality chest compressions. The responsibility of this team member is to compress for 2 minutes and be the on-deck compressor for 2 minutes.
- **On-deck compressor.** Responsible for relieving the active compressor at the 2-minute point without any interruption in compressions. Other functions include assisting with application of a mechanical adjunct to circulation (if available), checking on vital signs, and preparing the patient for transport.
- **Other support personnel.** Responsible for analyzing the ECG and delivering shocks, gaining IV/IO access, providing documentation for the PCR, and supporting family members.

Code Team Leader Roles

Every resuscitation team needs a leader to organize the efforts of the group. Clearly the code team leader must know all of the specific skills and be able to perform each skill expertly. Occasionally, the code team leader will serve as the backup for a team member who may be having difficulty inserting an ET tube or gaining IV/IO access. The code team leader is often responsible for making sure everything gets done at the right time in the right way.

The responsibilities of the code team leader may include all of the following:

- Obtaining the patient's history and performing the physical exam.
- Interpreting the ECG.
- Keeping track of the time.
- Making a medication decision following the algorithm.
- Clearly delegating tasks to code team members.
- Completing documentation after the resuscitation attempt.
- Talking with medical control.
- Controlling the resuscitation scene.
- Fostering the concepts of CRM.

Code team leaders must also model excellent behavior and leadership skills for their team and all others who may be involved in the resuscitation. The code team leader should help train future team leaders, seek to improve the effectiveness of the entire team through continuous quality improvement, and practice after the resuscitation to help prepare for the next code.

■ Plan for a Code

The following plan is merely one example of a plan for a field code; it is not the only way. Obviously, different communities have different resources that arrive at different times in different ways. The point is that you need a plan and you need to practice this plan diligently.

This example focuses on an out-of-hospital EMS agency and its response to a cardiac arrest in a private home, assuming a five-person team that could arrive on different units (eg, EMT unit, paramedic unit, EMS field supervisor with a mechanical chest compression device or other adjunct to circulation) at different times in the first few minutes. Roles for the adult scenario include Compressor 1, Compressor 2, Ventilator, Code Team Leader, and the EMS Field Supervisor:

- **Compressor 1.** Responsible for performing high-quality chest compressions (delivers at a rate between 100 and 120 per minute, presses hard and fast, and allows full chest recoil); stays in position and compresses for 2 minutes and then rests for 2 minutes (for the duration of the time the patient is pulseless); may assist with application of the mechanical chest compression device or other adjunct to circulation, provided Compressor 2 is continuing uninterrupted compressions.

- **Compressor 2.** Responsible for performing high-quality chest compressions (delivers at a rate between 100 and 120 per minute, presses hard and fast, and allows full chest recoil); stays in position and compresses for 2 minutes and then rests for 2 minutes (for the duration of the time the patient is pulseless); may assist with application of the mechanical chest compression device or other adjunct to circulation, provided Compressor 1 is continuing uninterrupted compressions.
- **Ventilator.** Responsible for providing ventilations (via bag-mask device, oropharyngeal airway, oxygen) at a ratio of 30:2, ensuring visible chest rise with each ventilation (1 second in duration); may need to briefly suction the patient as necessary, and then as appropriate will switch over to the ATV; assists with the transition from BLS airway to advanced airway (not a high priority). After an advanced airway is placed, the ventilator ventilates once every 6 seconds to achieve visible chest rise over a 1-second duration for each ventilation.
- **Code Team Leader.** Responsible for initial ECG analysis and defibrillation with a single shock; responsible for overall timing of the code and reassessment after 2 minutes of cycles of CPR with the interruption not to exceed 10 seconds. (Some EMS systems use a metronome set at 110 beats per minute to keep the rate of compressions on track; other agencies employ CPR feedback devices that are a part of the monitor/defibrillator.) After the initial shock (or ascertaining "no shock" rhythm), the code team leader proceeds to establish IV/IO access (no medications down the tube), then begins administration of a vasopressor every 3 to 5 minutes (1 mg epinephrine 0.1 mg/mL [1:10,000]); helps to transition the airway from BLS to an advanced airway (ie, ET tube, Combitube, King LT,

or LMA), and continues with single shocks every 2 minutes if patient is still in VF or pVT; makes the decision with input from the code team and medical control that the resuscitation should be terminated if ROSC is not achieved in the first 15 to 30 minutes.

If ROSC is achieved, then the code team leader administers the appropriate antidysrrhythmic (eg, amiodarone, lidocaine), ensures appropriate ventilations, and assists the team in preparing for transport. After the field code is completed, the code team leader works with the entire team to debrief the code based on all available feedback. Some EMS systems measure the **compression fraction**, which is an indication of how well the team is minimizing pauses in CPR. It is calculated by dividing the amount of time compressions are delivered by the amount of time compressions are indicated. The goal is to have a compression fraction has high as possible with a target of at least 60% (Class IIb).

- **EMS Field Supervisor.** Brings in the Thumper or other adjunct to circulation and works with one of the compressors to transition the patient to mechanical CPR compressions with minimal interruption. Assists the medic with IV or IO, advanced airway placement, and preparation of medications, and contacts medical control, per local protocols.

Managing the field code is complex, but not impossible. Have confidence and expect patients to survive if you come on the scene and someone is already performing CPR. Remember, the paradigm has changed since the early years of EMS and the first edition of this textbook. Today, with all five links of the out-of-hospital chain of survival in place, you should expect patients to survive more than 40% of the time!

YOU are the Paramedic   SUMMARY

1. **What links of the out-of-hospital chain of survival are present that would make you optimistic about the potential for ROSC?**

All five links in the out-of-hospital chain of survival are present. Early access to 9-1-1 following a witnessed arrest contributed to immediate response of an advanced life support (ALS) unit. Early cardiopulmonary resuscitation (CPR) was provided at the scene by a layperson who had recently completed CPR training. Early defibrillation was available due to the close proximity of an automated external defibrillator (AED) at the golf course.

2. **On the basis of the events occurring prior to your arrival and your own analysis of the ECG, what are your next steps as code team leader?**

Based on finding CPR in progress, you are aware that at least five cycles or 2 minutes of compressions have been performed since the AED delivered a shock to the patient. You have found the patient to be in a shockable rhythm, so delivering another shock is appropriate. Once additional ALS resources are available, you can delegate preparation of medications for administration. You should also be tracking times throughout the incident, interventions performed, and assessment findings.

3. What alternative medications are indicated for VF/pVT and at what dosages?

Aside from amiodarone 300 mg IV/IO bolus with repeat dose of 150 mg, lidocaine may be used in some emergency medical services (EMS) systems with an initial dose of 1 to 1.5 mg/kg IV/IO bolus and repeat dose of 0.5 to 0.75 mg/kg IV/IO bolus. Epinephrine 1 mg of 0.1 mg/mL (1:10,000) concentration is used as the vasopressor during an arrest.

4. If the rhythm had been analysed as torsades de pointes, then what medication might be beneficial and at what dosage?

For a patient with torsades de pointes, magnesium sulfate 1 to 2 g IV over 1 to 2 minutes might be helpful. It is indicated in refractory VF and pVT, especially torsades de pointes. Hypomagnesemia may cause these types of cardiac dysrhythmias.

5. Why is intubation not an early intervention consideration in the patient in cardiac arrest?

Studies that assess the value of intubation are inconclusive. High-quality compressions with minimal disruption should be the primary focus during resuscitation. You can effectively administer oxygen using a bag-mask device. Skill degradation affects your ability to intubate correctly and rapidly. Multiple or extended attempts to intubate can disrupt effective compressions, thereby decreasing the potential for successful return of spontaneous circulation (ROSC). If successful, rapid intubation is questionable, then consider alternative advanced airway options.

6. What is the importance of ETCO$_2$ monitoring in the patient in cardiac arrest?

Carbon dioxide levels rise in cardiac arrest due to anaerobic metabolism. As effective CPR is delivered, these levels can begin to normalize and assist you in monitoring the effectiveness of CPR. In the out-of-hospital environment, potential for dislodgement of an ET tube is high with movement and transferring of the patient. Monitoring ETCO$_2$ levels and waveform capnography can provide for early detection of proper and improper tube placement, as well as potential obstructions in the ET tube such as secretions or disconnection from the automatic transport ventilator.

7. If resuscitative efforts are eventually successful, then what is the significance of transporting the patient in cardiac arrest to a facility capable of advanced cardiac care?

Considering the links in the out-of-hospital chain of survival, your goal is to continue to seek an optimal outcome for the patient. Based on a patient's recent medical history, a cardiac event may have resulted in the arrest. Assuming you are successful in achieving resuscitation with ROSC, a facility capable of interventional cardiac procedures (cardiac catheterization lab) may offer more definitive treatment if this is the case.

8. What is the significance of completing ALS care prior to transport?

Survival of cardiac arrest is linked to optimizing on-scene care. Preparation for transport and moving of patients to the ambulance can significantly compromise the quality of the CPR being delivered. By providing full ALS care at the scene, you are ensuring high-quality compressions can be delivered with minimal disruption during the heart's most receptive period to resuscitation. You are also better able to secure your airway, obtain intravenous access, and prepare and deliver first-line medications as indicated. Most of these interventions are more difficult to perform in the confines of the ambulance and there is often less room for additional personnel to assist in carrying out the resuscitative efforts safely.

9. What is the significance of good documentation for improvement of survival in out-of-hospital cardiac arrests?

Data collection for the purposes of research and providing quality improvement in patients in cardiac arrest includes information you document on your patient care report. The receiving hospital may participate in the American Heart Association's Get With The Guidelines program or the Cardiac Arrest Registry to Enhance Survival program. Familiarize yourself with the recommended guidelines for reporting data for out-of-hospital cardiac arrest. By participating, your community can compare its data with other progressive communities. Quality improvement and medical review allow for the ability to optimize the performance of your EMS system in managing these patients.

YOU are the Paramedic **SUMMARY** (continued)

EMS Patient Care Report (PCR)

Date: 06-28-18	Incident No.: 201032591		Nature of Call: Cardiac arrest		Location: 1 Golf Club Drive
Dispatched: 1415	**En Route:** 1416	**At Scene:** 1420	**Transport:** 1448	**At Hospital:** 1458	**In Service:** 1525

Patient Information

Age: 54
Sex: M
Weight (in kg [lb]): 78.2 kg (172 lb)

Allergies: No known drug allergies
Medications: OTC acid-reducers and pain relievers
Past Medical History: Indigestion per wife
Chief Complaint: Cardiac arrest

Vital Signs

Time: 1426	BP: Not obtainable	Pulse: 0	Respirations: 0	SpO$_2$: Not obtainable
Time: 1432	BP: Not obtainable	Pulse: 0	Respirations: 0	SpO$_2$: Not obtainable
Time: 1436	BP: Not obtainable	Pulse: 0	Respirations: 0	SpO$_2$: Not obtainable
Time: 1441	BP: 86/60	Pulse: 80	Respirations: 10 via bag-mask device	SpO$_2$: Not obtainable
Time: 1447	BP: 88/54	Pulse: 68	Respirations: 10 via bag-mask device	SpO$_2$: 99%
Time: 1453	BP: 100/68	Pulse: 72	Respirations: 10, ventilator assisted	SpO$_2$: 99%

EMS Treatment (circle all that apply)

Oxygen @ __15__ L/min via (circle one): NC NRM (Bag-mask device)	(Assisted Ventilation)	(Airway Adjunct)	(CPR)
(Defibrillation)	Bleeding Control	Bandaging	Splinting	(Other: Epinephrine and amiodarone)

Narrative

EMS requested to above location for a man not breathing and without a pulse. On arrival, pt found lying supine on the ground with CPR in progress. Several bystanders and local volunteer emergency responders on scene with AED attached to the pt. Pt confirmed to be in VF. CPR continued with bag-mask ventilations using high concentration oxygen at 10/min. Defibrillated pt with 200 J at 1423. IV line established 18 gauge in left AC. Epinephrine 1 mg 0.1 mg/mL (1:10,000) administered IV at 1427. Confirmed rhythm to be pVT and defibrillated pt with 200 J at 1427. Amiodarone 300 mg administered IV at 1429. Confirmed rhythm to be pVT and defibrillated with 200 J at 1431. Pt intubated with size 7.5 ET tube orally in first attempt at 1433. Placement confirmed via cord visualization, auscultation, and ETCO$_2$ with waveforms. Tube secured at 27 cm mark with tube holder device. Epinephrine 1 mg 0.1 mg/mL (1:10,000) IV administered at 1433. Confirmed rhythm to be VT and defibrillated with 200 J at 1434. Amiodarone 150 mg administered IV at 1439. Pt had ROSC at 1440. Ventilations continued via ATV at 1441. EMS advised pt's wife of receiving facility. Pt will be transported to for evaluation and treatment. Pt reassessed en route with changes. Report called to ED prior to arrival which included pt's current condition and ETA. ECG transmission of 12-lead showing STEMI. Medical control advises to transport pt directly to cardiac cath lab. On arrival, pt was transferred to the cardiac procedure table and report given to RN and cardiologist. Physician signature obtained for medications delivered under ACLS protocol.**End of report**

Prep Kit

▶ Ready for Review

- Use the five links in the out-of-hospital chain of survival as a guide to manage cardiac arrest: recognition and activation of the emergency response system, immediate high-quality cardiopulmonary resuscitation (CPR), rapid defibrillation, basic and advanced emergency medical services care, and advanced life support (ALS) and postarrest care.
- The *Guidelines for Cardiopulmonary Resuscitation and Emergency Cardiac Care* from the American Heart Association and International Liaison Committee on Resuscitation continue to emphasize the importance of providing high-quality CPR beginning with compressions (push hard and fast, and allow full chest recoil).
- Advanced airways are only considered during the field code if a basic airway is not adequate or the airway needs to be better protected due to a patient who is vomiting. The focus of care should be CPR with high-quality compressions.
- The principles of basic life support are the same for infants, children, and adults. Anyone between the ages of 1 month and 1 year is considered an infant. A child is between age 1 year and adolescence (signs of puberty or secondary sexual characteristic development, such as axillary hair in boys or breast development in girls). Adulthood is from onset of puberty and older.
- You must first assess the patient's circulation. If the patient has no pulse, then provide artificial circulation by beginning with chest compressions at a rate of 100 to 120 per minute and a depth appropriate for the patient's age.
- CPR can be performed with one or two rescuers. Two-rescuer CPR or a team approach is always the first choice. When a rescuer is performing adult CPR alone or with another rescuer, the ratio of compressions to ventilations is 30:2.
- Defibrillation needs to be carried out as soon as possible in the presence of two shockable rhythms—ventricular fibrillation (VF) and pulseless ventricular tachycardia (pVT)—because the likelihood of its success declines rapidly with time.
- When you use a manual defibrillator, you interpret the cardiac rhythm and determine whether defibrillation is needed. An automated external defibrillator (AED) interprets the cardiac rhythm for you and determines if defibrillation is indicated.
- Defibrillation is indicated for patients in nontraumatic cardiac arrest who are older than 1 month. If you are using an AED on a child between age 1 year and the onset of puberty, then use pediatric-sized pads and a dose-attenuating system (energy reducer) if available.
- The Advanced Cardiac Life Support Algorithm separates the treatment approach into two basic pathways: shockable rhythms (VF or pVT) or nonshockable rhythms (asystole or pulseless electrical activity).
- For all arrests, regardless of the rhythm, consider the reversible causes ("Hs and Ts") and manage them appropriately.
- For asystole or pulseless electrical activity, do not deliver shocks.
- Certain devices may be used as mechanical adjuncts to circulation in certain situations to help improve the quality of compressions when you are providing CPR. These devices include the load-distributing band, the mechanical chest compression device, the mechanical piston device, and the impedance threshold device.
- For postresuscitative care, if an effective cardiac rhythm is restored in the field, then transport immediately. Goals of postresuscitative care include stabilizing the cardiac rhythm, normalizing the blood pressure, and elevating the patient's head to a 30 degree angle if blood pressure allows.
- Follow the ALS termination of resuscitation rule regarding the cessation of resuscitative efforts in an adult in out-of-hospital cardiac arrest where ALS providers are present.
- Teamwork divides tasks while multiplying the chances for a successful resuscitation.
- The principles of crew resource management can help a code team to work effectively and to enhance situational awareness. These principles include flat management hierarchy, communication, appreciative inquiry, and the sterile cockpit.
- Whether you are a code team member or a code team leader, you should know both your own role and the roles of the other members of your code team during the resuscitation attempt.

▶ Vital Vocabulary

active compression-decompression CPR A manual technique that involves compressing the chest and then actively pulling it back up to its neutral position or beyond (decompression); may increase the amount of blood that returns to the heart and, thus, the amount of blood ejected from the heart during the compression phase.

asynchronous In cardiopulmonary resuscitation, when two rescuers perform ventilations and compressions individually; ventilations are not timed and do not require waiting for the other rescuer to pause.

Prep Kit (continued)

automated external defibrillator (AED) A defibrillator that can analyze the patient's heart rhythm and determine whether a defibrillating shock is needed to terminate ventricular fibrillation or ventricular tachycardia.

automatic transport ventilator (ATV) A portable mechanical ventilator attached to a control box that allows the variables of ventilation (such as rate and tidal volume) to be set.

code team leader The code team member who has the responsibility for managing the rescuers or team members during a cardiac arrest, as well as choreographing the effort of the group.

code team member A member of the resuscitation team trying to revive the patient.

compression fraction An indication of how well the team is minimizing pauses in cardiopulmonary resuscitation; it is calculated by dividing the amount of time compressions are delivered by the amount of time compressions are indicated.

defibrillation The use of an unsynchronized direct current electric shock to terminate ventricular fibrillation or ventricular tachycardia.

manual defibrillation A mode available on automated external defibrillators, allowing the paramedic to interpret the cardiac rhythm and determine whether defibrillation is indicated (rather than the monitor making the determination).

return of spontaneous circulation (ROSC) The return of spontaneous heart beat and blood pressure during the resuscitation of a patient in cardiac arrest.

SMART A mnemonic used to describe the objectives of a community-based program to improve the survival of patients in out-of-hospital cardiac arrest: Specific, Measurable, Attainable and Achievable, Realistic and Relevant, and Timely.

targeted temperature management (TTM) A procedure intended to lower body temperature in patients who are in a coma after return of spontaneous circulation; ideally performed in the hospital setting; formerly called therapeutic hypothermia.

► References

1. Chatalas H, Plorde M, eds. *Division of Emergency Medical Services 2014 annual report to the King County Council.* Seattle, WA: Emergency Medical Services Division of Public Health Department—Seattle and King county. 2014. http://www.kingcounty.gov/depts/health/emergency-medical-services/~/media/depts/health/emergency-medical-services/documents/reports/2014AnnualReport.ashx. Accessed June 8, 2015.

2. Nichol G, Thomas E, Callaway CW, et al. Regional variation in out-of-hospital cardiac arrest incidence and outcome. *J Am Med Assoc.* 2008;300(12):1423-1431.

3. Mozaffarian D, Benjamin EJ, Go AS, et al.; on behalf of the American Heart Association Statistics Committee and Stroke Statistics Subcommittee. Executive summary: heart disease and stroke statistics—2016 update: a report from the American Heart Association. *Circulation.* 2016;133:447-454.

4. Out-of-hospital Chain of Survival. © 2016 American Heart Association, Inc. All rights reserved. http://cpr.heart.org/AHAECC/CPRAndECC/AboutCPRFirstAid/CPRFactsAndStats/UCM_475731_CPR-Chain-of-Survival.jsp. Accessed August 19, 2016.

5. Be CPR Smart. © 2016 American Heart Association, Inc. All rights reserved. http://www.becprsmart.org/content.aspx?page=issue. Accessed September 26, 2016.

6. Perkins GD, Jacobs IG, Nadkarni VM, et al.; for the Utstein Collaborators. Cardiac arrest and cardiopulmonary resuscitation outcome reports: update of the Utstein Resuscitation Registry Templates for out-of-hospital cardiac arrest: a statement for healthcare professionals from a task force of the International Liaison Committee on Resuscitation (American Heart Association, European Resuscitation Council, Australian and New Zealand Council on Resuscitation, Heart and Stroke Foundation of Canada, InterAmerican Heart Foundation, Resuscitation Council of Southern Africa, Resuscitation Council of Asia); and the American Heart Association Emergency Cardiovascular Care Committee and the Council on Cardiopulmonary, Critical Care, Perioperative and Resuscitation. *Circulation.* 2015;131:1286–1300.

7. McNally B, Robb R, Mehta M, et al. Out-of-hospital cardiac arrest surveillance—Cardiac Arrest Registry to Enhance Survival (CARES), United States, October 1, 2005–December 31, 2010. Centers for Disease Control and Prevention. *Morb Mortal Wkly Rep.* 2011 Jul 29;60(SS08);1-19.

8. Committee on the Treatment of Cardiac Arrest: Current Status and Future Directions; Board on Health Sciences Policy; Institute of Medicine; Graham R, McCoy MA, Schultz AM, eds. Washington, DC: *National Academies Press*; 2015 Sep 29, Table 2-1: Types of reported OHCA Incidence Among Adults in 2013.

9. Herlitz J, Svensson L, Holmberg S, et al. Efficacy of bystander CPR: Intervention by lay people and by health care professionals. *Resuscitation.* 2005;66(3):291–295.

Prep Kit (continued)

10. Wik L, Steen PA, Bircher NG. Quality of bystander cardiopulmonary resuscitation influences outcome after prehospital cardiac arrest. *Resuscitation.* 1994;28(3):195–203.

11. Aufderheide TP, Sigurdsson G, Pirrallo RG, et al. Hyperventilation-induced hypotension during cardiopulmonary resuscitation. *Circulation.* 2004;109:1960-1965.

12. Atkins DL, Berger S, Duff JP, et al. Part 11: pediatric basic life support and cardiopulmonary resuscitation quality: 2015 American Heart Association Guidelines Update for Cardiopulmonary Resuscitation and Emergency Cardiovascular Care. *Circulation.* 2015;132(suppl 2):S519.

13. Wyckoff MH, Aziz K, Escobedo MB, et al. Part 13: neonatal resuscitation: 2015 American Heart Association Guidelines Update for Cardiopulmonary Resuscitation and Emergency Cardiovascular Care. *Circulation.* 2015;132(suppl 2):S543.

14. Brownstein D, Shugerman R, Cummings P, et al. Prehospital endotracheal intubation of children by paramedics, *Ann Emerg Med.* 1996;28(1):34-39.

15. Nakayama DK, Gardner MJ, Rowe MI. Emergency endotracheal intubation in pediatric trauma. *Ann Surg.* 1990;211(2):218-223.

16. Katz SH, Falk JL. Misplaced endotracheal tubes by paramedics in an urban emergency medical services system. *Ann Emerg Med.* 2001;37(1):32-37.

17. Link MS, Berkow LC, Kudenchuk PJ, et al. Part 7: adult advanced cardiovascular life support: 2015 American Heart Association Guidelines Update for Cardiopulmonary Resuscitation and Emergency Cardiovascular Care. *Circulation.* 2015;132(suppl 2):S444-S464. Published November 3, 2015.

18. Institute of Medicine of the National Academies. Strategies to improve cardiac arrest survival: a time to act. Report Brief. http://www.nationalacademies.org/hmd/~/media/Files/Report%20Files/2015/Cardiac-Arrest/CardiacArrestReportBrief.pdf. Published June 2015. Accessed September 1, 2016.

19. The National Academies of Sciences, Engineering, and Medicine. Health and Medicine Division. Our web address & division name. http://www.nationalacademies.org/hmd/About-HMD/Division-Name.aspx. Accessed August 30, 2016.

20. Mittal et al. Monophasic vs. biphasic shocks for transthoracic defibrillation. *J Am Coll Cardiol.* 1999 Nov 1;34(5):1595-1601.

21. Callaway CW, Donnino MW, Fink EL, et al. Part 8: post-cardiac arrest care: 2015 American Heart Association Guidelines Update for Cardiopulmonary Resuscitation and Emergency Cardiovascular Care. *Circulation.* 2015;132(suppl 1):S465-S482.

22. Bobrow BJ, Vadeboncoeur T, Stolz U, et al. The influence of scenario-based training and real-time audiovisual feedback on out-of-hospital cardiopulmonary resuscitation quality and survival from out-of-hospital cardiac arrest. *Ann Emerg Med.* 2013;62(1):47-56.e1.

23. Brooks SC, Anderson ML, Bruder E, et al. Part 6: alternative techniques and ancillary devices for cardiopulmonary resuscitation: 2015 American Heart Association Guidelines Update for Cardiopulmonary Resuscitation and Emergency Cardiovascular Care. *Circulation.* 2015;132(suppl 2):S436–S443.

24. American Heart Association. Highlights of the 2015 American Heart Association guidelines update for cardiopulmonary resuscitation and emergency cardiovascular care. https://eccguidelines.heart.org/index.php/circulation/cpr-ecc-guidelines-2/. Published October 15, 2015. Accessed May 11, 2016.

25. Hopkins CL, Burk C, Moser S, et al. Implementation of pit crew approach and cardiopulmonary resuscitation metrics for out-of-hospital cardiac arrest improves patient survival and neurological outcome. *J Am Heart Assoc.* 2016;5(1):e002892.

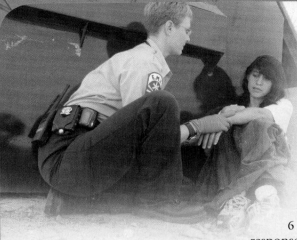

Assessment
in Action

At 0310 hours you are dispatched to a single-family residence. Dispatch information indicates you are responding to an 82-year-old woman who is not breathing and has no pulse. Dispatch has also requested the assistance of the nearest fire department as well as your field supervisor. Emergency medical responders (EMRs) are estimated to be on scene within 6 minutes and are capable of basic life support (BLS), whereas the response time of your advanced life support (ALS) unit will be approximately 8 minutes. You begin to consider the potential outcome for this patient. Dispatch advises you that they are providing hands-only cardiopulmonary resuscitation (CPR) instructions to bystanders via mobile phone.

On arrival you note that the engine company is on scene while the field supervisor pulls in behind you. You are met at the door of the residence by a woman who states she is the patient's daughter. She advises you that when she arrived home at approximately 0300 hours, she found her mother on the couch not breathing. She quickly called 9-1-1 but would not provide CPR as dispatch requested because, as she said, "I was afraid I might hurt my mother." You assess the scene and find the two EMRs performing high-quality CPR on an older woman who has been placed on the floor in the living room. The automated external defibrillator (AED) is already attached. As the code team leader who has practiced this scenario many times, you begin delegating tasks to ensure all efforts are coordinated and interruptions to compressions are minimized. Your partner, also a paramedic, is instructed to take over the role of ventilator while your field supervisor moves to connect your cardiac monitor. You ask the EMRs to continue their compressions while you obtain a patient history and begin tracking times. The patient's daughter tells you that her mother had a hip operation a week ago and takes aspirin 81 mg daily, hydrocodone/acetaminophen (Lorcet) 10 mg every 4 hours for pain, and levothyroxine (Synthroid) 0.5 mg every day. Your supervisor notes that the patient's cardiac rhythm is asystole and that the EMRs have reported the AED advised "No shock indicated" when the rhythm was analyzed.

1. Which of the following factors is NOT a component of high-quality CPR?

   A. Early intubation and emergency drugs
   B. Complete chest recoil after each compression
   C. Compression depth of 2 inches (5 cm) not to exceed 2.4 inches (6 cm)
   D. Compression rate between 100 and 120 per minute

2. How often should the compressor be rotated during resuscitation of a patient in out-of-hospital cardiac arrest?

   A. Every 5 minutes
   B. After every five cycles (2 minutes) of compressions
   C. When the compressor is completely exhausted
   D. Every 10 minutes

3. Which of the following factors would influence you to shock first before initiating chest compressions?

   A. A bystander tells you the patient just "stopped breathing" as you arrived.
   B. Dispatch advises you that CPR is in progress while you are responding.
   C. You witness the patient arrest after connecting the cardiac monitor/defibrillator.
   D. The patient has an automatic implantable cardioverter defibrillator (AICD).

Assessment *in Action* (continued)

4. Which of the following is a contraindication for defibrillation in the patient in cardiac arrest?

   A. The patient is submerged in water or very wet.
   B. The patient has a pacemaker or an AICD.
   C. The patient is an infant or child.
   D. The patient has significant blood loss.

5. The patient was just defibrillated. What is the next step?

   A. Administer 1 mg of epinephrine.
   B. Administer a 10-mL fluid bolus.
   C. Begin chest compressions.
   D. Prepare for a second shock.

6. Which of the following interventions is NOT appropriate for the patient in asystole or pulseless electrical activity?

   A. Administration of a vasopressor
   B. High-quality CPR
   C. Defibrillation
   D. Consideration of possible reversible causes

7. On the basis of this patient's recent medical history and considering the "Hs and Ts", which of the following conditions may have been a potential cause of her cardiac arrest?

   A. Hyperkalemia
   B. Tension pneumothorax
   C. Pulmonary embolism
   D. Hypothermia

8. During resuscitation, how does scene choreography and teamwork improve chances of a successful resuscitation?

9. Current AHA guidelines offer rules for termination of both BLS and ALS support. Considering these rules and your findings for this patient, what next steps and decisions should you consider?

10. If you suspect the patient may have overdosed on her pain medications, then how might you have handled that situation?

Management and Resuscitation of the Critical Patient

National EMS Education Standard Competencies

Shock and Resuscitation

> Integrates a comprehensive knowledge of the causes and pathophysiology of shock, respiratory failure, or arrest into the management of these conditions, with an emphasis on early intervention to prevent arrest.

Knowledge Objectives

1. List examples of peri-arrest conditions that critical patients can present with in the field. (p 1983)
2. Describe the process of determining a differential diagnosis in the field assessment of a critical patient. (pp 1983-1985)
3. Discuss the rapid decision making involved in the assessment and management of a critical patient. (pp 1985-1987)
4. List examples of bias that can affect your critical decision making. (p 1985)
5. Describe the body's physiologic response to changes in perfusion. (pp 1988-1991)
6. Discuss the pathophysiology of shock and peri-arrest situations. (pp 1991-1993)
7. Describe the effects of decreased perfusion at the capillary level. (pp 1993-1994)
8. Define shock in relation to aerobic and anaerobic metabolism. (pp 1994-1996)
9. Predict shock based on mechanism of injury. (pp 1997-1998)
10. Relate pulse pressure changes to perfusion status. (p 1999)
11. Relate orthostatic vital sign changes to perfusion status. (p 1999)
12. Discuss the progression of shock. (pp 1998-2000)
13. Discuss the pathophysiologic changes associated with compensated shock. (p 1999)
14. Discuss the pathophysiologic changes associated with decompensated (hypotensive) shock. (p 1999)
15. Differentiate between compensated and decompensated shock. (p 1999)
16. Discuss the assessment findings associated with compensated shock. (pp 2000-2002)
17. Discuss the assessment findings associated with decompensated shock. (pp 2000-2002)
18. Discuss the assessment findings associated with shock and the peri-arrest situations. (pp 2000-2002)
19. Identify the need for intervention and transport of the patient with compensated shock. (pp 2001-2002)
20. Identify the need for intervention and transport of the patient with decompensated shock. (pp 2001-2002)
21. Identify the need for intervention and transport of the patient with shock or other peri-arrest situations. (pp 2001-2002)
22. Discuss the treatment plan and management of compensated shock. (pp 2003-2005, 2015)
23. Discuss the treatment plan and management of the patient with decompensated shock. (pp 2003-2005, 2015)
24. Discuss the treatment plan and management of shock and other peri-arrest situations. (pp 2003-2005, 2015)
25. Describe the pathophysiology, assessment, and management of specific types of shock, including cardiogenic, obstructive, distributive, and hypovolemic shock. (pp 2005-2015)

Skills Objectives

1. Defend the importance of teamwork, experience, and practice in preparation to manage the critical patient. (pp 1982, 1984)
2. Demonstrate rapid decision making based on the working diagnosis of the critical patient with a peri-arrest condition. (pp 1985-1987)

Introduction

The expert application of critical thinking and decision making is essential when you are confronted with a patient in critical condition. This process involves conducting a rapid assessment, providing lifesaving treatment, and developing a **differential diagnosis**, which is a list of the potential diagnoses based on the patient's assessment findings. To treat the patient, a working diagnosis must be selected as the most likely condition prompting the need for medical care from the list of potential diagnoses generated by the differential diagnosis based on assessment and continued reassessment of the patient. If you use this process consistently, then it will become routine when you need it most. It takes a great deal of practice to make the "right" decisions for each unique situation; eventually, however, making decisions quickly and working as part of a team will become an integral part of who you are.

When the patient's condition is critical, it is essential that you are well trained to make the *right* decisions, taking the *right* amount of time to do the *right* assessment, and provide the *right* care to the patient. In addition, on the basis of the patient's condition, transport to the *right* hospital for the most appropriate definitive care can be lifesaving. This approach involves crew resource management, situational awareness, team leadership and teamwork skills, prioritization, protocol compliance, use of the right equipment and resources, and collaboration with other public safety personnel and family members. A critical patient's survival is dependent on all of these *rights* coming into alignment.

This chapter discusses the approach that you should take when you are confronted with a critical patient. Managing critical patients often involves confronting premorbid or peri-arrest conditions. This chapter also takes a close-up look at perfusion, the function that fails in patients who are in shock. Next, it looks at the physiologic causes of shock and describes each of its major forms. Finally, it discusses the assessment and emergency management of shock in general and of each type of shock.

Developing Critical Thinking and Decision-Making Abilities

Emergency medical services (EMS) educators tell their students that excellent decision-making abilities come with experience. This is true, provided that the student acquires the right "entry-level" knowledge and skills, followed by the appropriate guided experience. According to the paramedic curriculum design, the training is developed to prepare a competent entry-level paramedic. The internship experience is a good first step to help students pull together the didactic education, lab skills, and clinical experiences to function as a paramedic in the field. An *excellent* internship experience guided by an experienced mentor (preceptor) will bring students to the competent entry-level milestone. State and national certification/registration/licensure follows, and from there, the paramedic has a "license to practice and learn" from continued experiences.

YOU are the Paramedic — PART 1

You are the paramedic on an advanced life support unit dispatched to an apartment at a senior residence complex. The dispatcher informs you a home health aide found the patient, a 77-year-old man, unresponsive in his bed this morning. You are told the patient is breathing and has a pulse. When you arrive at the apartment complex at 0915 hours, you are escorted by the security officer to the elevator to get to the fifth floor. The security officer tells you he has not seen the patient, Mr. Oliver, for his last two shifts. Due to the nature of the call, you are bringing your electrocardiogram (ECG) monitor/defibrillator, primary care (ABCs) bag, and intravenous (IV)/medication kit with you.

You are met at the apartment by the home health aide. She tells you she routinely visits Mr. Oliver twice a week to help with cleaning and cooking. This morning when she arrived, security personnel were needed to gain access to his apartment because he did not open the door when she knocked. She explains that she found Mr. Oliver in bed unresponsive. She says he was sick the last time she saw him 3 days ago and that she encouraged him to see his physician. She follows you to his bedroom. As you move through the apartment, you conduct a scene size-up. The apartment appears relatively neat and clean. You see no dirty dishes or other evidence of a recent meal. All furniture is upright, and you note no evidence of a disturbance. When you reach the bedside, your general impression is of a thin, older adult man who appears to be asleep. He has audible respirations that sound congested, and his skin appears pale and mottled. Your partner prepares the oxygen while you assess the patient's mental status. He responds only to painful stimuli. You request an engine company and your paramedic supervisor to be dispatched to your location for additional assistance.

1. What should your next course of action be for this patient?
2. Discuss the role of intuition in forming a differential diagnosis and explain how bias can affect the diagnosis.

▶ Critical Patients

When caring for **critical patients** who require your critical thinking skills, you will be confronting premorbid conditions, major trauma, or conditions relating to the peri-arrest period. The **peri-arrest period** is the time either just before or just after cardiac arrest, when the patient is critical and care must be taken to prevent progression or regression into cardiac arrest. Examples of peri-arrest conditions include unstable dysrhythmias (symptomatic bradycardia, symptomatic supraventricular tachycardia, ventricular tachycardia, and complete atrioventricular block), shock, syncope, myocardial ischemia, or heart failure. **Premorbid conditions** are conditions that precede the onset of a disease. In the context of emergency medicine, the "disease" is life-threatening trauma or medical conditions that need to be rapidly identified and managed. Typically, premorbid conditions are sorted into those occurring in adults presumed to be healthy and, more frequently, those occurring in unhealthy adults, as shown in Table 40-1 .

Many adult patients have other preexisting conditions (comorbidities) that can contribute to their placement in the critical patient category. These comorbidities are especially dangerous when a patient experiences trauma such as a full-thickness burn over 20% of the total body surface area or when the head, chest, or abdomen are involved with significant hemorrhage, leading to shock. Other conditions that would contribute to placement in the critical patient category include acute coronary syndrome, heart failure, renal failure, uncontrolled hypertension, uncontrolled diabetes, obesity, electrolyte imbalance, electrocution, drowning or submersion, hypothermia, drug toxicity, stroke, near-fatal asthma, anaphylaxis, and pulmonary embolus Figure 40-1 . The epidemiology and pathophysiology of these conditions are discussed in detail in other chapters of this text.

▶ The EMS Approach to Diagnosis

Common complaints of critical patients may include altered mental status, difficulty breathing, severe pain, and chest pain. The EMS approach to determining a **working diagnosis** involves following the standard approach discussed in Chapter 12, *Critical Thinking and Clinical Decision*

Table 40-1	**Adult Premorbid Conditions Directly Affecting EMS**	
Condition	**Healthy Adult**	**Unhealthy Adult**
Heart failure	Unlikely	X
Coronary artery disease	Unlikely	X
Drug toxicity	X	X
Electrolyte imbalance	X	X
Obesity	Unlikely	X
Pulmonary embolus	X	X
Renal failure	Unlikely	X
Stroke	Unlikely	X
Uncontrolled hypertension	Unlikely	X
Uncontrolled diabetes	Unlikely	X

© Jones & Bartlett Learning.

Making, and emphasized throughout this text. To arrive at a working diagnosis, after considering the most serious life threats and managing them, your approach involves considering or ruling out various conditions (ie, your differential diagnosis). This process leaves you with the working diagnosis, as illustrated in **Figure 40-2**.

For example, you have a patient who has a chief complaint of altered mental status, and you need to consider

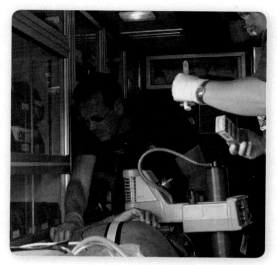

Figure 40-1 A critical patient being managed in the field.
© Mark C. Ide.

the differential diagnosis. To start this process, you will need to consider each of the potential causes. There are many approaches that you may use to work through the differential diagnosis. One approach is represented by the acronym M-T SHIP:

M: Medication overdose/noncompliance (ie, barbiturates, narcotics, alcohol), metabolic causes (ie, B_{12} or thiamine deficiency)

T: Tumor, trauma, toxins (ie, lead, mercury, carbon monoxide, toxidromes)

S: Seizures (ie, status epilepticus, postictal state), stroke

H: Hypoxia (ie, pulmonary, cardiac, anemia, or carbon dioxide retention), hyperthermia/hypothermia, hyperglycemia/hypoglycemia, hypertensive crisis, hypovolemia, hyperkalemia/hypokalemia (and other electrolyte imbalances)

I: Infection and uremia (ie, renal or hepatic dysfunction)

P: Psychiatric or behavioral disorders

By determining whether trauma was involved, whether or not the patient has a history of diabetes, or whether there is fever or infection, this list can be narrowed down

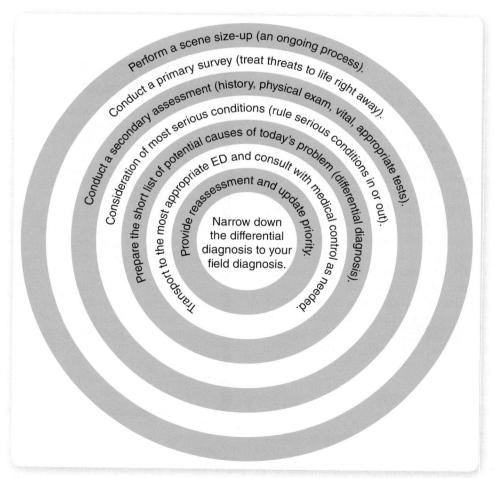

Perform a scene size-up (an ongoing process).

Conduct a primary survey (treat threats to life right away).

Conduct a secondary assessment (history, physical exam, vital, appropriate tests).

Consideration of most serious conditions (rule serious conditions in or out).

Prepare the short list of potential causes of today's problem (differential diagnosis).

Transport to the most appropriate ED and consult with medical control as needed.

Provide reassessment and update priority.

Narrow down the differential diagnosis to your field diagnosis.

Figure 40-2 Practice and experience will help the paramedic to consistently "hit the target."
© Jones & Bartlett Learning.

considerably. Further questioning will also narrow down the differential diagnosis.

Suppose your patient has a chief complaint of chest pain and you need to consider the differential diagnosis. The patient could have ischemic chest pain indicating a possible cardiac condition such as an acute coronary syndrome, aortic dissection, coronary spasm, pericarditis, myocarditis, or hypertrophic cardiomyopathy. Gastrointestinal (GI) system causes of the chest pain may be heartburn, esophageal spasm, hiatal hernia, and gallbladder or pancreatic problems. Or, the patient could be experiencing musculoskeletal problems such as costochondritis, sore muscles, injured ribs, or a pinched nerve. There are also a number of respiratory causes of chest pain, such as pulmonary embolism, pleurisy, pneumothorax, and asthma. Finally, the chest pain may be due to a panic attack, shingles, or cancer in the chest.

Evaluating the patient through history taking and physical examination while considering a targeted differential diagnoses list will guide you to the most serious problems that could lead to the cause of the chest pain and help you to arrive at your working diagnosis. With experience you will come to refine the questions and examinations needed to quickly assess the patient.

▶ The Role of Intuition in Critical Decision Making

Some paramedics describe a sense they get when the situation is much worse than it initially appears from reviewing the patient's vital signs. Others describe having a "gut feeling" when they first look at a patient who gives a poor general impression, such as a patient who is so diaphoretic that the ECG electrodes will not stick to the skin.

The **intuition** that comes with experience is hard to teach. Intuition is described as pattern recognition and pattern matching, based on your own past experiences. Intuition can keep you out of trouble by forewarning you, or it can get you in trouble by leading you to make treatment decisions based on inaccurate assumptions. In medicine, intuition may be used to "up-triage" the patient rather than "down-triage" the patient. For example, if your instinct tells you the patient is more serious than he or she seems, treat the patient as such; however, if your instinct tells you otherwise, you will need to investigate the complaint thoroughly before downgrading the response.

How could your intuition potentially lead you astray? Just because you are good at pattern recognition in one field, or level of training, does not mean you are automatically good at pattern recognition in a field in which you have less experience. Be cautious not to misuse analogies and make a decision based on intuition that draws on incorrect experiences. In highly complicated, ambiguous situations, complexities can obscure pattern-recognition ability.

When decisions are being made based on intuition, it is often difficult for the team leader to communicate to the other team members his or her thought process. Therefore, it may be difficult for the team members to stay onboard with the line of thinking (or treatment plan in this case). The organizational scholar Karl Weick has proposed a simple five-step process for communicating intuitive decisions and obtaining feedback from team members to ensure all involved have a clear understanding[1]:

1. Here is what I think we are dealing with.
2. Here is what I think we should do.
3. Here is why.
4. Here is what we should keep our eyes on.
5. Now talk to me. Are there any other concerns?

▶ Bias in Decision Making

There are a number of biases that can lead to faulty decision making. One of the most prevalent biases is confirmation bias. A **confirmation bias** is a tendency to gather and rely on information that confirms your existing views and avoids or downplays information that does not confirm your preexisting hypothesis or differential diagnosis. Another bias is an **anchoring bias**, which involves allowing an initial reference point to distort your estimates. Your brain allows you to begin at that reference point and adjust from there, even if the initial reference point was possibly incorrect. For example, if dispatch indicates a stroke and you become anchored in this thought process, you may fail to check for and possibly treat a hypoglycemic condition.

Be careful about making a misjudgment based on overconfidence. Overconfidence errors occur when you assume you know what is going on with the patient. To avoid this situation, always search for information that would refute the differential diagnosis you have arrived at, and make sure you have looked at all of the angles of the problem. *Never assume anything.* You may have transported this patient multiple times for being intoxicated, but today could be the day he has fallen and experienced a subdural hematoma.

Last, when you are treating a patient who exhibits the "classic" presentation of a specific condition, do not assume the patient has that condition without obtaining all of the necessary information and data. Similarly, do not dismiss the possibility of a condition just because the patient does not present with classic signs and symptoms. In all cases, you must consider the spectrum of the differential diagnosis. For example, the classic presentation of acute myocardial infarction (AMI) in a male patient involves crushing substernal chest pain radiating down the left arm accompanied by nausea and shortness of breath. It may be easy to omit AMI from the differential diagnosis when these classic symptoms aren't encountered in a patient; however, as you've learned in your training, many women, older adults, and people with diabetes experiencing an AMI do not experience chest pain. Be careful not to prematurely jump to conclusions when you are assessing a critical patient.

A Snapshot of Critical Decision Making

It is 0500 hours and you have been dispatched to the home of a 62-year-old woman whose son called 9-1-1. The son states he woke up and found his mother sitting in the living room complaining of pressure in the center of her chest. Because of the complaint of chest pain and the patient's age, this is a priority dispatch and your medic unit, a backup unit, and the supervisor are quickly en route. The traffic is light and your equipment is ready. As you pull up in front of the home, you are met at the doorway by the son, who quickly leads you to his mother.

The scene appears to be safe, but you realize you will need to pay attention to the environment you are entering and all potential hazards. The police, who respond on most of your calls, are just pulling up outside the residence. You introduce yourselves to the patient and ask about the chief complaint. The woman, Judith, explains that she has been to her primary physician twice, who felt that her chest pain was caused by stress and acid reflux. She has been taking antacids, but they have not alleviated the crushing sensation beneath her breastbone, accompanied by nausea and tingling in her left arm. The pain is a 7 out of 10, and it began this morning at around 0430 hours. You explain to Judith that you have a few more questions to ask her while your partner administers oxygen to her using a nasal cannula and obtains her vital signs. You know that oxygen is helpful and she is breathing well on her own with an oxygen saturation (SpO_2) of 92%, but you need to know if her blood pressure is where it should be and if her pulse rate is regular. Once you have determined that she has no cardiac history or allergies and that she does not take an anticoagulant, you give her four tablets of baby aspirin to chew, not swallow, per your protocols. You quickly ask the OPQRST (Onset, Provocation/palliation, Quality, Region/Radiation, Severity, Timing) questions to elaborate on the chief complaint of chest pain.

Once you have determined that she is tachycardic and has slight hypertension, you listen to her breath sounds while your partner obtains a 12-lead ECG. Although you might normally obtain a 3-lead ECG, you know this patient requires a 12-lead ECG. In your system, your medical director wants you to obtain the 12-lead ECG just prior to administering nitroglycerin. There is a slight crackling in the bases of her lungs. Your partner transmits the ECG results to the nearest hospital with a coronary catheterization lab.

The patient has ST-segment elevation in three contiguous leads (II, III, and AVF). Because of these findings, she fits the ST segment elevation myocardial infarction (STEMI) protocol for a possible inferior wall myocardial infarction (MI). Thus, you need to provide immediate transport since *time is muscle!* The criterion for percutaneous coronary intervention (PCI) is within a 90-minute window. Your partner starts an IV line to administer morphine sulfate

and metoprolol. You explain to the patient's son that it is in his mother's best interest to take her to the hospital that is 2 miles (3 km) beyond the local hospital because it has a coronary catheterization lab.

Your EMS supervisor arrives with another paramedic, and they bring in the stair chair and place the stretcher outside the front door. Just as you are lifting the patient from the couch to the stair chair, she passes out. As you try to arouse her by shouting her name, you notice the ECG changes from sinus tachycardia to ventricular fibrillation (VF). Instinctively, you and your partner move the patient to the floor. In the absence of a pulse, you begin chest compressions while the defibrillator pads are placed on the patient. The EMT from the backup unit kneels at the patient's head, sizes and inserts an oropharyngeal airway, and starts ventilations with the bag-mask device connected to supplemental oxygen. Once the pads are in place, VF is identified, the defibrillator is charged up to 200 joules, compressions are stopped briefly and the patient is cleared, and the first shock is delivered. Immediately thereafter, cardiopulmonary resuscitation (CPR) compressions resume.

At this point, all EMS personnel have a specific task because there will be five cycles of CPR (at a 30:2 ratio of compressions to ventilations), taking 2 minutes per cycle. You need to make sure each task occurs at the right time, including the following:

1. Get the mechanical CPR device (Thumper, Auto-Pulse, Lucas-2) ready to deploy with no interruption in manual chest compressions for more than 10 seconds.
2. Ensure the basic life support ventilations are effective, producing visible chest rise (and not too often) and switching over to the automatic transport ventilator.
3. Start an IV line. If this is not going to be easy, switch to plan B, and prepare for intraosseous (IO) infusion with the IO bone drill. IV access is needed because you will administer 1 mg of epinephrine (0.1 mg/mL [1:10,000]) every 3 to 5 minutes until her pulse returns.
4. Ensure there will be a fresh person to supply compressions for the second 2 minutes in case there is a delay in applying the mechanical CPR device. The quality of the compressions is crucial to the success of this resuscitation.
5. Draw up 300 mg of amiodarone because an antidysrhythmic will need to be administered soon.
6. Reanalyze and reshock the patient again at the 2-minute point.

After the third shock, the patient appeared to have a rhythm but now remains pulseless. CPR continues and an antidysrhythmic is administered IO in her right tibia, since IV access was not successful at this point. A medic considers placing an endotracheal tube and readies the equipment while ventilations continue. Necessary actions

Table 40-2	The "H and T" Questions of Cardiac Arrest	
Reversible Causes of Cardiac Arrest	**Questions to Ask Your Team**
Hypovolemia	Does this patient have any evidence of internal or external bleeding or fluid loss?
Hypoxia	How well is the patient oxygenating? Could there have been a respiratory event that led to this cardiac arrest?
Hydrogen ion (acidosis)	Is there any reason for metabolic or respiratory acidosis in this patient?
Hypokalemia/hyperkalemia	Does this patient undergo renal dialysis? Might the electrolytes be altered (ie, is the patient on a liquid diet)?
Hypothermia	Does the patient feel cold to touch? If so, obtain the core body temperature.
Hypoglycemic/hyperglycemic	Does the patient have diabetes? What is the blood glucose level?
Tension pneumothorax	Does the patient have bilateral breath sounds? Is the patient becoming difficult to ventilate? Consider the need for chest decompression.
Tamponade (cardiac)	Is there penetrating trauma to the patient's heart? Consider the need for pericardiocentesis or ultrasound (in the emergency department).
Toxins	Consider substance abuse (ie, narcotics or opiates). Consider naloxone (Narcan) intravenously/intramuscularly/intranasally.
Thrombosis (pulmonary)	Does the patient have a history of blood clots? Does the patient smoke and/or take birth control? Has the patient had a recent long bone immobilization?
Thrombosis (coronary)	Does the patient have a large acute myocardial infarction developing? Is this patient a candidate for percutaneous coronary intervention (PCI)?
Trauma	Is there a mechanism of injury for life-threatening trauma?

© Jones & Bartlett Learning.

are taking place, so you take a moment to consider the causes of cardiac arrest. You know that you need to consider the reversible causes because they are your differential diagnoses in the case of a patient who is in cardiac arrest Table 40-2 .

Patient history reveals that Judith did not sustain any trauma or report symptoms of GI bleeding (ie, diarrhea; dark, tarry, smelly stool). Her systolic blood pressure (SBP) was initially slightly high, so it is not likely that she is hemorrhaging. She does not have diabetes and was initially alert, so low levels of blood glucose are unlikely. She did not have respiratory distress and was not cold to the touch, so pulmonary embolus and hypothermia are not likely. She did have STEMI, and with the vague presentation that older adult female patients often have, it is likely she is experiencing a massive AMI.

Just after the fourth shock, the patient wakes up. She is anxious and scared and her SpO_2 is 93%. You ask the EMT managing the airway to switch back to the nasal cannula because the endotracheal tube has not yet been placed. You tell Judith that she is sick and her condition warrants going to the hospital right away. You assure her that all of her needs are being taken care of and that her son is nearby and will be coming along. In the meantime, crew members are assigned to package and carry the patient on the Reeves stretcher out to your stretcher. One medic sets up an amiodarone drip and prepares to administer a mild sedative to calm the patient without affecting her respirations.

Once you are en route, you contact the emergency department (ED) to update the staff, and another 12-lead ECG is transmitted. You proceed to reassess the vital signs, document the incident, and discuss the situation with the patient. On arrival, because you have already transmitted the 12-lead ECG to the ED, the patient is admitted directly to the catheterization lab. Two arteries, each 90% blocked, are cleared, and stents are inserted by the interventional cardiologist.

Shock: The Critical Patient Evolving in Front of You

Shock is a state of collapse and failure of the cardiovascular system in which blood circulation slows and eventually ceases, leading to insufficient perfusion of organs and tissues. Shock is best explained as a normal compensatory mechanism of the body designed to maintain both the SBP and brain perfusion during times of distress. This response can accompany a broad spectrum of events (eg, heart attacks, falls, allergic reactions, motor vehicle crashes). If not treated promptly, shock will injure the body's vital organs and ultimately lead to death.

Anatomy and Physiology of Perfusion

Perfusion is the circulation of blood within an organ or tissue in adequate amounts to meet the cells' current needs for oxygen, nutrients, and waste removal. Perfusion requires a working cardiovascular system, adequate gas exchange in the lungs, adequate nutrients (ie, glucose) in the blood, and adequate removal of waste through the lungs. Because tissue perfusion is primarily a function of the cardiovascular system, an examination of that system is important in understanding shock, or **hypoperfusion**.

To keep the blood moving continuously through the body, the cardiovascular system requires three intact components **Figure 40-3** :

- A functioning pump: the heart
- Adequate fluid volume: the blood and body fluids
- An intact system of tubing capable of reflex adjustments (constriction and dilation) in response to changes in pump output and fluid volume: the blood vessels

The heart's contractility allows it to increase or decrease the volume of blood it pumps with each contraction, also known as **stroke volume**. The heart can also vary the speed (rate) at which it contracts by raising or lowering the pulse rate. **Cardiac output** is the volume of blood that the heart pumps per minute, and it is dependent on several factors. First, the heart must have adequate strength, which is largely determined by the heart muscle's **myocardial contractility**, or ability to contract. Second, the heart must receive adequate blood to pump. As the volume of blood flowing to the heart increases, the precontraction pressure in the heart builds up. This precontraction pressure is known as **preload**. Preload involves the initial stretching of the cardiac muscle prior to contraction; it is related to the chamber volume of blood just prior to contraction. As preload increases, the volume of blood within the ventricles increases, causing the heart muscle to stretch. When the muscle is stretched, myocardial contractility increases, leading to greater force of contraction and increased cardiac output. This concept is discussed in Chapter 30, *Bleeding*, as the Frank-Starling

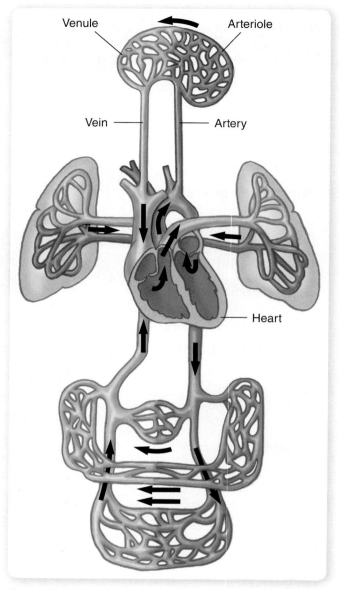

Figure 40-3 The cardiovascular system requires continuous operation of its three components: the heart (pump), the blood vessels (container), and the blood and body fluids (contents).

© Jones & Bartlett Learning.

mechanism. Lastly, the resistance to flow in the peripheral circulation must be appropriate. The force or resistance against which the heart pumps is known as **afterload**.

Blood pressure is usually carefully controlled by the body so that there is always sufficient circulation to the tissues and organs; it is also considered a rough measure of perfusion. Because the heart cannot pump out what is not in its holding chambers, blood pressure varies directly with cardiac output, systemic vascular resistance, and blood volume. **Systemic vascular resistance** is the resistance to blood flow within all of the blood vessels except the pulmonary vessels. Remember, blood pressure is the pressure of blood within the vessels at any one time. The SBP is the peak arterial pressure, or pressure generated every time the heart contracts; the diastolic blood pressure (DBP) is the pressure maintained within the arteries while the heart rests between heartbeats.

Perfusion depends on the efficiency with which blood and, subsequently, oxygen are distributed throughout the body. It is a function of blood pressure (BP), cardiac output (CO), heart rate (HR), stroke volume (SV), and systemic vascular resistance (SVR). It is represented by the following formulas:

$$CO = HR \times SV$$
$$BP = CO \times SVR$$

Mean arterial pressure (MAP) is a measure of the patient's blood pressure that takes into consideration the SBP and DBP. MAP is ultimately the blood pressure required to sustain organ perfusion; it is roughly 60 mm Hg in the average person. If the MAP falls significantly below 60 mm Hg for an appreciable amount of time, then the resulting lack of perfusion will cause ischemia of the organ or organs. Thus, the MAP needs to be greater than 60 mm Hg to ensure the brain, coronary arteries, and kidneys remain perfused. MAP is determined with this formula:

$$MAP = DBP + \frac{1}{3}(SBP - DBP)$$

Using the example of a patient who has a blood pressure of 120/60 mm Hg, the **pulse pressure** (difference between the SBP and DBP) would equal 60 mm Hg (120 mm Hg − 60 mm Hg = 60 mm Hg). To calculate the MAP, take one-third of the pulse pressure and add the DBP to it (20 + 60 = 80 mm Hg). **Table 40-3** shows an example of how these data affect the field provider.

The body is perfused via the cardiovascular system. Control of the cardiovascular system is a function of the

YOU are the Paramedic   PART 2

Your partner attempts to open the patient's airway with a head tilt–chin lift maneuver. On the basis of your scene assessment, there is no indication that Mr. Oliver has fallen or sustained trauma that would necessitate spinal immobilization. You suction the airway and remove loose but thick, light brown secretions. You note that this suctioning stimulates his gag reflex and induces coughing. You assess your patient's breathing, and it is slightly labored with a respiratory rate of 24 breaths/min. His SpO2 is 92%. Chest rise is equal bilaterally. Auscultation reveals crackles and rhonchi in all lung fields. You assess for a radial pulse and detect one that is weak, with a rate of 120 beats/min. Your impression of his skin is that it is pale, mottled, cool, and clammy to touch. The patient appears to be critical, and a rapid assessment is indicated before initiating transport.

Because the patient is nonverbal and unable to respond to your questions, you look to his home health aide for assistance. Your paramedic partner is assisting the patient's ventilations with a bag-mask device and supplemental oxygen at 15 L/min. You obtain a limited SAMPLE (Signs and symptoms, Allergies, Medications, Pertinent past medical history, Last oral intake, Events leading up to the illness or injury) history from his aide. She tells you that Mr. Oliver had a terrible cough 3 days ago and a temperature of 101°F (38°C). She says he also reported pain when he took a deep breath. She told him she was concerned he may have pneumonia and that he should call his doctor. She knows he has an allergy to shellfish. His medications are in the kitchen, and she tells you he took them regularly as far as she knows. She hands you her information sheet on Mr. Oliver's medical history. You note he has a history of hypertension and chronic bronchitis and that he had an AMI 5 years ago. The aide is unsure as to when he last ate but tells you he refused lunch during her last visit when he said he had no appetite. She is not sure how long he has been like this or when his condition changed, but he normally took a walk each morning at around 0800 hours. You recall the security officer telling you he did not see Mr. Oliver for his last two shifts.

Recording Time: 6 Minutes	
Appearance	Poor
Level of consciousness	Unresponsive
Airway	Partially obstructed by secretions, then patent after suctioning
Breathing	24 breaths/min, shallow and slightly labored, assisted with bag-mask device
Circulation	120 beats/min and weak, skin is pale, mottled, and cool

3. Describe the contributing factors that would lead you to label this patient as critical.
4. Discuss pathophysiologic changes associated with septic shock.

Table 40-3	**Mean Arterial Pressure (MAP)**

Formula: $MAP = DBP + \frac{1}{3}(SBP - DBP)$

Example: Blood pressure = 120/60 mm Hg
MAP calculation = $60 + 1/3(120 - 60)$
MAP = 80 mm Hg

Diastolic	Systolic								
	120	116	112	96	92	86	82	78	74
80	93	92	91	85	84	82	-	-	-
76	91	89	88	84	83	79	-	-	-
72	88	87	85	80	76	77	75	-	-
68	85	84	83	77	76	74	73	71	-
64	83	81	80	75	73	71	70	69	-
60	80	79	77	72	71	69	67	66	65
56	77	76	75	69	68	66	65	63	62

Abbreviations: DBP, diastolic blood pressure; SBP, systolic blood pressure

© Jones & Bartlett Learning.

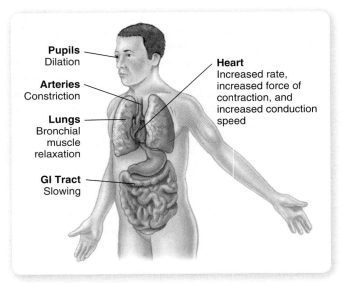

Figure 40-4 The sympathetic nervous system.
© Jones & Bartlett Learning.

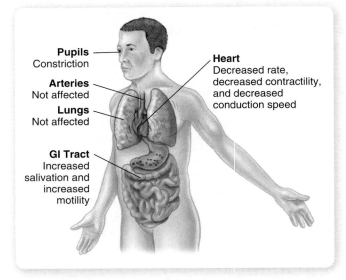

Figure 40-5 The parasympathetic nervous system.
© Jones & Bartlett Learning.

autonomic nervous system, which is composed of competing subsystems (see Chapter 8, *Anatomy and Physiology*). One of the subsystems, the sympathetic nervous system, known as the fight-or-flight system, prepares the body for physical activity during a stressful situation. This preparation includes increasing the pulse rate, blood pressure, and respiratory rate while dilating blood vessels in areas required for physical activity and constricting those in areas primarily involved with reproduction and restoration.

The autonomic nervous system is primarily controlled by the upper part of the medulla oblongata of the brain. Nerve signals caused by stimulation of the sympathetic nervous system travel between the brain and the body by way of nerves traveling through the spinal cord. These nerves leave the spinal cord between each pair of vertebrae and spread out to affect the tissues in those areas **Figure 40-4**. Another mechanism used by the sympathetic nervous system is the chemical release of epinephrine and norepinephrine from the adrenal glands into the bloodstream. These chemicals travel through the bloodstream to all parts of the body to activate a sympathetic response in those areas.

The other subsystem of the autonomic nervous system is the parasympathetic nervous system, which is primarily responsible for rest and regeneration **Figure 40-5**. The parasympathetic nervous system opposes every action of the sympathetic nervous system. Where the sympathetic system increases the pulse rate, blood pressure, and respiratory rate, the parasympathetic nervous system decreases

Words of Wisdom

The **Fick principle** states that movement and use of oxygen in the body depend on the following:
1. Adequate concentration of inspired oxygen (F_{IO_2} [fraction of inspired oxygen])
2. Appropriate movement of oxygen across the alveolar-capillary membrane into the arterial bloodstream
3. Adequate number of red blood cells to carry the oxygen
4. Proper tissue perfusion
5. Efficient offloading of oxygen at the tissue level

these functions. The parasympathetic nervous system also constricts blood vessels in muscular tissue and dilates those in the digestive system.

► Respiration and Oxygenation

As you learned in Chapter 8, *Anatomy and Physiology*, each time you take a breath, the alveoli receive a supply of oxygen-rich air. The oxygen then dissolves in the blood plasma and attaches to the blood's hemoglobin. The oxygen gas molecules from the oxygenated blood pass through the alveolar wall into the walls of a fine network of pulmonary capillaries that are in close contact with the alveoli. If the oxygenated blood is not properly circulated, then some of the cells and organs will not receive proper nutrients, possibly resulting in cellular death.

Oxygen and carbon dioxide pass rapidly across these thin tissue layers through diffusion. **Diffusion** is a passive process in which molecules move from an area with a higher concentration of molecules to an area of lower concentration. There are more oxygen molecules in the alveoli than in the blood. Therefore, the oxygen molecules move from the alveoli into the blood. Because there are more carbon dioxide molecules in the blood than in the inhaled air, carbon dioxide moves from the blood into the alveoli.

Just like oxygen, carbon dioxide is dissolved in the plasma and attaches to the blood's hemoglobin. The body takes the carbon dioxide, combines it with water, and creates carbonic acid. Carbonic acid concentrations become high just as the blood is moving toward the lungs. Once it reaches the lungs, the carbonic acid breaks down and the carbon dioxide is exhaled. All of this action takes place to maintain the delicate balance between the gases and maintain the pH of the body.

► Regulation of Blood Flow

Blood flow through the capillary beds is regulated by the capillary sphincters, circular muscular walls that constrict and dilate, acting as a gate to increase or decrease flow. These **sphincters** are under the control of the autonomic nervous system, which regulates involuntary functions such as sweating and digestion. Capillary sphincters also respond to other stimuli (ie, heat, cold, the need for oxygen, and the need for waste removal). Under normal circumstances, not all cells have the same needs at the same time. For example, the stomach and intestines have a high need for blood flow during and shortly after eating, when digestion is at a peak. Between meals, blood flow is lessened, and blood is diverted to other areas. The brain, by contrast, needs a constant and consistent supply of blood to function. This regulation of blood flow is determined by cellular need and is accomplished by vessel constriction or dilation, together with sphincter constriction or dilation.

■ Pathophysiology of Shock

Shock can result from inadequate cardiac output, decreased systemic vascular resistance, or the inability of red blood cells (RBCs) to deliver oxygen to tissues. If there is a disturbance in the transportation of oxygen and removal of carbon dioxide, then dangerous waste products will build up, leading to cellular death and eventually death of the entire organ. Because the body is built in a framework where every cell ultimately relates to the body, conditions such as inadequate perfusion will cause damage to the cells as well as the body Figure 40-6 . If the shock state persists, then it will ultimately lead to death. As mentioned, shock is a state of failure and ultimate collapse of the cardiovascular system that causes inadequate cellular oxygenation and hypoperfusion. To protect vital organs, the body attempts to compensate by shunting (directing) blood flow from organs that are more tolerant of low flow (ie, skin and intestines) to vital organs that cannot tolerate hypoperfusion (ie, heart, brain, and lungs). If the cause of shock is not promptly addressed, the patient will most likely progress from "compensated" to "decompensated" to death.

The cardiovascular system consists of three parts: the heart, the blood vessels or arteries, and the fluid (blood). These three parts can be referred to as the "perfusion triangle" Figure 40-7 . When a patient is in shock, one or more of the three parts is not working properly.

Blood is the vehicle for carrying oxygen and nutrients through the vessels to the capillary beds to tissue cells, where these supplies are exchanged for waste products created during metabolism. For this process to happen, the vessels (container) must be intact. Blood contains RBCs, white blood cells, platelets, and plasma. The functions of the blood components are discussed in Chapter 8, *Anatomy and Physiology*.

Blood clots are an important response from the body to control blood loss. There are three main mechanisms leading to blood clot formation. Clots form because a blockage in blood circulation results in retention of blood (ie, blood stasis); there is damage to the vessel wall (ie, a wound); or a disease process (eg, malignancy) or medication (eg, oral birth control pills) predisposes the blood to clotting. When injury occurs to tissues in the body, platelets begin to aggregate at the site of injury, causing the RBCs to become sticky and clump together. As the RBCs begin to clump, a substance in the body called fibrinogen reinforces the RBCs. This is the final step in the formation of a blood clot. However, clots are unstable and prone to rupture because blood is continually moving and exerting pressure.

The body's neural and hormonal mechanisms (ie, autonomic nervous system and hormones) are triggered when the body senses that the pressure in the system is falling and there is an increased need for perfusion of vital organs. The sympathetic side of the autonomic nervous system will assume more control (fight-or-flight response) of the body's functions during a state of shock. The parasympathetic nervous system controls involuntary functions by sending signals to the cardiac, smooth, and glandular muscles. When the autonomic nervous system releases epinephrine and norepinephrine, these hormones cause changes in certain body functions such as an increase

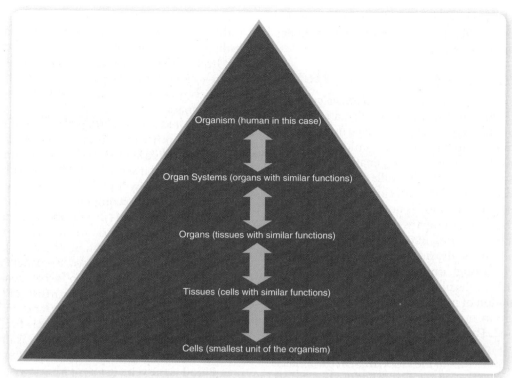

Figure 40-6 The relationship between the organism and the cells of the body.
© Jones & Bartlett Learning.

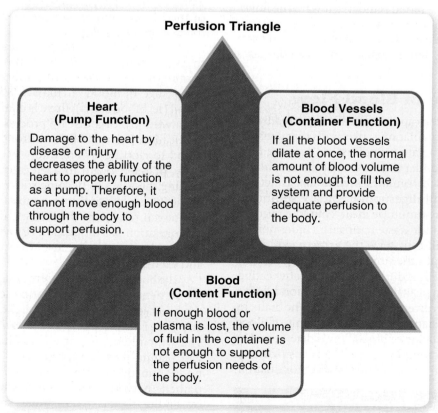

Figure 40-7 The heart, the blood vessels, and the blood and body fluids represent the perfusion triangle.
© Jones & Bartlett Learning.

in the pulse rate, an increase in the strength of cardiac contractions, and vasoconstriction in nonessential areas, primarily in the skin, muscles, and GI tract (peripheral vasoconstriction). Together, these actions are designed to maintain pressure in the system and, as a result, sustain perfusion of the vital organs (ie, brain, heart, lungs, kidneys, and liver).

Eventually, there is also a shifting of body fluids to help maintain pressure within the system. However, the response of the autonomic nervous system and hormones comes within seconds. It is this response that causes all the signs and symptoms of shock in a patient.

▶ Compensation for Decreased Perfusion

Central among the homeostatic mechanisms that regulate cardiovascular dynamics are those that maintain blood pressure. When any event results in decreased perfusion (ie, blood loss, MI, loss of vasomotor tone, or tension pneumothorax), the body must respond immediately to preserve vital organs. **Baroreceptors** located in the aortic arch and carotid sinuses (and in most of the large arteries of the neck and thorax) sense the decreased blood flow and activate the vasomotor center in the medulla oblongata, which oversees changes in the diameter of blood vessels, to begin constriction of the vessels and, therefore, increase blood pressure. Assisting in this process, **chemoreceptors** measure subtle shifts in the amounts of carbon dioxide in the arterial blood. In Chapter 8, *Anatomy and Physiology*, you learned that these sensors help regulate the respiratory rate and control the acid-base balance in the body.

Normally, stimulation occurs when the SBP is between 60 and 80 mm Hg in adults or even lower in children. A decrease in the SBP to less than 80 mm Hg stimulates the vasomotor center to increase the arterial pressure by constricting vessels. As the arterial pressure drops, the walls of the arteries are not stretched as much, thereby decreasing baroreceptor stimulation. Normally, baroreceptor stimulation prevents the vasoconstrictor center of the medulla from constricting the vessels, leading to vasodilation in the peripheral circulatory system and a decrease in pulse rate and contractility, causing a concomitant decrease in arterial pressure. With dropping pressure, the baroreceptors are not stimulated to allow for vasodilation, so the vessels constrict to raise the blood pressure. The sympathetic nervous system is also stimulated as the body recognizes a potential catastrophic event. This message is sent to the adrenal glands to release epinephrine and norepinephrine into the bloodstream. These two naturally occurring "medications" will cause tachycardia and increase the contractility of the heart. Additionally, they will cause venous and arteriolar constriction, resulting in a decrease in blood flow to the skin, muscles, the GI tract, and often the kidneys. This allows for a relative redistribution of blood to the brain and heart. Capillary hydrostatic pressure decreases in the "compensated phase" of shock, allowing fluid from the interstitial compartment to flow into the vessels.

Also, in response to hypoperfusion, the renin-angiotensin-aldosterone system in the kidneys is activated and antidiuretic hormone is released from the pituitary gland. Together, these mechanisms trigger salt and water retention and peripheral vasoconstriction. The result is an increase in the patient's blood pressure and maintenance of cardiac output. Depending on the severity of the insult, variable amounts of fluid will shift from the interstitial tissues into the vascular compartment. The spleen also releases some RBCs that are normally sequestered there to augment the blood's oxygen-carrying capacity. The overall response of the initial compensatory mechanisms is to increase the preload, stroke volume, and pulse rate, which usually results in an increase in cardiac output. This "autotransfusion" effect, along with the subtle effects in other response systems of the body (ie, osmosis, insulin and glucagon production in the pancreas, as well as the effects of the hormones arginine vasopressin, adrenocorticotropic hormone cortisol system, and somatotropin), allows the body to compensate adequately for a volume loss of up to 25%. Remember, shock is a *normal compensatory response* of the body, and disease can occur or become exacerbated when normal response systems are activated under abnormal conditions.

As hypoperfusion persists, the myocardial oxygen demand continues to increase. Eventually, the accelerated compensatory mechanisms are no longer able to keep up with the body's demand. Myocardial function then worsens, with decreased cardiac output and ejection fraction. Tissue perfusion decreases, leading to impaired cell metabolism. Often, the SBP decreases, especially in progressive hypoperfusion or "decompensated" shock. Fluid may leak from the blood vessels, as in the case of a severe allergic reaction, causing systemic and pulmonary edema.

As the patient decompensates, perfusion to the brain and coronary arteries decreases, and cells switch from aerobic to anaerobic metabolism. In **anaerobic metabolism**, cellular processes occur in the absence of oxygen; in contrast, in **aerobic metabolism**, all of the cells' processes occur with an adequate oxygen supply. This switch is a critical point, and lactic acidosis begins to develop from this inefficient form of metabolism, shifting the oxygen-hemoglobin dissociation curve to the right to increase tissue oxygen delivery. This shift in the curve also decreases cardiac function and makes the heart more susceptible to the effect of the circulating catecholamines (causing dysrhythmias). Other signs of hypoperfusion may also be present, such as dusky skin color, oliguria, and impaired mentation.

The body produces its own "medicines," epinephrine and norepinephrine, in the adrenal glands in response to hypoperfusion. These substances are released by the body as part of the global compensatory state. Release of epinephrine improves cardiac output by increasing the pulse rate and strength. The alpha-1 response to its release includes vasoconstriction, increased peripheral vascular resistance, and increased afterload from the arteriolar constriction. Alpha-2 effects ensure a regulated release of alpha-1. Beta responses from the release of epinephrine primarily affect the heart and lungs. Increases in pulse rate, contractility, conductivity, and automaticity occur in tandem with bronchodilation.

Effects of norepinephrine are primarily alpha-1 and alpha-2 in nature and center on vasoconstriction and increasing peripheral vascular resistance. The alpha and beta effects of epinephrine and norepinephrine are discussed in Chapter 13, *Principles of Pharmacology*. This vasoconstriction allows the body to shunt blood from areas of lesser need to areas of greater need, serving to keep the brain and other vital organs perfused in the early phases of shock. In an effort to maintain circulation to the brain, the body will shunt blood away from the following tissues, in this order: placenta, skin, muscles, gut, kidneys, liver, heart, lungs. This "planned shunting of blood" is referred to as the "pecking order." The skin and muscles can survive with minimal blood flow from vasoconstriction for a much longer period than can major organs such as the kidneys, liver, heart, and lungs. If the blood supply is inadequate to the major organs for more than 60 minutes, they often develop complications that will lead to death, such as renal failure and shock lung. This concept has been traditionally referred to as the "Golden Period," and it explains why it is so important for you to immediately address the cause of the shock.

Failure of compensatory mechanisms to preserve perfusion leads to decreases in preload and cardiac output. Myocardial blood supply and oxygenation decrease, reducing myocardial perfusion. As cardiac output further decreases, coronary artery perfusion also decreases, leading to myocardial ischemia. As all of these changes are occurring, other organ systems are affected too. The normal functions of the liver and pancreas are impacted by the low perfusion state, inhibiting insulin release. This is why patients in shock have been described as being in a diabetic-like state. GI motility is decreased, causing stress ulcers to develop. When kidney perfusion is diminished, so is urine production; if reperfusion does not occur within 45 minutes to 1 hour, kidney failure will result. Normal urine output is roughly 30 to 40 mL/h. An output of less than 500 mL per day is considered oliguria and can lead to acute kidney insufficiency, an indicator of the severity of acute underlying illness; it is also associated with mortality in sepsis and pneumonia.

▶ Shock-Related Events at the Capillary and Microcirculatory Levels

As perfusion decreases, cellular ischemia occurs. Minimal blood flow passes through the capillaries, causing the cells to switch from aerobic metabolism to anaerobic metabolism, which can quickly lead to metabolic acidosis. With less circulation, the blood stagnates in the capillaries. The precapillary sphincter relaxes in response to the buildup of lactic acid, vasomotor center failure, and

increased amounts of carbon dioxide. The postcapillary sphincters remain constricted, causing the capillaries to become engorged with fluid.

> ### Words of Wisdom
>
> The Frank-Starling mechanism states that the length of the fibers constituting the heart's muscular wall determines the force of the heartbeat.[2] In other words, an increase in diastolic filling increases the force of the contraction, whereas a decrease in diastolic filling decreases the force of the contraction. Decreased perfusion in shock is partially the result of decreased cardiac contractility, which may be the result of loss of fluid, increased container size, or a damaged pump.

The capillary sphincters—circular muscular walls that constrict and dilate—regulate blood flow through the capillary beds. These sphincters are under the control of the autonomic nervous system, which regulates involuntary functions such as sweating and digestion. Capillary sphincters also respond to other stimuli such as heat, cold, increased demand for oxygen, and the need for waste removal. Thus, regulation of blood flow is determined by cellular need and is accomplished by vessel constriction or dilation, working in tandem with sphincter constriction or dilation.

The body can tolerate anaerobic metabolism for only a limited time. You learned in Chapter 8, *Anatomy and Physiology*, that anaerobic metabolism is much less efficient than aerobic metabolism and leads to systemic acidosis and depletion of the body's normally high adenosine triphosphate (ATP) reserves. During anaerobic metabolism, incomplete glucose breakdown leads to an accumulation of pyruvic acid. Pyruvic acid cannot be converted to acetyl coenzyme A without oxygen, however, so it is transformed in greater amounts to lactate and other acid by-products. Acidosis develops because ATP is hydrolyzed to adenosine diphosphate and phosphate with the release of a proton. Hydrogen ions accumulate, decreasing the pool of bicarbonate buffer. Lactate also buffers protons, and lactic acid accumulates in the body.

At the same time, ischemia stimulates increased carbon dioxide production by the tissues. The higher the body's metabolic rate, the higher the carbon dioxide level in hypoperfused states. The excess carbon dioxide combines with intracellular water to produce carbonic acid. Increased tissue acids will, in turn, react with other buffers to form more intracellular acidic substances. Thus, acidosis serves as an indirect measure of tissue perfusion. The acidic condition of the blood inhibits hemoglobin in the RBCs from binding with and carrying oxygen. This adds to the cellular oxygen debt, shifting the oxyhemoglobin dissociation curve to the right.

Sodium, which is usually more abundant outside the cells than inside them, is naturally inclined to diffuse into cells. Normally the sodium-potassium pump acts like a "bouncer" at the cell membrane, sending the sodium back out against the concentration gradient. This mechanism involves active transport and requires an ample supply of ATP to fuel the bouncer. Reduced levels of ATP, however, result in a dysfunctional sodium-potassium pump and alter the cell membrane function. Excessive sodium begins to diffuse into the cells, along with water, which ultimately depletes the interstitial compartment.

Intracellular enzymes that usually help digest and neutralize bacteria introduced into a cell are bound in a relatively impermeable membrane. Cellular flooding explodes cell membranes and releases these lysosomal enzymes, which then autodigest tissue. If enough cells are destroyed in this way, organ failure will become evident. The release of the lysosomes opens the floodgates for the onset of what is often called "irreversible" or "terminal" shock.

To compound these problems, accumulating acids and waste products act as potent vasodilators, further decreasing venous return and diminishing blood flow to the vital organs and tissues. The arterial pressure falls to the point at which even the "protected organs" such as the brain and heart are no longer perfused. When aortic pressures fall below a MAP of 60 mm Hg, the coronary arteries no longer fill, the heart is weakened by lack of blood flow and oxygen delivery to the heart tissue itself, and the cardiac output falls. Myocardial depressant factor is released from an ischemic pancreas, further decreasing the pumping action of the heart and slowing the cardiac output.

Eventually, the reduced blood supply to the vasomotor center in the brain results in slowing and then stopping of sympathetic nervous system activity. The metabolic wastes

YOU are the Paramedic PART 3

The engine crew arrive and brings the stretcher from your medic unit. Your supervisor arrives and obtains vital signs while you attempt to establish IV access. After a failed attempt, you switch to an IO attempt in the right tibia, since you would like to begin an infusion of normal saline as soon as possible. The patient's blood pressure is 68 mm Hg by palpation so you administer a fluid bolus of normal saline at 30 mL/kg per your local protocol. You attach the cardiac monitor and identify the rhythm as a sinus tachycardia at a rate of 118 beats/min and without ectopy. Your partner and the engine crew prepares the patient for transport while the home health aide gathers his medication at your request so that you can evaluate them and turn them over to hospital personnel. She also gathers pertinent identification for you to take. Once you have loaded your patient into the ambulance, you ask one of the firefighters from the engine to drive you to the closest appropriate facility so your partner can continue assisting ventilations while you and your supervisor provide care and assessment during transport.

You evaluate the patient's medications once transport has begun. His medications include lisinopril 10 mg daily, aspirin 81 mg daily, albuterol metered-dose inhaler two puffs three times daily and as needed, and furosemide 20 mg daily. After a quick count, you notice that it appears there are two more tablets of lisinopril than there should be if Mr. Oliver had been compliant with his medications. This discovery supports your concerns that he has been in bed for at least 24 hours. You reevaluate his vital signs as transport continues.

Recording Time: 10 Minutes	
Skin	Pale, cool, moist
Pulse	118 beats/min and weak
Blood pressure	68 mm Hg by palpation
Respirations	20 breaths/min, assisted with a bag-mask device
Oxygen saturation (Spo$_2$)	Not obtainable secondary to poor perfusion
Pupils	PERRLA
Temperature	96°F (36°C)

5. Discuss the phase of shock this patient may be in.
6. Describe how you should manage this patient with suspected shock.

are released into the slower-flowing blood. The blood's sluggish flow, coupled with its acidity, leads to platelet agglutination and formation of microthrombi. Because the capillary walls are stretched, they lose their ability to retain large molecules, allowing them to leak into the surrounding interstitial spaces. Hydrostatic pressure forces plasma into the interstitial spaces, further increasing the distance from the capillaries to the cells. In turn, oxygen transport decreases, increasing cellular hypoxia.

The continuing buildup of lactic acid and carbon dioxide acts as a potent vasodilator, leading to relaxation of the postcapillary sphincters. The accumulated hydrogen, potassium, carbon dioxide, and thrombosed (clotted) RBCs wash out into the venous circulation, increasing the metabolic acidosis. This has been referred to as the capillary "washout phase." The result is an even greater drop in cardiac output. Ischemia and necrosis ultimately lead to multiple-organ dysfunction syndrome, in which the various organ systems fail in succession.

Words of Wisdom

Capillary hydrostatic pressure tends to force fluids through capillary walls, whereas interstitial fluid hydrostatic pressure pushes fluid back into the cells.

Oncotic pressure pulls fluids from the surrounding tissue into the capillaries as a result of a difference in the concentration of solutes in the fluid inside the capillaries. Fluid leaves the capillaries as a result of hydrostatic pressure, while albumin and other large proteins remain inside, resulting in a greater concentration of solutes inside the capillaries. The oncotic pressure rises, pulling more water into the capillaries to balance the solute concentration. If capillary hydrostatic pressure is greater, fluid will leave the capillaries. If capillary oncotic pressure is greater, fluid will be pulled into the capillaries.

In conjunction with all this injury going on, the white blood cells and blood clotting system are impaired. The result is a decreased resistance to infection and the possible development of disseminated intravascular coagulation (DIC). DIC is a serious disorder whereby the proteins that normally control clotting become inappropriately active. Once again, a normal function becomes activated under abnormal circumstances. Research shows that 97% of patients who die from hemorrhagic shock have evidence of coagulation defects prior to fluid or blood administration. This finding of preexisting coagulation defects occurs most often in patients with head trauma and suggests preexisting DIC. The most frequent abnormality was elevated prothrombin (97%), followed by depressed platelet counts (72%), and elevated partial thromboplastin time (70%).[3] DIC has also been found to complicate septic shock.

▶ Multiple-Organ Dysfunction Syndrome

Multiple-organ dysfunction syndrome (MODS) is a progressive condition characterized by concurrent failure of two or more organs or organ systems that were initially unharmed by the acute disorder or injury that caused the patient's initial illness. Six organ systems are surveyed when you are diagnosing MODS: the respiratory, hepatic, renal, hematologic, neurologic, and cardiovascular systems. Each system is assigned a score to determine the patient's overall risk (ie, the Glasgow Coma Scale is used to score the patient's neurologic system function).

Consider this: if each type of tissue has its own **warm ischemic time**—that is, the time it can be deprived of oxygenated blood before it starts to die—then different tissue types (ie, nervous, muscle, epithelial tissue) will exhibit the effects of poor perfusion differently, depending on how long it takes to reestablish adequate perfusion. For example, the warm ischemic time of the brain and central nervous system (CNS) tissue is approximately 4 to 6 minutes, and the warm ischemic time for the skin and muscles is almost 2 hours. The Golden Period corresponds to the warm ischemic time of the rest of the vital organs (ie, liver, kidneys, heart, and lungs). When a patient has poor perfusion in the field and it is not adequately restored within the first hour, blood is diverted from other organs—first from the skin and muscles, then from the gut, next the liver, then the kidneys, and finally the heart and lungs—in an effort to keep the brain well perfused. This compensatory process is often the cause of the development of serious, often life-threatening complications of organ damage to the liver (liver failure), the kidneys (renal failure), the lungs (acute respiratory distress syndrome), and the heart (massive MI). Thus, what was initially a single injury causing the patient to lose significant amounts of blood or fluids can have a devastating impact on multiple organs and organ systems. This process is all directly related, *from the single cell to the entire organism*.

Patients with MODS have an overall mortality rate of 60% to 90%. Previously called multisystem organ failure, today MODS is considered the major cause of death following septic, traumatic, and burn injuries. MODS is classified as primary or secondary. Primary MODS is a direct result of an insult, such as a pulmonary contusion from striking the chest on the steering wheel during a vehicle crash. Secondary MODS encompasses the organ dysfunction that occurs as an integral component to the patient's response to cellular hypoperfusion (eg, renal failure following trauma).

MODS occurs when injury or infection (septic shock) triggers a massive systemic immune, inflammatory, and coagulation response, resulting in the release of numerous inflammatory mediators and activation of the following systems:

- **The complement system.** Normally, this group of plasma proteins functions to eliminate invading bacteria; that is, these components are part of the immune response. In MODS, an overactive complement system activates phagocytes and induces further inflammation and damage to cells.

- **The coagulation system.** Endothelial damage and coagulation, especially in the microscopic venules and arterioles, become uncontrolled in MODS, which results in microvascular thrombus formation and tissue ischemia.
- **The kallikrein-kinin system.** The release of bradykinin, a potent vasodilator, leads to tissue hypoperfusion and may contribute to hypotension.

The net outcome of overactivity in these systems is maldistribution of systemic and organ blood flow. Often the body attempts to compensate by accelerating tissue metabolism. The result is an oxygen supply-demand imbalance that leads to tissue hypoxia, tissue hypoperfusion, exhaustion of the cells' fuel supply (ATP), metabolic failure, lysosome breakdown, anaerobic metabolism, acidosis, and impaired cellular function. As MODS progresses, more organs begin to malfunction as a result of the cell and tissue hypoxia.

MODS typically develops within hours to days following resuscitation. The signs and symptoms include hypotension, insufficient tissue perfusion, uncontrollable bleeding (coagulopathy), and multisystem organ failure. A low-grade fever may develop from the inflammatory response, tachycardia, and dyspnea. It may also be difficult to oxygenate patients because of acute lung injury and acute respiratory distress syndrome.

In a 14- to 21-day period, renal and liver failure can develop, along with collapse of the GI and immune systems. If the patient does not respond to treatment of the underlying condition, then **cardiovascular collapse** and death typically occur within days to weeks of the initial insult.

MODS affects specific organs and organ systems in the following ways:

- **Heart.** Hypoperfusion may stun a healthy heart and result in dysrhythmias, muscle ischemia, infarction, and pump failure with ejection fractions falling far below 40%. Peripheral pulses are weak or absent. Extremities become cyanotic and cold.
- **Lungs.** Failure is evidenced by adult respiratory distress syndrome or noncardiogenic pulmonary edema. Hypoxic vasoconstriction of pulmonary beds increases pulmonary arterial pressures and produces pulmonary hypertension, putting a strain on the right ventricle. Pulmonary capillary blood flow reduction results in impaired gas exchange, a reduced partial pressure of oxygen (PaO_2) level, and an increased $PaCO_2$ level. Alveolar cells become ischemic and slow their production of surfactant, resulting in massive atelectasis and a reduction in pulmonary compliance. At the same time, pulmonary capillaries become permeable to water, resulting in interstitial and intra-alveolar edema at low pulmonary artery wedge pressure (PAWP) of less than 18 mm Hg. The PAWP measures pressures generated by the left ventricle and is used to assess left ventricular function, where normal PAWP is 8 to 12 mm Hg. The net results are respiratory failure, severe hypoxemia, and respiratory acidosis.

- **CNS.** Decreased cerebral perfusion pressure and cerebral blood flow result in confusion, reduced responses to verbal and painful stimuli, and, ultimately, unresponsiveness.
- **Kidneys.** A reduction in renal blood flow produces acute tubular necrosis, which in turn leads to oliguria (urine output of less than 20 mL/h). Toxic waste products cannot be excreted, so they are retained in the blood. Metabolic acidosis worsens as the kidneys become unable to excrete acids or retain bicarbonate.
- **Liver.** Impaired metabolic function and alterations in clotting factors produce coagulopathies such as DIC, in which clotting and bleeding occur at the same time. The liver fails to filter bacteria, leaving the patient vulnerable to infections. Failure to metabolize waste products, such as ammonia and lactate, causes markedly increased blood levels of these toxins. Cell death is evidenced by an increase in enzyme levels (including lactate dehydrogenase, aspartate aminotransferase, and alanine aminotransferase) in the blood. The net result is ischemic hepatitis (liver shock) or hypoxic hepatitis.
- **GI tract.** Hypoperfusion results in ischemic gut syndrome. Release of vasodilating endotoxins into the gut causes the gut to leak, which further contributes to the progression of shock.

Causes of Shock

Shock can result from many conditions—namely, bleeding, respiratory failure, acute allergic reactions, and overwhelming infection. In all cases, the damage occurs because of insufficient perfusion of organs and tissues. As soon as perfusion stops or becomes impaired, tissues start to die, affecting all local body processes. If the conditions causing shock are not promptly arrested and reversed, then death soon follows.

You should have a high index of suspicion for shock in many emergency medical situations. For example, you would expect hemorrhagic shock to accompany massive external or internal bleeding. You should also expect shock if a patient has any one of the following conditions:

- Multiple severe fractures
- Abdominal or chest injury
- Spinal injury
- Severe infection
- Massive myocardial infarction
- Anaphylaxis

Understanding the basic physiologic causes of shock will better prepare you to treat it. **Figure 40-8** describes the three basic mechanisms of shock—pump failure, low fluid volume, and poor vessel function.

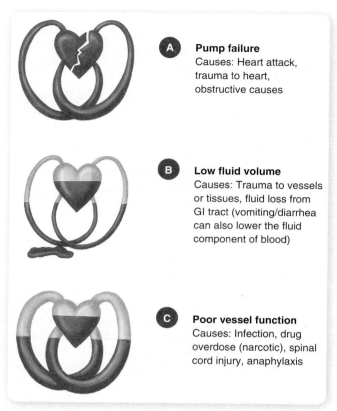

A **Pump failure**
Causes: Heart attack, trauma to heart, obstructive causes

B **Low fluid volume**
Causes: Trauma to vessels or tissues, fluid loss from GI tract (vomiting/diarrhea can also lower the fluid component of blood)

C **Poor vessel function**
Causes: Infection, drug overdose (narcotic), spinal cord injury, anaphylaxis

Figure 40-8 There are three basic causes of shock and impaired tissue perfusion. **A.** Pump failure occurs when the heart is damaged by disease, injury, or obstructive causes. The heart may not generate enough energy to move the blood through the system. **B.** Low fluid volume, often a result of bleeding, leads to inadequate perfusion. **C.** Poor vessel function causes inefficient perfusion. If blood vessels dilate excessively, the blood within them, even though it is of normal volume, is inadequate to fill the system and provide efficient perfusion.
© Jones & Bartlett Learning.

Words of Wisdom

Shock is a complex physiologic process that gives subtle signs to its presence before it becomes severe. These early signs relate closely to the events that lead to more severe shock, so it is important for you to know the underlying processes thoroughly. If you understand what causes shock, then you will be able to recognize it in many patients before it becomes out of control.

Certain categories of patients are at high risk to develop shock. They include patients known to have had trauma or bleeding; patients with massive MI; pregnant women; and patients with a possible source for septic shock (ie, burned patients and people with diabetes or cancer). Older adults are particularly at risk for shock, especially older adult patients with urinary tract infections. Increased age works against patients in that they normally have a decreased resting cardiac output, decreased cardiac reserves (as much as 50%), and atherosclerosis, which impairs vasoconstriction.

Words of Wisdom

More than one type of shock may be present at one time. Consider the patient who was in a motor vehicle crash who presents with hypovolemic shock from a ruptured spleen and other internal injuries as well as spinal shock from a severed spine. Or, consider the burn patient who is losing body fluid and has cells that are leaking and swelling tremendously.

The Progression of Shock

Shock occurs in two successive phases—compensated and decompensated (hypotensive). As discussed in Chapter 30, *Bleeding*, the Advanced Trauma Life Support classification developed by the American College of Surgeons Committee on Trauma describes four categories of hemorrhage and associated shock states; classes I and II are compensated shock, and classes III and IV are decompensated shock. Your goal is to recognize the clinical signs and symptoms of shock in its earliest phase and begin immediate treatment before permanent damage occurs. To do so, you must be aware of the subtle signs exhibited while the body is compensating effectively and treat the patient aggressively **Table 40-4** . Anticipate the potential for shock from the scene size-up and evaluation of the mechanism of injury (MOI). Recognize the signs of poor perfusion that precede hypotension, and do not rely on any one sign or symptom to determine the phase of shock the patient is going through. Always err on the side of caution when you are treating a patient who may be in shock. Rapid assessment and immediate transport are essential to preserve any chance of survival.

Altered mental status is a late indicator because a key purpose of the shock syndrome is to keep the brain well perfused. Sometimes "alert" patients may be agitated or

Table 40-4	Compensated Versus Decompensated Shock	
Compensated Shock	**Decompensated Shock**	
• Agitation, anxiety, restlessness • Sense of impending doom • Weak, rapid (thready) pulse • Clammy (cool, moist) skin • Pallor with cyanotic lips • Shortness of breath • Nausea, vomiting • Delayed capillary refill in infants and children • Thirst • Normal blood pressure	• Altered mental status (verbal to unresponsive)* • Hypotension • Labored or irregular breathing • Thready or absent peripheral pulses • Ashen, mottled, or cyanotic skin • Dilated pupils • Diminished urine output (oliguria) • Impending cardiac arrest	

*Mental status changes are late indicators.

© Jones & Bartlett Learning.

anxious during the compensated phase, but this presentation is not considered an altered mental status.

Compensated Shock

The earliest stage of shock, in which the body can still compensate for blood loss, is called **compensated shock**. In this phase, the patient's level of responsiveness is a better indicator of tissue perfusion than most other vital signs. Release of chemical mediators by the autonomic nervous system as it recognizes a potential catastrophic event causes the arterial blood pressure to remain normal or slightly elevated. There is an increase in the rate and depth of respirations as the body attempts to bring in more oxygen and remove more carbon dioxide. This effort helps to maintain the acid-base balance by creating respiratory alkalosis to offset the metabolic acidosis.

During the compensated phase of shock, blood pressure is maintained. Blood loss in hemorrhagic shock can be estimated to be at 15% to 30% at this point. A narrowing of the pulse pressure also occurs. The pulse pressure reflects the tone of the arterial system and is more sensitive to changes in perfusion than is the SBP or DBP alone. Patients in the compensated phase will also have a positive orthostatic tilt test result.

Decompensated Shock

The next stage of shock, when blood pressure is falling, is **decompensated shock** (also called uncompensated, progressive, or hypotensive shock). It occurs when blood volume drops by more than 30%. The compensatory mechanisms begin to fail, and signs and symptoms become much more obvious. The cardiac output falls dramatically, leading to further reductions in blood pressure and cardiac function. The signs and symptoms become more obvious as blood is shunted to the brain, heart, and kidneys. At this point, vasoconstriction can have a disastrous effect if allowed to continue. Cells in the nonperfused tissues become hypoxic, leading to anaerobic metabolism. Treatment at this stage will sometimes result in recovery.

Blood pressure may be the last measurable factor to change in shock. The body has several automatic mechanisms to compensate for initial blood loss and to help maintain blood pressure. Thus, by the time you detect a drop in blood pressure, shock is well developed. This is particularly true in infants and children, whose blood pressure may be maintained until their blood volume loss is more than 35% to 40%. Always consider it an emergency when treating a patient who is hypotensive and whom you suspect to be in shock, and start transport in less than 10 minutes, providing fluid resuscitation en route to the most appropriate ED.

Irreversible (Terminal) Shock

Irreversible shock refers to the point at which shock has progressed to what is considered a terminal stage.[5] Arterial blood pressure is abnormally low (typically in hemorrhagic shock there is a 40% or greater blood volume loss). A rapid deterioration of the cardiovascular system occurs that cannot be reversed by compensatory mechanisms or medical interventions. Life-threatening reductions in cardiac output, blood pressure, and tissue perfusion are observed. Blood is shunted away from the liver, kidneys, and lungs to keep the heart and brain perfused. Cells begin to die. Even if the cause of shock is treated and reversed, vital organ damage may be permanent, and the patient may eventually die. Providing aggressive treatment at this stage does not usually result in recovery; however, because it is difficult to determine who will or will not survive, you should provide aggressive treatment en route to the trauma center!

Patient Assessment of Shock

Scene Size-up

The general assessment plan of a patient who is suspected of having hypoperfusion or shock follows the plan reinforced throughout this text. Size up the scene for hazards, take standard precautions, and determine the number of patients and the need for additional or specialized resources.

The size-up also includes a quick assessment of the MOI or nature of illness (NOI). For a patient with suspected shock, this information can give you clues about the causes of nonhemorrhagic shock or the extent of any bleeding (whether internal or external); for example, a patient lying unconscious at the base of a building where a third-floor window is open suggests the possibility that the person fell or was pushed out.

Primary Survey

Start the primary survey by forming a general impression. How does the patient look to you? Some patients simply do not pass the "look test" and will need to be fast tracked based on the MOI/NOI and the poor impression you have. A patient who is blue or has a sweaty pale look will need your immediate attention. If patients do not greet you as you approach, then it may be because they are concentrating on breathing or their injuries or because they are in severe pain. Next, assess the patient's mental status using the AVPU mnemonic (Awake and alert, responsive to Verbal stimuli, responsive to Pain, Unresponsive). Introduce yourself and ask if they know their name, where they are, and the day of the week.

Next, you will need to quickly assess the patient for any threats to airway and breathing. If you suspect cardiac arrest or life-threatening external bleeding, then use the CABDE (Circulation, Airway, Breathing, Disability, and Exposure) approach. Otherwise, assess the ABCDEs (Airway, Breathing, Circulation, Disability, and Exposure). If the patient is conscious, listen to the patient speak. Patients with life-threatening airway problems cannot speak, or they speak in short one- or two-word sentences. Immediately manage any threats to the patient's airway or breathing. This may involve positioning the unconscious patient's airway (ie, head tilt–chin lift or jaw thrust); clearing the airway of secretions, blood, or vomitus; and administering oxygen. If you suspect there

YOU are the Paramedic PART 4

You become concerned that peripheral perfusion has become too diminished. You consult medical direction for orders to initiate a vasopressor to increase cardiac output. You receive orders for dopamine (Intropin) with an initial dose of 5 mcg/kg/min. You will monitor and titrate as needed to increase cardiac output and SBP. Your partner notes the patient's decreasing respirations and indicates he believes intubation is becoming necessary. Based on the history of chronic bronchitis, you also consider that your patient has end-stage chronic obstructive pulmonary disease (COPD) and a hypoxic drive that is failing due to the high concentrations of oxygen. Securing his airway and providing positive pressure ventilations should allow for controlling his breathing and ensuring adequate oxygenation in the presence of decreased peripheral perfusion. You obtain another set of vital signs prior to initiating intubation.

Recording Time: 15 Minutes	
Skin	Pink, cool, and dry
Pulse	100 beats/min
Blood pressure	72 mm Hg by palpation
Respirations	8 breaths/min and shallow without assistance via bag-mask device
Oxygen saturation (Spo$_2$)	Not obtainable due to poor perfusion
Pupils	PERRLA, but sluggish

7. Why should a patient's hypoxic drive not be a consideration when treating shock?

8. What are the anticipated benefits of dopamine administration for this patient?

is difficulty breathing, then examine the chest for flail segments, impaled objects that need to be stabilized, and holes that need to be sealed with an occlusive dressing. Assess the adequacy of the patient's ventilation with respect to volume and rate, and make a decision if it will be necessary for you to assist the patient with bag-mask ventilation and high-concentration oxygen. Once the airway is open and secure, and breathing is adequate, move on to assess circulation.

After assessing airway and breathing, assess circulation, disability, and exposure. If you suspect the patient does not have a pulse, then you would take the CABDE approach and perform chest compressions at this time. With a patient who has a pulse, your approach should be to determine whether the pulse is adequate to sustain life, for now, and then perform a rapid full-body scan to check for external blood loss that you can control.

In responsive patients, you will usually assess the pulse at the radius; in unconscious patients, you will typically check the carotid pulse in the neck. The radial pulse can give you clues about the phase of shock and the patient's ability to compensate for shock. Ask yourself, "Is the radial pulse strong and regular, or weak and thready, or irregular?" If the radial pulse is barely palpable, and yet the patient is sitting up and talking to you with a bullet hole in the abdomen, remember the purpose of the shock syndrome is to keep the brain perfused—but the reduction in the radial pulse is an indicator to you that the SBP is dropping fast. In such a case, you may then decide that you cannot take the time to measure the patient's blood pressure because you already know the patient is hypotensive (indicating decompensated shock) and instead, make the decision to provide immediate transport to the ED.

The rapid full-body scan to determine locations of uncontrolled external bleeding is designed to help you detect an injury that is life threatening and needs to be dealt with immediately. Otherwise, note the patient's skin CTC (color, temperature, and condition) as you move on to determine the priorities for the patient's condition. Your assessment of disability includes the mental status and the ability to move the extremities. Finally, cover the patient to retain his or her body heat. Shivering wastes energy that the patient will need during this ordeal.

At this point, all patients need to be prioritized. Patients who are in shock will usually be given high priority. If the shock originates from a medical condition, then the patient should be fast-tracked through your elaboration of the chief complaint using OPQRST to assess the body systems involved. If the patient has experienced some sort of trauma, the MOI should guide your assessment of the major body cavities and regions. For example, the patient was standing on a corner at a busy intersection when a truck cut the corner too tight and ran over both her legs. She may have stable vital signs and no immediate life threats, but beware: given the typical bleeding from a broken bone—and in this case, there are multiple

fractures in both the upper and lower legs—you should suspect significant blood loss for this patient.

History Taking

In a high-priority patient, history taking can be done en route to the ED along with the secondary assessment and the reassessment. Time is of the essence in shock patients; focus on getting to the ED and limit the on-scene care to the essential items that must be done before moving the patient (ie, ABCs and spinal immobilization). Unless the patient is pinned and there may be a delay in extrication, delay establishing IV/IO access until you are en route. Keep in mind that the interventions that add time to the scene time must be justified by the benefits they will produce for the patient.

Secondary Assessment

Shock is considered hypovolemic or hemorrhagic until proven otherwise. Table 40-5 summarizes the hemodynamic parameters in the differentiation of shock. The phase of shock in hypovolemic or hemorrhagic shock (compensated or decompensated) relates to the percentage of blood loss. In the other types of shock, the best indicator that the body is no longer able to compensate is a drop in the SBP or altered mental status.

Other indicators you need to pay attention to (in addition to mental status and vital signs) include the end-tidal carbon dioxide ($ETCO_2$) level, which is lowered in hypoperfused states, and lactic acid buildup. Lactate is a sign of metabolic distress and is an early indicator of severe sepsis (ie, lactate levels above 4 mmol/dL). Portable lactate monitors are tools traditionally used by elite athletes Figure 40-9. This tool is similar to a glucometer and has been incorporated into sepsis alert programs in cities such as Denver, Colorado. Sepsis alert programs use specific criteria for early sepsis recognition, allowing caregivers to provide more effective care.

Reassessment

This portion of patient assessment is important in patient care. The rule of thumb is to assess, intervene, then reassess. In this portion of the assessment, you revisit the primary survey, the vital signs, the chief complaint, and any treatment performed on the patient, including oxygen administration. You must reassess the patient to determine whether the interventions you performed are having any effect on the patient. This step prepares you to present the patient at the hospital with a complete, concise account of the patient encounter and care.

You must determine what interventions are needed for your patient at this point based on the findings of your

Table 40-5	**Differentiation of Shock**					
Characteristics						
Origin	**Etiology**	**BP**	**Pulse**	**Skin**	**Lungs**	**EMS Treatment**
↓ Pump performance	Cardiogenic	↓	↓ → ↑	Pale, cool, moist	Crackles	Dopamine infusion
↓ Fluid volume	Hypovolemic, hemorrhagic	↓	↑	Pale, cool, moist	Clear	IV fluids
Vessels or container dilates: maldistribution of blood; low peripheral resistance	Neurogenic	↓	↓	Flushed, dry, warm	Clear	IV fluids, atropine, dopamine infusion
	Septic	↓	↑	Flushed or pale, hot or cool, moist	Crackles if pulmonary origin	IV fluids, high-dose dopamine
	Anaphylactic	↓	↑	Flushed, warm, moist	May have wheezes; may be ↓ with no sounds	Epinephrine, diphenhydramine, albuterol, ipratropium, corticosteroids
Hemodynamic Parameters						
Parameter		**Hypovolemic**	**Cardiac**	**Neurogenic**		**Septic**
Mean arterial pressure		↓	↓	↓		↓
Pulse rate		↑	↑ or ↓	↓		↑
Central venous pressure		↓	Variable	↓		↑
Cardiac output		↓	↓	↓		↑ then ↓
Peripheral vascular resistance		↑	↑	↓		↑
pH		↓	↓	↓		↓
Pao_2		↓	↓	↓		↓
$Paco_2$		↓	↓	Increase and decrease the rate		↓

Abbreviations: IV, intravenous; Pao_2, partial pressure of oxygen, arterial; $Paco_2$, partial pressure of carbon dioxide, arterial; pH, potential of hydrogen

assessment. Focus on supporting the cardiovascular system by treating for shock early and aggressively to prevent the harmful effects of inadequate perfusion. Administer oxygen, as needed, and put the patient in the position dictated by local protocol for shock patients. Provide warmth, gain IV access, and administer fluid as needed based on patient presentation. Specific interventions are discussed in the emergency medical care section later in this chapter.

Patients who are in decompensated shock will need rapid interventions to restore adequate perfusion. Most of the interventions used to treat shock do not require a specific physician's order; however, that depends on local protocols. Determine, based on the signs and symptoms found in your assessment, whether your patient is in compensated or decompensated shock. Document these findings after you have treated for shock.

▶ Special Considerations for Assessing Shock

Healthy, fit, young adults usually are well prepared to combat a situation of life-threatening blood loss.

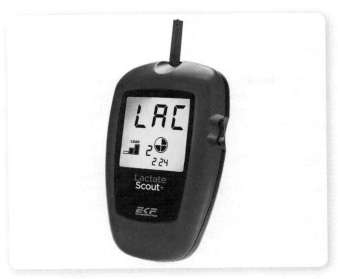

Figure 40-9 A lactate monitor.
Courtesy of EKF Diagnostics www.ekfdiagnostics.com.

When young adults stay fit through aerobic exercise, their cardiovascular systems are resilient and the heart's stroke volume is usually larger than that of the average patient. In addition, keeping their weight within the normal range for their height and consuming a diet low in salt, fats, and cholesterol help prepare the body to handle the effects of the epinephrine and norepinephrine released during compensated shock. Their blood vessels can handle the vasoconstriction of the body's pecking order without developing clots, and arteries are generally free of obstructions such as plaque. Being a nonsmoker also contributes to better oxygenation when extra cardiac output is needed to combat the challenges of shock.

Special Populations

When managing pediatric patients, remember their bodies can compensate well until they have blood volume loss of about 30% to 35%; then their condition declines rapidly. Their ability to compensate relies on an increasing pulse rate and systemic vascular resistance. This reaction causes the body to rapidly burn glucose. Unfortunately, children have little glucose in storage. The child is able to compensate through vasoconstriction and increase peripheral vascular resistance up to the point that not enough blood is perfused to the brain, heart, and lungs to stay alive. Treat pediatric patients aggressively and early if there is a significant MOI or any indication of developing shock. Never wait to see a drop in the SBP to be aggressive in the management of a child you suspect may be in the early phase of shock. Administer oxygen, manage body temperature, place the patient in the appropriate position, and initiate vascular access en route to the appropriate facility.

Special Populations

When you treat older adult patients, remember that their ability to manage blood volume loss is diminished. Vasoconstriction is less effective, and renal and vascular systems cannot effectively handle infusion of large fluid volumes. Thermoregulation is less effective in patients with a history of smoking or COPD. When older adult patients receive significant burns, their survival is about half that of a young adult because their bodies cannot handle the calories needed to heal a burn injury as well as the tremendous fluid volumes needed for resuscitation. Fluid therapy should be carefully managed by administering fluid boluses and reassessing the patient, including the breath sounds. Be aware the anemic patient starts off at a disadvantage for managing shock. Older adult patients may also have cardiovascular disorders or diabetes, affecting their body's ability to compensate when confronted with shock. Finally, these patients may be on blood-thinning medications (eg, warfarin) that prevent them from forming clots following major injuries; for example, a fractured leg can bleed significantly. Even minor bleeding, such as a nosebleed, can also be a serious issue when a patient is on blood-thinning medication.

■ Emergency Medical Care of a Patient With Suspected Shock

As with any patient, airway and ventilatory support take top priority when you are treating a patient with suspected shock. Maintain an open airway, and suction as needed. Administer high-flow supplemental oxygen via a non-rebreathing mask or assist ventilation with a bag-mask device. Consider early definitive management in patients who are unable to maintain their airways. Control any external hemorrhage, and try to estimate the amount of blood loss. Look for signs of internal hemorrhage, and consider the potential for loss in the area of suspected hemorrhage. For example, a patient may lose as much as a liter of blood in the tissues of the thigh in a closed, uncomplicated femur fracture. Consider the MOI, and maintain a high index of suspicion for occult injuries, especially when the patient has signs of shock (ie, tachycardia, dizziness, pallor, thirst) with no obvious cause.

IV fluid therapy can be helpful in supplementing the initial therapies; however, this should be done en route to the ED so as to not prolong the time at the scene, especially when you are managing a patient who is actively bleeding. While en route, establish IV access with two 16- to 18-gauge catheters and administer IV volume expanders to replace blood loss. Isotonic crystalloids, such as normal saline or lactated Ringer solution, should be used (synthetic solutions may also be used). If the patient is trapped or the extrication will be delayed, then it is reasonable to begin IV fluid resuscitation at the scene. Solutions of dextrose in water are not effective for resuscitation of trauma patients; as such, most EMS systems removed them from their protocols years ago. The goal of volume replacement is to maintain perfusion without increasing internal or uncontrollable external hemorrhage. For this reason, in the absence of traumatic brain injury, it is advisable to administer 250-mL boluses with reevaluation of blood pressure to a maximum of four doses in the prehospital environment prior to obtaining online consultation. The presence of radial pulses has been long thought to equate to an SBP of 80 to 90 mm Hg, which is generally sufficient to perfuse the brain and other vital organs. This belief has been contested by recent studies.[6] Some studies suggest a permissive hypotensive approach involving fluid therapy to maintain the SBP at approximately 80 mm Hg. This practice is thought to be safer for the patient than to attempt restoration of normotension, which may aggravate ongoing bleeding and also release clots that would cause problems in other parts of the circulatory system or vital organs.

If the patient exhibits signs of a tension pneumothorax, perform needle chest decompression to improve cardiac output and allow the mediastinum to shift back into its normal location so blood can enter the heart.

In cases of suspected cardiac tamponade, you must recognize the need for expeditious transport for pericardiocentesis or rapid ultrasound confirmation at the ED. Of course, always follow your local advanced life support (ALS) protocols because some paramedic systems have received additional training to provide these skills. Both of these conditions further impair circulation by compressing the heart and decreasing cardiac output.

Nonpharmacologic interventions for shock include proper positioning of the patient, prevention of hypothermia, and rapid transport. Apply the cardiac monitor, and be alert for dysrhythmias. When you are making your transport decision, consider the need for a regional trauma center. If travel time is lengthy, then air medical transport may be the best option. Provide psychological support en route; even unresponsive patients can sometimes hear and understand. Speak calmly and reassuringly to the patient throughout assessment, care, and transport.

In addition to the basic treatment of shock (ie, bleeding control, oxygen administration, warmth, and positioning), you will provide fluid therapy, airway management, and pharmacologic interventions (ie, antiemetics, pain relief, volume expanders, sympathomimetics), as guided by your local protocols.

▶ IV Therapy

IV lines are inserted for one of three purposes: (1) to provide a route for *immediate replacement* of fluid in patients who have significant fluid or blood loss, (2) to provide a route for *potential replacement* in patients who are at risk

of losing significant volumes of fluid or blood, and (3) to provide a route for the administration of medication. The IV fluids of choice will be normal saline or lactated Ringer solution.

Specifically, all patients in hypovolemic shock need IV fluid replacement. In addition, IV access should be obtained in patients who are likely to develop hypovolemic shock because they have one or more of the following conditions: profuse external bleeding, internal bleeding, vaginal bleeding, fracture of the pelvis or femur, severe or widespread burns, heat exhaustion, intractable vomiting or diarrhea, and neurogenic shock or septic shock.

In case of need for emergency administration of drugs, IV lines should also be inserted to keep a vein open. When a patient has poor cardiac output (as in shock), blood is shunted away from the skin and skeletal muscle. Thus, drugs administered subcutaneously or intramuscularly are absorbed at a low and unpredictable rate. Giving a drug directly into the vein ensures that the desired dose of the drug reaches the circulation. Patients who need a vein kept open include those at risk of cardiac arrest (it is easier to start the IV line before the arrest) and patients who may need parenteral medication, such as patients with seizures, diabetes, heart failure, or coma.

The IV flow rate is typically determined by local protocol. The decision on flow rates usually reflects the patient's presumptive diagnosis and the condition of his or her lungs (wet or dry) and takes into account whether the IV line was inserted to keep the vein open for future medication administration. Table 40-6 shows the blood pressure indicators that are often referenced when determining IV flow rates for patients with dry lungs (not pulmonary edema).

Volume Expanders and Plasma Substitutes

Hypovolemic shock should be treated with volume expanders to replace what has been lost or to "fill the container"

Table 40-6	IV Fluid Therapy
Adult SBP (mm Hg)	**Fluid Volume (presumes dry lungs)***
Normotensive (100 to 130)	Fluid challenge usually not needed
Hypotensive (80 to 90) or severe hypotension (50 to 80)	Fluid challenge of 250-mL bolus with reevaluation of blood pressure (maximum of 4 doses) in prehospital environment

Abbreviations: IV, intravenous; SBP, systolic blood pressure

*Fluid therapy for burn patients should follow the Consensus formula (see Chapter 32, *Burns*). In septic shock, the initial fluid bolus is 30 mL/kg.

© Jones & Bartlett Learning.

in relative hypovolemia. For cardiogenic shock, cautious use of volume expanders may increase preload and, subsequently, cardiac output. Positive cardiac inotropic drugs may be administered to increase the strength of contractions, along with rate-altering medications to further enhance perfusion. An example is epinephrine, which serves both purposes with its beta-1 effects.

The vasodilation that accompanies distributive shock creates relative hypovolemia. Treatment involves volume expanders and positive cardiac inotropic drugs. Volume expanders are also indicated for obstructive shock and spinal shock.

A variety of macromolecular solutions have colloidal and osmotic properties similar to those of plasma and are used to maintain circulatory volume in the emergency treatment of shock. Although such solutions cannot replace the RBCs, platelets, or plasma proteins lost in hemorrhage, they are more readily available than is whole blood or plasma in an emergency because they do not require typing and can be carried in the ambulance. Furthermore, during mass-casualty incidents, the supply of blood and blood products may not be adequate, and substitutes must be used. Plasma substitutes do not carry the risk of disease transmission, such as hepatitis or HIV. Available plasma substitutes and volume expanders include dextran (Gentran), plasma protein fractions, and polygeline (Haemaccel).

Dextran is a high-molecular-weight glucose polymer that stays in the vascular space because of its large size. Because it tends to coat RBCs, this substance may cause clotting problems if given in large quantities, and it can also interfere with the cross-matching of blood. For that reason, blood for type- and cross-matching should be drawn *before* administration of dextran. Dextran also interferes with platelet function, so it may increase bleeding. Given that virtually no prehospital research shows dextran to be superior to crystalloid solution administration, medical directors are not likely to approve its use in the field at this time.

Plasma protein fraction (Plasmanate) contains mainly albumin plus a small amount of serum globulin. It is an excellent plasma substitute but is expensive and has been reported to produce hypotensive reactions in some patients.

Polygeline, hetastarch (Hespan), and other starch solutions are constituted to resemble the osmotic and electrolyte composition of the plasma and do not interfere with clotting or blood typing. Many of these products have long shelf lives and may be ideally suited for prehospital use once research proves them effective in improving patient outcomes.

Crystalloids

Crystalloids are solutions that do not contain proteins or other large molecules; that is, they are noncolloids. Their effects in restoring volume in shock are usually quite transitory because the fluid rapidly equilibrates across the capillary walls into the tissues. For example, approximately 60% of infused normal saline, when given as a bolus, diffuses out of the intravascular space within 20 minutes of administration. Thus, when noncolloid solutions are used in the treatment of hemorrhagic shock, you need to administer two to three times the volume of blood loss.

Crystalloids are clearly the fluids of choice when only salt (sodium) and water loss has occurred, such as in dehydration. Debate continues, however, about the role of crystalloids versus colloids in the treatment of shock. Despite a great deal of research on the subject, no overwhelming evidence supports one therapeutic approach over the other. Until such evidence is forthcoming, practical considerations will continue to favor the use of crystalloids for initial fluid resuscitation in the field.

The crystalloids most commonly used for that purpose are normal saline and lactated Ringer solution. Normal saline is simply sodium chloride (0.9% NaCl) in water at a concentration isotonic with the extracellular fluid. Lactated Ringer solution is similarly constituted but includes small amounts of potassium and calcium. It contains 28 mEq of lactate as well, which is added as a buffer (the liver breaks lactate down into bicarbonate). Many trauma surgeons prefer lactated Ringer solution over normal saline because it may help decrease the acidosis in patients with severe hemorrhagic hypovolemia. However, this belief remains controversial, and either solution will benefit the patient.

There is a limit on the usefulness of crystalloids because they do not carry oxygen, change the viscosity of the blood by thinning it, and dissolve the clotting factors. Thus, initial fluid bolus of 1 liter may be required. Fluids are administered judiciously, as aggressive resuscitation before control of bleeding has been demonstrated to increase mortality.[7-10] Consider administering 250-mL boluses with reevaluation of blood pressure to a maximum of four doses in the prehospital environment prior to obtaining online consultation.

Pathophysiology, Assessment, and Management of Specific Types of Shock

The three primary classifications of shock coincide with the conditions that cause them: cardiogenic, distributive, and hypovolemic.

Cardiogenic shock results from a weakening pumping action of the heart. Distributive shock, which is characterized as a relative hypovolemia, can be further broken down into chemical and neural causes. Septic shock results from fluid shifts associated with massive infections and poisons resulting in vasodilation. Neurogenic shock results from blood vessel dilation caused by a brain or spinal/nerve injury, also causing vasodilation. There are also other conditions that decrease tissue perfusion, indirectly affecting the cardiovascular system. Among these are the conditions that obstruct the flow of oxygen into the bloodstream and into the starving tissue, leading to obstructive shock. Conditions that produce obstructive shock include tension pneumothorax, cardiac tamponade, pulmonary embolism, airway obstruction, and carbon monoxide poisoning. Whereas hypovolemic shock reduces the total fluid in the body, hemorrhagic shock, a form of hypovolemic shock, is a direct result of blood loss. Refer to Chapter 30, *Bleeding*, for more information on hemorrhagic shock. The nonhemorrhagic causes of hypovolemic shock (eg, severe burns, heatstroke, gastroenteritis), discussed in this chapter, are commonly grouped by how they reduce perfusion. These types of shock involve either a weakening of the pump, an increase in the size of the container, or a direct mechanical interference with the circulation. The initial management is the same for each type of shock and includes the following steps:

1. Manage the airway.
2. Administer supplemental oxygen if respiratory distress is present and/or SpO$_2$ is less than 94%.
3. Place the patient in a position of comfort.

4. Obtain vital signs, SpO$_2$, breath sounds, and a 12-lead ECG, and check lactate if available (>2.5 mmol/L is abnormal).
5. Obtain IV/IO access for medication or fluid bolus.
6. Maintain body heat.

Additional management may be necessary Table 40-7 .

Words of Wisdom

The Weil-Shubin classification considers shock from a mechanistic point of view.[11] From this perspective, two types of shock are distinguished: **central shock**, which consists of cardiogenic shock and obstructive shock, and **peripheral shock**, which includes hypovolemic shock and distributive shock.

Table 40-7	**Types of Shock**		
Type of Shock	**Examples of Potential Causes**	**Signs and Symptoms**	**Assessment and Treatment**
Cardiogenic	Inadequate heart function Disease of muscle tissue Impaired electrical system Disease or injury	Chest pain Irregular pulse Weak pulse Low blood pressure Cyanosis (lips, nailbeds) Cool, clammy, mottled or flushed skin Anxiety Rales Pulmonary edema Hepatomegaly	If lungs are clear and protocols allow, then administer a fluid challenge of 200 mL (to increase preload) Consider CPAP/BPAP

Obstructive	Mechanical obstruction of the cardiac muscle causing a decrease in cardiac output
	1. Tension pneumothorax
	2. Cardiac tamponade
		Dependent on cause:
		■ Dyspnea
		■ Rapid, weak pulse
		■ Rapid, shallow breaths
		■ Decreased lung compliance
		■ Unilateral, decreased, or absent breath sounds
		■ Decreased BP
		■ JVD
		■ Subcutaneous emphysema
		■ Cyanosis
		■ Tracheal deviation toward affected side
		■ Beck triad (cardiac tamponade):
		  • JVD
		  • Narrowing pulse pressure
		  • Muffled heart tones
			Dependent on cause:
			■ Administer fluid at a KVO rate
			■ Consider chest decompression (injured side for suspected tension pneumothorax)
			■ Consider immediate transport for pericardiocentesis for cardiac tamponade (a procedure that is NOT done in the field).

Type of Shock	Examples of Potential Causes	Signs and Symptoms	Assessment and Treatment
Septic	Severe bacterial infection	Warm, unstable skin temperatures Tachycardia Low BP	Administer fluid boluses to maintain radial pulses Consider sepsis alert program if protocol exists in your region. Consider medications depending on the existence of warm versus cold shock
Neurogenic	Cervical or thoracic spinal cord injury, which causes widespread blood vessel dilation	Bradycardia (slow pulse) or normal pulse Low BP Signs of neck injury	Administer warmed IV fluids to maintain radial pulses Consider vasopressors, steroids, or vagal blocker per local protocols
Anaphylactic	Extreme life-threatening allergic reaction	Develop within seconds Mild itching or rash Burning skin Vascular dilation Generalized edema Coma Rapid death	Determine cause of anaphylaxis Administer epinephrine IM or a vasopressor Administer fluid at a KVO rate Consider bronchodilator or antihistamine
Psychogenic (fainting)	Temporary, generalized vascular dilation Anxiety, bad news, sight of injury or blood, prospect of medical treatment, severe pain, illness, tiredness	Rapid pulse Normal or low BP	Determine duration of unresponsiveness Suspect head injury if patient is confused or slow to respond
Hypovolemic	Blood or fluid loss	Rapid, weak pulse Low BP Change in mental status Cyanosis (lips, nailbeds) Cool, clammy skin Increased respiratory rate	Control external bleeding Provide fluid resuscitation en route After initial fluid resuscitation, consider use of vasopressors to maintain BP
Respiratory insufficiency	Severe chest injury, airway obstruction	Rapid, weak pulse Low BP Change in mental status Cyanosis (lips, nailbeds) Cool, clammy skin Increased respiratory rate	Seal hole in chest Stabilize impaled objects Assure adequate ventilation; consider positive pressure ventilation Administer fluid at a KVO rate

Abbreviations: BP, blood pressure; CPAP/BPAP, continuous positive airway pressure/bilevel positive airway pressure; IM, intramuscularly; JVD, jugular venous distention; KVO, keep vein open

Note: For management of patients with adrenal insufficiency, refer to Chapter 23, *Endocrine Emergencies*.

© Jones & Bartlett Learning.

▶ Cardiogenic Shock

Cardiogenic shock occurs when the heart is unable to circulate sufficient blood to maintain adequate peripheral oxygen delivery. Circulation of blood throughout the vascular system requires the constant pumping action of a normal and vigorous heart muscle. Many diseases can cause destruction or inflammation of this muscle. Within certain limits, the heart can adapt to these problems. However, if too much muscular damage occurs, then the heart no longer functions effectively. Filling is impaired because of a lack of pressure to return blood to the heart (preload), or outflow is obstructed by a lack of pumping function. In either case, direct pump failure is the cause of shock. In the case of ischemic heart disease, pump failure is generally due to a loss of 40% or more of the functioning myocardium.

The most common cause of cardiogenic shock is an AMI accompanied by 40% dysfunction of the left ventricle. Anterior infarcts more commonly lead to cardiogenic shock than do inferior ones. Studies show that 74% of the patients who develop cardiogenic shock as a complication of AMI do so within the first 24 hours.[12] Other causes of cardiogenic shock may be right ventricular failure, valvular disorders, cardiomyopathies, ventricular septal defects, papillary muscle rupture, myocardial insufficiency, and sustained dysrhythmias. Some experts consider VF to be the ultimate form of cardiogenic shock. The causes may be classified as intrinsic or extrinsic, with the aforementioned examples being intrinsic causes. These conditions manifest with poor contractility, decreased cardiac output, or impaired ventricular filling. Extrinsic causes of cardiogenic shock include pericardial tamponade, effusion, pulmonary emboli, and tension pneumothorax. Cardiogenic shock may occur in approximately 7% to 10% of patients admitted to the hospital following an AMI.[13-15] Populations at the greatest risk of developing cardiogenic shock are older adult patients, patients with a history of

diabetes mellitus, and patients with a history of AMI with an ejection fraction of less than 35%. Ejection fraction is the portion of the blood ejected from the ventricle during systole. Normal ejection fraction is 55% to 70% of the blood in the heart leaving the left ventricle, as measured with an echocardiogram, magnetic resonance imaging, or computed tomography of the heart, or during cardiac catheterization.

The diagnosis of cardiogenic shock may be difficult to make in the field. Once the diagnosis has been made in a definitive setting, newer treatment modalities have greatly improved the long-term prognosis. Such modalities include medications such as super aspirins, blood thinners, inotropic agents, and fibrinolytics and surgical procedures such as angioplasty and stenting, coronary artery bypass, and insertion of a ventricular assist device.

Prolonged efforts to stabilize the condition of a patient in cardiogenic shock in the field are not recommended. Because this is a time-sensitive patient, you should expedite transport as quickly as possible. Place the patient in a position of comfort, secure the airway, monitor the SpO_2, and administer supplemental oxygen (if SpO_2 is less than 94% or there is respiratory distress). Consider continuous positive airway pressure or bilevel positive

YOU are the Paramedic   PART 5

You prepare to intubate your patient nasally due to the presence of spontaneous respirations and a positive gag reflex. The patient is intubated with lubrication without difficulty using the Beck Airway Airflow Monitor (BAAM) device on the tube. You confirm tube placement by auscultation and initiation of $ETCO_2$ monitoring. The tube is secured and connected to the automatic transport ventilator (ATV). You reassess all vital signs including cardiac rhythm and decide to obtain a 12-lead ECG to see if the patient may have also had an MI. Your patient continues to be in a sinus tachycardia. You are aware that dopamine is a sympathomimetic and may precipitate ventricular dysrhythmias, so you continue to monitor your patient closely. Once you have completed your reassessment, you contact the receiving facility to report on your patient. On arrival, you carefully transfer your patient to the ED stretcher in the assigned room. You provide a bedside report as the patient is transitioned to the hospital's equipment and monitors. You complete your patient care report while your partner prepares the ambulance for the next call.

Recording Time: 20 Minutes	
Skin	Pale and cool
Pulse	104 beats/min
Blood pressure	76/48 mm Hg
Respirations	12 breaths/min via ET tube using an ATV
Oxygen saturation (SpO$_2$)	99% on 100% oxygen
End-tidal carbon dioxide (ETCO$_2$)	42 mm Hg

9. What is the benefit of assessing lung compliance in the ventilated shock patient?
10. Discuss how your assessment findings for this patient led you to a differential diagnosis of septic shock.

airway pressure (CPAP/BPAP). Apply ECG electrodes, document the initial rhythm, and obtain a 12-lead ECG. IV access should consist of administration of a crystalloid solution. Auscultate the lungs; if they are clear and protocols allow, try a fluid challenge of 200 mL to increase the preload, and evaluate the effects on the blood pressure and breath sounds.

Some EMS systems advocate the use of dopamine at low doses in the beta range (5 mg/kg per minute) if the patient has a MAP of less than 60 mm Hg. Elevating the blood pressure by using high-dose dopamine in the alpha range may be temporarily ordered by medical control at the expense of other target organs. In such a case, anticipate rapid tachycardia that could adversely impact ventricular filling. Combination drug therapy is often needed at the hospital (eg, dopamine plus dobutamine, or norepinephrine) while awaiting cardiac catheterization, hemodynamic monitoring catheters, and insertion of an intra-aortic balloon pump.

▶ Obstructive Shock

Obstructive causes of shock are those not directly associated with fluid loss, pump failure, or vessel dilation. **Obstructive shock** occurs when blood flow in the heart or great vessels becomes blocked. Two of the most common examples of obstructive shock causes in trauma are tension pneumothorax and cardiac tamponade. Others include a pulmonary embolus, which can block the oxygen from entering the bloodstream through the alveoli, or carbon monoxide poisoning, which can block the oxygen from loading into the RBCs as they pass through the lungs.

Tension Pneumothorax and Cardiac Tamponade

Tension pneumothorax is caused by damage to the lung tissue. This damage allows air normally held within the lung to escape into the chest cavity. If a pneumothorax is allowed to continue untreated, then a sufficient amount of air will accumulate within the chest cavity and begin applying pressure to the structures of the mediastinum. When the trapped air begins to shift the chest organs toward the uninjured side, a pneumothorax becomes known as a tension pneumothorax. A pneumothorax is a respiratory problem, but a tension pneumothorax is a serious and life-threatening condition because the kinking of the vena cava that occurs as the mediastinum shifts can precede cardiac arrest. Usually the only action that can prevent eventual death from a tension pneumothorax is decompression of the injured side of the chest, relieving the pressure in the chest cavity and allowing the heart to expand fully again. Fortunately, needle chest decompression is a skill many providers are allowed to perform. The decision to decompress the chest should always be based on good evidence that a tension pneumothorax exists with decreased perfusion.

Cardiac tamponade is another traumatic condition that leads to obstructive shock. It is caused by blunt or penetrating trauma, tumors, or pericarditis and can progress quickly. Cardiac tamponade occurs when blood leaks into the tough fibrous membrane known as the pericardium, causing an accumulation of blood within the pericardial sac.

Blood accumulates quickly within the pericardium. This accumulation of leaked blood leads to compression of the heart. Because the pericardium has minimal ability to stretch, each contraction of the heart allows more blood accumulation between the heart and the sac. This accumulated blood prevents the heart from opening up to allow complete refilling. Continued pressure within the pericardial sac obstructs the flow of blood into the heart, resulting in decreased outflow from the heart. Vital clues that a cardiac tamponade is present include muffled heart sounds and SBP and DBP starting to merge (ie, the SBP drops and the DBP rises). You may also note electrical alternans and a small QRS on the ECG as this condition is developing.

The treatment for cardiac tamponade is pericardiocentesis, which involves inserting a needle attached to a syringe into the chest far enough to penetrate the pericardium and then withdrawing fluid. This technique is risky, however, and medical control rarely allows it to be performed by paramedics. Early recognition, rapid transport, and calling ahead to alert the ED are imperative to the patient's survival from this life-threatening condition. As always, follow your local ALS protocols.

▶ Distributive Shock

Distributive shock occurs when there is widespread dilation of the **resistance vessels** (small arterioles), the **capacitance vessels** (small venules), or both. As a result, the circulating blood volume pools in the expanded vascular beds and tissue perfusion decreases. The four most common types of distributive shock are septic shock, neurogenic shock, anaphylactic shock, and psychogenic shock.

Septic Shock

Sepsis comes from the Greek word *sepein*, meaning "to putrefy." **Septic shock** has been defined as the presence of sepsis syndrome plus an SBP of less than 90 mm Hg or a decrease from the baseline blood pressure of more than 40 mm Hg. There has been considerable confusion over the years about defining the sickest of the septic patients, and the term was further defined in 2016 by consensus. Thus, septic shock is defined as a subset of sepsis in which underlying circulatory, cellular, and metabolic abnormalities are associated with a greater risk of mortality than in sepsis alone. The clinical criteria include hypotension requiring use of vasopressors to maintain MAP of at least 65 mm Hg and having a serum lactate greater than 2 mmol/L persisting despite adequate fluid resuscitation.[16]

Sepsis occurs as a result of widespread infection, usually due to gram-negative bacterial organisms; gram-positive bacteria, fungi, viruses, and rickettsia can also be causative agents. Complex interactions occur between the pathogen and the body's defense systems. Initially, the body's defense mechanisms may keep the infection under control. The infection activates the inflammatory-immune response, which invokes humoral, cellular, and biochemical pathways. This response results in increased microvascular permeability (leaky capillaries), vasodilation, third-space fluid shifts, and microthrombi formation. In some patients, an uncontrolled and unregulated inflammatory-immune response occurs, resulting in hypoperfusion to the cells owing to opening of arteriovenous shunts, tissue destruction, and organ death. Left untreated, the result is MODS and, often, death.

Septic shock is a complex problem. First, there is an insufficient volume of fluid in the container, because much of the blood has leaked out of the vascular system (hypovolemia). Second, the fluid that leaks out often collects in the respiratory system, interfering with ventilation. Third, a larger-than-normal vascular bed is asked to contain the smaller-than-normal volume of intravascular fluid.

Septic shock presents similarly to hemorrhagic shock in that the patient will have a rapid weak, thready pulse; shallow, rapid respirations; and altered mental status. One major difference is that patients with septic shock often present with warm or hot skin due to the elevated core body temperature associated with the infection. Core body temperature is considered unstable at less than 96.8°F (36°C) or greater than 101.3°F (38.5°C).

The proper treatment of septic shock requires complex hospital management, including antibiotics. If you suspect a patient has septic shock, then take appropriate standard precautions and transport as promptly as possible. Administer high-flow oxygen during transport. Ventilatory support may be necessary to maintain adequate tidal volume. If the patient is normotensive after initial fluid therapy, then administer dopamine to maintain the blood pressure and renal perfusion. If the patient remains hypotensive and vasodilated in "warm" shock, norepinephrine is the appropriate intervention. If administering these drugs is permitted by medical control in your region, the dosages should be spelled out in the local protocols. If the patient remains hypotensive and vasoconstricted in "cold" shock, then administering epinephrine is the most appropriate course of action. Consider medications depending on the existence of warm versus cold shock. Provide blankets to conserve body heat. Gain IV or IO access immediately and administer fluid boluses (30 mL/kg) of crystalloid to maintain radial pulses, in accordance with local protocols.[18] As this is an unstable patient, frequent reassessment of hemodynamic status will be necessary while en route to the ED.

Neurogenic Shock

Neurogenic shock usually results from spinal cord injury. Less commonly, it may derive from medical causes such as brain conditions, tumors, or pressure on the spinal cord. The effect of these conditions is loss of normal sympathetic nervous system tone and vasodilation.

In neurogenic shock, the muscles in the walls of the blood vessels are cut off from the nerve impulses that cause them to contract. As a consequence, all vessels below the level of the spinal injury dilate widely, increasing the size and capacity of the vascular system and causing blood to pool. There may actually be visible lines of demarcation on the skin found in the patient with spinal shock. The available 11 to 13 pints (5 to 6 L) of blood in the body can no longer fill this enlarged vascular system. Perfusion of organs and tissues becomes inadequate, even though no blood or fluid loss, and shock occurs. The patient experiences relative hypovolemia, which leads to hypotension (SBP usually between 80 and 100 mm Hg). In addition, relative bradycardia occurs because the sympathetic nervous system is not stimulated to release catecholamines. The skin is pink, warm, and dry because of cutaneous vasodilation. There is no release of epinephrine and norepinephrine, which would otherwise produce the classic sign of pale, cool, diaphoretic skin. Instead, a characteristic sign of neurogenic shock is the absence of sweating below the level of injury.

The term **spinal shock** refers to the local neurologic condition that occurs after a spinal injury produces motor and sensory losses (which may not be permanent). Damage to the spinal cord, particularly at the upper cervical levels, may cause significant injury to the autonomic nervous system, which controls the size and muscular tone of the blood vessels. Swelling and edema of the cord begin within 30 minutes after an insult, creating a "physiologic" transaction with nerve conduction disruption. Secondary cord injury, aside from the initial lesions, often develops over the first few days due to the ischemic spinal cord tissue. Severe pain may be present just above the level of injury

Controversies

A recent analysis of a series of nine studies in which septic shock was assessed and early treatment begun in the prehospital setting has revealed that further research is still required in this area. The authors state that there is little robust evidence addressing the impact of prehospital interventions on outcomes in sepsis. That which is available is of very low quality and indicates that prehospital interventions have limited impact on outcomes in sepsis beyond improving process outcomes and expediting the patient's passage through the emergency care pathway. Evidence indicating that prehospital antibiotic therapy and fluid resuscitation improve patient outcomes is lacking. Well-conducted studies addressing key clinical interventions, such as antibiotic administration and fluid resuscitation, are required.[17] Nonetheless, there is evidence that early in-hospital treatment is lifesaving. If you suspect sepsis in the field, notify the emergency department en route so that they can be prepared to initiate a sepsis protocol on arrival.

owing to a zone of heightened sensitivity. Spinal shock is characterized by flaccid paralysis, flaccid sphincters, and absent reflexes. There is an absence of all pain, temperature, touch, proprioception, and pressure below the level of the lesion; absent or impaired thermoregulation; absent somatic and visceral sensations below the lesion; bowel distention; and loss of peristalsis. The level of the injury to the cord is related to the severity of neurogenic shock development. Injury above the T1 level can disrupt all the spinal tracts that control the entire sympathetic system. Injuries from T1 to L3 may only partially interrupt sympathetic outflow. The higher the level of the injury, the more severe it is and the more likely it is that the patient will develop spinal shock.

The care of a patient with suspected neurogenic shock is similar to the general management approach for any patient with shock. In addition, the patient should be immobilized to minimize further movement and injury to the spine. Specific concerns relate to keeping the patient warm because a spinal injury can disrupt the thermoregulatory mechanisms and leave the patient vulnerable to hypothermia.

Another specific concern relates to the issue of fluid therapy. You should determine the necessity for IV fluids based on the patient's hemodynamic status. Maintain adequate hydration and volume status to keep the SBP at 90 mm Hg or higher. General hemodynamic resuscitation includes volume loading with normal saline IV fluid boluses in 20-mL/kg increments up to 4 pints (2 L) through a large-bore (18-gauge) IV catheter. If possible, use warm fluid to prevent hypothermia.

In pure neurogenic shock not associated with hypovolemic shock or still present after concomitant injuries have been stabilized, administering vagal blockers (eg, atropine, 0.5 mg, by rapid IV push [up to a maximum of 3 mg] if the pulse remains severely bradycardic) and vasopressor agents (eg, a dopamine drip beginning at 10 mcg/kg per minute and titrating to 20 mcg/kg per minute) may be more effective than overhydrating the patient would be. Monitor the patient's response to vasopressors; it may be less than expected owing to the compromise of the sympathetic nervous system.

Anaphylactic Shock

Anaphylaxis occurs when a person reacts violently to a substance to which he or she has been sensitized. **Sensitization** refers to the development of a heightened reaction to a substance. An allergic reaction typically does not occur, or occurs in a milder form, during sensitization. Do not be misled by a patient who reports no history of allergic reaction to a substance following a first or second exposure: each subsequent exposure after sensitization tends to produce a more severe reaction.

In **anaphylactic shock**, there is no loss of blood, no vascular damage, and only a slight possibility of direct cardiac muscular injury. Instead, the patient experiences widespread vascular dilation, resulting in relative

hypovolemia. In other words, relative to the now larger container, the normal blood volume is less. The combination of poor oxygenation and poor perfusion, however, may easily prove fatal.

In anaphylaxis, immune system chemicals, such as histamine and other vasodilator proteins, are released when exposed to an allergen **Figure 40-10**. Their release causes the severe bronchoconstriction that accounts for wheezing if the patient is actually moving enough air. Anaphylaxis is also accompanied by urticaria (hives). The results are widespread vasodilation, which causes distributive shock, and blood vessels that continue to leak. Fluid leaks out of the blood vessels and into the interstitial space, resulting in hypovolemia and potentially causing significant swelling. In some cases, this swelling may occlude the upper airway, resulting in a life-threatening condition **Figure 40-11**.

Recurrent large areas of subcutaneous edema of sudden onset, usually disappearing within 24 hours and mainly seen in young women (frequently as a result of allergy to food or drugs), are called **angioedema**.

When a patient experiences shock due to a severe allergic reaction, you need to act fast. Remove the inciting cause if possible. Resolve any immediate life threats to the ABCs, which may require aggressive airway management (ie, intubation and/or rapid sequence intubation) and supplemental oxygen administration. Evaluate the patient's ventilatory status and the need for bag-mask ventilation.

Provide cardiovascular support with IV fluid challenges of crystalloid solution. Reverse the target-organ effect by administering epinephrine or a vasopressor such as dopamine in high doses. Consider the need for a bronchodilator such as albuterol (Proventil) or ipratropium (Atrovent). Impede further mediator release with an antihistamine such as diphenhydramine (Benadryl). If the patient has an epinephrine injector, take it to the hospital. All paramedics carry epinephrine in their drug boxes, and you should administer epinephrine intramuscularly as early as possible (prior to intubation).

Psychogenic Shock

A patient who is experiencing **psychogenic shock** has had a sudden reaction of the nervous system that produces a temporary, generalized vascular dilation, resulting in syncope (vasovagal syncope). Blood pools in the dilated vessels, reducing the blood supply to the brain; as a result, the brain ceases to function normally, and the patient faints. There are many causes of syncope, and it is important to realize that some are of a serious nature while others are not. Causes of syncope that are potentially life threatening result from events such as an irregular heartbeat or a brain aneurysm. Always consider all the potential causes of syncope before you decide it was just a simple vasovagal syncope. Syncope is discussed in detail in Chapter 18, *Neurologic Emergencies*. Non–life-threatening events that cause syncope may be the receipt of bad news

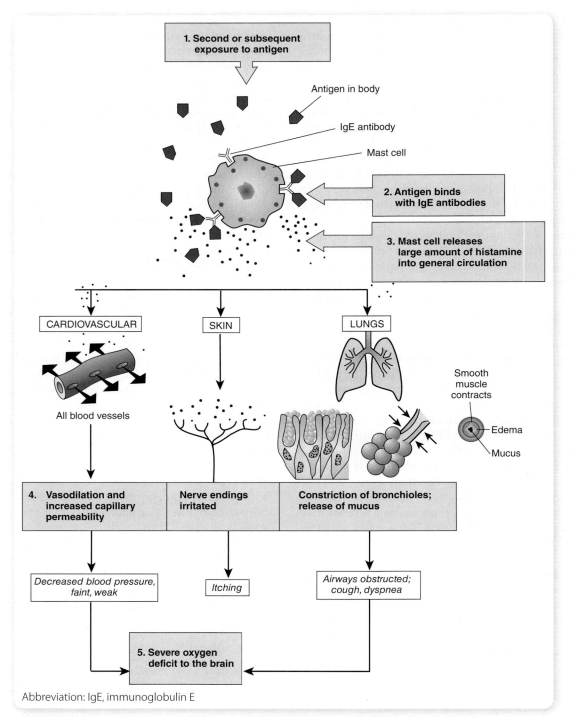

Figure 40-10 The effects of anaphylaxis (type I hypersensitivity reaction).
© Jones & Bartlett Learning.

or experiencing fear or unpleasant sights (such as the sight of blood).

In an uncomplicated case of fainting, once the patient collapses and becomes supine, circulation to the brain is usually restored and with it, a normal state of functioning. Remember, psychogenic shock can significantly worsen other types of shock. If the attack has caused the patient to fall, then check for injuries, especially in older adult patients. You should also assess the patient thoroughly for any other abnormality. If, after regaining consciousness, the patient is unable to walk without weakness, dizziness, or pain, then you should suspect another problem, such as head injury. You should transport this patient promptly.

Record your initial observations of vital signs (including orthostatic) and level of consciousness. Obtain

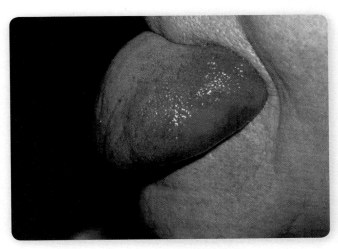

Figure 40-11 In anaphylaxis, interstitial fluid may cause significant swelling. In some cases, this swelling may occlude the upper airway, resulting in a life-threatening condition.

© SPL/Photo Researchers, Inc.

an ECG. In addition, try to learn from bystanders whether the patient complained of anything before fainting and how long he or she was unresponsive.

▶ Hypovolemic Shock

As discussed in Chapter 30, *Bleeding*, when shock comes about because of inadequate blood volume, it is termed **hypovolemic shock**. There are hemorrhagic and nonhemorrhagic causes of hypovolemic shock. Volume can be lost as blood (internal or external hemorrhagic shock), plasma (due to burns; nonhemorrhagic shock), or electrolyte solution (due to excessive GI fluid losses (vomiting, diarrhea), or profuse sweating; nonhemorrhagic shock).

Nonhemorrhagic hypovolemic shock will be discussed in this chapter. See Chapter 30, *Bleeding*, for information about hemorrhagic shock.

Nonhemorrhagic shock occurs when the fluid loss is contained within the body, as in dehydration, burn injury, crush injury, and anaphylaxis. With severe thermal burns, for example, intravascular plasma leaks from the circulatory system into the burned tissues that lie adjacent to the injury. By comparison, crushing injuries may result in the loss of blood and plasma from damaged (crushed) vessels into injured tissues.

Abnormal losses of fluids and electrolytes (dehydration) may occur through a variety of mechanisms, including the following:

- GI losses, especially through vomiting and diarrhea
- Increased loss as a consequence of fever, hyperventilation, or high environmental temperatures (through the lungs)
- Increased and excessive sweating
- Internal losses ("third-space" losses), as in peritonitis, pancreatitis, and ileus

- Plasma losses from burns, drains, and granulating wounds

Other causes of body fluid deficits include ascites, diabetes insipidus, acute renal failure, and osmotic diuresis secondary to hyperosmolar states (ie, diabetic ketoacidosis).

Most of the typical symptoms and signs of shock result from inadequate tissue oxygenation and the body's attempts to compensate for volume loss. The earliest signs of shock are restlessness and anxiety: the patient looks scared! The decline in tissue perfusion may not be enough to produce obvious asphyxia, but it *is* setting off alarms all over the body, to which the patient responds with a feeling of apprehension—a "gut" feeling that something is not right. If the patient is conscious, then the patient may report being thirsty, reflecting the deficit of fluids in the body; at the same time, the patient may feel nauseated and even vomit. The diversion of blood flow away from low-priority peripheral tissues causes the skin to become pale, cold, and clammy; sometimes it has a mottled appearance. Meanwhile, the heart speeds up to circulate the remaining RBCs more rapidly, producing a rapid, weak pulse—rapid because the heart is beating faster, weak because the blood vessels are now narrow and the volume moving through them is decreased.

In each case, the fluid loss has a unique electrolyte composition, and long-term therapy aims to restore the deficient body chemicals. For treatment in the field, however, all excessive fluid losses can be considered to lead to dehydration.

Symptoms of dehydration include loss of appetite (anorexia), nausea, vomiting, and sometimes fainting when standing up (postural syncope). Physical examination of a dehydrated patient reveals poor skin turgor (the skin over the forehead or sternum will "tent" when pinched); a shrunken, furrowed tongue; and sunken eyes. The pulse will be weak and rapid, rising more than 15 beats/min when the patient is raised from a recumbent to a sitting position (a maneuver that may cause the patient to feel faint). When fluid and electrolyte depletion is severe, shock and coma may be present.

A dehydrated patient needs replacement of fluid and electrolytes. Consider administering 20 mL/kg in 250-mL boluses, checking blood pressure after each bolus. Keep the patient in the position that optimizes circulation to the brain (follow local protocol).

The priorities in treating a patient in hypovolemic shock are the same as in treating any other patient—namely, the ABCs. Establish and maintain an open airway. Keep suction at hand to clear the mouth and pharynx if the patient should vomit. Administer supplemental oxygen, and assist ventilation as needed. Keep the patient warm.

En route to the ED, establish at least one, and preferably two, large-bore peripheral IV lines (18 gauge), using an over-the-needle catheter. If required by protocol, then draw blood (two red-top blood collection [Vacutainer] tubes and one purple-top tube) so the ED personnel may obtain a hematocrit, type- and cross-match, and other tests immediately on your arrival. Unless local medical policy favors a different resuscitation fluid, administer normal saline or lactated Ringer solution. For guidance, refer to your local protocol. Consider administering 20 mL/kg in 250-mL boluses, checking blood pressure after each bolus. If warmed fluids are available, then consider giving that as well.

Do not give the patient anything by mouth because he or she is likely to vomit. If vomiting occurs, then administering an antiemetic should be appropriate, especially if you have a long, bumpy ride to the ED. Keep the patient at normal temperature, covering the patient with a blanket and warming the patient compartment of the ambulance; patients in hypovolemic shock are often unable to conserve body heat effectively and are easily chilled. Place the patient in a position with the head elevated to a 15° to 30° angle and the legs elevated to a 30° angle on pillows (injuries permitting).

Monitor the ECG rhythm because any critically ill or injured patient is likely to have dysrhythmias. Also monitor the patient's mental status, pulse rate, blood pressure, SpO_2, and $ETCO_2$. In a patient with substantial vasoconstriction, the blood pressure sounds may be difficult to hear, especially under field conditions. If you can feel a pulse over the femoral artery but not over the radial artery, the SBP is most likely between 70 and 80 mm Hg. The pulse oximetry and $ETCO_2$ findings may help you assess perfusion status and the need for ventilation intervention, although they are not entirely reliable with poor perfusion states. Depending on local practice, medical control may order sodium bicarbonate to treat acidosis or a vasopressor (such as dopamine [Inotropin], metaraminol, or norepinephrine) to enhance vasoconstriction.

As bleeding or fluid loss continues, blood pressure finally falls in the shock patient. Do not wait until blood pressure falls before you suspect shock and begin treatment! Falling blood pressure is a *late* sign in shock (decompensated shock), signaling the collapse of all compensatory mechanisms and the fact that the patient may already have a volume fluid loss of 30% or more. Furthermore, blood pressure measured at the arm provides you with little information about perfusion of vital organs; it tells only about perfusion of the arms.

The goal in treating shock is to save the brain, lungs, and kidneys; these organs must remain perfused if the patient is to survive and return to a healthy life. The best indication of brain perfusion is the patient's state of consciousness. If the patient is alert, then the brain is being perfused adequately despite what the blood pressure findings show. If the patient has an altered mental status, perfusion of the brain is inadequate. Kidney perfusion can be gauged by urine output in a catheterized patient. Adequately perfused kidneys put out at least 30 mL to 50 mL of urine per hour; poorly perfused kidneys shut down and stop putting out any urine.

In the field—where patients will not ordinarily have urinary catheters—you can estimate the patient's peripheral perfusion by testing for capillary refill, although this is not the most reliable indicator. To determine how well the *vital* organs are being perfused, you must rely on the patient's state of consciousness.

▶ Respiratory Insufficiency

A patient with a severe chest injury, such as flail chest, or obstruction of the airway may be unable to breathe in an adequate volume to maintain appropriate tissue oxygenation. As a result, the ventilation process of respiration is affected; enough oxygen cannot be inspired to meet the metabolic demand.

An insufficient concentration of oxygen in the blood can produce shock as rapidly as vascular causes can, even if the volume of blood, the volume of the vessels, and the action of the heart are all normal. Without oxygen, the organs in the body cannot survive, and their cells promptly start to deteriorate.

Certain types of poisoning may affect the ability of cells to metabolize or carry oxygen. Carbon monoxide has a 200 to 250 times greater affinity for hemoglobin than oxygen has. If a patient is in an environment where he or she inhales carbon monoxide, then it will bind to the hemoglobin, forming carboxyhemoglobin, rather than allowing oxygen to bind. This results in a hypoxic state if not corrected. Cyanide impairs the ability of cells to metabolize oxygen within the cell, and cellular asphyxia may occur.

Anemia occurs when there is an abnormally low number of RBCs. RBCs contain hemoglobin, an iron-containing pigment. Hemoglobin transports oxygen from the lungs to the tissues. Each hemoglobin molecule is able to carry four molecules of oxygen. Anemia may be the result of either chronic or acute bleeding, a deficiency in certain vitamins or minerals, or an underlying disease process. If anemia is present, tissues may be hypoxic because the blood may not be able to carry adequate oxygen, even though the hemoglobin is fully saturated. In this situation, a pulse oximeter may indicate that there is adequate saturation, even though the tissues are hypoxic. This type of hypoxia is known as *hypoxemic hypoxia*.

When you are treating a patient who is in shock as a result of inadequate respiration, you must immediately seal any hole or stabilize any impaled object in the chest that is affecting ventilation and must then secure and maintain the airway. Clear the mouth and throat of anything obstructing the air passages, including mucus, vomitus, and foreign material. Assess the SpO_2, $ETCO_2$, and vital signs, and determine the need to assist ventilations with a bag-mask device and supplemental oxygen. Determine the most appropriate transport destination based on the patient's condition and local protocols.

■ Transport of Shock Patients

If you suspect a patient is in shock, then transport is inevitable; the questions you should be asking yourself are when, where, and how. Remember, scene time should be limited to 10 minutes or less. Preplanning will help determine where the patient should be taken and how to get the patient to the ED. Know how to access aeromedical transport in your community. Consideration for the priority of the patient and the availability of a regional trauma center should be your concerns, and local transport protocols may specifically deal with these issues. Patients who are suspected to be in shock, whether compensated or decompensated, may benefit from early surgical intervention and should be transported to a facility with appropriate capabilities. Patients with cardiogenic shock may need to go to a hospital with comprehensive cardiac care capabilities such as an interventional catheterization lab or a heart surgery program. If a facility of this type is not readily available, then medical control should help you make the transport decision. In some communities, reaching a hospital with advanced cardiac care capabilities will involve transport to a local facility and transfer (often aeromedical) to a tertiary care facility with the appropriate facilities and staff to handle the patient's complex needs.

YOU are the Paramedic   SUMMARY

1. **What should your next course of action be for this patient?**

   After conducting a scene size-up and forming a general impression of this patient, you recognize that you are dealing with a critical patient. There was no sign of trauma, and indications lead you to believe that this patient has been sick for several days. His altered mental status is a possible indication of the critical nature of his condition. Conduct a primary survey to identify and treat immediate life threats. Perform a rapid full-body scan during your secondary assessment to identify clues that will help determine the working diagnosis and initiate appropriate treatment.

2. **Discuss the role of intuition in forming a differential diagnosis and explain how bias can affect that diagnosis.**

   Intuition is safest to use in making treatment decisions that heighten your index of suspicion and result in increased care as opposed to downgrading your response to the patient's condition. It is important to remember that the more complex the patient, the greater the risk of obscuring patterns and matching them incorrectly. If you remain aware of the potential biases—confirmation bias, anchoring bias, and arbitrary bias—then it is easier to avoid being trapped by them.

3. **Describe the contributing factors that would lead you to label this patient as critical.**

   The patient would be labeled as a critical patient due to a peri-arrest condition. The peri-arrest period is prior to and following cardiac arrest. Shock, especially in its decompensation phase, is one of the conditions that can progress to cardiac arrest. While assessing this patient, you have determined he has a history of acute coronary syndrome and COPD and takes medication that supports these findings.

4. **Discuss pathophysiologic changes associated with septic shock.**

   When the body is stressed, the autonomic nervous system redirects blood flow toward the vital organs. Inadequate circulatory support to other areas of the body will lead to inadequate tissue perfusion or hypoperfusion. Pale or mottled skin discoloration is a good indicator of hypoperfusion. As shock progresses due to a failure to correct the precipitating cause, the vital organs become hypoperfused. As systemic vascular resistance begins to fall, cardiac output drops. This eventually leads to systemwide collapse of perfusion, including that to the myocardium, which further worsens the body's ability to compensate. In septic shock, the initial changes are due to widespread vasodilation due to infection that has activated the inflammatory-immune response. Fluid shifts and microvascular permeability decreases the available volume of fluid for circulation. Leakage in the pulmonary system creates congestion that reduces the ability for adequate gas exchange. Inadequate volume leads to decreased preload, which further compromises adequate cardiac output and perfusion status.

5. **Discuss the phase of shock this patient may be in.**

   Based on assessment findings, this patient may be in decompensated shock. Compensatory mechanisms have begun to fail as indicated by a reduction in blood pressure and cardiac function. System vasoconstriction is occurring as noted by the pale, cool, and mottled skin. These nonperfused tissues are becoming hypoxic. Because there is clear indication that reductions in cardiac output, blood pressure, and tissue perfusion are occurring, consideration should be given to the potential that this patient is entering irreversible shock.

6. Describe how you should manage this patient with suspected shock.

After establishing a patent airway and suctioning as needed, provide high-flow supplemental oxygen. In the patient who is unable to maintain his or her own airway, assist ventilations via a bag-mask device or the placement of an advanced airway. Gain IV access and support the circulation by administering isotonic fluids (ie, normal saline) to help improve blood pressure and tissue perfusion. Establish an available IV access port to allow for rapid medication administration as indicated. Consider administering vasopressors appropriate to the patient's condition. Nonpharmacologic interventions such as body positioning and prevention of hypothermia should also be employed. Cardiac monitoring allows for early identification of possible dysrhythmias and changes in cardiac function.

7. Why should a patient's hypoxic drive not be a consideration when treating shock?

In healthy people, peripheral chemoreceptors detect levels of carbon dioxide in the blood ($PaCO_2$) and respond by increasing the respiratory rate when there is too much. In some patients with chronic bronchitis or emphysema, the patient maintains a higher than normal level chronically. The chemoreceptors no longer are sensitive to the excessive carbon monoxide, and the CNS does not respond to these higher levels. The amount of oxygen in the blood (PaO_2) becomes the new mechanism for determining the need to alter respiratory rates. As levels rise with the administration of high concentrations of oxygen, the CNS may slow or cease respirations. Although this outcome is possible, the acutely ill patient, such as a patient in shock, should still receive high concentrations of oxygen in response to hypoxia due to diminished perfusion.

8. What are the anticipated benefits of dopamine administration for this patient?

Dopamine's action on alpha and beta-1 adrenergic receptors can result in increased blood pressure and, specific to beta-1 receptors, may have a positive inotropic effect on the heart. Cardiac output, stroke volume, and myocardial contractility should increase without excessive increases in myocardial oxygen demand. Dopamine also has less chronotropic effects than other sympathetic agonists, such as isoproterenol and epinephrine.

9. What is the benefit of assessing lung compliance in the ventilated shock patient?

Decreased lung compliance can be seen in patients with traumatic chest injuries such as chest wall trauma or in the presence of a tension pneumothorax due to increased pressures in the chest. Patients with acute respiratory distress syndrome (ARDS) may also have decreased compliance due to the formation of interstitial fluid accumulation in the lungs. Surfactant is lost and alveolar sacs collapse, creating impaired gas exchange. ARDS may be seen in the acute sepsis or shock patient, so assessment for lung compliance is beneficial to aid in identification of the presence of ARDS.

10. Discuss how your assessment findings for this patient led you to a "field" diagnosis of septic shock.

Assessment of this patient revealed an older man (77 years old) with a recent history of cough and fever. He had comorbid factors that included chronic bronchitis. Complaints on deep breathing led you to suspect a potential for pneumonia. He had not been seen for at least 24 hours, indicating less mobility than usual and a possible decrease in appetite based on his refusal of lunch at least 3 days ago. His clinical presentation of shock signs and symptoms in conjunction with your review of potential causes leads you to conclude infection as the underlying condition. You are aware an untreated infection in the older patient in addition to comorbid conditions increases the likelihood of progression to sepsis.

EMS Patient Care Report (PCR)

Date: 11-03-18	Incident No.: 201064376		Nature of Call: Unresponsive patient		Location: 4950 Waters Way, Apartment 512
Dispatched: 0915	**En Route:** 0916	**At Scene:** 0924	**Transport:** 0934	**At Hospital:** 0950	**In Service:** 1015

Patient Information

Age: 77 **Sex:** M **Weight (in kg [lb]):** 64.5 kg (142 lb)	**Allergies:** Shellfish **Medications:** Lisinopril 10 mg daily, ASA 81 mg daily, albuterol MDI 2 puffs TID and PRN, furosemide 20 mg daily **Past Medical History:** HTN, AMI 5 years ago, chronic bronchitis **Chief Complaint:** Altered mental status

Vital Signs

Time: 0930	BP: Not yet obtained	Pulse: 120	Respirations: 24 breaths/min, assisted	Spo₂: Not obtainable
Time: 0936	BP: 68 by palpation	Pulse: 118	Respirations: 20 breaths/min, assisted	Spo₂: Not obtainable
Time: 0941	BP: 72 by palpation	Pulse: 100	Respirations: 8 spont.	Spo₂: Not obtainable
Time: 0947	BP: 76/48	Pulse: 104	Respirations: 12 ATV	Spo₂: 99%

EMS Treatment (circle all that apply)

Oxygen @ __15__ L/min via (circle one):

NC   NRM   ⟨**Bag-mask device**⟩

⟨**Assisted Ventilation:** 12 breaths/min⟩

⟨**Airway Adjunct:** Oral ET tube⟩

CPR

Defibrillation	**Bleeding Control**	**Bandaging**	**Splinting**	⟨**Other:** Dopamine 5 mcg/kg/min drip; airway suction; saline IV⟩

Narrative

EMS requested to above location for a man who is unresponsive. On arrival, pt found lying supine in his bed. Home health aide is on scene. Pt confirmed to be responsive only to painful stimuli. No signs of trauma noted on scene. Building security notes pt has not been seen outside of his apartment for at least 24 hours. Pt's airway noted to be partially obstructed by secretions. Bag-mask assisted ventilations with high concentrations of oxygen initiated after opening and suctioning airway. Pt found with audible respirations and suctioning reveals thick, light brown sputum. Medications assessed and patient identification as well as medications gathered for transport. SAMPLE history obtained from aide on scene. Cardiac monitor reveals sinus tachycardia without ectopy. IV attempt was unsuccessful × 1, IO established in the right tibia. Fluid bolus of NS initiated at 30 mL/kg (1,800 mL). Pt transferred to unit for transport. Once en route, pt noted to have decreased respiratory effort and perfusion. Medical control contacted for orders for administering vasopressor. Dopamine drip initiated using premix bag at rate of 12 drops per minute. Pt intubated with 7.0 ET tube nasally and secured at 28-cm mark. Placement confirmed via auscultation and ETCO₂ monitoring and waveforms. Pt transport continued without further incident and report called to receiving facility. No changes noted to cardiac rhythm during transport. On arrival at the ED, pt transferred to stretcher in Room 6 and report given to RN at bedside. Pt placed in stretcher with all rails up and placed on ventilator by respiratory therapist. Signature for medication order obtained from Dr. Jackson.**End of report**

Prep Kit

► Ready for Review

- The paramedic needs to develop expertise in rapidly developing a differential diagnosis of the critical patient found in a peri-arrest condition or during a peri-arrest period.
- The novice paramedic can benefit from working with an experienced paramedic to help develop skills in intuition and become comfortable in making critical decisions when they are needed most.
- Hypoperfusion occurs when the level of tissue perfusion decreases below normal.
  - Early decreased tissue perfusion may result in subtle changes, such as aberrant mental status, long before a patient's vital signs appear abnormal.
  - Shock refers to a state of collapse and failure of the cardiovascular system that leads to inadequate circulation, creating inadequate tissue perfusion.
- The body is perfused via the cardiovascular system. Control of the cardiovascular system is a function of the autonomic nervous system, which is composed of competing subsystems.
- Tissue perfusion requires three intact mechanisms: a pump (heart), fluid volume (blood and body fluids), and tubing capable of reflex adjustments (constriction and dilation) in response to changes in pump output and fluid volume (blood vessels). If any one of those mechanisms is damaged, tissue perfusion may be disrupted, and shock will ensue.
- Shock occurs in two successive phases (compensated and decompensated). This progression is also referred to as the four grades of hemorrhage or four classes of shock, with classes I and II being compensated shock, and classes III and IV being decompensated shock.
- As with any patient, airway and ventilatory support take top priority when you are treating a patient with suspected shock.
- If a patient is suspected to be in shock, then transport is inevitable; the questions to be asked are when, where, and how.
  - The priority of the patient and the availability of a regional trauma center should be your concerns. Local transport protocols may specifically deal with these issues.
  - Patients who have suspected shock, whether compensated or decompensated, will benefit from early medical or surgical intervention and should be transported to a facility with those capabilities.
- Never wait for the blood pressure to drop; always treat shock aggressively in its compensated phase.
- The nonhemorrhagic causes of hypovolemic shock are commonly grouped by how they reduce perfusion. These types of shock involve either a weakening of the pump, an increase in the size of the container, or a direct mechanical interference with the circulation.
- Prevention of shock and its deadly effects begin with your immediate assessment of the mechanism of injury, primary survey findings, and the patient's clinical picture. Be alert, and search for early signs of shock.

► Vital Vocabulary

aerobic metabolism Metabolism that can proceed only in the presence of oxygen.

afterload The pressure in the aorta against which the left ventricle must pump blood.

anaerobic metabolism Metabolism that takes place in the absence of oxygen.

anaphylactic shock A severe hypersensitivity reaction that involves bronchoconstriction and cardiovascular collapse.

anchoring bias A type of bias in which an initial reference point distorts your estimates.

angioedema Recurrent large areas of subcutaneous edema of sudden onset, usually disappearing within 24 hours, which is seen mainly in young women, frequently as a result of allergy to food or drugs.

baroreceptors Receptors in the blood vessels, kidneys, brain, and heart that respond to changes in pressure in the heart or main arteries to help maintain homeostasis.

capacitance vessels The smallest venules.

cardiac output The volume of blood pumped through the circulatory system in 1 minute.

cardiogenic shock A condition caused by loss of 40% or more of the functioning myocardium; the heart is no longer able to circulate sufficient blood to maintain adequate oxygen delivery.

cardiovascular collapse Failure of the heart and blood vessels; shock.

central shock A condition that consists of cardiogenic shock and obstructive shock (Weil-Shubin classification).

chemoreceptors Sense organs that monitor the levels of oxygen and carbon dioxide and the pH of

Prep Kit (continued)

cerebrospinal fluid and blood and provide feedback to the respiratory centers to modify the rate and depth of breathing based on the body's needs at any given time.

compensated shock The early stage of shock, in which the body can still compensate for blood loss. The systolic blood pressure and brain perfusion are maintained.

confirmation bias A type of bias that occurs with the tendency to gather and rely on information that confirms your existing views and to avoid or downplay information that does not conform to your preexisiting hypothesis or field diagnosis.

critical patient A patient who is in premorbid condition, has experienced major trauma, or is in the peri-arrest period.

decompensated shock The late stage of shock, when blood pressure is falling.

differential diagnosis The process of weighing the probability of one disease versus other diseases by comparing clinical findings that could account for a patient's illness; also refers to the list of possible conditions considered based on the patient's signs and symptoms.

diffusion A process in which molecules move from an area of higher concentration to an area of lower concentration.

distributive shock A condition that occurs when there is widespread dilation of the resistance vessels, the capacitance vessels, or both.

Fick principle A principle that states the movement and use of oxygen in the body are dependent on an adequate concentration of inspired oxygen, appropriate movement of oxygen across the alveolar-capillary membrane into the arterial bloodstream, adequate number of red blood cells to carry the oxygen, proper tissue perfusion, and efficient offloading of oxygen at the tissue level.

hypoperfusion A condition that occurs when the level of tissue perfusion decreases below that needed to maintain normal cellular functions; also called shock.

hypovolemic shock A condition that occurs when the circulating blood volume is inadequate to deliver adequate oxygen and nutrients to the body.

intuition Pattern recognition and pattern matching, based on your own past experiences.

irreversible shock The point at which shock has progressed to a terminal stage, resulting in death.

mean arterial pressure (MAP) The blood pressure required to sustain organ perfusion; roughly 60 mm Hg in the average person.

multiple-organ dysfunction syndrome (MODS) A progressive condition usually characterized by combined failure of several organs, such as the lungs, liver, and kidneys, along with some clotting mechanisms, which occurs after severe illness or injury.

myocardial contractility The ability of the heart to contract.

neurogenic shock Circulatory failure caused by paralysis of the nerves that control the size of the blood vessels, leading to widespread dilation; seen in patients with spinal cord injuries.

nonhemorrhagic shock Shock that occurs as a result of fluid loss contained within the body, such as in dehydration, burn injury, crush injury, and anaphylaxis.

obstructive shock Shock that occurs when there is a block to blood flow in the heart or great vessels, causing an insufficient blood supply to the body's tissues.

orthostatic hypotension A drop in systolic blood pressure when moving a patient from a sitting to a standing position.

perfusion The delivery of oxygen and nutrients to the cells, organs, and tissues of the body.

peri-arrest period The period either just before or just after cardiac arrest when the patient is critical and care must be taken to prevent progression or regression into cardiac arrest.

peripheral shock A condition that consists of hypovolemic shock and distributive shock (Weil-Shubin classification).

preload The initial stretching of the cardiac muscle prior to contraction. It is related to the chamber volume of blood just prior to the contraction.

premorbid condition A condition preceding the onset of disease.

psychogenic shock A sudden reaction of the nervous system that produces a temporary, generalized vascular dilation, resulting in syncope (vasovagal syncope).

pulse pressure The difference between the systolic blood pressure and the diastolic blood pressure.

resistance vessels The smallest arterioles.

sensitization Developing a sensitivity to a substance that initially caused no allergic reaction.

Prep Kit (continued)

septic shock Shock caused by severe infection, usually a bacterial infection.

shock An abnormal state associated with inadequate oxygen and nutrient delivery to the metabolic apparatus of the cell; also called hypoperfusion.

sphincter A circular muscular wall of capillaries that constricts and dilates, acting as a gate to increase or decrease blood flow.

spinal shock The local neurologic condition that occurs after a spinal injury produces motor and sensory losses (which may not be permanent).

stroke volume The amount of blood that the left ventricle ejects into the aorta per contraction.

systemic vascular resistance The resistance to blood flow within all of the blood vessels except the pulmonary vessels.

warm ischemic time The amount of time that specific tissues of the body are deprived of oxygen typically as a result of an injury or arterial occlusion.

working diagnosis The one diagnosis from a differential list used to base the patient's treatment plan.

► References

1. Weick K, Sutcliffe K. *Managing the Unexpected: Resilient Performance in an Age of Uncertainty*. 2nd ed. San Francisco, CA: John Wiley & Sons; 2007.

2. Frank O. Zur dynamik des herzmuskels. *J Biol*. 1895;32:370-447. Translation from German: Chapman CP, Wasserman EB. On the dynamics of cardiac muscle. *Am Heart J*. 1959;58:282-317.

3. Chang, R, Cardneas JC, Wade CE, Holcomb JB. Advances in the understanding of trauma-induced coagulopathy. *Blood*. 2016;128(8):1043-1049.

4. Orthostatic hypotension. WebMD website. http://www.webmd.com/a-to-z-guides/hypotension-orthostatic. Updated August 27, 2014. Accessed May 10, 2017.

5. Healey MA, Samphire J, Hoyt DB, et al. Irreversible shock is not irreversible; a new model of massive hemorrhage and resuscitation. *J Trauma*. 2001;50(5):826-834.

6. Rezaie O. Is ATLS wrong about palpable blood pressure estimates? ALiEM: Academic Life in Emergency Medicine website. https://www.aliem.com/2013/is-atls-wrong-about-palpable-blood-pressure/. Published March 31, 2013. Accessed January 23, 2017.

7. National Association of Emergency Medical Technicians (NAEMT). *Prehospital Trauma Life Support*. 8th ed. Burlington, MA: Jones & Bartlett Learning, LLC; 2016:241.

8. Solomonov E, Hirsh M, Yahiya A, et al. The effect of vigorous fluid resuscitation in uncontrolled hemorrhagic shock after massive splenic injury. *Crit Care Med*. 2000;28(3):749-754.

9. Krausz MM, Horn Y, Gross D. The combined effect of small volume hypertonic saline and normal saline solutions in uncontrolled hemorrhagic shock. *Surg Gynecol Obstet*. 1992;174:363-368.

10. Bickell WH, Bruttig SP, Millnamow GA, et al. The detrimental effects of intravenous crystalloid after aortotomy in swine. *Surgery*. 1991;110(3):529-536.

11. Weil MH, Shubin H. Proposed reclassification of shock states with special reference to distributive defects. *Adv Exp Med Biol*. 1971;16:13-23.

12. Hochman JS, Buller CE, Dzavik V, et al. Cardiogenic shock complicating AMI etiologies, management and outcome—overall findings of the SHOCK Trial Registry. *Circulation*. 1998; 98(suppl 1):1-778.

13. Killip T, Kimball JT. Treatment of myocardial infarction in a coronary care unit. A two-year experience with 250 patients. *Am J Cardiol*. 1967;20:457-464.

14. Goldberg RJ, Gore JM, Alpert JS, et al. Cardiogenic shock after acute myocardial infarction. Incidence and mortality from a community-wide perspective, 1975 to 1988. *N Engl J Med*. 1991;325:1117-1122.

15. Braunwald EB, ed. *Heart Disease: A Textbook of Cardiovascular Medicine*. Philadelphia, PA: WB Saunders; 1997:1233-1245.

16. Singer M, Deutschman CS, Seymour CW, et al. The Third International Consensus Definitions for Sepsis and Septic Shock (Sepsis-3). *JAMA*. 2016;315:801-810.

17. Smyth MA, Brace-McDonnell SJ, Perkins GD. Impact of prehospital care on outcomes in sepsis: a systematic review. *West J Emerg Med*. 2016 Jul;17(4):427-437.

18. Rhodes A, Evans L, Alhazzani W, et al. Surviving sepsis campaign: international guidelines for management of sepsis and septic shock: 2016. *Critical Care Med*. 2017;45(3):486-552.

Assessment in Action

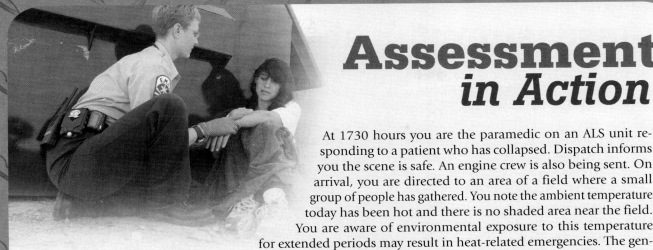

At 1730 hours you are the paramedic on an ALS unit responding to a patient who has collapsed. Dispatch informs you the scene is safe. An engine crew is also being sent. On arrival, you are directed to an area of a field where a small group of people has gathered. You note the ambient temperature today has been hot and there is no shaded area near the field. You are aware of environmental exposure to this temperature for extended periods may result in heat-related emergencies. The general impression of your patient as you approach is a petite young woman who is pale and silent with her eyes closed. You are approached by a woman who informs you she is the coach of the ladies' track team and they have been practicing for the past few days. Your patient, Jennifer, was running but then stopped, vomited, and collapsed to the ground. Your assessment of the scene does not reveal any structures or objects that she may have hit during her collapse, but you do note a small amount of vomitus near the patient.

You move to the patient's side to continue your primary survey, and the patient opens her eyes when you call her name. You ask her age and she tells you she is 18 years old. Assessment of her breathing reveals a respiratory rate of 28 breaths/min, and they are slightly labored. She has a radial pulse rate that is tachycardic at 120 beats/min, and her skin is mottled, cool, and dry. There are no obvious signs of trauma, but there are positive signs and symptoms of dehydration, including sunken eyes and poor skin turgor, as well as syncope, nausea, and vomiting. These findings indicate an immediate life threat, and you begin delegating care by assuming the role of team leader. She is a high-priority patient, and a short scene time and rapid transport to definitive care is appropriate.

While your partner applies a nonrebreathing mask and administers high-concentration oxygen at 15 L/min, emergency responders begin to prepare the patient for transport. You obtain a SAMPLE history and continue with a secondary assessment. The patient tells you she has been running all day trying to improve her times for an upcoming competition. This morning she felt nauseated so she did not eat or drink much during lunch. Her last full meal and fluid intake were at approximately 0800 hours. She is allergic to penicillin and takes 10 units of insulin at 0730 hours daily for her diabetes. You remind your partner to check her blood glucose level when obtaining vital signs. Her vital signs are a pulse rate of 120 beats/min and weak; respirations, 22 breaths/min and slightly labored; blood pressure, 108/64 mm Hg; oxygen saturation, 98% on high concentrations of oxygen; and blood glucose level, 66 mg/dL.

1. Which form of shock is this patient experiencing?

   A. Septic shock
   B. Neurogenic shock
   C. Cardiogenic shock
   D. Hypovolemic shock

2. Total blood volume in the patient is approximately how many liters?

   A. 3
   B. 6
   C. 8
   D. 10

3. Which phase of shock does this patient appear to be in?

   A. Compensated
   B. Decompensated
   C. Irreversible
   D. Terminal

4. Which of the following signs and symptoms of the patient in the scenario are NOT consistent with those of shock due to dehydration?

   A. Feelings of anxiety and restlessness
   B. Thirst
   C. Pale, cool, and moist skin
   D. An elevated body temperature

Assessment *in Action* (continued)

5. Which of the following is a concern for IV fluid therapy in this patient with significant dehydration?

   A. Heart failure
   B. Hypertension
   C. Increased external hemorrhage
   D. Extravasation

6. Which of the following is NOT a compensatory mechanism that the patient likely experienced as she developed shock?

   A. Increase in preload and cardiac output
   B. Maintenance of brain perfusion
   C. Increase in available oxygen
   D. Increase in urine output

7. Which of the following was likely the last factor to change as the patient's dehydration worsened?

   A. Mental status
   B. Blood pressure
   C. Skin condition
   D. Pulse rate

8. Why is it important to consider the preexisting medical conditions of the critical patient?

9. What physiologic changes associated with shock place the patient at risk for multiple-organ dysfunction syndrome (MODS)?

10. What sign indicates a patient whom you suspect is in shock from dehydration is progressing from compensated to decompensated shock?

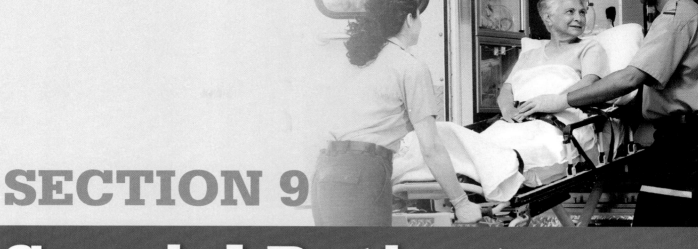

SECTION 9

Special Patient Populations

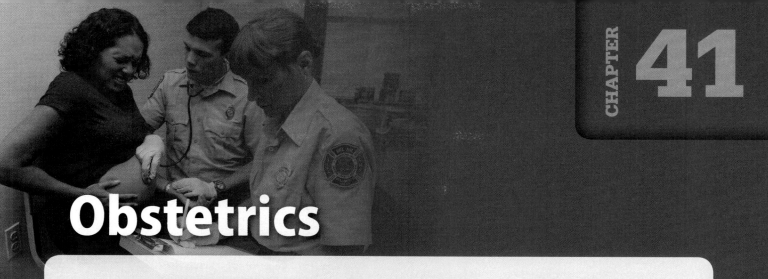

CHAPTER 41

Obstetrics

National EMS Education Standard Competencies

Special Patient Populations

Integrates assessment findings with principles of pathophysiology and knowledge of psychosocial needs to formulate a field impression and implement a comprehensive treatment/disposition plan for patients with special needs.

Obstetrics

> Recognition and management of
  • Normal delivery (pp 2045-2049)
  • Vaginal bleeding in the pregnant patient (pp 2040-2043)
> Anatomy and physiology of normal pregnancy (pp 2027-2032)
> Pathophysiology of complications of pregnancy (pp 2036-2040)
> Assessment of the pregnant patient (pp 2032-2036)
> Psychosocial impact, presentations, prognosis, and management of
  • Normal delivery (pp 2045-2049)
  • Abnormal delivery
    • Nuchal cord (pp 2047, 2055)
    • Prolapsed cord (p 2055)
    • Breech delivery (pp 2054-2055)
  • Third-trimester bleeding
    • Placenta previa (pp 2042-2043)
    • Abruptio placenta (pp 2042-2043)
  • Spontaneous abortion/miscarriage (pp 2040, 2043)
  • Ectopic pregnancy (pp 2042, 2043)
  • Preeclampsia/eclampsia (p 2037)
  • Antepartum hemorrhage (pp 2041-2042, 2043)
  • Pregnancy-induced hypertension (p 2037)

Trauma

Integrates assessment findings with principles of epidemiology and pathophysiology to formulate a field impression to implement a comprehensive treatment/ disposition plan for an acutely injured patient.

Special Considerations in Trauma

Recognition and management of trauma in
> Pregnant patient (pp 2057-2060)

> Pediatric patient (see Chapter 43, *Pediatric Emergencies*)
> Geriatric patient (see Chapter 44, *Geriatric Emergencies*)

Pathophysiology, assessment, and management of trauma in the
> Pregnant patient (pp 2057-2060)
> Pediatric patient (see Chapter 43, *Pediatric Emergencies*)
> Geriatric patient (see Chapter 44, *Geriatric Emergencies*)
> Cognitively impaired patient (see Chapter 45, *Patients With Special Challenges*)

Knowledge Objectives

1. Describe the process of conception and fetal development, from ovulation to the fetal stage. (pp 2028-2029)
2. Discuss the various functions of the placenta. (p 2028)
3. Understand the normal changes that occur in the various body systems during pregnancy. (pp 2029-2032)
4. Be aware of special considerations involving pregnancy in different cultures and with teenage patients. (p 2032)
5. Describe commonly used obstetric terminology. (p 2032)
6. Discuss the process of assessing a patient who is experiencing an emergency related to pregnancy, or who is in labor. (pp 2032-2036)
7. Describe the indications of an imminent delivery. (pp 2034, 2044)
8. Discuss complications related to pregnancy, including substance abuse, supine hypotensive disorder, heart disease, hypertensive disorders, seizures, diabetes, respiratory disorders, hyperemesis gravidarum, renal disorders, Rh sensitization, and infections. (pp 2036-2040)
9. Discuss bleeding during pregnancy, including third-trimester bleeding and its potential causes and management. (pp 2040-2043)
10. Differentiate between the three stages of labor. (pp 2043-2044)

11. Explain the steps involved in normal delivery management. (pp 2047-2048)
12. Explain the necessary care of the baby as the head appears. (p 2048)
13. Describe the procedure followed to cut and tie the umbilical cord. (p 2048)
14. Describe delivery of the placenta. (pp 2048-2049)
15. Discuss management of complications of labor, including premature rupture of membranes, preterm labor, fetal distress, and uterine rupture. (p 2051)
16. Discuss management of high-risk pregnancy considerations, including precipitous labor and birth, post-term pregnancy, meconium staining, fetal macrosomia, multiple gestation, intrauterine fetal death, amniotic fluid embolism, hydramnios, and cephalopelvic disproportion. (pp 2051-2053)
17. Discuss management of complications of delivery, including cephalic presentation, breech presentation, shoulder dystocia, nuchal cord, and prolapsed umbilical cord. (pp 2053-2055)
18. Discuss management of postpartum complications, including uterine inversion, postpartum hemorrhage, pulmonary embolism, and postpartum depression. (pp 2056-2057)

19. Discuss concerns related to trauma in the pregnant patient, including assessment and management of the woman and the unborn fetus. (pp 2057-2060)

Skills Objectives

1. Demonstrate how to listen to fetal heart sounds. (p 2036)
2. Demonstrate the procedure to assist in a normal cephalic delivery. (pp 2045-2049)
3. Demonstrate care procedures of the infant as the head appears during delivery. (p 2048)
4. Demonstrate the steps to follow in postdelivery care of the infant. (p 2048)
5. Demonstrate how to cut and tie the umbilical cord. (p 2048)
6. Demonstrate how to assist in delivery of the placenta. (pp 2048-2049)
7. Demonstrate the postdelivery care of the mother. (p 2049)
8. Describe how to assist with a breech delivery in the field. (pp 2054-2055)
9. Describe how to assist with shoulder dystocia in the field. (pp 2054-2055)

Introduction

When you are responding to an obstetric (OB) or maternity call, keep several key issues in mind. First, pregnancy itself is not a disease that needs treatment; rather, it is the natural continuation of the human species. Women have been having children without the benefit of a 9-1-1 response, emergency departments (EDs), epidurals, and pain medications since time began. For the most part, childbirth is a happy event for all involved. Emotions during this event can range from extreme excitement to panic; therefore, you must bring a sense of professional calm and control to the scene. Second, the number of patients increases to a minimum of two—the pregnant woman and the fetus—or perhaps more if more than one fetus is expected.

Whereas childbirth and pregnancy are both naturally occurring states, they have the potential for serious complications, including maternal and fetal death. With the advent of modern medicine, maternal and infant mortality rates have been significantly reduced, and close medical monitoring usually discovers problems well before childbirth.

YOU are the Paramedic PART 1

Your unit is dispatched as a second unit for a motor vehicle crash. The first unit on scene advises you that the incident involves a critical trauma patient—a pregnant woman (20 weeks' gestation) was the driver of one of the vehicles. When you arrive on scene, you find that a rear-end collision occurred. You are directed to your patient, who is sitting in the vehicle that struck the rear of the first car. You don your safety equipment and approach the patient.

1. What is your primary concern after scene safety is established?
2. Which questions are in your mind given your knowledge that the patient is pregnant?

■ Anatomy and Physiology Review

As discussed in Chapter 8, *Anatomy and Physiology*, the female reproductive organs include two ovaries, two uterine (fallopian) tubes, the uterus (womb), the cervix, the vagina (birth canal), the mammary glands, and the external genitalia. The ovaries are the beginning point for reproduction. These paired glands are found next to the uterus, one ovary on each side. They are similar to the testes in the male. Each ovary contains approximately 200,000 follicles, and each follicle contains an oocyte (egg). The human female is born with all the eggs she will ever release (approximately 400,000). Each month, during the menstrual cycle, several of these follicles attempt the process of maturation, but typically only a single follicle ultimately matures and releases an ovum; the other follicles die off and are reabsorbed by the body.

The processes that the follicle goes through and the actual release of the oocyte (ovulation) are stimulated by the release of specific hormones in the female body. An oocyte matures when the corresponding follicular cells respond to **follicle-stimulating hormone (FSH)** released by the anterior pituitary gland, after the pituitary is first stimulated by the release of gonadotropin-releasing factor (GnRF) from the hypothalamus. As the preovulatory phase of the menstrual cycle progresses, the anterior pituitary gland releases luteinizing hormone (LH), which stimulates the release of the egg (or at this point, the **ovum**).

LH continues to be excreted throughout the ovarian cycle and subsequent pregnancy, should it occur. What is left of the follicle after the egg has been released becomes the **corpus luteum**, which in turn secretes estrogen, progesterone, and **inhibin**. All three of these hormones inhibit secretion of FSH from the anterior pituitary gland, thereby preventing the further development of follicles. In addition, at the end of the pregnancy, the uterus and the **placenta** produce prostaglandins; they have hormone-like effects and, along with oxytocin, signal the uterus to contract, thereby beginning the process of labor.

After its release from the follicle, the ovum passes from the ovaries to the uterus through the fallopian tubes. Ciliary motion sweeps the egg into the fallopian tube, and smooth muscle contractions and the inner mucosa move the ovum through the tube to the uterus. If the egg encounters a sperm cell along the way, it may become fertilized. Fertilization can occur at any time within about a 24-hour window following ovulation.

If the ovum is *not* fertilized, it dies and degenerates 36 to 48 hours after being released. The endometrium then breaks down and is shed as menstrual flow on about the 28th day of the cycle (ie, about 14 days after ovulation). (Chapter 22, *Gynecologic Emergencies*, covers the menstrual cycle in detail.)

If an egg is fertilized, the glands of the endometrium immediately increase in size and secrete the materials on which the egg will implant and grow. The corpus luteum

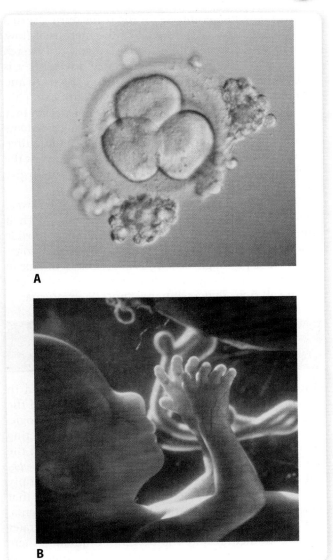

Figure 41-1 A. Embryo. **B.** Fetus.

continues to secrete hormones to support the pregnancy for 90 days. The fertilized egg proceeds to the uterus where, if implantation occurs, the fertilized egg develops into an embryo and then a **fetus** Figure 41-1 .

The uterus is a muscular, inverted pear-shaped organ that lies between the urinary bladder and the rectum. The uterus is where the fertilized ovum normally implants, where the fetus develops, and where the act of labor takes place. The uterus consists of three layers of muscle fibers: the **perimetrium** (outer protective layer), the **myometrium** (middle layer), and the endometrium (inner lining). The contractions of these muscles help expel the fetus during childbirth. The interior of the body of the uterus is the **uterine cavity**, and the interior of the cervix is the **cervical canal**.

The narrowest portion of the uterus, called the cervix, opens into the vagina. The vagina is a highly muscular, tubular organ lined with mucous membranes. Its functions include being the receptacle for the penis during sexual intercourse, the passage for exit of the menstrual flow, and the passage for childbirth. The vagina can stretch widely to accommodate the delivery of a fetus. If it is unable to stretch far enough, however, the tissues in and around the perineum may tear, causing significant pain and bleeding. In the hospital setting, the physician may make an incision in the perineal skin called an **episiotomy** to avoid these complications. In the prehospital setting, you are limited to providing gentle pressure against the newborn's head to prevent an explosive birth and to give the tissues time to expand.

The mammary glands (breasts) are modified sweat glands that are mainly composed of adipose tissue. Their primary purpose is lactation, or milk secretion, to provide nourishment to the newborn. Milk is carried to the surface of each breast through lactiferous ducts that terminate in a nipple. Breast enlargement, tenderness, and milk excretion are all signs that a woman is most likely pregnant.

Conception and Fetal Development

Once an egg has been fertilized and implanted in the endometrium of the uterus, both the egg and the pregnant woman begin to undergo major physiologic, hormonal, and chemical changes. The egg, on entering the uterus, begins absorbing uterine fluid through the cell membrane. As the fluid fills the interior of the egg, cell division increases rapidly, and the cells multiply on the outside of the egg surface, forming layers that will eventually generate the fetal membrane, placenta, and embryo. The egg, now called a **blastocyst**, migrates to the endometrial wall and becomes implanted there approximately 1 week after conception. The inner mass of cells of the blastocyst develops into the fetus; part of the outer blastocyst layer develops into the placenta and fetal membranes.[1] On implantation, the egg adheres to the endometrium, and enzymatic activity from the egg dissolves endometrial tissue and provides nourishment for its development. Occasionally, the mechanism of implantation may result in vaginal bleeding that is spotty and painless, but of concern to the patient who does not yet realize that she is pregnant.

The implantation and subsequent actions of the blastocyst trigger the development of placental tissues. Their formation stimulates the release of human chorionic gonadotropin (hCG) hormone, which in turn sends signals to the corpus luteum that pregnancy has begun. The corpus luteum then begins to produce hormones designed to support the pregnancy until the placenta is sufficiently developed to assume this function. By the second week after conception, the blastocyst has evolved into an embryonic disc, and the amniotic sac and placenta are starting to differentiate into their specialized duties. The developing placenta produces projections that tap into the external tissue layer of the blastocyst, where spaces called *lacunae* form. These spaces are filled with maternal blood. The connection from the placenta to the blastocyst allows both the embryo to draw on the maternal circulation for oxygenation and nutrition and embryonic waste products to be shunted safely away; thus, it serves as the beginning of the umbilical cord.

In the third week after conception, the egg, now officially recognized as an *embryo*, is ready to begin the process of forming specialized body systems. The rudiments of the central nervous system, cardiovascular system, spine, and portions of the skeletal anatomy begin to appear. At the end of this week, an S-shaped tubular heart begins to beat, and blood cells produced in the yolk sac begin to circulate. The pregnant woman, by this point, may notice that she has missed her period and begin to suspect that she is pregnant.

Around the fourth week of pregnancy, the placenta begins to develop. Essentially an enlarged endocrine gland, the placenta carries out a number of crucial functions during pregnancy. It serves as an early liver for the developing fetus, taking care of the synthesis of glycogen and cholesterol; it metabolizes fatty acids; and it produces antibodies that protect the fetus. The placenta also provides the following functions:

- Respiratory gas exchange. The placenta functions as the fetal lungs, enabling the fetus to exchange its carbon dioxide–laden blood for oxygen-rich blood.
- Transport of nutrients from maternal to fetal circulation.
- Excretion of wastes, some of which pass into the maternal circulation and others of which are excreted into the amniotic fluid.
- Transfer of heat from the woman to the fetus.
- Hormone production. About 10 to 12 weeks after conception, the placenta is sufficiently developed to assume responsibility for the production of hCG, a hormone that maintains the pregnancy and stimulates changes in the woman's breasts, vagina, and cervix that prepare her for delivery and motherhood.
- Formation of a barrier against harmful substances in the pregnant woman's circulation, such as chemicals or microorganisms. When the placenta blocks a drug from reaching the fetal bloodstream, it means that the drug "does not cross the placenta." The placenta is not able to exclude every harmful substance from reaching the fetus, however, so you need to be very careful when administering medications to women during pregnancy.

The **umbilical cord** connects the placenta to the fetus via the fetal umbilicus (navel) **Figure 41-2** .

The fetal circulation differs from the circulation of the pregnant woman. The umbilical *vein* carries oxygenated blood from the placenta to the fetus, while the umbilical *arteries* carry arteriovenous blood to the placenta. Because

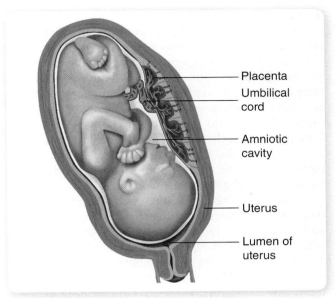

Figure 41-2 The umbilical cord and other structures of the pregnant uterus.

© Jones & Bartlett Learning.

the fetus obtains its oxygen via the placenta, the fetal circulation bypasses the fetus's lungs until birth. A duct connects the umbilical vein and the inferior vena cava (ie, the ductus venosus), another duct connects the pulmonary artery and the aorta (ie, the ductus arteriosus), and an opening (ie, the foramen ovale) separates the right and left atria of the fetal heart. At birth, the neonate's lungs begin to function, and the arteriovenous shunts close.

The **amniotic sac** is a membranous bag that encloses the fetus in a watery fluid called **amniotic fluid**. The volume of amniotic fluid reaches about 500 to 1,000 mL (1 L) at term, but this volume is constantly changing throughout the pregnancy. Amniotic fluid provides the fetus with a weightless environment in which to develop. In the latter stages of pregnancy, the fetus swallows amniotic fluid and passes wastes out into the fluid. In this way, amniotic fluid assists in fetal excretory function.

The fourth through the eighth weeks of embryonic development are critical for normal development of the fetus. During this period, the major organs and other body systems are forming and are most susceptible to damage. Some prescription drugs and even over-the-counter medications may have side effects that harm the fetus. Women who use illicit drugs, smoke tobacco, drink alcohol, or are exposed to other toxic substances during their pregnancy also increase the risk that their fetus will develop birth defects.

The **gestational period** is the time that it takes for the fetus to develop in utero. It normally lasts 38 weeks, with significant developmental progress occurring each week. The due date can be calculated by identifying the first day of the last menstrual cycle, adding 1 year, subtracting 3 months, and adding 7 days. Because the placental tissues usually start sending hormonal signals to the corpus

Words of Wisdom

Fetal alcohol spectrum disorders (FASDs) are a group of conditions that can occur as a result of the ingestion of alcohol during pregnancy. FASDs includes conditions such as fetal alcohol syndrome (the most severe form of FASD), partial fetal alcohol syndrome, alcohol-related birth defects, alcohol-related neurodevelopmental disorder, and neurobehavioral disorder associated with prenatal alcohol exposure.[2] The scope of disabilities and possible birth defects from FASDs varies and depends on factors such as the amount of alcohol consumed, the frequency of exposure, and the stage of fetal development during alcohol consumption, among others.

Fetal alcohol syndrome classically requires the following three abnormalities are present:

1. Poor growth—in utero or after the baby is born and into childhood.
2. Facial abnormalities—specifically shortened palpebral fissures, low-set ears, under development of the midfacial region, and a smooth philtrum (the area between the upper lip and nose) with or without a thin upper lip.
3. Dysfunction of the central nervous system— microcephaly, cognitive impairment, attention-deficit disorder/attention-deficit/hyperactivity disorder, and other behavioral problems later in life).[3]

FASDs are completely preventable if a woman abstains from all forms of alcohol use (eg, beer, wine, liquor) during pregnancy.

luteum to start changing the internal environment in the second week after conception, this dating method adds 2 weeks to the entire calculation, leading to 40 total weeks of pregnancy from conception to birth (prenatal period).

Physiologic Maternal Changes During Pregnancy

When a woman conceives, carries a fetus to term, and then gives birth, several physiologic changes occur within her body. Many of these changes can alter the normal response to trauma or exacerbate or create medical conditions that can threaten the health of both the woman and her fetus. In particular, hormonal changes associated with pregnancy precipitate physiologic changes, and the rapidly changing internal environment puts stress on the woman. Metabolic demands increase during pregnancy, and the enlarging uterus with its significant vascularity creates mechanical changes as well.

The most significant physiologic changes occur in the uterus. Before a woman's first pregnancy, the uterus measures about 3 inches (7.5 cm) long by 2 inches (5 cm) wide and is approximately 1 inch (2.5 cm) thick. After

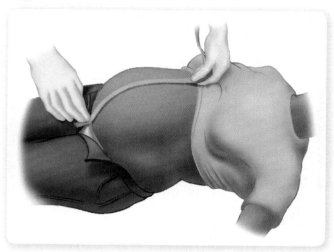

Figure 41-3 Measuring the fundus.
© Jones & Bartlett Learning.

pregnancy has stretched the uterus, it will rarely return to its previous dimensions. In the nonpregnant patient, the uterus weighs up to 70 g (2.5 oz) and has a capacity of approximately 10 mL (one third of an ounce). By the end of a full term pregnancy, the uterus weighs approximately 1,100 to 1,200 g (2.4 to 2.6 lb) and has a capacity of approximately 5,000 mL.[4]

Measurement of the fundus of the uterus (the top portion, opposite the cervix) can identify possible developmental problems. The fundus is measured in centimeters by running a measuring tape vertically from the top of the pubic bone to the top of the fundus **Figure 41-3**. The length in centimeters roughly corresponds to length of gestation. For example, if the patient is 32 weeks pregnant, the measurement would be 13 inches (32 cm). If the length does not match the expected value, it could indicate uterine growth problems or breech position (if shorter) or the possibility of twins (if longer).

As the pregnancy continues, the uterus enlarges and increases in weight. This weight places pressure on the lower end of the intestine and the woman's rectum and often results in constipation. The smooth muscles in the gastrointestinal (GI) tract relax due to increased progesterone levels, which causes a decrease in GI motility (ie, a decrease in moving the stomach contents to the duodenum). This decreased motility sometimes can also cause heartburn and burping. Because the stomach is not being emptied as quickly as in a nonpregnant woman, the pregnant patient is at higher risk of vomiting during an emergency, which may potentially result in airway compromise.

Physiologic changes also occur to the urinary system as the kidneys increase in size and volume. Kidney volume can increase as much as 30% during pregnancy. The ureters also increase in diameter, with the right side being more dilated than the left side in most cases. These changes result in increased urinary frequency for the pregnant woman and an increased chance of urinary tract infection

if she does not empty her bladder frequently. Increased pressure on the urinary bladder from the enlarging uterus also causes increased urinary frequency.

Most women also experience changes in their skin, hair, and eyes from the hormones released during pregnancy. Increased hair and nail growth and changes in texture are common. Some women also develop a "pregnancy mask"—brown and yellow color changes to the face (around the eyes, cheeks, and nose). The skin may darken around the areola, axilla, and genitalia. A dark line of pigment down the midline of the abdomen, called *linea nigra*, also develops in many women.

Pregnancy affects a woman's circulatory system in several ways. The average woman has approximately 8.5 to 10.5 pints (4 to 5 L) of blood available as total circulating volume. Blood volume increases by about 30% to 50% over prepregnancy levels, increasing rapidly during the first half of pregnancy, and then stabilizing or decreasing slightly by term.[5] The increase in the level of blood volume depends on such factors as patient size, single versus multiple gestation, **gravidity** (total number of times a woman has been pregnant regardless of those pregnancies' outcomes, including the current pregnancy) and **parity** (number of live births). The greater blood volume is needed to meet the metabolic needs of the developing fetus, to adequately perfuse maternal organs (especially the uterus and kidneys), and to help compensate for blood loss during delivery. At term, the uterus normally contains 15% to 16% of the woman's total circulating blood volume. During vaginal delivery, a woman may lose as much as 500 mL of blood (1,000 mL in case of cesarean section). The uterus, as it contracts, tends to shunt blood back into the maternal circulation (autotransfusion), thereby preserving maternal circulatory hemostasis.

As blood volume increases, so does the number of red blood cells (RBCs)—by as much as 33% over the normal count. The increase in RBCs heightens the pregnant woman's need for iron, which is why most women take **prenatal** vitamins. If the woman does not take iron supplements, the fetus will rob the maternal stores to meet its own needs for iron, resulting in anemia for the woman—and possibly leading to preterm labor and spontaneous abortion. Women who live in socioeconomically deprived areas and lack access to prenatal health care are the most likely to experience pregnancy-related anemia.

A woman's white blood cell (WBC) count also increases during pregnancy without an infection being present. Levels of clotting factors similarly increase, as do concentrations of fibrinogen levels.[5] These issues are important considerations if you have to deal with obstetric hemorrhage or thromboembolic disease.

The size of the pregnant woman's heart increases slightly due to the increased cardiac workload during pregnancy.[4] Cardiac output increases by 30% to 50% more than the prepregnancy level, reaching its maximum capacity at about 22 weeks' gestation and then declines to about 20% near term.[5] As the uterus enlarges and the diaphragm becomes elevated, the internal maternal organs begin to shift their positions in the abdomen to make room. The heart is displaced upward, forward, and to the left with a slight rotation in its long axis, which causes the apex of the heart to shift laterally (remember this point when you are auscultating the S_3 and S_4 heart sounds). In addition, the intensity of the "lub-dub" S_1 heart sound increases, while the S_2 heart sound generally remains normal. Systolic and diastolic murmurs are common.

A pregnant woman's heart rate gradually increases during pregnancy, by an average of 15 to 20 beats/min by term. Electrocardiogram (ECG) changes that can occur during pregnancy include ectopic beats and supraventricular tachycardia, which is often considered normal. Other changes include a slight left-axis deviation and lead III changes such as low-voltage QRS, T-wave inversion or flattening, or even occasional Q waves.

As the gestation proceeds, a woman's sensitivity to body positioning increases as well. Generally, after 20 weeks' gestation, resting or lying supine can cause the weight of the uterus to compress the inferior vena cava, thereby decreasing venous return to the heart.[6] Pressure by the fetus on the common iliac vein creates this problem as well. Over time, if pressure is not relieved, cardiac output decreases, blood pressure drops, and lower extremity edema occurs. Echocardiography is the standard way to measure cardiac output in pregnancy; however this is not done in the prehospital environment. Systolic and diastolic pressure may decrease until approximately 24 weeks' gestation.[5] Blood pressure may begin to increase from 24 weeks until birth, and usually returns to the normal prepregnancy level gradually.

Late in pregnancy, venous pressure increases progressively in the lower extremities. The enlarged uterus contributes to slowed venous return, pooling, dependent edema, hemorrhoids, and varicose veins in the legs.[5] Pregnant women who are bedridden or who spend a great deal of time lying down are in particular danger of experiencing deep venous thrombosis, which can lead to pulmonary embolism. This slow blood return to the heart also causes delayed absorption of subcutaneously or intramuscularly (IM) injected medications.

When the patient goes into labor, her birthing position may also stress the cardiovascular system. In the United States, the standard position is the lithotomy position, in which the woman is supine (on her back) with her knees spread apart, or her feet in stirrups **Figure 41-4** .

The workload of the heart increases significantly during both gestation and labor. For a healthy woman, this presents no undue complications. For a woman with heart disease or other forms of cardiac compromise, however, the increased work can result in ventricular failure or pulmonary edema, culminating in heart failure. Be sure to document the patient's cardiac history. The pain and pressures of labor can further stress the heart, resulting in cardiac arrest.

During pregnancy, the respiratory system experiences stresses as well. The uterus pushes the diaphragm up toward the abdominal cavity, resulting in an approximately

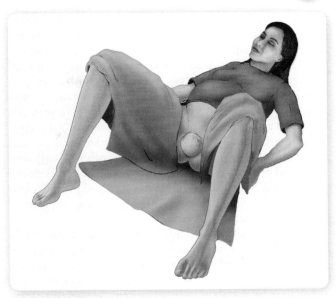

Figure 41-4 Lithotomy position.
© Jones & Bartlett Learning.

1½-inch (4-cm) displacement of the diaphragm. To compensate for this change, the rib margins flare outward, increasing the lower thoracic diameter and the total thoracic circumference by as much as 2½ inches (6 cm). This alteration allows the respiratory system to maintain intrathoracic volume. The abdominal muscles tend to lose their tone during pregnancy, which allows respiration to be more diaphragmatic.

As maternal oxygen demand increases, the respiratory physiology changes to accommodate this need. The hormone progesterone, which is produced early in pregnancy by the corpus luteum and later by the placenta, decreases the threshold of the medullary respiratory center to carbon dioxide. It also acts on the bronchi, causing them to dilate, and regulates mucus production, causing an overall decrease in airway resistance. Maternal oxygen consumption increase by 20% to 40% above nonpregnant levels because of the oxygen requirements of the fetus and placenta and the increased oxygen requirement of maternal organs.[7] By 8 weeks' gestation, increasing levels of progesterone cause the tidal volume to increase by 30% to 50% of the nonpregnant level.[7] The increase in tidal volume causes minute ventilation to increase by as much as 50% over prepregnancy values and Pa_{CO_2} to drop by about 5 mm Hg. The latter change is accompanied by a decrease in blood bicarbonate and a slight increase in plasma pH levels, which in turn affects acid-base balance. In the pregnant state, respiratory alkalosis is balanced by metabolic acidosis. The acid-base changes become quite marked during actual labor, but return to normal approximately 3 weeks **postpartum** (after delivery). Minute ventilation is also affected by a slight increase in the maternal respiratory rate, which typically rises to about 10 L/min.

At term, the displacement of the diaphragm by the fully enlarged uterus causes a decrease in expiratory reserve volume, functional residual capacity, and residual volume. Tidal volume and inspiratory reserve volume increase. Structural changes within the respiratory mucous membranes result in increased vascularity and edema.

The maternal metabolism undergoes phenomenal changes during pregnancy—most obviously, weight gain and alterations in physical structure. Weight gain is partly due to increased blood volume and increases in intracellular and extracellular fluid (6 to 7 pounds [2.7–3.2 kg]), uterine growth (3 pounds [1.5 kg]), placental growth (2 pounds [0.9 kg]), fetal growth (7 pounds [3.2 kg]), and increased breast tissue (2 to 3 pounds [0.9–1.4 kg]). Some weight gain is also attributable to increased proteins and fat deposits, with the average weight gain in pregnancy being 27 pounds (12.3 kg).

Increased joint laxity as manifested by increased lordosis and pubic symphyseal laxity may be due to release of the hormone relaxin during pregnancy, which causes collagenous tissues to soften and produces a generalized relaxation of the ligamentous system, especially along the spine.

Pregnancy increases the demand for carbohydrates, a change that seems to be based on fetal demand for glucose. Because the insulin molecule is too large to pass through the placental barrier, several hormones are used to compensate for the increased carbohydrate requirement. During pregnancy, chemical diabetes can develop in women who are predisposed to a diabetic state, but return to a normal carbohydrate metabolism postpartum. During pregnancy, the pancreas secretes insulin in greater amounts and at a faster pace, while cellular sensitivity to insulin declines. The increased production of insulin results from increased levels of free cortisol and progesterone. Estrogen has the effect of blunting the action of insulin, whereas progesterone decreases the utilization of insulin by the cells. The net effect is to make glucose available to the fetus in the form of increased energy production from fat. In a healthy woman, these systems work a very fine balancing act to maintain homeostasis. In obese women or women who have been diagnosed with or are predisposed to diabetes, this balance is much harder to achieve.

■ Cultural Values Considerations

The United States is among the most culturally diverse nations in the world. This diversity may be a factor when you are assessing and treating an obstetric patient from a culture different than yours. Some cultures may not permit a male health care provider, especially in the prehospital setting, to assess or examine a pregnant patient. Different cultures may view pregnancy differently than you do, assuming diverse social, psychologic, and emotional perspectives. Some may see pregnancy as a means of achieving status and recognition within the family unit, where others may experience a drop in self-esteem. Your responsibility is to the patient and is limited to providing care and transport. You should respect these differences and honor requests from these patients.

▶ Adolescent Pregnancy

The United States has very high teenage pregnancy rates compared with other developed countries.[8] During your career, you are likely to respond to many pregnant teens who may or may not be in labor. Adolescents present their own challenges to the emergency medical services (EMS) community in terms of their physical and psychologic development, even when pregnancy is not a contributing factor for a female teenager.

Pregnant teens may or may not know that they are pregnant or may be in denial of their situation. As you begin to assess all female teenagers, you should remember that pregnancy is a possibility as you would for any woman of childbearing age. The pregnancy itself may or may not be related to the nature of the call, but you should consider it when you are assessing the patient, talking to the patient, obtaining a history, and providing treatment. Respect the teenager's privacy and need for independence. If possible, question all teenagers and perform your assessment away from parents.

■ Patient Assessment

Special terminology is used when referring to a pregnant patient. As mentioned, *gravidity* refers to the number of times a woman has been pregnant, regardless of the outcome of each pregnancy. *Parity* refers to delivery of an infant carried for more than 20 weeks' gestation who is alive. The following are some other commonly encountered obstetric terms:

- **Primigravida**: A woman who is pregnant for the first time.
- **Primipara**: A woman who has had only one delivery.
- **Multigravida**: A woman who has had two or more pregnancies, irrespective of the outcome.
- **Multipara**: A woman who has had two or more deliveries. A woman who has had more than five deliveries is referred to as a "grand multipara."
- **Nullipara**: A woman who has never delivered.

For example, a woman who has had four pregnancies but carried only one of them to term—the three others ended in miscarriage—would be classified as gravida 4, para 1. The medical shorthand annotation would be G4P1. You could also write the preceding case history as G4A3P1, showing abortive history.

▶ Scene Size-up

As with every emergency call, your safety is the top priority when dealing with an obstetric case. Take standard precautions—gloves and eye protection at a minimum—especially if delivery has already begun or is imminent. If the call will result in a field delivery, you should also don a mask and gown.

Consider calling for additional or specialized resources. Remember, you may end up with two patients who will require hands-on care.

You will also encounter pregnant patients who are not in labor, so it is important to determine the mechanism of injury or nature of illness in a pregnant patient. Because a pregnant woman's balance may be altered by the weight and size of the fetus and hormones that relax the musculature, falls and spinal immobilization must be considered.

Primary Survey

The primary survey with a pregnant patient is the same as with any patient—assess the ABCDEs (Airway, Breathing, Circulation, Disability, and Exposure), and manage life threats.

The general impression is a good across-the-room assessment that should tell you whether the patient is in active labor and allows you to identify any life threats. The chief complaint may be "The baby is coming!" Take a moment to confirm whether the fetus will be delivered in the next few minutes or whether you have more time to continue to evaluate the situation. When trauma or another medical problem such as vaginal bleeding or seizure is the presenting complaint, evaluate it first and then assess the impact of this problem on the fetus. Use the AVPU (Awake and alert, responsive to Verbal stimuli, responsive to Pain, Unresponsive) scale to determine the patient's level of consciousness.

During an uncomplicated birth, life-threatening conditions with the mother's airway and breathing usually are not an issue. In contrast, a motor vehicle crash, an assault, or any number of medical conditions in a pregnant woman may create a life threat and, sometimes, result in a complicated delivery. In these situations, assess the patient's airway and breathing to ensure they are adequate. If needed, provide airway management and oxygen as appropriate.

Recall that normal changes in pregnancy result in increased overall blood volume, increased heart rate, and changes in blood clotting in the woman. These changes can have a significant impact on a pregnant patient who is bleeding, regardless of the cause. Quickly assess for any potentially life-threatening bleeding, and begin treatment immediately. Blood loss after delivery is expected, but significant bleeding is not. Assess the skin for color, temperature, and condition, and check the pulse rate to determine whether it is too fast or too slow. If signs of shock are apparent, control the bleeding, give oxygen, and keep the patient warm. A minimum of one intravenous (IV) line should be established in preparation for a fluid bolus if needed.

If delivery is imminent, prepare to deliver at the scene. The ideal place for the delivery is in the security of your ambulance or the privacy of the woman's home. The area should be warm and private, with plenty of room to move around.

If the delivery is not imminent, prepare the patient for transport and perform the remainder of the assessment en route to the ED. Administer oxygen. Pregnant women in the last two trimesters of pregnancy should be transported in the left lateral recumbent position to displace the weight of the uterus from the superior vena cava. Although the left lateral recumbent position is an accepted treatment and transportation option, if the woman does not develop supine hypotension and is more comfortable in a supine position, it is acceptable to use a supine position. If spinal immobilization is absolutely indicated, secure the woman to the backboard and elevate the right side of the board with rolled towels or blankets to prevent supine hypotensive syndrome. Provide rapid transport for pregnant patients who have significant bleeding and pain, are hypertensive, are having a seizure, or have an altered mental status.

Special Populations

Blood pressure is a late finding in hypoperfusion and even more so in a pregnant patient because a greater volume of blood can be lost before hypotension develops.

History Taking

Proper medical history taking and physical assessment are important parts of treating the obstetric patient. Investigate the history of the present illness (using OPQRST [Onset, Provocation/palliation, Quality, Region/radiation, Severity, Timing]), and obtain a past medical history (using SAMPLE [Signs and symptoms, Allergies, Medications, Pertinent past medical history, Last oral intake, Events leading up to the illness or injury]). Specifically, you want to know whether the patient is pregnant, how many times she has been pregnant (gravida), and how many times she has had a live birth (para). The first question can generally be bypassed if the patiently is obviously pregnant. Asking a woman who is near term if she is pregnant (the unspoken implication is that she is obese) is not a good way to develop trust, but if in doubt, ask. The number of times pregnant may also need to be clarified, because many women do not count abortions or miscarriages as pregnancies, and tend to think only of actual deliveries. Also ask about the length of gestation and the woman's estimated due date or date of confinement.

Has the woman had a baby before? Labor in a first-time mother usually proceeds more slowly and takes longer (average of 16 hours) than in subsequent pregnancies, allowing more time for transport.

Ask the patient whether she has experienced complications with any of her pregnancies, or whether she has had any obstetric or gynecologic complications. Has she ever had a cesarean section? If so, is a cesarean delivery planned for the current pregnancy or does the patient intend to have a vaginal birth after cesarean? Complications of vaginal birth after cesarean can include uterine rupture. Is the patient currently under a physician's care? Has she been taking prenatal vitamins? When was her last visit to her physician? Has her physician indicated any concerns about this pregnancy?

Has the patient undergone a recent ultrasonographic exam? What were the findings? Did the ultrasonogram reveal more than one fetus or any abnormal presentations? Is the patient taking any current medications? Any over-the-counter drugs, recreational drugs, or herbal supplements? Does the patient have any allergies?

What is your general impression of the patient's overall health? Has she been smoking, consuming alcohol, or used any illicit drugs during the pregnancy? If yes, how recently?

Is the patient currently experiencing pain? If yes, what is the quality and duration? Where is it located and does it radiate? Was the onset gradual or sudden? When did the pain start, and does anything relieve it? Has the patient experienced this type of pain before? When? Is the pain occurring regularly? Is it sporadic or constant?

Has the patient noticed any vaginal bleeding or spotting? If so, what was the amount of bleeding (how many pads has she gone through)? How long did the bleeding last? What color was the blood—red or brown? What was the patient doing prior to the bleeding? Did she use sanitary pads to absorb the bleeding? How many pads? Did the bleeding stop? Has the patient passed any clots or tissue? If so, try to obtain samples to give to providers in the ED. Has the patient experienced any other type of vaginal discharge? What was the amount, color, and duration of that discharge? Was any identifiable or disagreeable odor associated with the discharge?

If the patient is in active labor, has her water broken? Does she feel the need to move her bowels or push? That sensation occurring during labor is caused by the fetus's head in the woman's birth canal pressing against the rectum; it indicates that delivery is imminent. If the woman reports an urge to move her bowels, *do not allow her to go to the toilet.*

What are the contractions like? Some women experience Braxton-Hicks contractions throughout the pregnancy, so it is important to distinguish false labor from the real thing. The pains of true labor are regularly spaced and increase in intensity over time. Table 41-1 distinguishes false labor from true labor.

How frequent are the contractions? If they are more than 5 minutes apart, you generally have enough time to get the woman to a nearby hospital. Contractions that are less than 2 minutes apart signal impending delivery, especially in a multipara.

The answers to those questions should give you a good idea of whether there will be time to transport

Table 41-1	**False Labor Versus True Labor**	
Parameter	**True Labor**	**False Labor**
Contractions	Regularly spaced	Irregularly spaced
Interval between contractions	Gradually shortens	Remains long
Intensity of contractions	Gradually increases	Stays the same
Effects of analgesics	Do not abolish the pain	Often abolish the pain
Cervical changes	Progressive effacement and dilation	No changes

© Jones & Bartlett Learning.

the woman to the hospital. To double-check, *inspect* the woman for **crowning**—crowning indicates that the fetus will be born within the next few minutes.

Secondary Assessment

Your physical exam should be based on the patient's chief complaint. Just because a woman is pregnant, you should not rule out the possibility of asthma, heart attack, or allergic reactions, for example. No matter what the chief complaint, the full-body exam should also include fetal heart tones and heart rate. By feeling the abdomen, you can roughly palpate the fetal position. Ask the patient when she last felt the baby move or if there has been any change in how much the baby has been moving. Pay close attention to the vital signs of both patients—the woman and the fetus. If the patient tells you she has abdominal pain, ask her to describe the pain; this information will help determine whether she is having contractions.

Special Populations

If you note a scar above a woman's pubic hair line Figure 41-5 , it may mean that she has delivered in the past by cesarean section. Ask whether she knows of any reason why she would not be able to deliver her baby vaginally, and report her response to medical control. Women who have previously delivered by cesarean section are not precluded from having a normal vaginal delivery, but attempting to do so may increase their risk for uterine rupture.

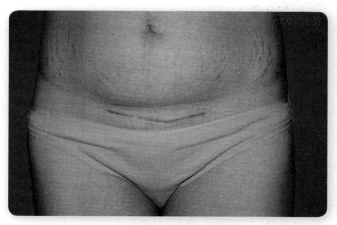

Figure 41-5 A scar from a cesarean section.
© Jones & Bartlett Learning.

Inspect the vaginal area for crowning or vaginal bleeding or discharge. Crowning indicates that you will need to deliver the fetus on scene. If there is no crowning, ask the woman how far apart the contractions are, and then time them. Ask the patient if her water has broken, and, if so, how long ago.

If you see bleeding or discharge, determine when it started and check the patient's abdomen for tenderness and rigidity. Normal abdomens are not rigid during pregnancy. Assessment of the serial vital signs will tell you if the woman or her fetus is in distress.

If the patient's water has broken, ask about the color of the fluid and whether it had an odor. A brown or black color or a strong odor may indicate meconium staining, discussed later in this chapter. Meconium can be aspirated into the fetus's lungs, resulting in potentially life-threatening

sepsis. Its presence requires special techniques discussed later in this chapter.

As noted earlier, some women may experience Braxton-Hicks contractions, or intermittent uterine contractions that occur every 10 to 20 minutes. Usually seen in the third trimester of pregnancy, this condition is also known as false labor. Because you have no way of telling in the field whether a patient's contractions are from a miscarriage or another complication of pregnancy, the patient needs to be transported.

Imminent Delivery

If delivery is imminent, you will not have time to perform an extensive physical examination, but you should attempt to do the following:

- **Assess the woman's vital signs.** If the woman's blood pressure is elevated or her hands and face look puffy, test the deep tendon reflexes at the knees ("knee jerks") for hyperactivity. Any of those signs—elevated blood pressure, facial edema, or hyperactive reflexes—strongly suggest that the woman has preeclampsia, and you must be prepared to deal with seizures before, during, or after delivery.
- **Try to estimate the gestational age.** Palpate the abdomen to estimate the height of the uterus. If the top of the uterus (the fundus) is palpable just above the symphysis pubis, the gestational age is 12 to 16 weeks; if the fundus is palpable at the level of the woman's umbilicus, the gestational age is 20 weeks; if the fundus reaches all the way to the xiphoid, the fetus is at or near term.

YOU are the Paramedic　　　PART 2

Your patient is sitting in the driver's seat of the vehicle. She is still wearing her seat belt, which is positioned across the widest part of her abdomen. The airbag has deployed from the steering wheel. The patient is responsive, alert, and oriented. She reports a cramping-type pain in her pelvis.

Recording Time: 1 Minute	
Appearance	Awake
Level of consciousness	Alert, oriented
Airway	Open
Breathing	Adequate
Circulation	Adequate

3. Is the location of the seat belt concerning to you?
4. Which steps will you take in your further assessment of this patient?

■ **Listen for fetal heart tones.** A fetal heart rate less than 120 beats/min suggests fetal distress in most pregnancies. If you have a Doppler stethoscope available, place the doppler probe over the pregnant woman's abdomen at the 4 o'clock position, approximately 2 inches from the woman's umbilicus. You may have to move the doppler probe around the abdomen until you can hear the fetal heart tones. Palpate the woman's pulse at the same time as you count the fetal heart rate. If the fetal heart rate is identical to the maternal pulse, you are probably listening to an echo of the maternal heartbeat and not the fetal heart. Change the position of the doppler probe and try again. Some modern ambulances may be equipped with Doppler stethoscopes, which make assessment of fetal heart sounds possible.

If the patient's history and physical assessment indicate that there is ample time to reach the hospital, place the woman in the left lateral recumbent position, remove any of her underclothing that might obstruct delivery (if delivery suddenly appears to be imminent en route to the hospital), and begin transport.

If you conclude that there is *not* enough time to get the patient to the hospital, prepare to assist in delivery of the fetus at the scene. In a crowded or public place, try to find an area of maximum privacy and cleanliness in which to work. In the patient's home, deploy nervous bystanders in such a way as to keep them occupied, preferably elsewhere. The pregnant woman may find it reassuring to have another woman or her partner present. Your own behavior, if calm and reassuring, will be the most effective sedative for the patient and bystanders alike.

Reassessment

Ongoing examination should include an assessment of the woman's serial vital signs and the fetal heart rate and heart tones. Also, time the contractions and perform a full-body exam of the woman (if you have not already done so) to avoid missing other possible injuries and complications. Check any interventions and transport to an appropriate facility.

If your assessment determines that delivery is imminent, notify staff at the receiving hospital. Provide an update on the status of the mother and newborn after delivery. On the rare occasion that the delivery does not occur within 30 minutes or you determine that a complication is occurring that cannot be treated in the field, notify the hospital staff of your findings and provide rapid transport. For a pregnant patient with complaints unrelated to childbirth (such as trauma or difficulty breathing), be sure to include the pregnancy status of the patient in your radio report.

■ Pathophysiology, Assessment, and Management of Complications Related to Pregnancy

Several medical conditions and situations may adversely affect the health of both the woman and the developing fetus. Pregnancy has the tendency to aggravate preexisting medical conditions and give rise to new ones.

▶ Substance Abuse

When a pregnant woman is a drug addict, the illicit drugs she uses pass through the placenta barrier and enter into the fetal circulation. The fetus may then develop birth defects and also become an addict. When you are delivering the fetus of a woman with a history of drug abuse, be aware that the newborn may have signs of withdrawal after it is born—for example, respiratory depression, bradycardia, tachycardia, seizures, and cardiac arrest. Treatment should revolve around cardiorespiratory support.

▶ Supine Hypotensive Syndrome

When the pregnant uterus compresses the inferior vena cava, venous blood return to the heart is diminished or, in some cases, occluded. This problem occurs mainly when a pregnant patient is in the supine position (hence the term **supine hypotensive syndrome**) but can also occur when the woman is sitting.[9] This condition is usually seen in the third trimester, when the uterus is at its largest and patient mobility is significantly impaired. It also occurs in women who have venous varicosities. Women are at risk for this syndrome during labor, but may also experience difficulties in sleep states, particularly if they fall asleep on their back. Left uncorrected, supine hypotensive syndrome can result in significant maternal hypotension and potentially lead to fetal distress because the maternal hypotension translates into placental hypoperfusion. Nausea, dizziness, tachycardia, and anxiety are early signs, progressing to breathing difficulty and syncopal episodes. Predisposing factors may include hypovolemia, from either blood loss or dehydration.

Management includes placing the patient in the left lateral recumbent position (tilting the backboard if needed) and treating underlying causes (ie, giving IV fluids, if the patient is hypovolemic). In addition, you must monitor the patient's blood pressure and other vital signs and obtain an ECG.

▶ Cardiac Conditions

Heart disease is of major concern when you are dealing with a pregnant patient. When you are obtaining the patient's medical history, find out the nature and treatment of any heart conditions. Which cardiac medications has the patient been taking? Has she previously been diagnosed with dysrhythmias or heart murmurs? Has she had a history of rheumatic fever, or was she born with a congenital heart defect? Such heart defects may be benign under normal conditions, but the added stresses of pregnancy could create major problems. Has the patient experienced any episodes of dizziness, light-headedness, or syncopal episodes with the pregnancy? Such episodes can be indicative of dysrhythmias that can become critical during the stresses of labor.

Peripartum Cardiomyopathy

Peripartum cardiomyopathy (PPCM), also known as postpartum cardiomyopathy, is an uncommon form of heart failure that happens during the last month of pregnancy or up to five months after giving birth. Risk factors include:

- Obesity
- History of cardiac disorders, such as myocarditis (inflammation of the heart muscle)
- Use of certain medications
- Smoking
- Alcoholism
- Multiple pregnancies
- African American descent
- Poor nourishment

PPCM can easily be confused with eclampsia. Although the two conditions have similar presentations, they are very different. The only way to differentiate PPCM from eclampsia however is to test for proteinuria, which is impossible in the field.

▶ Hypertensive Disorders

A major cause of mortality and morbidity in pregnant women is hypertension. Blood pressure is generally lower during the gestational period compared to prepregnancy level, but women who are hypertensive or borderline hypertensive may have their hypertension exacerbated by pregnancy.

Chronic hypertension is defined as a blood pressure that is equal to or greater than 140/90 mm Hg, which exists prior to pregnancy, occurs before the 20th week of pregnancy, or persists postpartum. Diastolic pressure greater than 110 mm Hg places the patient in an increased risk category for stroke and other cardiovascular dangers. Chronic hypertension can also retard growth and development of the fetus, impair liver and renal function, cause pulmonary edema, or progress to life-threatening grand mal seizures.

Gestational hypertension (formerly known as pregnancy-induced hypertension) develops after the 20th week of pregnancy in women with previously normal blood pressures and resolves spontaneously in the postpartum period. It is more commonly experienced by women who are obese or glucose intolerant. Pregnancy-induced hypertension may be an early sign of preeclampsia.

Women younger than 18 years who are experiencing their first pregnancy, women with advanced maternal age (defined as 35 years of age or older), and women with risk factors of chronic hypertension, renal disease, and diabetes are all at increased risk for **preeclampsia**.[10] Race also tends to play a factor in the development of this disorder, with African American women being most susceptible.[10] In addition, women who have experienced preeclampsia in a prior pregnancy are at increased risk to develop the disorder with subsequent pregnancies.[11] Preeclampsia manifests after the 20th week of pregnancy, with the onset of a triad of symptoms: edema, usually of the face, ankles, and hands; gradual onset of hypertension; and protein in the urine. Severe preeclampsia is identified when the systolic pressure exceeds 160 mm Hg or the diastolic pressure exceeds 110 mm Hg, or when severe symptoms are present, such as headache, dizziness, nausea and vomiting, agitation, rapid weight gain, and visual disturbances (floating spots of light). If severe preeclampsia is present, it may require the administration of magnesium sulfate to prevent seizures along with the administration of emergency antihypertensive medications. These may include labetalol (Normodyne, Trandate) or hydralazine (Alazine, Apresoline).[11] If left untreated, preeclampsia may progress to **eclampsia**. This occurs when the patient experiences a seizure in the presence of signs and symptoms consistent with preeclampsia. Eclampsia also requires the administration of magnesium sulfate in addition to antihypertensive medications when indicated.

While preeclampsia usually resolves with delivery, both preeclampsia and eclampsia can still be seen up to 10 days postpartum. The majority of postpartum cases are seen in the first 24 hours after delivery.[11]

Other conditions that may accompany preeclampsia include liver or renal failure, cerebral hemorrhage, abruptio placenta, and HELLP (Hemolysis, Elevated Liver enzymes, Low Platelets) syndrome. HELLP syndrome may occur in 4% to 12% of patients with severe preeclampsia or eclampsia. It is a distinct clinical entity and treatment in the field is limited to treating the presence of preeclampsia and/or eclampsia, with rapid transport to a medical facility.[11]

▶ Seizures

When a seizure occurs in pregnancy, two patients are involved—the pregnant woman and the fetus. Seizures can be caused by hypertension, toxemia, preeclampsia, or a preexisting seizure disorder. Treatment for a pregnant patient is especially difficult because diazepam (Valium) and phenobarbital—the drugs commonly used to treat seizures—can cross the placental barrier, causing fetal distress. In pregnant patients with seizure, magnesium sulfate is the recommended treatment, especially in the patient with eclampsia. In addition, high-flow supplemental oxygen is needed for both patients to counteract the hypoxia that occurs in seizures. Potential complications in such cases may include abruptio placenta, hemorrhage, disseminated intravascular coagulation, and death.

Diabetes

Gestational diabetes mellitus is the inability to process carbohydrates during pregnancy. Increased maternal insulin production may lead to an imbalance between the supply of the woman's insulin and her glucose production. The patient may be asymptomatic or may exhibit the same signs observed in patients with diabetes mellitus: polyuria, polydipsia, and polyphagia. Treatment consists of diet control and oral hypoglycemic medications. As gestational diabetes mellitus may occur early in the pregnancy, it is recommended that patients undergo a fasting glucose test as part of routine prenatal testing.

Diabetes may be markedly affected by pregnancy. Because the hormones of pregnancy alter the body's insulin-regulating mechanisms, patients with diabetes may experience wildly fluctuating blood glucose levels, manifested as hyperglycemic or hypoglycemic episodes. Unfortunately, oral hypoglycemic agents can cross the placental barrier and affect the fetus, so women with insulin-dependent diabetes may need to adjust their daily doses of these agents during pregnancy.

Pregnant patients with a history of diabetes or who present with an altered mental status or seizures should have their blood glucose level checked with a glucometer. Prehospital management should include high-flow oxygen, IV fluids, and administration of dextrose if indicated by a low blood glucose reading. Patients who are hyperglycemic should receive oxygen and IV fluid therapy per local protocol.

Respiratory Disorders

One of the most common complaints of pregnant patients is shortness of breath or general dyspnea. This condition is often precipitated by hormone-related anatomic changes to the respiratory system and is generally only of minor concern and discomfort to the patient. Careful patient assessment and a thorough SAMPLE history, however, may reveal an underlying condition that is being aggravated by the pregnancy.

Asthma is one of the most common conditions that can complicate pregnancy. It can either be aggravated as a preexisting illness or occur for the first time during pregnancy, triggered by the effects of stress or respiratory irritants on an already-sensitized respiratory system. Acute asthma attacks render the fetus and woman vulnerable to progressive hypoxia. Maternal complications of an asthma attack may include premature labor, preeclampsia, respiratory failure, vaginal hemorrhage, or eclampsia. Fetal complications may include premature birth, low birth weight, growth retardation, and potentially fetal death. Low birth weight and premature labor are common outcomes, with preterm delivery occurring in as many as 1 out of 10 patients with asthma and before 37 weeks' gestation.[12]

Hyperemesis Gravidarum

Nearly all pregnant women experience the infamous—but normal—"morning sickness," especially during the first several weeks of pregnancy. **Hyperemesis gravidarum** is a condition of persistent nausea and vomiting during pregnancy.[13] Its prolonged vomiting leads to dehydration and malnutrition, which have negative effects on the woman and fetus. The exact cause of this condition is unknown, but suspected culprits include increased hormone levels (especially estrogen and hCG), stress, and changes to the GI system. Hyperemesis gravidarum is most common in first-time pregnancies, with multiple gestations, and in women who are obese. Symptoms include severe and persistent vomiting, in excess of three or four times daily. Vomiting is usually projectile and generally consists of bile and possibly blood. Severe nausea, pallor, and possibly jaundice may also be seen.

Prehospital treatment of hyperemesis gravidarum includes the following:

- Check blood glucose level.
- Start an IV line of normal saline, administer 250 mL of fluid, and reassess.
- If protocols allow, administer diphenhydramine IV or deep IM. This drug has both sedative and antiemetic effects and is contraindicated if the patient is taking monoamine oxidase (MAO) inhibitors.
- If protocols allow, administer ondansetron IV or PO.[14,15]
- Check orthostatic vital signs, and obtain an ECG.
- Transport. Severe cases will ultimately require hospitalization.

Renal Disorders

As pregnancy progresses, a woman's kidneys increase in length by 0.4 to 0.6 inches (1–1.5 cm), and her ureters become longer, wider, and more curved. Although these changes increase the capacity of the ureters, they can also lead to urinary stasis, resulting in urinary tract infections. Such infections can be mild, but they may also progress to states that result in low fetal birth weight and retarded fetal development, premature labor, or even intrauterine fetal death.

Pressure on the bladder as the uterus enlarges can also result in increased urinary frequency. The renal plasma flow rate and the glomerular filtration rate increase significantly during pregnancy. Patients with preexisting renal disease are likely to experience compounding of associated problems, and those without a diagnosis of renal disease may experience renal malfunctions or failure due to hypertensive disorders or conditions such as hyperemesis gravidarum.

Rh Sensitization

Rh factor is a protein found on the RBCs of most people. When this factor is absent, the person is said to be Rh negative. When a woman who is Rh negative becomes pregnant by a man who has the Rh factor (Rh positive) and the fetus inherits this factor, the fetal blood can pass into the woman's circulation and produce maternal antibody (isoimmunization) to the factor. Rh disease is rarely a problem in first pregnancies, but in subsequent pregnancies the antibody will aggressively cross the placental barrier to attack the fetal RBCs, which the woman's body identifies as foreign proteins. This attack can result in death of the fetus or cause hemolytic disease (erythroblastosis fetalis) in a newborn. Newborns with hemolytic disease may present with jaundice, anemia, and hepatomegaly.

▶ Infections

Viral and parasitic infections in pregnancy can cause significant problems for the pregnant woman and the fetus. Infections early in pregnancy can affect the formation of the fetus's organ systems; infections later in pregnancy can result in neurologic impairments, growth disturbances, and heart and respiratory conditions. The most commonly encountered infections include varicella zoster virus, human parvovirus B19 (fifth disease), toxoplasmosis, and cytomegalovirus.

Urinary Tract Infections

Group B *Streptococcus* (GBS) is the leading cause of life-threatening infections in newborns during their first week of life.[16] In the United States, all pregnant patients seeking prenatal care are screened for GBS infection between 35 and 37 weeks' gestation. This infection is caused by *Streptococcus agalactiae*, bacteria that live in the genitourinary and GI tracts of healthy people, generally without causing any ill effects. In pregnancy, the bacteria can proliferate, resulting in urinary tract infection, infection of the uterus, and stillbirth. If the infection is passed on to the newborn, it can cause respiratory problems, pneumonia, septic shock, and meningitis. Infant illness generally manifests within the first 7 days after birth, but can occur several months later.

Human Immunodeficiency Virus

As discussed in Chapter 26, *Infectious Diseases*, **human immunodeficiency virus (HIV)** is a bloodborne pathogen that can be transmitted from mother to infant in the birthing process. In the United States, all pregnant women who receive prenatal care are tested for HIV infection. In the United States, the rate of infection from mother to child is only 1% to 2% because infected mothers are treated with antiretroviral drugs beginning in the second trimester of pregnancy.[17]

Cholestasis

Cholestasis is a disease of the liver that can occur during pregnancy. Hormones affect the gallbladder by slowing down or blocking the normal bile flow from the liver. Bile, which aids the process of digestion by breaking down fats, is produced in the liver and stored in the gallbladder.

When its normal flow is altered, bile acids build up in the liver and then spill out into the bloodstream.

The most common symptom of cholestasis is profuse, painful itching, particularly of the hands and feet. Patients may also report fatigue or depression, nausea, and right upper quadrant pain. They may also notice color changes in waste elimination—dark urine and abnormally colored stools (light gray, yellow, light brown, or white). Women who are carrying multiple fetuses are at a higher risk for the development of cholestasis, as are women who have a familial history of cholestasis or who have had previous liver damage.

Cholestasis is relatively benign and transitory for the pregnant woman, but can have serious effects on the fetus. Because the fetus relies on the woman's liver to remove bile acids from the blood, any impediment to this process puts stress on the developing fetal liver. Preterm birth and stillbirth are potential complications of untreated cholestasis.

TORCH Syndrome

The acronym TORCH stands for toxoplasmosis, other agents, rubella, cytomegalovirus, and herpes simplex. **TORCH syndrome** refers to infections that occur in neonates as a result of organisms passing through the placenta from the woman to the fetus. While the woman may show no symptoms, neonates show similar symptoms regardless of which of the five infections they have.

Toxoplasmosis is an infection caused by a parasite that pregnant women may get from handling or eating contaminated food or exposure from handling cat litter (cat ingests contaminated food and then passes the infection on in the feces). Depending on when the infection occurs, early versus late pregnancy, there is a chance of the fetus becoming infected. Persons with this infection may not have any signs and symptoms and not know they have the infection. Pregnant women are encouraged not to change cat litter boxes and to eat meat only if it has been thoroughly cooked. Some women may have their physician perform a blood test to detect the condition if they have risk factors.

If the pregnant woman becomes infected early in the pregnancy, there is a decreased chance of spread to the fetus, although signs and symptoms are usually more severe for the fetus if the transmission occurs early in the pregnancy. Newborns usually do not show any signs of the infection but may develop learning, visual, and hearing disabilities as they grow older.

Cytomegalovirus

Cytomegalovirus (CMV) is a member of the herpesvirus family. This common viral infection has no known cure, and the virus can remain dormant in the body for years. An estimated 80% of the US population has been exposed to CMV.[18] In its active stages, CMV may produce symptoms including prolonged high fever, chills, headache, malaise, extreme fatigue, and an enlarged spleen. People with an increased risk for developing active infection and more serious complications (such as fever, pneumonia, liver infection, and anemia) include those with immune disorders, people receiving chemotherapy, and pregnant women. Newborns who acquire CMV are susceptible to lung problems, blood problems, liver problems, swollen glands, rash, and poor weight gain.

■ Pathophysiology, Assessment, and Management of Bleeding Related to Pregnancy

▶ Pathophysiology

Abortion

Abortion is defined as expulsion of the fetus, from any cause, before the 20th week of gestation (some sources consider any loss of the pregnancy up to the 28th week of gestation to be an abortion). Most abortions occur during the first trimester, before the placenta is fully mature.

Abortions can be broadly classified as spontaneous or elective (induced). A **spontaneous abortion** (miscarriage) occurs naturally, and affects an estimated 10% to 25% of all pregnancies.[19] Causes may include acute or chronic illness in the pregnant woman, maternal exposure to toxic substances (illicit drugs), abnormalities in the fetus, or abnormal attachment of the placenta. In many cases, the cause of a spontaneous abortion cannot be found.

An **elective abortion** is brought about intentionally. When you are obtaining a medical history that includes an abortive history, you must be dispassionate and professional regardless of your personal convictions. You may encounter patients who are experiencing complications following an elective abortion, such as vaginal bleeding or sepsis from parts of the fetus remaining in the uterus. You may also encounter patients who have "self-medicated" in an attempt to induce an abortion and are experiencing toxic effects of the herbal remedy as well as a threatened or progressing abortion. Herbal preparations work by making the uterus and bloodstream too toxic for the fetus to survive, which in turn may be too toxic for the woman to survive.

You will most likely find yourself attempting to manage an abortion that is occurring spontaneously. The specific management of such a case depends to some extent on the stage of the abortion when the patient presents for treatment. All pregnant patients presenting with vaginal bleeding or abdominal pain should be transported and evaluated by a physician.

Some women experience recurrent miscarriages or **habitual abortions**, which is defined as three or more consecutive pregnancies that end in miscarriage. Habitual abortion is seen in less than 1% of patients.[20] Causes include chromosomal and endocrine disorders, ovarian issues, uterine malformations, cervical conditions (incompetence), infections, and lifestyle factors.

A **threatened abortion** is an abortion that is attempting to take place. It is generally characterized by vaginal bleeding during the first half of pregnancy—usually in the

YOU ▶ are the Paramedic · PART 3

Your patient confirms that she is 20 weeks pregnant and has been followed by her doctor throughout the pregnancy. She is expecting no complications. This is her second child; the first child is not in the vehicle with her, but rather is being cared for by her grandmother.

Recording Time: 5 Minutes	
Respirations	20 breaths/min
Pulse	100 beats/min
Skin	Pink, warm, dry
Blood pressure	130/72 mm Hg
Oxygen saturation (Spo₂)	98% on room air
Pupils	PERRLA

5. Which trimester is this patient in?

6. Do you have any additional concerns because this is the patient's second pregnancy?

first trimester. The patient may present with abdominal discomfort or report menstrual cramps. Severe pain is rarely a presenting complaint because uterine contractions are not rhythmic. The cervix remains closed. A threatened abortion can progress to an incomplete abortion, or it may subside, allowing the pregnancy to go to term. The treatment for a threatened abortion is usually complete bed rest, often in a hospital environment, so that the woman's condition can be monitored. Your role in this case is usually transport and emotional support.

An **imminent abortion** is a spontaneous abortion that cannot be prevented. The patient will generally present with severe abdominal pain caused by strong uterine contractions. Vaginal bleeding, often massive, will be present, as well as cervical dilation because the uterus is preparing to expel the products of conception. When you are treating a patient who is experiencing a spontaneous abortion, your goals are to maintain blood pressure and prevent hypovolemia. Treatment consists of establishing an IV line of normal saline to maintain blood pressure, 100% supplemental oxygen via a nonrebreathing mask at 15 L/min, obtaining an ECG, and providing emotional support with rapid transport. Be alert for signs of shock.

An **incomplete abortion** occurs when part of the products of conception are expelled but some remain in the uterus. (For example, the fetus is expelled but the placenta remains, or only part of the fetus is expelled.) Because the cervix has dilated to expel the fetus, vaginal bleeding will be present, which may be slight or profuse, but will be continuous. Be alert for signs and symptoms of shock, and start an IV line of normal saline. If products of conception are protruding from the vagina, consult medical control for instructions; gentle removal of protruding tissues may prevent or relieve signs of shock. You will most often encounter this situation when you find the patient on the toilet, having attempted a bowel movement, with the fetus in the toilet still attached to the umbilical cord hanging from the vagina. The fetus should be gently collected, and emotional support provided to the patient. Fundal massage may be beneficial in stimulating the placenta to deliver. All products of conception need to be collected and presented to the receiving facility. Do not deter the patient from viewing the fetus if she wishes, but be prepared for a strong emotional reaction. A **complete abortion** has occurred when all the products of conception have been expelled.

In a **missed abortion**, the fetus dies during the first 20 weeks of gestation but remains in utero. There is no field management of a missed abortion other than providing transport and emotional support. Management at the hospital will consist of a dilation and curettage (D&C), in which the cervix will be manually dilated and the endometrial lining scraped and suctioned. You should suspect a missed abortion when the patient presents with a history of threatened abortion. The typical history will be a cessation of vaginal bleeding followed by a gradual diminishing of the signs of pregnancy, such as uterine and breast enlargement. The woman may also report having had a brown vaginal discharge, possibly accompanied by a rank smell. On examination, the uterus may feel like a hard mass in the abdomen, and fetal heart sounds cannot be heard. Missed abortion is generally caused by maternal disease or abnormalities with the embryo, uterus, placental, or fetal chromosomes. It almost always occurs because of a problem with the fetus, but occasionally a healthy fetus can be expelled by a diseased or damaged uterus. A missed abortion generally precedes a spontaneous abortion.

Septic abortion was once the leading cause of maternal death worldwide. In medical literature, a common complication of childbirth was puerperal fever, which was caused by a streptococcal infection of the genital tract. The incidence of puerperal fever declined significantly in the early 20th century when physicians began routinely washing their hands between patients. Septic abortion occurs when the uterus becomes infected—often by common vaginal bacterial flora—following any type of abortion. The patient will generally give a history of fever and bad-smelling vaginal discharge, usually starting within a few hours after abortion. Physical examination will generally reveal fever and abdominal tenderness.

In severe cases, the infection will have progressed to septicemia, resulting in septic shock. For this life-threatening emergency, prehospital management consists of establishing an IV line of normal saline, administering 100% supplemental oxygen via a nonrebreathing mask, ECG monitoring, and rapid transport. The fluid administration rate should maintain the patient's blood pressure at an acceptable level.

> ### Words of Wisdom
>
> Any vaginal bleeding during the third trimester of pregnancy must be regarded as a dire medical emergency until proven otherwise.

Third-Trimester Bleeding

Abortion accounts for the majority of cases involving vaginal bleeding that results in an emergency call. Any detachment of the ovum or embryo from the uterine wall will result in bleeding. The patient may report light or heavy bleeding, normally accompanied by cramping abdominal pain. She may also report the passage of tissue or clots. Vaginal bleeding is a serious sign at any stage of pregnancy, but the complications of bleeding increase as the gestation time lengthens.

Third-trimester bleeding presents the greatest danger of hemorrhage, which becomes more acute as the woman approaches term. A complicating factor of third-trimester bleeding is the large volume of blood present within the pregnant woman's body and the compensatory mechanisms that are functioning as a result of pregnancy. A pregnant woman can lose a full 40% of her circulating volume before significant signs and symptoms of hypovolemia become apparent.

Ectopic Pregnancy

Ectopic pregnancy is a life-threatening condition. In an ectopic pregnancy, a fertilized ovum becomes implanted somewhere other than in the uterus, usually in one of the fallopian tubes. The fetus will not develop to term, even though all the normal signs and symptoms of pregnancy are usually present.

In a case involving ectopic pregnancy, you are typically dispatched to a patient with abdominal pain. The patient is in severe pain (from the threatened rupture of the tube), and may be in hypovolemic shock. It is important for you to be understanding, empathetic, and supportive. All female patients of child-bearing age with severe, lower abdominal pain should be considered as experiencing an ectopic pregnancy. Treatment for shock and rapid transport are your priorities. Ectopic pregnancy is discussed in detail in Chapter 22, *Gynecologic Emergencies*.

> ### Special Populations
>
> A pregnant woman may lose a large amount of blood before she shows signs of shock. Do not wait for signs and symptoms.

Bleeding and the Placenta

Major causes of significant hemorrhage before delivery are abruptio placenta and placenta previa.

Abruptio placenta refers to a premature partial or incomplete separation of a normally implanted placenta from the wall of the uterus **Figure 41-6**. It most commonly occurs during the last trimester of pregnancy, but can take place in the second trimester as well. Abruptio placenta affects about 1 of every 100 pregnancies that go to term.[21,22] Although the exact cause of abruptio placenta is unknown, hypertension, trauma, drug use, alcohol use, diabetes, and having multiple pregnancies increase the risk for this condition.[21,22]

The patient with abruptio placenta will present with a sudden onset of severe abdominal pain, often radiating into the back; there will also be decreased fetal movement and decreased fetal heart tones. The patient may report vaginal bleeding, although in some cases the blood does not emerge through the cervix and the bleeding may remain concealed within the endometrium. Physical examination may reveal signs of shock, often out of proportion to the apparent volume of blood loss. The abdomen will be tender and the uterus rigid to palpation. Other complications include severe hemorrhaging. If the hemorrhaging cannot be controlled after delivery, a hysterectomy may be necessary.

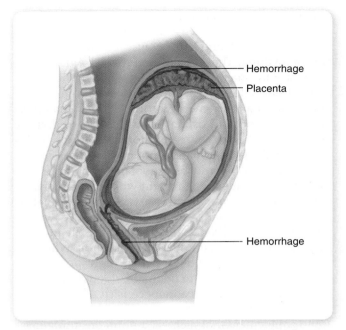

Figure 41-6 In abruptio placenta, the placenta partially or completely separates prematurely from the wall of the uterus.

© Jones & Bartlett Learning.

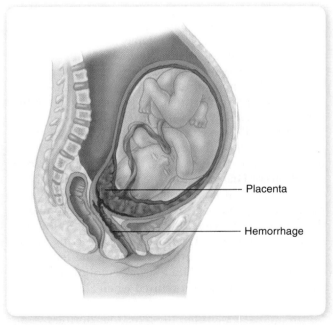

Figure 41-7 In placenta previa, the placenta develops over and covers the cervix.

© Jones & Bartlett Learning.

In **placenta previa**, the placenta is implanted low in the uterus and, as it grows, it partially or fully obscures the cervical canal **Figure 41-7**. This condition is the leading cause of painless vaginal bleeding in the second and third trimesters of pregnancy, with the majority of problems occurring near term because the cervix begins to dilate in preparation for delivery. Maternal age and multiparity are risk factors. Placenta previa occurs in about 1 of every 200 births,[23] with a maternal mortality rate of less than 1%.[24] Complications may include disseminated intravascular coagulation, hemorrhage, and low fetal birth weight.

The chief complaint of a woman with placenta previa is usually painless vaginal bleeding, with the loss of bright red blood. Because the blood supply to the fetus is not immediately jeopardized, fetal movements continue and fetal heart sounds remain audible. On gentle palpation, the uterus is soft and nontender. (Do *not* try to palpate the abdomen deeply in any woman with third-trimester bleeding; if she does have placenta previa, deep palpation may induce heavy bleeding.)

▶ Assessment and Management

When a pregnant patient presents with the chief complaint of vaginal bleeding, try to determine as much as possible about the nature of the bleeding. When did it start? Which activity was the woman engaged in at the onset? Was she active or at rest? How much blood has been lost (how many pads soaked)? Is the patient experiencing abdominal pain? What is the nature and quality of the pain: sharp, cramping, dull, or achy? Use OPQRST to elaborate on the chief complaint of labor pain. Rate its severity on a scale of 0 to 10.

During the physical examination, identify any changes in orthostatic vital signs. Orthostatic changes suggest a significant blood loss, which may differ from the physical evidence of bleeding, which may be slight. Look for a positive Grey Turner sign or Cullen sign, which can help correlate the presence of internal bleeding.

You do not need to identify the underlying cause of the bleeding to treat it. Regardless of the source of hemorrhaging, prehospital management is the same:

1. Keep the patient in a left lateral recumbent position.
2. Administer 100% supplemental oxygen via a nonrebreathing mask at 15 L/min.
3. Provide rapid transport to a definitive care facility, notifying the facility of the patient's condition en route.
4. Start an IV line of normal saline with an 18-gauge IV catheter. Begin infusing a 250-mL bolus of fluid and then reevaluate. Continue with such boluses as indicated up to 20 mL/kg. If blood pressure has not yet reached 90 mm Hg systolic, obtain medical direction and prepare to administer additional fluid boluses. An additional IV line may also be indicated.
5. Obtain an ECG and obtain baseline vital signs. Do not attempt to examine the woman internally or pack the vagina with trauma pads.
6. Use loosely placed trauma pads over the vagina in an effort to stop the flow of blood.

■ Normal Childbirth

Pregnant women may call 9-1-1 when going into labor. The chances that complications will occur increase significantly when an unplanned delivery occurs outside the hospital. In such a case, you will likely be working in an uncontrolled, nonsterile environment, so having a good working knowledge of potential complications and strategies to resolve them is mandatory.

▶ Stages of Labor

The following discussion focuses on the stages of normal labor. **Labor** refers to the mechanism by which the products of conception—that is, the fetus and the placenta—are expelled from the pregnant woman's uterus. It is called labor because it is *hard work*.

Labor progresses through several well-defined stages. The time for each stage depends, in part, on whether the woman is going through her first pregnancy or has had previous deliveries. The premonitory signs of labor, which often are unnoticed, include the woman beginning to feel a relief of pressure in her upper abdomen (**lightening**) and a simultaneous increase of pressure in her pelvis as the fetus starts its descent toward the birth canal. A plug of mucus, sometimes mixed with blood (called the **bloody show**), is expelled from the dilating cervix and discharged from the vagina, though this event may occur weeks before labor actually starts.

The **first stage of labor** begins with the onset of labor pains—crampy abdominal pains that may radiate into the small of the back and reflect the contractions of the uterus. Those early contractions come at 5- to 15-minute intervals, and they serve to maneuver the fetus into position and prepare the cervical opening for the delivery of the fetus. The latent phase occurs when the cervix begins to dilate and efface. As the uterus contracts, its less muscular lower segment is pulled upward over the presenting part, resulting in **effacement** (thinning and shortening) of the cervix. Effacement is accompanied by progressive cervical dilation—that is, stretching of the cervical opening until it is wide enough to accommodate passage of the fetus. The first stage of labor lasts until the cervix is fully dilated, an average of about 12 hours in a nullipara and anywhere up to 8 hours in a multipara.

During the active phase, there is a noticeable increase in the intensity of the contractions, which become more painful. Contractions occur more regularly, last longer, and are closer together. Cervical dilation occurs to approximately 7 centimeters in this phase. The transition phase begins when the cervix is fully dilated to 10 centimeters, at which point the woman may feel an urge to bear down, push, or have a bowel movement. Toward the end of this first stage of labor, the amniotic sac often ruptures, with a gush of fluid pouring out of the vagina.

The **second stage of labor** begins as the head of the fetus descends and flexes (chin to chest) to enter the birth canal. The fetus must go through several positional changes to pass through the pelvic ring and completely through the birth canal. The next position is internal rotation, in which the head is rotated so that the face is toward the woman's rectum. Extension occurs next, as the head of the fetus tilts to a position such that the crown of the head can be seen at the vaginal opening. Crowning is considered the beginning of the second stage of labor. The baby's head then rotates to the side (restitution) to align the head again with the shoulders. The final external rotation occurs with the movement of the shoulders that results in expulsion of the fetus's body.

The woman's contractions in this stage are more intense and more frequent, occurring 2 to 3 minutes apart. Her pulse rate increases, and sweat appears on her face. She tends to bear down with each contraction and, because of the pressure of the fetus's head against her rectum, she may feel as if she has to move her bowels. The cervix is fully dilated and effaced, and the presenting part of the fetus (the part that emerges from the woman first—normally the head) begins bulging out of the vaginal opening (crowning). When crowning occurs, delivery is imminent. The second stage of labor concludes when the newborn is fully delivered. Altogether, the second stage of labor takes 1 to 2 hours in a nullipara and about 30 minutes in a multipara.

> ### Words of Wisdom
>
> Never, never, never attempt to delay or restrain delivery in any fashion.

The **third stage of labor** (placental stage) is the period that involves separation of the placenta from the uterine wall. It lasts from the delivery of the newborn until the placenta has been fully expelled and the uterus has contracted. The placenta usually delivers spontaneously within 30 minutes after birth. Uterine contraction is necessary to squeeze shut all of the tiny blood vessels left exposed when the placenta separates from the uterine wall. **Table 41-2** summarizes the stages of labor.

Table 41-2	The Stages of Labor: Nullipara Versus Multipara	
Stage of Labor	Nullipara	Multipara
First stage	8 to 12 hours	6 to 8 hours
Second stage	1 to 3 hours	5 to 30 minutes
Third stage	5 to 60 minutes	5 to 60 minutes

© Jones & Bartlett Learning.

▶ Maternal and Fetal Responses to Labor

The body systems of the pregnant woman and the fetus respond differently during the strenuous stages of labor. Almost all of the responses are the direct result of the intense physical stressors that the woman experiences with each contraction. Contractions and the positional changes of the fetus through the birth canal are the primary causes of the fetal responses seen.

The woman experiences an increased workload on her heart during labor. Blood pressure, pulse, and cardiac output are all increased to ramp up her energy for childbirth. It is common to see an increase in systolic blood pressure of as much as 15 points during a contraction. Do not try to obtain a blood pressure reading during a contraction, as you will get a falsely high reading.

The woman's respiratory system also responds to labor by increasing her breathing rate to accommodate the increased demand for oxygen. During the second stage of labor, the woman's need for and consumption or use of oxygen approaches 100%. Pain from contractions and perineal stretching also drive increases in the respiratory rate during labor.

> ### Words of Wisdom
>
> If the fetus is coming fast, it is more important to control the delivery than to put on sterile drapes. When crowning occurs, place your sterile gloved hand over the emerging bony parts of the head, and by exerting minimal pressure, control the delivery of the head.

Typically, the woman's immune system responds to the stress and exertion of labor with an increase in WBC production. The renal system (kidneys) will preserve fluids and electrolytes. The increase in physical exertion increases the woman's body temperature; diaphoresis is common in laboring patients in an attempt to regulate their body temperature. The woman's body diverts blood flow to those areas most needed during labor so the GI system is essentially inactive, resulting in delayed stomach emptying and loose bowel movements. Nausea, vomiting, and diarrhea are common; be prepared to manage the airway to remove any vomiting that may occur.

The powerful uterine contractions also affect the body of the fetus. During a contraction, blood flow is greatly reduced, which can affect the hemodynamic status of the fetus. This results in decreased amounts of oxygen and nutrients reaching the fetus, as well as insufficient removal of waste from the fetus, and a decreased fetal heart rate during a contraction. Fetal acidosis represents the fetus's acid-base response to hypoxia and the buildup of lactic acid; this condition can be caused by a nuchal cord, multiple births, abnormal fetal position, a respiratory condition, shoulder dystocia, and other complications of childbirth.

▶ Preparing for Delivery

When birth is imminent and you may not have enough time to reach the hospital, you must assist in childbirth outside the hospital. In such cases, you generally do not have much time to make extensive preparations. You may have only a minute or two to get the woman into position, open the obstetric (OB) kit, and deliver the newborn. The sequence of actions in emergency childbirth needs to be well planned and well-rehearsed before you use it in the field.

Position the pregnant woman. If childbirth is to take place in the patient's home, the fetus is usually delivered with the woman lying supine in her bed or at least on a flat surface. Try to tilt her slightly with a pillow to help keep pressure off the inferior vena cava. Be aware that while placing the woman in the supine position makes things much easier for you assisting delivery, it makes things harder for the woman because she has to push against gravity. Some women prefer to sit at the edge of a chair or to squat for delivery—both positions that enable the woman to take advantage of gravity.

Controversies

Some medical personnel feel strongly that in-home delivery should take place on the stretcher if at all possible to facilitate quick removal should the situation take a turn for the worse.

Delivery modalities have changed dramatically in recent years. More women are opting for home deliveries versus in-hospital care, and natural childbirth is becoming more popular. The use of nurse-midwives, lay midwives, professional birth assistants, chiropractors, and doulas (an assistant who "mothers" the woman) during childbirth is gradually gaining acceptance within the medical community. With the proliferation of these professionals, alternative "pushing" positions are also becoming more popular. If the woman prefers to be in an alternative pushing position, you need to adapt to the circumstances and let her use whatever position she is most comfortable with as long as the alternative method does not endanger the woman.

Birthing Positions

Standing Birth. Birthing from a standing position is an ancient practice, and one that is still used in several areas of the world **Figure 41-8**. This position is sometimes used in the active birth model, in which the woman is allowed total freedom to move around and be active up to the point of delivery. Standing birth allows the woman

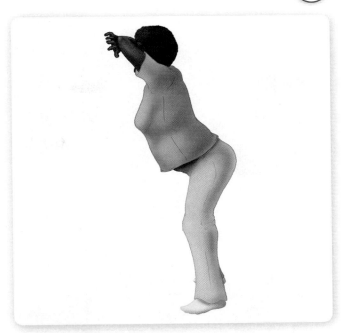

Figure 41-8 The standing position.
© Jones & Bartlett Learning.

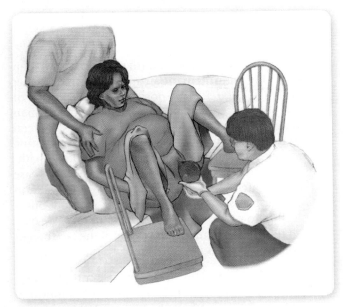

Figure 41-9 Semi-Fowler position.
© Jones & Bartlett Learning.

to take advantage of gravity and allows the pelvis to open to a maximal position. The fetal head is moved away from the sacral area as the woman arches her back, a movement that is not easily accomplished while supine.

Semi-Fowler Position. The semi-Fowler position is basically a modified lithotomy position, with the woman's torso propped up to a high Fowler or Fowler position **Figure 41-9**. Sitting up seems to help some women with pushing because they can lie back to rest in between contractions.

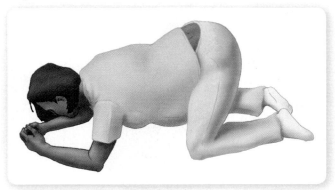

Figure 41-10 Kneeling birth position.
© Jones & Bartlett Learning.

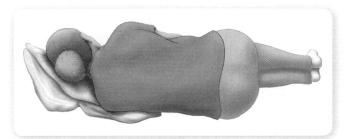

Figure 41-11 Left-Sims position.
© Jones & Bartlett Learning.

Kneeling Birth. In the kneeling birth position, the woman kneels with her buttocks in the air and usually rests on her elbows **Figure 41-10**. This position provides some of the same advantages as squatting: It enables the woman to arch her back to assist delivery, which allows the fetal head to move away from the sacrum, thereby facilitating the birth. Some women may use this method in a bathtub full of water (water birth), which is reputed to ease delivery. Unintentional submersion (of the woman and newborn) is a possible downside to this method, but is technically a low risk. The newborn continues to be oxygenated through the umbilical cord until the face breaks water, or the newborn is stimulated.

Side-Lying Position. This position is essentially a left-Sims position, with the upper torso possibly supported with pillows **Figure 41-11**. It ensures that the uterus and the fetus are moved away from the inferior aorta. Some midwives report a significantly reduced incidence of perineal tears using this method. While some women may prefer to have their legs widely spread during birth, the side-lying position allows the knees to be held together, which also purportedly reduces tearing, especially during the crowning stage.

The OB Kit and Preparation

Your sterile emergency OB kit should contain the following items **Figure 41-12**:

- Surgical scissors or a scalpel
- Umbilical cord clamps

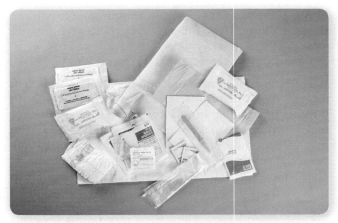

Figure 41-12 Your unit should contain a sterile obstetric kit.
© Jones & Bartlett Learning.

- A small rubber bulb syringe
- Towels, drapes, or sheets
- 4-inch × 4-inch (10-cm × 10-cm) gauze sponges and/or 2-inch × 10-inch (5-cm × 25-cm) gauze sponges
- Sterile gloves
- Infant blanket
- Sanitary pads
- A plastic bag
- Two items that need to be available but are not usually included in the OB kit are an infant-sized bag-mask device and goggles.

Take the following steps to prepare for the delivery:

- Open the sterile OB kit, making sure to maintain sterility by touching only the outside.
- Wash your hands thoroughly with a povidone-iodine or chlorhexidine scrub solution, if available.
- Put on a sterile gown and surgical mask, and wear eye protection.
- Put on sterile gloves, using a sterile donning technique.
- Maintain standard precautions. The chance of contamination from body fluid exposure is high.
- Prepare the woman for delivery by draping her with towels using the sterile towels in the OB kit. Have the woman lift her buttocks, and place the first towel beneath them. Wrap another sterile towel behind the patient's back and drape it over each thigh. Lay a third sterile towel or drape across the woman's abdomen. When you finish, everything should be covered with sterile drapes except the vaginal opening.

If the delivery of the fetus is imminent and you do not have time to place the sterile drapes, just concentrate on controlling the delivery. A safe and controlled delivery takes precedence over draping procedures.

Do not forget to attend to the emotional needs of the patient and family members who are bystanders. This job should be managed by your partner while you are getting prepared. Emotions tend to run high during deliveries, and additional stress may be experienced if the delivery is occurring in a crowded area. Your partner should take a position at the woman's head to help keep her calm and should administer oxygen if indicated (eg, with a high-risk pregnancy, hypotension or hypertension, or pain). Your partner should also ensure that an emesis basin and portable suction are at hand. If there is time, establish an IV line (especially if your protocols call for oxytocin administration after delivery), and apply the ECG monitor. Consider administering IV fluid boluses if the woman is hypotensive. Although not common, some protocols will direct you to administer analgesic pain medication. As always, follow your local protocol.

Encourage the woman to rest between contractions and to resist bearing down until you are ready to assist with the delivery. This may be challenging, because once the patient is ready to push, she is *going* to push. If she finds it difficult not to bear down, instruct her to pant during each contraction. Panting makes it nearly impossible to push because bearing down requires a closed glottis.

▶ Assisting Delivery

Follow these steps to assist with the delivery:

1. Control the delivery. When crowning occurs, place *gentle* pressure on the newborn's head with the palm of your gloved hand to prevent the head from delivering too quickly and tearing the woman's vagina.
2. As the newborn's head begins to emerge from the vagina, it will start to turn. Support the head as it turns **Figure 41-13**. Do *not* attempt to pull the newborn from the vagina! If the membranes cover the head after it emerges, tear the amniotic sac with your fingers or forceps to permit escape of amniotic fluid and enable the newborn to breathe.
3. Slip your middle finger alongside the newborn's head to check for a nuchal cord. In such a case, the umbilical cord becomes wrapped around part of the infant's body, generally the neck and as a single loop. In most cases, a nuchal cord is not a significant problem, but as the fetus descends during labor, cord compression may occur, causing the fetal heart rate to slow and resulting in fetal distress.
4. If you find a nuchal cord, try to slip it gently over the newborn's shoulder and head. Should this maneuver fail, and if the cord is wrapped tightly around the neck, place umbilical clamps 2 inches apart and cut the cord between the clamps.
5. If the airway appears to be obstructed, cradle and support the newborn's head in your hand, and clear the airway by suctioning with the bulb syringe.
6. Gently guide the head downward to allow delivery of the upper shoulder **Figure 41-14**. Do not pull on the newborn to facilitate the delivery.
7. Gently guide the head upward to allow delivery of the lower shoulder **Figure 41-15**.
8. Once the shoulders are delivered, the newborn's trunk and legs will follow rapidly **Figure 41-16**. Be prepared to grasp and support the newborn as it emerges, keeping in mind an important fact: *Newborns are wet and slippery.*
9. Once the newborn is delivered, maintain its body position at the same level as the vagina to prevent blood drainage from the umbilical cord.

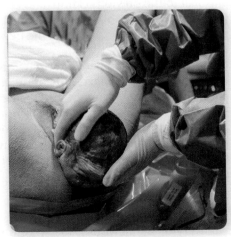

Figure 41-13 As the newborn's head begins to emerge from the vagina, it will start to turn. Support the head as it turns.
© University of Maryland Shock Trauma Center/MIEMSS.

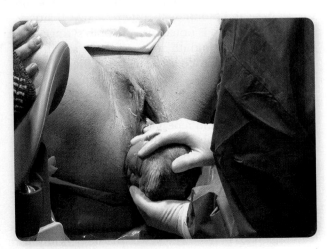

Figure 41-14 Gently guide the newborn's head downward to allow delivery of the upper shoulder.
© University of Maryland Shock Trauma Center/MIEMSS.

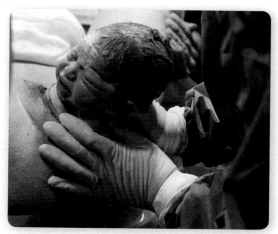

Figure 41-15 Gently guide the head upward to allow delivery of the lower shoulder.
© University of Maryland Shock Trauma Center/MIEMSS.

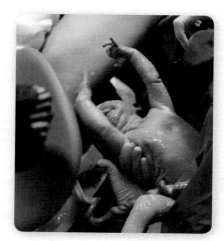

Figure 41-16 Once the shoulders are delivered, the newborn's trunk and legs will follow rapidly.
© University of Maryland Shock Trauma Center/MIEMSS.

10. Wipe any blood or mucus from the newborn's nose and mouth with a sterile gauze. If airway obstruction is noted, use the bulb syringe to suction the mouth and nostrils. Be sure to squeeze the bulb *before* inserting the tip, and only *then* place the tip in the newborn's mouth or nostril and release the bulb slowly. Withdraw the bulb, expel its contents into a waste container, and repeat suctioning as needed.
11. Dry the newborn with sterile towels (wet newborns lose heat faster than dry ones), and wrap the newborn with a dry blanket.
12. Record the time of birth for your patient care report.

In a normal delivery, the newborn will usually be breathing on his or her own. Newborns are typically born with a blue color, but after taking several breaths or crying they should turn a pink color, although their extremities may remain dusky.

Apgar Scoring

The **Apgar scoring system** (devised by Virginia Apgar, MD) is a useful means of evaluating the adequacy of a newborn's vital functions immediately after birth; such information will prove useful to those who take over the care of the newborn after your delivery. In this system, five parameters—heart rate, respiratory effort, muscle tone, reflex irritability, and color—are each given a score from 0 to 2 first at 1 minute and again at 5 minutes after birth. Most newborns are vigorous and have a total score of 7 to 10; they cough or cry within seconds of delivery and require no further resuscitation. Newborns with a score in the 4 to 6 range are moderately depressed; they may be pale or blue 1 minute after delivery, with poorly sustained respirations and flaccid muscle tone. These newborns will require resuscitation. Neonatal resuscitation is discussed in Chapter 42, *Neonatal Care*.

Cutting the Umbilical Cord

Once the newborn has been delivered and is breathing well, the umbilical cord can be clamped and cut because it is no longer necessary for the newborn's survival. Clamping of the cord should be delayed 30 seconds after delivery for most vigorous term and preterm (34–36 weeks) newborns, unless the newborn requires resuscitation.[25] The steps are as follows:

1. Handle the umbilical cord with care. It tears easily.
2. Once the cord has stopped pulsating, tie or clamp the cord about 4 inches (10 cm) from the newborn's navel, and then place the second tie (or clamp) 2 inches (5 cm) from the first tie. Cut the cord between the two ties or clamps.
3. Examine the cut ends of the cord to be certain there is no bleeding. If the cut end attached to the newborn is bleeding, tie or clamp the cord *proximal* to the previous clamp, and examine it again (do *not* remove the first clamp). There should not be any oozing from the newborn's end of the cord.
4. Once the cord is clamped and cut, wrap the newborn in a dry blanket. If the mother's condition is stable, you may give the newborn to her. This will give her a chance to bond and she may want to begin breastfeeding the newborn. The suckling reflex triggers the uterus to contract, which will speed the delivery of the placenta and reduce bleeding.

Delivery of the Placenta

With the delivery of the newborn, the second stage of labor is complete, and the third stage—delivery of the placenta—begins. The placenta is usually delivered within a few minutes of the newborn's arrival, although it may take as long as 30 minutes. During this time, you should

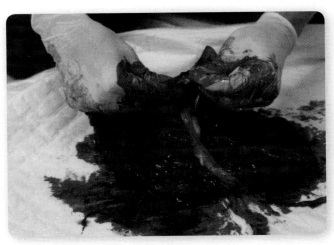

Figure 41-17 A whole placenta.
© Hattie Young/Photo Researchers, Inc.

reassess the mother and wait for the placenta to begin to separate spontaneously. *Never* attempt to speed delivery of the placenta by pulling on the umbilical cord.

The first sign that the placenta is separating from the uterine wall is usually the patient's report that her contractions are starting again. The uterus rises in the abdomen and feels hard to palpation. The end of the umbilical cord protruding from the vagina lengthens, and blood gushes from the vagina. When these signs occur, you should instruct the patient to bear down to expel the placenta.

One side of the placenta (fetal side) should be gray, shiny, and smooth; the other side (maternal side) should be dark maroon with a rough texture **Figure 41-17**. Place the placenta in a plastic bag from the OB kit and transport it with you to the hospital.

Examine the perineum for lacerations and apply pressure to any bleeding tears. Clean up and place a sanitary pad over the woman's vaginal opening, lower her legs, and prepare for transport. Do not wait for the placenta to be delivered before you begin your transport. Deliver the placenta en route.

Some women may request to keep the placenta. This is standard practice in some parts of the world, where consumption of the placenta is considered to help the mother quickly regain her strength after childbirth. Women from some cultures may want to keep the placenta to bury it and plant a tree over the spot, so that the tree and the child grow together. Follow your local protocols.

▶ Postpartum Care

After delivery of the newborn, obtain the mother's vital signs. Monitor the mother's condition closely for postpartum hemorrhage and shock, seizure activity, or respiratory difficulty. Assess the fundus (you should be able to palpate it easily around the mother's umbilicus—it should be firm). Massaging the fundus (after placenta delivery) will help control excessive postpartum hemorrhage (more than 500 mL). Determine whether the vaginal discharge following delivery—lochia—is the expected normal vaginal

discharge of blood and mucus. This discharge is usually red in the first few days and will decrease in amount and change to a brown color for several weeks after delivery. Finally, cover the mother with blankets to prevent mild hypothermia.

■ Emergency Pharmacology in Pregnancy

With pregnant patients, some concern always arises that pharmacologic agents might have dangerous effects on the fetus. However, these concerns are secondary when the life of the pregnant woman is at stake. As noted earlier, maternal physiology is altered in pregnancy, and these changes have an impact on pharmacologic therapies. Hepatic metabolism increases, as does renal excretion, which may cause IV-administered medications to pass quickly through the maternal system. Volume changes may affect distribution, such that higher doses are needed to realize appreciable systemic effects. Gastric absorption is slowed, so oral drugs may take longer than usual to achieve the desired effect.

Only a small number of medications are administered in the field for pregnancy-related problems.

▶ Magnesium Sulfate

Magnesium sulfate is classified as an electrolyte. This agent acts as a central nervous system depressant; in pregnancy, it is principally used in the management of eclampsia. Some physicians may order a magnesium sulfate infusion in patients with preeclampsia to prevent seizures.

Magnesium sulfate can cause respiratory depression, hypotension, and, potentially, circulatory collapse. This drug should be administered slowly because rapid infusion can potentiate these effects.

Administration of magnesium sulfate as a slow IV push may also be considered in the presence of seizures during or immediately following labor (eclampsia). (Hydralazine or labetalol can also be used to control blood pressure once seizures have stopped, if the patient is still hypertensive.) IM injection can be used to administer the drug as well, in which case the total dose should be placed in two separate syringes, with an equal dose in each syringe, and the two IM injections administered at different sites.

▶ Calcium Chloride

Classified as a supplement, calcium chloride is mainly used in the field for managing cases of hypocalcemia. If magnesium sulfate is administered to patients with eclampsia and causes respiratory depression to develop, calcium chloride (or calcium gluconate) can be given as an antidote to counter the effects of the magnesium sulfate.

Side effects of calcium chloride include nausea and vomiting, syncope, bradycardia, and dysrhythmias, and the drug may precipitate cardiac arrest. This agent is typically administered as an IV push with repeat doses per local protocol. This treatment may be repeated in 10-minute intervals as a buffer to magnesium toxicity.

▶ Terbutaline

Terbutaline is a tocolytic and sympathetic agonist. In pregnancy, this drug can be administered to suppress preterm labor through the action of uterine relaxation, a step that becomes necessary in the field in case of cord prolapse. Terbutaline can also be used to treat pregnancy-induced asthma because it has immediate bronchodilatory effects.

Side effects of terbutaline administration may include hypertension, nausea and dizziness, vomiting, chest pain, and cardiac dysrhythmias.

▶ Valium

Diazepam (Valium) is a benzodiazepine that is classified as a sedative/anticonvulsant. It is used principally in EMS to treat seizures. Its use is indicated in eclampsia when the patient's seizures do not respond to magnesium sulfate. Valium may also be ordered to treat anxiety in case of hypertensive crisis, such as in preeclampsia.

The principal side effects of diazepam administration include nausea and vomiting, respiratory depression, and hypotension. Ancillary side effects include headache and amnesia.

▶ Diphenhydramine

Diphenhydramine (Benadryl) is an antihistamine whose principal indication is treatment of allergic reactions. Because of its sedative and antiemetic properties, this agent is also useful in treating hyperemesis gravidarum. Its side effects include drowsiness, headache, tachycardia, and hypotension.

▶ Ondansetron

Ondansetron (Zofran) is an antiemetic used to treat nausea and vomiting. While it is classified into Pregnancy Class B, its widespread use in emergency settings has become common. Side effects of this medication include potential QT prolongation, therefore it is recommended that continuous ECG monitoring be available when administering this medication to pregnant patients.[26]

▶ Oxytocin

Oxytocin (Pitocin) is a naturally occurring hormone that triggers uterine contractions by acting on smooth muscle. This uterine stimulant can be used to induce labor, but is commonly used to control postpartum hemorrhage. In the prehospital setting, oxytocin should be used only to manage severe postpartum bleeding, and only after *all* products of conception have been expelled from the uterus (including additional fetuses).

YOU are the Paramedic — PART 4

The patient is still complaining of severe, cramping pain in her abdomen with a maximum intensity of 9/10. When you ask her if she has pain anywhere else, all she can focus on is her abdominal pain. You and your partner determine that the abdominal pain is a potential distracting injury and elect to place the patient in full spinal precautions. Once she is packaged, you and your partner move her to the back of the ambulance for further assessment. The patient still reports that her pain is unchanged, and still 9/10 intensity. The patient has no signs of bleeding. You see a seat belt burn on the patient's abdomen but the skin is not broken.

Recording Time: 10 Minutes	
Respirations	18 breaths/min
Pulse	98 beats/min
Skin	Pink, warm, dry
Blood pressure	130/72 mm Hg
Oxygen saturation (SpO$_2$)	98% on room air
Pupils	PERRLA

7. Given that spinal precautions are necessary, what should you do to the backboard to make this patient more comfortable?

8. Should you administer a pain medication to reduce the cramping pain that the patient is experiencing?

Side effects of this medication include nausea and vomiting, tachycardia, seizures, and cardiac dysrhythmias. Oxytocin can also induce coma or result in uterine rupture and hypertension if administered in excess.

Words of Wisdom

Any fetus who does not present head-first or buttocks-first during delivery must be managed at the hospital.

Pathophysiology, Assessment, and Management of Complications of Labor

▶ Premature Rupture of Membranes

When the amniotic sac ruptures or "opens" more than an hour before labor, the condition is called *premature rupture of the membranes*. In some instances, the sac will self-seal and heal itself. More commonly, though, labor will begin within 48 hours. If the pregnancy is term or near term, there is usually no concern. However, if the pregnancy is not yet term, there is a risk of infection. In this situation, you should provide emotional support to the patient and provide transport to the hospital.

▶ Preterm Labor

Labor—regular, intense uterine contractions that are accompanied by effacement—that begins after the 20th week but before the 37th week of gestation is considered preterm. The threat to the unborn fetus posed by preterm labor is a premature birth. Signs and symptoms of this type of labor are the same as with normal childbirth labor. If the pregnancy is not near term, the patient's physician may admit her to the hospital for medications, bed rest, and close monitoring.

▶ Fetal Distress

Many conditions may potentially cause fetal distress, including hypoxia, nuchal cord, trauma, abruptio placenta, fetal developmental disabilities, and a prolapsed cord. As a paramedic, you will find it difficult to assess for fetal distress in the field. Most pregnant women will be acutely aware of how much or how little the fetus is moving. You should rely on the information provided by the woman—for example, if she reports that the fetus is not moving or that the movement has markedly decreased. Remember that the best care for the fetus is quality care for the woman. Provide support to the woman and rapid transport.

▶ Uterine Rupture

Uterine rupture is a complication that occurs during labor. Patients at greatest risk are women who have had many children and those with a scar on the uterus (eg, from a previous cesarean section). Typically, you will find a woman in active labor who is reporting weakness, dizziness, and thirst. She may tell you that she initially had very strong and painful contractions, but then the contractions slackened off and she now has sharp, tearing pain. Physical examination will reveal signs of shock—sweating, tachycardia, and falling blood pressure. Significant vaginal bleeding may or may not be obvious. Treat the patient for shock and provide rapid transport.

Pathophysiology, Assessment, and Management of High-Risk Pregnancy Considerations

▶ Precipitous Labor and Birth

When EMS receives a call for a precipitous labor and birth, the newborn has usually been delivered prior to your arrival. This condition means that the entire labor time and actual birth of the newborn occurred in less than 3 hours. These types of births are not common in women who are pregnant for the first time, but the risk increases as the woman has more children. You should be prepared for this situation if the woman tells you that a prior delivery was precipitous. Contractions are usually more intense and, therefore, more effective. Assess the woman post delivery for tears and bleeding. Most newborns do not have any adverse effects, but there is a chance of infant facial bruising or an unusually misshaped head.

▶ Post-Term Pregnancy

A pregnancy is considered "post term" if the fetus has not been born after 42 weeks' gestation (normal pregnancy is 40 weeks' gestation). The cause of this condition is unknown. A post-term pregnancy is considered high risk because of the potential effects on the fetus, which may become malnourished because the placenta may no longer function as it should to provide nourishment to the fetus. There is also an increased chance for meconium aspiration. This condition has little to no effect on the woman.

Risk factors include previous post-term pregnancy and irregular menstrual cycles that increase the chance of a miscalculation of the due date. Because post-term fetuses may be larger than normal, there is a risk for a longer labor and a complicated delivery (see the section on cephalopelvic disproportion and shoulder dystocia). Generally, these deliveries should be performed by cesarean section.

► Meconium Staining

While in utero, the fetus passively ingests several elements—for example, lanugo (fine, downy hair), mucus, and amniotic fluid. This material is stored in the intestines and constitutes the first stool the fetus passes. This first stool, which is called **meconium**, is odorless, has a green-black color, and has a tar-like consistency. Unlike later feces, it is also sterile. In cases of fetal distress, or under the stresses of labor and delivery, the fetus may void the meconium into the amniotic fluid. If this occurs in utero, it may result in chemical pneumonia in the newborn. One condition that can cause such fetal distress is umbilical cord prolapse, if compression of the cord has occurred.

There is no way for you to ascertain whether meconium is present in the amniotic fluid until the amniotic sac breaks. Normally, the amniotic fluid should be clear. A yellow tint to the amniotic fluid suggests the meconium has been in the amniotic fluid for a while. A green-black color, especially with the presence of particulate matter, indicates recent passage of meconium and is a sign of danger.

If the newborn is depressed and you observe meconium in the airway, initiate ventilation in nonbreathing or ineffectively breathing newborns. If no airway obstruction is noted, normal neonatal resuscitation of the depressed newborn should be followed with warming, ventilation, and oxygenation.[27] If the newborn is moving vigorously and does not present as needing ventilation assistance, suctioning is not recommended.

► Fetal Macrosomia

Fetal macrosomia, also known as "big baby syndrome," refers to a large fetus—usually defined as weighing more than 4,500 grams (almost 9 pounds). Another term used for this condition is "large for gestational age."

Risk factors for this condition include gestational diabetes or poorly controlled diabetes in the pregnant woman. Other risk factors include excessive weight gain (woman), male fetus, post-term pregnancy, larger number of pregnancies, obesity (woman), and some genetic conditions (fetus).

Potential complications that you as the paramedic may face in the prehospital setting have to do with the size of the fetus in relation to the woman's anatomy, such as cephalopelvic disproportion and shoulder dystocia. Focus your treatment on supporting the woman and providing rapid transport, because most fetuses that are large for gestational age are delivered by cesarean section. If a field delivery should occur, encourage the woman to breastfeed the newborn, and check the newborn's blood glucose level because there is an increased risk of hypoglycemia.

► Multiple Gestation

After reaching an all-time high in 2014, the incidence of women carrying twins declined in 2015 in the United States, according to the Centers for Disease Control and Prevention.[28] The incidence of women carrying three or more infants reached its peak in 1998, but has been decreasing since then.[28] Multiple gestation is more likely when the woman uses fertility assistance or is an older mother.

Sometimes, there is a family history of twins or the woman may suspect that she is having twins due to an unusually large abdomen. More typically, multiples are diagnosed early in pregnancy with modern ultrasonographic techniques. With twins or multiples, always be prepared for more than one resuscitation, and call for assistance.

Twins are smaller than single newborns, and delivery is typically not difficult. Consider the possibility that you are dealing with twins if the first newborn is small or the woman's abdomen remains fairly large after the birth. You should also ask the woman about the possibility of multiples. If twins are present, the second one usually will be born within 45 minutes of the first. About 10 minutes after the first birth, contractions will begin again, and the birth process will repeat itself.

The procedure for delivering twins is the same as that for single newborns. Clamp and cut the cord of the first newborn approximately 30 seconds following birth and before the second newborn is delivered. The second newborn may deliver before or after the first placenta. There may be only one placenta, or there may be two. When the placenta has been delivered, check whether there is one umbilical cord or two. If two cords are coming out of one placenta, the twins are "identical." If only one cord is coming out of the placenta, then the twins are "fraternal," and there will be two placentas. Remember, if you see only one umbilical cord coming out of the first placenta, there is still another placenta to be delivered. If both cords are attached to one placenta, the delivery is over. Identical twins are of the same sex; fraternal twins may be of the same or different sexes.

Record the time of birth of each twin separately. Twins may be so small that they look premature; handle them very carefully, and keep them warm. In the case of twins, you should identify the first newborn delivered as "Baby A" by loosely tying an extra length of tape around a foot. With the delivery of more than two newborns, you can indicate the order of delivery by writing this information on a piece of tape and placing it on the blanket or towel that is wrapped around each newborn.

► Intrauterine Fetal Death

Unfortunately, in some cases you may find yourself delivering a fetus who died in the woman's uterus before labor. This response will be a true test of your medical, emotional, and social abilities. Grieving parents will be emotionally distraught and will require all your professionalism and support skills.

Intrauterine fetal death is the death of a fetus during the course of a normal pregnancy; it occurs in approximately 1% of all pregnancies.[29] Definitions vary by state and by source but, in general, it is considered death of the fetus after 20 weeks' gestation or when the fetus weighs

500 grams or more. Fetal deaths that occur at less than 20 weeks' gestation or with lower weights are considered miscarriages. Regardless of the definition, your treatment and care will focus on the woman.

The actual cause of intrauterine fetal death is usually difficult to determine, with the cause of death in many cases remaining unknown. If a cause is determined, it is usually attributed to a complication with the fetus, the placenta, or the woman. Risk factors for this condition include infections, genetic disorders, poorly controlled diabetes in the woman, hypertension, preeclampsia, eclampsia, Rh factor conditions, and multiple gestations.

The onset of labor can occur up to 2 weeks or longer after fetal death. Some women may already know that the fetus has died; others may not. In most cases, labor will progress normally. If an intrauterine infection has caused the demise, you may note an extremely foul odor. The delivered fetus may have skin blisters, skin sloughing, and a dark discoloration, depending on the stage of decomposition. The head will be soft and perhaps grossly deformed.

Do not attempt to resuscitate an obviously dead fetus. However, do not confuse such a newborn with a newborn who has experienced a cardiopulmonary arrest as a complication of the birthing process. You should attempt to resuscitate normal-appearing newborns.

▶ Amniotic Fluid Embolism

Amniotic fluid embolism is a life-threatening condition that is extremely rare and hardly ever seen in the hospital setting. Factors increasing the chance of this type of high-risk pregnancy include maternal age older than 35 years, eclampsia, abruptio placenta, placenta previa, uterine rupture, and fetal distress. Amniotic fluid embolism occurs when amniotic fluid and fetal cells enter the woman's pulmonary and circulatory system through the placenta via the umbilical veins. This transfer may occur owing to ruptured membranes and ruptured cervical or uterine veins. Regardless of the cause, the result is an exaggerated response from the pregnant woman's body (allergic reaction) that leads to coagulopathies, cardiac and respiratory collapse, and eventually death.

Signs and symptoms include a sudden onset of respiratory distress and hypotension. Many of these patients are very cyanotic and have seizures. They eventually go into cardiogenic shock, become unresponsive, and may experience cardiac arrest. If patients survive this initial reaction, they typically develop coagulopathies (their blood loses the ability to clot). Your treatment should focus on supporting the woman's vital systems (respiratory and circulatory) and providing rapid transport. Treatment for the fetus is aimed at successful resuscitation of the woman and probable cesarean section delivery in the hospital.

▶ Hydramnios

Hydramnios (also known as polyhydramnios) is a condition in which there is too much amniotic fluid. On average, most pregnancies will have approximately 1 pint (500 mL) of amniotic fluid. Multiple gestation (twins), fetal anemia, diabetes in the woman, and fetal conditions that cause the fetus to stop swallowing the fluid are all potential causes of hydramnios. This condition is usually detected on ultrasonographic exam, with patients then being closely followed by their obstetrician.

If you encounter a patient with this condition, you should be prepared for the possibility of a prolapsed cord and abruptio placenta due to the increased size of the uterus from the extra fluid. These patients also have an increased risk of postpartum hemorrhage (an overstretched uterus may not contract as efficiently to stop bleeding).

▶ Cephalopelvic Disproportion

In **cephalopelvic disproportion**, the head of the fetus is larger than the pelvis. Cephalopelvimetry (a radiographic measurement) is performed to obtain the dimensions of the fetal head. In most cases, a cesarean section will be required to prevent maternal and fetal distress. You should ask the patient about this complication before you attempt delivery in the field. Cephalopelvic disproportion may cause massive hemorrhage, along with other postpartum complications.

Pathophysiology, Assessment, and Management of Complications of Delivery

---

Most deliveries are normal: The fetus arrives headfirst, followed shortly by the placenta. Occasionally, however, complications arise. If you are to successfully deal with obstetric complications, you must know when to anticipate them, how to recognize them when they do occur, and which action to take to ensure that everyone makes it through the event successfully.

▶ Cephalic Presentation

With most deliveries, newborns present in the vertex or top-of-the-head position. The exact position of the newborn's head as it is exiting the birth canal can vary, however, and these positions define the different types of cephalic presentations. If the newborn's head is overly extended, you may encounter a face presentation. Face presentations are rare but can occur with a premature fetus, fetal macrosomia, and cephalopelvic disproportion. In a brow presentation, the head is extended, but only slightly. Occiput-posterior presentations (face up) can stall out and result in prolonged labor times. A military presentation occurs when the head is in a more neutral position—not flexed or only partially flexed—similar to a soldier in the military standing at attention. This head position causes a wider diameter of the head to attempt to exit through the birth canal, which can make for a more

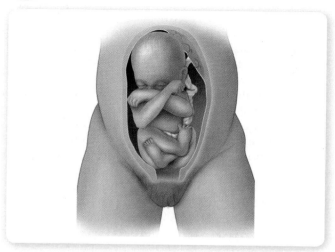

Figure 41-18 In a breech presentation, the buttocks are delivered first. These deliveries are usually slow, so you will often have time to transport the woman to the hospital.

© Jones & Bartlett Learning.

painful and difficult delivery. If you encounter one of these presentations and the newborn's head does not externally rotate into position or you are unable to complete the delivery, support the woman and the newborn and provide rapid transport.

▶ Breech Presentations

In a **breech presentation**, a part of the body other than the head leads the way. Usually, the buttocks emerges first (the word *breech* means "buttocks") **Figure 41-18**, but at other times one of the feet comes first. Breech presentations occur in 4% of all deliveries and are more common with premature births.[30] There are different types of breech presentations:

- **Frank**: Hips flexed and knees extended, with the buttocks as the presenting part
- **Incomplete**: One or both hips and knees extended, with one or both feet as the presenting part
- **Complete**: Hips and knees both flexed, with the buttocks as the presenting part

The best place for a breech presentation to be delivered is in the hospital. In the field, you may not always realize that you are dealing with a breech delivery until crowning occurs and you notice that the head is not the presenting part. At this point, it is usually too late to get the woman to the hospital.

If you have determined that the buttocks are the presenting part and delivery is imminent, proceed as follows:

- Position the woman with her buttocks at the edge of the bed or stretcher and her legs flexed.
- Allow the buttocks and trunk of the newborn to deliver spontaneously. *Do not pull on the newborn.*
- Once the newborn's legs are clear, support the newborn's body.

- Lower the newborn slightly so that it very nearly hangs by its own weight downward; that will help the head pass through the pelvic outlet. You can tell when the head is in the vaginal canal because you will be able to see the newborn's hairline at the nape of the neck just below the woman's symphysis pubis.
- When you can see the hairline, grasp the newborn by the ankles and lift him or her upward in the direction of the woman's abdomen. The head should then deliver without difficulty.
- If the head does not deliver within 3 minutes, the newborn is in danger of suffocation, and immediate action is indicated. Suffocation may occur when the newborn's umbilical cord is compressed by his or her head against the birth canal, which cuts off the supply of oxygenated blood from the placenta, and the face is pressed against the vaginal wall, which prevents the newborn from breathing on his or her own. Place your gloved hand in the vagina, with your palm toward the newborn's face. Form a V with your fingers on either side of the newborn's nose, and push the vaginal wall away from the face until the head is delivered.
- Remember: *This is a delivery, not an extrication.* Do not attempt to forcibly pull the newborn out or allow an explosive delivery. If the head does not deliver within 3 minutes of establishing the airway, provide rapid transport to the hospital, with the woman's buttocks elevated on pillows. Try to maintain the newborn's airway throughout transport. En route, alert the hospital so the personnel there can prepare for your arrival.

There are other abnormal ways in which the fetus may present for delivery; fortunately, most of them are quite rare. In a footling breech, one or both feet dangle down through the vaginal opening **Figure 41-19**. In a **transverse presentation** (transverse lie), the fetus lies crosswise in the uterus and one hand may protrude through the vagina. Even the fetus who is coming head-first may present with the face or brow (deflex) instead of the top of the head (vertex). With all of those abnormal presentations, the most important point for you to remember is *not to attempt delivery in the field.* Nearly all of these abnormal presentations will require delivery by cesarean section, so prehospital management is to provide rapid transport.

▶ Shoulder Dystocia

Another complication of delivery is **shoulder dystocia** or difficulty in delivering the shoulders. Women with diabetes, large fetuses, and post-term pregnancies are at increased risk for this complication. Shoulder dystocia occurs after the head has been delivered and the shoulder cannot get past

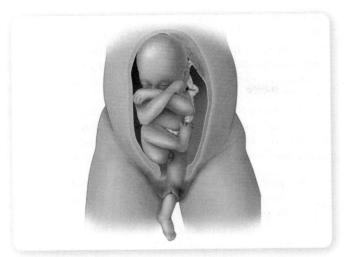

Figure 41-19 In very rare instances, a fetus's limb—usually a single arm or leg—presents first. This is a serious situation, and you must provide prompt transport for hospital delivery.

© Jones & Bartlett Learning.

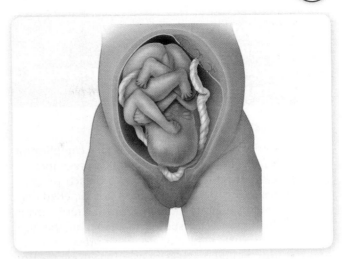

Figure 41-20 A prolapsed umbilical cord, though a rare situation, is very dangerous and must be cared for at the hospital.

© Jones & Bartlett Learning.

the woman's symphysis pubis; there is either difficulty in getting it to pass or it gets "stuck" behind the pelvic bones so that the fetus is unable to be delivered. This unexpected complication poses a life threat to the fetus if it is not delivered due to the increased chance of cord compression. As time passes and the shoulders are not clearing, the fetus cannot breathe (the lungs are still inside the birth canal) and/or the cord may become compressed between the fetus and the woman's tissue. The delivery needs to be completed for the fetus to breathe. The major concern for the newborn after delivery is damage to the brachial nerve plexus.

Several maneuvers may be attempted in an effort to widen the woman's pelvis or reposition the fetus to allow for a successful delivery. The McRoberts maneuver is one of the safest (for both woman and fetus) methods to use in the case of shoulder dystocia. To widen the woman's pelvis and flatten the lower back, hyperflex her legs tightly to her abdomen. It may be necessary to apply suprapubic pressure (on the woman's lower abdomen) and to *gently* pull on the fetus's head.

▶ Nuchal Cord

During delivery, the umbilical cord may potentially become wrapped around the newborn's neck—a condition termed a **nuchal cord**. Nuchal cords occur in 15% to 34% of all births.[31] As the fetus descends during labor, cord compression may occur, causing the fetal heart rate to slow and resulting in fetal distress. A nuchal cord rarely results in the death of a fetus, but it is one of the first things you should assess for when the fetus's head emerges.

If you observe that the umbilical cord is wrapped around the fetus's neck, slip your finger under the cord and gently attempt to slip it over the fetus's shoulder and head. If this attempt is not successful or if the cord is wrapped too tightly, carefully place umbilical clamps

2 inches (5 cm) apart and carefully cut the cord between the clamps in a motion going away from (not toward) the infant.

▶ Prolapsed Umbilical Cord

With a **prolapsed umbilical cord**, the cord emerges from the uterus ahead of the fetus **Figure 41-20**. With each uterine contraction, the cord is then compressed between the presenting part and the bony pelvis, shutting off the fetus's supply of oxygenated blood from the placenta. Fetal asphyxia may ensue if circulation through the cord is not rapidly reestablished and maintained until delivery. Cord prolapse, which occurs in approximately 1 in 10 deliveries,[32] is more likely when the presenting part does not completely fill the pelvic brim, such as in abnormal presentations or with small fetuses (premature births, multiple births).

Treatment of cord prolapse is clearly urgent. Take the following steps:

1. Position the woman supine with her hips elevated as much as possible on pillows.
2. Administer 100% supplemental oxygen via a nonrebreathing mask.
3. Instruct the woman to pant with each contraction, which will prevent her from bearing down.
4. With two fingers of your gloved hand, gently push the presenting part (not the cord) back up into the vagina until it no longer presses on the cord.
5. While you maintain pressure on the presenting part, have your partner cover the exposed portion of the cord with dressings moistened in warmed normal saline.
6. Try to maintain that position, with a gloved hand pushing the presenting part away from the cord, throughout *urgent transport* to the hospital.

Pathophysiology, Assessment, and Management of Postpartum Complications

▶ Uterine Inversion

Uterine inversion is a rare but potentially fatal complication of childbirth, occurring in 1 of every 2,000 pregnancies.[33] In this condition, the placenta fails to detach properly and adheres to the uterine wall when it is expelled. As a result, the uterus literally turns inside out. Uterine inversion usually occurs as a result of mismanaging the third stage of labor, such as placing excessive pressure on the uterus during fundal massage or exerting strong traction on the umbilical cord in an attempt to hasten delivery of the placenta.

The severity of inversion is graded based on how much the uterus has reversed itself; it ranges from incomplete inversion, to complete inversion, to prolapsed inversion, and finally to total inversion. With incomplete and complete inversions, the uterus does not protrude externally. You will most likely encounter a prolapsed or a total inversion. (The other forms are not readily identifiable in the field.) In a prolapsed inversion, the fundus of the uterus can be seen protruding from the vagina. In a total inversion, both the uterus and the vagina protrude inside out. This is a very painful condition, and hypovolemic shock may develop rapidly.

Management of uterine inversion is as follows:

1. Keep the patient recumbent.
2. Administer 100% supplemental oxygen via a nonrebreathing mask.
3. Start two IV lines with normal saline, and titrate fluid administration based on the woman's vital signs.
4. If the placenta is still attached to the uterus, do *not* attempt to remove it.
5. Carefully monitor the patient's vital signs, and treat for shock.
6. Consider giving oxytocin (Pitocin), 10 units IM, to help control exsanguinating hemorrhage, if your local protocol permits it.

Make *one* attempt to replace the uterus. Push the uterine fundus up and through the vaginal canal by applying pressure with the fingertips and the palm of your gloved hand. If this procedure fails, cover all protruding tissues with moist sterile dressings and provide rapid transport.

▶ Postpartum Hemorrhage

The average blood loss for women during the third stage of labor is approximately 0.3 pints (150 mL). When blood loss exceeds 1 pint (500 mL) during the first 24 hours after giving birth, this condition is considered postpartum hemorrhage (bleeding after birth). Postpartum hemorrhage can take one of two forms—early or late. Early postpartum hemorrhage, or bleeding within 24 hours of delivery, is the most common type of postpartum hemorrhage. Only a very small percentage of patients experience late postpartum hemorrhage, defined as bleeding that occurs from 24 hours to 6 weeks after delivery.

Anything that interferes with the contractions of the interlacing uterine muscle fibers after delivery of the placenta will promote postpartum hemorrhage. The following causes are particularly noteworthy:

- **Lacerations.** The mother may have tears or lacerations around the vaginal opening and in the perineum.
- **Prolonged labor or delivery of multiple babies.** Completion of a multiple gestation may lead to a "tired" uterus.
- **Retained products of conception.** Retained pieces or fragments of the placenta may cause bleeding, and the uterus cannot contract fully until it is empty.
- **Uterine atony.** The uterus loses the ability to contract after childbirth.
- **Grand multiparity.** After many pregnancies, the muscle tissue in the uterus is gradually replaced with fibrous tissue, which does not contract.
- **Multiple pregnancy.** The placental site is larger, and the overstretched uterine muscles do not contract as well.
- **Placenta previa.** Muscles in the lower segment of the uterus, where the placenta is implanted, do not contract efficiently.
- **A full bladder.** It may prevent proper placental separation and uterine contraction.

The only measures feasible in the field to manage postpartum hemorrhage are those that encourage uterine contraction and help restore circulating volume. Follow these guidelines when you encounter this type of situation:

1. Continue uterine massage: Gently but firmly knead and massage the uterus in a circular motion.
2. Encourage the woman to breastfeed.
3. If allowed by protocol, add 10 units of oxytocin to the IV bag (1,000 mL), and infuse at a rate of 20 to 30 mL/min.
4. Notify the receiving hospital of the woman's status and your estimated time of arrival.
5. Transport without delay.
6. Start another large-bore (18-gauge) IV line en route, and infuse normal saline wide open.
7. Do *not* attempt an internal examination of the vagina.
8. Do *not* attempt to pack the vagina with any form of dressing.
9. Manage *external* bleeding from perineal tears with firm pressure. It may be necessary to open the labia and place ice packs at the bleeding site.

► Pulmonary Embolism

One of the most common causes of maternal death during childbirth or postpartum is pulmonary embolism. An embolism may form from a number of sources, but a blood clot arising in the pelvic circulation is a frequent cause. Leakage of amniotic fluid into the maternal circulation (amniotic embolism), a clot arising from deep venous thrombosis (pregnancy-related venous thromboembolism), and water or air entering the vagina after a water birth (water embolism) are examples of potential embolic processes. Should the woman experience sudden dyspnea, tachycardia, atrial fibrillation, or hypotension in the postpartum state, you should suspect pulmonary embolism. The patient may report sudden, sharp chest or abdominal pain, or may experience syncope. Physical examination may reveal nothing unusual except for an increased pulse rate, tachypnea, and hypotension—signs that may be mistaken for shock. Management of a postpartum embolism is the same as management of a pulmonary embolism occurring in nonpregnant states: awareness/ recognition, high-flow oxygen, and rapid transport.

► Postpartum Depression

An estimated one out of every nine women experiences postpartum depression, or the "baby blues," and some would say that this mental health condition is the most common complication of pregnancy.[34] Symptoms of this disorder can appear at any time during the pregnancy and up to 1 year after birth. Adolescent mothers and those with lower income levels have an increased chance of having this condition.

Several factors have been identified that increase the risk for development of postpartum depression. They include a previous history of depression or family history; financial or marital/relationship issues; diabetes; a complicated pregnancy or delivery; major life-changing events such as job loss, divorce, or death of a family member; infertility issues; and multiple gestations.

You should be aware of the signs and symptoms of this type of depression so that you can provide the best care to your patient. Women with postpartum depression exhibit signs similar to those of other depressed people, including a lack of interest in caring for themselves, sleep disorders ranging from insomnia to sleeping all the time, overwhelming sadness and crying, and lack of an appetite. Some women may also have strong feelings of anger that may be directed toward their infant, may not have an interest in the infant, may experience strong feelings of guilt, and may even have thoughts of harming themselves or the infant. Postpartum depression is a serious condition that requires definitive treatment you will not be able to provide in the prehospital setting.

Your assessment and management of the woman in this situation may be a critical step in getting her the help she needs. Be aware of the signs and symptoms of postpartum depression so that you can recognize the condition in your patients. Maintain a professional approach and be a patient advocate. If at all possible, provide transport for the patient so she may seek and obtain the medical care she needs.

Words of Wisdom

What is good for the pregnant woman is good for the fetus.

■ Trauma and Pregnancy

Trauma is a serious complicating factor in pregnancy, partly because of the many physiologic changes that occur during pregnancy, but mostly because of the involvement of two patients—the woman and her fetus. Both patients are particularly vulnerable to trauma because of the unique features of pregnancy.

Special Populations

Throughout pregnancy, seat belts should be used whenever the woman is in a motor vehicle, with both the lap belt and the shoulder harness in place. The lap belt portion should be placed under the abdomen and over the iliac crests and the pubic symphysis. The shoulder harness should be positioned between the breasts.

Trauma is the leading cause of nonobstetric maternal death in the United States, with an estimated 8% of all pregnant women experiencing some type of trauma during their pregnancy, usually in the last trimester.[35] The major causes of injury to pregnant women are motor vehicle crashes, falls, domestic abuse, and penetrating injuries such as gunshot wounds.

► Pathophysiology and Assessment Considerations

In general, abdominal trauma occurs from the same mechanisms in pregnant women as in nonpregnant women. However, because the likelihood of domestic abuse increases greatly during a woman's pregnancy, you should be suspicious for evidence of this crime. Sexual assault is also a form of trauma that can occur during pregnancy; it is covered in Chapter 22, *Gynecologic Emergencies*.

The anatomic changes that occur during pregnancy have important implications when a woman experiences trauma. As the woman approaches term, her abdominal contents are compressed into the upper abdomen. The diaphragm is elevated by approximately 1½ inches (4 cm), so there is a higher incidence of abdominal injuries in association with chest trauma. Meanwhile, because the peritoneum is maximally stretched, significant abdominal trauma may occur without peritoneal signs.

In the first trimester of pregnancy, the uterus is well protected within the woman's bony pelvis and is rarely damaged from abdominal trauma. In the second and third trimesters of pregnancy, however, the uterus grows out from the pelvis and extends into the abdomen, making it more vulnerable to blunt and penetrating trauma. In motor vehicle crashes, for example, the use of a lap belt increases the likelihood of uterine damage because the lap belt compresses the uterus. Shoulder restraints, by contrast, decrease the chance of uterine injury. In penetrating injuries, the large uterus protects the other organs from injury. Because the uterus shields the other organs, pregnant women with penetrating wounds may have a better outcome, although the fetus is often injured by the trauma. In addition to abdominal tenderness, the examination of an injured pregnant woman may reveal an abnormal fetal position, an easily palpated fetus, inability to palpate the top of the uterus, or vaginal bleeding.

As early as the second trimester of pregnancy, the bladder is displaced upward (superior) and forward (anterior) so that it lies outside the pelvic cavity. It is therefore at increased risk of injury, particularly from a deceleration injury caused by a lap seat belt. Should you encounter a restrained pregnant patient in a motor vehicle crash, make a note of the seat belt placement. If the patient is found with the belt placed over the abdomen or on top of the uterine dome, this positioning should dramatically increase your index of suspicion for internal injuries to the woman and the fetus. The uterus also becomes more vulnerable to injury as it increases in size, and deceleration forces, such as those produced by vehicular trauma, may bring about abruptio placenta or uterine rupture.

A pregnant patient will show different signs and responses to trauma due to the pregnancy-related physiologic changes to her body. As noted earlier, pregnancy is accompanied by a significant increase in vascular volume. Normal vascular volume increases by nearly 50% during the first 6 months of pregnancy as a result of the pregnant woman having to perfuse her own circulation and that of the fetus. To meet this demand, normal cardiac output increases by approximately 40% as a result of the increasing pulse rate and stroke volume. The resting pulse rate increases by 15 to 20 beats/min over the rate in a nonpregnant patient, so the resting pulse may be as high as 100 beats/min by the end of the second trimester of pregnancy. This physiologic change makes it much more difficult to interpret tachycardia. Furthermore, because of the pregnant woman's vastly expanded blood volume, other signs of hypovolemia, such as a falling blood pressure, may not become evident until she has lost as much as 40% of her blood volume. Therefore, you need to be aggressive in managing a pregnant woman when the mechanism of injury suggests the potential for shock.

A relative redistribution of blood volume also occurs during pregnancy, with blood flow to the pelvic region increasing tenfold. Thus, if a pregnant woman sustains a pelvic fracture, her chances of bleeding to death are significantly higher than those of a nonpregnant woman. A large amount of blood volume can be lost before signs and symptoms of shock develop because other mechanisms are compensating for the loss.

Regarding respiration, the pregnant woman has a higher basal metabolism and, therefore, an increased need for oxygen. At the same time, she has more carbon dioxide to eliminate—hers and that produced by fetal metabolism. Her body responds by increasing her tidal volume and, therefore, her minute volume. In general, a respiratory rate that is less than 20 breaths/min is not considered adequate ventilation in the pregnant patient who experiences trauma. If she needs artificial ventilation, you should administer supplemental oxygen at a higher minute volume than usual.

During pregnancy, digestion slows and bowel motility decreases, resulting in the stomach staying full longer. With the gravid uterus placing pressure on the stomach, the chances of aspiration are dramatically increased.

> ## Special Populations
>
> A fetal heart rate of less than 120 beats/min likely means fetal distress. Other factors related to fetal distress include the length of time that a decreased fetal heart rate is sustained.

▶ Considerations for the Fetus Related to Trauma

The muscular wall of the uterus cushions the fetus from the direct effects of blunt trauma, but fetal injury can still occur as a result of rapid deceleration or secondary to impaired fetal circulation. The most common cause of fetal death from trauma is maternal death, but a woman will often survive an incident that proves fatal for the fetus. Blunt trauma resulting in abruptio placenta, for instance, has a good statistical outcome for pregnant women but often results in fetal death.

If the pregnant woman has sustained trauma and is bleeding massively, the maternal circulation will shunt blood away from the fetal circulation to maintain maternal homeostasis—maternal circulation takes precedence over the requirements of the fetus. Therefore, any injury that involves significant maternal bleeding will threaten the life of the fetus. The woman's increased heart rate is not an early sign of hypovolemic shock.

The best indication of the status of the fetus after trauma is the fetal heart rate. A normal fetal heart rate is between 120 and 160 beats/min. A rate slower than

120 beats/min means fetal distress and signals a dire emergency. Measurement of the fetal heart rate was discussed earlier in this chapter.

▶ Management of the Pregnant Patient With Trauma

Although trauma in a pregnant woman involves at least *two* patients, you can treat only one of them directly: the woman. During your assessment, determine the gestational age of the fetus if possible and relay this information to the receiving facility staff so they can better prepare to care for the newborn if needed. In general, what is good for the woman will be good for the fetus. For example, any effort to improve maternal perfusion will have a collateral effect of improving fetal circulation. The potential for injury to the fetus cannot be adequately assessed in the field, only presumed or suspected. Whereas a decreased fetal heart rate signals an emergency situation, a normal fetal heart rate does not guarantee that all is well. Even minor deceleration forces can cause significant injury to the fetus.

In general, the prehospital management of pregnant women with abdominal trauma is the same as that for nonpregnant patients. Airway, breathing, and circulation remain the highest priorities. However, because the large uterus can compress the vena cava (decreasing right atrial preload), a pregnant woman should be transported on her left side unless a spinal injury is suspected **Figure 41-21** . If you must transport a patient in the

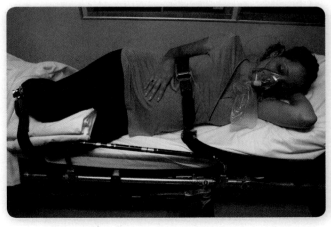

Figure 41-21 Whenever possible, transport a pregnant patient lying on her left side to allow for sufficient circulation through the vena cava.
© Jones & Bartlett Learning.

supine position, elevate her right hip approximately 6 inches (15 cm) to minimize the pressure of the vena cava. Be aware that because of the physiologic changes that occur in a woman's body during pregnancy, the fetus's circulation may be diminished even if the woman's vital signs appear normal. The fetus may be in shock before signs appear in the mother, so initiate early, aggressive fluid resuscitation.

Field treatment of a pregnant trauma patient is as follows:

1. Ensure an adequate airway. Regurgitation and aspiration are much more likely in a pregnant woman than in a patient who is not pregnant, so if the patient is unresponsive, provide early endotracheal intubation to isolate the airway. Provide cricoid pressure until the airway is secured.
2. Administer oxygen. A pregnant woman's oxygen needs are 10% to 20% higher than those in a nonpregnant woman, so provide 100% supplemental oxygen via a nonrebreathing mask if the patient is responsive.
3. Assist ventilations as needed, and provide a higher minute volume than usual. Because the uterus of a pregnant woman presses up against the diaphragm, ventilation will be more difficult. Once the patient is intubated, you may want to use a positive-pressure ventilator periodically to ensure visible chest rise (representing an adequate tidal volume).
4. Control external bleeding promptly. Splint any fractures.
5. Start one or two IV lines of normal saline. Use large-bore catheters and macrodrip sets. Administer a bolus if signs and symptoms of hemodynamic compromise are present, with the goal of maintaining blood pressure. Remember that a larger volume of fluid is necessary for the pregnant patient.
6. Notify the receiving hospital of the patient's status. Also indicate your estimated time of arrival.
7. Transport the woman in the lateral recumbent position. If she is on a backboard, tilt the backboard 30° to the left by wedging pillows beneath it. This will cause the uterus to shift, taking the weight off the inferior vena cava and improving venous return to the heart.

Maternal Cardiac Arrest

If cardiac arrest occurs, provide cardiopulmonary resuscitation (CPR) and advanced life support (ALS) care as you would for any patient with trauma, with one variation. Although CPR can be completed with a pregnant patient slightly tilted to the left lateral position, studies have shown that the quality of CPR is ineffective in this position.[36] The 2015 CPR and Emergency Cardiovascular Care (ECC) guidelines recommend positioning the pregnant patient with cardiac arrest in a supine position while another rescuer provides manual left uterine displacement **Figure 41-22** .[37] Additionally, the normal landmarks you would use for chest compressions may not be obvious in a pregnant patient in the third trimester—use the sternal notch as a guideline for hand placement (about 5 to 7 inches [13–18 cm] below the angle of Louis).

Once the patient arrives at the hospital, an emergency cesarean section may be performed. A cesarean section may be the only chance a term or near-term fetus has to survive. A pregnant patient with trauma who is in cardiac arrest requires rapid transport and early notification to the hospital. Even if the woman is *obviously* dead (eg, in case of decapitation), good CPR and ventilatory support may keep the fetus viable until a cesarean section can be performed.

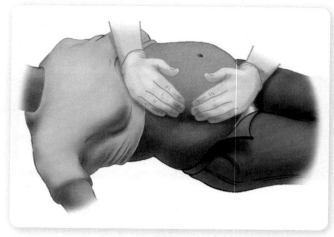

Figure 41-22 Manual left displacement of the uterus. The two-handed technique is shown. Alternately, one hand can be used if a partner is performing chest compressions.

© Jones & Bartlett Learning.

YOU are the Paramedic SUMMARY

1. What is your primary concern after scene safety is established?

Your immediate concern is the overall presentation of the patient. Does your rapid exam reveal any obvious life threats? Is she responsive? Does she have obvious breathing difficulty or evidence of injury? Does she appear pale, cyanotic, red, or gray? Is she alert and oriented or confused?

2. Which questions are in your mind given your knowledge that the patient is pregnant?

Focus on the patient's chief complaint. If the chief complaint is abdominal pain, you need to find out more about the pain itself. The OPQRST method works well for this purpose. How many weeks pregnant is the patient? Is the patient receiving prenatal care from a physician or nurse practitioner? These are important questions to answer in the care of this patient.

3. Is the location of the seat belt concerning to you?

As a general rule, all people, including pregnant women, should wear seat belts with the lap belt low on the hips. Because the seat belt is located visibly high on this patient, you would be wise to suspect a potential fetal injury. Even relatively minor trauma to the abdomen can cause injury to the placenta and uterus.

4. Which steps will you take in your further assessment of this patient?

You need to establish the status of the patient's pregnancy with more specific information such as the term and whether the patient expects any problems with her pregnancy. You should also perform all the steps in proper patient care just as you would for any patient. Apply spinal precautions, assess vital signs, and perform a secondary assessment including palpation of the abdominal quadrants.

5. Which trimester is this patient in?

This patient states that she is 20 weeks pregnant, which indicates her pregnancy is in the second trimester.

6. Do you have any additional concerns because this is the patient's second pregnancy?

Generally, a woman's second pregnancy or greater delivers more easily than a first pregnancy. This factor may be a concern with the patient in this scenario. Additionally, the patient should be able to tell you if something feels different or wrong because she has already delivered a child. If the patient has given birth previously, ask how the child was delivered. Was it natural childbirth or did the birth occur by cesarean section?

YOU are the Paramedic **SUMMARY** *(continued)*

7. Given that spinal precautions are necessary, what should you do to the backboard to make this patient more comfortable?

Consider raising the right edge of the backboard approximately 15% so the patient is lying in a left lateral position. This is especially important with patients who are 20 weeks pregnant or greater, due to the possibility of supine hypotension syndrome. You can accomplish this positioning by using pillows, rolled linen, or low-rise equipment that you will not need in the care of the patient. Remember that the backboard and patient still need to be secured to the stretcher.

8. Should you administer a pain medication to reduce the cramping pain the patient is experiencing?

At this point, you should avoid analgesia: Whatever you administer to the woman will also be administered to the fetus, which may or may not be in distress. It is best to wait until an assessment can be made in a hospital setting to determine the cause of the cramping.

EMS Patient Care Report (PCR)

Date: 05-15-18	**Incident No.:** 9745		**Nature of Call:** MVC		**Location:** Mason/3rd Ave
Dispatched: 1012	**En Route:** 1012	**At Scene:** 1015	**Transport:** 1030	**At Hospital:** 1042	**In Service:** 1100

Patient Information

Age: 28 **Sex:** F **Weight (in kg [lb]):** 98 kg (215 lb)	**Allergies:** No known drug allergies **Medications:** Prenatal vitamins **Past Medical History:** Denies **Chief Complaint:** Abdominal pain

Vital Signs

Time: 1020	**BP:** 130/72	**Pulse:** 100	**Respirations:** 20	**Spo$_2$:** 98% room air
Time: 1030	**BP:** 130/72	**Pulse:** 98	**Respirations:** 18	**Spo$_2$:** 98% on room air
Time: 1040	**BP:** 130/70	**Pulse:** 100	**Respirations:** 18	**Spo$_2$:** 98% on room air

EMS Treatment (circle all that apply)

Oxygen @ _____ L/min via (circle one): NC NRM **Bag-mask device**	**Assisted Ventilation**	**Airway Adjunct**	**CPR**
Defibrillation	**Bleeding Control**	**Bandaging**	**Splinting**	**Other:** Spinal immobilization

Narrative

Arrived to find 28-year-old alert and oriented × 4, 20-week pregnant female sitting in driver's seat of a midsize passenger car that struck another vehicle from behind. Moderate damage is noted to the front of this vehicle. Airbags have deployed in this vehicle. This pt was still restrained by her 3-point seat belt; the lap belt portion of the restraint was found high on the abdomen. There is a corresponding seat belt abrasion across the pt's abdomen. Pt is complaining of severe cramping pain in her pelvis. The pt states the pain has a maximum intensity of 9/10, and she is unable to describe whether or not she is injured anywhere else because of the severity of her abdominal pain. Due to the possibility of a distracting injury, full spinal precautions were applied. Pt removed from vehicle with good MSPs before and after spinal immobilization. Backboard raised approx 15 degrees so pt is left lateral to avoid potential inferior vena cava compression. Backboard and pt secured to stretcher and secured in ambulance. V/S stable, Spo$_2$ 98% RA, lungs CTA, skin pink/warm/dry to touch, PERRLA 4 mm, GCS 15. IV lock established in right forearm 18 ga. Trauma exam was unremarkable outside of initial findings. No change in pt condition during transport to trauma center at Regional Hospital. Report to RN Julia on arrival in the ED.**End of report**

Prep Kit

▶ Ready for Review

- The ovaries are the beginning point for reproduction. During the menstrual cycle, one follicle releases an ovum. If the ovum becomes fertilized, it develops into an embryo, and then into a fetus.
- The fallopian tubes are the structures that transport the ovum from the ovary to the uterus (a muscular, inverted pear-shaped organ). Once an egg is fertilized, it normally implants in the endometrium (the inner lining of the uterus).
- The fetus is enclosed in the amniotic sac, which contains amniotic fluid, allowing the fetus to develop in a weightless environment.
- The gestational period (the time that it takes for the infant to develop in utero) normally lasts 38 weeks.
- In the first trimester of pregnancy, the placenta, umbilical cord, specialized body systems, and limbs form. In the second trimester of pregnancy, the fetus gains weight and body systems become more specialized. In the last trimester of pregnancy, the fetus primarily puts on weight.
- Pregnancy is considered at term by week 37. Newborns born before 37 weeks' gestation are considered premature, and newborns born after 42 weeks' gestation are considered post term.
- Physiologic changes during pregnancy can alter a woman's normal response to trauma or exacerbate or create medical conditions that can threaten the health of both the woman and the fetus.
- When you are assessing a patient with an obstetric emergency, identify the length of gestation, estimated due date, any complications with this pregnancy or others, and the presence of any vaginal bleeding.
- There are many potential complications related to pregnancy, including substance abuse by the pregnant woman, and disorders that can develop during pregnancy or be exacerbated by pregnancy. Specific disorders include diabetes mellitus, heart disease, supine hypotensive syndrome, hyperemesis gravidarum, seizures, renal disorders, respiratory disorders, vaginal bleeding, placental problems, hypertensive disorders, and Rh sensitization.
- Preeclampsia is the most serious hypertensive disorder, manifesting after the 20th week of pregnancy. Symptoms include edema, gradual onset of hypertension, protein in the urine, severe headache, nausea and vomiting, agitation, rapid weight gain, and visual disturbances. Preeclampsia may lead to seizures and eclampsia.
- Abortion is expulsion of the fetus, from any cause, before the 20th week of gestation. It can cause bleeding during pregnancy.
- An incomplete abortion occurs when only some of the products of conception are expelled. In such patients, be alert for signs and symptoms of shock.
- Causes of bleeding during pregnancy include ectopic pregnancy or bleeding related to the placenta (abruptio placenta or placenta previa).
- Vaginal bleeding may cause shock. Keep the woman lying on her left side; administer supplemental oxygen; provide rapid transport, intravenous (IV) fluids, and ECG monitoring; and place sanitary pads over the vagina.
- Labor may begin with a bloody show, or release of mucus (sometimes with blood) from the vagina.
- The first stage of labor begins with the onset of contractions—crampy abdominal pains that may radiate into the lower back. The amniotic sac may also rupture.
- The second stage of labor begins when the fetus's head enters the birth canal. The woman's contractions become more intense and more frequent. When the fetus's head becomes visible at the vaginal opening (crowning), delivery is imminent.
- The third stage of labor occurs when the placenta is expelled.
- When you are assessing a pregnant patient, determine whether there is time to provide transport to the hospital.
- If delivery is imminent, quickly prepare a private clean area. Behave in a calm and reassuring way. Control the delivery. Clear the newborn's airway.
- Never pull on the umbilical cord to deliver the placenta. Gently massage the woman's abdomen to aid in delivery of the placenta.
- Pharmacology during pregnancy may include magnesium sulfate for eclampsia; calcium chloride to reverse respiratory depression following magnesium sulfate administration; terbutaline for asthma, as a uterine relaxant, and occasionally for cord prolapse; diphenhydramine for hyperemesis gravidarum; ondansetron for nausea and vomiting; and oxytocin for treatment of postpartum hemorrhage.
- Complications of labor include premature rupture of membranes, preterm labor, fetal distress, and uterine rupture.
- Complications related to high-risk pregnancy include precipitous labor and birth, post-term pregnancy, meconium staining, fetal macrosomia, multiple gestation, intrauterine fetal death, amniotic

Prep Kit (continued)

fluid embolism, hydramnios, and cephalopelvic disproportion.

- Meconium is the fetus's first stool. A yellow or green-black tint to the amniotic fluid indicates the presence of meconium. Suction the newborn if meconium staining is present with airway occlusion and the newborn is depressed (not vigorous).
- Complications of delivery include cephalic presentation, breech presentation, shoulder dystocia, nuchal cord, and prolapsed cord.
- Postpartum complications include uterine inversion, postpartum hemorrhage, pulmonary embolism, and postpartum depression.
- In the case of postpartum hemorrhage, massage the woman's abdomen, provide IV fluid resuscitation, and transport urgently.
- Pulmonary embolism can cause maternal death during childbirth or postpartum. Suspect this complication if the patient experiences sudden dyspnea, tachycardia, atrial fibrillation, or postpartum hypotension.
- The major causes of injury to pregnant women are motor vehicle crashes, falls, domestic abuse, and penetrating injuries such as gunshot wounds. Treatment of trauma in a pregnant woman is the same as treatment of a nonpregnant woman, except that the pregnant patient should be transported on her left side unless spinal injury is suspected.

▶ Vital Vocabulary

abortion Expulsion of the fetus, from any cause, before 20 weeks' gestation.

abruptio placenta A premature separation of the placenta from the wall of the uterus.

amniotic fluid A watery fluid that provides the fetus with a weightless environment in which to develop.

amniotic fluid embolism An extremely rare, life-threatening condition that occurs when amniotic fluid and fetal cells enter the pregnant woman's pulmonary and circulatory system through the placenta via the umbilical veins, causing an exaggerated allergic response from the woman's body.

amniotic sac The fluid-filled, baglike membrane in which the fetus develops.

Apgar scoring system A scoring system for assessing the status of a newborn that assigns a number value to each of five areas of assessment.

blastocyst The term for an oocyte once it has been fertilized and multiplies into cells.

bloody show A plug of mucus, sometimes mixed with blood, that is expelled from the dilating cervix and discharged from the vagina.

breech presentation A delivery in which the buttocks come out first.

cephalopelvic disproportion A situation in which the head of the fetus is larger than the woman's pelvis; in most cases, cesarean section is required for such a delivery.

cervical canal The interior of the cervix.

cholestasis A disease of the liver that occurs only during pregnancy, in which hormones affect the gallbladder by slowing down or blocking the normal bile flow from the liver; the most common symptom is profuse, painful itching, particularly of the hands and feet.

chronic hypertension A blood pressure that is equal to or greater than 140/90 mm Hg, which exists prior to pregnancy, occurs before the 20th week of pregnancy, or persists postpartum.

complete abortion Expulsion of all products of conception from the uterus.

corpus luteum The remains of a follicle after an oocyte has been released, and which secretes progesterone.

crowning The appearance of the newborn's body part (usually the head) at the vaginal opening at the beginning of labor.

cytomegalovirus (CMV) A herpesvirus that can produce the symptoms of prolonged high fever, chills, headache, malaise, extreme fatigue, and an enlarged spleen.

eclampsia Seizures that result from severe hypertension in a pregnant woman.

ectopic pregnancy An egg that attaches outside the uterus, typically in a fallopian tube.

effacement Thinning and shortening of the cervix; a normal process that occurs as the uterus contracts.

elective abortion Intentional expulsion of the fetus.

episiotomy An incision in the perineal skin made to prevent tearing during childbirth.

fetal macrosomia A situation in which a fetus is large, usually defined as weighing more than 4,500 grams (almost 9 pounds); also known as "large for gestational age."

fetus The developing, unborn infant inside the uterus.

Prep Kit (continued)

first stage of labor The stage of labor that begins with the onset of regular labor pains (crampy abdominal pains), during which the uterus contracts and the cervix effaces.

follicle-stimulating hormone (FSH) A hormone produced by the anterior pituitary gland that is important in the menstrual cycle.

gestational hypertension High blood pressure that develops after the 20th week of pregnancy in women with previously normal blood pressures, and that resolves spontaneously in the postpartum period; formerly known as pregnancy-induced hypertension.

gestational period The time that it takes for the fetus to develop in utero, normally 38 weeks.

gravidity The total number of times a woman has been pregnant, including the current pregnancy.

habitual abortion Three or more consecutive pregnancies that end in miscarriage.

human immunodeficiency virus (HIV) An infection that causes acquired immune deficiency syndrome (AIDS).

hydramnios A condition in which there is too much amniotic fluid; also known as polyhydramnios.

hyperemesis gravidarum A condition of persistent nausea and vomiting during pregnancy.

imminent abortion A spontaneous abortion that cannot be prevented.

incomplete abortion Expulsion of the fetus that results in some products of conception remaining in the uterus.

inhibin A protein that plays a key role in the menstrual cycle by triggering release of follicle-stimulating hormone.

labor The mechanism by which the fetus and the placenta are expelled from the uterus.

lightening In pregnancy, a feeling of relief of pressure in the upper abdomen; a premonitory sign of labor.

lochia The vaginal discharge of blood and mucus that occurs following delivery of a newborn; it usually lasts several days and then gradually decreases over the weeks following delivery.

meconium A dark green-black material in the amniotic fluid that indicates fetal distress, and that can be aspirated into the fetus's lungs during delivery; the fetus's first bowel movement.

missed abortion A situation in which a fetus has died during the first 20 weeks of gestation, but has remained in utero.

myometrium The middle layer of tissue in the uterus.

nuchal cord A situation in which the umbilical cord is wrapped around the fetus's neck; cord compression may occur during labor, causing the fetal heart rate to slow and resulting in fetal distress.

ovum A mature oocyte.

parity The number of live births a woman has had.

perimetrium The outer protective layer of tissue in the uterus.

placenta The tissue attached to the uterine wall that nourishes the fetus through the umbilical cord.

placenta previa A condition in which the placenta develops over and covers the cervix.

postpartum The period of time after a woman has given birth.

preeclampsia A condition of late pregnancy that involves gradual onset of hypertension, headache, visual changes, and swelling of the hands and feet; also called pregnancy-induced hypertension or toxemia of pregnancy.

prenatal The state of the pregnant woman before birth.

prolapsed umbilical cord A situation in which the umbilical cord comes out of the vagina before the newborn.

Rh factor A protein found on the red blood cells of most people; when a woman without this protein is impregnated by a man with this protein, the woman's body can create antibodies against the protein that attack future pregnancies.

second stage of labor The stage of labor in which the newborn's head enters the birth canal, during which contractions become more intense and more frequent.

septic abortion A life-threatening emergency in which the uterus becomes infected following any type of abortion.

shoulder dystocia A complication of delivery in which there is difficulty delivering the shoulders of a newborn; the shoulder cannot get past the woman's symphysis pubis.

spontaneous abortion Expulsion of the fetus that occurs naturally; also called miscarriage.

Prep Kit (continued)

supine hypotensive syndrome Low blood pressure resulting from compression of the inferior vena cava by the weight of the pregnant uterus when the woman is supine.

third stage of labor The stage of labor in which the placenta is expelled.

threatened abortion Expulsion of the fetus that is attempting to take place but has not occurred yet; usually occurs in the first trimester.

TORCH syndrome Infections that occur in neonates as a result of organisms passing through the placenta from the woman to the fetus; includes toxoplasmosis, other agents, rubella, cytomegalovirus, and herpes simplex.

toxoplasmosis An infection caused by a parasite that pregnant women may get from handling or eating contaminated food or exposure from handling cat litter; the fetus can become infected.

transverse presentation A delivery in which the fetus lies crosswise in the uterus; one hand may protrude through the vagina.

umbilical cord The conduit connecting the pregnant woman to the fetus via the placenta; it contains two arteries and one vein.

uterine cavity The interior of the body of the uterus.

uterine inversion A potentially fatal complication of childbirth in which the placenta fails to detach properly and results in the uterus turning inside out.

▶ References

1. Slone ME, Rowen JS, Smith MS, Nelson KA, Weiler AJ. Conception and prenatal development. In: *Maternal-Child Nursing*. 5th ed. St. Louis: Elsevier; 2018:195-213.

2. Williams JF, Smith VC; Committee On Substance Abuse. Fetal alcohol spectrum disorders. *Pediatrics*. 2015 Nov;136(5):e1395-406. https://www.ncbi.nlm.nih.gov/pubmed/26482673. Accessed May 4, 2017.

3. Beckmann CR B, et al. Ch. 6: Preconception and antepartum care. In: *Obstetrics and Gynecology*. 7th ed. Philadelphia, PA: Wolters Kluwer Health/Lippincott Williams & Wilkins; 2014:76.

4. McKinney ES, James SR, Murray SS, Nelson K, Ashwill J. *Maternal-Child Nursing*. 5th ed. Philadelphia, PA: Saunders; 2017:214.

5. Records K, Tanaka L. Physiology of pregnancy. In: Mattson S, Smith JE, eds. *Core Curriculum for Maternal-Newborn Nursing*. 5th ed. St. Louis, MO: Elsevier; 2011:83-107.

6. Lavonas EJ, Drennan IR, Gabrielli A, Heffner AC, Hoyte CO, Orkin AM, Sawyer KN, Donnino MW. Part 10: special circumstances of resuscitation: 2015 American Heart Association Guidelines Update for Cardiopulmonary Resuscitation and Emergency Cardiovascular Care. *Circulation*. 2015;132(suppl 2):S502.

7. Antony KM, Racusin DA, Aagaard K, Dildy III GA. Maternal physiology. In: Gabbe SG, Niebyl JR, Simpson JL, et al., eds. *Obstetrics: Normal and Problem Pregnancies*. 7th ed. Philadelphia, PA: Elsevier; 2017:38-63.

8. Teen pregnancy in the United States. Centers for Disease Control and Prevention website. April 26, 2016. https://www.cdc.gov/teenpregnancy/about/. Accessed March 31, 2017.

9. Kinsella SM, Lohmann G. Supine hypotensive syndrome. *Obstet Gynecol*. 1994;83(5 Pt 1):774-788.

10. August P, Sabai BM. Preeclampsia: clinical features and diagnosis. February 2017. https://www.uptodate.com/contents/preeclampsia-clinical-features-and-diagnosis?source=search_result&search=preeclampsia&selectedTitle=1~150. Accessed March 30, 2017.

11. Beckmann CR, et al. Ch. 22: Cardiovascular and respiratory disorders. In: *Obstetrics and Gynecology*. 7th ed. Philadelphia, PA: Wolters Kluwer Health/Lippincott Williams & Wilkins; 2014:206-210.

12. Preterm birth. Centers for Disease Control and Prevention website. November 20, 2016. https://www.cdc.gov/reproductivehealth/maternalinfanthealth/pretermbirth.htm. Accessed March 30, 2017.

13. American Pregnancy Association. Hyperemesis gravidarum: Signs, Symptoms and Treatment. http://americanpregnancy.org/pregnancy-complications/hyperemesis-gravidarum/. Accessed March 30, 2017.

14. Khan FH. Hyperemesis gravidarum in emergency medicine medication. January 8, 2016. http://emedicine.medscape.com/article/796564-medication. Accessed March 30, 2017.

15. Smith JA, Refuerzo JS, Ramin SM. Treatment and outcome of nausea and vomiting of pregnancy. *UpToDate* website. March 27, 2017. https://www.uptodate.com/contents/treatment-and-outcome-of-nausea-and-vomiting-of-pregnancy?source=search_result&search=Hyperemesis%20Gravidarum&selectedTitle=1~118. Accessed March 30, 2017.

Prep Kit *(continued)*

16. Group B strep (GBS): fast facts. Centers for Disease Control and Prevention website. June 15, 2016. https://www.cdc.gov/groupbstrep/about/fast-facts .html. Accessed March 31, 2017.

17. Centers for Disease Control and Prevention. Revised recommendations for HIV screening of pregnant women. *Morb Mortal Wkly Rep.* 2001;50(19):59-86.

18. Centers for Disease Control and Prevention. Sexually Transmitted Diseases Treatment Guidelines, 2015, Recommendations and Reports. *Morb Mortal Wkly Rep.* 2015;64(RR3):1-137.

19. Miscarriage: signs, symptoms, treatment, and prevention. American Pregnancy Association website. August 2016. http://americanpregnancy .org/pregnancy-complications/miscarriage/. Accessed March 31, 2017.

20. Qublan HS. Habitual abortion: causes, diagnosis, and treatment. *Rev Gynaecol Pract.* 2003;3(2):75-80.

21. Placental abruption. March of Dimes website. January 2012. http://www.marchofdimes.org /pregnancy/placental-abruption.aspx. Accessed March 31, 2017.

22. Ananth CV, Kinzler WL. Placental abruption: clinical features and diagnosis. *UpToDate* website. February 23, 2017. https://www .uptodate.com/contents/placental-abruption -clinical-features-and-diagnosis?source=search _result&search=Abruptio%20placenta%20 causes&selectedTitle=1~150#H1. Accessed March 31, 2017.

23. Placenta previa. March of Dimes website. January 2012. http://www.marchofdimes.org/complications /placenta-previa.aspx. Accessed March 30, 2017.

24. Lockwood CJ, Russo-Stieglitz K. Clinical features, diagnosis, and course of placenta previa. *UpToDate* website. November 30, 2016. https://www.uptodate .com/contents/clinical-features-diagnosis-and -course-of-placenta-previa?source=search _result&search=placenta%20previa&selectedTitle =2~104#H14. Accessed March 31, 2017.

25. Weiner GM, Zaichkin J. *Textbook of Neonatal Resuscitation (NRP).* 7th ed. Elk Grove Village, IL: American Academy of Pediatrics; 2016:36.

26. Koren G. Motherisk update. Is ondansetron safe for use during pregnancy? *Can Fam Physician.* 2012;58(10):1092-1093.

27. 2015 CPR & EEC guidelines. Part 13: neonatal resuscitation. American Heart Association website. https://eccguidelines.heart.org/index.php /circulation/cpr-ecc-guidelines-2/part-13-neonatal -resuscitation/. Accessed May 1, 2017.

28. Martin JA, Hamilton BE, Osterman MJK, Driscoll AK, Mathews TJ. Births: final data for 2015. *Natl Vital Stat Rep.* 2017;66(1). https://www.cdc.gov /nchs/data/nvsr/nvsr66/nvsr66_01.pdf. Accessed May 1, 2017.

29. Facts of stillbirth. Centers for Disease Control and Prevention website. March 7, 2017. https://www.cdc .gov/ncbddd/stillbirth/facts.html. Accessed April 4, 2017.

30. Breech births. American Pregnancy Association website. http://americanpregnancy.org/labor-and -birth/breech-presentation/. Accessed April 4, 2017.

31. Henry E, Andres RL, Christensen RD. Neonatal outcomes following a tight nuchal cord. *J Perinatol.* 2013;33(3):231-234. http://www.medscape.com /viewarticle/780171_1. Accessed April 4, 2017.

32. Umbilical cord prolapse. American Pregnancy Association website. August 2015. http:// americanpregnancy.org/pregnancy-complications /umbilical-cord-prolapse/. Accessed April 4, 2017.

33. Hostetler DR, Bosworth MF. Uterine inversion. *J Am Board Fam Med.* 2000;13(2):120-123. http://www .medscape.com/viewarticle/405770_1. Accessed April 4, 2017.

34. Depression among women. Centers for Disease Control and Prevention website. February 15, 2017. https://www.cdc.gov/reproductivehealth /depression/. Accessed April 4, 2017.

35. Murphy NJ, Quinlan JD. Trauma in pregnancy: assessment, management, and prevention. *Am Fam Physician.* 2014;90(10):717-724. http://www.aafp .org/afp/2014/1115/p717.html. Accessed April 4, 2017.

36. Rees GA, Willis BA. Resuscitation in late pregnancy. *Anaesthesia.* 1988;43:347-349.

37. 2015 CPR & EEC guidelines. Part 10: special circumstances of resuscitation. American Heart Association website. https://eccguidelines.heart.org /index.php/circulation/cpr-ecc-guidelines-2/part -10-special-circumstances-of-resuscitation/. Accessed May 1, 2017.

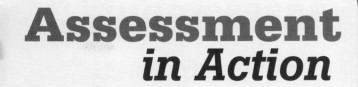

Assessment *in Action*

You are dispatched to a local residence for a patient with a severe headache. The dispatcher tells you this patient is 8 months pregnant and has a severe headache, dizziness, and "floating spots" in her visual fields. When you arrive at the residence, you find a 30-year-old woman who appears to be extremely overweight and in moderate distress. The patient tells you that her hands and feet have swollen a lot over the past day and she has had a severe headache. She has a past medical history of migraines, asthma, and kidney stones. She is at 34 weeks' gestation, and this is her second pregnancy. She experienced no complications with her prior pregnancy and she receives routine prenatal care. At her Ob/Gyn appointment last week she was told that there was a large amount of protein in her urine and her blood pressure was elevated. She was advised by her doctor to begin checking her blood pressure regularly at home. This morning when she checked it using her home cuff, she got a reading of 158/92 mm Hg.

1. The clinical presentation of this patient indicates that she may have:

   A. severe preeclampsia.
   B. eclampsia.
   C. HELLP syndrome.
   D. gestational hypertension.

2. At what blood pressure threshold does preeclampsia become a possible working diagnosis for this patient?

   A. ≥130 mm Hg systolic or ≥80 mm Hg diastolic
   B. ≥140 mm Hg systolic or ≥90 mm Hg diastolic
   C. ≥150 mm Hg systolic or ≥100 mm Hg diastolic
   D. ≥160 mm Hg systolic or ≥110 mm Hg diastolic

3. Which of the following characteristics put this patient at an increased risk for preeclampsia?

   A. This is the patient's second pregnancy.
   B. The patient is overweight.
   C. The patient is 30 years old.
   D. The patient has a history of migraines.

4. The pharmacologic treatment for this patient's condition is:

   A. amiodarone.
   B. calcium chloride.
   C. etomidate.
   D. magnesium sulfate.

5. What is the correct dosing for magnesium sulfate for this patient?

   A. Loading dose of 1 to 2 g in 50 to 100 mL of 5% dextrose in water (D_5W) over 5 to 60 minutes IV
   B. 25 to 50 mg/kg IV/IO of a 10% solution over 15 to 30 minutes to a maximum dose of 2 g
   C. 1 to 2 g of a 10% solution IV/IO over 5 to 20 minutes
   D. 1 to 4 g of a 10% solution IV/IO over 3 minutes; maximum dose of 30 to 40 g/day

6. If you suspected that this patient had been given too much magnesium sulfate, which of the following could be administered as an antagonist?

   A. Amiodarone
   B. Calcium chloride
   C. Etomidate
   D. Diphenhydramine

Assessment *in Action* (continued)

7. On arrival to the hospital, STAT labwork is evaluated and shows that the patient is now anemic with thrombocytopenia and altered liver function. What condition would you suspect is happening in addition to her original complaint?

   A. Placenta previa
   B. Abruptio placenta
   C. Oligohydramnios
   D. HELLP syndrome

8. What is false labor?

9. What are the three stages of labor, and during which stage is the fetus delivered?

10. At which point is a pregnancy considered "post term"?

CHAPTER 42

Neonatal Care

National EMS Education Standard Competencies

Special Patient Populations

Integrates assessment findings with principles of pathophysiology and knowledge of psychosocial needs to formulate a field impression and implement a comprehensive treatment/disposition plan for patients with special needs.

Neonatal Care

Anatomy and physiology of neonatal circulation (pp 2071-2072)
Assessment of the newborn (pp 2072, 2074-2075)
Presentation and management
> Newborn (pp 2071-2072, 2074-2075)
> Neonatal resuscitation (pp 2075-2086)

Knowledge Objectives

1. Explain terminology associated with infants, including newborn versus neonate. (p 2070)
2. List antepartum and intrapartum risk factors that can lead to a need for neonatal resuscitation. (p 2071)
3. Discuss the process of transitioning from a fetus to a newborn. (pp 2071-2072)
4. List causes of delayed transition in newborns. (pp 2071-2072)
5. Discuss measures to take to prepare for neonatal resuscitation. (pp 2071-2073)
6. List equipment for neonatal resuscitation. (pp 2071-2073)
7. Discuss the initial steps of assessment for neonates, including drying and warming, positioning, suctioning, and stimulation. (pp 2072, 2074-2078)
8. Explain how to measure essential parameters including pulse rate, color, and respiratory effort. (pp 2074-2076)
9. Discuss Apgar scores, including how and when to obtain them. (p 2075)
10. Discuss how to determine whether a neonate requires resuscitation. (pp 2075-2077)
11. Discuss methods used to improve oxygenation during neonatal resuscitation, including the use of positive end-expiratory pressure, free-flow oxygen, oral airways, and bag-mask devices. (pp 2076-2080)
12. Describe the technique for using a bag-mask device on a neonate. (pp 2079-2080)
13. Discuss when endotracheal intubation is required in a neonate. (p 2080)
14. Describe vascular access considerations in the neonate. (pp 2084-2085)
15. Discuss pharmacologic considerations pertaining to the neonate. (pp 2085-2086)
16. Describe family and transport considerations that apply to neonatal emergencies. (p 2086)
17. Discuss the pathophysiology, assessment, and management of specific emergencies, including apnea, bradycardia, acidosis, pneumothorax, meconium-stained amniotic fluid, low blood volume, diaphragmatic hernia, respiratory distress and cyanosis, and respiratory depression secondary to narcotics. (pp 2086-2090)
18. Discuss the pathophysiology, assessment, and management of premature or low birth weight infants. (pp 2090-2091)
19. Discuss the pathophysiology, assessment, and management of seizures in neonates. (pp 2091-2093)
20. Discuss the pathophysiology, assessment, and management of hypoglycemia in a neonate. (pp 2093-2094)
21. Discuss the pathophysiology, assessment, and management of vomiting in a neonate. (pp 2094-2095)
22. Discuss the pathophysiology, assessment, and management of diarrhea in a neonate. (pp 2095-2096)
23. Discuss the pathophysiology, assessment, and management of neonatal jaundice. (p 2096)
24. Discuss the pathophysiology, assessment, and management of emergencies related to thermoregulation, including fever and hypothermia. (pp 2096-2098)
25. Discuss the pathophysiology, assessment, and management of common birth injuries. (pp 2098-2099)
26. Discuss the pathophysiology, assessment, and management of cardiac conditions in newborns. (pp 2099-2103)

Skills Objectives

1. List the steps of neonatal resuscitation. (p 2076)
2. Describe the technique for performing endotracheal intubation in a neonate. (pp 2081-2082, Skill Drill 42-1)
3. Describe the technique for inserting an orogastric tube in a newborn. (pp 2081, 2083, Skill Drill 42-2)
4. Explain how to perform chest compressions on a neonate. (pp 2083-2084)
5. Describe the technique for cannulating the umbilical vein in a newborn. (pp 2084-2085)

Introduction

The care of a newborn or neonate must be tailored to meet the unique needs of this population. A **newborn** refers to an infant within the first few hours after birth; a **neonate** refers to an infant within the first month after birth. A healthy neonate is completely dependent on others for nourishment, warmth, and protection from the environment. Most parents recognize this need and instinctively wish to fulfill the role of nurturer and caregiver. However, when a newborn needs special support that necessitates intervention by trained caregivers, the parents may feel isolated and inadequate. It is important for you to support the needs of both the newborn and the parents or other caregivers by allowing them to be physically close as much as possible, explaining what is being done, and providing details of the plan for transport to the next level of care.

This chapter reviews the physiologic changes that occur in a newborn during birth, the care that should be provided during and immediately after birth, and the special needs of **premature** births or births complicated by other factors. It also reviews the steps involved in neonatal resuscitation and outlines the process of transporting an infant to a hospital or between hospitals.

General Pathophysiology and Assessment

Skilled care interventions to optimize cardiopulmonary function are routinely required in only 5% to

YOU are the Paramedic | PART 1

You are a crew member riding on Rescue 2 when a call for assistance from another ambulance comes in. Rescue 1 is on the scene with a mother who was doing housework when her amniotic sac ruptured. She contacted her obstetrician who instructed her to call 9-1-1, and Rescue 1 responded to her call. On arrival, you enter the residence and find the patient lying on the bed in the lithotomy position and yelling, "I need to push!" Personnel from Rescue 1 inform you that the patient says her water broke approximately 45 minutes ago and was green in color with a foul smell. Rescue 1 noted crowning on their arrival.

Maternal Assessment Recording Time: 1 Minute	
Appearance	Anxious, in pain
Level of consciousness	Alert (oriented to person, place, time, and event)
Airway	Patent
Breathing	Respirations, increased; adequate tidal volume
Circulation	Radial pulses present, increased and regular; no gross bleeding

1. What is the significance of the green amniotic fluid?
2. What further information would you like to obtain from the mother?

10% of deliveries in the United States.[1] Approximately 5% to 10% of newborns will require only minimal active interventions such as airway suctioning or positive pressure ventilation.[1] Chest compressions and/or emergency medications are required in an even smaller number of newborns, only being used in 1 to 3 per 1,000 births.[2]

In the United States, approximately 8% of newborns delivered each year weigh less than 5.5 pounds (2,500 g).[3] The most common cause of low birth weight is prematurity, and mortality in these infants increases as birth weight and gestational age decrease.[3] Table 42-1 and Table 42-2 outline risk factors for complications before and during birth.

Table 42-1	Antepartum (Before Birth) Risk Factors
<ul><li>Multiple gestation</li><li>Pregnant woman's age <16 yr or >35 yr</li><li>Preterm (<37 wks) gestation</li><li>Postterm (>42 wks) gestation</li><li>Hypertension, preeclampsia</li><li>Diabetes</li><li>**Polyhydramnios** (excessive amount of **amniotic fluid**)</li><li>Premature rupture of the membrane</li><li>Fetal malformation</li><li>Decreased fetal movement</li><li>Inadequate or no prenatal care</li></ul>	<ul><li>Prior history of perinatal morbidity or mortality</li><li>Maternal use of drugs/medications</li><li>Fetal anemia</li><li>**Oligohydramnios** (decreased volume of amniotic fluid during a pregnancy)</li><li>Maternal infections</li><li>Known malformations (high-risk OB patient)</li><li>Bleeding during pregnancy (abruption)</li></ul>

Abbreviation: OB, obstetric

© Jones & Bartlett Learning.

Table 42-2	Intrapartum (During Birth) Risk Factors
<ul><li>Premature labor</li><li>Rupture of membranes >18 h before delivery</li><li>Breech or abnormal presentation</li><li>**Prolapsed cord**</li><li>Chorioamnionitis</li><li>**Meconium**-stained amniotic fluid</li></ul>	<ul><li>Use of narcotics within 4 h of delivery</li><li>Prolonged labor (>24 h) or precipitous delivery</li><li>Significant bleeding</li><li>**Placenta previa**</li></ul>

© Jones & Bartlett Learning.

► Transition From Fetus to Newborn

In utero (ie, in the pregnant woman's womb), a fetus receives its oxygen from the placenta. The fetal lung is collapsed and filled with fluid, receiving only 10% of the total blood supply. As the fetus is delivered, a rapid series of events need to occur to enable the newborn to breathe. This process is called **fetal transition**.

Fetal circulation has three major blood flow deviations (shunts) from that of the adult. These shunts occur at the ductus venosus, **foramen ovale**, and ductus arteriosus Figure 42-1 . At birth, the shunts begin to close off during fetal transition. The adult remnants of these shunts are found at the ligamentum venosus, fossa ovale, and ligamentum arteriosus, respectively. Blood flow is no longer diverted and the neonate will have a physiologically mature circulatory pattern within hours to days after being born.[4]

The first breath is triggered by mild hypoxia and hypercapnia related to partial occlusion of the umbilical cord during normal delivery. Tactile stimulation and cold stress also promote early breathing. As the newborn's lungs become filled with air, the pulmonary vascular resistance drops, causing more blood to flow to the lungs, picking up oxygen to supply to the body. Any event that delays this decline in pulmonary pressure can lead to delayed transition, hypoxia, brain injury, and, ultimately, death Table 42-3 .

A newborn delivered at fewer than 37 completed weeks of **gestation** (the period of time from conception to birth) is considered **preterm**; a newborn born at 38 to 42 weeks of gestation is described as **term**; and a newborn born at more than 42 weeks of gestation is described as **postterm** (or postdates).

► Arrival of the Newborn

Use any time available before the fetus arrives to obtain a patient history and prepare the environment and equipment that may be necessary. Key questions you need to ask when you are at a scene involving a pregnant woman or a recent home birth include the woman's age; length of the pregnancy (preferably expressed in weeks); the presence and frequency of contractions; the presence or absence of fetal movement; whether there have been any pregnancy complications (eg, diabetes, hypertension, fever); whether membranes have ruptured, including the timing and the makeup of the fluid (clear, meconium stained, or bloody); if there are multiple fetuses, and the medications being taken (see the list of risk factors in Table 42-1 and Table 42-2). All of these questions will help you determine what resuscitation and equipment may be needed.

In the United States, 90% to 95% of all newborns require no active interventions at birth, and transition to extrauterine life without incident.[1] At a minimum, you will need warm, dry blankets, a bulb syringe, two small

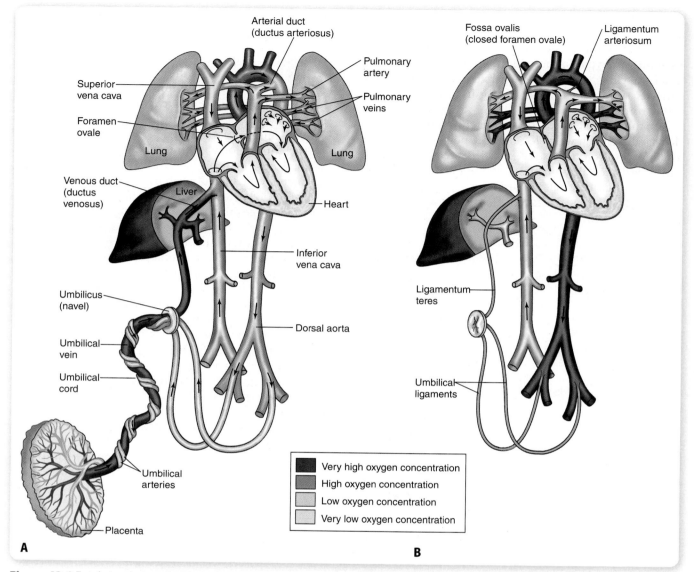

Figure 42-1 Fetal circulation. **A.** Oxygenated blood from the placenta reaches the fetus through the umbilical vein. Blood returns to the placenta via two umbilical arteries. Shunts (movements of blood from the normal path) occur at the ductus venosus, foramen ovale, and the ductus arteriosus. **B.** Fetal circulation following transition.

© Jones & Bartlett Learning.

Table 42-3	Causes of Delayed Transition in Newborns

- Hypoxia
- Meconium or blood aspiration
- Acidosis
- Hypothermia
- Pneumonia
- Hypotension
- Sepsis
- Birth **asphyxia**
- Pulmonary hypoplasia (underdevelopment)
- Respiratory distress syndrome

© Jones & Bartlett Learning.

clamps or ties, and a pair of clean scissors to cut the umbilical cord. However, any complications need prompt management. Even if a piece of equipment is in a sealed sterile wrap, having it near at hand will expedite its use once the newborn is delivered. Table 42-4 lists additional equipment that may be needed if more extensive resuscitation becomes necessary.

If the newborn is delivered in the ambulance, the foot of the stretcher, covered with clean, warm blankets, can be used for the initial stabilization steps. The newborn can then be placed on the mother's chest after you confirm adequate patency of the airway, breathing, and pulse rate. If more extensive resuscitation is needed, this area can be used as needed initially, optimally transitioning to a second ambulance equipped with a neonatal transport incubator to allow maintenance of

Table 42-4	Preparation of Area for Newborn Resuscitation, Including Resuscitation Equipment and Supplies
Equipment Category	**Equipment List**
Suction Equipment	• Bulb syringe, mechanical suction and tubing, suction catheters, 5F, 6F, 8F, 10F, 12F, or 14F • 8F feeding tube and 20-mL syringe
Ventilation Equipment	• Device for delivering positive pressure ventilation, capable of delivering up to 100% oxygen • Face masks, newborn and premature infant size (cushioned-rim masks preferred) • Compressed air source • Pulse oximeter and oximeter probe
Intubation Equipment	• Laryngoscope with straight blades, size 0 (preterm) and 1 (term) • Extra bulb, batteries for laryngoscope • Endotracheal tubes size 2.5, 3.0, 3.5, and 4.0 internal diameter • Stylet (optional) • Scissors • Tape or securing device for endotracheal tube • Capnograph or carbon dioxide detector • Laryngeal mask airway
Medications	• Epinephrine 0.1 mg/mL (1:10,000), 3- or 10-mL ampules • Isotonic crystalloid (normal saline or lactated Ringer solution), 100- or 250-mL bag • Normal saline for flushes • Dextrose, 10%, 250 mL
Umbilical Vessel Catheterization Equipment	• Sterile gloves • Scalpel or scissors • Antiseptic prep solution • Umbilical tape • Umbilical catheters, 3.5F, 5F (a sterile 3.5F feeding tube can be used in an emergency) • Three-way stopcocks for each catheter • Syringes: 1, 3, 5, 10, 20, and 50 mL • Needles: 25, 22, and 18 gauge or puncture device for needleless system
Miscellaneous	• Gloves and appropriate standard precautions • Radiant warmer or other heat source • Firm, padded resuscitation surface • Clock with second hand, timer optional • Warmed towels • Stethoscope, neonatal head • Tape, 1/2 or 3/4 in. • Cardiac monitor and electrodes or pulse oximeter and probe (optional for delivery room) • Oropharyngeal airways (0, 00, and 000 sizes or 30-, 40-, and 50-mm lengths)
For Very Preterm Newborns	• Size 00 laryngoscope blade (optional) • Reclosable, food-grade plastic bag (1-gal [4-L] size) or plastic wrap • Chemically activated warming pad (optional)

Modified from: Weiner GM, Zaichkin J. Lesson 2: preparing for resuscitation. In: *Textbook of Neonatal Resuscitation (NRP).* 7th ed. Elk Grove Village, IL: American Academy of Pediatrics; 2016:26-27.

a thermoneutral environment and observation of the newborn's color and tone.

When the newborn's head is delivered, suction the mouth and then the nose with a bulb syringe as needed to establish airway patency. Nasal suctioning helps clear the secretions and provides a stimulus to breathe. After delivery, keep the newborn at the level of the mother, with the head slightly lower than the body, while you clamp the umbilical cord in two places and then cut between the clamps **Figure 42-2**. See Chapter 41, *Obstetrics*, for information on cord clamping. Remember, for vigorous infants, cord clamping should occur 30 to 60 seconds after delivery.[5]

Special Populations

A delay in clamping the umbilical cord and keeping the newborn below the level of the placenta may cause more blood to flow into the newborn, which can in turn lead to **polycythemia** (an abnormally high red blood cell count). If the newborn is kept above the level of the placenta, reverse blood flow may occur and may cause anemia in the newborn.

If the umbilical cord comes out ahead of the newborn (more common with polyhydramnios, a condition characterized by extra amniotic fluid), the blood supply

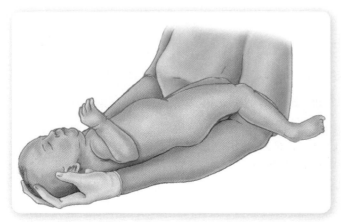

Figure 42-2 Positioning. Immediately after delivery, hold the newborn with the head slightly lower than the body to facilitate drainage of secretions.

through the umbilical cord to the fetus may be cut off. In this case, relieving pressure on the cord (by gently moving the presenting part of the newborn's body off the cord and pushing the cord back) can be lifesaving.

Your primary survey of the newborn may be done simultaneously with any treatment interventions. Note the time of delivery, and monitor the ABCs (Airway, Breathing, and Circulation). In particular, assess patency of the airway, respiratory rate, respiratory effort, tone, pulse rate, and color.

As you examine a newborn or neonate, be aware of normal and abnormal presentations. Inspect the skin for any abnormalities. Common findings, such as vernix (a white cheesy material), edema, and Mongolian spots (dark or blue pigmentation over the buttocks and lower lumbar regions in patients of African, Asian, Mediterranean, and Native American ancestry), are considered to be normal variants. Jaundice can appear in healthy newborns 2 to 5 days after birth and typically disappears after about 1 week. Jaundice that persists beyond 2 to 3 weeks should raise suspicion of biliary obstruction or liver disease. Examine the head for symmetry and abnormalities. Because the skull sutures are not fused at birth, it is common for the head to appear asymmetric immediately after birth. This normal variation allows the head to fit through the birth canal. In such cases, reassure the parents and explain to them the infant's head will typically become more symmetric within the next few days. Be aware that most young infants lack muscle strength in their necks and are unable to control the motion of their heads. Therefore, it is important to support the head and neck at all times when examining young infants.

Examine the eyes of the neonate for irregularities. A newborn who truly cannot open his or her eyes may have a congenital defect. Watch for abnormal eye movement, such as nystagmus (wandering or shaking eye movements) and strabismus (alternating convergence or divergence, creating a crossed-eye appearance). Look for abnormalities in the sclera and pupils. Subconjunctival hemorrhages are common and harmless in newborns. Examine for any drainage or ocular discharge, which may indicate a blocked tear duct. Inspect the newborn's umbilical cord to detect abnormalities. Normally, there are two thick-walled umbilical arteries and one larger but thin-walled **umbilical vein**, which is usually located in the 12-o'clock position. Note the presence of any abnormal abdominal findings, such as hernias.

The newborn is at risk for hypothermia because of significant heat loss through evaporation, a large surface area to volume ratio, limited ability to generate heat, and poor insulation from the environment. Ensure **thermoregulation** by placing the newborn on pre-warmed towels or a radiant warmer, drying the head and the body thoroughly, discarding the wet towels, and then covering the newborn with a dry towel. Cover the head with a cap to minimize heat loss. Position the newborn to ensure a patent airway, clear the airway of secretions as needed, and assess the newborn's respiratory effort. All newborns are cyanotic immediately after birth. If the newborn remains vigorous and begins to become pink in the first 5 minutes of life, ongoing observation and continued thermoregulation with direct skin-to-skin contact with the mother should be maintained while on the way to a local hospital. Bonding with the mother should be encouraged in a stable newborn.

Words of Wisdom

Do not milk the umbilical cord.

Patient Safety

Do not neglect to keep the newborn warm. However, as you warm an infant, be aware of the dangers of overwarming. It is possible to overwarm the neonate. In at least one case, paramedics were too aggressive with warming, resulting in the newborn having severe burns.[6]

▶ The Apgar Score

The **Apgar score**, named after Dr. Virginia Apgar, who developed the measure in 1953, helps record the condition of the newborn in the first few minutes after birth based on five signs (**Table 42-5**).[7] This score can help you

Table 42-5	The Apgar Score	
Condition	**Description**	**Score**
Appearance—skin color	Completely pink	2
	Body pink, extremities blue	1
	Centrally blue, pale	0
Pulse rate	>100	2
	<100, >0	1
	Absent	0
Grimace—irritability	Cries	2
	Grimaces	1
	No response	0
Activity—muscle tone	Active motion	2
	Some flexion of extremities	1
	Limp	0
Respiratory—effort	Strong cry	2
	Slow and irregular	1
	Absent	0

Reproduced from Apgar V. A proposal for a new method of evaluation of the newborn infant. *Curr Res Anesth Analg.* 1953 Jul-Aug;32(4):260-267. Reprinted by permission of Lippincott Williams & Wilkins.

determine the need for specific resuscitation measures and the effectiveness of your resuscitation efforts to facilitate the transition from fetus to newborn. Each sign is assigned a value of 0, 1, or 2. The Apgar score is the sum total of these values and is typically recorded at 1 and 5 minutes after birth. If the 5-minute Apgar score is less than 7, reassess the newborn's condition and assign an additional score every 5 minutes until 20 minutes after birth. If resuscitation is necessary, complete the Apgar score by determining the result of the resuscitation.

Words of Wisdom

Do not wait until you have measured the 1-minute Apgar score before you start resuscitation.

▶ Algorithm for Neonatal Resuscitation

If a problem arises, it is important for you to follow current neonatal resuscitation guidelines to optimize the outcome (**Figure 42-3**).[8] Because most babies respond to the initial basic steps of resuscitation and very few need medications, newborn resuscitation has been described as an inverted pyramid (**Figure 42-4**).[9]

Words of Wisdom

The Algorithm for Neonatal Resuscitation shown in Figure 42-3 should be considered a continuum of care. The interventions outlined in the first 60 seconds (the first minute) of care are important to execute quickly and efficiently. They should also be given enough time to work.

The Neonatal Resuscitation Provider course essentially divides the first 60 seconds of care into two sets of 30 seconds. At birth, providers should immediately perform initial interventions of drying, warming, suctioning, and stimulation.[10] Approximately 30 seconds after birth, providers should reassess the neonate's response to these initial interventions. If the response to the initial interventions is inadequate, then it is appropriate to administer supplemental oxygen, position the airway, and/or administer CPAP (depending on the situation and resources available).[11] After 30 seconds has elapsed, evaluate if this second set of interventions is effective by reassessing the newborn, and determine if it is necessary to proceed to more aggressive treatment. These two 30-second intervals of care make up the first 60 seconds of the newborn's life.

Finally, it is critical to note that if the newborn does not have adequate respiratory effort and a pulse above 100 beats/min within the first minute after birth, you must begin PPV. Ventilation of the newborn's lungs is the most important and effective treatment during neonatal resuscitation.[12]

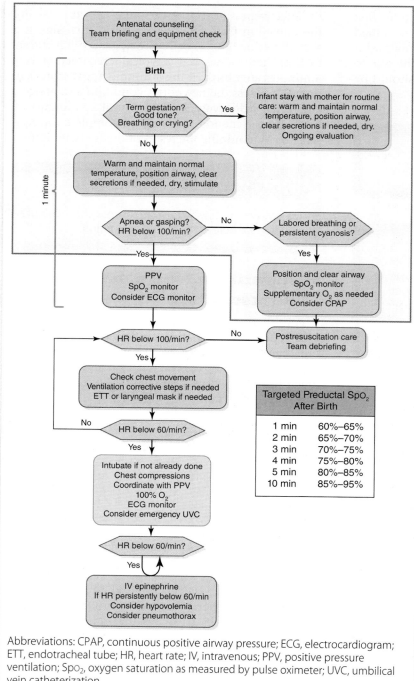

Abbreviations: CPAP, continuous positive airway pressure; ECG, electrocardiogram; ETT, endotracheal tube; HR, heart rate; IV, intravenous; PPV, positive pressure ventilation; SpO2, oxygen saturation as measured by pulse oximeter; UVC, umbilical vein catheterization

Figure 42-3 Algorithm for neonatal resuscitation. The shaded area outlines steps that apply to the distressed newborn.

Initial steps, reevaluation, and beginning ventilation should occur within the first 60 seconds. After delivery of the newborn, follow the initial steps of bulb suctioning of the mouth and nose, drying, and stimulating the newborn. If the newborn does not respond to these actions, further intervention is indicated. Assess the newborn's respiratory rate, respiratory effort, pulse rate, and color. Count the respiratory rate and pulse rate for 6 seconds and then multiply by 10 to quickly determine the rate per minute. The pulse rate can be determined either by auscultation or by feeling the base of the umbilical cord at the baby's abdomen because the umbilical artery should still have pulsatile flow **Figure 42-5**. Be sure to communicate the heart rate to other members of your resuscitation team. Many newborns become centrally pink but have blue hands and feet (**acrocyanosis**). This is considered normal. If the newborn has a normal breathing pattern and a pulse rate of greater than 100 beats/min but maintains **central cyanosis** of the trunk or of the mucous membranes, provide supplemental **free-flow oxygen**. If there is no other warming source available, keep the newborn on the mother's chest and continue to manage the airway.

If the baby is apneic (ie, has a 20-second or longer respiratory pause) or has a pulse rate of less than 100 beats/min after 30 seconds of drying and stimulation, begin positive pressure ventilation (PPV) by bag-mask device, being sure to use a newborn-sized bag-mask device. Use caution when you are squeezing the bag to avoid inadvertently delivering too much volume, potentially resulting in a pneumothorax. The size of breath provided should result in a physiologic chest rise. Room air is preferred when resuscitating term infants, and the addition of supplemental oxygen may not be necessary.[13]

In neonatal resuscitation, the pulse oximetry value should be obtained from a site that reflects the **preductal oxygen saturation**. The brachiocephalic artery is the first major vessel that arises from the ascending aortic arch, prior to the ductus arteriosus (referred to as "preductal"). Tissues perfused with blood from the brachiocephalic artery better reflect the oxygenation status of the heart and brain. The best pulse oximeter probe locations for obtaining a preductal oxygen saturation are the right hand or right earlobe.

If the neonate has not achieved the target preductal oxygen saturation value for their age **Table 42-6**, then additional oxygen may be necessary.

If the newborn's pulse rate is less than 100 beats/min, the next step in the algorithm is to check chest movement,

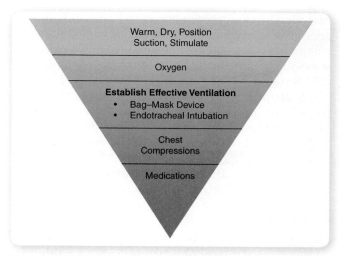

Figure 42-4 The neonatal resuscitation pyramid.

Modified from: 2015 Handbook of Emergency Cardiovascular Care for Healthcare Providers. American Heart Association; 2015:73.

Table 42-6	Target Oxygen Saturation Levels in Neonates After Birth	
Minutes	**Percent Oxygen Saturation**	
1	60% to 65%	
2	65% to 70%	
3	70% to 75%	
4	75% to 80%	
5	80% to 85%	
10	85% to 95%	

Data from: Web-based Integrated 2015 American Heart Association Guidelines for CPR & ECC. Part 13: neonatal resuscitation. © 2015 American Heart Association.

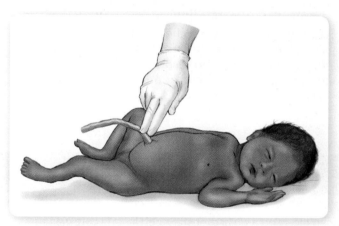

Figure 42-5 Feel for a pulse at the base of the umbilical cord.

© Jones & Bartlett Learning.

Words of Wisdom

Fewer than 1% of deliveries require treatment with chest compressions or emergency medications.[2] The most common etiology for bradycardia in a newborn is hypoxia, which is readily reversed by effective PPV. Profound hypoxia or shock is also the cause of cardiac arrest, which is almost always a secondary event after respiratory failure in these patients. Another less common etiology—but one that requires prompt intervention—is tension pneumothorax, which needs to be recognized and treated with needle decompression if resuscitation is to be successful.

take ventilation corrective steps if needed, and insert an ET tube or laryngeal mask as appropriate. Airway management is discussed in detail later in this chapter.

If the newborn's pulse rate is less than 60 beats/min, begin chest compressions in addition to PPV. Effective chest compressions should result in palpable pulses. Use a pulse oximeter when resuscitation is anticipated, if the newborn appears cyanotic, or if positive pressure ventilation or chest compressions are needed.

If ventilation and chest compressions do not improve the bradycardia, administer epinephrine, preferably via intravenous (IV) line.[14] In an emergency, epinephrine can be administered via endotracheal (ET) tube until IV access can be obtained, but absorption is less reliable via this route.[14,15] When no signs of life (pulse or respiratory effort) are present after 10 minutes of resuscitation, the chances of successful resuscitation are low and overall outcomes are associated with high early mortality and morbidity in surviving infants.[16-20]

■ Specific Intervention and Resuscitation Steps

▶ Drying and Stimulation

After you ensure the patency of the airway by bulb suctioning of the newborn's mouth and nose, dry and stimulate the newborn. Nasal suctioning is a stimulus for the newborn to breathe. Position the newborn on his or her back or side, with the neck in the sniffing position. If the airway is not clear, suction using a bulb syringe or suction

Words of Wisdom

Do not suction deep into the oropharynx. Do not suction for more than 10 seconds at a time.

catheter, with the head turned to the side. Remember to suction the mouth before the nose to prevent aspiration. Finally, flick the soles of the newborn's feet and gently rub the newborn's back. Avoid rubbing too roughly or slapping the newborn because these actions may lead to traumatic injury.

Words of Wisdom

When working with infants, always use weight-based dosing of medications.

Also, infants have small airways. Optimal positioning of the head and clearing any secretions that obstruct an airway are critical for all infants.

► Airway Management

Free-Flow Oxygen

If a newborn is cyanotic or pale, provide supplemental oxygen. Given that 5 g/dL of deoxygenated hemoglobin is needed before clinical cyanosis becomes apparent, a severely anemic hypoxic newborn will be pale, but not cyanotic. Therefore, provide oxygen to a pale newborn until an accurate oxygen saturation reading can be obtained using a pulse oximeter. Warm and humidify the oxygen if it will be provided for more than a few minutes. If PPV is not indicated (ie, the pulse rate is greater than 100 beats/min and the newborn has adequate respiratory effort), oxygen can initially be delivered through an oxygen mask or via oxygen tubing within your hand that is cupped and held close to the newborn's nose and mouth **Figure 42-6** . The oxygen flow rate should be set at 5 L/min. Do not blow oxygen directly into the newborn's eyes.

Oral Airways

Oral airways are rarely used for newborns, but they can be lifesaving if airway obstruction leads to respiratory failure. Some conditions that may require an oral airway are bilateral choanal atresia, Pierre Robin sequence, macroglossia (large tongue size), and other craniofacial defects that may affect the airway. In all the preceding cases, except for bilateral choanal atresia, an ET tube can be inserted down a nostril to a level below the base of the tongue. It is necessary to keep the newborn's mouth open to provide adequate ventilation when these conditions exist. Bilateral **choanal atresia** (bony or membranous

YOU ❯ are the Paramedic   PART 2

The mother tells you that this is her fifth pregnancy and she has been receiving regular prenatal care. Her due date was last week and her doctor has her scheduled to induce labor 2 days from now. She has not experienced any complications during her pregnancy. The only medication she takes is a daily prenatal vitamin.

As you take appropriate standard precautions and perform a visual inspection of the patient's vaginal area to confirm that crowning is present, your partner begins to check the obstetric (OB) kit that Rescue 1 opened prior to your arrival. Your exam confirms crowning of the newborn's head, which has a noticeable green stain on it. Rescue 1 applied oxygen to the mother via a nonrebreathing mask (NRM) at 12 L/min, and positioned her for delivery. Your partner confirms that the OB kit is intact and complete.

Maternal Assessment Recording Time: 2 Minutes	
Respirations	24 breaths/min; adequate tidal volume
Pulse	104 beats/min; strong and regular
Skin	Pink, warm, and moist
Blood pressure	128/74 mm Hg
Oxygen saturation (Spo$_2$)	97% via NRM at 12 L/min

3. Besides the OB kit, what additional equipment should you have available?
4. Should you stimulate the newborn immediately after birth?

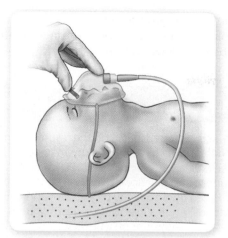

Figure 42-6 Free-flow oxygen can be delivered through an oxygen mask.
© Jones & Bartlett Learning.

Table 42-7	**Common Causes of Respiratory Distress**
• Lung or heart disease • Central nervous system disorders • Pneumothorax • Meconium aspiration • Lung immaturity/ respiratory distress syndrome • Shock and sepsis • Diaphragmatic hernia	• **Persistent pulmonary hypertension** • Mucous obstruction of nasal passages • Choanal atresia • Amniotic fluid aspiration • Pneumonia • Metabolic acidosis

Jones & Bartlett Learning.

obstruction of the back of the nose preventing air flow) can be rapidly fatal, but usually responds to placement of an oral airway (or a gloved finger until an adequate oral airway is located). The **Pierre Robin sequence** is a series of developmental anomalies including a small chin and posteriorly positioned tongue that frequently lead to airway obstruction. Positioning the patient prone (chest down) may relieve the obstruction. If not, insert an oral airway. As with infants and small children, use a tongue blade to depress the tongue and insert the oral airway without rotating it.

Words of Wisdom

Indications for artificial ventilation of the newborn:
- Apnea
- Pulse rate of less than 100 beats/min
- Persistent central cyanosis despite breathing 100% oxygen

Bag-Mask Ventilation

Bag-mask ventilation is indicated when a newborn is apneic, has inadequate respiratory effort, or has a pulse rate of less than 100 beats/min (bradycardia) after you clear the airway of secretions, relieve obstruction from the tongue, and dry and stimulate the newborn. Signs of respiratory distress that suggest a need for bag-mask ventilation include periodic breathing, intercostal retractions (sucking in between the ribs), nasal flaring, and grunting on expiration. Approximately 7% of neonates will experience some form of respiratory distress.[21] Recognizing and treating respiratory distress early can reduce mortality and morbidity in newborns. Table 42-7 summarizes the most common conditions leading to respiratory distress.

Three devices may be used to deliver bag-mask ventilation to a newborn:

1. You may use a self-inflating bag with an oxygen reservoir (an oxygen source is not necessary to provide PPV but is necessary to provide supplementary oxygen).
2. You may use a flow-inflating bag, though it needs a gas source to provide PPV; this technique is therefore more common in the operating room.
3. You may apply a T-piece resuscitator (also needs a gas source, mostly found in neonatal intensive care units).

In the field, you will most likely use a self-inflating bag for bag-mask ventilation. If available, always use the infant size (240 mL). Given that the breath size (tidal volume) of a newborn is only 3 to 6 mL/kg, only one-tenth of the bag's volume will be used for each breath—which explains why a larger bag can easily create problems. If a neonatal bag is not available and the newborn is in severe respiratory distress, has apnea, or has bradycardia, you can use a bag designed for adults or older children (750 mL or greater volume) as long as you carefully keep the delivered breath size appropriately small and monitor chest rise to avoid excessive volumes of delivered breaths.

When you are administering bag-mask ventilation with 100% oxygen, the face mask needs to provide an airtight seal, fitting over the newborn's mouth and nose, and extending down to the chin but not over the eyes Figure 42-7 . Pressure on the eyes, like deep suctioning, can lead to a vagal response and bradycardia. The newborn needs to have a patent airway, cleared of secretions, with his or her neck slightly extended in the sniffing position Figure 42-8 . The first few breaths after birth will frequently require higher pressures (possibly around 30 mm Hg) because the lungs are not yet expanded and are still full of fluid. To deliver these initial breaths, you may need to manually (cover with your finger) disable

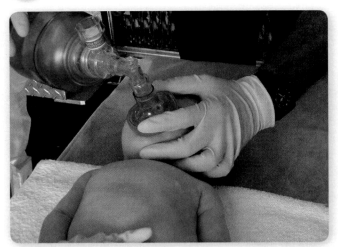

Figure 42-7 Bag-mask ventilation of the newborn. Hold the mask securely to the face with your thumb and index finger. Apply counter-pressure under the bony part of the chin with your middle finger.

Courtesy of Marianne Gausche-Hill, MD, FACEP, FAAP.

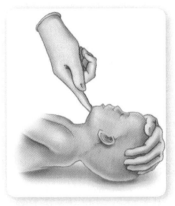

Figure 42-8 The sniffing position.

© Jones & Bartlett Learning.

the spring-loaded pop-off valve (it is usually set by the manufacturer at 30 to 40 cm H_2O). Subsequent breaths should be delivered with sufficient pressure to result in visible but not excessive chest rise, with the pop-off valve on.

In a newborn, it is important to provide the correct timing for ventilation at a rate of 40 to 60 breaths/min because breaths delivered at a higher rate can lead to hypocapnia, air trapping, or pneumothorax. To help with the timing, count "breath–two–three, breath–two–three" as you ventilate: Give a breath on "breath," and release on "two–three." Continue PPV as long as the pulse rate remains at less than 100 beats/min or the newborn's respiratory effort is ineffective. If prolonged PPV is needed (more than 1 minute), hook the system to a pressure manometer to aid in monitoring and minimizing excessive pressures (target peak inspiratory pressure less than 25 mm Hg in full-term newborns, less in preterm newborns).

The most common reasons for ineffective bag-mask ventilation are inadequate seal of the mask on the face

and incorrect head position. Other causes such as copious secretions, pneumothorax, or equipment malfunction need to be considered as well.

Intubation

Bag-mask ventilation provides successful resuscitation of most newborns. Intubation, however, may be necessary if the newborn requires resuscitation beyond simple interventions. The shaded area within Figure 42-3 outlines the steps pertaining to management of the distressed newborn.

Intubation is indicated in the following situations:

- Meconium-stained fluid is present and the newborn is not vigorous (ie, poor muscle tone, bradycardia, inadequate ventilation, no respiratory effort), a condition that may indicate in-utero hypoxia or stress. Note, routine tracheal suction is no longer recommended for a depressed newborn delivered through meconium-stained amniotic fluid.[25-27]

- Congenital **diaphragmatic hernia** (a congenital defect in which abdominal organs herniate through an opening in the diaphragm into the chest cavity) is known or suspected and respiratory support is indicated.
- Prolonged PPV is needed.
- Craniofacial defects impede the ability to maintain an adequate airway.

Before you begin ventilation, make sure that you have the following equipment available:

- Suction equipment (10F tubing, with 5F to 8F available, suction set to 100 mm Hg)
- Laryngoscope (check the light to ensure that the bulb is bright and screwed in tightly)
- Blades—straight: No. 1 for full-term newborns, No. 0 for preterm newborns
- Shoulder roll
- Adhesive tape, to tape the ET tube
- ET tube: 2.5 to 4.0 mm (2.5 mm if the newborn is delivered before 28 weeks of gestation, 3.0 mm if delivered at 28 to 34 weeks of gestation, 3.5 mm if delivered at 34 to 38 weeks of gestation, and 4.0 mm if delivered after 38 weeks of gestation)

Some paramedics use a stylet to provide rigidity to the ET tube. In such a case, you must secure the stylet (bending it over at the top of the ET tube so it cannot advance) and make sure that it does not extend beyond the ET tube, or tracheal perforation may occur. Intubation of the newborn is discussed in **Skill Drill 42-1**.

Complications of ET tube placement include oropharyngeal or tracheal perforation, esophageal intubation with subsequent persistent hypoxia, and right main-stem intubation, which can lead to atelectasis, persistent hypoxia, and pneumothorax. You can minimize these risks by ensuring optimal placement of the laryngoscope blade and carefully noting how far the ET tube is advanced.

Gastric Decompression

Gastric decompression using an orogastric tube is indicated when you are providing prolonged bag-mask ventilation (more than 5 to 10 minutes), if abdominal distention is impeding ventilation, and in the presence of a diaphragmatic hernia or a gastrointestinal congenital anomaly such as pyloric stenosis. Many diaphragmatic hernias are diagnosed prenatally by routine ultrasound; postnatally they are suspected clinically if there are decreased breath sounds on the left side (80% to 90% of diaphragmatic hernias are on the left), a scaphoid or concave abdomen (many of the abdominal contents are in the chest), and increased work of breathing.[28] **Skill Drill 42-2** shows gastric decompression in a newborn.

YOU are the Paramedic   PART 3

As the newborn's head delivers, you see green-stained fluid covering the infant's mouth and nose. You carefully suction the mouth and nose. The newborn continues to deliver without difficulty. Immediately following delivery, the infant has a weak cry and does not appear to be very vigorous. Due to the newborn's weak cry and poor tone, you quickly clamp and cut the cord so you can move the newborn to a warm blanket where the airway can be maintained and any necessary resuscitation can be carried out. You dry and stimulate the newborn to encourage more vigorous respiratory effort, and you suction the mouth and nose again to ensure the airway remains clear. The newborn continues to have weak respiratory effort and poor tone after 60 seconds of initial care. You note the heart rate to be 85 beats/min.

Newborn Assessment Recording Time: 1 Minute After Birth	
Respiratory effort	Weak and irregular; no cry
Pulse rate	85 beats/min, regular
Color	Cyanosis to the trunk and extremities
Apgar score	1-minute Apgar score deferred

5. What treatment is indicated for this newborn?
6. Why was the 1-minute Apgar score not obtained?
7. When is endotracheal intubation indicated in the newborn?

Skill Drill 42-1   **Intubating a Newborn**

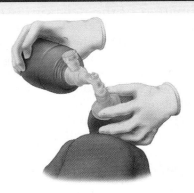

Step 1 Pre-oxygenate the newborn by bag-mask ventilation to an oxygen saturation greater than 95%. Administering 100% oxygen is not needed and can have deleterious effects in preterm infants.

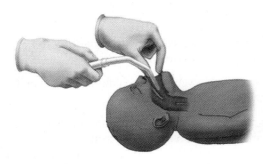

Step 2 Suction the oropharynx if there are copious secretions that prevent adequate ventilation. This can be a vagal stimulus, so pay close attention to the pulse rate and avoid repeated or vigorous suctioning. Provide bag-mask ventilation if bradycardia results.

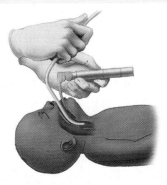

Step 3 Place the laryngoscope blade in the oropharynx. Visualize the vocal cords. Avoid applying torque to the blade because it increases the risk of trauma. Place the ET tube between the vocal cords until the black line on the ET tube is at the level of the cords. For full-term newborns, the ET tube is usually advanced until it is at 9 cm at the lip. For a premature newborn, you may need to advance the ET tube to only 6.5 to 7 cm at the lip. Limit the intubation attempt to 20 seconds, and initiate bag-mask ventilation if it is unsuccessful or if significant bradycardia develops.

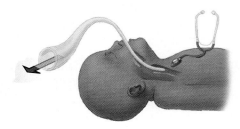

Step 4 Confirm ET tube placement. Observe chest rise, auscultate laterally in the epigastric region and high on the chest, note mist in the ET tube (seen when the patient exhales through the tube from condensation of humidified air leaving the lungs), note equal breath sounds on both sides, and observe for clinical improvement. Monitor $ETCO_2$ via waveform capnography and consider using pulse oximetry. This is often the earliest indicator of return of spontaneous circulation (ROSC). Pulse oximetry monitoring provides the peripheral oxygen saturation and reflects the response to adequate oxygenation and ventilation.

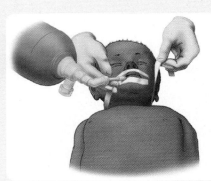

Step 5 Tape the ET tube in place on the face to minimize the risk of the tube dislodging. Monitor the newborn closely for complications such as tube dislodgement, tube occlusion by mucous plug or meconium, or pneumothorax.

Skill Drill 42-2 Inserting an Orogastric Tube in the Newborn

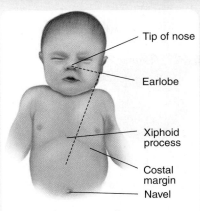

Tip of nose

Earlobe

Xiphoid process

Costal margin

Navel

Step 1 Measure for correct depth. Use an 8F feeding tube and measure the length from the bottom of the earlobe to the tip of the nose to halfway between the xiphoid process (lower tip of sternum) and the umbilicus.

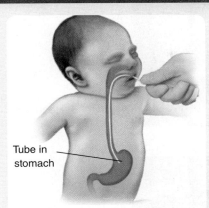

Tube in stomach

Step 2 Insert the tube through the mouth to the appropriate depth. Leave the nose open to allow for ventilation.

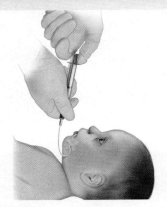

Step 3 Attach a 10-mL syringe and suction the stomach contents. Tape the tube to the newborn's cheek. Remove the syringe from the feeding tube to allow venting of air from the stomach. Intermittently suction the feeding tube.

© Jones & Bartlett Learning.

▶ Circulation

Chest Compressions

Chest compressions are indicated if the pulse rate remains at less than 60 beats/min despite positioning, clearing the airway, drying and stimulation, and 30 seconds of effective PPV.[29] Two people are needed to deliver effective chest compressions while continuing ventilation. Two different techniques are used Figure 42-9 .

1. **Thumb technique.** This is the preferred technique because it appears to generate superior peak systolic and coronary arterial perfusion pressure, while causing less fatigue in the rescuer.[8] Encircle the torso with both hands, with fingers under the newborn's back, supporting the spine. Place your two thumbs side by side or one over the other in a small preterm infant, over the lower third of the sternum. This area is between the xiphoid process and a line drawn between the nipples. Once the newborn's airway is secure or you have intubated, the chest compressions using this technique can be delivered from the head of the bed, allowing your colleague easier access to the umbilicus for insertion of an umbilical catheter.

2. **Two-finger technique.** Place the tips of your index and middle fingers of one hand over the lower third of the sternum. This area is between the xiphoid process and a line drawn between the nipples. Place the second hand behind the newborn's back to support the spine.

The depth of compression is one-third of the antero-posterior diameter of the chest. Your thumbs or fingers should remain in contact with the chest at all times. It is important for you to allow the chest to completely recoil after giving a compression. Liver laceration and rib fractures are possible risks when you are delivering chest compressions to a newborn. Refer to Chapter 39, *Responding to the Field Code,* for coverage of infant cardio-pulmonary resuscitation (CPR).

In newborns, the chest compressions and artificial ventilation should not be delivered simultaneously; rather, they should be coordinated to result in 90 compressions and 30 breaths/min. This equals a rate of 120 actions per minute, meaning that each action should occur every half second. The person doing the compressions takes over the counting out loud. The compressor counts "one-and-two-and-three-and-breathe-and." The person ventilating squeezes the bag or occludes the T-piece cap during "breathe-and" and releases during "one-and."

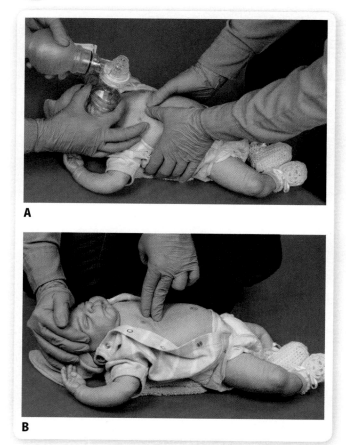

Figure 42-9 Chest compressions in the newborn. **A.** When using the thumb technique, position your thumbs side by side, placed between the xiphoid and an imaginary line drawn between the two nipples. Support the spine by encircling your fingers around the torso. **B.** When the newborn is large, use two fingers placed between the xiphoid and an imaginary line drawn between the nipples. Use the other hand to support the newborn's head.

© Jones & Bartlett Learning.

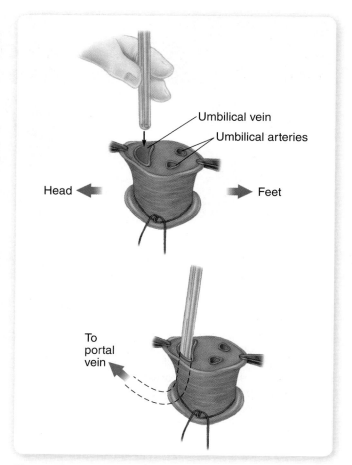

Figure 42-10 Location of the umbilical vein.

© Jones & Bartlett Learning.

To limit the number of pauses in compressions and maximize the chances of achieving return of spontaneous circulation, reassess for the presence of a pulse after 60 seconds of well-coordinated chest compressions and ventilations.[30] If the pulse rate is above 60 beats/min, you may stop chest compressions. Continue effective ventilation at the higher rate of 40 to 60 breaths/min after stopping the chest compressions. Recheck the pulse rate after 30 seconds. Once the pulse rate rises above 100 beats/min, gradually slow the rate and decrease the pressure of PPV.

Vascular Access

Emergent access becomes necessary when fluid administration is needed to support circulation, and when resuscitation medications (eg, epinephrine, sodium bicarbonate) and therapeutic drugs (eg, IV dextrose, antibiotics) must be administered intravenously. However, establishing peripheral access in a newborn can prove difficult.

If permitted by local protocol, the umbilical vein can be catheterized using an umbilical vein line in a newborn using the following steps:

1. Clean the umbilical cord with alcohol or another antiseptic such as povidone-iodine (Betadine). Drape the area with sterile towels, keeping the umbilical stump exposed. Place a sterile tie firmly, but not too tightly, around the base of the cord to control bleeding. Although the line must be placed quickly in a code situation, maintain sterile technique as much as possible.
2. Attach a 3-mL syringe and a stopcock to a sterile 3.5F to 5F umbilical vein line catheter (a comparable-size sterile feeding tube can be used in an emergency) and prefill the catheter. Turn the stopcock to off toward the patient.
3. Cut the cord with a scalpel between the clamp placed on the cord and the cord tie, keeping about 1 to 2 cm from the skin.
4. Insert a "low-UV line": The umbilical vein (UV) is a large, thin-walled vessel usually found at the 12 o'clock position, as compared with the two thick-walled, smaller umbilical arteries usually found at 4 and 8 o'clock **Figure 42-10**. Insert the catheter into this vein for a distance

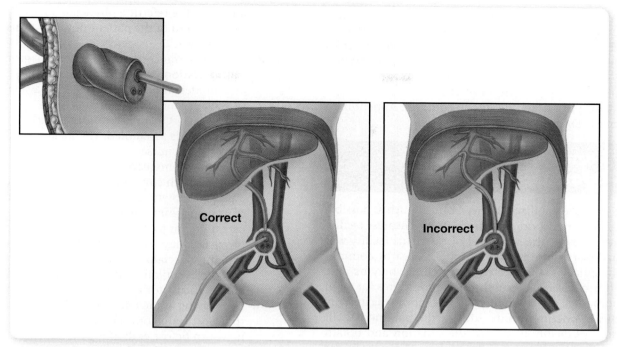

Figure 42-11 Umbilical vein catheterization. The illustration labeled *Correct* shows the proper depth of insertion; the illustration labeled *Incorrect* shows incorrect technique that has led to the catheter being inserted too far. The inset shows the cross section through the abdominal wall.

© Jones & Bartlett Learning.

of ¾ to 1½ inches (2 to 4 cm; less in preterm newborns) until blood can be aspirated. If the catheter is advanced too deep and into the liver, the infusion of hypertonic solutions may lead to irreversible damage **Figure 42-11** . If the catheter is advanced into the heart, dysrhythmias may develop.

5. Flush the catheter with 0.5 mL of normal saline and tape it in place.

A peripheral IV or intraosseous (IO) line can also be placed. Placement of an IO line is discussed in Chapter 14,

Medication Administration. Whereas the technique for placing an IO line is similar to that used with older children or adults, a smaller needle should be used in newborns to avoid exiting the far side of the bone.

◼ **Pharmacologic Interventions**

Medications are rarely needed in newborn resuscitation because most newborns can be resuscitated with effective ventilatory support. Medications in newborns are based on weight, so you may need to estimate the newborn's

Words of Wisdom

Special consideration for IV access: You may encounter newborns with exposed abdominal contents. A developmental defect may lead to the intestines appearing outside the abdomen. There are two types of abdominal wall defects seen.

1. *Gastroschisis* occurs when a portion of the abdominal organs (most often the intestines) have herniated through a weak area of the abdominal wall. The organs will not have a membrane covering them in this type of abdominal wall defect.[31,32]

2. *Omphalocele* occurs when a portion of the abdominal organs (most often the intestines) protrudes through the same outlet as the umbilical cord. There will be a thin membrane of skin overlying the organs in this type of

abdominal wall defect. Rarely this membrane can be ruptured or torn, creating what is known as a non-intact omphalocele, which may resemble gastroschisis.[31,32]

In these situations, while providing standard resuscitation, place the newborn from the waist down into a sterile, clear plastic bag immediately to keep the bowel clean and minimize heat/fluid loss. Intubate and secure the airway of the newborn to prevent distention and kinking of the intestinal loops. Monitor the color of the intestines through the clear bag (pink is an abnormal finding, blue/black is a normal finding) and position the newborn on his or her side to maintain the blood supply to the intestines. Place a peripheral IV or IO in these infants. Keep the intestines moist, using sterile saline as needed.

weight for dosing. A full-term newborn usually weighs 6.5 to 9 pounds (3 to 4 kg) and is 20 inches (50 cm) long; a newborn born at 28 weeks of gestation, on average, weighs 2.5 pounds (1 kg) and is approximately 14.75 inches (37.5 cm) long. A weight of 3 kg is often used for dose calculations in a full-term newborn.

Medication doses are discussed in the Appendix to Volume 1, *Emergency Medications*.

Family and Transport Considerations

Once you have stabilized the newborn as much as possible in the field, transport the patient to the nearest facility that can provide the next level of care. This facility will not necessarily be a tertiary hospital. A nearby community hospital, if it is located much closer, may be able to perform additional stabilization procedures for an ill newborn, such as placement of a chest tube for a clinically significant pneumothorax. Ideally, the paramedic will contact this facility to discuss the situation and obtain advice regarding care and disposition. Throughout the care process, communicate with the family regarding what is being done for the newborn and what care is planned to help allay their fears. Do not be specific about survival statistics. Many factors play into mortality and morbidity, and you do not want to be misleading. If family members have questions you cannot answer, be straightforward. Tell them that you do not have a definite answer, but you will help put them in touch with the people who do (ie, the center to which the newborn is being transferred).

During transport, continuously observe the newborn and perform frequent reassessments to ensure timely intervention should the newborn's status change. Attention to thermoregulation, respiratory effort, patency of airway, skin color, and pulse rate is vital. If the newborn is being transferred between facilities after the initial stabilization, continue to provide close observation and assessment of these factors to facilitate initiation of interventions should the newborn's condition change.

Because the average community hospital cannot provide the specially trained doctors and nurses or the specialized equipment needed for such care, it sometimes becomes necessary to transfer the critically ill newborn to a regional center, where the newborn may benefit from highly skilled personnel and sophisticated equipment. When efficient transport is available and referral facilities are staffed by appropriately educated nursing and medical staff, the mortality of high-risk infants born at community hospitals can be decreased to approaching that of advanced tertiary care centers.[33,34] In the well-organized regional referral system, transport of a high-risk newborn proceeds through the following several steps:

1. A physician at the referring hospital initiates a request for transport. A physician in the regional control center decides which intensive care nursery can accommodate the patient

and gives the referring physician advice on management of the patient until the transport team arrives.

2. A mode of transportation is chosen—ground transportation, helicopter, or fixed-wing aircraft, depending on the distance, availability of services, and weather conditions.

3. The transport team is mobilized, and equipment is assembled. The ideal team consists of a nurse with special training in neonatal intensive care, a respiratory therapist with similar special training, and a paramedic who has undertaken a period of apprenticeship in a neonatal intensive care unit. For particularly critical patients, a physician may also attend. The equipment is highly specialized, requiring appropriately designed ventilation and oxygenation units and an incubator meeting stringent criteria.

4. On arriving at the referring hospital, the transport team continues to stabilize the newborn before embarking on transport. Conditions such as hypoxemia, acidosis, hypoglycemia, and hypovolemia should be treated before leaving the referring hospital.

5. While stabilizing the newborn, the team collects information and materials including a copy of the mother's and newborn's charts and any radiographic studies taken of the newborn.

Words of Wisdom

Transport of a distressed newborn should be expedited to allow initiation of additional support not available in the field.

Pathophysiology, Assessment, and Management of Specific Conditions

The remaining sections in this chapter discuss specific neonatal emergencies and their assessment and management.

▶ Apnea

Apnea (respiratory pause greater than or equal to 20 seconds) is common in newborns delivered before 32 weeks of gestation, but is rarely seen in the first 24 hours after delivery, even in premature newborns. Apnea is defined as a respiratory pause of greater than 20 seconds. If it does not respond to stimulation and further steps such as PPV are not taken, apnea can lead to hypoxemia and bradycardia. Apnea often follows a period of hypoxia or hypothermia. Other causes include maternal or infant narcotic exposure, airway or respiratory muscle weakness, septicemia, prolonged or difficult labor and delivery, **gastroesophageal reflux**, central nervous system abnormalities including seizures, and metabolic disorders.

The pathophysiology of apnea depends on the underlying etiology. Apnea of prematurity is due to an underdeveloped central nervous system. Gastroesophageal reflux can trigger a vagal response, leading to apnea. Drug-induced apnea frequently results from direct central nervous system depression. Regardless of the cause, a newborn with apnea needs respiratory support to minimize hypoxic brain damage and other organ damage.

Assessment and Management

Assessment of an apneic newborn includes obtaining a careful history to elicit possible etiologic risk factors and performing a physical exam that focuses on neurologic signs and symptoms or signs of infection. At birth it is important to differentiate between **primary apnea** and **secondary apnea**. If the newborn has experienced a relatively short period of hypoxia, he or she will have a period of rapid breathing, followed by apnea and bradycardia. At this point, the use of drying and stimulation may cause a resumption of breathing and improvement in the pulse rate. If hypoxia continues during primary apnea, the newborn will gasp and enter secondary apnea. At this point, stimulation alone will not restart the newborn's breathing. Instead, PPV by bag-mask device is required. Follow the steps for neonatal resuscitation discussed earlier in the chapter.

▶ Bradycardia

Bradycardia in a newborn is most frequently a result of inadequate ventilation and often responds to effective PPV. If hypoxia continues, there could be persistent bradycardia. Other causes of bradycardia include hypothyroidism, acidosis, and congenital atrioventricular block in infants whose mothers have lupus. While increased intracranial pressure in older children can result in bradycardia, neonates have open fontanelles so they rarely present with increased intracranial pressure. Interventions can result in bradycardia as well. Prolonged suctioning or attempts at intubation, or vagal stimulation from an inadequately secured ET tube or orogastric tube, often result in bradycardia. The morbidity and mortality of bradycardia are determined by the underlying cause and how quickly it can be corrected.

Assessment and Management

Heart rate in a newborn is assessed via auscultation or by palpating the base of the umbilical cord. The Neonatal Resuscitation Algorithm (see Figure 42-3) addresses the steps to take when an infant with a heart rate below 100 beats/min is encountered.[4] Bradycardia in a neonate is often a result of inadequate ventilation and often responds to effective PPV (initially using room air, increasing to 100% oxygen while targeting an age-appropriate preductal SpO_2) if the heart rate is less than 100 beats/min.[24] Assess the patency of the airway. If hypoxia continues, there could be persistent bradycardia. Begin chest compressions for a heart rate that is less than 60 beats/min despite at least 30 seconds of effective PPV.[29] Administration of epinephrine is indicated when the newborn has a pulse rate of less than 60 beats/min after 30 seconds of effective ventilation and 60 seconds of chest compressions coordinated with ventilation.[13] A low umbilical vein catheter is the preferred access to administer medications during resuscitation. Administration of epinephrine via ET tube may be considered while IV access is being established. Dosing is discussed in the Appendix to Volume 1, *Emergency Medications*. Check the pulse rate about 1 minute after administering epinephrine (longer if administered via ET tube). In addition, ensure that ventilation is adequate and effective, that the ET tube is not dislodged, and that chest compressions are being given to adequate depth of one-third the anteroposterior diameter.

Focus on maintaining normothermia. Transport the patient to a facility that is able to handle high-risk neonates.

▶ Acidosis

If bradycardia persists after adequate ventilation, chest compressions, and volume expansion, suspect metabolic acidosis. Consider administering a bolus of normal saline to aid in improved perfusion and clearance of acid. There has been no evidence to support the routine use of sodium bicarbonate to correct metabolic acidosis. The best treatment is to identify and correct the underlying cause of the acidosis.[35]

▶ Pneumothorax Decompression

A pneumothorax can occur if an infant inhales meconium at birth, if the lung is weakened by infection, or if PPV is needed. If a newborn has signs of a significant pneumothorax—severe respiratory distress unresponsive to PPV with unilateral decreased breath sounds and (if the pneumothorax is on the left side) shift of heart sounds—a needle decompression of the pneumothorax may be necessary.

Assessment and Management

On the side of the suspected pneumothorax, clean the area around the second intercostal space, mid-clavicular line (usually just above the nipple), with alcohol. Prepare the equipment needed: a 22-g butterfly needle attached to extension tubing, a three-way stopcock, and a 20-mL syringe. Palpate the upper edge of the second rib and insert the needle above that rib as a second provider pulls back on the syringe (which is open to the patient). The nerves and blood vessels run below the ribs, so avoid piercing this area. Continue to slowly advance the needle until air is recovered. The butterfly needle is rigid, so be gentle so as to avoid further tearing the lung. If the 20-mL syringe becomes filled with air, turn the stopcock off to the newborn, push out the air from the syringe, open the stopcock to the newborn, and continue withdrawing air. Once no more air can be withdrawn, remove the needle.

> ### Words of Wisdom
>
> Before you resort to the use of a syringe, recheck the effectiveness of assisted ventilation.

If there is a symptomatic ongoing air leak, you can insert a 22-g angiocatheter in a similar location, remove the introducer needle, and attach the angiocatheter to the extension tubing. Note that the angiocatheter may further tear the lung during its initial placement and is more likely to kink than the butterfly needle.

Remove as much air as possible with the syringe. At this point, the tubing may be taped to the chest and briefly occluded while you place the end of the tubing that had been attached to the syringe in a small bottle of sterile water and release the tubing occlusion. This can relieve the pressure buildup from the pneumothorax until the patient can be transferred to a facility for placement of a chest tube. During transport, closely monitor the newborn for signs of a reaccumulation of the pneumothorax.

While you are performing the pneumothorax decompression, continue your reassessment—use proper positioning to maintain the airway and avoid aspiration, take steps to maintain thermoregulation, and ensure adequate communication with the family and with the medical team receiving the newborn. If the newborn is distressed, transport as rapidly as possible.

> ### Words of Wisdom
>
> Whereas positive pressure ventilation and chest compressions can be performed in a moving emergency vehicle, you should pull the vehicle over to the side of the road while placing and securing an advanced airway.

▶ Meconium-Stained Amniotic Fluid

Meconium-stained amniotic fluid is present in 10% to 15% of deliveries.[36] A small percentage of babies delivered in the presence of meconium-stained amniotic fluid may go on to develop meconium aspiration syndrome, which carries a high risk of mortality and morbidity.[36] Passage of meconium may occur either before or during delivery. It is more common in postterm newborns and in those who are small for their gestational age (weighing less than the 10th percentile for their age), and in newborns who are stressed before or during delivery. Newborns do not normally pass stool before birth, but if they do

and then inhale the meconium-stained amniotic fluid either in utero or at delivery, their airways may become plugged and hypoxia may ensue. This, in turn, can lead to atelectasis, persistent pulmonary hypertension (delayed transition from fetal to neonatal circulation), hypoxemia, and aspiration pneumonitis. Partial plugging of airways with meconium can lead to ball-valve effects, increasing the risk of pneumothorax, which may require needle aspiration. Any condition that leads to a delayed drop in pulmonary vascular resistance after birth, such as meconium aspiration, can result in right-to-left shunting across the foramen ovale or the **patent ductus arteriosus**, a condition referred to as persistent pulmonary hypertension of the newborn. Ensuring a clear airway, keeping the newborn warm, minimizing stimulation, and administering supplemental oxygen when needed to decrease the risk of the development of persistent pulmonary hypertension.

Once meconium aspiration has occurred, the newborn should be followed closely for signs of deterioration, including progressive hypoxia, hypercapnia, acidosis, and development of a pneumothorax.

Assessment and Management

When a newborn is delivered through meconium-stained amniotic fluid, assess the newborn's activity level under a radiant warmer if available. If the newborn is crying and vigorous, employ standard interventions. If the newborn is depressed (poor muscle tone, bradycardia of less than 100 beats/min, inadequate ventilation, no respiratory effort), start PPV. If PPV is not effective, intubation and suctioning may be required to remove an obstruction.

If the newborn is not responding well to the care outlined in the neonatal resuscitation algorithm, suspect airway occlusion or pneumothorax. Take steps to minimize hypothermia by avoiding cold environments, covering the newborn with warm blankets when possible, and placing the newborn, once stabilized, skin-to-skin on the mother, again covered with a blanket. Frequent reassessment of the newborn is indicated to ensure that his or her condition has not changed. If the newborn has prolonged hypoxia after significantly delayed resuscitation, the outcome will likely be poor. When you are transporting a newborn with these respiratory symptoms, stay in communication with a facility skilled at managing high-risk newborns to help with management and identification of an appropriate transport destination. To help support the family, explain what is being done for the newborn but do not discuss chance of survival.

▶ Low Blood Volume

If the newborn has significant intravascular volume depletion owing to conditions such as abruptio placenta (separation of the placenta from the uterus, which leads to excessive bleeding), twin-to-twin transfusion, placenta previa, or septic shock, fluid resuscitation may be needed. Signs of hypovolemia include pallor, persistently low pulse rate, weak pulses, or no improvement in circulatory status despite adequate resuscitation efforts. In a newborn, place a low umbilical vein line as outlined earlier. In a neonate who is more than a few days old, place a peripheral IV or IO line. Consider administering a fluid bolus. Multiple boluses may be administered if the patient remains clinically hypovolemic.

> ### Special Populations
>
> A fluid bolus in a newborn consists of 10 mL/kg of normal saline, lactated Ringer solution, or O Rh-negative blood administered via IV over 5 to 10 minutes.

▶ Diaphragmatic Hernia

Diaphragmatic hernia—that is, an abnormal opening in the diaphragm, most commonly on the left side causing the abdominal contents to herniate into the chest cavity and the heart and mediastinum to be shifted to the contralateral side of the hernia—has an incidence between 1 in 2,000 and 1 in 5,000 live births, with females twice as likely to be affected than males.[28] This diagnosis is often made on prenatal ultrasound before birth. Postnatally, the diagnosis is suspected clinically in a newborn with respiratory distress, heart sounds shifted to the right, decreased breath sounds on the left side (which can also be signs of a pneumothorax), bowel sounds heard in the chest (most commonly on the left side; 85% of these hernias are left sided)[28], and scaphoid abdomen (ie, the abdomen, rather than being round, is sunken because the abdominal contents are in the chest cavity). The overall survival for infants born with diaphragmatic hernia is 67%.[28]

Assessment and Management

A newborn with a congenital diaphragmatic hernia may demonstrate few or no symptoms, or may present with severe hypoxia and increased work of breathing, depending on the size of the hernia, the degree of lung hypoplasia, and associated anomalies such as cardiac disease. If there is significant mediastinal shift, the contralateral side can also have significant pulmonary hypoplasia. Although the NRP currently advocates initiating resuscitation using room air in full-term newborns, an exception to this rule is the newborn with a severe congenital diaphragmatic hernia who should be resuscitated with 100% oxygen if hypoxic. If a newborn has a diaphragmatic hernia, bag-mask ventilation will introduce air that distends the intestines in the chest cavity, further compromising the newborn's ability to ventilate. If PPV is needed in such a newborn, place an ET tube and deliver a peak ventilatory pressure of 25 mm Hg or less to minimize barotrauma—these newborns have poorly developed lungs and are at high risk of a pneumothorax developing even at fairly low peak inspiratory pressures. These infants are at increased risk of persistent pulmonary hypertension in addition to lung hypoplasia and may remain hypoxic in spite of supplemental oxygen.

Put an orogastric tube in place and provide intermittent suctioning to minimize intestinal distention. Monitor the patient's heart rate continuously throughout transport. Ultimately, a newborn with a diaphragmatic hernia will require surgical correction, so transport the newborn to a facility with a neonatal intensive care unit and a pediatric surgical team.

▶ Respiratory Distress and Cyanosis

Prematurity is the single most common cause of respiratory distress and cyanosis in the neonate. These conditions occur more frequently in newborns younger than 30 weeks of gestation or weighing less than 2.5 pounds (1,200 g). Women with multiple gestations and pregnancy complications are at increased risk as well.

There are many etiologies of respiratory distress and cyanosis in the neonate. Respiratory causes include airway obstruction, aspiration (meconium, amniotic fluid, maternal blood at delivery, gastroesophageal reflux, and foreign body), pneumonia, pneumothorax, tracheoesophageal fistula, congenital diaphragmatic hernia, or immature lungs. Any process that results in a delay in drop of pulmonary vascular resistance after birth (including all of the previously described conditions as well as acidosis, stress, and hypoxia) can lead to shunting of blood across the patent ductus arteriosus and patent foramen ovale, resulting in persistent pulmonary hypertension and cyanosis. Central nervous system depression can lead to ineffective respirations and subsequent cyanosis. Septic shock and severe metabolic acidosis often present with increased work of breathing and cyanosis. Cardiac anomalies typically result in cyanosis without increased work of breathing.

Assessment and Management

Remember to address the ABCs—ensure the airway is patent, breathing is adequate, and a pulse is present. Assess respiratory rate, respiratory effort (including periodic breathing, intracostal retractions, nasal flaring, grunting, choking, or gagging) and breath sounds. Ask the parents if they have noted increased symptoms with feeding attempts. Is the newborn cyanotic or pale? (Remember that a hypoxic newborn that is severely anemic will look pale, not cyanotic.)

Treatment focuses on establishing a patent airway (suction mouth, nose, and oropharynx as needed), ensuring adequate oxygen delivery by providing supplemental oxygen if needed, establishing effective ventilation, including providing PPV as needed, and ensuring adequate circulation, including chest compressions if bradycardia of less than 60 beats/min persists once supplemental oxygen and adequate ventilation have been established. Keep in mind that occasionally resuscitative efforts do not result in improvement in cyanosis or bradycardia due to an underlying pneumothorax. In this situation, needle thoracentesis can be a life-saving intervention. Remember to keep the family updated regarding the newborn's condition and what is being done to help him or her, and maintain communication with the receiving hospital for advice and to allow them to prepare for your arrival.

▶ Respiratory Depression Secondary to Narcotics

In the case of a drug-addicted mother, administration of naloxone (Narcan) to the newborn to reverse the narcotic effect may precipitate seizures that can potentially cause death, so this intervention is no longer recommended as a first-line drug in resuscitation. In the case of a newborn experiencing respiratory suppression from the mother's chronic use of narcotics, provide ventilatory support and transport immediately. If respiratory depression is the result of the mother being treated acutely with narcotics, and there is no chronic narcotic exposure, naloxone may be administered to the newborn via the IV (preferred) or intramuscular route to reverse the narcotic effect.

▶ Premature and Low Birth Weight Infants

Newborns delivered before 37 completed weeks of gestation are considered premature Figure 42-12 . While prematurity is often idiopathic, there are maternal conditions associated with preterm labor and delivery. These include maternal infection, including urinary tract infection, chorioamnionitis, maternal illness leading to dehydration, placental insufficiency, polyhydramnios, preeclampsia/eclampsia, and pregnancy-induced hypertension. In addition to the increased overall mortality when a fetus is delivered prematurely, there are a number of morbidities associated with prematurity. These include respiratory distress syndrome, respiratory suppression and

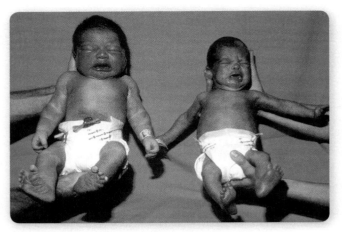

Figure 42-12 Premature newborns (right) are smaller and thinner than full-term newborns (left).
© American Academy of Orthopaedic Surgeons.

apnea, hypothermia, sepsis, and central nervous system compromise, including intraventricular hemorrhage and periventricular leucomalacia (increased in newborns with hypoxemia and fluctuations in blood pressure and serum osmolarity).

Newborns weighing less than 5.5 pounds (2,500 g) are considered low birth weight. The most common etiology for low birth weight is prematurity. A number of factors can predispose a woman to deliver prematurely, including genetic factors, infection, cervical incompetence (early opening of cervix), abruption (blood under the placenta), multiple gestations (eg, twins, triplets), previous delivery of a premature infant, drug use, and trauma. Other factors that may contribute to low birth weight include chronic maternal hypertension, smoking, placental anomalies, and chromosomal abnormalities. If a newborn is delivered

YOU ▶ are the Paramedic   PART 4

You provide positive pressure ventilation with room air (21% oxygen) for 30 seconds and then reassess the newborn. The assessment reveals a strong respiratory effort with adequate tidal volume and a strong rapid pulse rate palpated at the umbilical cord. The baby has excellent muscle tone and responds well when stimulated.

Newborn Assessment Recording Time: 2 Minutes After Birth	
Respiratory effort	48 beats/min; strong, rapid, and regular; good cry
Pulse rate	156 beats/min; regular
Color	Pink trunk but cyanosis to the extremities
Apgar score	9

8. What should you do for the newborn at this time?

prior to 24 weeks of gestation or weighs less than 1 pound (500 g) and is born outside of a center that is equipped to manage such deliveries, the newborn is unlikely to survive. If a premature infant is born after 32 weeks of gestation or weighs at least 3 pounds (1,500 g) and is provided warmth and cardiorespiratory support as needed until transfer to a center with a neonatal intensive care unit, survival is close to that of an infant born at term. The degree of immaturity can be estimated by physical characteristics such as skin appearance (more thin and translucent in more premature newborns). If you observe signs of life, attempt resuscitation until the newborn can be transported to an appropriate facility.

Approximately 12% of births in the United States are preterm (less than 37 weeks of gestation).[37] Morbidity and mortality in this population are, in large part, related to the degree of prematurity. Infants born at less than 28 weeks of gestation or who weigh less than 2 pounds (1,000 g) at birth have the highest risk of neonatal and infant mortality.[37] Preterm infants account for 75% of all perinatal mortality and 50% of long-term neurologic impairment in children in the United States.[37]

Assessment and Management

The degree of prematurity is the most predictive indicator of significant morbidity and mortality. Significant respiratory distress occurs most frequently in premature infants,[25] and newborns with lower birth weights will become hypothermic more quickly than full-term newborns. In addition to physical features of prematurity (maturity of skin, size of infant, degree of respiratory distress), the family can give additional information related to dating (last menstrual period, estimated date of confinement assigned by the obstetrician, ultrasound dating) and information related to other maternal or fetal complications.

If a newborn is delivered prematurely in the field, providing cardiorespiratory support and a thermoneutral environment will optimize his or her survival and long-term outcome. Premature newborns are at higher risk for respiratory distress owing to surfactant deficiency. Their thermoregulation can be improved with careful environmental control (eg, warm blankets, plastic wrap, or plastic bag up to neck). The lungs of a premature newborn are weak, so use only the minimum pressure necessary to move the chest when you are providing PPV. Brain injury can result from hypoxemia, rapid changes in blood pressure, or infusion of hyperosmolar solutions, leading to intraventricular hemorrhage. Premature newborns are also at risk of **retinopathy of prematurity** (abnormal vascular development of the retina), which may be worsened by long-term oxygen exposure. Because hypoxia causes irreparable brain damage, however, do not withhold oxygen from a cyanotic premature newborn.

The management of premature newborns focuses on clearing the airway, providing gentle stimulation, and administering supplemental oxygen if needed based on oxygen saturation and PPV if needed for ineffective or absent respiratory effort. Provide peak inspiratory pressures to maintain physiologic chest rise because excessive pressures increase the risk of pneumothorax. Finally, initiate chest compressions if effective ventilation does not result in adequate heart rate. As always, maintaining a warm environment for the newborn is critical.

Because it can be difficult to assess gestational age or predicted morbidity or mortality in the field, if there are signs of life, maintain resuscitative efforts until you can transfer the patient to a facility that can continue support.

▶ Seizures in the Newborn

Seizures strongly suggest the presence of neurologic disorder in the newborn. A seizure is defined clinically as a paroxysmal alteration in neurologic function (ie, behavioral and/or autonomic function). The degree of myelination will affect the manner of seizure presentation and observed clinical signs. Seizures are more common in premature newborns. The incidence in this population can be as high as 57.5 per 1,000 infants who weigh less than 3 pounds (1,500 g) at birth, compared with 2.8 per 1,000 infants who weigh between 5.5 pounds and 9 pounds (2,500 g and 3,999 g) at birth.[38] In the field, seizures are identified by direct observation; in the hospital, an electroencephalogram (EEG) is used to confirm the diagnosis of seizures.

Newborns may exhibit normal motor activity that can sometimes be mistaken for seizures. These myoclonic, dysconjugate eye movements or sucking movements are often seen when the newborn is drowsy or asleep. In addition, jitteriness is often confused with a seizure **Table 42-8**. Jitteriness is characteristically a disorder of

Table 42-8	Jitteriness Versus Seizures in the Newborn	
Characteristic	**Jitteriness**	**Seizures**
Ocular phenomenon (deviation or fixation of the eyes)	Not seen	Commonly associated
Stimulus sensitive (may be triggered by a stimulus)	Yes	No
Dominant movement	Tremor	Clonic jerking
Application of gentle pressure to limb	Stops jitteriness	Does not stop seizures
Autonomic phenomenon	Not associated	Common association

© Jones & Bartlett Learning.

the newborn and is rarely seen at a later age. Jitteriness is most commonly seen with hypoxic-ischemic encephalopathy, hypocalcemia, hypoglycemia, and drug withdrawal. Clinically, gastroesophageal reflux and choking episodes can also mimic seizures.

Seizures, by contrast, represent a relative medical emergency. They are usually related to a significant underlying abnormality—one that often requires specific therapy. Seizures may also interfere with cardiopulmonary function, feeding, and metabolic function. Finally, prolonged seizures may even cause brain injury.

Types of Seizures. There are five types of neonatal seizures, distinguished as follows:[39]

- **Subtle seizure.** A seizure characterized by eye deviations; blinking; chewing; tonguing; mouthing; primitive extremity movements such as rowing, pedaling, swimming, or stepping; episodes of high blood pressure; and apnea. This type of seizure is more common in premature than in full-term infants.
- **Clonic seizure.** May be classified as either a focal seizure if one body part is involved, or a multifocal seizure if multiple body parts are involved. The body parts involved may be contralateral to one another (ie, jerking of the left arm and kicking of the right leg.) Due to the immaturity of the newborn's nervous system, symmetric, bilateral generalized clonic seizures are not typically seen during the neonatal period as the neurons lack sufficient myelination to elicit this type of movement.
- **Tonic seizure.** May be classified as focal or generalized. The persistent posturing of one limb, the neck, or the trunk with horizontal eye deviation is characteristic of a focal tonic seizure. Generalized tonic seizures are more common and typically involve a tonic flexion of the arms with tonic extension of the legs.
- **Spasms.** Characterized by a single, brief (1- to 2-second) sudden movement resembling a tic or jerk. Spasms are short in duration, differentiating them from tonic seizure activity.
- **Myoclonic seizure.** Categorized as focal, multifocal, and generalized. The jerks in myoclonic seizures are much more rapid (less than 50 milliseconds) and do not have rhythm, in contrast to clonic seizure activity. Focal myoclonic seizure activity often involves flexion of the arms. Multifocal myoclonic seizure activity involves twitching of multiple body parts, asynchronously. Generalized myoclonic seizure activity involves bilateral jerking with flexion of the arms, and occasionally flexion of the legs.

Causes of Seizures. **Table 42-9** lists the most common (and important) causes of neonatal seizures. The time

Table 42-9	**Causes of Neonatal Seizures**

- Hypoxic-ischemic encephalopathy
- Intracranial infections (meningitis)
- Hypoglycemia
- Other metabolic disturbances
- Epileptic syndromes
- Intracranial hemorrhage
- Development defects
- Hypocalcemia
- Meningitis
- Encephalopathy
- Drug withdrawal

© Jones & Bartlett Learning.

of onset for **hypoxic-ischemic encephalopathy**, hypoglycemia, and other metabolic disturbances is up to 3 days after delivery. With all other causes listed in Table 42-9, seizures may begin 3 days or longer after birth.

Hypoxic-ischemic encephalopathy, usually secondary to perinatal asphyxia (lack of oxygen to tissues), is the single most common cause of seizures in both term and preterm newborns.[40] Seizures secondary to hypoxic-ischemic encephalopathy occur within 12 hours of birth and may become more severe during the first 48 to 72 hours of life.[39] Metabolic abnormalities include disturbances in the levels of glucose, calcium, magnesium, or other electrolytes. Other metabolic disturbances include abnormalities of amino acids, organic acids, blood ammonia, and certain toxins.

Hypocalcemia, another cause of neonatal seizures, has two major peaks of incidence. The first peak occurs at 2 to 3 days after delivery and is most commonly seen in low birth weight newborns and in newborns of diabetic mothers. Late-onset hypocalcemia is rare in the United States but may be seen in infants who consume cow's milk or synthetic formulas high in phosphorus.[41]

Another cause of seizures in the neonate is hypoglycemia, discussed in the next section.

Other metabolic disturbances are uncommon in newborns, although hyponatremia, hyperammonemia, other amino acid and organic acid abnormalities, or seizures from drug withdrawal (eg, narcotic analgesics, sedative hypnotics, tricyclic antidepressants, cocaine, or alcohol) may be seen.

Assessment and Management

When you evaluate a newborn with seizures, you must include a quick evaluation of prenatal and birth history and perform a careful physical exam. You may observe a quiet, often hypotonic infant. The newborn may be lethargic or apneic. Hypoglycemia must be recognized quickly and treated promptly. In these patients, blood glucose measurement and administration of dextrose may be lifesaving in the field. Obtain the newborn's baseline vital signs and oxygen saturation readings, and administer additional oxygen, assisted ventilation, blood pressure evaluation, and IV access as necessary. A 10% dextrose solution may be given as an IV bolus (2 mL/kg) if the newborn's blood glucose level is less than 40 mg/dL and the infant is symptomatic, with a recheck of the blood glucose level in about 30 minutes.[42,43] IV administration of dextrose often needs to be followed by a 10% dextrose infusion.

Consult with medical control if you are considering giving the newborn anticonvulsant medication. Benzodiazepines such as lorazepam (Ativan) and midazolam (Versed) are commonly used to terminate neonatal seizures and may be administered either rectally or intravenously; IV diazepam (Valium) and rectal diazepam (Diastat) may be used for those routes, respectively, as well.

Monitor the newborn's respiratory status and oxygen saturations carefully. Maintain the newborn's normal body temperature and keep the family informed about the care you are providing as transport gets under way.

▶ Hypoglycemia

In full-term or preterm newborns, hypoglycemia is a blood glucose level of less than 45 mg/dL. This condition represents an imbalance between glucose supply and utilization. Glucose levels may be low due to inadequate intake or storage or increased utilization of glucose. Most newborns remain asymptomatic until the glucose level falls below 20 mg/dL for a significant period of time. Because the brain relies on glucose as its primary fuel, hypoglycemia may result in seizures and severe, permanent brain damage. Table 42-10 lists risk factors for hypoglycemia in the newborn.

The fetus receives glucose from the mother and deposits glycogen in the liver, lung, heart, and skeletal muscle in utero. The newborn then begins to use those glycogen stores to meet glucose needs after birth; most full-term newborns will have sufficient glycogen stores to meet their glucose needs for 8 to 12 hours. Disorders related to decreased glycogen stores (small for gestational age, prematurity, postmaturity), to increased use of glucose (hypoxia, hypothermia, sepsis), or increased insulin in the fetus (newborn of a diabetic mother, large for gestational age) place the newborn at increased risk for hypoglycemia. Metabolic adaptations to maintain normal glucose levels are regulated by counterregulatory hormones such as glucagon, epinephrine, cortisol, and growth hormone. Frequently, stressed newborns will become hypoglycemic.

YOU ▶ are the Paramedic — PART 5

You and your partner prepare the newborn for transport, while Rescue 1 personnel continue to provide care for the mother. You calmly explain to the mother that her baby had some difficulty breathing immediately after birth, but appears to be okay now. You also explain that it would be best to transport the baby separately, just in case the respiratory difficulty returns. After allowing the mother to hold the newborn for a few moments to bond, Rescue 1 loads her for transport just as the father pulls into the driveway. You provide him with instructions on how to safely follow the ambulance, and you load the newborn into the ambulance to begin transport to the hospital.

En route to the hospital you continually reassess the newborn and note that there is no additional respiratory difficulty. You take measures to keep the baby warm, and call in to report to the emergency department (ED). You arrive just as Rescue 1 is wheeling the mother into the Labor and Delivery entrance, and you make your way to the ED so the newborn can be assessed prior to being admitted into the Mother/Baby unit for observation and rooming with the mother.

Newborn Assessment Recording Time: 15 Minutes After Birth	
Respirations	46 breaths/min; adequate tidal volume
Pulse	154 beats/min; strong and regular
Skin	Pink, warm, and moist
Blood pressure	Not obtained
Oxygen saturation (Spo$_2$)	96% on room air
Apgar score	10, obtained 5 minutes after birth

9. What are the five components that make up the Apgar score?

10. Why was the newborn's original Apgar score calculated as 9?

Table 42-10	Risk Factors for Hypoglycemia in the Newborn	
Risk Factor	**Specific Indicators**
Disorders of fetal growth and maturity	• **Small for gestational age** • Smaller of discordant twins (weight difference >25%) • Large for gestational age • Low birth weight infant (birth weight <5.5 lbs [2.5 kg])
Prematurity	• Less than 37 weeks of gestation or less than 5.5 lbs (2.5 kg)
Disorders of maternal glucose regulation	• Insulin-dependent diabetic mother • Gestational diabetic mother • Morbid obesity in mother
Neonatal conditions with disturbed oxidative metabolism	• Perinatal distress (eg, 5-minute Apgar score <5) • Hypoxemia due to cardiac or lung disease • Shock, hypoperfusion, sepsis, cold stress
Severe anemia	• Pallor (in the absence of hypovolemia)
Congenital anomalies and genetic disorders	• Visible anatomic deformities/abnormalities

© Jones & Bartlett Learning.

Assessment and Management

In the first 1 to 2 hours of life, the blood glucose level of healthy neonates may be 30 mg/dL and rise to above 45 mg/dL 12 hours after birth.[44]

Symptoms of hypoglycemia can be quite nonspecific. They may include cyanosis, apnea, irritability, poor sucking or feeding, limpness or floppiness (**hypotonia**), irregular respirations, eye rolling, hypothermia, and decreased response to stimuli. These symptoms may also be associated with lethargy, tremors, twitching or seizures, and coma. Newborns may also have tachycardia, tachypnea, or vomiting.

In these cases, blood glucose measurement and administration of dextrose may be lifesaving in the field. Check the blood glucose level in all sick newborns (by heel stick), and evaluate the newborn's vital signs. After you establish good oxygenation, ventilation, and circulation, manage the hypoglycemia. Establish IV access as necessary. Medical control personnel may order the administration of a dextrose solution if the newborn's blood glucose level

is less than 40 mg/dL. This intervention may be followed by an IV infusion of dextrose based on the newborn's gestational age. Medication doses are discussed in the Appendix to Volume 1, *Emergency Medications*. Recheck the blood glucose level in about 30 minutes. As always, maintain normal body temperature—hypothermia places additional stress on glucose demand.

▶ Vomiting

Vomiting is common in newborns. Between 70% and 85% of infants will have a vomiting episode within the first two months of life.[45] Vomiting will resolve without any treatment in 95% of these infants by age 1 year.[45] Vomiting ranges from "spitting up" to severe, bloody, or bilious projectile vomiting. Most episodes of vomiting are benign and do not result in weight loss, dehydration, or other ill effects. Bilious and/or bloody emesis (vomiting) indicates a pathologic condition that needs medical attention. Persistent vomiting is a warning sign and can cause excessive loss of fluid, dehydration, and changes in electrolyte levels (ie, sodium, potassium, and glucose).

Vomiting mucus, occasionally blood streaked, in the first few hours of life is not uncommon. Persistent vomiting or bilious vomiting suggests obstruction in the upper digestive tract or increased intracranial pressure. Vomitus containing dark blood is often a sign of a life-threatening illness; it indicates bleeding in the gut. Sometimes, vomitus may be accompanied by bloody or tarry stool, another worrisome sign. Aspiration of vomitus can cause respiratory insufficiencies or obstruction of the airway.

Causes of Vomiting. A newborn's presenting symptoms may give a clue to the site of obstruction or other problem that is causing the vomiting. One possible cause is esophageal atresia (a failure to develop the distal lumen) with or without a congenital tracheoesophageal fistula. Its incidence is 1 case per 2,500 to 4,500 live births.[46] Newborns are seen with excessive frothing soon after birth and may choke when attempting to feed because the swallowed milk is returned promptly.

Another possible cause of vomiting, gastroesophageal reflux, is common in infants. Gastroesophageal reflux is most commonly seen in infancy, with its incidence peaking in the 1- to 4-month age group.[47] The infant may vomit either immediately or a few hours after a feeding. The vomiting may not be forceful. In uncomplicated gastroesophageal reflux, the vomitus is not bile stained or bloody. Gastroesophageal reflux in infants and young children can present as typical or atypical crying and/or irritability, apnea and/or bradycardia, poor appetite, vomiting, wheezing, stridor, weight loss or poor growth (failure to thrive), hoarseness and/or laryngitis, or as a brief resolved unexplained event (an episode when the infant becomes pale or cyanotic; chokes, gags, or has an apneic spell; or has loss of muscle tone).

In **infantile hypertrophic pyloric stenosis (IHPS)**, marked hypertrophy and hyperplasia of the two (circular and longitudinal) muscular layers of the pylorus occur. As a consequence, the pylorus becomes thickened and obstructs the end of the stomach. The incidence of IHPS is 1 to 3 cases per 1,000 live births, with the firstborn male 4 to 6 times more likely to have the condition compared to the firstborn female in a family.[48] The usual age of presentation is approximately age 3 weeks (range, 1 to 18 weeks). In IHPS, the stomach muscles contract forcibly to overcome the obstruction. Affected infants usually present with projectile vomiting, dehydration, malnutrition, and electrolyte changes. The vomitus in this case is not bile stained, but it can be brown or coffee in color due to blood, resulting from gastritis or a Mallory-Weiss tear at the gastroesophageal junction.

Malrotation is a congenital anomaly of rotation of the midgut. In this condition, the small bowel is found predominantly on the right side of the abdomen; the cecum is found in the epigastrium–right hypochondrium. Malrotation predisposes the infant to midgut volvulus and secondary obstruction of the blood supply to the intestines. In cases of malrotation with midgut volvulus, the vomitus is bile stained and may be feculent (like feces/stool) if the obstruction is distal in the intestines. With symptomatic malrotation, 75% to 85% of cases occur in infants younger than age 1 year, and more than 50% of cases occur in infants younger than age 1 month.[49] When this condition is noted prior to one year of age, males are twice as likely to be diagnosed than are females.[50] After one year of age, this disparity largely disappears, and there is no notable difference in the prevalence between males and females.[50] Various studies have demonstrated that mortality in patients who receive surgical correction for malrotation ranges from 0% to 14%.[51-53] The factors that reduced mortality in these cases were earlier diagnosis and earlier corrective surgery. With the advent of new corrective surgical procedures, the morbidity and mortality have decreased significantly.[51-53]

Intestinal atresia or **intestinal stenosis** include congenital conditions where parts of the bowel may not have developed well (atresia) or may be narrow (stenosis). Conditions that affect the upper bowel—ie, duodenum, jejunum, and upper small bowel—may present with bilious vomiting within the first day or two after birth. Obstruction to the lower bowel (distal small intestine and large intestine) often presents as feeding intolerance and abdominal distention.

Another cause of vomiting is Hirschsprung disease. In this disease, the last segment of colon fails to relax and it causes mechanical obstruction. The infant usually has a history of not passing meconium in the first 24 hours of life. Meconium plugs may also cause the infant to not pass stool in the first 24 hours. They may be occasionally associated with Hirschsprung disease or cystic fibrosis.

Vomiting may also happen in conjunction with asphyxia, meningitis (infection of the layers covering the brain and spine), and hydrocephalus (large head size is a clue). It is often sudden, unexpected, and forceful in such cases, and it may be accompanied by persistent irritability.

Meningitis and hydrocephalus may also be associated with increased intracranial pressure (ICP).

Use of drugs during pregnancy can lead to several withdrawal symptoms in newborns, including vomiting. The drugs that most commonly cause vomiting in newborns are barbiturates.

Assessment and Management

On physical exam, you may note a distended stomach that has been caused by vomiting. Suspect an infection if the newborn has a fever or hypothermia, or a history of contact with people who are ill. You may also note temperature instability, apnea/bradycardia, abdominal tenderness/guarding, and minimal or absent bowel sounds.

Initial management steps for a newborn with vomiting start with the ABCs. Maintain a patent airway, while staying aware that a vomiting newborn can aspirate the vomitus and compromise the airway. Keep the newborn's face turned to one side to prevent further aspiration. Suction or clear the vomitus from the airway with the help of a suction catheter or suction bulb. Ensure adequate oxygenation, administering either free-flow supplemental oxygen or bag-mask ventilation as necessary. Bradycardia may be caused by vagal stimulus and is usually transient; it may resolve with stimulation and free-flow oxygen. Consider using a nasogastric or orogastric tube to decompress the stomach and reduce emesis or vagal effects of distention.

Antiemetics should not be administered in the field. The newborn may be dehydrated, however, and need fluid resuscitation. Dry mucous membranes, tachycardia, or a sunken fontanelle are clues that the patient needs hydration. Normal saline (10 mL/kg per bolus) may be required in that case.

On transport, place the newborn on his or her side, identify a facility capable of managing a high-risk newborn, and explain to the family what is being done for the newborn.

▶ Diarrhea

A normal number of stools per day for an infant is five to six, especially if the infant is breastfeeding, when infants often produce stool after every feeding. Diarrhea is an excessive loss of electrolytes and fluid in the stool. The global incidence of diarrhea is 2.9 episodes per person each year.[54] Some risk factors that increase the chances of contracting a diarrheal illness include close contact settings, such as day-care centers.[55] Diarrhea represents a common cause for hospitalization in the neonatal and pediatric populations, particularly when oral rehydration attempts fail.[55]

The most common cause of acute diarrhea in children is viral infection (especially rotavirus infection during the winter months). Less frequently encountered causes include poisoning due to insecticides, organophosphates, and carbamates. Diarrhea related to these agents is accompanied by profuse sweating, lacrimation, hypersalivation, and abdominal cramps, or more serious conditions such as **intussusception**, malrotation, increased ICP, and metabolic acidosis. Other causes of diarrhea include gastroenteritis, lactose intolerance, neonatal abstinence syndrome, thyrotoxicosis, and cystic fibrosis.

Severe cases of diarrhea can cause dehydration and subsequent electrolyte imbalance. Combinations of physical signs—such as ill general appearance, poor vital signs, capillary refill of greater than 2 seconds, dry mucous membranes, absent tears, weight loss, and low urine output—are good objective predictors of the degree of dehydration.

Assessment and Management

Assessment includes estimating the number and volume of loose stools, decreased urinary output, and degree of dehydration based on skin turgor, mucous membranes, presence of sunken eyes, and other signs. Patient management, as always, begins with the ABCs. The newborn's airway and ventilation may be compromised if he or she is severely dehydrated and is obtunded, so ensure adequate oxygenation and ventilation. Perform chest compressions in addition to PPV in a newborn if the pulse rate is less than 60 beats/min.

Fluid therapy may be indicated when a newborn has diarrhea. Normal saline (10-mL/kg boluses) may be needed immediately to provide fluid resuscitation to the newborn.

▶ Neonatal Jaundice

Jaundice in the newborn results from the immaturity of the liver to conjugate and excrete bilirubin from red blood cell breakdown in the first week of life. This transient hyperbilirubinemia has therefore been called "physiologic jaundice." Neonatal jaundice is considered pathologic when:

- Jaundice is clinically visible in the first 24 hours after birth
- Total serum bilirubin increases by more than 5 mg/dL per day
- Total bilirubin exceeds 12 mg/dL in full-term infants
- Conjugated bilirubin makes up greater than 20% of total serum bilirubin concentration
- Clinical jaundice persists for more than 1 week in full-term infants or for more than 2 weeks in preterm infants

Jaundice can result from hemolysis (ABO incompatibility, Rh incompatibility), various types of red blood cell disorders, polycythemia, or excessive bruising in the newborn, among other causes.

Additionally, cholestasis can present after the first 2 weeks of life. Causes of cholestasis in the neonate include hepatitis, metabolic disorders, and prolonged total parenteral nutrition, among other causes.

Severe hyperbilirubinemia can lead to kernicterus, a form of developmental delay from the deposition of bilirubin in neuronal tissues.

Assessment and Management

It is clinically difficult to determine the extent of the problem just based on the distribution of the yellow color. Initial evaluation includes total and direct bilirubin measurement at the hospital; therefore, transport is essential. Additional assessment includes blood type and Rh of both mother and infant, antiglobulin (Coombs) test on the infant, hematocrit value, and reticulocyte count. These tests are not available in the field. A neonate with significant clinical jaundice can be started on IV fluids in the field to help decrease the level of bilirubin and minimize the long-term neurologic effects. Any newborn with jaundice must be specifically communicated to medical control. The treatment for most cases of neonatal hyperbilirubinemia is phototherapy. Light helps break down the unconjugated bilirubin and aids in its excretion. In extreme cases, patients may require exchange transfusion. Phototherapy and other modes of treatment will be available at the medical center. Treatment will need to be started early in sick neonates and preterm infants as bilirubin-induced encephalopathy may develop at lower bilirubin levels than in healthy term infants.

For newborns with potential cholestasis, because it is not toxic, management includes diagnostic testing and then treatment of the cause; therefore, transport the patient to a facility where this can occur.

■ Pathophysiology, Assessment, and Management of Conditions Related to Thermoregulation

Thermoregulation is the body's ability to balance heat production and heat loss so as to maintain a normal body temperature. This ability is limited in the newborn. The average normal temperature of a newborn at birth is 99.5°F (37.5°C). For the neonate, the thermoneutral temperature range is 97.9°F to 99°F (36.6°C to 37.2°C).

Nonshivering thermogenesis, the production of heat by metabolism, is the primary source of heat production in the newborn. Brown fat (deposited in the fetus after 28 weeks of gestation, and principally stored around the scapula, kidneys, adrenal glands, neck, and axilla) is a thermogenic tissue unique to the newborn.

Heat loss occurs when heat is lost to the environment, through any of the following four mechanisms, as discussed in Chapter 38, *Environmental Emergencies* **Figure 42-13** .

▶ Fever

Fever is defined as a rectal temperature of greater than 100.4°F (38°C). Oral and axillary temperatures are, respectively, 1°F (0.6°C) and 2°F (1.1°C) lower than the rectal temperature on average.

A newborn's temperature regulation system is relatively immature, so fever may not always be a presenting

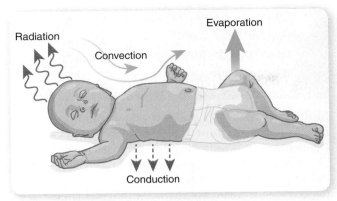

Figure 42-13 Heat loss occurs when heat is lost to the environment through any of the following four mechanisms: evaporation, convection, conduction, and radiation.

© Jones & Bartlett Learning.

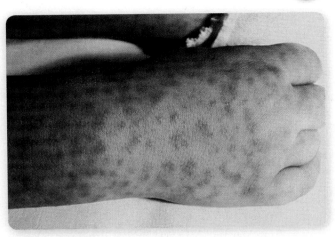

Figure 42-14 A newborn with a fever may also have petechiae or pinpoint pink or red skin lesions.

Courtesy of Centers for Disease Control and Prevention.

feature with infection or illness. In fact, newborns may become hypothermic with infection. Neonates may also become hypoglycemic during a fever because their enteral intake decreases, and they may even develop lactic acidosis because of anaerobic metabolism. Also, hypoglycemia may be a symptom of septicemia. No matter what the presenting symptoms are, it is important to identify newborns with serious bacterial infection (eg, bacteremia, urinary tract infection, meningitis, bacterial gastroenteritis, and pneumonia) or serious viral infection (eg, herpes simplex) for which treatment is available. Neonates who appear well but present with fever carry an approximately 7% chance of having a serious underlying bacterial infection.[56]

Overheating may also cause fever. Infants can easily become too hot when dressed in many layers of clothing, over-bundled in a heated car, or placed in direct sunlight, even through a window, or near heating vents at home. Fever related to dehydration is an important consideration in breastfeeding infants, especially in the first week after birth. These infants have often lost more than 10% of their weight and may have a history of difficulty in initiating breastfeeding.

Newborns have limited ability to control their temperature. They do not sweat when they are hot to allow cooling, and they do not shiver to raise their temperature when they are cold. Term infants may produce sweat over their brow but not the rest of their body. Premature infants do not produce sweat. Moreover, many newborns with serious life-threatening infections may actually see their core temperature drop; these newborns are at a higher risk for hypoglycemia and metabolic acidosis. A careful examination will reveal irritability, somnolence, and decreased feeding. The newborn may feel warm to touch. Some newborns with fever, however, may be initially asymptomatic.

Assessment and Management

When fever is suspected, examine the newborn for the presence of rashes, especially petechiae or pinpoint

pink or red skin lesions **Figure 42-14**. Obtain a careful history regarding general activity, feeding, voiding, and stooling. Note increased respiratory rate, along with increased work of breathing. Obtain the newborn's vital signs and ensure adequate oxygenation and ventilation, providing free-flow supplemental oxygen if necessary. Perform chest compressions, if indicated. Administration of antipyretic agents such as acetaminophen or ibuprofen is controversial in the prehospital setting; do not give ibuprofen to a newborn. To cool the newborn, remove additional layers of clothing and improve ventilation in the environment.

▶ Hypothermia

Hypothermia is a drop in body temperature to less than 95°F (35°C). Hypothermia in the newborn occurs in all climates, but is more common during the winter months. Moderate hypothermia is associated with an increased risk of death in low birth weight newborns. Infants may die of cold exposure at temperatures adults find comfortable. **Table 42-11** lists risk factors for hypothermia.

Table 42-11	**Risk Factors for Hypothermia**

- All newborns in the first 8 to 12 h after birth
- Home delivery
- Prolonged resuscitation
- Infant who is small for gestational age
- Infant with central nervous system problems
- Prematurity
- Sepsis
- Inadequate measures to keep the infant warm during transport

© Jones & Bartlett Learning.

Newborns have an increased surface area-to-volume ratio, making them extremely sensitive to environmental conditions, especially when wet after delivery. An increase in metabolic function in an attempt to overcome the heat loss can cause hypoglycemia, metabolic acidosis, **pulmonary hypertension**, and hypoxemia. Every hypothermic newborn should also be assessed for infection.

Assessment and Management

Hypothermic newborns are cool to the touch, initially in the extremities; as their temperature drops, however, the skin becomes cool all over. The newborn may also be pale and have acrocyanosis. The hypothermic newborn may present with decreased respiratory effort, apnea, bradycardia, cyanosis, irritability, and a weak cry. As a newborn's temperature drops, he or she may become lethargic and obtunded. In severely hypothermic newborns, the face and extremities may appear bright red. Sclerema—hardening of the skin associated with reddening and edema—may be seen on the back, limbs, or all over the body. Thermal shock, disseminated intravascular coagulopathy, and death may occur in more serious cases.

Take the preventive measures discussed earlier in the chapter, such as warming your hands, drying the newborn thoroughly, placing a prewarmed cap on the newborn's head, and placing the newborn skin-to-skin with the mother if possible. Continue the rewarming process until the newborn's temperature reaches the normal range or his or her feet are no longer cold. Do not use hot water bottles—they may cause burns because blood circulation is poor in the cold skin of newborns. If the newborn is hypoglycemic, you may administer $D_{10}W$. Warm IV fluids can assist in rewarming the newborn. Once stabilized, it is ideal if possible to place the critically ill newborn in a prewarmed incubator; however, these are most often not available in the prehospital environment. Instead, cover the newborn with warm blankets and place him or her on mother's chest. Ensure the ambulance heat is turned up. Consider heat packs, but *never* place them directly on the skin.

Recent studies in newborns with hypoxic-ischemic injury indicate improved outcomes when the newborn is provided mild therapeutic hypothermia within 6 hours of birth.[57-59] This approach is not recommended in the field, although it is prudent to prevent hyperthermia. Maintain the newborn at the lower margin of normal temperature (axillary temperature no higher than 97.7°F [36.5°C]).

Special Populations

Newborns are susceptible to conjunctivitis from sexually transmitted diseases passed on by the mother, irritation to antibiotic eye drops at birth, or an infection from a clogged tear duct.

Pathophysiology, Assessment, and Management of Common Birth Injuries in the Newborn

Birth trauma includes both avoidable and unavoidable injuries to the newborn resulting from mechanical forces (ie, compression, traction) during the delivery process. The overall incidence of birth injuries in singleton vaginal deliveries is estimated to be around 2%.[60,61] The incidence is slightly lower at 1.1% in cesarean deliveries.[60,61] Most birth injuries are self-limiting and have a favorable outcome. Recognition of risk factors and anticipation of a potentially difficult delivery may allow you to avoid trauma to the neonate during the birth process.

A difficult birth or injury to the newborn can occur because of the newborn's size or position during labor and delivery. Conditions associated with a difficult birth include **primigravida** (first pregnancy), prolonged labor, cephalopelvic disproportion (the size and shape of the maternal pelvis are not adequate for the vaginal delivery of the newborn), prolonged or rapid labor, abnormal presentation (eg, breech), large size (birth weight exceeding 9 pounds, or 4,000 g), shoulder dystocia, prematurity, or low birth weight.

Birth trauma includes a variety of injuries. For example, abrasions, lacerations, bruises, and subcutaneous fat necrosis can occur with deliveries that involve instruments (eg, a vacuum or forceps). Molding of the head and overriding parietal bones are part of the normal process of labor, but occasionally excessive molding may be seen.

Caput succedaneum is swelling of the soft tissue of the newborn's scalp as it presses against the dilating cervix. This type of scalp swelling is common. The swelling usually disappears in the first day or two after birth.

A cephalohematoma is an area of bleeding between the parietal bone and its covering periosteum. It often appears several hours after birth as a raised lump on the newborn's head, is limited by the boundaries of the bone, and may take 2 weeks to 3 months to resolve. If the bleeding is severe, jaundice may be seen as the red blood cells break down. Newborns born by instrumental vaginal delivery are more likely to have a cephalohematoma. There is no need to drain a scalp hematoma in the prehospital setting. Supportive care and rapid transport are recommended.

Linear skull fractures are occasionally seen with difficult births (spontaneous vaginal deliveries or deliveries using instruments). Nondisplaced fractures can be managed conservatively. Care should be observed to avoid pressure to the involved area. Displaced fractures warrant neurosurgical evaluation.

Brachial plexus injuries typically occur in deliveries complicated by shoulder dystocia and have an incidence ranging from 0.04% to 0.3% of live births.[60-62] The most common brachial plexus injury is **Erb palsy** (involvement of C5, C6). **Klumpke paralysis** (involvement of C8 to T1) is rare and results in the weakness of the intrinsic muscles of the hand.[63]

Although branches of the facial nerve may be injured in forceps delivery, most facial nerve palsy is unrelated to trauma. Physical findings include asymmetric faces with crying (lack of movement on the affected side makes the face appear to be "pulled" to the opposite side). Full resolution of cranial nerve injuries may take several weeks. Additionally, subconjunctival and retinal hemorrhage are possible results of birth trauma.

Diaphragmatic paralysis may occur as an isolated finding when the cervical roots supplying the phrenic nerve are injured or in association with a brachial plexus injury. The newborn may experience respiratory distress with hypoxemia, hypercapnia, and acidosis.

Laryngeal nerve injury appears to result from an intrauterine posture in which the head is rotated and flexed laterally. The newborn presents with stridor or a hoarse cry. Bilateral injury may be associated with severe respiratory distress needing respiratory support. The paralysis often resolves in 4 to 6 weeks, but may occasionally take as long as 6 to 12 months to clear up.

Spinal cord injury may result from excessive traction (in a breech delivery) or rotation and torsion (in a vertex delivery). The clinical presentation is stillbirth or rapid neonatal death with failure to establish an adequate airway.

The clavicle is the most frequently fractured bone in the newborn; such a bone injury is most often an unpredictable, unavoidable complication of normal birth. Risk factors may include large size, mid-forceps delivery, and shoulder dystocia (ie, the newborn's shoulders get stuck in the birth canal). The newborn may present with pseudoparalysis as he or she tries not to move the affected extremity to minimize pain. Examination will show crepitus and palpable bony irregularity. There may be lack of movement of the arm freely on the side of the fractured clavicle.

Loss of spontaneous arm or leg movement is an early sign of long bone fracture. The femur and humerus are the most commonly affected long bones. The fractures are treated by splinting. Radial nerve injury may be present when the humerus is fractured. Remember to always assess distal pulse, motor function, and sensation before and after splinting.

Intra-abdominal injury is uncommon and may be overlooked as a cause of death in a newborn. Possible intra-abdominal injuries include liver contusion or fracture, rupture of the spleen, or adrenal hemorrhage. Hemorrhage is the most serious complication, and the liver is the organ most commonly injured. The bleeding may be catastrophic or insidious, and the patient presents with circulatory collapse. Consider intra-abdominal bleeding in every newborn presenting with shock, or unexplained pallor, plus abdominal distention. Finally, hypoxia and shock could be caused by birth trauma.

Pathophysiology, Assessment, and Management of Congenital Heart Disease

Various congenital heart diseases or malformations of the heart may cause cardiac emergencies in newborns; therefore, it is useful for you to be familiar with them. **Figure 42-15** shows the locations of pulmonary stenosis, atrial septal defect, and ventricular septal defect, which will be discussed next.

▶ Pathophysiology

Congenital heart disease (CHD) refers to abnormalities of the heart during development. It is the most common birth defect and occurs in 8 per 1,000 live births.[64] Approximately one-quarter of these conditions are considered critical[65-67]—forms of CHD that are usually associated with hypoxia in the newborn period and require intervention during the first months of life.

Among children with congenital malformations, congenital heart disease is the leading cause of death. Many of these children had an undiagnosed CHD that was not identified until an autopsy was performed.[64] There have been great improvements in surgical care of these infants, and in early diagnosis of critical congenital heart disease by prenatal ultrasound and early pulse oximetry screening. With the advent of prenatal ultrasonography, many congenital heart problems are diagnosed in utero

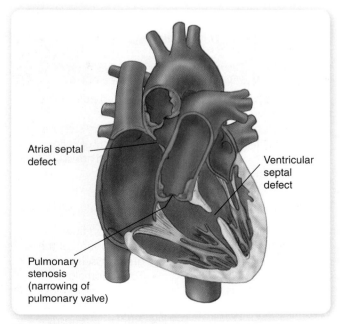

Figure 42-15 Locations of various congenital heart malformations.

© Jones & Bartlett Learning.

and preparations made for treatment well in advance, but patients may lack prenatal care or decompensate while waiting for evaluation and repair.

Neonates and infants can present with varying degrees of cardiorespiratory compromise depending on the particular cardiac lesion. Patients with these congenital defects typically present in the neonatal period with increasing respiratory distress, poor perfusion, cyanosis, and eventual cardiovascular collapse if their defect goes unrecognized. Early recognition, emergent stabilization, and transport to an appropriate cardiac care center are crucial in the outcome of newborns with these conditions.

It is well recognized that visual detection of cyanosis is difficult. A painless, noninvasive way to detect cyanosis is to measure oxygen saturation of hemoglobin in arterial blood. Pulse oximetry has been found to be a noninvasive and accurate method to detect oxygenated versus deoxygenated blood. Monitoring oxygen saturation has been shown to have the highest sensitivity and highest specificity with the right hand and one foot, using cutoff values of less than 95% or a greater than 3% difference between the two. The best outcomes are found when a physical exam is paired with pulse oximetry screening beyond 24 hours of age.

In 2011, the Department of Health and Human Services and the American Academy of Pediatrics recommended pulse oximetry screening for full-term healthy newborns in an effort to diagnose CHD early in the neonatal period.[68] Because some disorders may present with significant cardiopulmonary compromise without apparent cyanosis, the recommended term is *critical CHD* rather than the term *cyanotic heart disease*, which is sometimes used (Table 42-12).

Table 42-12	**Congenital Heart Diseases**
Increased pulmonary blood flow	Decreased pulmonary blood flow
▪ Atrial septal defect	▪ Pulmonary stenosis
▪ Ventricular septal defect	▪ Tetralogy of Fallot
	▪ Tricuspid atresia
▪ Patent ductus arteriosus	
▪ Atrioventricular canal	
Obstruction of blood flow from the heart	Mixed blood flow
▪ Coarctation of the aorta	▪ Transposition of the great vessels
▪ Aortic stenosis	▪ Total anomalous pulmonary venous return
	▪ Truncus arteriosus
	▪ Hypoplastic left heart syndrome

Noncyanotic Disease

Noncyanotic congenital heart diseases (also called pink defects) include atrial septal defects, ventricular septal defects, patent ductus arteriosus, and coarctation of the aorta. With these abnormalities, oxygenated blood is shunted from the left (systemic) side of the heart to the right (pulmonary) side. This defect is called a left-to-right shunt.

Atrial Septal Defect. Septal defects can exist in the atria or the ventricles within the heart. When an **atrial septal defect** is present, an abnormal opening (hole or defect) exists in the wall (septum) separating the atrial chambers of the heart. This opening allows some of the oxygenated blood from the left atrium (at higher pressure) to flow through the hole to the right atrium (at lower pressure) instead of flowing through the left ventricle, out the aorta, and to the body. The failure of the foramen ovale to close after birth allows for this process to take place. The foramen ovale exists in utero, during which time it enables the fetus to receive oxygen-rich blood from the placenta—essential because the fetus's lungs are nonfunctioning. After the fetus is born, a drop in circulatory pulmonary pressure occurs, allowing the foramen ovale to close. In a patient with an open foramen ovale, hemodynamic status can be dependent on how much blood flow is being shunted.

The increased volume of blood flowing to the right atrium and ventricle due to atrial septal defect causes enlargement of these chambers. If the defect is not repaired, pulmonary hypertension usually develops in adulthood. Infants and children with atrial septal defect are usually asymptomatic, although height and weight are often below normal and endurance may be limited. A characteristic murmur is present with atrial septal defect. Patients are at risk for atrial dysrhythmias, probably from atrial enlargement and stretching of conduction fibers. Small atrial septal defects (less than 8 mm) often close on their own by 18 months of age. Large defects can lead to failure to thrive, frequent respiratory infections, or heart failure. These lesions often require surgery, usually before school age.

Ventricular Septal Defect. In a **ventricular septal defect**, an abnormal opening exists in the wall separating the right and left ventricles. This opening allows some of the oxygenated blood to flow from the left ventricle through the hole to the right ventricle and pulmonary artery instead of being pumped into the aorta; when the left ventricle contracts, this forces some of the blood flow back into the right ventricle. Because less blood is pumped out of the left ventricle, stroke volume is reduced, affecting cardiac output. Because the right ventricle is under greater pressure and must pump extra blood, it may enlarge. If the right ventricle is unable to accommodate the increased workload, the right atrium may also enlarge. Another result of ventricular septal defect is an increase in the right ventricle pressure, which subsequently results in pulmonary hypertension developing in the patient.

If the opening is small, the patient is usually asymptomatic and growth and development are unaffected. If the opening is of moderate to large size, delayed growth and development (height usually is normal but weight may be decreased), decreased exercise tolerance, and repeated pulmonary infections often occur. Signs of heart failure (eg, tachypnea, grunting respirations, tachycardia, diminished pulses, fatigue with feeding, and diaphoresis) and a characteristic murmur may be present.

Infants and children with a ventricular septal defect are at risk for bacterial endocarditis and must take antibiotics before certain dental and surgical procedures. Many small defects close on their own during the first year of life. Moderate and large defects may require surgical closure.

Patent Ductus Arteriosus. Patent ductus arteriosus exists when the ductus arteriosus fails to close after birth. In the fetus, an open ductus arteriosus allows blood flow to bypass the right ventricle and lungs due to the fetus's lungs being filled with fluid. The ductus arteriosus connects the pulmonary artery and the aorta; after birth, it is supposed to evolve into the ligamentum arteriosum **Figure 42-16** . The ductus arteriosus normally closes within a few hours of birth. Persistence of the ductus arteriosus beyond 10 days of life is considered abnormal.

In patent ductus arteriosus, oxygenated blood traveling through the aorta is shunted from the aorta, across the duct, to the pulmonary artery (instead of flowing from the aorta and on to the body), where it mixes with deoxygenated blood. The workload of the left atrium and ventricle is increased because of the additional blood that is recirculated through the lungs to these heart chambers. At the same time, less blood is delivered to the lungs to be oxygenated.

Patient signs and symptoms depend on the size of the ductus and how much blood flow it carries. The patient with a small shunt may be asymptomatic. Signs and symptoms associated with a large shunt may include fatigue, failure to thrive, poor feeding, bounding peripheral pulses, a characteristic murmur, and increased work of breathing.

An untreated patent ductus arteriosus may cause the patient to subsequently develop heart failure.

Coarctation of the Aorta. Coarctation of the aorta (CoA) is a narrowing of the aorta, the largest oxygen-carrying artery in the human body. The aorta is pinched or constricted in the area of the ductus arteriosus, just beyond the aorta's branching vessels to the head and arms. Because a segment of the aorta is narrowed, the left ventricle must work harder to force blood through the narrowed area to the lower part of the body. This results in increased blood pressure proximal to the defect (head and arms) and decreased blood flow distal to it (the body and legs). In cases of severe narrowing, the left ventricle may not be strong enough to perform this extra work, resulting in heart failure or poor perfusion. Coarctation of the aorta may be associated with other cardiac defects, typically those involving the left side of the heart.

Most patients with coarctation of the aorta are asymptomatic until later in childhood, at which time the child presents with a heart murmur or hypertension. Physical findings may include dyspnea, poor feeding, and poor weight gain; high blood pressure and bounding pulses in the arms; lower blood pressure with weak or absent femoral pulses and cool lower extremities; chest pain; muscle weakness; and possibly differential cyanosis (eg, the lower half of the body is cyanotic). Infants may show signs of heart failure. Dizziness, frequent headaches, fainting, and nosebleeds may be present in the older child as a result of hypertension. Surgical repair is recommended within the first 2 years of life.

Cyanotic Disease

Cyanotic heart lesions (also called blue defects) are congenital abnormalities in which deoxygenated blood from the right (pulmonary) side of the heart mixes with oxygenated blood from the left (systemic) side and enters the systemic circulation, bypassing the pulmonary circulation. This defect is called a right-to-left shunt. Examples of cyanotic disease include truncus arteriosus, tricuspid atresia, hypoplastic left heart syndrome, tetralogy of Fallot, transposition of the great arteries, and total anomalous pulmonary venous return.

Pulmonary Stenosis. Pulmonary stenosis is a disease in which the pulmonic valve located near the right ventricle of the heart becomes damaged. When this exists, the patient will have a decrease in blood flow to the lungs and will present with jugular vein distention, cyanosis, or right ventricular hypertrophy. Pulmonary stenosis is typically associated with CHD but can also result from rheumatic heart disease.

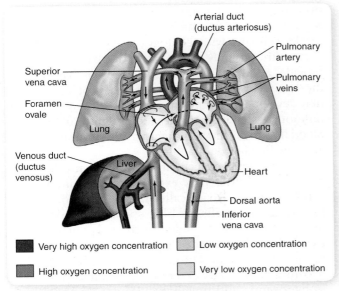

Superior vena cava

Foramen ovale

Lung

Venous duct (ductus venosus)

Liver

Arterial duct (ductus arteriosus)

Pulmonary artery

Pulmonary veins

Lung

Heart

Dorsal aorta

Inferior vena cava

■ Very high oxygen concentration ▢ Low oxygen concentration

▢ High oxygen concentration ▢ Very low oxygen concentration

Figure 42-16 If the ligamentum arteriosum does not fully evolve after birth, the patient may develop heart failure.

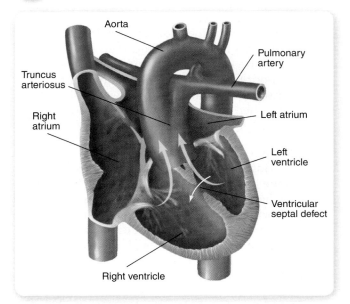

Figure 42-17 In truncus arteriosus, the pulmonary artery and the aorta are combined into one vessel.

© Jones & Bartlett Learning.

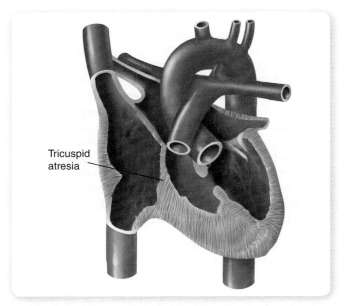

Figure 42-18 Tricuspid atresia, or lack of the tricuspid valve, results in an undersized or absent right ventricle.

© Jones & Bartlett Learning.

Truncus Arteriosus. In a normal circulatory system, the pulmonary artery and the aorta are two separate vessels. In **truncus arteriosus**, these vessels are combined into one (Figure 42-17). This merger greatly increases the blood flow coming into the lungs, ultimately causing these patients to have heart failure. Early in life, the patient will demonstrate slightly lower oxygen levels, which eventually result in cyanosis. Affected patients will require surgical intervention.

Tricuspid Atresia. In **tricuspid atresia**, the patient lacks the tricuspid valve, which normally separates the right atrium and the right ventricle. The lack of the tricuspid valve results in an undersized or absent right ventricle (Figure 42-18). Patients who present with this condition will have a significantly decreased blood flow coming into the lungs—a condition leading to severe hypoxemia and ultimately resulting in death. Treatment may require a Fontan procedure, which redirects the inferior vena cava and hepatic vein into the pulmonary circulation.

Hypoplastic Left Heart Syndrome. **Hypoplastic left heart syndrome** is the complete underdevelopment of the left side of the heart. The mitral and aortic valves may be closed or severely underdeveloped, the aorta extremely small, and the left ventricle very small. All of these inadequacies result in the left side of the heart being unable to fulfill the circulation needs of the body. Patients with this condition will present with a murmur or cyanosis. A heart transplant is necessary to resolve the cardiovascular insufficiencies resulting from hypoplastic left heart syndrome.

Tetralogy of Fallot. **Tetralogy of Fallot** is a combination of four heart defects: a ventricular septal defect, pulmonary

stenosis, right ventricular hypertrophy, and an overriding aorta (the aorta lies directly over the ventricular septal defect). As discussed earlier, ventricular septal defect allows some oxygenated blood to flow from the left ventricle to the right ventricle and pulmonary artery instead of being pumped into the aorta; pulmonary stenosis causes the heart to have to pump harder due to the lack of blood flow to the lungs. Right ventricular hypertrophy is a thickening of the right ventricle that occurs so that the body can efficiently pump blood to the lungs. In a normal circulatory system, the aorta is connected to the left ventricle. In tetralogy of Fallot, the aorta is connected between the left and right ventricles over the ventricular septal defect. All of these defects result in poor oxygenation.

Most infants with tetralogy of Fallot are pink at birth because they usually have a patent ductus arteriosus that provides additional pulmonary blood flow. However, as the ductus closes in the first hours or days of life, cyanosis may develop or become more severe. Clubbing occurs as pulmonary stenosis becomes more significant, reducing blood flow to the lungs. A characteristic murmur is present after the first few days of life.

When arterial oxygen saturation suddenly decreases, an infant or child may experience a tetralogy spell. Tetralogy spells also are called tet spells, hypoxic spells, hypercyanotic spells, or blue spells. A hypoxic spell usually results from sudden, increased constriction of the outflow tract to the lungs, further restricting pulmonary blood flow. During a hypoxic spell, the child becomes increasingly cyanotic and irritable in response to hypoxemia and breathes quite deeply and rapidly (hyperpnea). If left untreated, a severe spell may result in syncope, seizures, stroke, or death. In infants, a hypoxic spell often occurs in the morning after crying, feeding, or a bowel movement.

Emergency care for a hypoxic spell includes keeping the infant or child as calm as possible. An infant having a hypoxic spell should be picked up and held in a knee-chest position (ie, place the infant on the caregiver's shoulder with the knees tucked up underneath). This provides a calming effect and reduces venous return. The older child having a hypoxic spell often squats to recover. Squatting compresses the superior vena cava and increases systemic vascular resistance, directing blood through the pulmonary stenosis and into the lungs (rather than across the ventricular septal defect). Give oxygen, IV fluids, and medications as ordered by medical direction. Morphine may be ordered to suppress the respiratory center and resolve the hyperpnea.

Open heart surgery is required to correct tetralogy of Fallot.

Transposition of the Great Arteries. In transposition of the great arteries, the positions of the pulmonary artery and the aorta are reversed. The aorta is connected to the right ventricle, so deoxygenated blood returning to the right atrium from the body is pumped out to the aorta and back to the body without first going to the lungs for oxygenation. The pulmonary artery is connected to the left ventricle, so oxygenated blood returning from the lungs to the left atrium goes back to the lungs by the pulmonary artery without being sent to the body **Figure 42-19** .

An infant born with transposition of the great arteries can survive only if one or more associated defects permits oxygenated blood to reach the systemic circulation, such as an atrial septal defect, ventricular septal defect, or patent ductus arteriosus that allows mixing of oxygenated and deoxygenated blood.

Cyanosis is usually present soon after birth. At birth, a patent ductus arteriosus may permit sufficient mixing of oxygenated and deoxygenated blood to prevent severe cyanosis. However, as the ductus closes in the first hours or days of life, cyanosis becomes increasingly severe. A murmur may be present depending on the type of associated cardiac defects, but many infants do not have a murmur. Signs of heart failure and hypoglycemia may be present, as well as shortness of breath and clubbing of fingers and toes.

Patients with transposition of the great arteries may require surgical intervention to correct the defect.

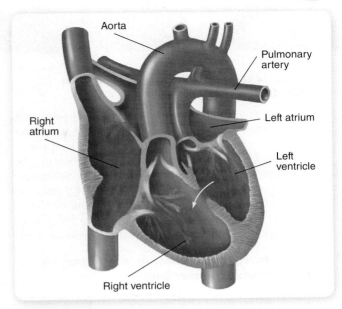

Figure 42-19 Transposition of the great arteries.
© Jones & Bartlett Learning.

Special Populations

Children and adolescents with cyanotic disease may not have normal baseline oxygenation; it is best to ask the family what the normal pulse oximetry value should be.

Total Anomalous Pulmonary Venous Return. Total anomalous pulmonary venous return is a rare congenital defect in which the four pulmonary veins do not connect to the left atrium. Instead, the pulmonary veins connect to the right atrium, resulting in diminished oxygen and an increased load on the right ventricle. These patients will present with signs and symptoms shortly after birth.

▶ General Assessment and Management

Critical CHD commonly presents in the neonatal period. Rapid detection and transport are critical because the conditions of patients can become unstable very quickly. Communication with medical control is crucial to having adequate services available for diagnosis and treatment upon arrival at the emergency facility.

YOU are the Paramedic SUMMARY

1. **What is the significance of the green amniotic fluid?**

   Amniotic fluid should be clear and odorless. The presence of a green or green-black staining indicates that the fetus has passed fetal stool (meconium). This can be a sign of fetal distress, and is an indicator that the delivery may be high-risk. When signs of a potential high-risk delivery are present, additional help should be requested if possible (as Rescue 1 did in this case). If the fetus inhales the meconium into his or her lungs, it can cause a severe pneumonia leading to respiratory distress, respiratory failure, or death.

2. **What further information would you like to obtain from the mother?**

   At this point in time you should address two major points. The first one is "will the delivery occur on-scene or is there time to transport to the hospital?" Ask the mother whether she feels the need to push or have a bowel movement. If she answers "yes" to either question, check for crowning; an urge to push signifies that the fetus will likely deliver soon. The second question that you need to ask is "are there any other risk factors present that might require resuscitation of the newborn once he or she is born?" Four important questions to consider when determining resuscitation risk factors include: what is the expected gestational age of the infant, is the amniotic fluid clear, how many babies are expected, and does the mother know of any additional risk factors that she has discussed with her obstetrician.

3. **Besides the OB kit, what additional equipment should you have available?**

   Because you already detected the presence of meconium, you must have your resuscitation equipment available and ready to go. At a minimum, make sure that your suction and positive pressure ventilation/intubation equipment are functioning properly. Most importantly, the infant may require resuscitation so make sure that additional assistance is available. In this case the first arriving unit (Rescue 1) made a good decision to call for help, and prepared for imminent delivery by taking out and readying the OB kit while awaiting arrival of Rescue 2.

4. **Should you stimulate the newborn immediately after birth?**

   Yes, the resuscitation of this newborn should be done in the same manner as that for any other newborn. Dry and stimulate the infant, and if the infant does not have adequate respiration by 30 seconds, begin PPV by bag-mask device on room air. Suctioning may be required to clear the airway. All of this should occur before the 60-second mark.

5. **What treatment is indicated for this newborn?**

   This newborn's pulse rate is 85 beats/min. If the newborn has a pulse rate below 100 beats/min and has a weak respiratory effort after drying and stimulation, positive pressure ventilation via a bag-mask device is necessary. Make sure that you ventilate at a rate of 40 to 60 breaths/min and use only enough pressure to cause chest rise.

6. **Why was the 1-minute Apgar score not obtained?**

   The 1-minute and 5-minute Apgar scores should only be performed when they can be obtained without delaying resuscitation. In this case, the neonate had weak respiratory effort and poor tone. It is more important to initiate newborn care and resuscitation than to obtain the 1-minute Apgar score in this particular scenario. *Do not delay resuscitation efforts to calculate an Apgar score!* You can obtain an Apgar score once the newborn is stabilized.

7. **When is endotracheal intubation indicated in the newborn?**

   Endotracheal intubation is *not* routinely required during the resuscitation of a newborn. However, there are certain circumstances when intubation is necessary. These include: (1) a congenital diaphragmatic hernia is suspected and respiratory support is needed; (2) the newborn does not respond to bag-mask ventilation despite corrective measures; and (3) prolonged positive pressure ventilation is required. Epinephrine is best administered via IV line or IO line, but the endotracheal route may be used if there is no intravenous or intraosseous access.

8. **What should you do for the newborn at this time?**

   Because the newborn now has a good respiratory rate and pulse rate, and you cut and clamped the cord after your last reassessment, you should now make sure that the newborn stays warm. Wrap the newborn in clean, dry towels or the swaddler that is contained in the OB kit, and place the hat on the newborn's head. If the mother and newborn are stable, place them securely in the ambulance with skin-to-skin contact and nursing encouraged if it may be safely performed.

9. **What are the five components that make up the Apgar score?**

   When you assess the newborn to calculate an Apgar score, the five key parameters to evaluate are: appearance, pulse rate, grimace or irritability, activity, and respirations.

10. **Why was the newborn's original Apgar score calculated as 9?**

    This infant has a pink trunk with cyanosis in the extremities noted (acrocyanosis), and receives a score of 1 for color. The heart rate is above 100 beats/min and is scored at 2. The infant responds well when stimulated and receives a score of 2 for reflex irritability. The baby has excellent muscle tone and good crying respirations, both worth 2 points. All of these together form a combined total of 9 points for the Apgar score.

YOU are the Paramedic **SUMMARY** *(continued)*

Maternal Patient Care Report

EMS Patient Care Report (PCR)

Date: 07-06-18	**Incident No.:** 187444	**Nature of Call:** Possible childbirth	**Location:** 8901 NW Pembroke Road

Dispatched: 0910	**En Route:** 0911	**At Scene:** 0917	**Transport:** 0952	**At Hospital:** 1012	**In Service:** 1020

Patient Information

Age: 29 years **Sex:** F **Weight (in kg [lb]):** 78 kg (172 lb)	**Allergies:** None **Medications:** Prenatal vitamins **Past Medical History:** None **Chief Complaint:** Water broke

Vital Signs

Time: 0919	**BP:** 128/74	**Pulse:** 104	**Respirations:** 24	**Spo$_2$:** 97% via NRM at 12 L/min
Time: 0940	**BP:** 124/70	**Pulse:** 94	**Respirations:** 18	**Spo$_2$:** 99% via NRM at 12 L/min
Time: 1000	**BP:** 122/74	**Pulse:** 86	**Respirations:** 18	**Spo$_2$:** 99% via NRM at 12 L/min

EMS Treatment (circle all that apply)

Oxygen @ __12__ L/min via (circle one): NC **(NRM)** Bag-mask device	**Assisted Ventilation**	**Airway Adjunct**	**CPR**
Defibrillation	**Bleeding Control**	**Bandaging**	**Splinting**	**Other:** OB kit, IV

Narrative

Dispatched to the home of a 29-year-old female for possible childbirth. Arrived on scene to find the pt sitting on the edge of her bed, clutching her abdomen and grimacing in pain. Pt states that her "water broke about 45 minutes ago and when she saw that it was green she called her OB who told her to call 9-1-1." There is a large puddle of green fluid on the floor beside the bed. Pt states that she feels like she has to go to the bathroom and wants to begin pushing. Pt states that she is 41 weeks' pregnant with her fifth child. Pt denies other PMH. Pt states that she was scheduled to be induced 2 days from now. Pt states that she has had routine prenatal care with no known complications. Pt takes prenatal vitamins and denies any medication allergies. Pt placed on O$_2$ 12 L/min via nonrebreathing mask. Pt placed in supine position with legs flexed toward the abdomen to facilitate inspection of the vaginal area. Crowning is noted upon inspection at 0922. At this time it was determined that delivery was imminent and this was a high-risk birth. Additional assistance was requested and Rescue 2 was dispatched to the location. OB kit and neonatal resuscitation equipment are prepared. Following delivery and stabilization of mother and baby, the mother held the baby prior to transport being initiated. Due to the high-risk nature of this delivery and initial resuscitation efforts required, the decision to transport mother and baby in separate ambulances was made to ensure that adequate care could be administered should either patient begin to deteriorate. Separate PCR filed by Rescue 2 that transported newborn. En route to Grand View Hospital an 18-gauge IV was placed in the mother's left AC and a 1,000 mL bag of normal saline was hung at a rate of 200 mL/h. Physical assessment findings: Pt AAO × 4. PERRLA. No JVD or tracheal deviation noted. Chest symmetrical with bilateral chest rise and clear lung sounds. Abdomen soft and non-tender following delivery. PMS × 4. Hospital contacted and report given to labor and delivery. No further orders were given. Mother remained stable through transport. The placenta was delivered as rescue was entering the parking lot of the hospital. Mother was brought to labor and delivery. Report given to Dr. Aarons and Judy ARNP. Cleared for service at 1020.**End of report**

YOU are the Paramedic **SUMMARY** (continued)

Newborn Patient Care Report

EMS Patient Care Report (PCR)

Date: 07-06-18	**Incident No.:** 596833	**Nature of Call:** Possible childbirth		**Location:** 8901 NW Pembroke Road	
Dispatched: 0922	**En Route:** 0923	**At Scene:** 0929	**Transport:** 0954	**At Hospital:** 1012	**In Service:** 1020

Patient Information

Age: Newborn **Sex:** F **Weight (in kg [lb]):** Approx. 4 kg (8 lb)	**Allergies:** None **Medications:** None **Past Medical History:** None **Chief Complaint:** Childbirth

Vital Signs

Time: 0933	**BP:** N/A	**Pulse:** 85	**Respirations:** N/A	**O₂:** N/A
Time: 0935	**BP:** N/A	**Pulse:** 156	**Respirations:** 48	**O₂:** N/A
Time: 0941	**BP:** N/A	**Pulse:** 154	**Respirations:** 46	**Spo₂:** 95% on room air
Time: 0948	**BP:** N/A	**Pulse:** 154	**Respirations:** 46	**Spo₂:** 96% on room air
Time: 1000	**BP:** N/A	**Pulse:** 154	**Respirations:** 46	**Spo₂:** 96% on room air

EMS Treatment (circle all that apply)

Oxygen @ _____ L/min via (circle one): NC NRM ⬭Bag-mask device on room air⬭	**Assisted Ventilation**	**Airway Adjunct**	**CPR**	
Defibrillation	**Bleeding Control**	**Bandaging**	**Splinting**	⬭**Other:** Suction, warming⬭

Narrative

See separate narrative filed by Rescue 1 for information regarding the mother. Rescue 2 was called to assist Rescue 1 with a possible high-risk childbirth. Arrived to find Rescue 1 personnel providing care for the mother. Rescue 1 personnel reported that meconium-stained amniotic fluid was present and they noted crowning on their initial vaginal examination. A significant urge to push was described by the mother. Rescue 1 personnel continued to care for the mother and Rescue 2 personnel initiated steps to prepare for imminent high-risk delivery. Rescue 1 personnel had prepared the OB kit and resuscitation equipment prior to the arrival of Rescue 2. Repeat vaginal exam of the mother at 0930 confirmed that crowning was present and delivery was imminent. At approximately 0933 the baby's head was delivered and the mouth and nose were suctioned with a bulb syringe, while Rescue 1 personnel continued to provide care for the mother. Moderate amounts of thick green meconium were removed from the oral cavity. Upon delivery the baby was noted to have a weak respiratory effort and cyanosis to the trunk and extremities. Umbilical cord was clamped and cut. After 30 seconds of positive pressure ventilation with room air, the baby was noted to have a good cry, pink trunk with acrocyanosis present, and a pulse rate of 156 beats/min. Breath sounds are clear and equal. 2-minute Apgar score was 9. The baby was dried with a towel and wrapped in the silver swaddler. 5-minute Apgar score was 10.

　　Due to the high-risk nature of this delivery and initial resuscitation efforts required, the decision to transport mother and baby in separate ambulances was made to ensure that adequate care could be administered should either patient begin to deteriorate. Both patients were stable at the time of transport, and mother was allowed to hold the baby prior to Rescue 1 initiating her transport to the hospital. The father arrived on scene as transport of the baby was initiated by Rescue 2, and he was given instructions to safely follow the ambulance to the transport destination. Baby placed on stretcher and secured with blanket roll and straps. Hospital contacted and report given to labor and delivery. No further orders were given. Baby remained stable through transport. Baby was brought to labor and delivery. Report given to Dr. Aarons and Judy ARNP. Cleared for service at 1020.**End of report**

Prep Kit

▶ Ready for Review

- The care of a newborn or neonate must be tailored to meet the unique needs of this population. The rate of complications increases as birth weight and gestational age decrease.
- Initial steps of neonatal resuscitation include positioning and stimulating the newborn to breathe, and assessing heart rate and oxygenation. In a newborn, resuscitation efforts are focused on establishing the airway and ensuring adequate ventilation. The airway is cleared if necessary.
- At birth, a fetus must transition from receiving oxygen from the placenta to receiving oxygen via breathing. A rapid series of events must occur to enable the newborn to breathe. Anything that delays this decline in pulmonary pressure can lead to delayed transition, hypoxia, brain damage, and, ultimately, death.
- While a delivery is occurring, use any time available to obtain a patient history and prepare the environment and equipment that may be necessary for neonatal resuscitation.
- Your primary survey of the newborn may be done simultaneously with any treatment interventions. Note the patency of the airway, respiratory rate, respiratory effort, pulse rate, color, and capillary refill.
- Initial stabilization efforts include warming the newborn; positioning; clearing the airway if necessary; drying the newborn's head, face, and body; and stimulating the newborn. Additional steps that may be required include providing supplemental oxygen, monitoring oxygen saturation, assisting ventilation by providing positive pressure, intubating, providing chest compressions, and administering medications as needed.
- The Apgar score is used to determine the need for and the effectiveness of resuscitation. It includes a score for appearance, pulse rate, grimace or irritability, muscle activity, and respiratory effort. This score is obtained at 1 and 5 minutes after birth.
- It is important to follow the neonatal resuscitation algorithm developed by American Heart Association.
- Initial steps, reevaluation, and beginning ventilation should occur within the first 60 seconds.
- Thermoregulation is limited in the newborn; therefore, you must take an active role in keeping the newborn's body temperature in the normal range. Place the newborn directly on the mother's chest. Dry the head and the body with towels. Cover the newborn with a dry towel; cover the head with a prewarmed cap. Position the newborn to ensure a patent airway.
- If the newborn has a normal breathing pattern and a pulse rate of greater than 100 beats/min but maintains central cyanosis of the trunk or of the mucous membranes, provide supplemental free-flow oxygen.
- In neonates with apnea, poor respiratory effort, or a pulse rate of less than 100 beats/min after 30 seconds of drying and stimulation, begin positive pressure ventilation (PPV) by bag-mask device.
  - Resuscitation should begin with room air (21% oxygen).
  - If the newborn's respiratory effort has not improved after 30 seconds of PPV, intubation should be considered.
  - Supplemental oxygen should be administered when the preductal oxygen saturation level is below the target range.
  - Supplemental oxygen should be weaned and discontinued if possible once the target preductal oxygen saturation has been achieved.
- If the newborn's pulse rate is less than 60 beats/min, begin chest compressions in addition to PPV. Effective chest compressions should result in palpable pulses.
- If ventilation and chest compressions do not result in improvement, consider pharmacologic intervention.
- Airway management in the newborn follows these steps: If a newborn is cyanotic or pale, administer warmed, humidified free-flow oxygen. If the newborn has an airway obstruction, for example from a congenital malformation, insert an oral airway. If these measures are not effective and the newborn is apneic, has inadequate respiratory effort, or is bradycardic, perform bag-mask ventilation. If this is not effective, endotracheal intubation is required.
- Gastric decompression using an orogastric tube is indicated for prolonged bag-mask ventilation (more than 5 to 10 minutes), if abdominal distention is impeding ventilation, and in the presence of a diaphragmatic hernia or a gastrointestinal congenital anomaly like a tracheoesophageal fistula.
- Chest compressions are indicated if the pulse rate remains less than 60 beats/min despite positioning, clearing the airway, drying and stimulation, and 30 seconds of effective PPV.
- Emergent vascular access becomes necessary when fluid administration is needed to support circulation, when resuscitation medications must be administered intravenously, and when therapeutic drugs must be given intravenously. Vascular access in a newborn

Prep Kit (continued)

occurs via the umbilical vein. Most newborns can be resuscitated with effective ventilatory support.

- Neonatal medication doses are based on estimated weight.
- Once the newborn is stabilized as much as possible in the field, provide transport to the nearest facility that can provide the next level of care.
- Ongoing communication with the family is a must. Do not be specific about survival statistics. If you do not have an answer, put the family in touch with the people who do.
- Bradycardia in a newborn is usually caused by hypoxia, which is readily reversed by effective PPV. Another cause is a tension pneumothorax that requires needle decompression. If ventilation and chest compressions do not improve the bradycardia, administer epinephrine via an IV line or ET tube.
- A small percentage of babies delivered in the presence of meconium-stained amniotic fluid may go on to develop meconium aspiration syndrome, which carries a high risk of mortality and morbidity. If the newborn is depressed, start PPV. If PPV is not effective, intubation and suctioning may be required to remove an obstruction.
- Diaphragmatic hernia is an abnormal opening in the diaphragm. If PPV is needed in a newborn with this condition, endotracheal intubation will be necessary, along with an orogastric tube to minimize intestinal distention. Surgical correction is required for this condition.
- Newborns born before 37 weeks of gestation are considered premature. Provide cardiorespiratory support and a thermoneutral environment to optimize their survival and long-term outcome.
- Seizures are a very distinctive sign of neurologic disease in the newborn. Quickly evaluate prenatal and birth history, and perform a careful physical exam. Consult with medical control if you are considering administering anticonvulsant medication.
- Non-bilious vomiting is common in newborns. Keep the newborn's face turned to one side to prevent further aspiration. Suction or clear the vomitus from the airway with the help of a suction catheter or suction bulb. Ensure adequate oxygenation. Consider fluid resuscitation. Transport the newborn on his or her side.
- In an infant with diarrhea, estimate the number and volume of loose stools, decreased urinary output, and degree of dehydration. Ensure adequate oxygenation and ventilation. Perform chest compressions in addition to PPV in a newborn if the pulse rate is less than 60 beats/min. Administer fluid therapy.

- If fever is suspected, observe the newborn for the presence of rashes. Obtain a careful history and vital signs. Ensure adequate oxygenation and ventilation. Remove additional layers of clothing and improve ventilation in the environment. Perform chest compressions, if indicated. Do not administer antipyretic agents.
- Birth trauma includes both avoidable and unavoidable injuries to the newborn resulting from mechanical forces during the delivery process. A difficult birth or injury to the newborn can occur because of the newborn's size or position during labor or delivery.
- Various congenital heart diseases or malformations of the heart may cause cardiac emergencies in newborns.

▶ Vital Vocabulary

acrocyanosis A decrease in the amount of oxygen delivered to the extremities. The hands and feet turn blue because of narrowing (constriction) of small arterioles (tiny arteries) toward the end of the arms and legs.

amniotic fluid A clear, slightly yellow liquid that surrounds the fetus during pregnancy; contained in the amniotic sac.

Apgar score Scale used to assess the status of a newborn 1 and 5 minutes after birth (range, 0 to 10).

asphyxia Condition of severely deficient supply of oxygen to the body leading to end organ damage.

atrial septal defect A hole in the atrial septal wall that allows oxygenated and deoxygenated blood to mix; patients with this hole have a higher incidence of stroke.

central cyanosis Blue discoloration of the skin due to the presence of deoxygenated hemoglobin in blood vessels near the skin surface.

choanal atresia A narrowing or blockage of the nasal airway by membranous or bony tissue; a congenital condition, meaning it is present at birth.

cleft lip An abnormal defect or fissure in the upper lip that failed to close during development. It is often associated with cleft palate.

cleft palate A fissure or hole in the palate (roof of the mouth) that forms a communicating pathway between the mouth and nasal cavities.

Prep Kit (continued)

coarctation of the aorta Pinching or narrowing of the aorta that obstructs blood flow from the heart to the systemic circulation.

congenital heart disease (CHD) The most common birth defect; associated with hypoxia in the newborn period requiring intervention during the first months of life.

diaphragmatic hernia Passage of loops of bowel with or without other abdominal organs, through a developmental defect in the diaphragm muscle; occurs as the bowel from the abdomen "herniates" upward through the diaphragm into the chest (thoracic) cavity.

Erb palsy Lack of movement at the shoulder due to nerve injury resulting from the stretching of the cervical nerve roots (C5 and C6 most commonly) during delivery of the newborn's head during birth. The effect is usually transient, but can be permanent.

fetal transition The process through which the fluid in the fetal lungs is replaced with air, the ductus arteriosus constricts, and the newborn begins adequate oxygenation of its own blood.

foramen ovale An opening in the septum of the heart that closes after birth.

free-flow oxygen Oxygen administered via oxygen tube and a cupped hand on the patient's face.

gastroesophageal reflux A condition in which stomach acid rises into the esophagus on a regular or frequent basis, potentially causing irritation and damage; a common cause of vomiting.

gestation Period of time from conception to birth. For humans, the full period is normally 9 months (or 40 weeks).

hypoplastic left heart syndrome Underdevelopment of the aorta, aortic valve, left ventricle, and mitral valve; this defect involves the entire left side of the heart.

hypotonia Low or poor muscle tone (floppiness).

hypoxic-ischemic encephalopathy Damage to cells in the central nervous system (the brain and spinal cord) from inadequate oxygen.

infantile hypertrophic pyloric stenosis (IHPS) Marked hypertrophy and hyperplasia of the two (circular and longitudinal) muscular layers of the pylorus, resulting in the pylorus becoming thick and obstructing the end of the stomach.

intestinal atresia A congenital condition in which part of the bowel does not develop.

intestinal stenosis A congenital condition in which part of the bowel is narrow.

intussusception An event where one part of the intestine folds into another part of the intestines leading to a blockage.

Klumpke paralysis An injury of childbirth affecting the spinal nerves C8 to T1 of the brachial plexus. It can be contrasted to Erb palsy, which affects C5 and C6.

malrotation A congenital anomaly of rotation of the midgut, the small bowel is found predominantly on the right side of the abdomen. Results in increased incidence of intestinal volvulus.

meconium A dark green fecal material that accumulates in the fetal intestines and is discharged around the time of birth.

multifocal seizure Seizure activity that involves more than one site, is asynchronous, and is usually migratory.

neonate Infant during the first month after birth.

newborn Infant within the first few hours after birth.

oligohydramnios Decreased volume of amniotic fluid during a pregnancy; a risk factor associated with abnormalities of the urinary tract, postmaturity (birth after a prolonged pregnancy), and intrauterine growth retardation.

patent ductus arteriosus A situation in which the ductus arteriosus, which assists in fetal circulation, does not transition as it should after birth to become the ligamentum arteriosum; the result is that the connection between the pulmonary artery and the aorta remains, allowing some oxygenated blood to move back into the heart rather than all of it moving out of the aorta and into the systemic circulation.

persistent pulmonary hypertension Delayed transition from fetal to neonatal circulation.

Pierre Robin sequence A condition present at birth marked by a small lower jaw (micrognathia). The tongue tends to fall back and downward (glossoptosis), and there is a cleft soft palate.

placenta previa Abnormal location of the placenta in the lower part of the uterus, near or over the cervix.

polycythemia Abnormally high red blood cell count.

polyhydramnios An excessive amount of amniotic fluid. May cause preterm labor.

postterm Any pregnancy that lasts more than 42 weeks.

preductal oxygen saturation The pulse oximetry value obtained during neonatal resuscitation, which

Prep Kit (continued)

evaluates the oxygenation status of blood from the brachiocephalic artery, prior to the ductus arteriosus. Tissues perfused with blood from the brachiocephalic artery better reflect the oxygenation status of the heart and brain. This value is best obtained from the right hand or earlobe.

premature Underdeveloped; the condition of an infant born too soon. Refers to infants delivered before 37 weeks from the first day of the last menstrual period.

preterm Describes an infant delivered at less than 37 completed weeks.

primary apnea Apnea caused by oxygen deprivation; usually corrected with stimulation, such as drying or slapping the newborn's feet. Primary apnea is typically preceded by an initial period of rapid breathing.

primigravida First pregnancy.

prolapsed cord When the umbilical cord presents itself outside of the uterus while the fetus is still inside; an obstetric emergency during pregnancy or labor that acutely endangers the life of the fetus; can happen when the amniotic sac breaks and with the gush of amniotic fluid the cord comes along.

pulmonary hypertension Elevated blood pressure in the pulmonary arteries from constriction; causes problems with the blood flow in the lungs, and makes the heart work harder.

pulmonary stenosis Narrowing of the pulmonary valve.

retinopathy of prematurity A disease of the eye that affects premature infants, thought to be caused by disorganized growth of retinal blood vessels resulting in scarring and retinal detachment; can lead to blindness in serious cases.

secondary apnea When asphyxia continues after primary apnea, the infant responds with a period of gasping respirations, falling pulse rate, and falling blood pressure. Positive pressure ventilation is indicated to reverse secondary apnea.

small for gestational age An infant whose size and weight are considerably less than the average for infants of the same age.

term Describes a newborn delivered at 38 to 42 weeks of gestation.

tetralogy of Fallot A cardiac anomaly that consists of four defects: a ventricular septal defect, pulmonary stenosis, right ventricular hypertrophy, and an overriding aorta.

thermoregulation The process by which the body maintains temperature through a combination of heat gain by metabolic processes and muscular movement and heat loss through respiration, evaporation, conduction, convection, and perspiration.

total anomalous pulmonary venous return A rare congenital defect in which the four pulmonary veins do not connect to the left atrium; instead, the pulmonary veins connect to the right atrium, resulting in diminished oxygen and an increased load on the right ventricle.

transposition of the great arteries A defect in which the great vessels are reversed; the aorta is connected to the right ventricle, and the pulmonary artery is connected to the left ventricle.

tricuspid atresia The absence of a tricuspid valve, which normally separates the right atrium and the right ventricle.

truncus arteriosus A condition in which the pulmonary artery and the aorta are combined into one.

umbilical vein The blood vessel in the umbilical cord used to administer emergency medications.

ventricular septal defect A hole in the septum separating the ventricles, allowing blood from the left ventricle to flow into the right ventricle.

▶ References

1. Kliegman RM, Stanton BF, St. Geme JW, Schor NF. Chapter 100: delivery room emergencies. In: *Nelson Textbook of Pediatrics*. 20th ed. Philadelphia, PA: Elsevier; 2016:844.
2. Weiner GM, Zaichkin J. Lesson 1: foundations of neonatal resuscitation. In: *Textbook of Neonatal Resuscitation (NRP)*. 7th ed. Elk Grove Village, IL: American Academy of Pediatrics; 2016:3.
3. Kliegman RM, Stanton BF, St. Geme JW, Schor NF. Chapter 97: the high risk infant. In: *Nelson Textbook of Pediatrics*. 20th ed. Philadelphia, PA: Elsevier; 2016:822.
4. Weiner GM, Zaichkin J. *Textbook of Neonatal Resuscitation (NRP)*. 7th ed. Elk Grove Village, IL: American Academy of Pediatrics; 2016.
5. Weiner GM, Zaichkin J. Lesson 3: initial steps of newborn care. In: *Textbook of Neonatal Resuscitation (NRP)*. 7th ed. Elk Grove Village, IL: American Academy of Pediatrics; 2016:36.
6. Rockefeller S. Rexburg family sues city after paramedics severely burn newborn baby. East Idaho

Prep Kit (continued)

News website. https://www.eastidahonews
.com/2016/10/local-family-sues-city-after
-paramedics-burn-newborn-baby/. Updated
October 23, 2016. Accessed April 20, 2017.

7. The Virginia Apgar Papers: Biographical
information. U.S. National Library of Medicine
website. https://profiles.nlm.nih.gov/ps/retrieve
/Narrative/CP/p-nid/178. Accessed April 6, 2017.

8. Wyckoff MH, Aziz K, Escobedo MB, et al.
Part 13: neonatal resuscitation: 2015
American Heart Association guidelines update
for cardiopulmonary resuscitation and emergency
cardiovascular care. *Circulation.* 2015;132
(suppl 2):S544.

9. American Heart Association. *2015 Handbook
of Emergency Cardiovascular Care for Healthcare
Providers.* Dallas, TX: American Heart Association;
2015:73.

10. Weiner GM, Zaichkin J. Lesson 3: initial steps of
newborn care. In: *Textbook of Neonatal Resuscitation
(NRP).* 7th ed. Elk Grove Village, IL: American
Academy of Pediatrics; 2016:39.

11. Weiner GM, Zaichkin J. Lesson 3: initial steps of
newborn care. In: *Textbook of Neonatal Resuscitation
(NRP).* 7th ed. Elk Grove Village, IL: American
Academy of Pediatrics; 2016:42.

12. Weiner GM, Zaichkin J. Lesson 3: initial steps of
newborn care. In: *Textbook of Neonatal Resuscitation
(NRP).* 7th ed. Elk Grove Village, IL: American
Academy of Pediatrics; 2016:44.

13. Wyckoff MH, Aziz K, Escobedo MB, Kapadia VS,
Kattwinkel J, Perlman JM, Simon WM, Weiner
GM, Zaichkin, JG. Part 13: neonatal resuscitation:
2015 American Heart Association Guidelines
Update for Cardiopulmonary Resuscitation and
Emergency Cardiovascular Care. *Circulation.*
2015;132(suppl 2):S547.

14. Wyckoff MH, Aziz K, Escobedo MB, et al. Part 13:
neonatal resuscitation: 2015 American Heart
Association guidelines update for cardiopulmonary
resuscitation and emergency cardiovascular care.
Circulation. 2015;132(suppl 2):S549.

15. Weiner GM, Zaichkin J. Lesson 3: initial steps of
newborn care. In: *Textbook of Neonatal Resuscitation
(NRP).* 7th ed. Elk Grove Village, IL: American
Academy of Pediatrics; 2016:187.

16. Wyckoff MH, Aziz K, Escobedo MB, et al. Part 13:
neonatal resuscitation: 2015 American Heart
Association guidelines update for cardiopulmonary
resuscitation and emergency cardiovascular care.
Circulation. 2015;132(suppl 2):S543.

17. Jain L, Ferre C, Vidyasagar D, et al.
Cardiopulmonary resuscitation of apparently
stillborn infants: survival and long-term outcome.
J Pediatrics. 1991;118(5):778-782.

18. Haddad B, Mercer BM, Livingston JC, et al. Outcome
after successful resuscitation of babies born with
Apgar scores of 0 at both 1 and 5 minutes. *Am
J Obstet Gynecol.* 2000;182(5):1210-1214.

19. Harrington DJ, Redman CW, Moulden M,
Greenwood CE. The long-term outcome in surviving
infants with Apgar zero at 10 minutes: a systematic
review of the literature and hospital-based cohort.
Am J Obstet Gynecol. 2007;196:463.e1-463.e5.

20. Kasdorf E, Laptook A, Azzopardi D, et al.
Improving infant outcome with a 10 min
Apgar of 0. *Arch Dis Child Fetal Neonatal Ed.*
2015;100:F102-F105.

21. Reuter S, Moser C, Baack M. Respiratory distress in
the newborn. *Pediatr Review.* 2014;35(10):417-428.

22. Kliegman RM, Stanton BF, St. Geme JW, Schor NF.
Chapter 100: delivery room emergencies. In: *Nelson
Textbook of Pediatrics.* 20th ed. Philadelphia, PA:
Elsevier; 2016:845.

23. Weiner GM, Zaichkin J. Lesson 3: initial steps of
newborn care. In: *Textbook of Neonatal Resuscitation
(NRP).* 7th ed. Elk Grove Village, IL: American
Academy of Pediatrics; 2016:49.

24. Weiner GM, Zaichkin J. Lesson 3: initial steps of
newborn care. In: *Textbook of Neonatal Resuscitation
(NRP).* 7th ed. Elk Grove Village, IL: American
Academy of Pediatrics; 2016:47.

25. Kliegman RM, Stanton BF, St. Geme JW, Schor NF.
Chapter 100: delivery room emergencies. In: *Nelson
Textbook of Pediatrics.* 20th ed. Philadelphia, PA:
Elsevier; 2016:846.

26. Delivery of a newborn with meconium-stained
amniotic fluid. Committee Opinion No
689. American College of Obstetricians and
Gynecologists. *Obstet Gynecol.* 2017;129:e33-e34.

27. Weiner GM, Zaichkin J. Lesson 3: initial steps of
newborn care. In: *Textbook of Neonatal Resuscitation
(NRP).* 7th ed. Elk Grove Village, IL: American
Academy of Pediatrics; 2016:51.

28. Kliegman RM, Stanton BF, St. Geme JW, Schor NF.
Chapter 101: respiratory tract disorders. In: *Nelson
Textbook of Pediatrics.* 20th ed. Philadelphia, PA:
Elsevier; 2016:862.

29. Weiner GM, Zaichkin J. Lesson 6: chest
compressions. In: *Textbook of Neonatal Resuscitation
(NRP).* 7th ed. Elk Grove Village, IL: American
Academy of Pediatrics; 2016:166.

30. Weiner GM, Zaichkin J. Lesson 6: chest
compressions. In: *Textbook of Neonatal Resuscitation
(NRP).* 7th ed. Elk Grove Village, IL: American
Academy of Pediatrics; 2016:171.

31. Kliegman RM, Stanton BF, St. Geme JW, Schor NF.
Chapter 100: delivery room emergencies. In: *Nelson
Textbook of Pediatrics.* 20th ed. Philadelphia, PA:
Elsevier; 2016:847.

Prep Kit (continued)

32. Kliegman RM, Stanton BF, St. Geme JW, Schor NF. Chapter 105: the umbilicus. In: *Nelson Textbook of Pediatrics.* 20th ed. Philadelphia, PA: Elsevier; 2016:890.

33. Kliegman RM, Stanton BF, St. Geme JW, Schor NF. Chapter 97: the high-risk infant. In: *Nelson Textbook of Pediatrics.* 20th ed. Philadelphia, PA: Elsevier; 2016:831.

34. Lee SK, Zupancic JAF, Pendray M, et al. Transport risk index of physiologic instability: a practical system for assessing infant transport care. *J Pediatrics.* 2001;139(2):220-226.

35. Weiner GM, Zaichkin J. Lesson 8: post-resuscitation care. In: *Textbook of Neonatal Resuscitation (NRP).* 7th ed. Elk Grove Village, IL: American Academy of Pediatrics; 2016:221.

36. Kliegman RM, Stanton BF, St. Geme JW, Schor NF. Chapter 101: respiratory tract disorders. In: *Nelson Textbook of Pediatrics.* 20th ed. Philadelphia, PA: Elsevier; 2016:859.

37. Beckmann CR. Chapter 15: preterm labor. In: *Obstetrics and Gynecology.* 7th ed. Philadelphia, PA: Wolters Kluwer Health/Lippincott Williams & Wilkins; 2014:157.

38. Kliegman RM, Stanton BF, St. Geme JW, Schor NF. Chapter 593: seizures in childhood. In: *Nelson Textbook of Pediatrics.* 20th ed. Philadelphia, PA: Elsevier; 2016:2849.

39. Kliegman RM, Stanton BF, St. Geme JW, Schor NF. Chapter 593: seizures in childhood. In: *Nelson Textbook of Pediatrics.* 20th ed. Philadelphia, PA: Elsevier; 2016:2849-2850.

40. Kliegman RM, Stanton BF, St. Geme JW, Schor NF. Chapter 593: seizures in childhood. In: *Nelson Textbook of Pediatrics.* 20th ed. Philadelphia, PA: Elsevier; 2016:2850.

41. Kliegman RM, Stanton BF, St. Geme JW, Schor NF. Chapter 593: seizures in childhood. In: *Nelson Textbook of Pediatrics.* 20th ed. Philadelphia, PA: Elsevier; 2016:2851.

42. Kliegman RM, Stanton BF, St. Geme JW, Schor NF. Chapter 92: hypoglycemia. In: *Nelson Textbook of Pediatrics.* 20th ed. Philadelphia, PA: Elsevier; 2016:787.

43. Kliegman RM, Stanton BF, St. Geme JW, Schor NF. Chapter 107: the endocrine system. In: *Nelson Textbook of Pediatrics.* 20th ed. Philadelphia, PA: Elsevier; 2016:898.

44. Adamkin DH. Postnatal glucose homeostasis in late-preterm and term infants. *Pediatrics.* 2011;127(3):575-579.

45. Czinn SJ, Blanchard S. Gastroesophageal reflux disease in neonates and infants: when and how to treat. *Paediatr Drugs.* 2013;15(1):19.

46. Cassina M, Ruol M, Pertile R, et al. Prevalence, characteristics, and survival of children with esophageal atresia: a 32-year population-based study including 1,417,724 consecutive newborns. *Birth Defects Res A Clin Mol Teratol.* 2016;106(7):542-548.

47. Kliegman RM, Stanton BF, St. Geme JW, Schor NF. Chapter 323: gastroesophageal reflux disease. In: *Nelson Textbook of Pediatrics.* 20th ed. Philadelphia, PA: Elsevier; 2016:1787.

48. Kliegman RM, Stanton BF, St. Geme JW, Schor NF. Chapter 329: pyloric stenosis and other congenital anomalies of the stomach. In: *Nelson Textbook of Pediatrics.* 20th ed. Philadelphia, PA: Elsevier; 2016:1797.

49. Kliegman RM, Stanton BF, St. Geme JW, Schor NF. Chapter 330: intestinal atresia, stenosis, and malrotation. In: *Nelson Textbook of Pediatrics.* 20th ed. Philadelphia, PA: Elsevier; 2016:1803.

50. Bensard DD. Intestinal malrotation. Medscape website. http://emedicine.medscape.com /article/930313-overview#a6. Updated March 2, 2017. Accessed April 19, 2017.

51. Messineo A, MacMillan JH, Palder SB, Filler RM. Clinical factors affecting mortality in children with malrotation of the intestine. *J Pediatr Surg.* 1992;27(10):1343-1345.

52. Rescorla FJ, Shedd FJ, Grosfeld JL, Vane DW, West KW. Anomalies of intestinal rotation in childhood: analysis of 447 cases. *Surgery.* 1990;108(4):710-715;discussion 715-716.

53. Wallberg SV, Qvist N. Increased risk of complications in acute onset intestinal malrotation. *Dan Med J.* 2013;60(12):A4744.

54. Kliegman RM, Stanton BF, St. Geme JW, Schor NF. Chapter 340: acute gastroenteritis in children. In: *Nelson Textbook of Pediatrics.* 20th ed. Philadelphia, PA: Elsevier; 2016:1863.

55. Kliegman RM, Stanton BF, St. Geme JW, Schor NF. Chapter 340: acute gastroenteritis in children. In: *Nelson Textbook of Pediatrics.* 20th ed. Philadelphia, PA: Elsevier; 2016:1867.

56. Kliegman RM, Stanton BF, St. Geme JW, Schor NF. Chapter 177: fever without a focus. In: *Nelson Textbook of Pediatrics.* 20th ed. Philadelphia, PA: Elsevier; 2016:1280.

57. Ambalavanan N, Carlo WA, Shankaran S, et al. Predicting outcomes of neonates diagnosed with hypoxemic-ischemic encephalopathy. *Pediatrics.* 2006;118(5):2084-2093.

58. Bonifacio SL, Glass HC, Vanderpluym J, et al. Perinatal events and early magnetic resonance imaging in therapeutic hypothermia. *J Pediatr.* 2011;158(3):360-365.

59. Chaudhary R, Farrer K, Broster S, McRitchie L, Austin T. Active versus passive cooling during neonatal transport. *Pediatrics.* 2013;132(5):841-846.

Prep Kit (continued)

60. Alexander JM, Leveno KJ, Hauth J, et al. Fetal injury associated with cesarean delivery. *Obstet Gynecol.* 2006;108(4):885-890.

61. Demissie K, Rhoads GG, Smulian JC, et al. Operative vaginal delivery and neonatal and infant adverse outcomes: population based retrospective analysis. *Brit Med J.* 2004;329(7456):24-29. Erratum in: *Brit Med J.* 2004;329(7465):547.

62. Foad SL, Mehlman CT, Ying J. The epidemiology of neonatal brachial plexus palsy in the United States. *J Bone Joint Surg Am.* 2008;90(6):1258-1264.

63. Volpe JJ. Injuries of extracranial, cranial, intracranial, spinal cord, and peripheral nervous system structures. In: *Neurology of the Newborn.* 5th ed. Philadelphia, PA: Saunders; 2008:959.

64. Kliegman RM, Stanton BF, St. Geme JW, Schor NF. Chapter 424: epidemiology and genetic basis of congenital heart disease. In: *Nelson Textbook of Pediatrics.* 20th ed. Philadelphia, PA: Elsevier; 2016:2182.

65. Tennant PW, Pearce MS, Bythell M, Rankin J. 20-year survival of children born with congenital anomalies: a population-based study. *Lancet.* 2010;375(9715):649-656.

66. Canfield MA, Honein MA, Yuskiv N, et al. National estimates and race/ethnic-specific variation of selected birth defects in the United States, 1999-2001. *Birth Defects Res A Clin Mol Teratol.* 2006;76(11):747-756.

67. Bird TM, Hobbs CA, Cleves MA, Tilford JM, Robbins JM. National rates of birth defects among hospitalized newborns. *Birth Defects Res A Clin Mol Teratol.* 2006;76(11):762-769.

68. Kliegman RM, Stanton BF, St. Geme JW, Schor NF. Chapter 425: evaluation and screening of the infant or child with congenital heart disease. In: *Nelson Textbook of Pediatrics.* 20th ed. Philadelphia, PA: Elsevier; 2016:2187.

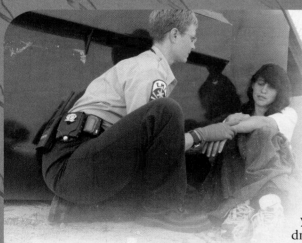

Assessment in Action

You and your partner just delivered a newborn who is premature at 27 weeks' gestation. During your newborn assessment you observe a slow, weak respiratory effort, slow pulse rate, and cyanosis of the trunk and extremities. An additional rescue unit arrives and assumes care of the mother, allowing you and your partner to treat the newborn. After 30 seconds of drying and stimulation there is no change in your assessment.

1. What intervention should be performed immediately?

   A. Chest compressions
   B. Endotracheal intubation
   C. Administration of epinephrine
   D. Positive pressure ventilation

2. Which of the following is the correct ventilation rate for this newborn?

   A. 10 to 20 breaths/min
   B. 20 to 40 breaths/min
   C. 40 to 60 breaths/min
   D. 60 to 80 breaths/min

Assessment *in Action* (continued)

3. If the newborn does not respond to positive pressure ventilation, at what point during resuscitation should chest compressions be started?

    A. If the newborn's pulse rate remains below 60 beats/min following 30 seconds of positive pressure ventilation via a bag-mask device

    B. If the newborn's pulse rate remains below 60 beats/min following 30 seconds of positive pressure ventilation via an endotracheal tube

    C. If the newborn's pulse rate remains below 60 beats/min following 30 seconds of drug administration

    D. If the newborn's pulse rate remains below 60 beats/min following 30 seconds of free-flow oxygen at 5 L/min

4. If the newborn's heart rate does not respond to positive pressure ventilation, how deep should you compress the chest when performing cardiopulmonary resuscitation on the newborn?

    A. Two-thirds the anteroposterior diameter of the chest

    B. One-half the anteroposterior diameter of the chest

    C. One-third the anteroposterior diameter of the chest

    D. One-quarter the anteroposterior diameter of the chest

5. What is the compression-to-ventilation ratio if providing neonatal cardiopulmonary resuscitation to the newborn?

    A. 15:2
    B. 30:2
    C. 3:1
    D. 5:1

6. If the newborn's heart rate does not respond to effective positive pressure ventilation and chest compressions, what is the recommended dose and concentration of epinephrine for the newborn?

    A. 0.3 mg/kg; 0.1 mg/mL (1:10,000) via ET tube

    B. 0.03 mg/kg; 0.1 mg/mL (1:10,000) via umbilical venous line or IV line

    C. 0.3 mg/kg; 1 mg/mL (1:1,000) via IV line

    D. 0.03 mL/kg; 1 mg/mL (1:1,000) via umbilical venous line or ET tube

7. Which intervention is most likely to establish adequate heart rate in the newborn?

    A. Ventilatory support
    B. Chest compressions
    C. Fluid replacement
    D. Medication administration

8. What are some of the factors that can cause a woman to deliver prematurely?

9. What are the indications for artificial ventilation of the newborn?

10. Pulmonary stenosis, a disease in which the pulmonic valve located near the right ventricle of the heart becomes damaged, is typically associated with what?

Pediatric Emergencies

National EMS Education Standard Competencies

Special Patient Populations

Integrates assessment findings with principles of pathophysiology and knowledge of psychosocial needs to formulate a field impression and implement a comprehensive treatment/disposition plan for patients with special needs.

Pediatric Emergencies

Age-related assessment findings, and age-related and developmental stage related assessment and treatment modifications for pediatric-specific major or common diseases and/or emergencies:

> Foreign body (upper and lower) airway obstruction (pp 2138-2140)
> Lower airway reactive disease (pp 2142-2144)
> Respiratory arrest distress/failure (pp 2137-2138)
> Shock (pp 2156-2160)
> Seizures (pp 2168-2169)
> Sudden infant death syndrome (SIDS) (pp 2186-2187)
> Gastrointestinal disease (pp 2172-2174)
> Bacterial tracheitis (pp 2141-2142)
> Asthma (pp 2142-2143)
> Bronchiolitis (pp 2143-2144)
> Respiratory syncytial virus (RSV) (p 2143)
> Pneumonia (p 2144)
> Croup (pp 2140-2141)
> Epiglottitis (p 2141)
> Hyperglycemia (p 2175)
> Hypoglycemia (p 2175)
> Pertussis (p 2144)
> Cystic fibrosis (p 2144)
> Bronchopulmonary dysplasia (pp 2144-2145)
> Hydrocephalus and ventricular shunts (pp 2170-2171)

Patients With Special Challenges

> Recognizing and reporting abuse and neglect (pp 2183-2186 and see Chapter 44, *Geriatric Emergencies*)

Health care implications of
> Abuse (pp 2183-2186 and see Chapter 44, *Geriatric Emergencies*, and Chapter 45, *Patients With Special Challenges*)
> Neglect (pp 2183-2186 and see Chapter 44, *Geriatric Emergencies*, and Chapter 45, *Patients With Special Challenges*)
> Homelessness (see Chapter 45, *Patients With Special Challenges*)
> Poverty (see Chapter 45, *Patients With Special Challenges*)
> Bariatrics (see Chapter 45, *Patients With Special Challenges*)
> Technology dependent (see Chapter 45, *Patients With Special Challenges*)
> Hospice/terminally ill (see Chapter 45, *Patients With Special Challenges*)
> Tracheostomy care/dysfunction (see Chapter 45, *Patients With Special Challenges*)
> Home care (see Chapter 45, *Patients With Special Challenges*)
> Sensory deficit/loss (see Chapter 45, *Patients With Special Challenges*)
> Developmental disability (see Chapter 45, *Patients With Special Challenges*)

Trauma

Integrates assessment findings with principles of epidemiology and pathophysiology to formulate a field impression to implement a comprehensive treatment/disposition plan for an acutely injured patient.

Special Considerations in Trauma

Recognition and management of trauma in the
> Pregnant patient (see Chapter 41, *Obstetrics*)
> Pediatric patient (pp 2187-2192)
> Geriatric patient (see Chapter 44, *Geriatric Emergencies*)

Pathophysiology, assessment, and management of trauma in the
> Pregnant patient (see Chapter 41, *Obstetrics*)
> Pediatric patient (pp 2187-2192)
> Geriatric patient (see Chapter 44, *Geriatric Emergencies*)
> Cognitively impaired patient (see Chapter 45, *Patients With Special Challenges*)

Knowledge Objectives

1. Explain some of the challenges inherent in providing emergency care to pediatric patients and why effective communication with both the patient and his or her family members is crucial to a successful outcome. (p 2118)
2. Describe the developmental stages of children, including examples of each stage. (pp 2118-2120)
3. Describe differences in the anatomy, physiology, and pathophysiology of the pediatric patient as compared with the adult patient and their implications for the health care provider. (pp 2120-2125)
4. Describe challenges in dealing with stressed parents or caregivers of ill and injured children. (p 2125)
5. Describe the steps in the primary survey for providing emergency care to a pediatric patient, including the elements of the Pediatric Assessment Triangle, hands-on ABCDEs, and transport decision considerations. (pp 2125-2133)
6. Describe the steps in the secondary assessment, including the systematic assessment, which may include a full-body examination or a focused assessment on the body part or body system specifically involved. (pp 2133-2136)
7. Describe the different causes of pediatric respiratory emergencies; the signs and symptoms of increased work of breathing; the differences among respiratory distress, respiratory failure, and respiratory arrest; and the emergency medical care strategies used in the management of each. (pp 2136-2138)
8. Explain upper airway emergencies in a pediatric patient, including anaphylaxis, croup, epiglottitis, and bacterial tracheitis; their possible causes, signs, and symptoms; and steps in the management of a child who is experiencing these conditions. (pp 2138-2140, 2145-2155)
9. List the steps in the management of foreign body airway obstruction of an infant and a child. (pp 2139-2140)
10. Explain lower airway emergencies in a pediatric patient, including asthma, infection with RSV, bronchiolitis, pneumonia, and pertussis; their possible causes, signs, and symptoms; and steps in the management of a child who is experiencing these conditions. (pp 2142-2144, 2145-2155)
11. Discuss other respiratory conditions, including cystic fibrosis and bronchopulmonary dysplasia; their possible causes, signs, and symptoms; and steps in the management of a child who is experiencing these conditions. (pp 2144, 2145-2155)
12. Discuss the most common causes of shock (hypoperfusion) in a pediatric patient, its signs and symptoms, and emergency medical management in the field. (pp 2156-2160)
13. Describe the procedure for establishing intravenous access in the pediatric patient. (p 2157)
14. List the steps to establish an intraosseous infusion in pediatric patients. (pp 2157-2159)
15. Describe common pediatric heart rhythm disturbances and management of each dysrhythmia. (pp 2160-2165)
16. Discuss the most common causes of altered mental status in a pediatric patient, its signs and symptoms, and emergency medical management in the field. (pp 2167-2168)
17. List the common causes of seizures in a pediatric patient, the different types of seizures, and their emergency medical management in the field. (pp 2168-2169)
18. List the common causes of meningitis, patient groups who are at the highest risk for contracting this infection, its signs and symptoms, special precautions, and emergency medical management in the field. (pp 2169-2170)
19. Discuss the types of gastrointestinal emergencies that might affect pediatric patients, including biliary atresia, viral gastroenteritis, appendicitis, ingestion of foreign bodies, gastrointestinal bleeding, intussusception, Meckel diverticulum, pyloric stenosis, and malrotation with volvulus. (pp 2172-2174)
20. Discuss the pathophysiology, assessment, and management of endocrine emergencies, including hyperglycemia, hypoglycemia, and congenital adrenal hyperplasia. (pp 2174-2176)
21. Describe conditions in which the pituitary produces inadequate amounts of some or all of its hormones. (p 2176)
22. Describe special considerations in patients with childhood immunodeficiencies. (p 2177)
23. Discuss hematologic disorders, including sickle cell disease, thrombocytopenia, hemophilia, von Willebrand disease, and leukemia and lymphoma; signs and symptoms; special precautions; and emergency medical management in the field. (pp 2177-2179)
24. Discuss toxicologic emergencies in pediatric patients, including common sources, assessment findings, and techniques for emergency medical management, including decontamination and antidotes. (pp 2179-2181)
25. Describe special considerations during the management of a pediatric behavioral or psychiatric emergency, including safety precautions and assessment and management techniques. (pp 2181-2182)
26. Discuss the common causes of a fever emergency in a pediatric patient and management techniques. (pp 2182-2183)
27. Describe child abuse and neglect and its possible indicators, and discuss the medical and legal

responsibilities when caring for a pediatric patient who is a possible victim of child abuse. (pp 2183-2185)

28. Discuss SIDS, including its risk factors, patient assessment, and special management considerations related to the death of an infant patient. (pp 2186-2187)
29. Discuss the common causes of pediatric trauma emergencies and the differences in injury patterns in adults, infants, and children. (pp 2187-2188)
30. Describe the procedure for performing needle decompression in the pediatric patient. (pp 2188-2189)
31. List the steps to immobilize both an infant and a child. (pp 2190-2191)
32. Describe the indications for fluid and pain management for a pediatric trauma patient. (pp 2191-2192)
33. Discuss the significance of burns in pediatric patients, common causes, and general assessment and management techniques. (pp 2192-2193)
34. Describe the needs of technology-assisted children, including the various types of medical technology used. (pp 2193-2195)
35. Describe injury patterns and the potential areas for intervention and prevention. (pp 2195-2196)

Skills Objectives

1. Demonstrate the steps for inserting an oropharyngeal airway in a child. (p 2146, Skill Drill 43-1)
2. Demonstrate the steps for inserting a nasopharyngeal airway in a child. (p 2147, Skill Drill 43-2)
3. Demonstrate how to perform bag-mask ventilation for an infant or child. (pp 2148-2150, Skill Drill 43-3)
4. Demonstrate how to perform endotracheal intubation of a pediatric patient. (pp 2152-2153, Skill Drill 43-4)
5. Describe how to insert an orogastric tube and a nasogastric tube in a pediatric patient, including how to prepare the patient and the equipment and how to assess the placement of the tubes. (pp 2154-2155)
6. Demonstrate how to establish intraosseous access in pediatric patients. (pp 2158-2159, Skill Drill 43-5)
7. Demonstrate how to perform needle decompression in a child. (pp 2188-2189)
8. Demonstrate how to immobilize a child who has been involved in a trauma emergency. (p 2190, Skill Drill 43-6)
9. Demonstrate how to immobilize an infant who has been involved in a trauma emergency. (pp 2190-2191, Skill Drill 43-7)

YOU are the Paramedic PART 1

You and your partner are sitting down for lunch when dispatch sends you to an apartment for a sick child. You are met at the door by a 14-year-old girl. She is crying and saying she cannot wake up her brother. She brings you into the living room, where you see a 3-year-old boy lying supine on the couch. The girl tells you she and her brother were watching television and fell asleep. When she woke up, she discovered that she could not awaken her brother. The girl became scared and called 9-1-1.

Recording Time: 1 Minute	
Appearance	Toddler lying on the couch who appears to be asleep
Level of consciousness	U (unresponsive to verbal or painful stimuli)
Airway	Open
Breathing	Adequate rate and volume; no retractions or audible sounds
Circulation	Pale, cold, dry skin, with mottled extremities; absent radial pulses and weak central pulses

1. Using the Pediatric Assessment Triangle (PAT) as a guide, what is your general impression of the child?
2. Which information would you like to get from the sister?

Introduction

Children differ anatomically, physiologically, and emotionally from adults. In addition, the types of illnesses and injuries they sustain and their responses to them vary across the pediatric age span. Sick or injured children present unique challenges in evaluation and management. Their perceptions of their illness or injury, their world, and you differ from the perceptions of adults. Depending on their ages, they may not be able to report what is bothering them. Fear or pain may make children difficult to assess as well. When interacting with pediatric patients, you will also have to work with concerned parents and caregivers who may be stressed or frightened and acting irrationally. In addition, you must always consider abuse as a possible cause of illness or injury. In the midst of this chaos, you are expected to be an island of calm and authority, carrying out your job systematically, carefully, and confidently.

The manner in which you approach a sick or injured child will depend on the child's age and developmental level. Childhood extends from the neonatal period, just after birth, until age 18 years. An enormous amount of physical and psychologic development occurs in these 18 years. The child's anatomy, physiology, and stage of psychosocial development will all influence your assessment and treatment. For these reasons, you must tailor your approach to accommodate the developmental and social issues unique to pediatric patients.

This chapter addresses some of the special considerations that will enhance your effectiveness in caring for an ill or injured child. It begins by discussing the approach to pediatric patients, with an eye toward their developmental level and the anatomic or physiologic differences unique to this age group. This information is used to outline an approach to pediatric assessment,

review specific pediatric emergencies, and address their prehospital management. Finally, the chapter details the skills needed to care efficiently and effectively for pediatric patients, regardless of the diagnosis.

Developmental Stages

The growth and development of infants, toddlers, preschoolers, school-age children, and adolescents are discussed in Chapter 10, *Life Span Development*. Refer to that chapter to familiarize yourself with pediatric physical and psychosocial stages of development. Infancy and toddlerhood have their own specific phases that are discussed in detail in the next section.

▶ Neonate and Infant

The first month of life is called the neonatal period, whereas infancy refers to the first 12 months of life. Neonates do not do much other than eat, sleep for as much as 16 hours per day, and cry in an attempt to communicate. This can be a particularly difficult time for new parents, adjusting to a demanding schedule. See Chapter 42, *Neonatal Care*, for more information about infants that are younger than age 1 month. As infants reach the 2- to 6-month threshold, they begin to hold their heads up and seek attention. At 6 to 12 months, infants begin to crawl and babble. A great deal of development occurs in this interval Table 43-1 .

Because infants cannot communicate their feelings or needs verbally, it is especially important to respect a caregiver's perception that "something is wrong." Persistent crying, irritability, and lack of eye contact may be a symptom of a serious problem such as a bacterial infection, a cardiac problem, depressed mental status, or an electrolyte disturbance. Nonspecific concerns about a young infant's behavior, feeding, sleep pattern, or arousability may be tip-offs to a serious underlying illness or injury.

Table 43-1	Infant Development		
	Birth to 2 Months	**2 to 6 Months**	**6 to 12 Months**
Physical Development	■ Controls gaze ■ Turns head	■ Can recognize caregivers ■ Makes eye contact ■ Uses both hands ■ Rolls over ■ Most sleep through the night	■ Sits without support ■ Crawls ■ Puts things in mouth ■ Teething begins ■ Eats soft foods
Cognitive Development	■ Begins crying to communicate needs ■ Crying peaks at 6 weeks	■ Increased awareness ■ Explores own body	■ Babbles (learns first word by 12 months) ■ Remembers objects ■ Curious about what objects do
Emotional Development	■ Trust develops in parents	■ Uses expressions of joy, anger, fear, surprise ■ Seeks attention	■ Separation anxiety develops ■ Start of tantrums ■ Self-determination while eating

Table 43-2	Toddler Development	
	12 to 18 Months	**18 to 24 Months**
Physical Development	• Crawls • Walks • Front teeth emerge ahead of molars • Undergoes sensory development	• Has improved gait and balance • Runs • Climbs • Head grows more slowly than body
Cognitive Development	• Imitates others • Makes believe • Understands more than expressed • Knows major body parts • Knows 4 to 6 words	• Begins to understand cause and effect • Labels objects • Speech picks up to approximately 100 words by 24 months
Emotional Development	• Demonstrates basic reasoning • Understands object permanence • Demonstrates separation anxiety	• Demonstrates attachment to certain objects, such as a pacifier, doll, or blanket

© Jones & Bartlett Learning.

You should also pay particular attention to the child's stage of development because increased mobility in an infant or toddler can often lead to injury. Any behaviors out of line with development (eg, a 2-month-old infant who reportedly sustained injuries from rolling off of a couch) should increase your suspicion for the possibility of abuse; the history should match the child's developmental stage.

Consider the best location for performing your assessment and keep the child warm to avoid hypothermia. Support the head and neck of young infants. Although separating a 2-week-old infant from a parent will not cause distress, an older infant in stable condition will be calmest in a parent's arms. Make sure your hands and stethoscope are warm; a startled, crying infant will be difficult to examine. Be opportunistic with your exam, use a soft voice, and smile. If the child is quiet, listen to the heart and lungs first. If a young infant starts crying, letting the infant suck on a pacifier or gloved finger may quiet the child enough to allow you to complete your assessment. Jingling keys or shining a penlight may distract an older infant long enough for you to finish an exam. Do not provide small objects that pose a risk of aspiration.

Words of Wisdom

Keep infants and young children close to their parents during your assessment to help them feel safe and to improve your ability to perform the assessment.

▶ Toddler

The toddler period includes the ages from 1 to 2 years. It includes the "terrible twos," a behavioral manifestation of the child's struggle between the continued dependence on caregivers for food, shelter, and love and the emerging drive for independence Table 43-2 . Children in this age group are not capable of reasoning, and they have a poorly developed sense of cause and effect. Language development is occurring rapidly, along with the ability to explore the world by crawling, walking, running, and climbing. Many toddlers will develop associations—possibly negative—with health care providers. Painful procedures may make lasting impressions.

Your assessment of a toddler begins with observation of the child's interactions with the caregiver, vocalizations, and mobility, measured through the PAT, which is described in detail later. Examine a toddler in stable condition on the parent's lap so as to avoid separation anxiety. Get down to the child's level, sitting or squatting for the exam. Talk to the child throughout the assessment. You may need to be creative to perform a good exam on a toddler with stranger anxiety: Use a parent to lift the shirt so that you can count the respiratory rate, or have the parent press on the child's abdomen to see if that appears painful. Use play and distraction techniques whenever possible; listening to a doll's chest first may buy you a few minutes of cooperation. Offer toddlers limited choices when possible because they like to be in control. If you ask yes-or-no questions, the answer is likely to be "No!" Consider saving the more upsetting parts of the exam, such as palpating a tender abdomen or examining an injured extremity, for last. Be flexible in your approach; some toddlers will not let you complete an orderly head-to-toe exam.

▶ Preschool-Age Child

During the preschool years (3 to 5 years), the child is becoming rapidly verbal and active. He or she can understand directions and be engaged with an activity or set of goals. Generally, a preschooler will be able to tell you what hurts and may have a story to share about the illness or injury. Preschoolers will understand as you explain what you are going to do, but choose your words carefully because preschoolers are very literal. Saying "I'm going take your pulse" may lead preschoolers to believe that you are taking something from them and wonder if you plan to give it back! Speak to them in plain language about what you are going to do and provide lots of reassurance. This is the stage of monsters under the bed and many other fears. At this age, they often believe that their thoughts or wishes can cause injury or harm to themselves or to others. They may believe that an injury is the result of a bad deed they did earlier in the day.

By age 4 years, the child develops 20/20 vision and performs normal running and walking, in addition to throwing, catching, and kicking as a school-age child would. Right- or left-handedness is also discovered.

As you perform your assessment, take advantage of the child's curiosity, rich fantasy life, and desire to cooperate. Respect the child's modesty by keeping him or her covered. If the child is in medically stable condition, offer to take turns in listening to the heart and lungs. Let the preschooler play with or hold equipment that is safe. To help give the child some sense of control, offer simple choices and avoid procedures on the dominant hand or arm. Tantrums may occur when preschool-age children feel they cannot control the situation or its outcomes. Avoid yes-or-no questions. Set limits on behavior if the child acts out; children at this age know what acceptable behavior is. Appeal to their thinking and you should be able to talk a preschooler through an orderly exam.

▶ School-Age Child (Middle Childhood)

As a child enters the school-age period (6 to 12 years), he or she becomes much more analytic and capable of abstract thought. School is important at this stage, and concerns about popularity and peer pressure occupy a great deal of time and energy. At this age, the child can understand cause and effect. Children with chronic illness or disabilities can become self-conscious because of concerns about fitting in with their peers. At this stage, children begin to understand that death is final, which may increase their anxieties about illness or injury. School-age children will have their own stories to tell about the illness or injury and may have their own ideas about the care to be given. By age 8 years, the child's anatomy and physiology are similar to those of adults. Girls develop breasts between ages 8 and 13 years, and their menstrual period begins between ages 9 and 16 years. Boys experience an increase in the size of their testicles around age 10 years. Children at this age may be self-conscious about their body image.

During assessment of a school-age child, ask the child about the history leading to calling 9-1-1 and let the child describe the symptoms, rather than focusing on the caregiver. Explain what you plan to do in simple language, and answer the child's questions. Give the child

appropriate choices and control whenever possible, and provide ongoing reassurance and encouragement.

School-age children can understand the difference between emotional and physical pain. They also have concerns about the meaning of pain. Give them simple explanations about what is causing their pain and what will be done about it. Respect the modesty of these patients and keep them covered as much as possible during your examination. Games and conversation may distract them. Asking about school will often allow them to warm up to you. Ask them to describe their favorite place, their pets, or their toys. Ask the caregiver's advice in choosing the right distraction.

Rewarding the school-age child after a procedure can be helpful in his or her recovery, but reward a child only for completing the procedure.

▶ Adolescence

The adolescent years, from 13 to 18 years, can be difficult. Adolescents are struggling with issues of independence, body image, sexuality, and peer pressure. Friends are key support figures, and this is a time of experimentation and risk-taking behaviors. Adolescents begin to understand who they are, and they develop morals and the ability to reason. Relationships may shift from same sex to those with the opposite sex. With respect to cardiopulmonary respiration (CPR) and foreign body airway obstruction procedures, once secondary sexual characteristics have developed (breasts or facial/axillary hair), the child should be treated as an adult.

During the assessment, you must address and reassure the patient. Failure to do so can result in the adolescent feeling left out of his or her own care, which can alienate the patient, making it difficult for you to get an accurate assessment or give appropriate treatment. Encourage the patient's questions and involvement. Address all concerns and fears. Also, provide accurate information; a teen may become alienated and uncooperative if you are suspected of being misleading.

When you perform the physical exam, respect the patient's privacy. If possible, address the adolescent without a caregiver present, especially about sensitive topics such as sexuality or drug use. If the adolescent's friends are on scene, he or she may want them to remain during the assessment. Let the patient have as much control over the situation as appropriate. Of course, do not let down your guard regarding scene safety.

■ Pediatric Anatomy, Physiology, and Pathophysiology

Anatomic and physiologic differences can create difficulties with your assessment of the child if you do not understand them. This section provides an overview of the anatomic and physiologic differences of children.

Special Populations

Because of their proportionately large heads, children are more vulnerable to head injuries than adults are.

▶ The Head

When you are looking at infants or young children, you will note that children have heads that are large relative to the rest of their bodies. In fact, an infant's head is already two-thirds the size it will be in adulthood. The large surface area means more mass relative to the rest of the body—an important factor in the high incidence of head injuries in young patients, who tend to lead with their head in a fall.

Because of the proportionally larger occiput, special care must be taken when you are positioning the child's airway. In seriously injured children younger than 2 years, place a thin layer of padding under the shoulders or upper torso to obtain a neutral position. In seriously ill children older than 2 years, a folded sheet placed under the occiput may be required to obtain a sniffing position. The large head also means more surface area for heat loss. Always keep the child's head covered to conserve warmth.

During infancy, the anterior and posterior fontanelles are open. The fontanels are areas where the infant's skull bones have not fused together, thereby allowing for compression of the head during the birthing process and for rapid growth of the brain. By the time the child reaches 4 months, the posterior fontanels close; by the time the child reaches 2 years, the anterior fontanels close.

The fontanels are an important anatomic landmark when you are assessing a sick or injured infant. Bulging fontanels suggest increased intracranial pressure (ICP); sunken fontanels suggest dehydration. These conditions will be discussed later in this chapter.

▶ The Neck and Airway

Children have short, stubby necks, which can make it difficult for you to feel a carotid pulse or see jugular veins. Not surprisingly, the airway of a young child is also much smaller than that of an adult. That smaller diameter makes the airway more prone to obstruction, either by foreign body inhalation, inflammation with infection, or the child's disproportionally large tongue. During the first few months of life, infants are obligate nose breathers, and nasal obstruction with mucus can result in significant respiratory distress. Their epiglottis is long, floppy, U-shaped, and narrow, extending at a 45° angle into the airway, making it difficult to visualize the vocal cords during intubation. Finally, the narrowest part of a young child's airway occurs at the level of the cricoid cartilage below the vocal cords, rather than at the vocal cords as in adults; this issue should influence your choice of endotracheal (ET) tubes.

You must have a thorough understanding of the anatomic and physiologic differences in the child's airway to provide appropriate management. With the aforementioned anatomic differences, it is important for you to remember the following:

- Keep the nares clear with suctioning in infants younger than 24 months. Nasal congestion is enough to cause respiratory distress in infants and toddlers.
- The tracheal cartilage in a child is softer and more collapsible as compared with that in an adult; avoid hyperextension of the child's neck. Hyperextension may result in reverse hyperflexion and kinking of the trachea; it may also displace the tongue posteriorly, creating an airway obstruction.
- Keep the airway clear of all secretions; even a small amount of particulate matter may result in an airway obstruction.
- Use care when you are managing the child's airway, such as when you are inserting airway adjuncts; the jaw is smaller than an adult's jaw and the soft tissues are delicate and prone to swelling. In many cases, the child's airway can be maintained by correct positioning, thereby negating the use of airway adjuncts (ie, oral or nasal airways).

▶ The Respiratory System

Proportionally, tidal volume in children is slightly smaller than in adults. However, the metabolic oxygen demand of children is doubled. In addition, their functional residual capacity is smaller, resulting in proportionally smaller oxygen reserves. Functional residual capacity is the volume of air remaining in the lungs following exhalation, also referred to as oxygen reserve.

An infant breathes faster than an older child breathes. The child's lungs will grow and develop better abilities to handle the exchange of oxygen as the child ages. A respiratory rate of 30 to 60 breaths/min is normal for newborns, whereas teenagers are expected to have rates closer to the adult range **Table 43-3**.

The higher respiratory rate and oxygen demand needed to meet the higher metabolic rate of infants and children put them at higher risk for effects from inhaled toxins. Compared to adults, children typically inhale a proportionally larger amount of toxic fumes from the same environment and therefore become symptomatic sooner.

Infants have little use of their chest muscles to make their chests expand during inspiration; they use the diaphragm (belly breathers). Anything that puts pressure on the abdomen of an infant or young child can block the movement of the diaphragm and cause respiratory compromise. Young children also experience muscle fatigue much more quickly than do older children, which can lead to respiratory failure if a child has had to breathe hard for long periods.

Table 43-3	**Pediatric Respiratory Rates**
Age	**Respirations (breaths/min)**
Neonate (0 to 1 month)	30 to 60
Infant (1 month to 1 year)	30 to 53
Toddler (1 to 2 years)	22 to 37
Preschooler (3 to 5 years)	20 to 28
School-age child (6 to 12 years)	18 to 25
Adolescent (12 to 15 years)	12 to 20

Data from: American Heart Association (AHA). Vital signs in children. In: AHA. *Pediatric Advanced Life Support*. Dallas, TX: AHA; 2015.

Table 43-4	**Pediatric Pulse Rates**	
Age	**Awake Rate (beats/min)**	**Asleep Rate (beats/min)**
Neonate (0 to 1 month)	100 to 205	90 to 160
Infant (1 month to 1 year)	100 to 180	90 to 160
Toddler (1 to 2 years)	98 to 140	80 to 120
Preschooler (3 to 5 years)	80 to 120	65 to 100
School-age child (6 to 12 years)	75 to 118	58 to 90

Data from: American Heart Association (AHA). Vital signs in children. In: AHA. *Pediatric Advanced Life Support*. Dallas, TX: AHA; 2015.

You must be aware that infants and children, especially during respiratory distress, are susceptible to hypoxia because of their decreased functional residual capacity, increased oxygen demand, and easily fatigued respiratory muscles. Infants and children will develop hypoxia rapidly with apnea and ineffective bagging and can spiral into cardiovascular collapse and arrest. Hypoxia is the most common cause of bradycardia and cardiovascular collapse in children. Use a larger bag if needed to ventilate a pediatric patient, but use only enough pressure to achieve visible chest rise so as to avoid pneumothorax. The bag's volume should have no less than 450–500 mL. The goal is to maintain a pediatric oxygen saturation level of greater than 94%. Special considerations are necessary with children who have uncorrected cardiac disease, as some of these patients may have baseline oxygenation rates that are less than 90% on room air. Similarly, oxygen saturation levels for patients with certain congenital cardiac defects can be in the 75% to 80% range. Increased oxygenation could lead to harm in these patient groups; this state is best clarified with the parent.

▶ The Cardiovascular System

It is important for you to know the normal pulse rate ranges when you are evaluating children because this is the primary method for the child's body to compensate for decreased oxygenation (Table 43-4). Children rely mainly on their pulse rate to maintain adequate cardiac output. An infant's pulse rate can be 200 beats/min or more if the body needs to compensate for injury or illness.

Children have limited but vigorous cardiac reserves. Proportionally, they have a larger circulating blood volume per kilogram of body weight compared with adults; however, their absolute blood volume is less, approximately 70 mL/kg. Constriction of the child's blood vessels (vasoconstriction) provides the ability to keep vital organs well perfused.

Because a child has a relatively large circulating blood volume compared with an adult, injured children can maintain their blood pressure for longer periods than adults can, even though they are still in shock (hypoperfusion). In other words, a proportionally larger volume of blood loss must occur in the child before hypotension develops.

Suspect shock when an infant or child presents with tachycardia. Bradycardia, however, usually indicates severe hypoxia and must be managed aggressively. Remember that hypotension, when it occurs in a child, is an ominous sign and often indicates impending cardiopulmonary arrest.

Constriction of the blood vessels can be so profound that blood flow to the periphery of the body diminishes. Signs of vasoconstriction can include weak peripheral pulses, delayed capillary refill in children younger than 6 years (capillary refill less than 2 seconds is normal for children), and pale, cool extremities.

Special Populations

When you are assessing a sick or injured child, be aware that bradycardia is most often the result of hypoxia; therefore, treatment is aimed at ensuring adequate oxygenation and ventilation. In addition, despite the presence of a normal blood pressure, a child may still be in shock.

The Heart

Circulation in the fetus is much different from that in the newborn, and large right-sided forces on the electro-cardiogram (ECG) are normal in young infants. During the first year of life, the ECG axis and voltages shift to reflect left ventricular dominance. Cardiac output is rate dependent in infants and young children. They have relatively poor ability to increase stroke volume, which is reflected in their normal pulse rates (higher in newborns than in older children and adults) and in rate response to physiologic stress and hypovolemia.

The mediastinum of pediatric patients is more mobile than that of adults. This is important to remember when you are dealing with pediatric trauma or abuse cases because these patients are at a high risk of injury to mediastinal organs that may not be immediately evident on exam. Cardiac tamponade can present with muffled heart tones, whereas cardiac contusions can cause dysrhythmias.

▶ The Nervous System

The nervous system continually develops throughout childhood. Until the nervous system is fully developed, the neural tissue and vasculature are fragile, easily damaged, and prone to bleeding from injury. The brain and spinal cord are not as well protected by the developing skull and spinal vertebrae. As a consequence, it takes less force to cause brain and spinal cord injuries in children than in adults.

The subarachnoid space in a child is relatively smaller than that of an adult, providing less cushioning effect for the brain. Bruising and damage to the brain may be the result of head momentum such as is seen with "shaken baby syndrome." The pediatric brain also requires nearly twice the cerebral blood flow as an adult's brain, making even minor injuries significant. This requirement increases the risk of hypoxia. Head injuries are greatly exacerbated by hypoxia and hypotension, causing ongoing damage.

The brain continues to develop after birth. As the brain matures, the infant's responses to the environment, outside stimuli, and even pain become more organized and purposeful. The rapidity of brain development can be appreciated by comparing the abilities and interactions of a 4-day-old infant, whose repertoire is limited to eating, sleeping, and defecating, with those of a 4-month-old infant, who smiles socially, rolls over, and plays with a rattle, and with those of a 12-month-old infant, who walks, is beginning to talk, and expresses preferences for people and activities.

The Spinal Column

The vertebral column develops along with the child. When the child is younger, the cervical spine fulcrum (or bending point) is higher, closer to C1-C2, because the head is heavier and proportionally larger than the adult head. As the child grows, the fulcrum descends to "adult level," around C5 through C7. An infant who sustains blunt head trauma involving acceleration-deceleration forces is at high risk for a fatal, high cervical spinal injury. By comparison, a school-age child who experiences the same injury will likely sustain a lower cervical spinal injury and may be paralyzed.

Fortunately, vertebral fractures and spinal cord injuries in young children are uncommon. Spinal ligaments and joint capsules are more lax in children than in adults, leading to increased mobility and the phenomenon of cord injury in the absence of identifiable vertebral bony fracture or dislocation. Vertebral bodies are also aligned anteriorly and can slide forward, potentially causing cord damage with significant forward flexion.

> ### Words of Wisdom
>
> Spinal cord injuries with normal-appearing radiographs are referred to as SCIWORA (spinal cord injury without radiographic abnormalities). Children are more prone to SCIWORA-type injuries because of ligamentous laxity that is not present in adults.

Thoracic and lumbar spinal injuries are also encountered relatively infrequently until a child is pursuing adult activities, such as driving and diving. Nevertheless, these injuries are seen in children in association with specific mechanisms—for example, seat belt–associated lumbar spine injuries (often associated with abdominal injury) and compression fracture due to axial loading in a fall. When you are confronted with a significant mechanism of injury (MOI), the safest course is to assume that the child has a cervical spine injury and transport with spinal immobilization precautions.

▶ The Abdomen and Pelvis

The abdominal organs of an infant or child are susceptible to injury for several reasons. The abdominal wall is thin, so the organs are closer to the surface of the abdomen. Compared to adults, children have proportionally larger solid organs, less subcutaneous fat, and less protective abdominal musculature. The appearance of abdominal distention in a healthy infant is due to two factors: the weak abdominal wall muscles and the larger size of the solid organs.

In young children, the liver and the spleen are lower in the abdomen and are less protected by the rib cage. These organs have a rich blood supply, so injuries to them can result in significant blood loss. The kidneys are also more vulnerable to injury in children for the following reasons:

- They are more mobile and less well supported than in adults.
- They are large in proportion to the abdomen.
- The lower ribs do not shield them from injury.

- Underdevelopment of the abdominal wall muscles and a lack of extensive fat around them provide less protection for these organs.

Finally, the duodenum and pancreas are more likely to be damaged in handlebar injuries. As the child grows, the organs become more proportional in size and better protected.

Words of Wisdom

Even seemingly insignificant forces can cause serious internal injury in children. Multiple organ injuries are common in pediatric patients.

Pelvic fractures are uncommon in young children and are generally seen only with high-energy MOIs. The risk for pelvic fracture increases in adolescence, when the skeleton and MOIs become more like those of adults.

▶ The Musculoskeletal System

Reaching adult height requires active bone growth. The growth plates (**ossification centers**) of a child's bones are made of cartilage, are relatively weak, and are easily fractured. As a consequence, the bones of growing children are weaker than their ligaments and tendons, making fractures more common than sprains. Joint dislocations without associated fractures are not common. Bones finish growing at differing times, but most growth plates will be closed by late adolescence. Growth plate fractures can be seen with low-energy MOIs and may lack the degree of tenderness, swelling, and bruising usually associated with a broken bone.

Slipped capital femoral epiphysis (SCFE), for example, is a problem in the hip that affects the epiphysis of the femur. It occurs in children and adolescents. It is also more prominently found in overweight children compared with children of normal weight. SCFE is considered a pediatric disease. Unless there are signs of trauma, SCFE is a gradual-onset condition. The most common signs are difficulty in walking and a noticeable limp. Sometimes the patient will not be able to bear any weight on the limb. There may be pain at the hip, and normal flexion and rotation will be painful and limited.

Stabilize all sprains or strains and suspect fractures; growth plate injuries may result in poor bone growth. Immobilize the injured part in the same way as you would for an adult, and use cold packs to reduce swelling.

▶ The Chest and Lungs

A child's chest wall is quite thin, with less musculature and less subcutaneous fat to protect ribs and organs. A child's ribs, however, are more pliable and flexible than those of an adult. This increased laxity and flexibility can lead to significant intrathoracic injury with minimal external

findings. Children often have fewer rib fractures and flail chest events, but injuries to the thoracic organs may be more severe because the pliable rib cage and fragile lung tissue are more easily compressed during blunt trauma. As a consequence, children are more vulnerable than adults are to pulmonary contusions, cardiac tamponade, and diaphragmatic rupture. The lungs are also prone to pneumothorax from excessive pressures during bag-mask ventilation.

Be sure to look for signs of chest injuries in a child with suspected chest trauma, but note that the signs of pneumothorax or hemothorax in children are often subtle. You may not see signs such as jugular vein distention, and it may be difficult to determine tracheal deviation. Also, be suspicious of bruising to the chest and torso in nonambulatory children; this finding is highly suspicious for nonaccidental trauma and should be investigated further.

Special Populations

Because the chest of a child is small and the chest wall is thin, breath sounds are easily transmitted from one side of the chest to the other. As a result, breath sounds may be heard despite the presence of a pneumothorax or hemothorax, or with an esophageal intubation. To minimize the possibility of sound transmission from one side of the chest to the other, listen under each armpit (axillary region) and in the midclavicular line under each clavicle. Alternate from side to side, compare your findings, and confirm tube placement with capnography.

▶ The Integumentary System

In comparison with adults, infants and children have thinner and more elastic skin, a higher ratio of body surface area (BSA) to weight, and less subcutaneous (fatty) tissue. These factors contribute to the following risks:

- Increased risk of injury following exposure to temperature extremes
- Increased risk of hypothermia (can complicate resuscitative efforts) and dehydration
- Increased severity of burns (Many burns that would ordinarily be classified as minor or moderate in adults are classified as severe in children.)

Special Populations

Because of their thinner skin and proportionally higher ratio of BSA to weight, burns are more severe in children and, therefore, are a leading cause of death in the pediatric age group.

▶ Metabolic Differences

Infants and children have limited stores of glycogen and glucose that are rapidly depleted as a result of injury or illness. You should maintain a high index of suspicion for hypoglycemia and check blood glucose levels in any patient with lethargy, seizures, or decreased activity. Because it takes glucose to produce energy and energy is required to maintain body temperature, children are susceptible to hypothermia. The risk of hypothermia is further increased because of the child's high BSA-to-weight ratio. Significant hypovolemia and electrolyte derangements can result from severe vomiting and diarrhea.

It is crucial to keep the child warm during transport and take measures to prevent the loss of body heat. To conserve body heat, be sure to cover the child's head; because of its proportionally large size, this structure is a source of significant heat loss.

Parents of Ill or Injured Children

The majority of children you will treat will have at least one parent or caregiver present. Thus, in many pediatric calls, you will be dealing with more than one "patient"—even if only the child is ill or injured. Serious illness or injury to a child is one of the most stressful situations caregivers can face. Some may react to this stress by becoming angry—at the fact that their child is sick, at the person or situation that caused the injury, or at you simply because they need someone to blame! Other parents will be frightened or guilty about the circumstances that led to the illness or injury. Establishing a rapport with caregivers is vital, however, because they will be a source of important information and assistance. Children look to their parents when they are frightened and often mimic their response, so helping calm a parent may also help the patient cope.

Approach stressed caregivers in a calm, quiet, and professional manner. Enlist their help in caring for the child. Along the way, explain what you are doing and provide honest reassurance and support. Above all, do not blame the parent for what has happened. Finally, transport at least one caregiver with the child.

If the parent is extremely emotional, provide support, but remember that your first priority is the child. Do not let a distraught or aggressive parent interfere with your care. If necessary, enlist the help of other family members or law enforcement personnel.

Pediatric Patient Assessment

Just as your general approach to a pediatric patient differs somewhat from your approach to an adult patient, so, too, will your assessment. In particular, you may need to adapt your assessment skills. Ensure you have age-appropriate equipment and review age-appropriate vital signs in anticipation of potential developments.

Scene Size-up

On the way to the scene, prepare for a pediatric scene size-up, the use of pediatric equipment, and an age-appropriate physical assessment. If possible, collect information from dispatch on the age and sex of the child, the location of the scene, and the nature of illness (NOI) or MOI.

As with any call, the scene size-up begins with ensuring that you and your partner have taken the appropriate standard precautions. On arriving at the scene, observe for any hazards or potential hazards that may pose a threat to you, your partner, or the patient. Resist the temptation to hastily approach the patient because you know the patient is a child. Personal safety must always remain your priority.

As you enter the scene, note the position in which the child is found. Observe the area for clues to the MOI or NOI; these observations will help guide your assessment and management priorities.

At a trauma scene when the child is unable to communicate because of his or her developmental age or is unresponsive, assume that the MOI was significant enough to cause head or neck injuries. Spinal immobilization with a cervical collar should be performed if you suspect the MOI to be severe. Remember the need to pad under the pediatric patient's head and/or shoulders to facilitate a neutral position for airway management.

Note the presence of any pills, medicine bottles, alcohol, drug paraphernalia, or household chemicals that would suggest toxic exposure or possible ingestion by the child. If the child has been injured—as in a motor vehicle crash, a fall, or a vehicle-pedestrian incident—carefully observe the scene or vehicle (if involved) for clues to the potential severity of the child's injuries.

Other important assessments that can be made during the scene size-up include the following:

- Orderliness, cleanliness, and safety of the home
- General appearance of other children in the family
- Presence of any medical devices used for the child (such as a home ventilator)
- Indications of parental substance abuse

Determine whether additional resources are necessary, including law enforcement, fire equipment, extrication equipment, special rescue services, additional medical personnel, or special transport services (eg, aeromedical transport).

Primary Survey

Using the Pediatric Assessment Triangle to Form a General Impression

After ensuring scene safety, the first step in the primary survey of any patient begins with your general impression

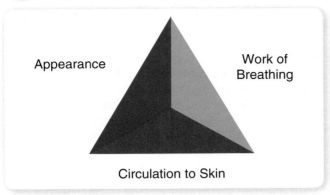

Figure 43-1 The Pediatric Assessment Triangle.

Used with permission of the American Academy of Pediatrics, *Pediatric Education for Prehospital Professionals*, © American Academy of Pediatrics, 2000.

Table 43-5	**Characteristics of Appearance: The TICLS Mnemonic**
Characteristic	**Features to Look For**
Tone	Is the child moving or resisting examination vigorously? Does the child have good muscle tone? Or, is the child limp, listless, or flaccid?
Interactiveness	How alert is the child? How readily does a person, object, or sound distract the child or draw the child's attention? Will the child reach for, grasp, and play with a toy or exam instrument, like a penlight or tongue blade? Or, is the child uninterested in playing or interacting with the caregiver or prehospital professional?
Consolability	Can the child be consoled or comforted by the caregiver or by the prehospital professional? Or, is the child's crying or agitation unrelieved by gentle reassurance?
Look or gaze	Does the child fix his or her gaze on a face, or is there a "nobody home," glassy-eyed stare?
Speech or cry	Is the child's cry strong and spontaneous, or weak, muffled, or hoarse?

Modified from: American Academy of Pediatrics. Pediatric assessment. In: Fuchs S, Klein BL, eds. *Pediatric Education for Prehospital Professionals*. Rev 3rd ed. Burlington, MA: Jones & Bartlett Learning; 2016:6.

of how the patient looks (the "sick–not sick" classification). An assessment tool called the **Pediatric Assessment Triangle (PAT)** Figure 43-1 has been developed to help emergency medical services (EMS) providers form a "from-the-doorway" general impression of pediatric patients. Providers with experience in treating ill and injured children intuitively use some version of the PAT to make the important distinction between sick and not-sick patients. The PAT standardizes this approach by including three elements—the child's appearance, work of breathing, and circulation—that collectively paint an accurate clinical picture of the patient's cardiopulmonary status and level of consciousness. This quick assessment is conducted before assessing the ABCDEs (Airway, Breathing, Circulation, Disability, and Exposure) and does not require touching the patient. It applies a rapid, hands-off systematic approach to observing an ill or injured child and helps establish urgency for treatment or transport.

Special Populations

Use the PAT to help with your from-the-doorway general impression of pediatric patients.

Appearance

The first element of the PAT is the child's appearance. In many cases, appearance is the most important factor in determining the severity of illness, the need for treatment, and the response to therapy. Appearance reflects the adequacy of ventilation, oxygenation, brain perfusion, body homeostasis, and central nervous system function. The TICLS (pronounced "tickles") mnemonic highlights the most important features of a child's appearance: Tone, Interactiveness, Consolability, Look or gaze, and Speech or cry Table 43-5 .

To assess appearance, observe the child from a distance, allowing the child to interact with the caregiver

as he or she chooses. Walk through the characteristics of the TICLS mnemonic while observing the child from the doorway. Delay touching the patient until you have developed your general impression, because the child may become agitated by your touch. Unless a child is unconscious or critically ill, take your time in assessing his or her general appearance by observation before you begin the hands-on assessment and obtain vital signs. Figure 43-2 and Figure 43-3 demonstrate examples of an infant with a normal appearance and one with an abnormal appearance.

An abnormal appearance may result from numerous underlying physiologic abnormalities. A child may show evidence of inadequate oxygenation or ventilation, as in respiratory emergencies; inadequate brain perfusion, as from cardiovascular emergencies; systemic abnormalities

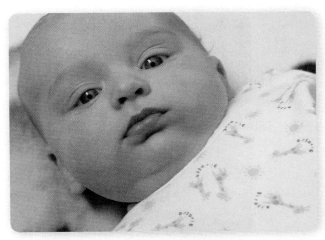

Figure 43-2 A child with a normal appearance. An infant or child who is not very sick will make good eye contact.

© Photos.com/Getty.

Table 43-6	Characteristics of Work of Breathing
Characteristic	**Features to Look For**
Abnormal airway sounds	Snoring, muffled or hoarse speech, stridor, grunting, or wheezing
Abnormal posturing	Sniffing position, tripod position, refusal to lie down
Retractions	Supraclavicular, intercostal, or substernal retractions of the chest wall; head bobbing in infants
Flaring	Flaring of the nares on inspiration

© Jones & Bartlett Learning.

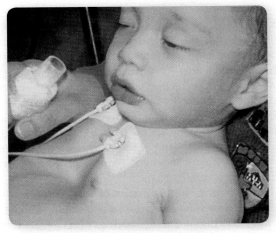

Figure 43-3 A child with an abnormal appearance. A limp child unable to maintain eye contact may be critically ill or injured.

Courtesy of Health Resources and Services Administration (HRSA), Maternal and Child Health Bureau (MCHB), Emergency Medical Services for Children (EMSC) Program.

or metabolic derangements, such as with poisoning, infection, or hypoglycemia; or acute or chronic brain injury. In any event, a child with a grossly abnormal appearance is seriously ill and requires immediate life support interventions and transport. The remainder of the PAT—work of breathing and circulation—plus the hands-on portion of the primary survey (assessment of the ABCDEs) may help you identify the cause of the abnormal appearance and determine the severity of a child's illness and the need for treatment and transport.

Work of Breathing

A child's work of breathing is often a better assessment of his or her oxygenation and ventilation status than auscultation of lung sounds or determining the child's respiratory rate. The work of breathing reflects the child's attempt to compensate for abnormalities in oxygenation and ventilation, and, therefore, is a proxy for effectiveness of gas exchange. The hands-off assessment of work of breathing includes listening for abnormal airway sounds and looking for signs of increased breathing effort Table 43-6 .

Some abnormal airway sounds can be heard without a stethoscope and can indicate the likely physiology and anatomic location of the breathing problem. For example, snoring can indicate obstruction at the level of the oropharynx, muffled or hoarse voice can indicate obstruction at the level of the glottis or supraglottic structures, and stridor (a harsh sound during inspiration, high-pitched due to partial upper airway obstruction) can indicate obstruction at the level of the glottis or subglottic structures. Such an upper airway obstruction may result from croup, bacterial upper airway infections, lodged foreign body, bleeding, or edema.

Lower airway obstruction is suggested by abnormal grunting or wheezing. Grunting is a form of auto-PEEP (positive end-expiratory pressure), a way to distend the lower respiratory air sacs, or alveoli, to promote maximum gas exchange. **Grunting** involves exhaling against a partially closed glottis. This short, low-pitched sound is best heard at the end of exhalation and is often mistaken for whimpering. Grunting suggests moderate to severe hypoxia and is seen with lower airway conditions such as pneumonia and pulmonary edema. It reflects poor gas exchange because of fluid in the lower airways and air sacs. Wheezing is a musical tone caused by air being forced through constricted or partially blocked small airways. It often occurs during exhalation only but can occur during inspiration and expiration during severe asthma attacks. Although this sound is often heard only by auscultation, severe obstruction may result in wheezing that is audible even without a stethoscope.

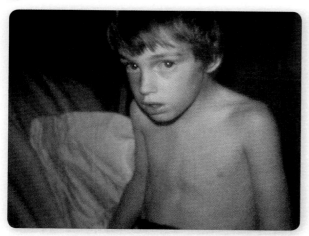

Figure 43-4 A child in the sniffing position is trying to align the airway to increase patency and improve airflow.

Courtesy of Health Resources and Services Administration (HRSA), Maternal and Child Health Bureau (MCHB), Emergency Medical Services for Children (EMSC) Program.

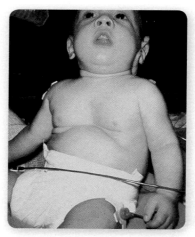

Figure 43-6 Retractions can occur in the suprasternal, intercostal, and substernal areas and indicate increased work of breathing.

Courtesy of Health Resources and Services Administration (HRSA), Maternal and Child Health Bureau (MCHB), Emergency Medical Services for Children (EMSC) Program.

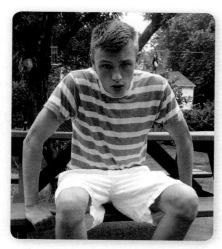

Figure 43-5 A child in the tripod position is maximizing his or her accessory muscles of respiration. A patient in the tripod position will sit leaning forward on outstretched arms with the head and chin thrust slightly forward.

© Jones & Bartlett Learning.

Abnormal positioning and retractions are physical signs of increased work of breathing that can easily be assessed without touching the patient. A child who is in the **sniffing position** is trying to align the axes of the airways to improve patency and increase airflow **Figure 43-4**; such a position often reflects a severe upper airway obstruction. The child who refuses to lie down or who leans forward on outstretched arms (**tripoding**) is creating the optimal mechanical advantage to use accessory muscles of respiration **Figure 43-5**.

Retractions represent the recruitment of accessory muscles of respiration to provide more "muscle power" to move air into the lungs in the face of airway or lung disease or injury. To optimally observe retractions, expose the child's chest. Retractions are a more useful measure of work of breathing in children than in adults because a child's chest wall is less muscular, so the inward excursion

of skin and soft tissue between the ribs is more apparent. Retractions may be evident in the supraclavicular area (above the clavicle), the intercostal area (between the ribs), or the substernal area (under the sternum) **Figure 43-6**. Another form of retractions that is seen only in infants is head bobbing, the use of neck muscles to help breathing during severe hypoxia. The infant extends the neck as he or she inhales, then allows the head to fall forward during exhalation. Nasal flaring is the exaggerated opening of the nostrils during labored inspiration and indicates moderate to severe hypoxia.

Combine the characteristics of work of breathing—abnormal airway sounds, abnormal positioning, retractions, and nasal flaring—to make your general assessment of the child's oxygenation and ventilation status. Together with the child's appearance, the child's work of breathing suggests the severity of the illness and the likelihood that the cause is in the airway or is a respiratory process.

Circulation to Skin

The goal of rapid circulatory assessment is to determine the adequacy of cardiac output and core perfusion. When cardiac output diminishes, the body responds by shunting circulation from nonessential areas (eg, skin) toward vital organs. Therefore, circulation to the skin reflects the overall status of core circulation. Visually scan the child's skin and mucous membranes, looking for pallor, mottling, and cyanosis.

Pallor or paleness may be the initial sign of poor circulation or even the only visual sign in a child with compensated shock. It indicates reflex peripheral vasoconstriction that is shunting blood toward the core. Pallor may also indicate anemia or hypoxia.

Mottling reflects vasomotor instability in the capillary beds demonstrated by patchy areas of vasoconstriction and vasodilation. It may also be a child's physiologic response to a cold environment.

Cyanosis, a blue discoloration of the skin and mucous membranes, is the most extreme visual indicator of poor perfusion or poor oxygenation. **Acrocyanosis**, blue hands or feet in an infant younger than 2 months, is distinct from cyanosis; it is a normal finding when a young infant is cold. True cyanosis is seen in the skin and mucous membranes and is a late finding of respiratory failure or shock.

Combine the three pieces of the PAT to estimate the severity of the child's condition and the likely underlying pathologic cause **Table 43-7** . On the basis of the findings from the PAT, you will determine whether the pediatric patient is in stable condition or requires urgent care. If the pediatric patient is in unstable condition, assess the ABCDEs, treat any life threats, and transport the pediatric patient immediately to an appropriate facility. If the pediatric patient is in stable condition, then you have time to perform the entire patient assessment process.

Hands-on Primary Survey

After using the PAT to form a general impression of the patient, you will need to complete the rest of the primary survey; that is, you must assess the child's ABCDEs and mental status and prioritize the care and need for transport. Threats to the ABCs are managed as they are found, providing a prioritized sequence of life support interventions to reverse critical physiologic abnormalities. The steps are the same as with adults, albeit with differences related to the child's anatomy, physiology, and signs of distress. If you suspect the child is experiencing life-threatening external bleeding or cardiac arrest, which is rare, the order is CAB because hemorrhage control or chest compressions would be the priority. You will also assess disability (D) and expose (E) the patient for examination.

Early in your assessment of a young child, you will need to estimate the child's weight, because much of your care will depend on the child's size. The best way to estimate a child's weight is with a pediatric length-based resuscitation tape measure, which will also provide appropriate medication doses and equipment sizes **Figure 43-7** . The pediatric length-based resuscitation tape measure can estimate weight and height in pediatric patients weighing up to 75 pounds (34 kg).

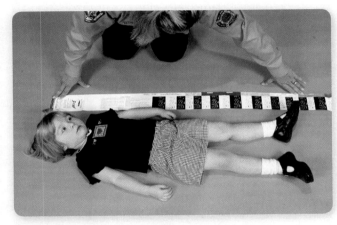

Figure 43-7 Use of a length-based resuscitation tape is one way to estimate a child's weight and identify the correct size for pediatric equipment and medication doses.
© Jones & Bartlett Learning. Courtesy of MIEMSS.

Table 43-7	Categorization of the Pediatric Assessment Triangle Findings		
Physiologic Abnormality	**Appearance**	**Work of Breathing**	**Circulation to Skin**
Cardiopulmonary failure	Abnormal	Abnormal	Abnormal
Compensated shock	Normal	Normal	Abnormal
Decompensated (hypotensive) shock	Abnormal	Normal or abnormal	Abnormal
Primary brain dysfunction or systemic problem	Abnormal	Normal	Normal
Respiratory distress	Normal	Abnormal	Normal
Respiratory failure	Abnormal	Abnormal	Normal or abnormal

Modified from: Dieckmann RA. Pediatric assessment. In: Fuchs S, Yamamoto L, eds. *APLS: The Pediatric Emergency Medicine Resource.* 5th ed. Burlington, MA: Jones & Bartlett Learning; 2012:2-37; Santillanes G. General approach to the pediatric patient. In: Marx JA, Hockberger RS, Walls RM, eds. *Rosen's Emergency Medicine: Concepts and Clinical Practice.* 8th ed. Philadelphia, PA: Saunders; 2014:2087-2095.

To use the pediatric length-based resuscitation tape measure, follow these steps:

1. Measure the child's length, from *head to heel*, with the tape (with the red portion at the head).
2. Note the weight in kilograms that corresponds to the child's measured length at the heel.
3. If the child is longer than the tape, use adult equipment and medication doses.
4. From the tape, identify appropriate equipment sizes.
5. From the tape, identify appropriate medication doses.

Patient Safety

Children are at particularly high risk of medication errors, secondary to incorrect dosages, for several reasons. Often, estimations of weight in children can be significantly different from actual weight due to EMS providers' inability to accurately estimate weight even when using length-based resuscitation tapes. Additionally, many more medication doses are based on weight in children than in adults, so they require weight-based calculations to arrive at the correct total dose—a process that is prone to calculation errors by providers. Finally, some medications come in more than one concentration (eg, antidysrhythmics and vasopressors), which can add to dosing confusion. If there is a caregiver with the child, ask them how much the child weighs and how recent that information is.

To reduce the risk of medication errors, use available resources such as reference cards, charts, or smartphone applications rather than commit difficult formulas or medication dosages to memory. In addition, ensure the tools you use are up to date with current resuscitation guidelines. Additional information on pediatric drug dosages is discussed in Chapter 14, *Medication Administration*.

Airway

The PAT may suggest the presence of an airway obstruction based on abnormal airway sounds and increased work of breathing. As with adults, determine whether the airway is open and the patient has adequate chest rise with breathing. Check for mucus, blood, or a foreign body in the mouth or airway. If there is potential obstruction from the tongue or soft tissues, position the airway and suction as necessary. Determine whether the airway is patent, partially obstructed, or totally obstructed. If suctioning is required, do not keep the suction tip or catheter in the back of a child's throat too long because young patients are sensitive to vagal stimuli and the pulse rate may plummet.

Breathing

The breathing component of the primary survey involves calculating the respiratory rate, auscultating breath sounds, and checking pulse oximetry for oxygen saturation. Verify the respiratory rate per minute by counting the number of chest rises in 30 seconds and then doubling that number. Healthy infants may show periodic breathing, or variable respiratory rates with short periods of apnea (less than 20). As a consequence, counting for only 10 to 15 seconds may give a falsely low respiratory rate. Interpreting the respiratory rate requires knowing the normal values for the child's age and putting the respiratory rate in context with the rest of the primary survey. Rapid respiratory rates may reflect high fever, anxiety, pain, or excitement. Normal rates, by contrast, may occur in a child who has been breathing rapidly with increased work of breathing and is becoming fatigued. Serial assessment of respiratory rates may be especially useful because the trend may be more accurate than any single value.

Auscultate the breath sounds with a stethoscope over the midaxillary line to hear abnormal lung sounds during inhalation and exhalation. Listen for extra breath sounds such as inspiratory crackles, wheezes, or rhonchi; rhonchi often indicate harsh breath sounds or sounds that may be transmitted from the upper airways. If you cannot determine whether the sounds are being generated in the lungs or the upper airway, hold the stethoscope over the nose or trachea and listen. Also, listen to the breath sounds for adequacy of air movement. Diminished breath sounds may signal severe respiratory distress. Auscultation over the trachea may also help distinguish stridor from other sounds.

Check the pulse oximetry reading to determine the oxygen saturation level while the child breathes ambient air. You can place the pulse oximetry probe on a young child's finger just as you would with an adult. In infants or young children who try to remove the probe, it may be helpful to place the probe on a toe, possibly with a sock covering it. A pulse oximetry reading of greater than 94% saturation while breathing room air indicates good oxygenation.

As with the respiratory rate, evaluate the pulse oximetry reading in the context of the PAT and remainder of the primary survey. A child with a normal pulse oximetry reading, for example, may be expending increasing amounts of energy and increasing the work of breathing to maintain his or her oxygen saturation. The primary

Words of Wisdom

Consider pulse oximetry readings in terms of the environmental context and the physiologic status of the child. Peripheral vasoconstriction from hypothermia or poor perfusion may alter these readings. Always correlate the pulse oximetry waveform with the patient's pulse rate and ECG reading.

survey would identify the respiratory distress and point to the need for immediate intervention despite the normal oxygen saturation level.

Circulation

The information obtained from the PAT about circulation to the skin directs the next step of the primary survey. Integrate this assessment of circulation with the pulse rate and quality, as well as skin CTC (color, temperature, and condition plus capillary refill time), to obtain an overall assessment of the child's circulatory status. This information needs to be placed in context within the PAT and the remainder of the primary survey because cool extremities and delayed capillary refill are commonly seen in a child in a cool environment.

Obtain the child's pulse rate by listening to the heart or feeling the pulse for 30 seconds and doubling the number. As with respiratory rates in pediatric patients, it is important to know normal pulse rates based on age. Interpret the pulse rate within the context of the overall history and primary survey. Tachycardia may indicate early hypoxia or shock or a less serious condition such as fever, anxiety, pain, or excitement.

Feel for the pulse to ascertain the rate and quality of pulsations. If you cannot find a peripheral (distal) pulse (ie, radial or brachial), feel for a central pulse (ie, femoral or carotid). Check the femoral pulse in infants and young children and the carotid pulse in older children and adolescents. Start CPR if there is no pulse or if a pulse is present but the rate is less than 60 beats/min with signs of poor perfusion (ie, pallor, mottling, cyanosis) despite support of oxygenation and ventilation.

After checking the pulse rate, do a hands-on evaluation of skin CTC. Check whether the hands and feet are warm or cool to the touch. It is common for neonates to have acrocyanosis immediately after birth. Whereas in the adult population cyanosis in the extremities indicates severe hypoxia, in the neonate population it may be a normal variant, particularly if the ambient temperature is cool.

Evaluate capillary refill time, also called the blanching test, in an uninjured limb to assess the patient's level of perfusion in conjunction with other assessments of circulation. Keep in mind, though, that capillary refill can be affected by the patient's body temperature, position, preexisting medical conditions, or medication. Conditions unrelated to circulation, such as age, cold exposure, frostbite, and vasoconstriction, may also slow capillary refill. Injury to bones and muscles of the extremities may cause local circulatory compromise, resulting in hypoperfusion.

To assess capillary refill in older infants and children younger than 6 years, press the skin or nail bed using moderate pressure and determine how long it takes for the color to return.[1] In newborns and young infants, press the forehead, chin, or sternum to determine capillary refill time. Blood will be forced from the capillaries in the nail bed. Release the pressure, and the nail bed will remain blanched for a brief period. As the underlying capillaries refill with blood, the normal color of the nail bed will be

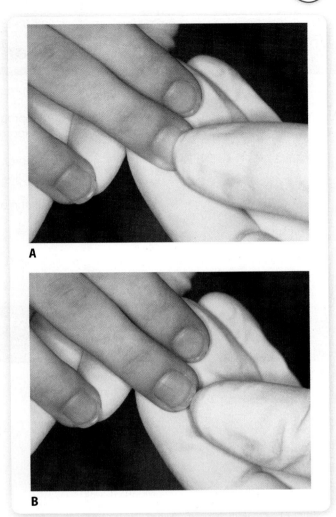

A

B

Figure 43-8 A. To test capillary refill, compress the fingertip for 5 seconds using moderate pressure. **B.** Release the fingertip, and count the number of seconds it takes for the normal color to return to the nail bed.

© Jones & Bartlett Learning. Courtesy of MIEMSS.

restored. With adequate perfusion, color in the nail bed should be restored within 2 seconds—about the length of time it takes to say "capillary refill" at a normal rate of speech **Figure 43-8**. Suspect poor peripheral circulation if the capillary refill takes more than 2 seconds or the nail bed remains blanched.

You may sometimes hear abnormal heart sounds that are considered normal variants in the pediatric population. For example, the presence of an S_3 in a child is considered a benign finding, as long as the patient has no other signs of cardiac compromise. A split S_2 is also relatively common among young children and is considered benign when the split is associated with respiratory patterns. If the split S_2 is fixed regardless of the respiratory pattern, further evaluation is necessary, since such a finding is typically associated with a septal defect. The point of maximum impulse is not always palpable in infants and is affected by respiratory patterns, a full stomach, and the infant's position.

Table 43-8	**AVPU Scale**		
Category	**Stimulus**	**Response Type**	**Reaction**
Alert	Normal environment	Appropriate	Normal interactiveness for age
Verbal	Simple command or sound stimulus	Appropriate Inappropriate	Responds to name Nonspecific or confused
Painful	Pain	Appropriate Inappropriate	Withdraws from pain Makes sound or moves without purpose or localization of pain
		Pathologic	Posturing
Unresponsive			No perceptible response to any stimulus

Abbreviation: AVPU, Awake and alert, responsive to Verbal stimuli, responsive to Pain, Unresponsive

© Jones & Bartlett Learning.

Table 43-9	**Pediatric Glasgow Coma Scale (GCS)**				
Activity	**Score**	**Infant**	**Score**	**Child**	
Eye opening	4	Open spontaneously	4	Open spontaneously	
	3	Open to speech or sound	3	Open to speech	
	2	Open to painful stimuli	2	Open to painful stimuli	
	1	No response	1	No response	
Verbal	5	Coos, babbles	5	Oriented conversation	
	4	Irritable cry	4	Confused conversation	
	3	Cries to pain	3	Cries; inappropriate words	
	2	Moans to pain	2	Moans; incomprehensible words/sounds	
	1	No response	1	No response	
Motor	6	Normal spontaneous movement	6	Obeys verbal commands	
	5	Localizes pain	5	Localizes pain	
	4	Withdraws from pain	4	Withdraws from pain	
	3	Abnormal flexion (decorticate)	3	Abnormal flexion (decorticate)	
	2	Abnormal extension (decerebrate)	2	Abnormal extension (decerebrate)	
	1	No response (flaccid)	1	No response (flaccid)	

Modified from: Davis RJ et al. Head and spinal cord injury. In: Rogers MC, ed. *Textbook of Pediatric Intensive Care.* Baltimore, MD: Williams & Wilkins; 1987; James H, Anas N, Perkin RM. *Brain Insults in Infants and Children.* New York, NY: Grune & Stratton; 1985; and Morray JP et al. Coma scale for use in brain-injured children. *Critical Care Medicine.* 1984;12:1018.

Disability

The assessment of the pediatric patient's level of consciousness can be done using the AVPU (Awake and alert, responsive to Verbal stimuli, responsive to Pain, Unresponsive) scale Table 43-8 , modified as necessary for the child's age, or the Pediatric Glasgow Coma Scale Table 43-9 .

After evaluating the patient's response with the AVPU scale, assess the pupillary response to a beam of light to assess brainstem response. Note whether the pupils are dilated, constricted, reactive, or fixed. Next, evaluate motor activity, looking for symmetric movement of the extremities, seizures, posturing, or flaccidity. Combine this information with the PAT results to determine the child's neurologic status.

Exposure

Proper exposure of the child is necessary to complete the primary survey. The child will need to be at least partially undressed to assess the work of breathing and circulation. However, it is also important to perform a rapid exam of the entire body to look for unsuspected injuries and anatomic abnormalities. Be careful to avoid heat loss, especially in infants, by covering the child as soon as possible. Keep the temperature in the ambulance high, and use blankets when necessary.

Transport Decision

After completing the primary survey and beginning resuscitation when necessary, you must make a crucial decision: whether to immediately transport the child to the emergency department (ED) or to continue the additional assessment and treatment on scene. Immediate transport is imperative if the emergency call is for trauma and the child has a serious MOI, a physiologic abnormality, or a potentially significant anatomic abnormality or if the scene is unsafe. In these cases, manage all life threats and then begin transport. Attempt to obtain vascular access on the way to the ED. If the emergency call is for an illness, the decision to stay or go is less clear-cut and depends on the following factors: expected benefits of treatment, EMS system regulations, comfort level, and transport time.

History Taking

If the child seems to be in physiologically unstable condition based on the primary survey, you may decide to begin transport immediately and conduct history taking and the secondary assessment in the ambulance en route to the ED. The goal of history taking is to elaborate on the chief complaint (ie, OPQRST [Onset, Provocation/palliation, Quality, Region/radiation, Severity, Timing]) and obtain a patient history (ie, SAMPLE [Signs and symptoms, Allergies, Medications, Pertinent past medical history, Last oral intake, Events leading up to the illness or injury]) Table 43-10 .

Secondary Assessment

Whereas the primary survey addresses immediately life-threatening pathologic problems, the secondary assessment includes a systematic assessment of the patient that may include a full-body examination or a focused assessment of the body part or body system specifically involved. A complete set of baseline vital signs, using monitoring devices as appropriate, should also be obtained at this time.

Tailor the exam to the child's age and developmental stage. For a full-body examination, infants, toddlers, and preschool-age children should be assessed starting at the feet and ending at the head; this strategy tends to gain trust and decreases the child's fear. Infants are usually not overly distressed by being manipulated by adults, so the basic head-to-toe approach to assessment is reasonable with them. Children ages 1 to 3 years can be challenging to care for, however, and as a rule will strenuously object to being touched or otherwise manipulated by a stranger. The toe-to-head approach is a good strategy in this age group. Decide which aspects of the exam must be performed, set some reasonable ground rules for the exam, and then examine the patient accordingly. Practice ways to safely and adequately hold young patients to facilitate the assessment. If possible, have family members assist with this task.

Children ages 4 to 5 years are typically much less of a management challenge for you. They are usually

Table 43-10	SAMPLE Components for Pediatric History Taking
Component	**Features**
Signs and symptoms	Onset and nature of symptoms of pain or fever Age-appropriate signs of distress
Allergies	Known medication reactions or other allergies
Medications	Exact names and doses of ongoing drugs (including over-the-counter, prescribed, herbal, and recreational drugs) Timing and amount of last dose Time and dose of analgesics or antipyretics
Past medical history	Previous illnesses or injuries Immunizations History of pregnancy, labor, delivery (infants and toddlers)
Last oral intake	Timing of the child's last food or drink, including bottle or breastfeeding
Events leading to illness or injury	Key events leading to the current incident Fever history

© Jones & Bartlett Learning.

cooperative and helpful with the exam, and the standard head-to-toe approach can usually be employed. School-age children tend to be cooperative as well and should be actively engaged in the examination process. Take the time to explain what you are doing during the examination.

Evaluating adolescents can be a bit more demanding because these patients prefer to preserve their autonomy, and they may be concerned about involving parents or peers in some situations. They also tend to be concerned with bodily integrity, so be prepared to reassure them things are okay if a physical finding is not worrisome.

When you assess any child, some general principles apply. No matter how stressful or disturbing the situation, remain calm, patient, and gentle. Be honest; if something is likely to hurt, say so—but do not elaborate. If at all possible, attempt to keep children and parents together. Many children have a normal fear of separation; in the setting of acute illness or injury, these anxieties will only be heightened. Remember, pediatric patients in the prehospital setting are often trauma victims. Appropriately assess for injury, and treat any illness or injury accordingly. Do not neglect a child's pain.

The extent of the examination will depend on the situation and may include the following elements:

- **Head.** Look for bruising, swelling, and hematomas. Significant blood can be lost between the skull and the scalp of a small infant. Assess the anterior fontanel in patients younger than 2 years. Temporary bulging of the anterior fontanel may be seen during periods of crying, coughing, or vomiting. The presence of a bulging fontanel in a quiet infant suggests elevated ICP caused by meningitis, encephalitis, or intracranial bleeding. A sunken fontanel suggests dehydration.
- **Pupils.** Note whether the pupils are equal, round, and reactive to light and accommodation (PERRLA). The response of the pupils is a good indication of how well the brain is functioning, particularly when trauma has occurred.
- **Nose.** Inspect the nose for the drainage of blood or fluid. Note if nasal flaring is present. Young infants prefer to breathe through their nose, so nasal congestion with mucus can cause respiratory distress. Gentle bulb suction of the nostrils may bring relief.
- **Ears.** Look for any drainage from the ear canals. Leaking blood suggests a skull fracture. Check for bruises behind the ear or Battle sign, a late sign of skull fracture. The presence of pus may indicate an ear infection or perforation of the eardrum. Bruising on the ear can be a sign of child abuse.
- **Mouth.** In the trauma patient, look for active bleeding and loose teeth. Listen for hoarseness and note the presence of drooling. Note the smell of the breath. Some ingestions are associated with identifiable odors, such as hydrocarbons. Acidosis, as in diabetic ketoacidosis (DKA), may impart an acetone-like smell to the breath.
- **Neck.** Examine the trachea for swelling or bruising. Note the use of accessory muscles and the presence of a stoma. Suspect bacterial or viral meningitis if the child cannot move his or her neck and has a high fever.
- **Chest.** Examine the chest for penetrating injuries, lacerations, bruises, or rashes. Note the presence of vascular access devices. If the pediatric patient is injured, feel the clavicles and every rib for tenderness or deformity. An infant with rib fractures will often display paradoxical crying; that is, he or she may cry when held and be calm when not touched.
- **Back.** Inspect the back for lacerations, penetrating injuries, bruises, or rashes.
- **Abdomen.** Inspect the abdomen for distention. Gently palpate the abdomen and watch closely for guarding or tensing of the abdominal muscles, which may suggest infection, obstruction, or intra-abdominal injury. Note any tenderness or masses. Look for any seat belt abrasions or bruising. Be suspicious of bruising on the abdomen of a nonambulatory child; this finding is highly suspicious for nonaccidental trauma. In an infant, a common finding is a range of active tinkling bowel sounds when the stethoscope is placed on the belly. Because patients react to cold stimuli, warming the diaphragm of your stethoscope before placing it on the skin might yield a more accurate result. You can percuss an infant's abdomen as you would an adult's; however, you might note a more tympanic sound.
- **Extremities.** Assess for symmetry. Compare both sides for color, warmth, size of joints, swelling, and tenderness. Put each joint through full range of motion while watching the eyes of the pediatric patient for signs of pain, unless there is obvious deformity of the extremity suggesting a fracture.
- **Capillary refill (in children younger than 6 years).** Normal capillary refill time should be 2 seconds or less. Cold temperatures will increase capillary refill time, making it a less reliable sign.
- **Level of hydration.** Assess skin turgor, noting the presence of **tenting**, a condition in which the skin slowly retracts after being pinched and pulled away slightly from the body. In infants, note whether the fontanels are sunken or flat. Ask the parent or caregiver how many diapers the infant has soiled over the last 24 hours. Determine whether the child is producing tears when crying; note the condition of the mouth. Is the oral mucosa moist or dry?

Words of Wisdom

Blood pressure is just one component of the overall assessment of pediatric patients. Determination of physiologic stability should be based on all data collected from the PAT, physical exam, and initial vital signs.

It may be difficult to obtain an accurate measurement of blood pressure in a young child or infant because of a lack of cooperation and need for proper cuff size. Nevertheless, you should attempt to measure the blood pressure on the upper arm or thigh, making sure the cuff has a width two-thirds the length of the upper arm or thigh. One formula for determining the lower limit of acceptable blood pressure in children ages 1 to 10 years is this: minimal systolic blood pressure = 70 + (2 × age in years). For example, a 2-year-old toddler should have a minimal systolic blood pressure of 74; a lower reading indicates hypotension. (Table 43-11 shows normal minimal systolic blood pressure values for different ages.) Given the technical difficulty of trying to measure the blood pressure in a pediatric patient, make one attempt in the field; if unsuccessful, move on to the rest of the assessment.

Special Populations

For children ages 1 to 10 years, calculate the lower limit of acceptable systolic blood pressure with the following formula:

Minimum systolic = 70 + (2 × age in years)

Today, assessment of pain is recognized as part of vital signs assessment, and management of pediatric pain and anxiety should be a routine part of field care. This effort requires a thorough understanding of nonpharmacologic techniques, drugs, potential drug contraindications and complications, and management of the complications.

Table 43-11	Normal Blood Pressure for Age	
Age	**Systolic Blood Pressure (mm Hg)**	**Diastolic Blood Pressure (mm Hg)**
Neonate (0 to 1 month)	67 to 84	35 to 53
Infant (1 month to 1 year)	72 to 104	37 to 56
Toddler (1 to 2 years)	86 to 106	42 to 63
Preschooler (3 to 5 years)	89 to 112	46 to 72
School-age child (6 to 12 years)	97 to 120	57 to 80
Adolescent (12 to 15 years)	110 to 131	64 to 83

Data from: American Heart Association (AHA). Vital signs in children. In: AHA. *Pediatric Advanced Life Support.* Dallas, TX: AHA; 2015.

Inadequate treatment of pain has many adverse effects on the child and family. Pain causes misery for the child and caregivers, and it interferes with your ability to accurately assess physiologic abnormalities. Children who do not receive appropriate analgesia may be more likely to have exaggerated pain responses to subsequent painful procedures.

Assessment of pain must consider developmental age. The ability to identify pain improves with the age of the child. In infants and preverbal children, it may be difficult to distinguish crying and agitation due to hypoxia, hunger, or pain. Further assessment and discussion with caregivers about their perceptions of the child's pain are essential to identify pain in this age group. Pain scales using pictures of facial expressions, such as the Wong-Baker FACES scale, may prove helpful **Figure 43-9** .

Remaining calm and providing quiet, professional reassurance to parents and child are crucial for managing pediatric pain and anxiety. A calm parent will help keep the child calm and more at ease. Distraction techniques with toys or stories may prove helpful in reducing pain, as may visual imagery techniques and music. Sucrose pacifiers may reduce pain in neonates. Pharmacologic methods for reducing pain—such as acetaminophen, opiates, benzodiazepines, and nitrous oxide—are available to paramedics in a number of EMS systems. The benefit of such analgesic or anxiolytic medication must be weighed against the risks of its administration (respiratory depression, bradycardia, hypoxemia, and hypotension are potential adverse effects of sedatives), including the potential route of administration. Medications that are given intravenously are often most effective at reducing pain, but they require establishing intravenous (IV) access, which itself is a painful procedure. Pediatric IV therapy considerations are discussed in Chapter 14, *Medication Administration.*

You must not discount the possibility of child abuse when assessing a child. Conflicting information from the parents or caregivers, bruises or other injuries that are not consistent with the MOI described, or injuries that are not consistent with the child's age and developmental abilities should increase your index of suspicion for abuse. Observe and note the parents' or caregivers' interaction with the

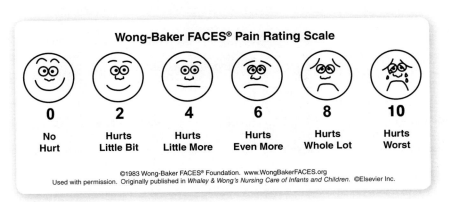

Wong-Baker FACES® Pain Rating Scale

0	2	4	6	8	10
No Hurt	Hurts Little Bit	Hurts Little More	Hurts Even More	Hurts Whole Lot	Hurts Worst

©1983 Wong-Baker FACES® Foundation. www.WongBakerFACES.org
Used with permission. Originally published in *Whaley & Wong's Nursing Care of Infants and Children.* ©Elsevier Inc.

Figure 43-9 The Wong-Baker FACES scale.

child. Do they appear to be appropriately concerned, angry, or indifferent? Does the child seem comforted by their presence or scared by them? Child abuse will be discussed in greater detail later in this chapter.

Special Populations

Consider pain to be a vital sign in pediatric patients. Assess and reassess pain along with the other vital signs. Treat pain accordingly.

Reassessment

The elements in the reassessment include the PAT, patient priority, vital signs (every 5 minutes if the patient is in unstable condition and every 15 minutes if in stable condition), assessment of the effectiveness of interventions (eg, medications administered, splints applied, bleeding controlled), and reassessment of the focused exam areas. Perform the reassessment on all patients to observe their response to treatment, to guide ongoing treatments, and to track the progression of identified pathologic and anatomic problems. New problems may be identified on reassessment. The reassessment may also guide the choice of an appropriate transport destination and your radio or telephone communications with medical oversight or ED staff.

■ Pathophysiology, Assessment, and Management of Respiratory Emergencies

Respiratory problems are among the medical emergencies that you will most frequently encounter in children. Pediatric patients with a respiratory chief complaint will span the spectrum from mildly ill to near death. In pediatrics, respiratory failure and arrest precede the majority of cardiopulmonary arrests; by contrast, a primary cardiac event is the usual cause of sudden death in adults. Early identification and intervention can stop the progression from respiratory distress to cardiopulmonary failure and help to avert much pediatric morbidity and mortality.

The entire tracheobronchial tree of a child is smaller than that of an adult. The smaller diameter of pediatric airways makes small amounts of swelling or bronchospasm much more significant than the same amount of narrowing in an adult airway. This simple fact complicates the entire spectrum of respiratory illness in the pediatric population.

YOU ▸ are the Paramedic   PART 2

Using the PAT, you classify the child as sick. You suspect shock on the basis of his abnormal appearance, abnormal circulation, and normal work of breathing. The child's oxygen saturation on room air is 91%. Your partner applies 100% oxygen via a nonrebreathing mask and places the patient on the cardiac monitor, which shows a sinus tachycardia. On questioning the sister, you learn that the child has had a stomachache with vomiting and diarrhea for the past few days and has not eaten or drunk anything since the night before. She says that he never gets sick.

Recording Time: 5 Minutes	
Respirations	22 breaths/min unlabored; clear breath sounds
Pulse	180 beats/min, regular; absent radial pulses and weak central pulses
Skin	Pale, cool, and dry; mottled extremities
Blood pressure	68/42 mm Hg
Oxygen saturation (Spo₂)	99% at 12 L/min of oxygen on nonrebreathing mask
Capillary refill	5 seconds

3. What is the significance of the child's blood pressure?
4. What should your treatment consist of at this point?

▶ Respiratory Arrest, Distress, and Failure

Infants have a limited ability to compensate for respiratory insults and often expend huge amounts of energy to breathe. At times, infants are intubated to take over the work of breathing even when adequate physiologic parameters are being maintained. In older children, increasing compensatory skills develop, and juvenile patients with asthma can sometimes compensate for days, with adequate oxygen saturation, before tiring out and literally dying of fatigue.

Many infants and children with respiratory conditions have respiratory distress (difficulty breathing), some have respiratory failure (which invariably leads to decompensation), and a few are in respiratory arrest. If the child in respiratory arrest can be resuscitated before cardiac arrest occurs, survival with a return to full function is likely. Any respiratory compromise in children must be monitored closely and the child transported to the closest ED. If a pediatric-specific ED is available, consult medical direction or your local transport protocols for advice.

When you are faced with a respiratory emergency, the first step is to determine the severity of the disease: is the patient in respiratory distress, respiratory failure, or respiratory arrest? Keep the anatomic and physiologic respiratory differences in mind as you approach the child.

Respiratory distress entails increased work of breathing to maintain oxygenation and/or ventilation; that is, it is a compensated state in which increased work of breathing results in adequate pulmonary gas exchange. Signs of respiratory distress—which is classified as mild, moderate, or severe—include the following:

- Pallor or mottled color
- Irritability, anxiety, restlessness
- Respiratory rate faster than normal for age
- Retractions (suprasternal, intercostal, subcostal)
- Abdominal breathing
- Nasal flaring
- Inspiratory stridor
- Grunting
- Mild tachycardia

A patient in **respiratory failure** can no longer compensate for the underlying pathologic or anatomic problem by increased work of breathing, so hypoxia and/or carbon dioxide retention occur. Signs of respiratory failure may include decreased or absent retractions owing to fatigue of the chest wall muscles, altered mental status owing to inadequate oxygenation and ventilation of the brain, and an abnormally low respiratory rate Table 43-12. Respiratory failure is a decompensated state, requiring urgent intervention to ensure adequate oxygenation and ventilation and prevent respiratory or cardiopulmonary arrest. Do not be afraid to assist ventilations at this point if you judge the tidal volume or respiratory effort to be inadequate.

Table 43-12	Signs of Impending Respiratory Failure
Assess	**Sign**
Mental status	Agitation, restlessness, confusion, lethargy (VPU components of the AVPU scale)
Skin color	Central cyanosis despite oxygen administration, pallor
Respiratory rate	Tachypnea → bradypnea → apnea
Respiratory effort	Severe retractions and accessory muscle use, nasal flaring, grunting, paradoxical abdominal motion, tripod positioning
Auscultation	Stridor, wheezing, crackles, or diminished air movement
Blood oxygen saturation	Low despite supplemental oxygen administration
Pulse rate	Tachycardia → bradycardia

Abbreviation: AVPU, Awake and alert, responsive to Verbal stimuli, responsive to Pain, Unresponsive
© Jones & Bartlett Learning.

Special Populations

Initiate aggressive airway management and ventilatory support with a bag-mask device and supplemental oxygen as soon as possible for a child with respiratory failure.

Respiratory arrest means the patient is not breathing spontaneously. Administer immediate bag-mask ventilation with supplemental oxygen to prevent progression to cardiopulmonary arrest. Resuscitation of a child from respiratory arrest is often successful, whereas resuscitation of a child in cardiopulmonary arrest may or may not be.

Your determination of whether the patient is in respiratory distress, respiratory failure, or respiratory arrest will drive your next steps, by indicating the urgency for treatment and transport. You can obtain the SAMPLE history at the scene or during transport, depending on the patient's stability. Table 43-13 lists key questions to ask during a respiratory emergency.

Most pediatric patients with a primary respiratory complaint will have respiratory distress and require only supportive care. Allow the child to assume a position of comfort, and provide supplemental oxygen. The choice of oxygen delivery method will depend on the severity of illness and the child's developmental level. Young children may become agitated by a nasal cannula or face

Table 43-13	SAMPLE Components for Pediatric Respiratory Emergencies	
Component	**Features**	
Signs and symptoms	Shortness of breath, hoarseness Stridor, wheezing, cough, chest pain, choking, rash/hives Cyanosis	
Allergies	Known medication or food allergies; smoke exposure	
Medications	Names and doses of ongoing medications; recent use of corticosteroids	
Past medical history	History of asthma, chronic lung disease, heart problems, prematurity; prior hospitalizations and intubation for breathing problems; history of choking or anaphylaxis; immunizations	
Last oral intake	Timing of last food, including bottle or breastfeeding	
Events leading to illness or injury	Fever history or recent illness; history of injury to chest; history of choking on food or object	

© Jones & Bartlett Learning.

mask. Because crying and thrashing increase metabolic demands and oxygen consumption, you must weigh the benefits of this therapy against the potential cost. Allowing a caregiver to deliver blow-by oxygen to a calm toddler may be your best choice, if the child does not show signs of respiratory failure.

As a child becomes fatigued, respiratory distress may progress to respiratory failure. As part of your reassessment, electronically monitor the patient's pulse rate, respiratory rate, and oxygen saturation level. A significant change or trend in any of these variables requires prompt attention. You should also perform frequent reassessment to evaluate the effects of your treatment.

Consider the following when caring for a child with a respiratory emergency[2]:

- Give supplemental oxygen; escalate from a nasal cannula to a simple face mask to a nonrebreathing mask as needed to maintain normal oxygenation.
- Perform ECG monitoring if there are no signs of clinical improvement after treating respiratory distress.

- Establish IV access if you have clinical concerns about dehydration or if you anticipate the need to administer IV medications.
- The child's airway should be managed in the least invasive way possible. Supraglottic airway devices and intubation should be performed only if bag-mask ventilation fails.

Special Populations

Respiratory distress, respiratory failure, and respiratory arrest exist along a continuum. Intervene early to prevent progression to respiratory arrest in pediatric patients.

▶ Upper Airway Emergencies

Upper airway emergencies in children may be caused by foreign body aspiration or obstruction, anaphylaxis, croup, epiglottitis, and bacterial tracheitis.

Foreign Body Aspiration or Obstruction

Infants and toddlers explore their environment by putting objects into their mouths, resulting in a high risk of foreign body aspiration. Any small object or food item has the potential to obstruct a young child's narrow trachea. Peanuts, hot dogs, grapes, balloons, and small toys or pieces of toys are frequent offenders. Swallowed foreign bodies can also cause respiratory distress in infants and young children because a rigid esophageal foreign body can compress the relatively pliable trachea. In addition, the tongue, owing to its large size relative to the upper airway, frequently causes mild upper airway obstruction in a child with a decreased level of consciousness and diminished muscle tone. Pencil erasers, candy, and beans frequently obstruct children's nostrils; these items often remain in the nose for a day or two before the child has pain and a foul-smelling nasal discharge.

Words of Wisdom

The soft latex of a deflated balloon can be sucked into a child's airway past the cricoid ring, where you are unlikely to be able to remove it. Because of this hazard, do not blow up a glove and give it to a child as a toy.

In the absence of a fever, cough, or respiratory congestion, suspect foreign body aspiration when a child has a sudden onset of respiratory distress accompanied by coughing, gagging, stridor, or wheezing. An awake patient with stridor, increased work of breathing, and good color on the PAT has mild upper airway obstruction. Auscultation may reveal fair to good air entry, and the presence of unilateral wheezing may tip you off to a foreign body lodged in a main stem bronchus. In contrast, a patient with severe airway obstruction is likely to be cyanotic and unconscious when you arrive, owing to profound hypoxia. If the child has spontaneous respiratory effort, you will hear poor air entry, but you may *not* hear stridor owing to minimal airflow through the trachea. A typical SAMPLE history for foreign body aspiration reveals a previously healthy child with sudden onset of coughing, choking, or gagging while eating or playing.

Initial management of mild airway obstruction involves allowing the patient to assume a position of comfort, providing supplemental oxygen as tolerated, and transporting the child to an appropriate medical facility. Avoid agitating the child because this stimulus could worsen the situation. Continuous monitoring and frequent reassessments are needed to ensure the problem does not progress to severe airway obstruction. In cases of a severe airway obstruction, the patient is unable to cough or make any sound. Rapid intervention is needed to clear the obstruction.

Removing a Foreign Body Airway Obstruction in Responsive Infants. For a responsive infant, deliver five back slaps and five chest thrusts (**Figure 43-10**):

1. Hold the infant facedown, with the body resting on your forearm. Support the infant's head and face with your hand, and keep the head lower than the rest of the body.
2. Deliver five back slaps between the shoulder blades using the heel of your hand.
3. Place your free hand behind the infant's head and back, and bring the infant upright on your thigh, sandwiching the infant's body between your two hands and arms. The infant's head should remain below the level of the body.
4. Give five quick chest thrusts in the same location and manner as for chest compressions, using two fingers placed on the lower half of the sternum. For larger infants, or if you have small hands, you can place the infant in your lap and turn the infant's whole body as a unit between back slaps and chest thrusts.
5. Check the airway. If you can see the foreign body now, remove it. If you cannot, repeat the cycle as often as necessary. Do not stick your fingers in the infant's mouth to remove a foreign body unless you can actually visualize the object.
6. If the infant becomes unresponsive, begin CPR with compressions, remembering to look in the airway before ventilations each time.

Removing a Foreign Body Airway Obstruction in Unresponsive Infants. As with the adult and the child, if the infant loses consciousness, start CPR beginning with 30 chest compressions (15 compressions if two rescuers

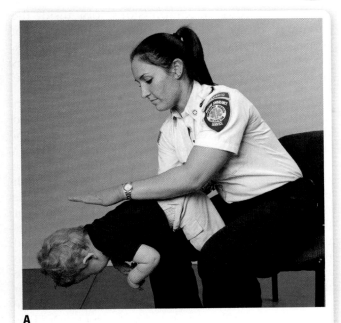

A

B

Figure 43-10 Perform back slaps and chest thrusts to clear a foreign body airway obstruction in a responsive infant. **A.** Deliver five quick back slaps between the shoulder blades, using the heel of your hand. **B.** Give five quick chest thrusts, using two fingers placed on the lower half of the sternum.

© Jones & Bartlett Learning. Photographed by Glen E. Ellman.

Words of Wisdom

According to current resuscitation guidelines, an infant is younger than age 1 year; a child is a person from age 1 year until the onset of puberty (age 12 to 14 years).[3]

are present). After 30 compressions, look inside the mouth. If you see the object, remove it. If not, attempt to give 2 breaths. Continue the process of compressions, always looking in the mouth, and attempting ventilations until the obstruction is relieved. Then, assess for a pulse.

Removing a Foreign Body Airway Obstruction in Children.
Performing abdominal thrusts (also called the Heimlich maneuver) is the most effective method of dislodging and forcing an object out of the airway of a responsive adult or child. This method aims to increase the pressure in the chest, creating an artificial cough that may force a foreign body from the airway. Use this maneuver until the obstructing object is expelled or the child becomes unresponsive. If the child becomes unresponsive, carefully position him or her supine and perform 30 chest compressions (15 compressions if two rescuers are present). After 30 compressions, look inside the mouth. If you see the object, remove it. If not, attempt to give 2 breaths. If the first breath does not produce visible chest rise, reopen the airway and reattempt to ventilate. If both breaths fail to produce visible chest rise, continue chest compressions. If you are unable to relieve a severe airway obstruction in an unresponsive patient with the basic techniques previously discussed, you should proceed with direct laryngoscopy (visualization of the airway with a laryngoscope) for the removal of the foreign body. Insert the laryngoscope blade into the patient's mouth. If you see the foreign body, carefully remove it from the upper airway with Magill forceps, a special type of curved forceps. Refer to Chapter 15, *Airway Management*, for more information on this procedure.

Anaphylaxis

Anaphylaxis is a potentially life-threatening allergic reaction, triggered by exposure to an antigen (foreign protein). Food—especially nuts, shellfish, eggs, and milk—and bee stings are among the most common causes, although anaphylaxis to antibiotics and other medications can occur as well. Exposure to the antigen stimulates the release of histamine and other vasoactive chemical mediators from white blood cells, leading to multiple organ system involvement. Onset of symptoms generally occurs immediately after the exposure and may include hives, respiratory distress, circulatory compromise, and gastrointestinal symptoms (vomiting, diarrhea, abdominal pain). See Chapter 25, *Immunologic Emergencies*, for more information about the sequence of events in anaphylaxis.

Although a child with mild anaphylaxis may experience only hives and some wheezing, a child with severe anaphylaxis may be in respiratory failure and shock when you arrive. The PAT may reveal an anxious child. With severe anaphylaxis, the child may be unresponsive due to respiratory failure and shock. He or she may have increased work of breathing due to upper airway edema or bronchospasm and poor circulation. The primary survey will usually reveal hives, with other findings potentially including swelling of the lips and oral mucosa, stridor,

and/or wheezing. If the child has a known allergy, the SAMPLE history may reveal recent contact with or ingestion of the potentially offending agent (including consumption of prepared foods containing traces of eggs, nuts, and milk at day care or school).

The "gold standard" treatment for anaphylaxis is epinephrine. Epinephrine's alpha-agonist effect decreases airway edema by vasoconstriction and improves circulation by increasing peripheral vascular resistance. Its beta-agonist effect causes bronchodilation, resulting in improved oxygenation and ventilation. Epinephrine should be given by the intramuscular (IM) route.[4] This dose may be repeated as necessary every 5 to 15 minutes. If several doses are needed, the child may require a continuous IV epinephrine drip. In addition to epinephrine, treatment of anaphylaxis should include supplemental oxygen, fluid resuscitation for shock, diphenhydramine (Benadryl), and bronchodilators for wheezing.

Many children with a history of anaphylaxis will have been treated with IM epinephrine by a caregiver before EMS activation. Given the short half-life of this drug, the child should be transported, even if asymptomatic on your arrival.

Evidence-Based Medicine

Recently, the US Food and Drug Administration updated the administration instructions for epinephrine autoinjectors.[5] The duration of the injection time has been shortened to reduce the risk of injury to a moving or uncooperative child. It is now recommended that the leg be held firmly in place during the injection and that the epinephrine autoinjector be held in place for approximately 3 seconds, as opposed to the originally recommended 10 seconds.[6]

Croup

Croup (laryngotracheobronchitis) is a viral infection of the upper airway. The virus is transmitted by respiratory secretions or droplets from coughing, sneezing, and breathing. Croup primarily affects children between 6 months and 6 years of age,[7] with most cases occurring in the fall and winter months. The viruses that lead to croup have an affinity for the **subglottic space**—the narrowest part of the pediatric airway—and cause edema and progressive airway obstruction. Turbulent airflow through the narrowed subglottic airway produces the hallmark sign of croup—stridor. The SAMPLE history usually reveals several days of cold symptoms and low-grade fever, followed by the onset of a barky cough, stridor, and trouble breathing. The cough and respiratory distress are often worse at night.

The severity of croup may range from mild to severe. With mild croup, there is an absence of stridor at rest, minimal respiratory distress, and an occasional cough. With moderate croup, the child's behavior and mental status are normal but inspiratory stridor and retractions are present at rest and the amount of respiratory distress is increased. With severe croup, mental status changes are present accompanied by significant respiratory distress and decreasing air entry, indicating impending respiratory failure.[8]

> ## Special Populations
>
> The presence of hypoxia in a child with croup is a potentially ominous finding, indicating significant subglottic edema. Assess and transport the patient quickly.

The initial management of croup is the same as that for most respiratory emergencies. Allow the child to assume a position of comfort, and avoid agitating him or her. The use of humidified oxygen or mist therapy is not indicated.[2] A steroid, such as dexamethasone, may be administered IV or IM to reduce inflammation. For patients with stridor at rest, moderate to severe respiratory distress, poor air exchange, hypoxia, or altered appearance, nebulized epinephrine is the treatment of choice. It works by causing vasoconstriction and decreasing upper airway edema. Nebulized epinephrine is available in two formulations: racemic epinephrine and L-epinephrine. Although only a small amount of epinephrine is absorbed via the nebulized route, adverse effects may include tachycardia, agitation, tremor, and vomiting.

In the case of croup and respiratory failure, nebulized epinephrine alone may not be adequate and assisted ventilation may be necessary. Assisted ventilation with bag-mask ventilation will often succeed in overcoming the upper airway obstruction. Advanced airway placement is rarely needed in croup. If performed, choose an ET tube one-half to one full size smaller than normal for age or size to accommodate the subglottic edema. Children requiring nebulized epinephrine or assisted ventilation need to be transported immediately to an appropriate treatment facility.

> ## Words of Wisdom
>
> Bag-mask ventilation is the mainstay of treatment for most upper airway emergencies.

Epiglottitis

Epiglottitis is a life-threatening condition that causes the epiglottis and supraglottic tissues to swell. The pus-filled flap of tissue then partially or completely occludes the glottic opening. Although this disease can affect any age group, it is most prevalent in 2- to 7-year olds. Its incidence has fallen sharply since 1988, when administration of the *Haemophilus influenzae* type b (Hib) vaccine to children became routine.

The classic presentation of epiglottitis is easily distinguished using the PAT. A child with epiglottitis looks sick and will be anxious, will sit upright in the sniffing position with the chin thrust forward to allow for maximal air entry, and may be drooling because of an inability to swallow secretions. The work of breathing is increased, and pallor or cyanosis may be evident. Stridor heard on auscultation over the neck, a muffled voice, decreased or absent breath sounds, and hypoxia are all signs of a significant airway obstruction. The SAMPLE history will reveal a sudden onset of high fever and sore throat. Because symptoms progress rapidly, children with epiglottitis are generally sick for only a few hours before they come to medical attention. Remember to ask about immunizations as part of the pertinent medical history for patients suspected of having epiglottitis.

Your goal is to get the child with epiglottitis to an appropriate hospital with a maintainable airway. Because of the risk for acute airway obstruction and respiratory arrest, minimize your on-scene time. Allow the patient to assume a position of comfort, and provide supplemental oxygen only if tolerated by the patient. Do not attempt to look in the mouth or insert an IV line because doing so can agitate the child and worsen his or her respiratory distress. Be prepared with a bag-mask device and an ET tube one to two sizes smaller than anticipated for the child's age and length in the event of complete obstruction during transport and the need for assisted ventilation. ET intubation of a child with epiglottitis is difficult because of the extreme distortion of the airway anatomy. Alert personnel at the receiving facility to the suspected diagnosis and the patient's condition, because they will need to mobilize a team for the management of this difficult airway.

Some uncommon conditions can also cause upper airway obstruction, including retropharyngeal abscess, peritonsillar abscess, tracheitis, and diphtheria. Presentation may include fever, stridor, difficulty handling secretions, and respiratory distress. Regardless of the underlying diagnosis, assessment and management will be the same as for croup.

Bacterial Tracheitis

Bacterial tracheitis is an acute bacterial infection of the subglottic area of the upper airway. Bacterial tracheitis is complicated by copious thick, pus-filled secretions. Children typically present with cough, stridor, and respiratory distress of varying degrees with a history of a preceding viral infection. Toddlers are at increased risk of complications due to their relatively narrow airway diameter and may present in extremis. Patients are often febrile and may prefer the sniffing position to increase airway diameter.

Allow the patient to assume a position of comfort, and provide supplemental oxygen as tolerated by the patient. Do not attempt to look in the mouth because doing so can precipitate complete airway obstruction, and do not insert an IV line. Try to keep the patient as calm and comfortable as possible. You should be prepared with a bag-mask device and an ET tube one to two sizes smaller than anticipated for the child's age and length in the event of complete obstruction during transport and the need for assisted ventilation. Alert the receiving facility of the potential need for intubation of a difficult airway.

► Lower Airway Emergencies

The underlying pathophysiology in upper airway emergencies involves restriction of airflow *into* the lungs (inhalation). By contrast, the pathophysiology of lower airway respiratory emergencies involves restriction of airflow *out* of the lungs (exhalation).

Even relatively minor viral infections that affect the airway can cause significant respiratory distress in small children. One millimeter of swelling in an adult airway might be annoying and cause a scratchy throat, but the same amount of swelling in a young child's airway can cause respiratory distress.

Asthma

Asthma is the most common chronic illness of childhood.[9] Recent studies indicate that the incidence and mortality of this disease are increasing. While it has long been erroneously thought that infants do not get asthma, researchers and rescuers increasingly recognize that even infants can have reactive airway disease caused by specific triggers.

With asthma, bronchospasm, mucus production, and airway inflammation lead to obstruction and poor gas exchange. As the obstruction becomes more severe, air trapping, inadequate ventilation, more severe hypoxemia, and hypoventilation with respiratory acidosis occur. Respiratory failure becomes imminent. Triggers for asthma attacks may include upper respiratory infections, environmental allergies, exposure to cold, changes in the weather, and secondhand smoke. Clinical signs include frequent cough, wheezing, and more general signs of respiratory distress.

The primary survey for a child with an acute exacerbation of asthma will vary based on the degree of obstruction and the presence or absence of respiratory fatigue. A child with mild to moderate respiratory distress will be awake and alert, sometimes preferring a seated posture. Although increased work of breathing may be evident by retractions and nasal flaring, circulation will seem normal. Decreasing alertness, assumption of the tripod position, deep retractions, and cyanosis are signs of severe respiratory distress and impending respiratory failure. The primary survey will reveal shortness of breath as evidenced by inability to speak in full sentences, increased respiratory rate, prolonged expiration phase, and wheezes noted on auscultation. Expiratory wheezing alone may be heard in patients with mild to moderate asthma attacks, but wheezing may be heard on inspiration and expiration in patients with moderate to severe disease. Decreased air movement and the absence of wheezes in a patient

with asthma suggest severe lower airway obstruction and respiratory fatigue and signal the need for immediate treatment to prevent respiratory arrest.

The SAMPLE history for a patient suspected of having asthma should reveal the frequency and severity of previous asthma attacks, as reflected by ED visits and hospitalizations. While taking the patient's history, keep in mind factors that increase the risk of asthma-related death, which include the following[9]:

- A history of near-fatal asthma requiring intubation and mechanical ventilation
- Hospitalization or an emergency care visit for asthma in the past year
- Currently using or having recently stopped using oral corticosteroids (a marker of event severity)
- Not currently using inhaled corticosteroids
- Overuse of short-acting beta-agonists
- Poor adherence with asthma medications
- Food allergy in a patient with asthma

The medication history should identify any preventive treatment (controller medications) and any rescue medications administered by the caregiver before your arrival. Inhaled steroids are the most common controller medications used in pediatrics, whereas inhaled albuterol is the most common beta-2 agonist drug used as a rescue medication.

The initial management of an asthma exacerbation remains basic respiratory care: allow the patient to remain in a position of comfort, and administer supplemental oxygen. The gold standard treatment consists of bronchodilators—that is, beta-agonists that act to relax smooth muscles in the bronchioles, thereby decreasing bronchospasm and improving air movement and oxygenation. Listen to breath sounds before and after administration to assess the child's response to treatment.

Bronchodilators may be delivered by nebulizer or metered-dose inhaler (MDI) with a spacer-mask device. Unit doses of 2.5 mg of albuterol premixed with 3 mL of normal saline are often used for nebulization and represent an acceptable starting dose for most young children. For a larger child or a child of any age who is in severe distress, consider administering 5 mg of albuterol as the initial dose. Children with moderate to severe respiratory distress can be given treatments as often as needed during transport, including back-to-back nebulizer treatments. Although albuterol is a relatively safe medication, its potential adverse effects include tachycardia, tremor, and mild hyperactivity. An isomer of albuterol, levalbuterol, reportedly has fewer adverse effects.

Children with moderate to severe respiratory distress may also benefit from treatment with inhaled ipratropium (Atrovent), an anticholinergic bronchodilator. Studies have shown that the combination of albuterol and ipratropium (which may be mixed and delivered together by nebulizer) is more effective than albuterol given alone. The dose of ipratropium given is based on the patient's weight: a 0.25-mg unit dose nebulized or one puff by MDI for children weighing less than 10 kg (22 pounds); a 0.5-mg unit dose nebulized or two puffs by MDI for children weighing more than 10 kg (22 pounds). Additionally, IM dexamethasone at 0.6 mg/kg (maximum dose of 16 mg) given early can shorten acute exacerbations of asthma and prevent or shorten hospitalizations, particularly if administered within the first hour of presentation.[10]

If a child is in severe respiratory distress, has an altered mental status, or has markedly diminished air movement on auscultation, a dose of epinephrine may be required. Epinephrine will cause immediate relaxation of bronchial smooth muscles, opening the airways to allow bronchodilators to work. The dose is 0.01 mg/kg of 1 mg/mL (1:1,000) epinephrine injected IM; single doses should not exceed 0.3 mg.[10] Initiate bronchodilator therapy immediately after administering the epinephrine.

Assisted ventilation can be problematic for patients with an asthma exacerbation. High inspiratory pressures force air into the lungs, but exhalation is compromised by bronchospasm, mucus production, and inflammation, which can lead to air trapping and a high risk of pneumothorax and cardiovascular collapse. Assisted ventilation should be undertaken only if the patient has respiratory failure and has failed to respond to IM epinephrine and high-dose bronchodilators. If this therapy is performed, use slow rates to allow time for adequate exhalation. Your goal is adequate oxygenation.

Respiratory Syncytial Virus Infection

Respiratory syncytial virus (RSV) is the leading cause of lower respiratory tract infections in infants, older people, and immunocompromised people; it is a common and contagious virus that causes bronchiolitis and pneumonia in children. This virus spreads in the hospital environment and in the community. In the community setting, outbreaks generally occur in late fall, winter, and early spring.

Transmission may occur in two ways: (1) by direct contact with large droplets, which do not travel more than 3 feet (1 m), or (2) by indirect contact with contaminated hands or contaminated items. Research has shown that RSV on hands will die within 1 hour; however, the virus has been shown to survive on other surfaces for as long as 30 hours. The incubation period ranges from 2 to 8 days. Most EDs can identify RSV by means of a nasal swab.

Signs and symptoms include those of upper respiratory infection—sneezing, runny nose, nasal congestion, cough, and fever. The disease progresses to the lower respiratory tract, leading to pneumonia, bronchiolitis, and tracheobronchitis. Hypoxemia and apnea are often seen in infants and are usually the leading cause for a child's hospitalization.

Prevention of RSV transmission relies on proper use of personal protective equipment. Gloves should be worn when caring for an RSV-infected patient, and their removal must be followed by good handwashing. The use of alcohol-based foams or gels is acceptable. Post-transport cleaning of the vehicle is important, but special cleaning solutions are not required.

Postexposure treatment consists of supportive care. If you have been exposed, your designated infection control officer will monitor your health status. Health care providers in whom RSV infection develops should be placed on work restrictions. In particular, they should not care for immunocompromised patients.

Bronchiolitis

Bronchiolitis is an inflammation or swelling of the small airways (bronchioles) in the lower respiratory tract due to viral infection. The most common cause of this disease is infection with RSV, although a newer virus, metapneumovirus, and some other respiratory viruses have also been found to cause this illness. Transmission of bronchiolitis generally occurs by inhaling droplets of infected mucus or respiratory secretions. Infections with these viruses occur with highest frequency during the winter months, and they primarily affect infants and children younger than 2 years. A highly contagious disease, bronchiolitis has a severity that ranges from mild to moderate respiratory distress with hypoxia and respiratory failure. Infants are at particularly high risk for episodes of apnea associated with RSV infection, which may not be associated with severe respiratory distress.

The signs and symptoms of bronchiolitis can be difficult to distinguish from those of asthma. One clue is the child's age: asthma is rare in children younger than 1 year. An infant with a first-time wheezing episode occurring in late fall or winter likely has bronchiolitis. Mild to moderate retractions, tachypnea, diffuse wheezing, diffuse crackles, and mild hypoxia are characteristic findings during the primary survey. As is true in a patient with asthma, a sleepy patient with bronchiolitis or one with severe retractions, diminished breath sounds, or moderate to severe hypoxia (oxygen saturation less than 90%) is in danger of respiratory failure and requires immediate transport. Infants in the first months of life or who have a history of prematurity, underlying lung disease, congenital heart disease, or immunodeficiency are at greatest risk for respiratory failure and arrest.

The management of infants and young children with bronchiolitis is supportive. Leave the patient in a position of comfort (eg, in the caregiver's arms, if the child does not seem to be in respiratory failure), and provide supplemental oxygen. Thick nasal and oral secretions should be suctioned to clear the airway. Because the bronchioles are usually too deep in the airway to be surrounded by any smooth muscle, aerosol bronchodilators rarely help patients with this condition. In fact, one definition of bronchiolitis is wheezing that is unresponsive to bronchodilators. Although bronchodilator therapy has not proved effective in the majority of cases, nebulized racemic epinephrine (0.5 mL of a 2.25% solution for inhalation) should be administered to children in severe respiratory distress if suctioning and oxygen administration fail to result in clinical improvement.[11] Continuous positive airway pressure (CPAP) should be administered, if available, for severe respiratory distress. Assist breathing with a bag-mask device if signs of respiratory failure are present. Supraglottic devices and ET intubation should be used only if bag-mask ventilation fails.[11]

Pneumonia

Pneumonia is a common disease process that infects the lower airway and the lung. Although it can occur at any age, in pediatric patients it is commonly seen in infants, toddlers, and preschoolers. In infants and toddlers, pneumonia is often caused by a virus. As children get older, however, the incidence of bacterial pneumonia increases. Children with pneumonia typically have a recent history of a cough or cold, or a lower airway infection (ie, bronchiolitis). Maintain a high index of suspicion when called for children with any drop in oxygen saturation, particularly when accompanied by a fever or abnormal breath sounds.

Often pediatric patients will present with unusually rapid breathing or will breathe with grunting or wheezing sounds. Additional signs and symptoms include nasal flaring, tachypnea, crackles, chest pain, and hypothermia or fever. The patient may also exhibit unilateral diminished breath sounds. Assess the work of breathing by observing for signs of accessory muscle use. Pneumonia in the infant population may not be tolerated as well as in the older child or adult populations because infants have an increased oxygen demand and less reserve amounts.

For a pediatric patient with suspected pneumonia, your primary treatment will be supportive: monitor the patient's airway and breathing status, and administer supplemental oxygen if required. Take standard precautions and consider placing a mask on the child if tolerated. Vascular access is generally not indicated for children with pneumonia; however, if the child's condition warrants medication therapy, establish IV or intraosseous (IO) access en route to the hospital.

Pertussis

Pertussis, also known as whooping cough, is a highly contagious disease caused by a bacterium that is spread through respiratory droplets. As the result of vaccinations, this potentially deadly disease is less common in the United States. Unfortunately, immunization rates have fallen in recent years because of apathy, lack of access to medical care, and the growing fear of some parents that immunization has negative consequences. As a result, the incidence of pertussis infection is on the rise in the United States.

The typical signs and symptoms of pertussis are similar to those of a common cold: coughing, sneezing, and a runny nose. As the disease progresses, the coughing becomes more severe and can take on a "staccato" or repetitive/episodic characteristic, and children can develop the distinctive whoop sound heard during the inspiratory phase between coughing episodes. The cough can last as long as 6 weeks, earning pertussis the title "the 100-day cough." It can be so severe that it can cause post-cough vomiting (posttussive emesis), conjunctival hemorrhages, and cyanotic hypoxia. In very young infants, pertussis can also present with apnea.

To treat these pediatric patients, keep the airway patent and transport to the ED. Because pertussis is a contagious disease, take standard precautions, including wearing a mask and eye protection.

▶ Other Respiratory Conditions

Cystic Fibrosis

Cystic fibrosis (CF) is a genetic disease that primarily affects the respiratory and digestive systems. It is the most common life-shortening hereditary disease among people of European descent. People with CF chronically produce copious amounts of thick mucus in their respiratory and digestive tracts, which makes them susceptible to recurrent respiratory infections and requires them to maintain a relatively strict regimen of aerosol treatments, mucus management, and pulmonary exercise. People with CF have frequent respiratory illnesses that require hospitalization.

Pediatric patients may present with tachypnea, chest pain, and crackles, though it may be difficult to separate acute exam findings from chronic disease. Assess the work of breathing by observing for signs of accessory muscle usage, tachypnea, and nasal flaring. Apply supplemental oxygen as needed. Vascular access is generally not needed.

Bronchopulmonary Dysplasia

Bronchopulmonary dysplasia is a spectrum of lung conditions found in full-term and preterm infants who required long periods of high-concentration oxygen and ventilator support, ranging from mild reactive airway to debilitating chronic lung disease. While efforts to save premature infants during the past several decades have improved the ability to save smaller and smaller infants, some of the survivors are left with severely damaged lungs, occasionally requiring long-term ventilator support. Children with bronchopulmonary dysplasia may use home ventilators, have tracheostomies, or have fragile lungs and many pulmonary complications. These patients are at high risk for recurrent pulmonary infections, including pneumonias, bronchiolitis, and tracheitis. Because many patients will be on home oxygen, it is important to ask caregivers about baseline oxygen requirements, tracheostomy secretions, and ventilator settings, and to note any acute changes that have occurred with illness.

As in all pediatric patients with respiratory symptoms, upper airway obstruction in children with bronchopulmonary dysplasia can cause distress, so remembering the ABCs of airway management is important. Positioning the airway with a head tilt–chin lift or jaw-thrust maneuver, or with a nasopharyngeal or oropharyngeal airway, may help overcome the obstruction and distress. Bag-mask ventilation and positive airway pressure should also be considered. CPAP or bilevel positive airway pressure may be beneficial, but ultimately patients with broncho-pulmonary dysplasia may require intubation for severe distress or respiratory failure. When intubating such a patient, consider the patient's size and weight when choosing an ET tube; the size needed may be smaller than you would typically pick if you considered only the child's chronologic age. A length-based resuscitation tape measure may be helpful in selecting the appropriate ET tube size.

Although administering oxygen may lead to lung damage in premature infants and subsequently cause bronchopulmonary dysplasia, children with desaturations require oxygen therapy. If bronchospasm is present, bronchodilators such as albuterol may be tried, though improvement may not be seen because the mechanism could be related to the underlying lung disease. Ipratropium may be beneficial in some patients with bronchopulmonary dysplasia. Steroids such as dexamethasone can be considered acutely, but they should be avoided if overwhelming infection is a concern.

► General Assessment and Management of Respiratory Emergencies

Infants and young children with severe tachypnea and retractions, in association with hypoxia, bradycardia, or altered mental status, are in respiratory failure and need immediate intervention to prevent respiratory arrest. A respiratory rate too slow for age in a child with a history of respiratory distress should also raise concerns for respiratory fatigue and failure.

Airway Management

Managing any respiratory emergency starts with the airway. Check for obstruction, and position the airway using the head tilt–chin lift or jaw-thrust maneuver **Figure 43-11**. In a child younger than 2 years, place a thin layer of padding under the shoulders or upper torso to align the airway **Figure 43-12**.

An airway adjunct may be helpful if the patient is unresponsive and cannot maintain a patent airway. The use of a nasal or oral airway will help to maintain an open airway and improve bag-mask ventilation, and it may avert the need for an advanced airway (such as an ET tube, laryngeal mask airway, King LT airway, or Combitube). When you are placing the adjunct airway, make sure to start by choosing the appropriately sized equipment.

Oropharyngeal Airway

An oropharyngeal (oral) airway is designed to keep the tongue from blocking the airway, and it makes suctioning

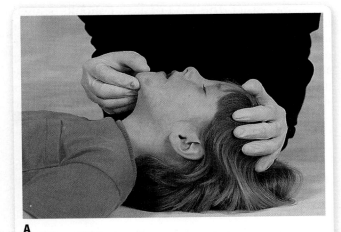

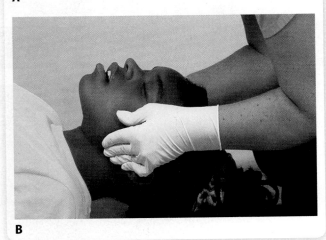

Figure 43-11 A. Use the head tilt–chin lift maneuver to open the airway of a child without trauma. **B.** For a child with suspected spinal injury, use the jaw-thrust maneuver to open the airway.

© Jones & Bartlett Learning. Courtesy of MIEMSS.

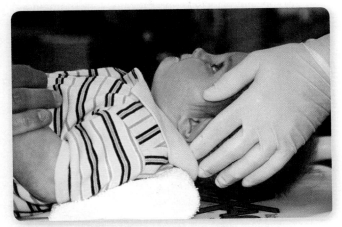

Figure 43-12 Padding, such as a shoulder roll, is often required in children younger than 2 years to achieve a neutral airway position.

© American Academy of Orthopaedic Surgeons.

the airway easier. This kind of airway should be used for pediatric patients who are unresponsive and cannot maintain their own airway spontaneously. It should *not* be used for conscious patients or patients with a gag reflex; an oropharyngeal airway may stimulate vomiting, thereby increasing the risk of aspiration. In addition, this adjunct should *not* be used for children who have ingested a caustic (corrosive) or petroleum-based product. **Skill Drill 43-1** shows the preferred technique for inserting an oropharyngeal airway in a child.

Take care to avoid injuring the hard palate as you insert the airway. Rough insertion can cause bleeding that may aggravate airway problems and cause vomiting. If the oropharyngeal airway is too small, the tongue may be pushed back into the pharynx, obstructing the airway. If it is too large, it may obstruct the larynx.

Nasopharyngeal Airway

A nasopharyngeal airway is usually well tolerated and is not as likely as the oropharyngeal airway to cause vomiting. The nasopharyngeal airway is used for conscious patients and patients with altered levels of consciousness. In pediatric patients, it is typically used in association

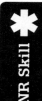

Skill Drill 43-1 **Inserting an Oropharyngeal Airway in a Pediatric Patient**

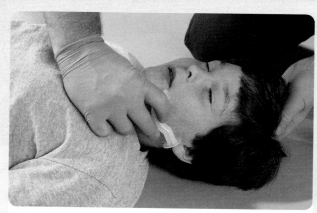

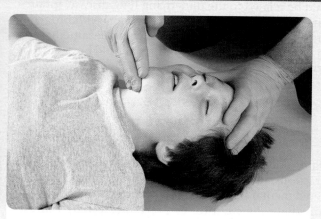

Step 1 Determine the appropriate size airway by measuring from the corner of the mouth to the angle of the jaw or by using a length-based resuscitation tape to measure the patient. Place the airway next to the face, with the flange at the level of the central incisors and the bite block segment parallel to the hard palate. The tip of the airway should reach the angle of the jaw.

Step 2 Position the patient's airway. For medical patients, use the head tilt–chin lift maneuver, avoiding hyperextension. If the patient has a traumatic injury, use the jaw-thrust maneuver and provide in-line spinal stabilization.

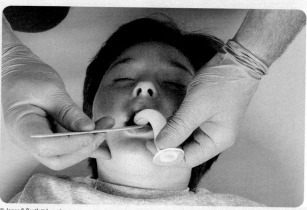

Step 3 Open the mouth by applying pressure on the chin with your thumb. Insert the airway by depressing the tongue with a tongue blade on the base of the tongue and inserting the airway directly over the tongue blade. If a tongue blade is not available, point the airway tip toward the roof of the mouth to depress the tongue. Gently rotate the airway into position as it passes through the mouth toward the curve of the tongue. Insert the airway until the flange rests against the lips. Reassess the airway after insertion.

with respiratory failure. It is also a good choice for maintaining an airway in patients who are experiencing a seizure or who are in a postictal state. This type of airway is rarely used for children younger than 1 year because of the small diameter of their nares, which tend to become easily obstructed by secretions. Follow the steps in (Skill Drill 43-2) to insert a nasopharyngeal airway in a child.

Several problems are possible with the nasopharyngeal airway. A diameter that is too small may become obstructed by mucus, blood, vomitus, or the soft tissues of the pharynx. If the airway is too long, it may stimulate the vagus nerve and slow the pulse rate; it may also enter the esophagus, causing gastric distention. Inserting the airway in responsive patients may cause spasm of the larynx and result in vomiting. A nasopharyngeal airway should not be used when the patient has facial trauma because the airway may tear soft tissues and cause bleeding into the

airway. Similarly, a nasopharyngeal airway should not be used for a patient with moderate to severe head trauma because it could increase ICP.

Oxygenation

As part of your breathing assessment, you will assess the patient's ventilatory and oxygenation status. All patients with respiratory emergencies should receive supplemental oxygen. The two most common ways to deliver oxygen to pediatric patients are the blow-by technique and the nonrebreathing mask.

The **blow-by technique** does not deliver high concentrations of oxygen to the patient, so it is best used when only a small amount of supplemental oxygen is needed or when the patient cannot tolerate wearing the mask needed for higher oxygen delivery. You can use oxygen tubing, a mask, a cup, or a similar device to deliver blow-by

---

Skill Drill 43-2 Inserting a Nasopharyngeal Airway in a Pediatric Patient

NR Skill

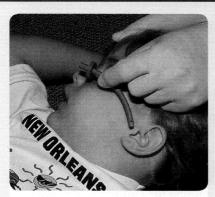

Step 1 Determine the appropriately sized airway. The external diameter of the airway should not be larger than the diameter of the naris, and there should be no blanching (turning white) of the naris after insertion. Place the airway next to the patient's face to make sure the length is correct. The airway should extend from the tip of the nose to the tragus of the ear (ie, the small cartilaginous projection in front of the opening of the ear). Position the patient's airway, using the techniques described for the oropharyngeal airway.

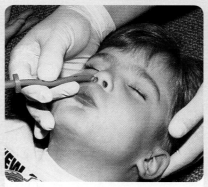

Step 2 Lubricate the airway with a water-soluble lubricant. Insert the tip into the right naris with the bevel pointing toward the nasal septum.

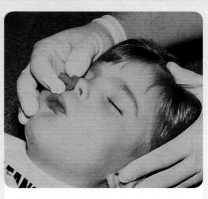

Step 3 Carefully move the tip forward, following the curvature of the nose, until the flange rests against the outside of the nostril. If you are inserting the airway on the left side, insert the tip into the left naris upside down, with the bevel pointing toward the septum. Move the airway forward slowly until you feel a slight resistance, and then rotate the airway 180°. Reassess the airway after insertion.

oxygen **Figure 43-13**. The child or caregiver can hold the device near the patient's face. Do not use a Styrofoam cup because it may blow fluorocarbons into the child's airway. The idea is to increase the oxygen concentration immediately around the patient's mouth and nose.

For children in significant respiratory distress or respiratory failure or for older children, a nonrebreathing mask is the preferred method of oxygen delivery. At a flow rate of 10 to 15 L/min, a nonrebreathing mask can deliver up to 95% oxygen to the patient **Figure 43-14**.[12]

Bag-Mask Ventilation

If the patient's respiratory effort is not improved with airway positioning or insertion of an airway adjunct, you should start assisted ventilation using a bag-mask device.

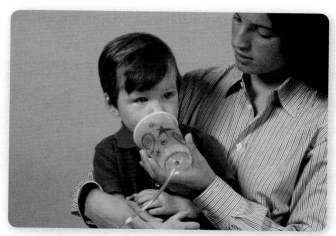

Figure 43-13 The blow-by oxygen technique can be used for a child with mild respiratory distress who will not tolerate a facial mask. Make a small hole in the base of a 6- to 8-ounce (180- to 240-mL) cup. Connect the oxygen tubing to an oxygen source, and hold the cup about 1 to 2 inches (3 to 5 cm) from the child's mouth.

© Jones & Bartlett Learning.

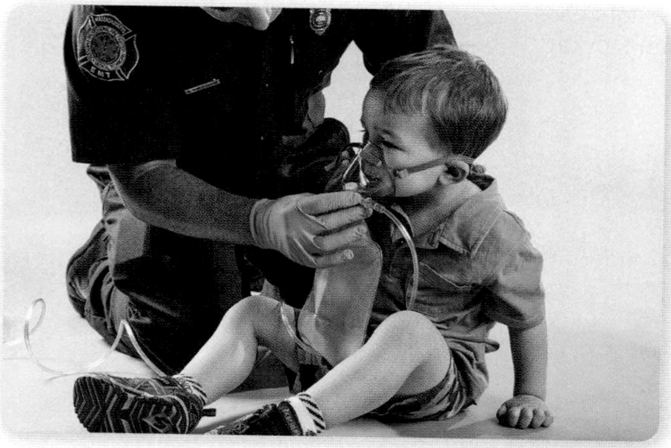

Figure 43-14 A pediatric nonrebreathing mask is the oxygen delivery method of choice for children who can tolerate it.

© Jones & Bartlett Learning.

Bag-mask ventilation is always the first step in assisted ventilation, and it represents definitive airway management for many patients. Proficiency in bag-mask ventilation is a vital skill for all EMS providers and may avert the need for ET intubation, a procedure with a much higher complication rate. You may need to try a variety of mask sizes to find the one that gives the optimal seal. Do not hesitate to change providers, hand position, or technique if difficulty with ventilation continues.

> ### Words of Wisdom
>
> Limit ventilation volume to just that necessary to cause the chest to rise.

Avoid excessive tidal volumes and rate to minimize the risk of gastric distention, vomiting, and aspiration. Deliver breaths at a rate of 12 to 20 breaths/min for infants and children (one breath every 3 to 5 seconds), squeezing the bag only until you see the chest rise. Do not overdistend the chest.

Assist the ventilation of an infant or child using a bag-mask device in the following way:

1. Ensure that you have the appropriate equipment in the right size. The mask should extend from the bridge of the nose to the cleft of the chin, avoiding compression of the eyes **Figure 43-15**. The mask is transparent, so you can observe for cyanosis and vomiting. The mask volume should be small to decrease dead space and avoid rebreathing. For infants and young children, the bag should contain at least 450 to 500 mL of air.[3] Use an infant bag rather than a neonatal bag for children older than 1 year. Older children and adolescents may need an adult-size bag. Make sure there is no pop-off

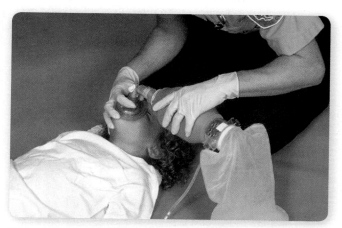

Figure 43-15 Ensure that you have the proper mask size for bag-mask ventilation.

© Jones & Bartlett Learning.

valve on the bag; if there is one, make sure you can hold it shut as necessary to achieve adequate chest rise.

2. Maintain a good seal with the mask on the face. An inadequate mask-to-face seal will result in inadequate tidal volume delivery and a decreased concentration of delivered oxygen. Consider the use of airway adjuncts (nasopharyngeal and oropharyngeal airways) in tandem with bag-mask ventilation.

3. Ventilate at the appropriate rate and volume using a slow, gentle squeeze (1 second per breath), until the chest visibly rises. Do not hyperventilate.

Errors in technique, including providing too much volume with each breath, squeezing the bag too forcefully, and ventilating at an excessive rate, can result in gastric distention (and the associated risks of vomiting and aspiration) and decreased venous return to the heart (preload)

because of increased intrathoracic pressure. An inadequate mask-to-face seal or improper head position can lead to inadequately delivered tidal volume and hypoxia.

Perform one-person bag-mask ventilation for an infant or child by following the steps in **Skill Drill 43-3**. By comparison, two-person bag-mask ventilation requires two rescuers—one to maintain an adequate mask-to-face seal and maintain the patient's head position and one to ventilate the patient. This technique is usually more effective at maintaining a tight seal and delivering adequate tidal volume. Because it is not possible to perform a one-handed jaw-thrust maneuver and also maintain spinal immobilization, ventilating the trauma patient is a two-person skill.

Supraglottic Airways

Several supraglottic airways are available for use in the pediatric patient. These devices are used to provide positive pressure ventilation to apneic patients and to maintain

Skill Drill 43-3 **Performing One-Person Bag-Mask Ventilation on a Pediatric Patient**

NR Skill

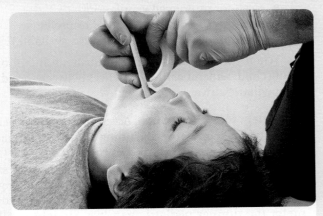

Step 1 Open the airway and insert the appropriate airway adjunct.

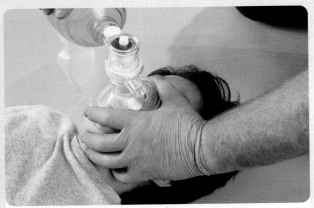

Step 2 Hold the mask on the patient's face by using the one-handed head tilt–chin lift technique (E-C grip) method. To use the E-C method, form a C with your thumb and index finger along the mask, while your other three fingers form an E along the mandible. With infants and toddlers, support the jaw with only your third finger. Do not compress the area under the chin, because you may push the tongue into the back of the mouth and block the airway. Keep your fingers on the mandible. Ensure the mask forms an airtight seal on the face. Maintain the seal while checking that the airway is open.

(continued)

Skill Drill 43-3 Performing One-Person Bag-Mask Ventilation on a Pediatric Patient *(continued)*

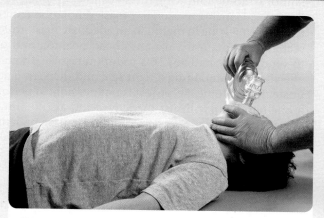

Step 3 Squeeze the bag, using the correct ventilation rate: 12 to 20 breaths/min for infants and children (1 breath every 3 to 5 seconds). Allow 1 second per ventilation, providing adequate time for exhalation.

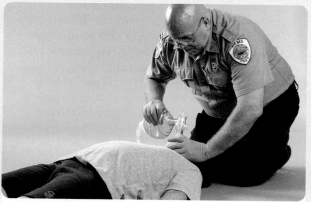

Step 4 Assess the effectiveness of ventilation by watching the bilateral rise and fall of the chest.

© Jones & Bartlett Learning.

a patent airway in unresponsive patients who are breathing spontaneously but who require advanced airway management. Refer to Chapter 15, *Airway Management*, for more information about these devices.

Endotracheal Intubation

ET intubation is defined as passing an ET tube through the glottic opening and sealing the tube with a cuff inflated against the tracheal wall. Consider ET intubation only if adequate oxygenation and ventilation cannot be achieved with good bag-mask technique or if transport times are long. Intubation has the advantage of providing a definitive airway and carrying a decreased risk of aspiration, but studies have shown significant failure and complication rates when using this technique in the prehospital setting. Potential complications include damage to teeth and oral structures, aspiration of gastric contents, bradycardia due to a vagal response, bradycardia due to hypoxemia from prolonged attempts, increased ICP, and incorrect placement. Incorrect placement of the ET tube into the right main stem bronchus may result in hypoxia and inadequate ventilation. A potentially catastrophic complication is an unrecognized esophageal intubation.

Indications for ET intubation in pediatric patients are the same as those in adults:

- Cardiopulmonary arrest
- Respiratory failure or arrest
- Traumatic brain injury
- Unresponsiveness

- Inability to maintain a patent airway
- Need for prolonged ventilation
- Need for ET administration of resuscitative medications (if no IV or IO access available)

When you are preparing to intubate an infant or a young child, remember the differences between the adult and pediatric airways Table 43-14 .

Equipment for ET Intubation. Access to pediatric-specific equipment is mandatory, including a range of laryngoscope blades in sizes 0 to 3 and ET tubes in sizes 2.5 (for field deliveries of premature infants) to 6.0. ET tube size selection is based on the child's age. Any size of laryngoscope handle can be used, although many paramedics prefer the thinner pediatric handles. Straight (Miller or Wis-Hipple) blades make it easy to lift the floppy epiglottis to provide a direct view of the vocal cords. If a curved (Macintosh) blade is used, the tip of the blade is positioned in the vallecula to lift the jaw and epiglottis to visualize the vocal cords.

The appropriately sized blade extends from the patient's mouth to the tragus of the ear. Acceptable means of measuring include using the length-based resuscitation tape measure or following these general guidelines:

- Premature newborn: size 0 straight blade
- Full-term newborn to 1 year: size 1 straight blade
- 2 years of age to adolescent: size 2 straight blade
- Adolescent age or older: size 3 straight or curved blade

Table 43-14	**Differences in the Pediatric Airway**

- Infants and small children (up to age 5 or 6 years) have a larger, rounder occiput, which causes the head of an infant or small child who lies supine to be in a flexed position.

- In children, the tongue is proportionally larger and the mandible is proportionally smaller—differences that increase children's propensity for airway obstruction.

- The epiglottis in a child is more floppy and U-shaped, so it must be lifted, or positioned, out of the way to visualize the vocal cords.

- The trachea in a child is smaller, shorter, and narrower than an adult's, and it is positioned more anteriorly and superiorly.

- The narrowest portion of the child's airway is the cricoid ring, which is below the vocal cords (subglottic), and the anatomy below the vocal cords is funnel-shaped. This difference makes a cuff less necessary for occluding the trachea; the developing cartilage of the cricoid ring could be injured by inflation of a cuffed ET tube.

Abbreviation: ET, endotracheal

© Jones & Bartlett Learning.

Length-based resuscitation tapes are more accurate than age-based formula estimates for determining the correct ET tube size in patients up to about 77 pounds (35 kg). If an uncuffed ET tube is used for intubation, use a 3.5-mm tube for infants up to 1 year of age and a 4-mm tube for children between 1 and 2 years of age.[13] For children older than 2 years, use this formula to estimate uncuffed ET tube size[13]:

$$4 + (\text{age in years} \div 4) = \text{Uncuffed tube size (in mm)}$$

If using a cuffed ET tube, use a 3-mm tube for infants and a 3.5-mm tube for children between 1 and 2 years of age.[13] For children older than 2 years, use this formula to estimate cuffed ET tube size[13]:

$$3.5 + (\text{age in years} \div 4) = \text{Cuffed tube size (in mm)}$$

Always have a tube that is one size smaller and one that is one size larger than expected available for situations in which there is variability in upper airway diameter.

For patients who are younger than 8 to 10 years, you may choose to use uncuffed ET tubes, although a noninflated cuffed tube is acceptable. A cuff at the cricoid ring may be unnecessary to obtain a seal in young children. Furthermore, there is the possibility of ischemia and damage to the mucosa of the trachea at this location when cuffs are inflated at high pressures.

The appropriate depth for insertion is 2 to 3 cm beyond the vocal cords. This depth should be recorded as the mark at the corner of the child's mouth. Uncuffed tubes often include a black glottic marker at the tube's distal end that you can use as a guide. When you see this line go through the vocal cord, stop. For cuffed tubes, when the cuff is just below the vocal cords, stop. Another guideline is to insert the tube to a depth that is equal to three times the inside diameter of the ET tube. The depth of insertion is important to avoid right main stem intubation or unplanned extubation.

Pediatric stylets will fit into tubes sized 3 to 6 mm, whereas adult stylets are used for tubes 6 mm or larger. The use of a stylet is based on personal preference. If you use a stylet, insert it into the ET tube, stopping at least 1 cm from the end of the tube; a stylet that protrudes beyond the end of the tube can damage the oral mucosa and vocal cords. With the stylet in place, bend the ET tube into a gentle upward curve. In some cases, bending the tube into the shape of a hockey stick is beneficial.

Preparing for and Performing Endotracheal Intubation. Pediatric patients should be preoxygenated (but not hyperventilated) with a bag-mask device and 100% supplemental oxygen for at least 2 to 3 minutes before you attempt intubation using the "squeeze, release, release" technique. Adequate preoxygenation cannot be overemphasized. During this time, you must also ensure the child's head is in the proper position—the neutral position for patients with suspected spinal trauma or the sniffing position for patients without trauma. Insert an airway adjunct if one is needed to ensure adequate ventilation.

Because bradycardia can occur during intubation, you should apply a cardiac monitor if one is available. Use a pulse oximeter before, during, and after the intubation attempt to monitor the patient's pulse rate and oxygen saturation. Have suction handy.

To perform ET intubation in an infant or a child, follow the steps listed in **Skill Drill 43-4**.

Documentation & Communication

Vital signs, especially pulse rate and oxygen saturation, should be recorded before and after each intubation attempt. Record the size of the ET tube and the depth of insertion as measured at the patient's lip.

If an intubated child deteriorates, use the DOPE mnemonic (Displacement, Obstruction, Pneumothorax, Equipment failure) to identify the potential problem, and institute an appropriate intervention **Table 43-15**.

Skill Drill 43-4 Performing Pediatric Endotracheal Intubation

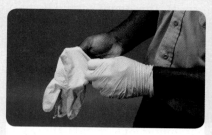

Step 1 Take standard precautions (gloves and face shield).

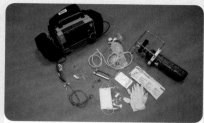

Step 2 Check, prepare, and assemble your equipment.

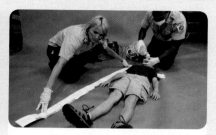

Step 3 Measure the length of the child using a length-based resuscitation tape to aid in determining needed equipment sizes.

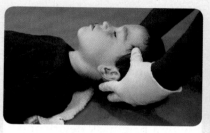

Step 4 Manually open the child's airway.

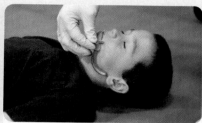

Step 5 Measure for proper size and then insert an oropharyngeal or nasopharyngeal airway.

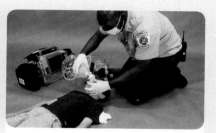

Step 6 Ventilate the patient with a bag-mask device at a rate of 12 to 20 breaths/min with sufficient volume to produce visible chest rise. Attach the pulse oximeter and note the child's oxygen saturation level. Preoxygenate the child for at least 2 to 3 minutes with 100% oxygen.

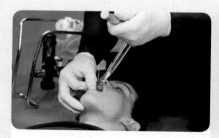

Step 7 Place the patient's head in a neutral or sniffing position; add padding as needed to achieve proper positioning. Remove the airway adjunct, then insert the laryngoscope into the right side of the mouth, and sweep the tongue to the left. Lift the tongue with firm, gentle pressure. Avoid using the teeth or gums as a fulcrum.

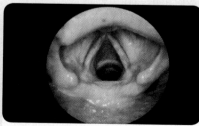

Step 8 Identify the vocal cords. If the cords are not yet visible, instruct your partner to perform the BURP maneuver (also called external laryngeal manipulation), if possible.

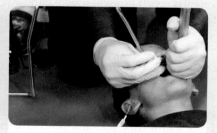

Step 9 Introduce the ET tube in the right corner of the child's mouth.

Skill Drill 43-4 Performing Pediatric Endotracheal Intubation (continued)

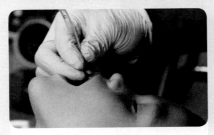

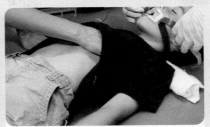

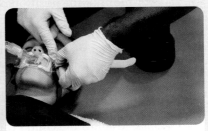

Step 10 Pass the ET tube through the vocal cords to approximately 2 to 3 cm below the vocal cords. Remove the laryngoscope from the patient's mouth. Inflate the cuff to the proper pressure and immediately remove the syringe if a cuffed tube is used.

Step 11 Attach an end-tidal carbon dioxide detector (waveform capnography preferred). Attach the bag-mask device, and auscultate for equal breath sounds over each lateral chest wall high in the axillae. Ensure absence of breath sounds over the epigastrium. Assess for hypoxia during the intubation attempt.

Step 12 Secure the ET tube with a commercial device or tape, noting the placement of the distance marker at the child's teeth or gums. Ventilate the patient at the proper rate and volume while monitoring capnography and pulse oximetry.

Step 1-7 and 9-12: © Jones & Bartlett Learning. Courtesy of MIEMSS; **Step 8:** © CNRI/Science Source.

Table 43-15	The DOPE Mnemonic for Troubleshooting Acute Deterioration in an Intubated Child
Displacement	■ Reauscultate breath sounds and any sounds over the epigastrium. ■ If breath sounds are louder on the right, slowly withdraw the tube until they are equal bilaterally. ■ If breath sounds are absent and you hear epigastric gurgling, immediately remove the ET tube, suction as needed, and ventilate with a bag-mask device and 100% oxygen.
Obstruction	■ If thick pulmonary secretions are interfering with your ability to effectively ventilate an intubated child, perform tracheobronchial suctioning. ■ Consider tube obstruction if ventilation compliance is decreased (ie, it is difficult to squeeze the bag).
Pneumothorax	■ Suspect a pneumothorax if breath sounds are louder on the *left* side and decreased or absent on the right; such findings are not consistent with right main stem bronchus intubation. ■ Ventilation compliance may also be decreased in a child with a pneumothorax. ■ Prepare to perform needle decompression.
Equipment failure	■ Ensure that you are giving 100% oxygen. ■ Check the reservoir bag on the bag-mask device for tears, ensure the device is attached to a 100% oxygen source, and check the bag itself for tears. ■ Immediately replace defective or damaged equipment.

Abbreviation: ET, endotracheal

© Jones & Bartlett Learning.

Complications of Endotracheal Intubation. Complications associated with ET intubation in pediatric patients are essentially the same as those for adult patients:

- **Unrecognized esophageal intubation.** *Frequently* monitor the position of the tube, especially after *any* major patient move. Use continuous waveform capnography.
- **Induction of emesis and possible aspiration.** *Always* have a suctioning device immediately available.
- **Hypoxia resulting from prolonged intubation attempts.** Limit pediatric intubation attempts to *20 seconds*. Monitor the child's cardiac rhythm and oxygen saturation during intubation.
- **Damage to teeth, soft tissues, and intraoral structures.** Technique, technique, technique!

Special Populations

A single intubation attempt should be limited to 20 seconds. If the attempt is not successful after 20 seconds, resume bag-mask ventilation and preoxygenate the child for the next attempt.

Orogastric and Nasogastric Tube Insertion

During positive pressure ventilation, it is common to inflate the stomach, as well as the lungs, with air and liquid. Gastric distention slows downward movement of the diaphragm and decreases tidal volume, making ventilation more difficult and necessitating higher inspiratory pressures. It also increases the risk that the patient will vomit and aspirate stomach contents into the lungs. Invasive gastric decompression involves placement of a nasogastric (NG) tube or an orogastric (OG) tube to decompress the stomach by removing the contents with suction, making assisting ventilation easier. Gastric decompression with an NG or OG tube is contraindicated in unresponsive children with a poor or absent gag reflex and an unsecured airway. Instead, you should perform ET intubation first to decrease the risk of vomiting and aspiration.

Preparation of Equipment. To perform NG or OG tube insertion, you will need an appropriately sized NG or OG tube, a 30- to 60-mL syringe with a funnel-tipped adapter for manual removal of stomach contents through the tube, mechanical suction, adhesive tape, and a water-soluble lubricant. To prepare the patient and the equipment for NG or OG tube placement, take the following steps:

1. Select the proper size of tube. Use a pediatric length-based resuscitation tape measure to determine the proper size, or use a tube size twice the uncuffed ET tube size that the child would need. For example, a child who needs a

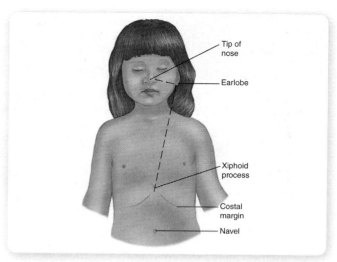

Figure 43-16 Technique for measuring the distance to insert a nasogastric or orogastric tube.

© Jones & Bartlett Learning.

5-mm uncuffed ET tube requires a 10-F OG or NG tube.

2. Measure the tube on the patient. The length of the tube should be the same as the distance from the lips or tip of the nose (depending on whether the OG or NG route is used) to the earlobe *plus* the distance from the earlobe to the xiphoid process **Figure 43-16**.
3. Mark this length on the tube with a piece of tape. When the tip of the tube is in the stomach, the tape should be at the lips or nostril.
4. Place the patient in a supine position.
5. Assess the gag reflex. If the patient is unresponsive and has a poor or absent gag reflex, perform ET intubation before gastric tube placement.
6. In a trauma patient, maintain in-line stabilization of the cervical spine if a neck injury is possible. Choose the OG route of insertion if the patient has a severe head or midfacial injury.
7. Lubricate the end of the tube.

OG Tube Insertion. Follow these steps to insert an OG tube in an infant or child:

1. Insert the tube over the tongue, using a tongue blade if necessary to facilitate insertion.
2. Advance the tube into the hypopharynx, then insert it rapidly into the stomach.
3. If the child begins coughing or choking or has a change in voice, immediately remove the tube; it may be in the trachea.

NG Tube Insertion. Follow these steps to insert an NG tube in an infant or child:

1. Insert the tube gently through the naris, directing the tube straight back along the nasal floor. Do not angle the tube superiorly. If the

tube does not pass easily, try the opposite naris or a smaller tube. Never force the tube.

2. Advance the tube into the stomach.
3. If NG passage is unsuccessful, use the OG approach.

Assessing Placement of OG and NG Tubes. Follow these steps to confirm successful placement of an NG or OG tube:

1. Check tube placement by aspirating stomach contents. Use a syringe with an appropriate adapter to quickly instill 10 to 20 mL of air through the tube while auscultating over the left upper quadrant. If you hear a rush of air (or gurgling) over the stomach, the placement is correct.
2. If correct placement cannot be confirmed, remove the tube.
3. Secure the tube to the bridge of the nose or to the cheek, using adhesive tape.
4. Aspirate air from the stomach, using a 30- to 60-mL catheter-tipped syringe, or connect the tube to mechanical suction at a low, continuous suction of 20 to 40 mm Hg or at the intermittent setting.

Complications of OG or NG Tube Insertion. As with ET intubation, you must be aware of the potential complications associated with the placement of an NG or OG tube—namely, placement of the tube into the trachea, resulting in hypoxia; vomiting and aspiration of stomach contents; airway bleeding or obstruction; and passage of the tube into the cranium. The last complication can occur if you insert an NG tube into a patient with severe head or midfacial trauma because the tube may be passed through the fracture and into the brain.

▶ Cardiopulmonary Arrest

Most pediatric out-of-hospital cardiopulmonary arrests are the result of respiratory failure leading to shock or ischemia caused by inadequate myocardial blood flow resulting from hypovolemia, sepsis, or cardiogenic shock.[14] For these patients, treatment of respiratory failure or shock may prevent the arrest. About 25% of pediatric out-of-hospital cardiac arrests are the result of sudden dysrhythmias (ie, pulseless ventricular tachycardia or ventricular fibrillation).[15] In these situations, the delivery of high-quality CPR, recognition of a shockable rhythm, and prompt defibrillation are crucial.

The signs, symptoms, and treatment of cardiopulmonary arrest are discussed later in this chapter. The following section addresses methods of maintaining and improving circulation in the infant or child, including IV and IO vascular access and IV fluid resuscitation.

YOU ▶ are the Paramedic PART 3

You ask your partner to obtain a blood glucose level while you prepare to start an IV line. A quick look for a peripheral vein yields nothing, so you choose to insert an IO needle into the proximal tibia. You successfully insert the IO needle and confirm placement by aspirating bone marrow and observing free flow of fluids into the bone without swelling behind the insertion site. According to the pediatric length-based resuscitation tape measure, the child weighs approximately 14 kg (31 pounds) and requires 280 mL of normal saline for a fluid bolus. As you start administering the initial fluid bolus, your partner tells you the blood glucose level is 28 mg/dL.

Recording Time: 9 Minutes	
Respirations	22 breaths/min; adequate depth and volume
Pulse	180 beats/min, regular; absent peripheral pulses and weak central pulses
ECG	Sinus tachycardia
Skin	Pale, cool, and dry; some mottling of the extremities
Blood pressure	74/50 mm Hg
Oxygen saturation (Spo₂)	99% at 12 L/min on nonrebreathing mask
Pupils	PERRLA

5. What are the potential complications of IO needle insertion?
6. How should you manage the blood glucose level?

■ Pathophysiology, Assessment, and Management of Shock

Shock is defined as inadequate delivery of oxygen and nutrients to tissues to meet metabolic demand. The types of shock that you may encounter are the same in adults and children: hypovolemic, distributive, and cardiogenic.

Besides determining the cause of shock, you must quickly determine whether the child is in a compensated or decompensated state. In compensated shock, although the child has critical abnormalities of perfusion, his or her body is (for the moment) able to mount a physiologic response to maintain adequate perfusion to vital organs by shunting blood from the periphery, increasing the pulse rate, and increasing the vascular tone. A child in compensated shock will have a normal appearance, tachycardia, and signs of decreased peripheral perfusion, such as cool extremities with prolonged capillary refill. Timely intervention is needed to prevent a child in compensated shock from decompensating.

Decompensated shock is a state of inadequate perfusion in which the body's own mechanisms to improve perfusion are no longer sufficient to maintain a normal blood pressure. Remember, decompensated shock includes hypotension. Hypotension is relative to the age of the child, as indicated in Table 43-11. In addition to being profoundly tachycardic and showing signs of poor peripheral perfusion, a child in decompensated shock may have an altered appearance, reflecting inadequate perfusion of the brain. Because children typically have strong cardiovascular systems, they are able to compensate for inadequate perfusion by increasing the pulse rate and peripheral vascular resistance more efficiently than adults. Hypotension is, therefore, a late and ominous sign in an infant or a young child, and urgent intervention is needed to prevent cardiac arrest.

Initial management involves allowing the child to assume a position of comfort and administering supplemental oxygen. After completing the primary survey, make a transport decision based on the severity of the problem. Start resuscitation on scene for any child who shows signs of decompensated shock. Whereas rapid transport is imperative, the risk of deterioration to cardiac arrest is too high to permit a "load-and-go" approach.

▶ Hypovolemic Shock

Hypovolemia is the most common cause of shock in infants and children,[15] with loss of volume occurring due to illness or trauma. Because of their small blood volume (70 mL/kg body weight), a combination of excessive fluid losses and poor intake in an infant or a young child with gastroenteritis ("stomach flu") can result in shock relatively quickly. The same vulnerability exists with hemorrhage from trauma.

Initially, the patient with hypovolemic shock will have a normal mental status or may appear slightly anxious. Early indicators of shock include tachycardia, pale or mottled skin, narrowing of the pulse pressure, and cool extremities. As shock progresses, the patient becomes restless and less alert, the respiratory rate increases, capillary refill is delayed, the skin becomes cold, and hypotension ensues. Further assessment may identify signs of dehydration such as sunken eyes, dry mucous membranes, and poor skin turgor. In an injured child, the site of bleeding may be identified.

Allow the child to remain in a position of comfort, administer supplemental oxygen, and keep the child warm. Apply direct pressure to stop any external bleeding. Volume replacement is the mainstay of treatment for hypovolemic shock, whether medical or traumatic in origin.

Special Populations

Shock in children is most likely due to hypovolemia. Isotonic fluid resuscitation is the mainstay of treatment.

If the child is in compensated shock, you can attempt to establish IV or IO access en route to the hospital. As with all procedures, gather all the equipment necessary before beginning this step. Catheters—preferably an over-the-needle catheter—are available in pediatric sizes of 20, 22, and 24 gauge. A butterfly needle is a temporary alternative if an over-the-needle catheter is unavailable; this stainless steel needle stays in the vein, predisposing it to infiltration.

Many of the sites used for IV access in adults are the same for children. The most commonly used sites are the dorsum of the hand and the antecubital fossa. In children, veins in the foot may also be used **Figure 43-17**. Scalp veins and the external jugular veins are used less commonly.

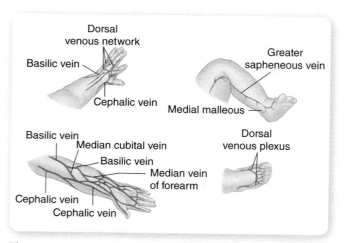

Figure 43-17 Commonly used sites for intravenous access in infants and children include the hands, antecubital fossa, saphenous veins at the ankle, and feet.

© Jones & Bartlett Learning.

The procedure for establishing IV access in the pediatric patient is as follows:

1. Choose the appropriate fluid, and examine the bag for clarity and expiration date. Make sure that no particles are floating in the fluid and that the fluid is appropriate for the child's condition and is not expired.

2. Choose the appropriate drip set, and attach it to the fluid. A macrodrip set (eg, 10 gtt/mL) should be used for a child who needs volume replacement; a microdrip set (eg, 60 gtt/mL) should be used for a child who needs a medication infusion.

3. Fill the drip chamber by squeezing it.

4. Flush or "bleed" the tubing to remove any air bubbles by opening the roller clamp. Make sure no errant bubbles are floating in the tubing.

5. Tear the tape before venipuncture, or have a commercial device available.

6. Apply gloves before making contact with the patient. Secure the appropriate limb to minimize movement during the procedure (ie, use of an arm board). Palpate a suitable vein. Veins should be "springy" when palpated. Stay away from areas that are hard when palpated.

7. Apply the constricting band above the intended IV site. It should be placed approximately 4 to 8 inches (10 to 20 cm) above the intended site.

8. Clean the area using aseptic technique. Use an alcohol pad to cleanse in a circular motion from the inside out. Use a second alcohol pad to wipe straight down the center.

9. Choose the appropriately sized catheter and twist the catheter to break the seal. Do not advance the catheter upward because doing so may cause the needle to shear the catheter. Examine the catheter and discard it if you discover any imperfections. Occasionally you will find "burrs" on the edge of the catheter.

10. Insert the catheter at an angle of approximately 45° with the bevel up while applying distal traction with your other hand. This traction will stabilize the vein and help to keep it from "rolling" as you insert the catheter.

11. Observe for "flashback" as blood enters the catheter. The clear chamber at the top of the catheter should fill with blood when the catheter enters the vein. If you note only a drop or two, you should gently advance the catheter farther into the vein.

12. Occlude the catheter to prevent blood from leaking out while you are removing the stylet. Hold the hub while withdrawing the needle so as not to pull the catheter out of the vein.

13. Immediately dispose of all sharps in the proper container.

14. Attach the prepared IV line. Hold the hub of the catheter while connecting the IV line.

15. Remove the constricting band.

16. Open the IV line to ensure fluid is flowing and the IV is patent. Observe for any swelling or infiltration around the IV site. If the fluid does not flow, check whether the constriction band has been released. If infiltration is noted, immediately stop the infusion and remove the catheter while holding pressure over the site with a piece of gauze to prevent bleeding.

17. Secure the catheter with tape or a commercial device. Wrap the IV tubing with extra gauze to prevent the child from pulling out the IV catheter.

Once IV access is established, fluid resuscitation should begin with isotonic fluids *only*, such as normal saline or lactated Ringer solution. Begin with 20 mL/kg of isotonic fluid, and then reassess the patient's status. The use of warm IV fluids (when possible) can counteract the effects of systemic hypothermia from environmental exposure, blood loss, or open wounds. Multiple fluid boluses may be necessary during transport.

Volume resuscitation should be addressed separately from treatment of hypoglycemia. In a child with shock due to medical illness, perform a bedside glucose check; treat with dextrose-containing fluid only for a documented low blood glucose level. Hypoglycemia is less likely in shock due to acute injury. Dextrose dosing can be found in the Appendix to Volume 1, *Emergency Medications*.

If a child is in decompensated shock, begin initial fluid resuscitation at the scene. Evaluate sites for IV access. If this is unsuccessful, begin an IO infusion. When an IO needle is placed correctly, it will rest in the medullary canal, the space within the bone that contains bone marrow. An IO infusion is contraindicated if a secure IV line is available or if a fracture (or possible fracture) exists in the same bone in which you plan to insert the IO needle. Anything that can be administered through an IV line can be administered through an IO line (such as isotonic fluids, medications).

Special Populations

A child with decompensated shock from hypovolemia needs fluid resuscitation. Do not waste time with multiple IV insertion attempts. Insert an IO needle, and begin fluid therapy.

The IO needles are usually double needles, consisting of a solid-bore needle inside a sharpened hollow needle **Figure 43-18** . This double needle is pushed into the bone (usually the proximal tibia) with a screwing, twisting action away from the joint to avoid disruption of the growth plate. Once the needle pops through the bone, the solid needle is removed, leaving the hollow steel needle in place. Standard IV tubing is attached to this catheter.

The IO lines require full and careful immobilization because they rest at a 90° angle to the bone and are easily

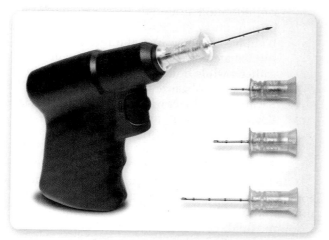

Figure 43-18 Standard pediatric intraosseous needle.
Courtesy of VidaCare Corporation (www.vidacare.com).

dislodged. Stabilize the IO needle, thereby ensuring adequate flow, in the same manner that you would any impaled object. As with any invasive procedure, several complications may be associated with IO infusion: compartment syndrome, failed infusion, growth plate injury, bone inflammation caused by infection (osteomyelitis), skin infection, and bony fracture. Proper technique will help to minimize these complications.

Follow the steps in Skill Drill 43-5 to establish an IO infusion in pediatric patients.

As with IV administration, administer 20 mL/kg boluses of isotonic fluid via IO infusion to treat hypovolemia, reassessing after each bolus and repeating as needed based on physiologic response. As much as 60 mL/kg may be needed during transport to improve the child's blood pressure, pulse rate, mental status, and peripheral perfusion. Rapidly transport the patient to an appropriate treatment facility.

▶ Distributive Shock

In distributive shock, decreased vascular tone develops, resulting in vasodilation and third spacing of fluids due to increased vascular permeability (leakage of plasma out of the blood vessels and into the surrounding tissues).

Skill Drill 43-5 Performing Pediatric IO Infusion

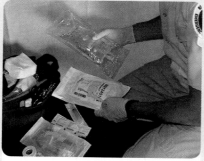

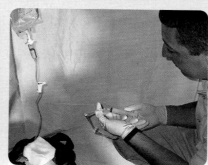

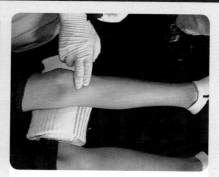

Step 1 Check selected IV fluid for proper fluid, clarity, and expiration date. Look for any discoloration or particles floating in the fluid. If any are found, discard the fluid and choose another bag of fluid. Select the appropriate equipment, including an IO needle, syringe, saline, and extension set. A three-way stopcock may also be used to facilitate easier fluid administration.

Step 2 Select the proper administration set. Connect the administration set to the bag. Prepare the administration set. Fill the drip chamber, and flush the tubing. Ensure no air bubbles remain in the tubing. Prepare the syringe and extension tubing.

Step 3 At any time before the IO puncture, cut or tear the tape and prepare bulky dressings. *Before* the IO puncture, take standard precautions. Identify the proper anatomic site for IO puncture. To miss the epiphyseal (growth) plate, you should measure two fingerbreadths below the knee on the medial side of the leg.

Skill Drill `43-5` **Performing Pediatric IO Infusion** (continued)

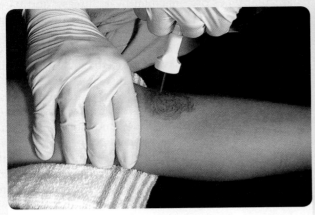

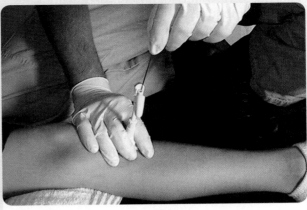

Step 4 Cleanse the site using aseptic technique (ie, in a circular manner from the inside out). Stabilize the tibia. Place a folded towel under the knee, and hold it so that you keep your fingers away from the puncture site. Insert the needle at a 90° angle to the leg. Advance the needle with a twisting motion until you feel a "pop."

Step 5 Unscrew the cap, and remove the stylet from the needle.

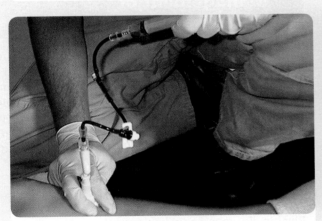

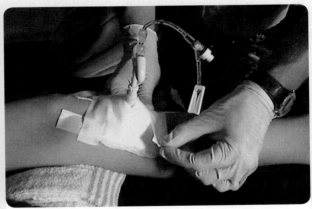

Step 6 Remove the stylet from the catheter. Attach the syringe and extension set to the IO needle. Pull back on the syringe to aspirate blood and particles of bone marrow to ensure placement. If you are not able to aspirate marrow but the IO flushes easily with no signs of infiltration (swelling around insertion site), then continue to flush. Slowly inject saline to ensure proper placement of the needle. Watch for infiltration, and stop the infusion immediately if any is noted. It is possible to fracture the bone during insertion of the IO needle; if this happens, you should remove the IO needle and switch to the other leg. Connect the administration set, and adjust the flow rate as appropriate. Fluid does not flow well through an IO needle, and boluses are given by administering the fluid using the syringe and a three-way stopcock.

Step 7 Secure the needle with tape, and support it with a bulky dressing. Be careful not to tape around the entire circumference of the leg because doing so could impair circulation and create compartment syndrome. Dispose of the needle in the proper container.

This results in a drop in effective blood volume and functional hypovolemia. Distributive shock may be due to sepsis, anaphylaxis, adrenal insufficiency, and spinal cord injury; sepsis accounts for the bulk of pediatric cases.

Early in distributive shock, the child may have warm, flushed skin and bounding pulses as a result of peripheral vasodilation. In contrast, the symptoms and signs of *late* distributive shock will look much like hypovolemic shock. Fever is a key finding in septic shock, whereas urticarial rash and wheezing may be noted in anaphylaxis, and neurologic deficits are apparent in shock due to spinal cord injury.

First-line treatment of pediatric patients in distributive shock is volume resuscitation, because the child is in a state of relative hypovolemia. In a child with apparent sepsis who remains persistently hypotensive despite administration of a total of 60 mL/kg of isotonic fluid, vasopressor support to improve vascular tone may be considered. If anaphylaxis is present, provide emergency medical care as discussed earlier in this chapter. The decision about timing of IV access and transport for patients in distributive shock considers the same factors as for patients in hypovolemic shock.

Adrenal insufficiency can lead to distributive shock. Patients may have a preexisting condition (eg, Addison disease) or may have adrenal suppression from chronic steroid use (eg, to treat autoimmune disease or a malignancy). These patients will benefit from fluids but will need stress-dose steroids to maintain circulation; medical direction may order that 2 mg/kg IV (maximum of 125 mg) be given for this purpose.[16]

▶ Cardiogenic Shock

Cardiogenic shock is the result of pump failure: intravascular volume is normal, but myocardial function is poor. This type of shock is uncommon in the pediatric population but may be present in children with underlying congenital heart disease, myocarditis, cardiomyopathy, or rhythm disturbances. It is important to recognize cardiogenic shock based on the child's history or from the primary survey, because the treatment for this type of shock differs from that for hypovolemic or distributive shock.

A child in cardiogenic shock will appear listless or lethargic (like a child in hypovolemic or distributive shock) but is likely to show signs of increased work of breathing owing to heart failure and pulmonary edema. Circulation will be impaired, and the skin will look pale, mottled, or cyanotic and often feels clammy. The primary survey may reveal an abnormal pulse rate or rhythm or findings of a murmur or gallop. You may feel hepatomegaly (an enlarged liver), which results from pooling of blood in the portal circulation and the leakage of fluid into the tissues of the liver. The caregiver may describe the infant sweating with feeding and, in many cases, will recount a history of congenital heart disease.

If you suspect cardiogenic shock, allow the child to remain in a position of comfort (often sitting upright), administer supplemental oxygen, and transport. The transport destination is a crucial decision, because the facility needs to be capable of providing pediatric critical care. Supplemental oxygen may not increase oxygen saturation in children with particular types of congenital heart disease, and parents will often alert you to this fact. Consider establishing IV access en route to the receiving facility. Treat dysrhythmias if they are present and contributing to shock. Unless you are sure of the diagnosis of cardiogenic shock (ie, the child has a history of congenital heart disease, is afebrile, and has no history of volume loss), err on the side of fluid resuscitation. If you suspect cardiac dysfunction, administer a single isotonic fluid bolus slowly, and monitor the patient carefully to assess its effect. Increased work of breathing, a drop in oxygen saturation, or worsening perfusion after a fluid bolus will confirm your suspicion of cardiogenic shock. Although inotropic agents may be needed to improve cardiac contractility and improve perfusion, they are rarely administered in the field. See Chapter 40, *Management and Resuscitation of the Critical Patient*, for more information on cardiogenic shock.

Pathophysiology, Assessment, and Management of Cardiovascular Emergencies

Cardiovascular emergencies are relatively rare in children. When such problems arise, they are often related to respiratory insufficiency or respiratory arrest, hypovolemia, or infection, rather than a primary cardiac cause, unless the child has congenital heart disease. Through the primary survey, you can quickly identify a cardiovascular emergency, understand the likely cause, and institute potentially life-saving treatment.

▶ Dysrhythmias

Rhythm disturbances can be classified based on whether the pulse rate is normal for age, too slow (bradydysrhythmias), too fast (tachydysrhythmias), or absent (pulseless). The signs and symptoms associated with a rhythm disturbance are often nonspecific; for example, the patient or caregiver may report fatigue, irritability, vomiting, chest or abdominal pain, palpitations, and shortness of breath. If you suspect a rhythm disturbance, quickly move through the primary survey, supporting the patient's ABCs as necessary. An ECG will help you to identify the underlying rhythm, thereby allowing you to decide which specific management steps should be initiated. Address reversible causes of dysrhythmias such as hypoxemia. The decision to stay on scene to obtain additional history and perform a secondary assessment will be dictated by the child's overall physiologic status.

Bradydysrhythmias

In children, a bradydysrhythmia most often occurs secondary to hypoxia. Because of this, airway management, supplemental oxygen, and assisted ventilation as needed are always first-line treatment. Less common causes of bradycardia include hypothermia, congenital or acquired heart block, and toxic ingestion of beta-blockers, calcium-channel blockers, or digoxin. Elevated ICP can also cause bradycardia and should be considered in children with ventricular shunts, a history of head injury, or suspected child abuse without a consistent injury history. As you provide emergency care, attempt to identify and treat the underlying cause of the bradycardia.

A bradydysrhythmia can cause cardiovascular compromise. Possible signs and symptoms include acute changes in mental status, dizziness, fatigue, hypotension, light-headedness, respiratory distress or failure, shock, and syncope. Initiate electronic cardiac monitoring as part of the primary survey.

With a sinus bradycardia, the heart rate is slower than the lower range of normal for the patient's age. Healthy, athletic adolescents may have sinus bradycardia as an incidental finding.

Atrioventricular (AV) blocks can be congenital or acquired. First-degree block, evidenced by a consistently prolonged PR interval, is often an incidental finding seen on the ECG. No intervention is needed for the first-degree block, but treatment may be needed if the underlying rhythm is slow and accompanied by signs of cardiovascular compromise. Second-degree AV block may involve a progressive prolongation of the PR interval with a subsequent drop of the QRS complex (type I) or a random drop of the QRS complex (type II). Type II second-degree blocks may progress to third-degree AV blocks, in which the atrial and ventricular rates are totally uncoordinated. These rhythms can lead to poor perfusion and cardiovascular compromise.

If the patient is asymptomatic, no further treatment is indicated in the field. Recommended treatment guidelines for pediatric bradycardia accompanied by poor perfusion appear in Figure 43-19.

If the child's heart rate is slower than 60 beats/min with signs of poor perfusion (eg, acute changes in mental

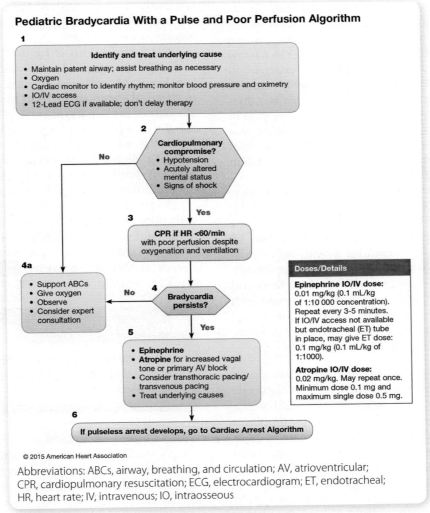

Figure 43-19 Algorithm for managing pediatric bradycardia with a pulse and poor perfusion.

status, hypotension, delayed capillary refill, abnormal skin color) despite oxygenation and ventilation, begin chest compressions and ventilations. For chest compressions to be effective, the patient should be placed on a firm, flat surface with the head at the same level as the body. If you need to carry an infant while providing CPR, your forearm and hand can serve as the flat surface. See Chapter 39, *Responding to the Field Code*, for more information about infant and child CPR.

> ### Special Populations
>
> The preferred medication for a symptomatic brady-cardia in an infant or child is epinephrine, unless the bradycardia is suspected to originate from increased vagal tone, primary AV block (ie, not secondary to factors such as hypoxia), or cholinergic drug toxicity.[13]

Tachydysrhythmias

In infants and children, a tachycardia is present if the heart rate is faster than the upper limit of normal for the patient's age.[17] Tachydysrhythmias are subdivided into two types based on the width of the QRS complex. A narrow complex (ie, supraventricular) tachycardia exists when the QRS complex is 0.09 second or less; a wide complex tachycardia exists when the QRS complex is greater than 0.09 second. Interpret the significance of a tachycardia in conjunction with your physical examination findings and the patient's history. Recommended treatment guidelines for pediatric tachycardia accompanied by poor perfusion appear in **Figure 43-20**.

Sinus tachycardia is common in children and may be caused by fever, pain, anxiety, increased activity, or exercise. It may also occur as a compensatory response to hypovolemia, hypoxia, or heart failure or may be medication-induced. Treatment for a sinus tachycardia is directed at the underlying cause (see Figure 43-20). For example, if a child appears well but has a fever and the monitor shows a sinus tachycardia, treatment with antipyretics is all that is necessary. If a child with a sinus tachycardia has a history of copious vomiting or diarrhea, fluid resuscitation is the appropriate treatment.

Narrow Complex Tachycardia. In children, supraventricular tachycardia (SVT) is the most frequent tachydysrhythmia requiring treatment.[17] With SVT, the ECG will reveal a regular ventricular rhythm with narrow QRS complexes that begins and ends abruptly. The heart rate is often 220 beats/min or faster in an infant or 180 beats/min or faster in a child and remains constant; that is, it does not vary with stimulation or activity. Generally, P waves cannot be discerned because of the rapid rate. In a child who does not have congenital heart disease, the history obtained often does not explain the rapid heart rate. An infant or young child may have a history of poor feeding or "not acting right" and present with fussiness and pallor.

An older child may complain of dizziness, palpitations, and chest pain or pressure. Signs of shock may be present depending on the duration and rate of the tachycardia.

The treatment of SVT depends on the patient's perfusion and overall stability. If the child is in stable condition, consider attempting a vagal maneuver while obtaining IV access. Record the patient's cardiac rhythm before, during, and after a vagal maneuver. Ask an older child to hold his or her breath, blow into a straw with the end crimped over, or bear down as if having a bowel movement; in a younger child, place an exam glove filled with ice firmly over the midface, being careful not to obstruct the nose and mouth. Attempt these techniques only once.

If the child is hemodynamically stable and the SVT persists despite the use of a vagal maneuver, adenosine is the medication of choice to terminate the rhythm, assuming vascular access has been obtained (see Figure 43-20). Its administration may be followed by a brief episode of bradycardia, ventricular tachycardia (VT), ventricular fibrillation (VF), or asystole, before converting spontaneously to sinus rhythm. Persistence of any of these rhythms is rare, but be prepared to switch dysrhythmia algorithms if necessary.

For a child who is hemodynamically unstable with SVT, **synchronized cardioversion** is recommended. Synchronized cardioversion is the timed administration of electrical energy to the heart to correct a dysrhythmia. The dose of the initial synchronized cardioversion attempt is 0.5 to 1 joule per kilogram of body weight (J/kg). If the first shock is unsuccessful, increase the energy level to 2 J/kg. Because cardioversion is a painful procedure, sedation should be provided to an awake patient before the procedure when possible (follow your protocol).

An alternative approach to treating the child in SVT with poor perfusion is to give a dose of IV adenosine if vascular access is readily available. Do not delay synchronized cardioversion if vascular access is not already established, however. **Table 43-16** compares sinus tachycardia, SVT, and VT.

> ### Words of Wisdom
>
> Keep a laminated copy of the pediatric algorithms with you at all times for your reference during a cardiovascular emergency.

Wide Complex Tachycardia. A child with a wide QRS complex tachycardia with a palpable pulse is likely to be in VT—an uncommon, but potentially life-threatening rhythm in children. Its presence may reflect underlying cardiac pathology. SVT may sometimes manifest as a wide complex rhythm, and distinguishing between the two dysrhythmias can be challenging.

If a child with suspected VT is in hemodynamically stable condition, IV access is available, and the patient's

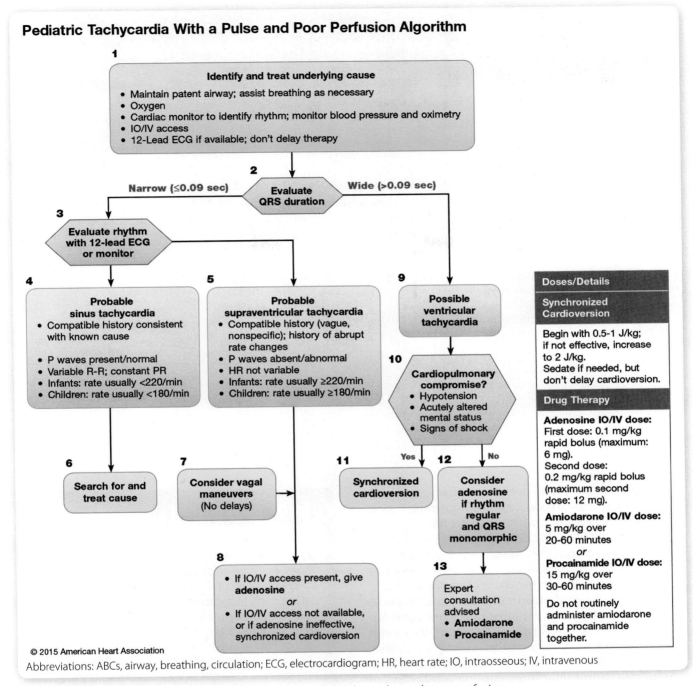

Figure 43-20 Algorithm for managing pediatric tachycardia with a pulse and poor perfusion.

Reprinted with permission. Web-based Integrated 2015 American Heart Association Guidelines for CPR and ECC—Part 12: Pediatric Advanced Life Support © 2015 American Heart Association, Inc.

ventricular rhythm is regular and monomorphic (ie, the QRS complexes are of similar shape), consider giving adenosine IV to help differentiate SVT from VT. If the rhythm persists, amiodarone is the medication of choice, although procainamide is an acceptable alternative. Do not give amiodarone *and* procainamide, because both prolong the QT interval. If a child with VT is hemodynamically unstable, perform synchronized cardioversion using the same energy level as that used for SVT (see Figure 43-20).

If a child with a tachydysrhythmia is or becomes pulseless, begin CPR and follow the pulseless arrest treatment guidelines. Prepare to immediately transport any child with a dysrhythmia to an appropriate receiving facility. Copies of rhythm strips or ECG tracings will be helpful to hospital personnel for diagnostic and therapeutic purposes.

Pulseless Arrest. The survival rate from pediatric cardiac arrest in the prehospital setting is poor; only about 5% to

Table 43-16	**Features of Sinus Tachycardia, Supraventricular Tachycardia, and Ventricular Tachycardia**			
Rhythm	**History**	**Heart Rate**	**QRS Duration**	**Treatment**
Sinus tachycardia	Fever Volume loss Hypoxia Pain Increased activity or exercise	<220 beats/min (infant) <180 beats/min (child)	Narrow: ≤0.09 s	Fluids Oxygen Splinting Analgesia
Supraventricular tachycardia (SVT)	Congenital heart disease Known SVT Nonspecific symptoms (eg, poor feeding, fussiness)	≥220 beat/min (infants) ≥180 beats/min (child)	Narrow: ≤0.09 s	Vagal maneuver Adenosine Synchronized cardioversion
Ventricular tachycardia	Acute systemic illness	>120 beats/min	Wide: >0.09 s	Consider adenosine if regular rhythm and monomorphic QRS Amiodarone or procainamide Synchronized cardioversion

© Jones & Bartlett Learning.

10% of patients survive to hospital discharge, and only about 2% to 5% have a good neurologic outcome.[18] Most out-of-hospital pediatric cardiac arrests are not witnessed; it has been estimated that only about 30% of children who experience an out-of-hospital cardiac arrest receive bystander CPR.[18] These statistics could be improved by strengthening the links in the chain of survival.

When you are confronted with a pediatric patient in cardiopulmonary arrest, the most important consideration is to provide high-quality CPR. Attach a monitor or defibrillator to determine the underlying cardiac rhythm. If the rhythm is pulseless VT or VF, defibrillation is indicated. Additional interventions include establishing vascular access, administering epinephrine, and considering the administration of an antidysrhythmic, such as amiodarone. If the cardiac rhythm is asystole or pulseless electrical activity (PEA), defibrillation is not indicated, and additional treatment is limited to establishing vascular access and administering epinephrine. After administering the medication, perform five cycles of CPR (approximately 2 minutes) before rechecking the rhythm. If asystole or PEA persists, continue with CPR and epinephrine. The steps for managing the pediatric patient in cardiac arrest follow the Pediatric Cardiac Arrest Algorithm **Figure 43-21** . Chapter 39, *Responding to the Field Code,* covers providing CPR to pediatric patients in detail.

Words of Wisdom

Commotio cordis is a condition in which a sudden blunt impact to the chest causes sudden death in the absence of cardiac damage.[19] It occurs most often in athletes between the ages of 8 and 18 years who are participating in sports involving projectiles such as a baseball, hockey puck, or lacrosse ball.[19] It has been suggested that commotio cordis occurs more often in younger patients because they have a narrow, pliable chest wall that facilitates transmission of energy from the site of impact to the myocardium.[20] Data available from 2006 through 2012 indicate a 58% survival rate, which is attributed to greater public awareness of this condition, the earlier commencement of CPR, and public-access defibrillation using increasingly available automated defibrillators.[21]

▶ Heart Failure

Heart failure occurs when the heart can no longer meet the metabolic demands of the body at normal physiologic venous pressures. Infants with heart failure typically present with tachypnea, respiratory distress (retractions), grunting,

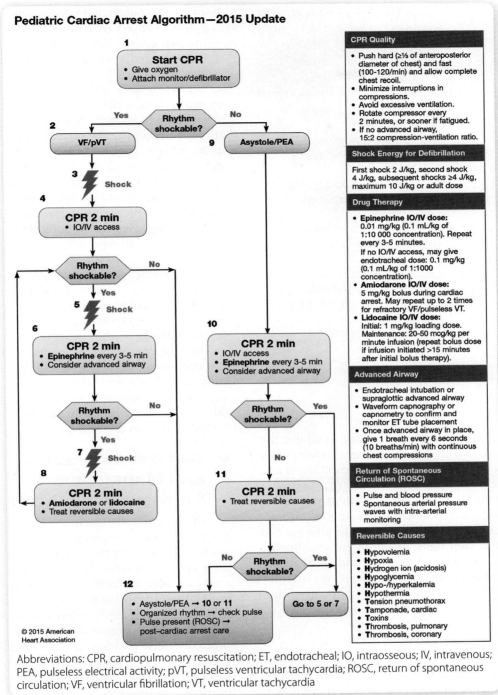

Figure 43-21 Pediatric Cardiac Arrest Algorithm.

Reprinted with permission. Web-based Integrated 2015 American Heart Association Guidelines for CPR and ECC—Part 12: Pediatric Advanced Life Support © 2015 American Heart Association, Inc.

and difficulty with feeding. Often, children with this condition demonstrate profuse sweating and increased work of breathing during feedings. Older children may have tachycardia, tachypnea, crackles on exam, or an enlarged liver.

Treatment of heart failure focuses on correcting hypoxia, reducing preload, reducing afterload, and improving myocardial contractility. You will need to work quickly to help relieve the patient's symptoms. The patient should be supported with oxygen; diuretics

and inotropic medications may be ordered by medical direction. IV fluids should be used judiciously because these patients are prone to worsening symptoms from fluid overload.

Myocarditis

Myocarditis is a condition resulting from inflammation of the heart muscle that results in myocardial dysfunction

Table 43-17	Signs and Symptoms of Myocarditis	
Infants	**Older Children, Adolescents**	
• Fever • Irritability or listlessness • Periodic episodes of pallor that precede tachypnea or respiratory distress • Diaphoresis • Poor feeding; sweating while feeding if heart failure is present • Mild cyanosis • Cool, mottled skin from decreased cardiac output • Rapid, labored breathing; grunting • Heart failure	• Low-grade fever • Palpitations (common) • Fatigue, exhaustion • Pallor • Decreased appetite • Muscle aches and pain • Chest pain (usually described as sharp, stabbing) • Dyspnea with activity • Orthopnea and shortness of breath at rest • Heart failure	

© Jones & Bartlett Learning.

and can lead to heart failure. In contrast to adults, the majority of children with myocarditis present with acute disease, usually resulting from a viral infection. Signs and symptoms of myocarditis are shown in **Table 43-17** .

Because of the high risk of dysrhythmias and hemo-dynamic compromise, the patient with suspected myocarditis should be transported with cardiac monitoring and close attention to vital signs, including pulse oximetry. Obtain vascular access, but give IV fluids judiciously because these patients are prone to fluid overload from inefficient heart function. Patients will often need inotropic support. Oxygen should be administered to all patients during transport.

Cardiomyopathy

Cardiomyopathy is a disease of the heart muscle in which contraction of myocardial muscle fibers are impaired. The three main types of cardiomyopathy are dilated, hypertrophic, and restrictive.

Dilated cardiomyopathy is characterized by progressive dilation of the ventricles with poor contraction of the myocardial muscle fibers, resulting in low cardiac output and symptoms of heart failure. This is the most common type of cardiomyopathy in children.[22] It is estimated that at least 30% to 50% of cases of dilated cardiomyopathy are inherited.[23] Other possible causes include infection, nutritional deficiency, and exposure to toxins. Common symptoms include fatigue, weakness, and signs of heart failure, including tachycardia,

dyspnea, and pulmonary congestion. Atrial and ventricular dysrhythmias are common. Because of ineffective ventricular contraction, blood pools within the heart chambers, predisposing the patient to systemic and pulmonary emboli.

In **hypertrophic cardiomyopathy**, the heart muscle is unusually thick, which means the heart must pump harder to get blood to leave the heart. This type of cardiomyopathy is an inherited disorder. Symptoms usually appear in the school-age years or during adolescence and may include chest pain, dysrhythmias, dyspnea with exertion, and syncope. Sudden death is possible. When hypertrophic cardiomyopathy occurs during infancy, signs and symptoms are those of heart failure. It is crucial for you to thoroughly investigate reports of unexplained syncope in all patients, but especially in the younger population and athletes.

With restrictive cardiomyopathy, ventricular filling is impaired because the walls of the ventricles are stiff as a result of endocardial disease, myocardial disease, or both.[22] Signs and symptoms are similar to those of heart failure. Tachydysrhythmias are common.

Because of the high risk of dysrhythmias and hemodynamic compromise, the patient should be transported with cardiac monitoring and frequent reassessment of vital signs. Obtain vascular access. Be prepared to treat heart failure and dysrhythmias according to local protocol or instructions from medical direction.

► General Assessment and Management of Cardiovascular Emergencies

As with all pediatric emergencies, when you are called to a scene for a suspected cardiac complaint, begin your assessment by using the PAT and then move to the primary survey and secondary assessment. For a suspected cardiovascular problem, an abnormal appearance may indicate inadequate brain perfusion and the need for rapid intervention. Tachypnea, without retractions or abnormal airway sounds, is common in an infant or child with a primary cardiac problem; it is a mechanism for blowing off carbon dioxide to compensate for metabolic acidosis related to poor perfusion. In contrast, when cardiac compromise progresses to heart failure, pulmonary edema leads to increased work of breathing and a fast respiratory rate. The presence of pallor, cyanosis, or mottling may give you clues to this problem.

For suspected cardiovascular compromise, combine information gathered during the primary survey to make a decision about the likely underlying cause, the patient's priority, and the need for immediate treatment or transport. If the patient's condition is stable enough that you can continue the assessment on site, do so. (**Table 43-18** reviews key elements of a cardiovascular SAMPLE history.) Repeat the PAT and assessment of ABCs after each intervention, and monitor trends over time.

Table 43-18	SAMPLE Components for a Child With Cardiovascular Problems
Components	**Features**
Signs and symptoms	Presence of vomiting or diarrhea; number of episodes Vomiting blood or bile; blood in stool External hemorrhage Presence or absence of fever Rash Respiratory distress or shortness of breath
Allergies	Known allergies History of anaphylaxis
Medications	Exact names and dosages of medications Use of laxative or antidiarrheal medications Long-term diuretic therapy Potential exposure to other medications or drugs Timing and dosages of analgesics or antipyretics
Past medical problems	History of heart problems History of prematurity Prior hospitalizations for cardiovascular problems
Last oral intake	Timing of the child's last food or drink, including bottle or breastfeeding
Events leading to injury or illness	Travel Trauma Fever history Symptoms in family members Potential toxic exposure

© Jones & Bartlett Learning.

Pathophysiology, Assessment, and Management of Neurologic Emergencies

Neurologic emergencies can be benign (eg, febrile seizure) or life threatening (eg, ventricular shunt failure). When such problems arise, it is important for you to obtain a thorough past medical history, including information about previous seizures, shunts, cerebral palsy, or any recent trauma or ingestions. Infants and children are particularly difficult to assess neurologically because they can often be uncooperative with your exam due to a lack of understanding or fear. Assess the child's general appearance, and seek the parents' impression of changes in behavior, as the parents will be attuned to more subtle changes in their child's demeanor and activity level.

▶ Altered Mental Status

Many conditions can interfere with brain activity and result in abnormal mental status, including metabolic problems, infectious diseases, intracranial structural abnormalities, trauma, hypoxia, and poisonings. A child with altered mental status displays changes in personality, behavior, or responsiveness inappropriate for age. The child may appear agitated, combative, sleepy, withdrawn, slow to respond, or completely unresponsive. Recall from Chapter 18, *Neurologic Emergencies* that the mnemonic AEIOUTIPS can be used to help remember common causes of altered level of consciousness. Without a good history, it may be difficult to determine the underlying cause of this condition, and you may find yourself simply identifying and treating concerning symptoms.

Run through the PAT and ABCDEs quickly to determine possible points of intervention. Assess the need to protect the airway. Pay special attention to possible disability and dextrose issues. Use the AVPU scale to identify the level of disability. In addition, check the patient's glucose level, because hypoglycemia (defined as a serum glucose concentration of less than 40 mg/dL in a newborn and less than 60 mg/dL in all other infants and children) is easily treatable.

History taking and the secondary assessment, whether performed at the scene or en route to the hospital, may also provide clues about the underlying cause. For example, a child with a history of epilepsy may be in a postictal state after an unwitnessed seizure; a child with diabetes may be hypoglycemic or in DKA. A history of toxic ingestion, recent illness, or injury may also reveal the cause of the altered mental status.

Regardless of the cause, the management of altered mental status is the same. Support the ABCs by carefully assessing the patient's airway and breathing. Provide assisted ventilation or airway support as needed. If the child is hypoglycemic, give glucose at a targeted dose of 0.5 to 1 g/kg as described earlier in this chapter. Always recheck the blood glucose level after giving IV glucose. The goal is to maintain a *normal* glucose level; hyperglycemia is associated with worse neurologic outcomes in patients with cerebral ischemia. For children with altered mental status and signs or symptoms suggestive of an opiate toxidrome, consider giving naloxone. Toxidromes are discussed in Chapter 27, *Toxicology*. All patients with altered mental status should be transported expeditiously to an appropriate medical facility. Assess for increased ICP and intervene as appropriate.

When you are intubating a pediatric patient with an altered mental status, etomidate 0.3 mg/kg is commonly used as an induction agent if septic shock is not suspected. It is considered a good choice if the patient is hypotensive because etomidate has less effect on blood pressure than other choices. Midazolam 0.1 mg/kg and ketamine 2 mg/kg are other options. Ketamine is a bronchodilator, so it is a good choice for patients with respiratory problems such as asthma, though it can cause increased bronchorrhea and may cause a transient drop in the blood pressure. Muscle relaxants such as succinylcholine 1 to 2 mg/kg and rocuronium 1 mg/kg can also be used in the pediatric population.

> **Patient Safety**
>
> Be cautious about using succinylcholine in patients who may have hyperkalemia as a result of medications such as thiazide diuretics or angiotensin-converting enzyme inhibitors, crush injuries, severe burns, renal diseases, Addison disease, or adrenal disease.

In patients in whom increased ICP is suspected, the administration of lidocaine prior to intubation may blunt the increase in ICP associated with intubation. Signs of increased ICP include Cushing triad: bradycardia, irregular respirations, and widened pulse pressure (systolic hypertension). If you suspect increased ICP, elevate the patient's head 30° if cervical spine injury is not suspected. Hyperventilation of the patient can lower ICP temporarily, but this practice must be used judiciously.

▶ Seizures

Seizures result from abnormal electrical discharges in the brain. Although many types of seizures exist, generalized seizures manifest as abnormal motor activity and an altered level of consciousness. Some children are predisposed to seizures because of underlying brain abnormalities, whereas others experience seizures as a result of trauma, metabolic disturbances, ingestion, or infection. Seizures associated with fever (febrile seizures) are unique to young children and are typically benign, though frightening to the parents.

The physical manifestation of a seizure will depend on the area of the brain firing the electrical discharges and the age of the child. Infants have immature brains, so seizures in this age group may be subtle. Repetitive movements such as lip smacking, chewing, and "bicycling" suggest seizure activity. Apnea and cyanosis can also be signs of underlying seizure activity.

The prognosis following a seizure is closely linked to the underlying cause. For example, a child with a febrile seizure will not have brain damage as a consequence of the event, whereas a child who has a seizure as a complication of a head injury or meningitis may experience long-term neurologic abnormalities. All types of seizures (but especially first-time seizures) are frightening to caregivers, and they often result in 9-1-1 calls.

Types of Seizures

The classification system for seizures is the same for children and adults (see Chapter 18, *Neurologic Emergencies*, for an in-depth discussion of seizures). Briefly, seizures that involve the entire brain are considered **generalized seizures**, whereas those that involve only one part of the brain are called **partial seizures**. The most common types of seizures are generalized **tonic-clonic seizures** (grand mal), which involve jerking of both arms and legs. **Absence seizures** (petit mal) are generalized seizures that involve a brief loss of attention without abnormal body movements. Partial seizures can be further subclassified into **simple partial seizures**, which involve focal motor jerking without loss of consciousness, and **complex partial seizures**, which feature focal motor jerking with loss of consciousness.

Febrile Seizures

Febrile seizures occur in about 2% to 5% of all children.[24] To make this diagnosis, the child must be between age 3 months and 6 years,[24] have a fever, and have no identifiable precipitating cause (such as head injury, ingestion, or meningitis). The strongest predictor for having a febrile seizure is a history of this diagnosis in a first-degree relative. The child's temperature usually increases rapidly to 101.8°F (38.8°C), and the seizure occurs during the temperature rise rather than after a prolonged elevation.

Simple febrile seizures are brief, generalized tonic-clonic seizures (lasting less than 15 minutes) that occur in a child without underlying neurologic abnormalities. **Complex febrile seizures** have a longer duration (lasting more than 15 minutes), are focal, or occur in a child with baseline developmental or neurologic abnormality. They may also be associated with serious illness.

The postictal phase after a febrile seizure is usually brief, so the child will often be waking up or back to baseline by the time you arrive at the scene. Depending on your agency's policy, a well-appearing child who has a history consistent with a simple febrile seizure may be transported either by EMS or by parents, but he or she always needs urgent physician evaluation.

The prognosis for children with simple febrile seizures is excellent. In rare cases, febrile seizures that last more than 30 minutes may cause scar tissue in the temporal lobe of the brain. In some of these patients, chronic epilepsy develops, which often can be effectively treated.[24]

> **Special Populations**
>
> Febrile seizures are unique to children. Reassure the parents that febrile seizures are common and that children who experience them typically recover completely.

Assessment of Seizures

When you are conducting the primary survey of a child with a history of seizures, you should give special attention to compromised oxygenation and ventilation and signs of ongoing seizure activity. Seizures place a child at risk for respiratory distress or failure because of airway obstruction (often from the tongue), aspiration, or depressed respiratory drive. Given the typical EMS response time, any child who is still having a seizure when you arrive has likely been having seizure activity for at least 8 to 10 minutes and should be considered to be in status epilepticus; therefore, you need to initiate treatment to stop the seizure in such cases. **Status epilepticus** has historically been defined as a seizure that lasts longer than 4 to 5 minutes or consecutive seizures without a return to consciousness between seizures. Refer to your local protocols for guidelines related to how long a seizure can continue before you should intervene. As part of history taking, ask about prior seizures; anticonvulsant medications; recent illness, injury, or suspected ingestion; duration of the seizure activity; and the character of the seizure.

Management of Seizures

Treatment of seizures at the scene will be limited to supportive care if the seizure has stopped by your arrival, but status epilepticus requires more extensive intervention. Provide 100% supplemental oxygen to the patient, and start bag-mask ventilation as indicated for hypoventilation. For a child with ongoing seizure activity, open the airway using the head tilt–chin lift or jaw-thrust maneuver. Proximal airway obstruction is common during a seizure or postictal state because the tongue and jaw fall backward owing to the decreased muscle tone associated with altered mental status. If the airway is not maintainable with positioning, consider inserting a nasopharyngeal airway. Suction for secretions or vomitus, and consider the lateral decubitus position in case of ongoing vomiting. Do not attempt to intubate a patient who is experiencing an active seizure: ET intubation in this setting is associated with serious complications and is rarely successful. More appropriate care includes using BLS airway management, stopping the seizure, and then considering the child's need for ALS airway support. Consider placing an NG tube to decompress the stomach if the patient requires assisted ventilation.

Assess the child for viable IV sites. Measure the serum glucose level, and treat any documented hypoglycemia.

Consider your options for anticonvulsant administration. Insertion of an IV line can be difficult in a child having a seizure, and alternative routes for medication delivery may be needed. The goal of medical therapy is to stop the seizure while minimizing anticonvulsant side effects.

First-line anticonvulsant treatment consists of a benzodiazepine—lorazepam, diazepam, or midazolam. All benzodiazepines can cause respiratory depression, so monitor oxygenation and ventilation carefully, especially when you give repeated doses or combinations of anticonvulsants. Lorazepam is an excellent choice for seizure management because of its rapid onset of action, lower risk of respiratory depression, and relatively long half-life. The half-life of diazepam is relatively short, and breakthrough seizures may occur with longer transport times. Midazolam may be administered by the IV, IM, and intranasal (using an atomizer) routes. Although it has excellent anticonvulsant effects, it has the shortest duration of action of the three benzodiazepines mentioned. Be prepared to repeat dosing for recurrent seizures.

Any child with a history suggestive of seizures requires physician evaluation to look for the cause. Although treatment at the scene is appropriate for a child in status epilepticus, detailed assessment should be performed during transport. Monitor cardiorespiratory status in any postictal child, and reassess frequently for recurrent seizure activity.

▶ Meningitis

Meningitis is an inflammation or infection of the meninges, the covering of the brain and spinal cord. It is most often caused by a viral or bacterial infection. Viral meningitis is more common in the summer, is usually caused by an enterovirus, and presents with associated gastrointestinal symptoms such as vomiting and diarrhea. Although children may look and feel quite ill, viral meningitis is rarely a life-threatening infection. By contrast, bacterial meningitis is potentially fatal. Children with bacterial meningitis can progress rapidly from appearing mildly ill to suffering a coma and even death. In the early stages of illness, it is difficult to tell which type of infection is present, so take the safe route: always proceed as if the child has bacterial meningitis.

The symptoms of meningitis vary depending on the age of the child and the agent causing the infection. In general, the younger the child, the more vague the symptoms. A newborn with early bacterial meningitis may have a fever as the only symptom. Young infants will often have a fever and perhaps localizing signs such as lethargy, irritability, poor feeding, and a bulging fontanel. Young children rarely show typical "meningeal signs" such as **nuchal rigidity** (neck stiffness with movement of the neck) until they are older. Verbal children will often report headaches and neck pain. An altered level of consciousness and seizures are ominous symptoms at any age. Projectile vomiting and photosensitivity are also common findings. Other signs may include Kernig sign (the patient cannot extend his or her leg at the knee when the thigh is flexed because of stiffness in the hamstrings) and Brudzinski sign (passive flexion of the leg on one side causes a similar movement in the opposite leg).

Neonates most often contract meningitis-causing bacteria during the birthing process. The bacteria that are a normal part of the mother's vaginal tract—*Escherichia coli*, group B *Streptococcus*, and *Listeria monocytogenes*—can produce serious infections in newborns. Neonatal

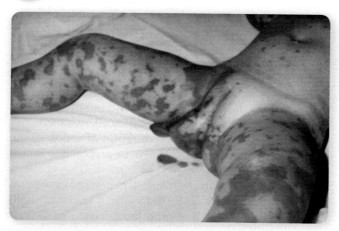

Figure 43-22 Purpura in a child with meningococcal sepsis.
Courtesy of Ronald Dieckmann, MD.

Table 43-19	SAMPLE Components for a Child With Suspected Meningitis	
Component	**Features**	
Signs and symptoms	Onset and duration of illness, including "cold symptoms"— runny nose, cough Onset and duration of fever Rash, headache, neck pain Photophobia, irritability	
Allergies	Known medication reactions or other allergies	
Medications	Exact names and doses of ongoing medications Timing and amount of most recent dose Time and dose of analgesics and antipyretics	
Past medical history	Previous illnesses or injuries Immunizations Perinatal history for young infants	
Last oral intake	Timing of the child's last food or drink, including bottle or breastfeeding	
Events leading to illness or injury	Any known exposures to children with illnesses and which kind of illnesses they have	

© Jones & Bartlett Learning.

meningitis is usually not seen beyond 3 months of age. Older infants and young children are at risk for contracting viral meningitis from enteroviruses, which are widespread during the summer and fall. Bacterial meningitis in this age group most often involves *Streptococcus pneumoniae* (also known as pneumococcus) and *Neisseria meningitidis* (also known as meningococcus), although pneumococcus infection is becoming less frequent because more young children are vaccinated against this bacterium. Meningitis from *H influenzae* is rare because an effective vaccine against this pathogen was introduced in the 1990s.

N meningitidis may also cause **sepsis** (an overwhelming bacterial infection in the bloodstream). Meningococcal meningitis with sepsis is typically characterized by a **petechial** (small, pinpoint red spots) or **purpuric** (larger purple or black spots) rash in addition to the other symptoms of meningitis (Figure 43-22).

Infection control is an important part of managing a child who may have meningitis. Meningococcus, in particular, is quite contagious. Protect yourself and others from contracting this illness by being vigilant about using standard and respiratory precautions. Wear a gown, gloves, and a mask if meningitis is a possibility and remember to place a mask on the patient.

Children with meningococcal sepsis and meningitis quickly become extremely sick, so you need to move quickly through your assessment. Form your general impression, and perform the primary survey as usual, while recognizing that the initial presentation of a child with meningitis can be highly variable. Look for fever, altered mental status, bulging fontanel, photophobia, nuchal rigidity, irritability, petechiae, purpura, and signs of shock. Perform a bedside glucose check because hypoglycemia may result from the hypermetabolic state. Helpful components of a SAMPLE history are shown in (Table 43-19).

For children in physiologically unstable condition, provide lifesaving interventions as needed and transport them quickly, ideally to a facility with a pediatric intensive care unit. En route, perform frequent reassessments, as one of the hallmarks of meningitis is rapid deterioration.

Monitor vital signs and changes in physical exam findings closely to anticipate a child's needs, and intervene early. Patient needs may include oxygen, airway management, and ventilation support. Medical control may order IV fluids based on patient signs and symptoms, and medications may be ordered en route if seizures occur or the patient shows signs of shock. See Chapter 26, *Infectious Diseases*, for more information about meningitis.

► Hydrocephalus

Hydrocephalus is a condition resulting from impaired circulation and absorption of cerebrospinal fluid (CSF), leading to increased size of the ventricles (fluid-filled spaces in the brain) and increased ICP. The CSF production rate is normally matched by the absorption rate, so that the net volume of fluid within the brain remains constant.

Hydrocephalus occurs in two main forms. Normal-pressure hydrocephalus is a rare condition that occurs in older adults. Its mechanism is unclear. The other type of hydrocephalus results in increased pressure within the cranial vault. The most common cause of increased ICP hydrocephalus is the slowed movement of CSF. Congenital malformations

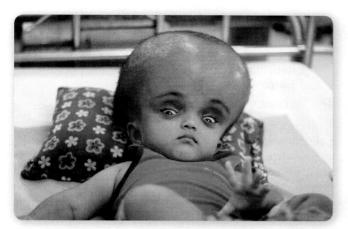

Figure 43-23 The "sunsetting sign" is so called because pressure on cranial nerves forces the eyes downward, leaving only a crescent visible beneath the sclera. This is a late sign of increased intracranial pressure hydrocephalus.
© Barcroft Media/Getty.

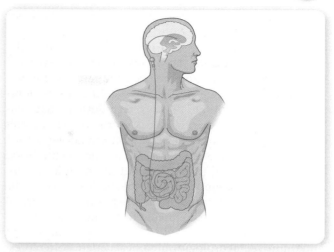

Figure 43-24 An intraventricular shunt is a tube that originates in the lateral ventricle within the brain. It travels under the skin, usually along the neck, and terminates in the chest or abdomen. It allows excess cerebrospinal fluid to be reabsorbed outside of the skull.
© Jones & Bartlett Learning.

in the aqueducts for CSF, tumors, trauma, intracranial hemorrhage, and meningitis are the most common reasons why the flow of fluid slows. Even though movement of CSF decreases, production does not; therefore, total CSF volume increases. Hydrocephalus is most commonly seen in children born with brain malformations, as a complication of prematurity, or following surgery for a brain tumor.

The signs and symptoms of increased ICP hydrocephalus can develop gradually, over months, or suddenly, over days. These signs and symptoms will also vary, however, depending on the cause and the age of the patient. An infant has a relatively soft skull, so the increased pressure results in increased head circumference. Infants also experience lethargy, irritability, vomiting, sun-setting eyes (a downward deviation of the eyes **Figure 43-23**), tense or bulging fontanels, and seizures.

Older children and adults do not have the flexibility of the skull that infants have, so their symptoms are slightly different. Headache, nausea, projectile vomiting, blurry or double vision, ataxia, poor coordination, and memory and personality impairments are seen in this population.

To decrease the increased ICP, patients will often have a cerebral shunt placed **Figure 43-24** . Ventriculoperitoneal (VP) or, less commonly, ventriculoatrial (VA) shunts are surgically inserted into the ventricles of the brain by neurosurgeons. VP shunts drain excess fluid from the ventricular system of the brain into the peritoneal cavity through a tube that exits the skull at a valve. VA shunts are similar, except the tubing terminates in the right atrium of the heart. The tubing can often be felt in the lateral portion of the neck. In thin or young children, coils of tubing may also be palpable in the abdomen. Draining off the extra CSF prevents herniation of the brain.

Complications of cerebral shunts include infections, blockages, and overdrainage. Excessive drainage can cause the brain to collapse because of its own weight, which causes tearing and intracranial hemorrhage; insufficient drainage causes increased ICP. Signs of a cerebral shunt malfunction include vomiting, headache, altered level of consciousness, visual changes, and—with infection—fever, redness, or tenderness over the shunt itself. In patients with VP shunts, peritonitis can also accompany VP shunt infections. For any of these conditions, management of increased ICP and immediate transport to a medical center with pediatric neurosurgical capabilities is required. In addition, as children grow, the length of the tube tends to become shorter than needed and must be replaced.

Care for these patients involves standard care. Be prepared for seizures and increased ICP. Because the patient is typically a child with multiple medical problems, the family can be a great resource. Use of invasive medical technology, including feeding tubes and ventilators, is common. Use the experience of the family in helping to care for these medically complicated children. Do not manipulate the VP shunt. The ED physician will access the shunt if needed. In patients without shunts, an emergency ventriculostomy can be done to relieve pressure within the skull.

▶ Traumatic Brain Injury

Head trauma is common in childhood. Most head trauma in children is minor and not associated with brain injury or long-term sequelae. However, a small number of children who appear to be at low risk may have an intracranial injury. A number of states have laws requiring *medical evaluation* prior to allowing children who have been concussed in a sporting event back into play, and only a physician, physician assistant, or nurse practitioner should clear the child to return to play. The goal of the evaluation of children with head trauma is to identify those with traumatic brain injury and prevent deterioration and secondary injury. Any child who presents with head injury should also be evaluated for signs of potential abuse.

An epidural hematoma is a hemorrhage into the space between the dura and the overlying skull. Epidural hematomas are uncommon in pediatric patients, but they may occur after a low-velocity fall.[25] Child abuse accounts for a significant number of cases of epidural hematomas in infants and children, whereas motor vehicle crashes account for most epidural hematomas in adolescents.[26] The low incidence of epidural hematoma in childhood has been attributed to the fact that the middle meningeal artery is not embedded in the bone surface of the skull until about 2 years of age; therefore, a fracture of the temporal bone is less likely to lacerate the artery.[26] Prompt diagnosis is crucial to successful management and improved neurologic outcomes. Patients often present with loss of consciousness or altered mental status. Patients also often report a severe headache accompanied by persistent vomiting, or ataxia. Infants may be difficult to console and have a cephalohematoma on exam. Older patients may have a lucid interval with minimal symptoms after head trauma, followed several hours later by rapid clinical deterioration.

By contrast, a subdural hematoma forms when there is hemorrhage into the potential space between the dura and the arachnoid membranes. Subdural hematoma is fairly common in infants, with a peak incidence between birth and 4 months of age. It often occurs as a result of birth trauma, falls, assaults, or violent shaking.[26] Any infant or toddler with a subdural hematoma should be suspected of having been abused until proven otherwise.

Suspect cervical spine injury and take cervical spine precautions. Hypoxia must be prevented to avoid secondary injury to brain tissue. Expect vomiting, and suction as needed. Administer supplemental oxygen if indicated. Be prepared to assist inadequate breathing. Vascular access is often indicated in patients with epidural hematomas but is less often needed for patients with subdural bleeding. Consult medical direction to determine the appropriate rate at which fluids should be infused. If hypotension is present, look for signs of internal bleeding. Treat seizures if present. Perform frequent neurologic checks, including vital signs, arousability, size and reactivity of the pupils to light, and extent and symmetry of motor responses. Repeated assessments are crucial to detect signs of increasing ICP. Transport the patient rapidly to the closest appropriate facility.

■ Pathophysiology, Assessment, and Management of Gastrointestinal Emergencies

Complaints of gastrointestinal origin are common in the pediatric population. The gut embryonically develops external to the body, then regresses into the abdominal cavity. Features of maldevelopment are responsible for certain pediatric gastrointestinal diseases such as Meckel diverticulum or malrotation with volvulus. Organs such as the liver mature over the first few months of life.

▶ Biliary Atresia

Children with severe liver disease, though rare, can also present with jaundice. Biliary atresia can present in the newborn period. In this disease, the biliary tract is malformed such that bilirubin cannot be excreted—a condition that leads to liver disease and failure. Some rare genetic disorders can also present as liver failure. These children may have esophageal varices, which can bleed profusely. Transport children with massive gastrointestinal bleeds to the nearest ED, obtain IV access, and administer fluid boluses with isotonic saline or lactated Ringer solution.

▶ Viral Gastroenteritis

A common source of gastrointestinal upset is acute viral gastroenteritis, an infection caused by a variety of viruses, or the ingestion of certain foods, such as milk or ice cream (lactose intolerance), or unknown substances. In most of these cases, you will encounter a pediatric patient who is experiencing abdominal discomfort with nausea, vomiting, and diarrhea. Many patients also have a fever. These findings can become a concern because both vomiting and diarrhea can quickly cause dehydration in children. If you suspect dehydration, place an IV line and administer 20 mL/kg of an isotonic fluid such as normal saline. Do not administer a bolus with one-half normal saline or fluids containing dextrose or potassium.

▶ Appendicitis

Appendicitis is common in pediatric patients and, if untreated, can lead to peritonitis (inflammation of the peritoneum, which lines the abdominal cavity) or shock. Patients with appendicitis will typically present with a fever and pain on palpation of the right lower abdominal quadrant. Patients often describe the pain as starting in the periumbilical region and migrating to the right lower quadrant over time, usually hours. Some patients with appendicitis have a fever or vomiting. In addition, rebound tenderness may be present, but it is not a finding specific to appendicitis.[27]

Constipation can also be a cause of severe abdominal pain in children. In patients with pain from this source, the pain often follows a meal and is intermittent. These patients have diffuse abdominal pain, but do not have guarding or rebound tenderness on examination. The severity of pain can often mimic the pain of appendicitis.

Never assume that you can distinguish between appendicitis and constipation based on history and physical examination in the field alone. Transport the patient to the ED for further evaluation.

▶ Ingestion of Foreign Bodies

The ingestion of foreign bodies is a common cause of gastrointestinal complaints in pediatric patients. Although most foreign bodies pass without trouble, if a foreign object gets lodged in the esophagus, patients will often present with gagging, vomiting, and difficulty swallowing. Worsening pain raises the concern for perforation of an organ, and difficulty breathing or choking raises the possibility of a foreign body airway obstruction. In this situation, keep the child in a calm, comfortable position, often on the parent's lap, and transport the child to the ED immediately.

▶ Gastrointestinal Bleeding

Gastrointestinal bleeding is rare in the pediatric population, and the causes of such bleeds are often different from those for adults. Because of the rapid transport times in the pediatric gastrointestinal tract, cases involving children with ingested, upper, or lower bleeding may present with hematochezia or bright red rectal bleeding. In adults, upper bleeding may present as melena or dark black, tarlike stools because of the digestion of the blood in the gastrointestinal tract.

In newborns, blood ingested during birth can present as rectal bleeding. This sort of bleeding is seen in the first few days of life and is harmless. Infants may have blood in their stool if maternal bleeding from the nipples occurs during breastfeeding. Maternal mastitis, an infection of the breast, is a common cause.

Children may also have rectal bleeding from ingested blood from epistaxis (nosebleeds), after surgery such as tonsillectomy, or after multiple episodes of forceful vomiting. Children with gastroenteritis and repetitive vomiting can get small tears of the esophagus called Mallory-Weiss tears. These mucosal tears can present as blood streaking of the emesis or blood in the stool. They are usually small, harmless, and self limited. Finally, children with constipation can have small anal fissures that present as rectal bleeding. The blood from fissures presents as blood streaking on the surface of the stool. Fissures can be painful but are also self limiting. Abusive trauma should always be part of the differential diagnosis of rectal bleeding in the pediatric population.

▶ Intussusception

Intussusception is a disease that most commonly occurs in children between ages 6 months and 6 years. It involves the telescoping of the bowel into itself, commonly the small intestine into the large intestine at the cecum. Patients present with intermittent severe abdominal pain and lethargy, and sometimes with bloody stools (or currant jelly–like stools). Intussusception is considered a surgical emergency, and patients should be transported to the ED for immediate evaluation.

▶ Meckel Diverticulum

Meckel diverticulum is one of the most common congenital malformations of the small intestines. Affected patients present with painless rectal bleeding or hematochezia. This condition presents with the "rule of 2s" because it occurs in 2% of the population, has a 2:1 male-to-female ratio, is located within 2 feet of the ileocecal valve, is commonly 2 cm in diameter and 2 inches in length, contains 2 types of ectopic tissue (pancreatic and gastric), and is more common before the age of 2.[27] Meckel diverticulum can cause concern because of the large volume of blood loss. If you suspect Meckel diverticulum, transport the patient to the ED for further evaluation.

▶ Pyloric Stenosis and Malrotation With Volvulus

In infants younger than 2 months, pyloric stenosis and malrotation with volvulus are two diseases that cause vomiting and need prompt attention. **Pyloric stenosis** occurs when the pylorus—the muscle that serves as a one-way valve for contents leaving the stomach—becomes hypertrophied. Infants with this condition classically present with nonbloody and nonbilious projectile vomiting occurring after feedings. Poor weight gain or weight loss, dehydration, and electrolyte abnormalities can be seen due to the amount of vomiting. Surgery is curative in these children.

Malrotation with volvulus occurs when the bowel becomes twisted around its mesenteric attachment to the abdominal wall. Patients present with bilious emesis (dark green), pain, and a distended, rigid abdomen. They may have blood in the vomitus or stool. This condition is considered a surgical emergency. Any bilious emesis within the first month of life warrants further evaluation for malrotation. Infants who are vomiting should be transported immediately to an ED with pediatric capabilities.

▶ General Assessment and Management of Gastrointestinal Emergencies

When obtaining a history for a child with gastrointestinal complaints, it is important to consider the patient's age, sex, and prematurity at birth (if any). Ask about current medication use, as well as a history of similar complaints in the past. For example, severe abdominal pain is a common complaint associated with a large number of differential diagnoses; however, recurrent abdominal pain that can mimic the pain of appendicitis can be seen with constipation or gastroenteritis. Patients on polyethylene glycol may have pain from constipation, whereas patients on H_2-blockers such as ranitidine may have gastritis or ulcer disease.

Physical examination findings in patients with gastrointestinal complaints include looking for pallor or jaundice. Scleral jaundice may also be present. Collectively, these may be signs of hepatic disease or blood breakdown or loss. Tachycardia is seen before hypotension in pediatric patients with significant dehydration or blood loss. Tachycardia should be treated with an IV fluid bolus of

20 mL/kg. The location and severity of abdominal pain should be assessed and reassessed at regular intervals for changes. Premature infants and those with symptoms in the first weeks of life require further evaluation at a center with pediatric capabilities.

Special consideration should be paid to patients with gastrostomy tubes (G-tubes) because these patients may require continuous feeds to maintain hydration. G-tubes can become dislodged by the child playing or pulling them, or when the balloon that secures the tube deflates. Many parents have been trained in replacing G-tubes. If a replacement tube is not available, insertion of a sterile urinary catheter or other similar catheter into the stoma is important. Stomas can become narrow within hours and completely close off after the tube is removed; reinsertion of the original tube into the stoma can help prevent this outcome. When replacing a G-tube or inserting another catheter through the abdominal wall stoma, consider the time since the tube was originally inserted and, therefore, the age of the tract the G-tube follows. Mature tracts, or those more than 6 months old, can safely be replaced. In contrast, immature G-tube tract tubes should not be replaced in the field because of the risks of perforating the tract and inserting the G-tube into the abdominal cavity rather than the stomach. To replace a G-tube, use a water-soluble lubricant on the end of the tube being inserted through the stoma. Apply gentle pressure to ensure that the tube slides into the stoma. If significant resistance is felt or if pain or bleeding occurs, then the attempt should be aborted. Tape the replacement to hold it in place, and transport the child to the ED for definitive replacement.

Because the pediatric population is sensitive to fluid loss, obtain a thorough history from the primary caregiver. In particular, ask questions such as the following:

- How many wet diapers has the child had today?
- Is your child tolerating liquids, and is he or she able to keep them down?
- How many times has your child had diarrhea and for how long?
- When he or she cries, are tears present?

The answers to these questions can help you determine just how dehydrated the pediatric patient may be.

When transporting a patient with a suspected gastrointestinal emergency, do not give the patient anything to eat or drink until a thorough assessment can be completed. Vascular access is often indicated in patients who show signs of clinical dehydration and need IV fluids. The patient should be kept comfortable on cardiorespiratory monitors with frequent assessment for change in hemodynamic status.

■ Pathophysiology, Assessment, and Management of Endocrine Emergencies

When you are caring for pediatric patients with endocrine-related emergencies, it is important to remember that children are not just "small adults." Children and young adults are much more commonly diagnosed with type 1

YOU ▶ are the Paramedic   PART 4

Prior to packaging the patient for transport, you administer 28 mL of 25% dextrose (D_{25}) solution. The child begins to move around as he is placed on the stretcher and is opening his eyes by the time you are ready to leave. Law enforcement personnel arrive to care for the sister as you are loading the child into the back of the ambulance.

Recording Time: 15 Minutes	
Respirations	20 breaths/min; adequate depth and volume
Pulse	160 beats/min, regular; weak peripheral pulses and strong central pulses
Skin	Pale, warm, and dry; decreased mottling of the extremities
Blood pressure	80/54 mm Hg
Oxygen saturation (Spo₂)	99% at 12 L/min on nonrebreathing mask
Pupils	PERRLA

7. What do you think was the cause of shock in this patient?

8. Which additional treatment should be given en route to the hospital?

diabetes; therefore, they are susceptible to DKA, a life-threatening event. Moreover, hypoglycemia can be particularly damaging to the developing brain. Children are at varying stages of cognitive development, depending on age and maturity; therefore, consistent maintenance of blood glucose levels within the normal range can be challenging.

A low socioeconomic status is associated with an increased incidence of DKA, poor blood glucose control, and lengthier hospital admissions. Children and adolescents have unique needs, and it is essential that the family be involved and supportive to increase compliance.

▶ Hyperglycemia

Hyperglycemia is an abnormally high blood glucose level. It can be the presenting problem in a child with new-onset diabetes mellitus, or it may occur as a complication in a child with a known history of diabetes. If not recognized or promptly treated, hyperglycemia can result in severe dehydration and DKA, both of which are potentially life threatening.

During your assessment of the child with suspected hyperglycemia, you will typically find that a dose of insulin was missed, a greater proportion of food was eaten compared with the dose of insulin, or the insulin pump malfunctioned. The patient's signs and symptoms will depend on how high the level of blood glucose is. During your assessment, ask about insulin administration; functioning of an insulin pump, including when the site of insertion was last changed; changes in urine output; changes in mental status; patterns on recent glucose checks; the presence of urine ketones (if the parents/patient check this); and any other symptoms, including headache, visual changes, seizures, abnormal speech, or the presence of vomiting and abdominal pain.

Management of hyperglycemia begins by administering 100% oxygen or assisted ventilation if needed. Monitor vital signs closely. Obtain IV access and administer isotonic fluids such as normal saline or lactated Ringer solution. A 10-mL/kg bolus may be administered if the patient is in shock; this treatment may be repeated as needed, up to 40 mL/kg total infusion, to maintain adequate perfusion.[28] Rapid IV fluid administration increases the risk of cerebral edema in a patient in DKA; therefore, if needed, IV fluids should be run slowly during transport to a hospital (such as 20 mL/kg over an hour). If patients report worsening of a headache or if their mental status deteriorates during fluid administration, fluids should be discontinued and the patient assessed and treated for increased ICP from cerebral edema and impending herniation.

Closely monitor the patient's ABCs and be prepared to adjust your treatment accordingly. Electrolyte imbalances (particularly of potassium) may lead to ECG abnormalities and dysrhythmias. Closely monitor the ECG. The patient in DKA desperately needs insulin; however, this drug is not administered in the prehospital setting. If an insulin pump is working, however, do not discontinue its use in the field. Immediate transport of the patient to the closest appropriate facility is crucial.

▶ Hypoglycemia

Hypoglycemia (low blood sugar) may occur in patients with diabetes, often because of treatment with insulin or oral hypoglycemic agents. Hypoglycemia is common in metabolically stressed children because a child is unable to store large quantities of glucose and mobilize what they can store. Prolonged hypoglycemia can lead to irreversible brain damage. In children, alcohol intoxication increases susceptibility to hypoglycemia and altered mental status because alcohol suppresses the ability of the liver to make glucose. The blood sugar level may become too low if the patient with diabetes has taken too much insulin, not eaten enough food, overexercised and burned off sugar faster than normal, or experienced significant physical or emotional stress.

Signs and symptoms of hypoglycemia are nonspecific. Early signs include headache, hunger, nausea, weakness, irritability, and agitation. Later signs include cool, pale, clammy skin; tachycardia; tachypnea; abdominal pain (stomachache); dizziness; sweating; pallor; confusion; tremors; seizures; and coma.

In addition to appropriate care to ensure an open airway, adequate breathing, and effective circulation, consider the following actions if the patient shows signs of hypoglycemia. Establish vascular access and give normal saline at a to-keep-open rate unless signs of shock are present. If signs of shock are observed or if the child is dehydrated, give a fluid bolus of normal saline at 20 mL/kg as instructed by medical direction. Reassess the child's response. Determine the child's blood glucose level. If the glucose level is low, treat with dextrose as described earlier in this chapter. Recall that the dextrose concentration and dosage are age dependent. If IV access cannot be established, medical direction may order glucagon IM or IN. If glucagon is given, place the child on his or her side after administration (unless contraindicated) because glucagon may cause nausea. Give oral glucose gel only if the patient can swallow, has a gag reflex, and is alert or can be roused to alertness. Repeat a blood glucose reading 10 to 15 minutes following the administration of glucose and frequently thereafter until the level stabilizes.

Special Populations

Although hypoglycemia is more common in children with diabetes, physical exertion, illness (particularly severe gastroenteritis), or injury can result in hypoglycemia in children without diabetes. Simply fasting for prolonged periods in a young infant or toddler can lead to profound hypoglycemia due to low glycogen and fat stores. Remember to assess blood glucose levels in all ill or injured children with an altered mental status or bizarre behavior.

► Congenital Adrenal Hyperplasia

Congenital adrenal hyperplasia (CAH) is an autosomal-recessive disorder of an enzyme responsible for the metabolism of cortisol (steroidogenesis) and aldosterone in the adrenal glands. The most common form is due to 21-hydroxylase deficiency. Males born with this disorder appear normal, although some may exhibit signs of puberty as a toddler, including increased musculature, penis growth, pubic hair, and a lowering of the voice. Females may be masculinized, with an enlarged clitoris that may resemble a penis. Patients sometimes undergo early pubertal development with pubic hair growth, early growth acceleration, and development of facial hair, and they may also exhibit short stature and severe acne.

Surgery can correct genital deformities early in life. Dexamethasone may be prescribed to a pregnant woman prior to the infant's delivery if the condition is diagnosed early in the first trimester of pregnancy.

When children with CAH become sick, their bodies may not be able to compensate because of the lack of cortisol—a factor that can lead to salt wasting from decreased aldosterone (decreased levels of mineralocorticoids). Although newborn screenings assess for CAH, this condition can sometimes be missed. Infants who present with salt-wasting crisis because of loss of urinary sodium may present with metabolic acidosis and hyperkalemia.

Clinically, infants with CAH may have vomiting, poor weight gain, and dehydration, and they may progress to shock in the first few weeks of life. Hypoglycemia may also be present. If this condition is suspected, hydrocortisone and IV boluses of normal saline (and glucose if hypoglycemic) are needed. Stress-dose steroids should be considered for patients with suspected CAH; contact medical control before administering these medications. For children on chronic steroid replacement, ask the parents if they have a stress-dose steroid regimen. Parents usually know the appropriate dose to give if their child becomes ill. If the parents do not know the appropriate dose, it is reasonable to give an extra dose of the child's home steroid dose, which is often tripled (or given three times a day rather than once a day) during acute illnesses. Consult with medical control. For children who appear in shock, IV hydrocortisone or methylprednisolone may be considered in consultation with medical control.

► Panhypopituitarism

The pituitary, which is located at the base of the brain, produces eight hormones. Examples include growth hormone, adrenocorticotropic hormone, follicle-stimulating hormone, thyroid-stimulating hormone, and antidiuretic hormone. **Hypopituitarism**, a condition in which the pituitary gland does not produce normal amounts of some or all of its hormones, can be congenital; occur secondary to tumor, infection, or stroke; or develop after trauma or radiation therapy. When they experience hyposecretion of any of these hormones, patients require replacement therapy.

Because several pituitary hormones affect the production of secretions of the adrenal glands, patients with panhypopituitarism can be at risk for adrenal crisis. **Panhypopituitarism** is the inadequate production or absence of the pituitary hormones, including adrenocorticotropic hormone, cortisol, thyroxine, luteinizing hormone, follicle-stimulating hormone, estrogen, testosterone, growth hormone, and antidiuretic hormone. When stressed or sick, patients with this condition can present with symptoms similar to those associated with CAH, including hypoglycemia, dehydration, poor weight gain or weight loss, vomiting, muscle cramping, weakness, dizziness, hypotension, and, if gradual in onset, tanning of the skin. These patients require IV fluid boluses with normal saline, glucose replacement, and replacement of steroids with IV hydrocortisone.

It is important for a pediatric endocrinologist to manage children diagnosed with panhypopituitarism. Often these conditions are a result of the hypothalamus—rather than the pituitary gland—functioning abnormally. These hormones control growth and sexual maturation. Once hormone therapy is initiated, children can generally live a normal life. Hormone replacement therapy will need to be continually monitored throughout the patient's life.

► Inborn Errors of Metabolism

Inborn errors of metabolism (IEMs) are a group of congenital conditions that cause either accumulation of toxins or disorders of energy metabolism in the neonate. These conditions are characterized by an infant's failure to thrive and by vague signs such as poor feeding. Because they are inherited, there may be a family history of the disorder; however, many are recessive, so a family history may not be obvious. Examples of these disorders appear in **Table 43-20**.

Usually identified in infancy, IEMs are grouped into two categories (with selected examples presented here):

- Disorders that result in toxic accumulations
  - Maple syrup urine disease—a genetic disorder that causes a buildup of the amino acids leucine, isoleucine, and valine
  - Phenylketonuria—the body's inability to break down the amino acid phenylalanine
- Disorders of energy production or use
  - Hereditary fructose intolerance—a lack of aldolase B, the enzyme responsible for breaking down fructose
  - Galactosemia—the inability to break down the simple sugar galactose

All IEMs present in childhood, though the presenting symptoms can vary significantly, from poor weight gain and failure to thrive, to loss of milestones in development, to recurring vomiting and diarrhea, skin problems, dental deformities, deafness, blindness, and various cancers. A neonate with sepsis or who is critically ill should be assessed for an IEM.

Table 43-20	Examples of Inborn Errors of Metabolism Disorders
Disordered Process	**Examples**
Carbohydrate metabolism	Glycogen storage diseases such as Pompe disease and von Gierke disease
Amino acid metabolism	Phenylketonuria and maple syrup urine disease
Fatty acid oxidation and mitochondrial metabolism	Medium-chain acyl-coenzyme A dehydrogenase deficiency
Porphyrin metabolism	Porphyria
Purine or pyrimidine metabolism	Lesch-Nyhan syndrome
Steroid metabolism and function	Congenital adrenal hyperplasia
Peroxisomal function	Zellweger syndrome
Lysosomal storage	Gaucher disease and Niemann-Pick disease

© Jones & Bartlett Learning.

Dietary restrictions and replacements can be implemented to control many of these disorders. For example, the labels of diet soda contain the following information to prevent people with phenylketonuria from consuming these beverages: "Warning, contains phenylketone."

Some patients with IEMs become hypoglycemic, particularly when they are sick or vomiting. They may also be hypermetabolic when ill, so the administration of boluses of glucose and the use of 10% dextrose (D_{10}) fluids may be necessary to maintain normoglycemia. Consider IEMs in patients with severe hypoglycemia who are resistant to initial therapy. If the patient has been diagnosed with an IEM, many geneticists give families specific care plans with instructions on emergent treatment.

■ Pathophysiology, Assessment, and Management of Hematologic, Oncologic, and Immunologic Emergencies

Hematologic, oncologic, and immunologic diseases are common in pediatric patients, ranging from cancers to bleeding disorders to immune deficiencies. Children may be immunosuppressed for several reasons, including cancer, congenital diseases of the immune system, chronic steroid use, chemotherapy, immunosuppressive medications after transplantation, and infections like human immunodeficiency virus (HIV). Because of the altered immunity, children may present with severe illness and even shock. Early recognition of shock and initiation of IV fluids can be extremely important for a positive long-term outcome.

Children have a great capacity for compensation when in shock due to their ability to increase cardiac output by greatly increasing heart rate; hypotension is a late finding. Tachycardia associated with a fever or hypothermia should indicate the possibility of sepsis. When these patients are ill, the oxygen-carrying capacity of hemoglobin is altered, resulting in decreased oxygen-carrying capacity. Oxygen supplementation is an important early intervention if a patient is suspected of being potentially septic. Special considerations besides sepsis in patients with childhood immunodeficiencies and cancer include acute chest syndrome associated with sickle cell crisis, stroke with sickle cell crisis, tumor lysis syndrome in chemotherapy patients, and an increased overall risk of infection, including bacterial infections, viral infections (varicella or shingles, herpes, and viremia), and fungal infections.

Patients with abnormal hematologic systems, including bleeding disorders or blood cancers, may also have either increased or decreased tendencies toward clotting of their blood. Because of these alterations, the primary survey of these patients needs to include evaluation of the ABCDEs, pain and location, shortness of breath, weakness or neurologic symptoms, bleeding or swelling, fever, or other concerns. Remember, hypoglycemia can cause altered mental status, especially in young children because of their relatively low glucose stores (as compared to adults). Decreases in blood glucose can occur quickly, so bedside glucose checks should be considered in these patients.

Patients with congenital or acquired immunodeficiencies are at high risk for recurrent infections and invasive disease. Bacterial, viral, and fungal organisms can quickly lead to severe morbidity and mortality. Patients should be quickly assessed for signs of sepsis and decompensation.

Examination of these patients should include a thorough lung, circulatory, and neurologic examination, and evaluation of the extremities for swollen joints that could be a sign of infection, hemarthrosis (bleeding into the joint), or a pain crisis. Delay in the capillary refill and diminished peripheral pulses can be an indicator of early sepsis and should be treated with aggressive boluses of isotonic fluids. Because some patients with hematologic, oncologic, and immunologic problems have indwelling catheters such as peripherally inserted central catheter lines, Broviacs, and Port-A-Caths, evaluation of the catheter site for erythema, swelling, and tenderness is imperative. These findings can be signs of central line infections and warrant early initiation of antibiotics after blood cultures are obtained.

▶ Sickle Cell Disease

Sickle cell disease is a genetically inherited autosomal-recessive disorder of red blood cells that causes the red blood cells to be misshapen, resulting in poor oxygen-carrying capability and potentially lodging of the red blood cells in blood vessels or the spleen. The lodging of red blood cells leads to vascular occlusion and subsequently to ischemia and painful crises. Sickle cell disease is discussed in detail in Chapter 24, *Hematologic Emergencies*.

Sickle cell vasoocclusive episodes can be precipitated by hypoxia, infection, fever, dehydration, cold environment, and acidosis. An infant experiencing a vasoocclusive crisis may present with fussiness, irritability, crying, poor feeding, and other nonspecific findings. Older children may report pain in specific locations of the body, including joints, the back, and the chest. Opioids are often started early in childhood and continued throughout adult life to manage the pain associated with vasoocclusive episodes; however, these medications are sometimes inadequate in controlling severe painful episodes. When obtaining the patient's history, ensure you ask about any medication taken since the onset of the present pain.

Treatment of patients includes giving oxygen to prevent further destruction of the red blood cells due to hypoxia. Medical direction may instruct you to give IV fluids to counter the patient's dehydration and flush damaged red blood cells from the organs and peripheral tissues. Opioids will likely be ordered for pain control.

▶ Bleeding Disorders

A bleeding or clotting disorder is a condition characterized by an abnormality in clotting of the blood. The development of a blood clot, called **thrombosis**, can occur in either arterial or venous blood vessels. The patient's symptoms depend on which part of the vascular system the clot occurs in, how large the clot is, and whether the clot becomes dislodged and travels to another part of the body.

Most bleeding is the result of trauma, but when a patient has a bleeding disorder, bleeding may be more severe or spontaneous. For all bleeding patients, the first thing for you to consider is how to best control the bleeding, if possible. Direct pressure, packing, and the judicious use of tourniquets may be necessary. As with all patients, significant blood loss in a patient with a bleeding disorder can lead to shock, so fluid replacement with boluses of isotonic fluids such as saline or lactated Ringer solution is necessary until the patient is at a hospital for definitive care and blood transfusions.

Bleeding may be drug induced, inherited, or acquired. Drugs such as aspirin and nonsteroidal anti-inflammatory drugs (eg, ibuprofen) can cause a decrease in platelet adhesion, making patients more prone to bleeding. Medications such as aspirin, warfarin (Coumadin), and heparin interfere with the clotting cascade and decrease the tendency to form a clot. Over-the-counter medications (ginkgo biloba, ginger, vitamin E, ginseng, and garlic) and some antibiotics can also increase bleeding tendencies. Though rare in young children, ethanol use or diseases that affect the liver can lead to bleeding by decreasing the liver's capacity to synthesize the factors needed in the clotting cascade. Bleeding disorders are discussed in detail in Chapter 24, *Hematologic Emergencies*.

Thrombocytopenia

Thrombocytopenia occurs when the blood contains an abnormally low number of platelets. Thrombocytopenia can have many causes, including infections, cancers such as leukemia, rheumatologic diseases such as lupus, and splenic sequestration. Some inherited conditions may also cause low platelet counts. In addition, many medications (including valproic acid used to treat seizures) and chemotherapy drugs can reduce the platelet count.

Besides spontaneous bleeding or prolonged bleeding with injury, patients with low levels of platelets may exhibit petechiae or purpura. Large bruises may develop from minimal injuries or with no history of injury. Physical abuse should always be considered in children with unexplained bruising until proven otherwise.

Treatment of patients with bleeding secondary to thrombocytopenia includes treating the underlying cause if present (eg, treating infections, stopping offending medications) and transfusing platelets if bleeding cannot be controlled with local measures. Consultation with a hematologist is required for these patients, so transport to a hospital with these capabilities should not be delayed.

Hemophilia

Hemophilia is a genetic disorder usually inherited from the mother. People with hemophilia have a significant decrease in one of their clotting factors (proteins in the blood that work with platelets to help blood clot). Without the clotting factor, it is more difficult for the body to stop bleeding. A child with severe factor deficiencies can experience hemorrhage after minor trauma, such as a bruise, or during the loss of a deciduous tooth.[29] Spontaneous bleeding into the joints (particularly the knees, elbows, and ankles) and IM hemorrhages are common. Intracranial hemorrhage is one of the major causes of death.[29] The family of a child with hemophilia who is 2 to 3 years of age is taught how to perform venipuncture and administer clotting factors. The child learns how to self-administer clotting factors between the ages of 8 and 12 years. An older child with this disease is often a reliable historian and will be able to relay his or her signs and symptoms and their onset.[29]

When caring for a child with hemophilia, it is essential to recognize signs of internal bleeding. Be alert for signs of cerebral bleeding, which may include headache, slurred speech, and an altered mental status. Also, be alert for signs of gastrointestinal bleeding, such as black, tarry stools. Provide supportive care, which may include supplemental oxygen if signs of hypoxia are present and IV fluids if hypotension is present.

von Willebrand Disease

von Willebrand disease is a bleeding disorder in which the patient is missing the von Willebrand factor (a protein essential for platelet adhesion), preventing the blood from clotting well. Most people with von Willebrand disease are undiagnosed. Several types of von Willebrand disease have been identified, which can range in severity from mild (presenting with nosebleeds) to severe with uncontrolled bleeding tendencies. In the field, treatment is aimed at controlling bleeding and transporting the patient to a hospital with hematology services.

▶ Leukemia/Lymphoma

In children, two forms of leukemia are generally recognized: acute lymphoblastic leukemia and acute myelogenous leukemia. At its onset, the child with leukemia often displays few symptoms. The condition may be diagnosed when a child has had a minor infection, such as a cold, but continues to be febrile, listless, and pale with little appetite. Parents typically seek medical attention for the child upon noticing weight loss, bruising without cause, and complaints of bone and joint pain.[26] At other times the diagnosis of leukemia is made following an unrelated event, such as a routine physical exam before playing sports.

Treatment of leukemia involves the use of IV chemotherapy and may involve radiation therapy. An immunosuppressed state often occurs secondary to the leukemic cells overtaking the bone marrow or the treatments they are receiving. These patients are susceptible to bacteremia, sepsis, and shock. Fluid therapy should be aggressive in pediatric patients who are tachycardic, as this can be the first sign of sepsis. Hypotension is a late sign of sepsis in the pediatric population.

Like patients with leukemia, patients with lymphoma generally require treatment involving some form of chemotherapy or radiation therapy. These patients may be in constant pain, requiring supportive care and pain management in transit to an appropriate receiving facility for definitive care.

■ Pathophysiology, Assessment, and Management of Toxicologic Emergencies

Toxic exposures account for a significant number of pediatric emergencies. Toxic exposures can take the form of ingestion, inhalation, injection, or application of a substance (see Chapter 27, *Toxicology*, for more information on specific exposures). A toddler or preschool-age child is most likely to have an unintentional exposure, the result of developmentally normal exploration. In this age group, ingestion tends to involve small quantities of a single cleaning product, cosmetic product, or plant, or a few pills. In contrast, toxic exposures in adolescents

Table 43-21	One Pill Can Kill: Potentially Lethal Toddler Ingestion
Medicine	**Lethal Dose**
Camphor	One teaspoon of oil
Chloroquine	One 500-mg tablet
Clonidine	One 0.3-mg tablet
Diphenoxylate/atropine	Two 2.5-mg tablets
Glyburide	Two 5-mg tablets
Imipramine	One 150-mg tablet
Lindane	Two teaspoons of 1% lotion
Oil of wintergreen	One teaspoon of oil
Propranolol	One or two 160-mg tablets
Theophylline	One 500-mg tablet
Verapamil	One or two 240-mg tablets

© Jones & Bartlett Learning.

typically result from recreational drug use or suicide attempts and often involve multiple agents. Although intentional exposures among adolescents lead to greater morbidity and mortality, the toxic effects of some medications are such that "one pill can kill" in small children Table 43-21 .

Evidence-Based Medicine

According to a study done over a 16-year period from 2000 through 2015, poison control centers in the United States received one call every 45 minutes for an opioid exposure in children and adolescents younger than 20 years. Of these reported incidents, the opioid hydrocodone was responsible for the largest number of exposures overall.[30]

▶ Assessment of Toxicologic Emergencies

The evaluation of a child who has experienced a potentially toxic exposure follows the standard assessment sequence. Identify the agents to which the child was exposed, the quantity, and the route and time of exposure. Findings of physical assessment will vary widely based on these factors. Make special note of vital signs, pupillary changes, skin temperature and moisture, and any unusual odors. Putting together these pieces of the puzzle may allow you to identify a toxidrome—a pattern of symptoms and signs typical of a particular poisoning.

When you are performing the primary survey, attend to the ABCDEs as indicated. A dextrose (glucose) check is essential because ingestion of some common substances can lead to hypoglycemia—namely, ethanol and other alcohols, insulin, oral hypoglycemic agents, and beta-blockers. Treat documented hypoglycemia as part of your resuscitation.

Special Populations

Any child with unexplained hyperpnea should be suspected to have salicylate poisoning.

If the child is in stable condition without physiologic abnormalities and without a serious toxic exposure, stay on scene to obtain additional history and perform a secondary assessment. See Table 43-22 for the SAMPLE history for a pediatric patient with a potential toxic exposure. During the secondary assessment, look for toxidromes by assessing the patient's mental status, pupillary changes, skin CTC, gastrointestinal activity (bowel sounds, emesis, or diarrhea), and abnormal odors. Perform frequent reassessments because the child's condition may change.

Children with potentially life-threatening toxic exposures may be asymptomatic on your arrival, and the dose of drug in an accidental toddler ingestion may be high. Always attempt to collect any pill containers or bottles and transport them with the patient to the hospital to assist the ED staff in making treatment decisions.

Words of Wisdom

Have the national Poison Center number (1-800-222-1222) in your clipboard for suspected poisonings.

▶ Management of Toxicologic Emergencies

The management of any potential toxic exposure begins with supportive care and attention to the ABCDEs. Other management options include reducing the absorption of the substance by performing decontamination, enhancing elimination of the substance, and providing an antidote. Pay special attention to the risks of environmental exposures for the EMS crew, who may also require decontamination measures.

If you are not sure if an exposure is dangerous or potentially toxic to a child, the national Poison Center

Table 43-22	SAMPLE Components for a Child With Toxic Exposure
Components	**Features**
Signs and symptoms	Time of suspected exposure Behavior changes in child Emesis and content of vomit
Allergies	Known drug reactions or other allergies
Medications	Identity of suspected toxin Amount of toxin exposure (count pills or measure volume) Pill or chemical containers on scene Exact names and doses of prescribed medications
Past medical problems	Previous illnesses or injuries
Last oral intake	Timing of the child's last food or drink Type and time of home treatment
Events leading to injury or illness	Key events leading to the exposure Type of exposure (inhaled, injected, ingested, or absorbed through the skin) Poison Center contact

© Jones & Bartlett Learning.

hotline is available 24 hours per day at 1-800-222-1222. This nationwide number puts you in contact with experts who can help manage the care of ingestions, exposures, inhalations, and other toxicologic emergencies.

Decontamination

If a toxic substance has been applied to the skin, reducing absorption involves removal of all clothing and a thorough washing of the skin. With ocular exposure, immediately wash out the eyes. For ingested toxins, options to reduce gastric absorption include dilution, gastric lavage, and activated charcoal.

Depending on the substance ingested, it may be useful to dilute the substance by having the child drink a glass of milk or water. This decision should be made in conjunction with a Poison Center consultant or your medical control physician or nurse, depending on your protocols. If the child has any airway or breathing concerns, do not allow the child to drink.

Although parents were once encouraged to keep syrup of ipecac available to induce vomiting in young children, this treatment is no longer recommended by the American Academy of Pediatrics.[31] Ipecac does not remove significant amounts of ingested toxins and can cause prolonged emesis; it should not be used in the prehospital management of pediatric toxic ingestion.

Today, the method most commonly used for gastrointestinal decontamination in the ED setting is administration of activated charcoal. Activated charcoal absorbs many ingested toxins in the gut, making less of the toxin available for systemic absorption if the charcoal is administered within the first hour after exposure. Be aware that some common toxins do not bind to charcoal—for example, heavy metals, alcohols, hydrocarbons, acids, and alkalis. Activated charcoal is also messy to administer and is rarely readily accepted by pediatric patients. For these reasons, and because of the risk of severe chemical pneumonia, if a child with altered mental status or vomiting aspirates the charcoal, this treatment may be best given in the hospital setting. If activated charcoal is administered in the field, the typical dose is 1 g/kg.[32]

When the toxicity is due to substances that are renally excreted, diuresis may be beneficial. IV fluid administration can increase diuresis, as can mannitol. Care must be taken with mannitol administration for this purpose, as this treatment can lead to hypotension. Some substances have enhanced excretion in an alkali environment, such as salicylates and methyl alcohol (antifreeze or wood alcohol). When the toxic emergency is due to one of these substances, the use of sodium bicarbonate to alkalinize the urinary pH can be beneficial. Dialysis is required for some overdoses and for overdoses that do not improve with other therapies such as alkalization of the urine. Examples of ingestions or overdoses for which dialysis is helpful include salicylates, lithium, methyl alcohol, ethylene glycol, and barbiturates such as phenobarbital.

If the toxic substance is inhaled, the patient's respiratory status should be assessed carefully. Bronchodilators may be needed for bronchial irritation and bronchospasm. Monitoring of oxygen saturation levels and intubation may be necessary, particularly with inhalational injuries associated with house fires. If soot is visible in the upper airway, if the patient has stridor, or if swelling of the upper airway is apparent, early intubation is indicated. Carbon monoxide inhalation injuries may be difficult to diagnose because the patient's oxygen saturation level will be near 100%—a result that occurs because the oximeter may misinterpret carboxyhemoglobin as oxyhemoglobin. Patients with suspected carbon monoxide poisoning should be placed on a nonrebreathing mask until their blood carboxyhemoglobin levels can be checked at the hospital.

Enhanced Elimination

Cathartics such as sorbitol or magnesium citrate are sometimes combined with activated charcoal to speed up elimination of the toxic substance. In general, though, cathartics are not recommended for young children because they have been known to cause significant diarrhea

Table 43-23	Common Antidotes
Poison	**Antidote**
Carbon monoxide	Oxygen
Organophosphate	Atropine/pralidoxime
Tricyclic antidepressants	Bicarbonate
Opiates	Naloxone
Beta-blockers	Glucagon
Calcium-channel blockers	Calcium
Benzodiazepine	Flumazenil
Acetaminophen	N-acetylcysteine

© Jones & Bartlett Learning.

with serious—sometimes life-threatening—electrolyte abnormalities.

Antidotes

Antidotes can be lifesaving but are available for only a few poisons. They work by reversing or blocking the effects of the ingested toxin. Table 43-23 lists some of the more commonly available antidotes; indications for their use are the same for young children as for adults. The dose depends on the weight of the child.

Special Populations

Autism can vary in severity and falls under a broader category known as pervasive developmental disorders (PDDs). PDDs cause delays in many areas of childhood development, such as the development of skills to communicate and interact socially, and the effects can be lifelong. See Chapter 45, *Patients With Special Challenges*, for more information on this condition.

Pathophysiology, Assessment, and Management of Psychiatric and Behavioral Emergencies

As a paramedic, you will encounter children with behavioral and psychiatric problems. The call may be for out-of-control behavior or for a suicide attempt. Unfortunately, EMS calls for behavioral emergencies are increasing, reflecting in part the limited community resources available for children with mental health problems. Of children between 13 and

18 years old, 21.4% either currently or in their life have had a seriously debilitating mental disorder.[33]

Many of these problems begin as simple complaints not easily recognized by health care providers. When not treated properly, such problems usually persist into adulthood. Given that suicide is the second leading cause of death in adolescents and the second leading cause of death in children between ages 10 and 14 years,[34] medical professionals have given increased attention to mood disorders, anxiety, and other behavioral problems in this population.

Children also are more likely to have coexisting problems (eg, attention-deficit/hyperactivity disorder, conduct disorder, and oppositional defiant disorder) along with the more traditional mental health disorders.

▶ Safety

When you are called to a home for a behavioral or psychiatric emergency, safety should be your first priority. Assess the scene for your own safety and for the safety of the patient. If weapons are involved or you cannot determine the degree of risk, call for law enforcement backup.

Approach the child calmly, letting him or her know you are there to help. Address the patient directly when you are obtaining the history, and explain clearly what you are doing and why. Some children are flight risks, so determine how best to deploy your squad so that they do not leave the scene. As always, answer questions as honestly as possible.

A small percentage of children cannot be safely talked down for transport and must be mechanically restrained for their own protection and the protection of the EMS crew. Applying these restraints may be a task for EMS or for law enforcement personnel. If you decide to apply restraints, carefully document the reason and keep the restraints in place until arrival at the ED. Try to avoid using chemical restraints (ie, tranquilizing drugs) in the prehospital setting.

▶ Assessment and Management of Psychiatric and Behavioral Emergencies

Mental health problems in children are difficult to diagnose because the lines between normal and abnormal behavior are blurred in this population. Diagnosis and treatment may be difficult when you try to distinguish among organic, genetic, and environmental causes. Cultural and ethnic factors also blur the line between normal and abnormal coping mechanisms.

The mental status assessment of the child is similar to that of an adult but also considers the child's developmental level. Abnormal findings in the developmental and mental status examinations often are related to adjustment disorders and stress rather than the more serious disorders. Your assessment of any child must include suicide risk.

The PAT will give you a general impression of the child's mental status and cardiovascular stability. A child who has attempted suicide by ingestion may have life-threatening medical complications that take precedence over his or her psychiatric concerns. In the absence of acute medical issues,

Table 43-24	SAMPLE Components for a Child With Behavioral Problems
Component	**Features**
Signs and symptoms	Out-of-control behavior Suicidal or homicidal thoughts or actions Harm to self, others, or pets Recent change in behavior Recent change in medication Auditory or visual hallucinations
Allergies	Known food or medication allergies and their reactions
Medications	List of all patient's medications and vitamins, prescribed and over the counter
Past medical history	History of any behavior or psychiatric problems Therapist, counselor, or psychiatrist contact information Prior psychiatric or behavioral hospitalizations Any medical illnesses
Last oral intake	Timing and identification of last food and drink
Events leading to behavioral problems	Ongoing or new stressors Argument or fight with boyfriend/girlfriend or family members

© Jones & Bartlett Learning.

the bulk of your assessment will be based on observation and history. In cases involving an agitated child, your hands-on assessment may be limited. **Table 43-24** lists specific SAMPLE questions for behavioral emergencies. As always, treat any existing medical problems or injuries by using standard protocols.

■ Pathophysiology, Assessment, and Management of Fever Emergencies

Fever is a common pediatric complaint but often not a true medical emergency. A symptom of an underlying infectious or inflammatory process, fever can have multiple causes. Most pediatric fevers are caused by viral infections that are often mild and self-limiting. In other cases, fever is a symptom of a more serious bacterial infection.

Your general impression and primary survey will help you determine the severity of illness. Remember, young children with a fever can look quite ill because increased body temperature causes increased metabolism, tachycardia, and tachypnea. Record temperature as part of the vital signs, but recognize that the height of the fever does not reflect the severity of the illness. If the patient is a young infant, a rectal temperature is most accurate, but recognition that fever is present is more important than the exact temperature. As you move through the primary survey, look for signs of respiratory distress, shock, seizures, stiff neck, petechial or purpuric rash, or a bulging fontanel in an infant. These signs may tip you off to the presence of pneumonia, sepsis, or meningitis, all of which can be life threatening and require prompt transport to an appropriate facility.

Young infants (younger than 2 months) should always be considered at risk for serious infection. Such infants have few ways of interacting with the world, and a fever (defined as body temperature greater than 100.4°F [38°C]) may be the only sign of a potentially life-threatening illness. Regardless of how well a child in this age group looks, he or she should be assessed and transported quickly to an ED for a full sepsis workup, including blood, urine, and CSF analysis. All children younger than 28 days with a fever, and most children younger than 2 months, will require admission to the ED.

History taking and the secondary assessment will help you determine the underlying cause of the fever and the severity of illness. Perform this assessment on scene if the child is in stable condition or en route to the ED if the child appears seriously ill. Ask about the presence of vomiting, diarrhea, poor feeding, headache, neck pain or stiffness, and rash. A history of infectious exposure may provide clues to the likely cause of the child's current illness. History taking may also identify a child at high risk for serious bacterial illness. For example, sickle cell disease, HIV infection, and childhood cancers may all lead to an immunocompromised state.

A child with a fever may require little intervention in the field. You should simply support the ABCs as needed. Although fever by itself is not dangerous, temperature control will make the child with a minor acute illness look and feel better. Consider treatment with acetaminophen or ibuprofen, but avoid aspirin in children. Use of aspirin in children has been linked with a rare illness called Reye syndrome, which can result in cerebral edema and liver failure. Other cooling measures should be limited to undressing the child. Transport the patient to an appropriate medical facility while performing ongoing reassessment for clinical deterioration.

Special Populations

Fever itself is generally not an emergency, but rather a symptom of an underlying process. Use your assessment skills to determine the child's severity of illness.

Child Abuse and Neglect

Sadly, child abuse is prevalent in our society. **Child abuse** is any improper or excessive action that injures or otherwise harms a child or infant; it includes physical abuse, sexual abuse, neglect, and emotional abuse. In the United States, a report of child abuse is made every 10 seconds.[35] In 2014, state agencies identified an estimated 1,580 children who died as a result of abuse and neglect—between four and five children per day.[35] More than 70% of the children who died as a result of child abuse or neglect were 2 years of age or younger; more than 80% were not yet old enough for kindergarten. Around 80% of child maltreatment fatalities involve at least one parent as perpetrator.[35]

Physical abuse involves the infliction of injury to a child. Sexual abuse occurs when an adult engages in sexual activity with a child; it can range from inappropriate touching to intercourse. Emotional abuse and child neglect are often difficult to identify and may go unreported. **Neglect** is refusal or failure on the part of the caregiver to provide life necessities, whereas emotional abuse may be described as lack of emotional support by the caregiver.

Abandonment occurs when a parent or guardian physically leaves a child without regard to the child's health, safety, or welfare. Abandoned children (called foundlings) may be found in a home where the parents or caregivers have left them without appropriate supervision, or they may be dropped off in a location to be found by someone else. In these situations, parents have relinquished consent authority, and EMS providers should render care without written or verbal consent. Safe-haven laws allow parents to leave a child without fear of legal implications, with these children then becoming wards of the state. Police stations, fire houses, hospitals, and specialized infant boxes are all locations where children may be left unharmed by caregivers. All 50 states have passed safe-haven laws, but the precise details vary from state to state; you should become familiar with the applicable laws where you practice.

Words of Wisdom

EMS providers are mandated reporters of suspected child abuse and neglect in all states.

Keep the possibility of child abuse in mind when you are called to assist with an injured child. The information you gather from the scene size-up and interviews may prove invaluable. If you suspect child abuse, you should act on your suspicions because child abuse involves a pattern of behavior. A child who is abused once is likely to be abused again—and next time, the abuse may be more serious or even fatal.

► Risk Factors for Abuse

No child asks to be abused, but certain risk factors make abuse more likely. Younger children are more often abused than are older children, perhaps as a function of their helplessness and limited ability to communicate their needs. Children who require extra attention, such as those with handicaps, chronic illnesses, or other developmental problems, are also more likely to be abused.

Child abuse occurs across all socioeconomic levels, although it is more prevalent in lower-socioeconomic families. Divorce, financial problems, and illness can contribute to the overall stress level of parents, placing them at higher risk to abuse their children. Drug and alcohol abuse can also interfere with a caregiver's ability to parent, and both are associated with higher rates of abusive behavior. Domestic violence in the home places a child at a much higher risk for child abuse.

► Suspecting Abuse or Neglect

When you are called to the home of an injured child and suspect abuse, trust your instincts. Look for "red flags" that could suggest child maltreatment:

- A history inconsistent with the type of injury sustained—for example, a child who fell from a tree but whose bruises are on the buttocks only
- An account of the injury that is inconsistent with the developmental abilities of the child—for example, a 2-month-old infant rolling off a bed
- An old injury that went unreported
- Inappropriate actions or language from the caregiver

Signs that should raise your level of suspicion for child maltreatment are summarized in the mnemonic CHILD ABUSE Table 43-25 .

► Assessment and Management of Abuse and Neglect

To recognize abuse, you first have to suspect it. Once you begin to question whether abuse is involved, it becomes important to carefully document what you see. Although it may be difficult to remain impartial when child abuse is suspected, such self-control is an important part of professionalism. Record what you see and hear—just the facts and objective findings—and do not editorialize. Be detailed in your incident report about the child's environment, noting the condition of the home and the

Documentation & Communication

If you suspect child abuse, take extra care with your documentation. Record conversations verbatim (in quotes), and document on your patient care report what you see and hear.

Table 43-25	CHILD ABUSE Mnemonic for Suspicion of Child Abuse
C	Consistency of the injury with the child's developmental age
H	History inconsistent with injury
I	Inappropriate parental concerns
L	Lack of supervision
D	Delay in seeking care
A	Affect (of the parent or caregiver and the child in relation to the caregiver)
B	Bruises of varying ages
U	Unusual injury patterns
S	Suspicious circumstances
E	Environmental clues

© Jones & Bartlett Learning.

interactions among the caregivers, the child, and the EMS crew. Record concerning comments verbatim in quotes, as well as the name of the person who made the comments and when.

In all states, prehospital personnel, including EMS providers, are mandated reporters, meaning you have an independent obligation under the law to report a suspicion of child abuse to **child protective services (CPS)** and law enforcement. Failure to make a report may be a crime. Review the specific law in your state. Reporting is done in conjunction with emergency physicians, social workers, and child protection teams at the ED. Involving police early is important to secure the crime scene and collect evidence that may be destroyed or lost. In cases where death occurs, the medical examiner will investigate the cause of death. The medical examiner should be notified of any death if the child is not being transported to the ED.

Do not approach the caregiver with your concerns, but make sure you pass these concerns on to staff at the ED. Be aware of local regulations; you may have a legal—and an ethical—obligation to ensure a report is made to the local CPS. The primary objective of CPS is to ensure the safety of children and keep children safe within their own families.

Although child abuse can generate an emotional response from the EMS crew, remember that your primary focus should be on trauma assessment and management and on ensuring the safety of the child. Base your general impression on the PAT, which may range from normal in a child with minor inflicted injuries to grossly abnormal in a child with severe internal or central nervous system injuries. In shaken baby syndrome, you may encounter a child with an abnormal appearance but no external signs of injury. In such a case, the child (typically an infant) receives a severe brain injury when a caregiver violently shakes him or her, often when the child is crying inconsolably. Given that few caregivers will admit to having hurt the child, be alert for a history that is inconsistent with the clinical picture.

Pay special attention to the child's skin while looking for bruises, especially in different stages of healing or in concerning locations. Active toddlers often have bruises on their shins from falls and active playing but rarely on their backs or buttocks. Bruises in identifiable patterns such as belt buckles, looped cords, or straight lines are rarely incurred accidentally. **Figure 43-25** and **Figure 43-26** are examples of bruises that are suggestive of physical abuse.

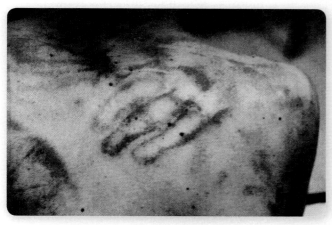

Figure 43-25 Bruises from child abuse. Look for bruises that look like finger or hand marks.

Courtesy of Moose Jaw Police Service.

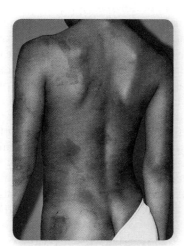

Figure 43-26 Multiple bruises or injuries that are in different stages of healing are concerns for abuse.

Courtesy of Ronald Dieckmann, MD.

> ### Words of Wisdom
>
> Use the TEN-4 bruising clinical decision rule (BCDR) to determine whether child abuse is a possibility. TEN stands for Torso, Ears, and Neck. The TEN-4 BCDR states that any bruising in the "TEN" region in a child younger than 4 years is concerning for child abuse, as is any bruise in a child younger than 4 months.[36]

Use the CHILD ABUSE mnemonic when you obtain additional history. Ask yourself, "Does the caregiver's explanation make sense? Could this child produce this bruise or injury through his or her normal activities?"

Mimics of Abuse

It can be difficult to distinguish some normal skin findings from inflicted injuries. For example, Mongolian spots **Figure 43-27** can mimic bruises. These birthmarks are generally found on the lower back and buttocks of children of Asian or African American descent; they may be mistaken for bruises because of their unique blue coloring. Other medical conditions can also mimic bruises, such as the purpura of meningitis and Henoch-Schönlein purpura, or the petechiae of idiopathic thrombocytopenic purpura and leukemia. Exposure to the sun can cause reactions with certain medications or fruits (limes, mangos), causing red-purple discolorations of the skin called phytophotodermatitis.

Certain cultural customs also produce skin markings that can mimic child abuse. Coining **Figure 43-28** and cupping **Figure 43-29** are traditional Asian healing practices, often used in the treatment of fever. Both techniques are thought to draw sickness from the body and help restore balance. Coining and cupping share the common feature of leaving marks on the skin that may

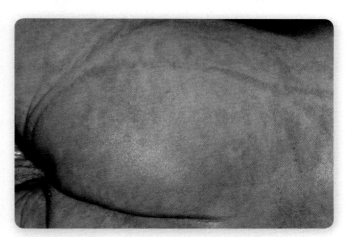

Figure 43-27 A Mongolian spot is a birthmark that can mimic a bruise. It may be on the back, buttocks, or extremities.

© Dr. P. Marazzi/Science Source.

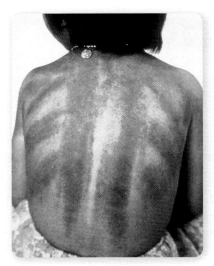

Figure 43-28 Coining, the practice of rubbing hot coins on the back as a treatment of medical illnesses, can leave impressive markings that can mimic child abuse.

Used with permission of the American Academy of Pediatrics, *Pediatric Education for Prehospital Professionals,* © American Academy of Pediatrics, 2000.

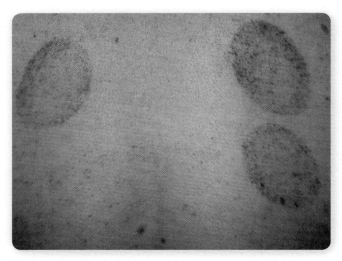

Figure 43-29 Round, flat, red circles on a child's back may be from the practice of cupping—placing warm cups on the skin to draw out illness from the body.

© Jones & Bartlett Learning.

appear to be bruises or a pathologic rash. If the family uses these traditional techniques on a child before seeking medical attention, the markings may raise the suspicion of child abuse or maltreatment. The marks may also appear to be a rash or bruising, which may lead to an incorrect diagnosis.[37] Although the skin markings can be impressive, the practice is not harmful and does not represent abuse.

Sudden Infant Death Syndrome

Sudden unexpected infant death (SUID) is the death of an infant younger than 1 year that occurs suddenly and unexpectedly, the cause of which is not immediately

obvious before investigation. Most SUIDs are reported as one of three types[38]:

1. **Sudden infant death syndrome (SIDS).** SIDS, formerly known as crib death, is the sudden death of an infant younger than 1 year that cannot be explained after a thorough investigation is conducted, including a complete autopsy, examination of the death scene, and a review of the clinical history. About 1,600 infants died of SIDS in 2015. SIDS is the leading cause of death among infants 1 to 12 months old.
2. **Unknown cause.** The sudden death of an infant younger than 1 year may remain undetermined because one or more parts of the investigation was not completed.
3. **Accidental suffocation and strangulation in bed.** The sudden death of an infant younger than 1 year can happen because of suffocation by soft bedding (for example, when a pillow or waterbed covers an infant's nose and mouth), overlay (when another person rolls on top of or against the infant while sleeping), wedging or entrapment (when an infant is wedged between two objects, such as a mattress and the wall), or strangulation (for example, when an infant's head and neck become caught between crib railings).

Whatever the cause, the sudden death of an apparently healthy infant is devastating to families and to the EMS crew who responds to the call.

▶ Assessment and Management of SIDS

The typical scenario for a SIDS call is that of a healthy infant who was put down for a nap and later found dead in bed. On arrival of EMS, the baby will be lifeless and, depending on discovery time, may have rigor mortis and dependent lividity (pooling of blood on the underside of the body). The presence of frothy or blood-tinged fluid in the mouth or nose or on the bedding is typical of SIDS. Be alert for clues to other potential causes of death, such as trauma, suffocation, or maltreatment.

Your decision to start resuscitative efforts, or to stop CPR that was started by first responders or family members, can be difficult in cases of suspected SIDS. Your actions will be guided by local protocols on declaring death in the field and by your assessment of the patient and the needs of the family. Although a victim of SIDS cannot be resuscitated, failure to initiate care may not be acceptable to the shocked family. Likewise, ED care will not change the outcome for the infant, but hospital-based social services for the family may be an important resource. In cases that meet the criteria for declaring death at the scene and nontransport, notify the coroner, medical examiner, or law enforcement personnel, as dictated by local protocol, so that appropriate scene investigation can be undertaken. You also have an important role in mobilizing support for the survivors—for example, a chaplain or minister, SIDS team, social worker, or other family members.

Despite the emotionally charged atmosphere, doing a thorough scene size-up and obtaining the pertinent history are important. A history of recent illnesses, chronic conditions, medications, or trauma may decrease the likelihood of SIDS as the cause of death. The presence of pillows, stuffed toys, window blind cords, or sheepskin in the baby's crib may make suffocation a possibility.

Special Populations

Whatever you suspect as the cause of death of a child, be compassionate and nonjudgmental in dealing with caregivers. Find out the child's name, and use it. Do not hesitate to tell the family how sorry you are. Families in this situation will often look to you for answers. Even when there is nothing to do medically, you can make a big impact by providing emotional support and care to the surviving family members.

■ Brief Resolved Unexplained Event

A **brief resolved unexplained event (BRUE)**, formerly known as an apparent life-threatening event (ALTE), is an episode during which an infant becomes pale or cyanotic; chokes, gags, or has an apneic spell; or loses muscle tone. These changes are sufficiently dramatic that the caregiver becomes frightened and may think that the baby is dying. BRUEs frequently prompt 9-1-1 calls. Their causes may include benign diagnoses, such as a brief episode of laryngospasm during feedings or gastroesophageal reflux, and serious diagnoses, such as sepsis, congenital heart disease, and seizures.

BRUEs were once thought of as existing along a spectrum with SIDS; hence they were called near-miss or aborted SIDS. More recent evidence demonstrates that although both events occur in early infancy, the two are not related.[39] It is common to find a distraught caregiver and a well-appearing baby on arrival at the scene of a BRUE call. Provide life support if the infant shows signs of cardiorespiratory compromise or altered mental status, and transport all infants with a history of a BRUE to an appropriate medical facility for evaluation. This is a challenging age group to assess, and overtriage is the safest path. Because BRUEs may be associated with serious underlying illness, failure to transport may be associated with grave consequences for the child.

■ Pathophysiology, Assessment, and Management of Pediatric Trauma Emergencies

Children's age-related anatomy and physiology make their injury patterns and responses to trauma different from those seen in adults. In addition, a child's developmental stage will affect his or her response to injury. For a young child, being strapped to a backboard may be as traumatic as the injury leading to the EMS call! Refer to the beginning of this chapter for a review of age-related anatomy and physiology and a discussion of how trauma affects children as a result of their anatomic and physiologic differences.

▶ Pathophysiology of Traumatic Injuries

Blunt trauma is the MOI in most pediatric injury cases. Because children have less muscle and fat mass than adults have, they have less protection against the forces transmitted in blunt trauma.

Falls are common in pediatric patients, and the injuries sustained will reflect the anatomy of the child and the height of the fall. For example, a 6-year-old child playing on the monkey bars is most likely to sustain an upper extremity fracture when falling onto an outstretched arm. Internal or head injuries would be uncommon with this mechanism. Conversely, an infant, with a big head and no protective reflexes, who falls out of a shopping cart will commonly have a skull fracture and could have an intracranial hemorrhage. Falls from a standing position usually result in isolated long bone injuries, whereas high-energy falls (eg, from a window, via ejection from a motor vehicle, in a vehicle-pedestrian collision) may result in multisystem trauma.

Injuries from bicycle handlebars typically produce compression injuries to the intra-abdominal organs. Duodenal hematomas and pancreatic injuries are common with this MOI, as are upper extremity injuries. You must also consider a head injury if the patient went over the handlebars, especially if not wearing a helmet.

Motor vehicle crashes can result in a variety of injury patterns depending on whether the child was properly restrained and where the child was seated in the car. For unrestrained passengers, assume multisystem trauma. Restrained passengers may sustain chest and abdominal injuries associated with seat belt use. If you see chest or abdominal bruising in a seat belt pattern, you should have a high suspicion for spinal fractures. Airbags pose a particular threat for head and neck injuries in young children.

A child who is the victim of a vehicle-pedestrian collision is likely to sustain multisystem trauma. Depending on the child's height and the height of the vehicle's bumper, a child may receive chest, abdominal, and lower extremity injuries at impact. Head and neck injuries may result from the fall when the child is thrown.

▶ Assessment and Management of Traumatic Injuries

The first steps in managing pediatric trauma are the same as for medical emergencies. Begin with a thorough scene size-up, addressing safety concerns, determining the MOI or NOI as you approach the scene, noting the number of patients, and taking standard precautions before coming into contact with the patient. Also determine whether additional resources are needed.

Use the PAT to form a general impression. If the PAT findings are grossly abnormal, quickly move on to the management of the ABCs to prevent death or disability. An abnormal appearance should make you think immediately of a head injury. With an isolated closed head injury, the child's breathing and circulation may be normal. Of course, abnormal appearance may also reflect inadequate oxygenation of the brain owing to shock or respiratory failure. Abnormalities in work of breathing will tip you off to chest or airway injury, and abnormal circulation signals the presence of a hemorrhage problem. If multisystem injuries are present, all three sides of the PAT may be abnormal.

Initiate life support interventions as you identify problems. Assess the airway for obstruction with teeth, blood, vomit, or edema, and suction as needed. For cervical spinal injury, open the airway using the jaw-thrust maneuver. If the child cannot maintain the airway, consider insertion of an NG or oropharyngeal airway. If you attempt ET intubation, maintain cervical spinal precautions. Establishing an emergency surgical airway in a child is fraught with complications, and the failure rate is high; for these reasons, tracheotomy should be reserved for the most expert surgeons in a controlled setting. The chances of needing to perform a needle cricothyrotomy in a child are remote. In younger children, identification of the cricothyroid membrane is difficult. Needle cricothyrotomy is described in Chapter 15, *Airway Management*.

Breathing assessment includes evaluation for symmetric chest rise and equal breath sounds. Provide 100% supplemental oxygen, give bag-mask ventilation as needed, and place an NG or OG tube for stomach decompression.

Pneumothorax is not common in pediatric blunt chest injury, but it may be present when the patient experiences penetrating trauma of the chest or upper abdomen. Remember, you are less likely to see jugular venous distention and feel tracheal deviation in a child. If the MOI suggests a possible tension pneumothorax and the child is in significant respiratory distress, perform needle decompression. Signs and symptoms of tension pneumothorax include the following:

- Tachycardia
- Difficult ventilation despite an open airway
- Absent or decreased breath sounds on the affected side
- Jugular vein distention (may not be present with associated hemorrhage)
- Hyperresonance to percussion on the affected side
- Tracheal deviation away from the affected side (this late sign is not always present)
- Pulsus paradoxus

Needle decompression is discussed in detail in Chapter 35, *Chest Trauma*. When performing this skill in a pediatric patient, you should first assess the child to ensure the presentation is due to a tension pneumothorax. Notably, tracheal deviation, hyperresonance, pulsus paradoxus, and even decreased breath sounds can be difficult to assess in a young child. Remember, tracheal deviation is a late finding, and tension pneumothorax can be present without it. Use a large-bore IV catheter, preferably 14 to 16 gauge, for these patients; locate the second or third intercostal space in the midclavicular line on the affected side; and insert the needle at a 90° angle, just superior to the third rib **Figure 43-30** .

Any trauma patient should be considered to be at risk for developing shock from visible external bleeding or internal bleeding. Assess the child's circulation by checking the pulse rate and quality, capillary refill, skin temperature, and blood pressure. In pediatric patients, the only sign of compensated shock might be an elevated pulse rate; children have a remarkable capacity for peripheral vasoconstriction and can maintain their blood pressure despite significant blood loss. If the MOI is concerning and the child is tachycardic, assume the presence of compensated shock and initiate volume resuscitation with 20 mL/kg of isotonic fluid (normal saline or lactated Ringer solution). Ideally, you will insert two peripheral IV lines, but an IO line may be best in a child with hemorrhagic shock. Control external bleeding as you would in any trauma patient. Once the ABCs are stabilized, continue your assessment of disability with the AVPU scale. Your assessment of appearance in the PAT will already have identified an altered level of consciousness. Check the child's pupils and motor function. Place a cervical collar, and immobilize the child on a long backboard as indicated.

If increased ICP is a concern, keep the head midline to facilitate jugular venous return to the heart. If the child is not in shock, elevate the backboard or head of the stretcher to 30°. Perform shock resuscitation with IV fluids; brain hypoperfusion will worsen the situation. If the child has acute signs of herniation such as a "blown" pupil or the Cushing triad, consider mild hyperventilation guided to an end-tidal carbon dioxide level of 30 to 35 mm Hg and administer mannitol.[40]

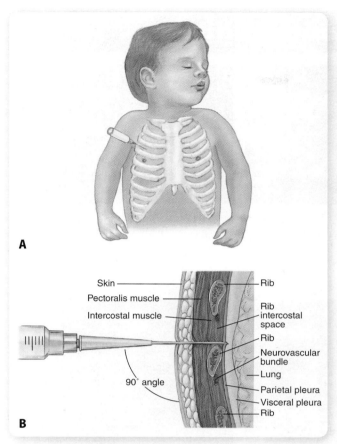

A

B

Skin — Rib
Pectoralis muscle — Rib intercostal space
Intercostal muscle — Rib
Neurovascular bundle
90° angle — Lung
Parietal pleura
Visceral pleura
Rib

Figure 43-30 If the mechanism of injury suggests a possible tension pneumothorax and the child is in significant respiratory distress, perform needle decompression: **A.** Find the second or third intercostal space at the midclavicular line on the affected side. **B.** Insert the needle at a 90° angle.
© American Academy of Orthopaedic Surgeons.

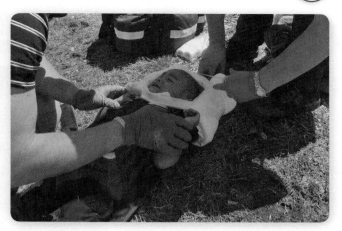

Figure 43-31 Cervical spinal stabilization with towels and tape for an infant or toddler.
© Mark C. Ide.

Assess "exposure"; that is, perform a rapid exam to identify all injuries. Log roll the child, and examine the back and buttocks. Once you have completed this exam, cover the child with blankets. Do not forget to cover the head, especially in infants and young children, and avoid drafts from heating or air conditioning units. Children have a relatively high ratio of skin surface area to body mass, increasing their risk for heat loss and hypothermia. Consider the use of warm IV fluids, warm oxygen, and a warm patient transport environment, and keep the patient covered. Also ensure you remove any wet clothing that could conduct heat away from the patient.

Treat any fractures—open or closed—as you would in an adult. Check out your equipment ahead of time to ensure you have splints appropriate for pediatric patients.

▶ Transport Considerations

After stabilization of the child, you are faced with the transport decision. Some traumas are load-and-go situations because of the severity of injuries and the child's unstable condition. Examples include trauma involving an ominous MOI regardless of how the child looks on scene, a child with an unstable or compromised airway, a child in shock, a child with difficulty breathing, and a child with a severe neurologic disability. For these situations, perform lifesaving procedures on scene or en route, and quickly transfer the patient to an appropriate trauma center according to local trauma triage protocols.

All trauma victims in whom spinal injury is suspected require appropriate spinal stabilization. The indications are the same for children and adults. You may have difficulty finding an appropriate size cervical collar for infants or young children. Do not attempt to place a collar that is too big on a small child; use towel rolls and tape to immobilize the head. Apply the tape across the temples and forehead, but avoid tape over the chin or throat because it may impair ventilation. Choose a pediatric immobilizer with a recess for the child's large occiput, or place a towel or small blanket under the shoulders and back to prevent neck flexion in infants and toddlers Figure 43-31 .

Immobilize a child by following the steps in Skill Drill 43-6 ; follow the steps in Skill Drill 43-7 to immobilize an infant. Secure the child firmly onto the backboard, but leave room for adequate chest expansion. Being immobilized is a frightening experience, especially for a young child who cannot understand your intent. Use developmentally appropriate language to explain what you are doing and why, and keep a parent close by when possible.

The identification of the nearest appropriate facility depends on local protocols and the capabilities of local EDs. In some areas of the country, you may be directed to take the patient directly to a pediatric trauma center or to arrange for air transport to a pediatric trauma center. In other areas of the country, children are evaluated primarily at local EDs and then transferred to a pediatric trauma center.

Skill Drill 43-6 Immobilizing a Child

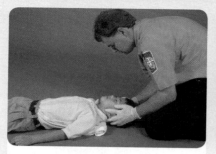

Step 1 Use a towel under the neck and shoulder area of a child to maintain the head in a neutral position.

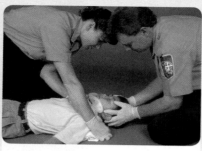

Step 2 Apply an appropriately sized cervical collar.

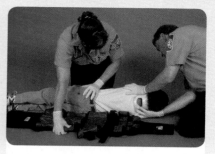

Step 3 Carefully log roll the child onto the immobilization device.

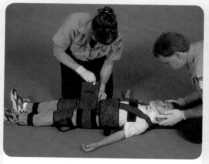

Step 4 Secure the child's torso to the immobilization device first.

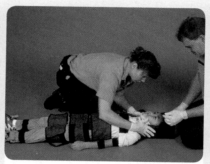

Step 5 Secure the child's head to the immobilization device.

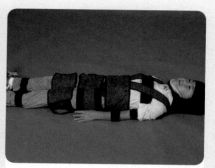

Step 6 Complete immobilization by ensuring that the child is strapped in properly.

© Jones & Bartlett Learning. Courtesy of MIEMSS.

Skill Drill 43-7 Immobilizing an Infant

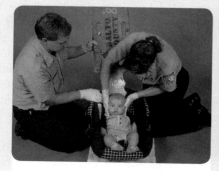

Step 1 Carefully stabilize the infant's head in a neutral position and lay the seat down into a reclined position on a hard surface.

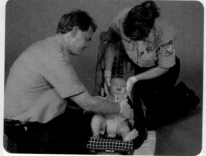

Step 2 Position a pediatric board or a similar device between the infant and the surface on which the infant is resting.

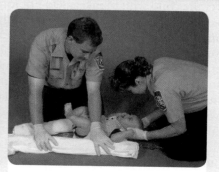

Step 3 Slide the infant onto the board.

Skill Drill 43-7 Immobilizing an Infant (continued)

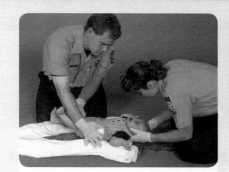 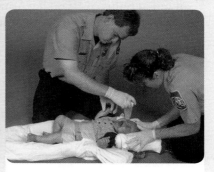

Step 4 Make sure the infant's head is in a neutral position by placing a towel under the infant's shoulders.

Step 5 Secure the torso first, and place padding to fill any voids.

Step 6 Secure the infant's head to the backboard.

© Jones & Bartlett Learning. Courtesy of MIEMSS.

► History Taking and Secondary Assessment

If the patient is in stable condition and does not meet the load-and-go criteria, obtain additional history as outlined in Table 43-26 and perform a more thorough physical exam. A full-body, back-to-front detailed physical exam should be performed on all trauma patients with significant MOI en route to the ED. For infants, this exam will include checking the anterior fontanel for bulging (a sign of increased ICP). Look for bruises, abrasions, or other subtle signs of injury that may have been missed during the primary survey. Be sure to revisit the primary survey during your reassessment on the way to the ED, because the patient's condition can change quickly.

► Fluid Management

Circulatory compromise is less common in children than in adults as the result of trauma; therefore, airway management and ventilatory support take priority over management of circulation. Tachycardia is usually the first sign of circulatory compromise in a child, but it can also be caused by agitation, being scared, or being restrained. Children are able to compensate for blood loss from any cause, including trauma, so hypotension is a late finding in pediatric trauma. Once a pediatric patient is hypotensive, the child is already in severe trouble. Thus, recognizing circulatory compromise and treating it early are even more important in the pediatric population than in the adult population.

Consider the following factors when you are establishing vascular access in the injured child:

- Large-bore IV catheters should be inserted into a large peripheral vein whenever possible.

Table 43-26	SAMPLE Components for Pediatric Trauma
Component	**Features**
Signs and symptoms	Time of event Nature of symptoms or pain Age-appropriate signs of distress
Allergies	Known medication reactions or other allergies
Medications	Timing and last dose of long-term medications Timing and dose of analgesics or antipyretics
Past medical history	Prior surgeries Immunizations, especially last tetanus
Last oral intake	Time of child's last food and drink, including bottle or breastfeeding
Events leading to the injury	Key events leading to the current incident Mechanism of injury Hazards at the scene

© Jones & Bartlett Learning.

In infants and young children, 20- or 22-gauge IV needles may be considered "large bore."

- Because definitive care can be provided only at the ED, never delay transport for the purpose of starting an IV line; this procedure should be performed en route.

- To maintain perfusion in a child, administer an initial bolus of 20 mL/kg using an isotonic crystalloid solution (ie, normal saline, lactated Ringer solution).
  - Frequently reassess the child's vital signs and provide additional IV fluid boluses of 20 mL/kg if no improvement is noted following the initial bolus. As much as 60 mL/kg may be needed during the resuscitation of a pediatric patient. If the patient weighs more than 50 kg, use adult resuscitation fluid volumes.
  - If the child's condition does not improve following two boluses of an isotonic crystalloid, blood loss is likely severe and the patient may need surgical intervention. Provide rapid transport with continuous monitoring of the child en route.

If the child is hypotensive and IV access cannot be obtained within 90 seconds, consider inserting an IO needle to gain access to the vascular system.

▶ Pain Management

Pain is often undertreated in young children. Whether or not a child can communicate with you verbally, do not overlook signs of pain in young trauma patients. Consider pain assessment as important as the vital signs, and use one of the many tools available to elicit the child's self-report of pain level. Tachycardia and inconsolability may be the only options a child has to express pain, and findings may be similar to those associated with early shock or plain old fear.

Pain treatment includes use of a calm, reassuring voice, distraction techniques, and, when appropriate, medications. Commonly used pain medications include morphine and fentanyl. Patients who are intubated should receive pain medication and sedation (such as diazepam and midazolam) if they are in hemodynamically stable condition. These medications, which may need to be redosed depending on transport time, can also be used in conjunction with narcotics for patients in stable condition. Side effects of narcotics and benzodiazepines include respiratory depression, hypoxemia, bradycardia, and hypotension.

You must weigh the risks and benefits when deciding to administer these medications. Children who are in shock and hemodynamically unstable condition are not good candidates for narcotics or sedatives; these medications may worsen their already precarious status. All children receiving such medications should be carefully monitored in terms of their pulse rate, respiratory rate, pulse oximetry, and blood pressure.

■ Pathophysiology, Assessment, and Management of Burns

The initial assessment and management of pediatric burn victims is similar to that of adults, with a few key differences. Notably, the higher ratio of skin surface to body mass of children makes them more susceptible to heat and fluid loss. Worrisome patterns of injury or suspicious circumstances should also raise concerns of child abuse.

▶ Assessment and Management of Burns

The assessment of scene safety is an important element in a burn call. Check for ongoing dangers such as fire, chemicals, or other hazardous materials. Your from-the-doorway assessment may identify signs of smoke inhalation, such as abnormal airway sounds and respiratory distress, or soot around the nose. Quickly move the patient and crew to a well-ventilated area.

An estimation of the percentage of BSA burned may affect your decision to start fluid resuscitation in the field and influence the transport destination. For adolescents, use the same rule of nines that you would use for adult burn victims; see Chapter 32, *Burns*. For younger children, this rule of nines is modified to account for a child's disproportionally larger head size. For infants, the head and trunk each account for 18% of BSA, the arms each count as 9%, and the legs each count as 13.5%. The size of a child's palm (not including fingers) represents about 1% total BSA; you can also use this rule of palm to assess the extent of the burn.

Special Populations

Use the rule of palm to estimate the percentage of BSA burned in a young child or infant: a child's palm is equal to 1% of total BSA.

Burns suggestive of abuse include those in which the mechanism or pattern observed does not match the history or the child's developmental capabilities. For example, a child who cannot stand independently is unlikely to pull a hot cup of coffee off a table. Splash burns—as from tipping over a pot of boiling water—should have an irregular configuration because the hot liquid runs down the child's body. Be suspicious if a burn has clear demarcation lines or appears on the buttocks.

Initial management begins with removal of burning clothing and support of the ABCs. If you observe signs of smoke inhalation, consider early intubation. Ensure you have a range of tubes available, because airway edema and sloughing may necessitate use of a smaller tube than that originally estimated.

All patients with moderate to severe burns should be provided with 100% supplemental oxygen, regardless of the presence or absence of signs of respiratory distress. Smoke inhalation may cause bronchospasm resulting in wheezing and mild respiratory distress. Consider using a bronchodilator such as albuterol or epinephrine IM.

If it is possible, insert an IV line and initiate fluid resuscitation during transport for patients with more than 5% of burned BSA. Start with 20 mL/kg of isotonic fluid, and reassess the need for additional boluses; large burns can lead to huge fluid shifts.

Clean burned areas minimally to avoid hypothermia, and cover them with clean, dry cloth. Avoid putting lotions or ointments on burned skin because they can trap heat and bacteria. Avoid heat loss by covering the burn and the patient as needed.

Analgesia is a crucial part of the early management of burns; these injuries can be incredibly painful. Assess and treat pain and anxiety as discussed previously. Carefully monitor any child given narcotics or benzodiazepines for signs of respiratory or hemodynamic compromise.

Once the patient's condition is stabilized, begin transport to an appropriate medical facility. Larger burns, full-thickness burns, and burns involving the face and neck are best treated at a regional burn center.

Children With Special Health Care Needs

Children with special health care needs include those with physical, developmental, and learning disabilities. The disabilities have a broad range of causes, including premature birth, traumatic brain injury, congenital anatomic anomalies, and acquired illnesses. Advances in technology and drugs have enabled an increasing number of children with disabilities to receive care in the community, leading to a corresponding increase in the number of EMS calls for this medically complex population.

▶ Technology-Assisted Children

Technology-assisted children constitute a subset of children with special health care needs who may require your assistance. Many children who use high-tech medical devices live at home. It is important to familiarize yourself with the various types of medical technology that you may encounter and have to troubleshoot.

Tracheostomy Tubes and Artificial Ventilators

Tracheostomy is a surgical procedure that involves creation of a **stoma**—in this case, a permanent connection between the skin of the throat and the trachea—through which a tracheostomy tube can be placed for long-term ventilatory

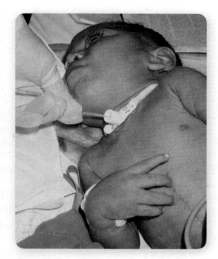

Figure 43-32 A tracheostomy is a surgical opening in the neck into the trachea, which creates an artificial airway.
Courtesy of Cindy Bissell.

needs **Figure 43-32**. A child might need a tracheostomy for a variety of reasons, including long-term ventilator support for chronic lung disease, inability to protect the airway because of neurologic impairment, or a congenital airway anomaly leading to airway obstruction. Caregivers have been trained in the use and care of their child's tracheostomy and are a source of valuable information. In general, they will have a spare tracheostomy tube available.

A child with a tracheostomy tube may breathe spontaneously with room air, if the function of the tube is simply to bypass mechanical upper airway obstruction. Alternatively, the child may be dependent on a home ventilator and supplemental oxygen if he or she has severe lung disease or problems with respiratory drive.

Although a tracheostomy tube is intended to provide a secure, permanent airway, problems can arise, as with any mechanical device. The most common problem is obstruction of the tracheostomy tube with secretions, resulting in respiratory distress or respiratory failure. The pediatric tracheostomy tube is often too small to have an inner cannula that can be removed if it becomes clogged with secretions (see Chapter 15, *Airway Management*). As a result, the tube is sometimes coughed out, and a well-meaning caregiver may cause trauma while trying to reinsert it.

If you are faced with a child with a tracheostomy tube and respiratory distress, start by assessing tube position and suctioning the tube. If the child is using a home ventilator, disconnect the circuit and provide bag-mask ventilation. If these measures do not improve the child's condition or if the child is cyanotic or in severe distress, you may need to remove and replace the tracheostomy tube, preferably using a tube of the same diameter and length. Confirmation of tube position is done in the same manner as for an ET tube.

In addition, a small ET tube can be inserted through the tracheostomy. A standard oral ET intubation can usually be performed. Make sure the ET tube comes to rest below

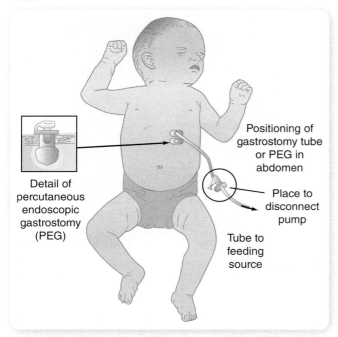

Figure 43-33 A gastrostomy tube passes through an opening in the skin directly into the stomach.
© Jones & Bartlett Learning.

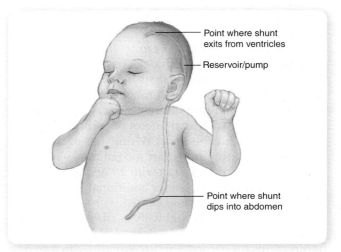

Figure 43-34 A ventricular shunt directs cerebrospinal fluid away from the ventricles in the brain to the abdomen to relieve pressure.
© Jones & Bartlett Learning.

the level of the tracheostomy, or cover the tracheostomy and ventilate the patient with a bag-mask device.

Gastrostomy Tubes

Gastrostomy tubes (G-tubes) are surgically placed directly into the patient's stomach through the skin **Figure 43-33**. They provide nutrition or medications directly into the stomach, bypassing the oropharynx and esophagus. Some children are unable to take food or medication by mouth and depend on a G-tube for all of their nutrition; for other patients, the tube is used to supplement intake and ensure adequate nutrition.

Problems such as obstruction, dislodgment, or leakage of a G-tube are not uncommon but rarely qualify as an emergency. Most of these calls can be managed by supportive care and transport. Urgent physician evaluation is needed if a G-tube has been pulled out because the opening on the abdominal wall tends to constrict quickly, making replacement difficult.

Central Venous Catheters

A **central venous catheter** may be inserted when a child needs long-term IV access for medications or nutrition. Such a device is placed surgically or by interventional radiologists into large central veins, such as the subclavian vein. Completely implanted central lines, with a port or reservoir accessible under the skin, may be left in place for months to years. For example, they are commonly placed in children with cancer who are undergoing long courses of chemotherapy. Partially implanted central lines have tubing external to the skin.

Complications associated with central venous catheters include infections, obstruction, and dislodged or broken catheters. Children with an infection of the central line may have redness, swelling, tenderness, or pus at the skin site of insertion; they may also have systemic signs of infection (such as fever) or signs of septic shock. Central line obstruction may be a medical emergency, depending on what is infusing through the line. If the child is not in urgent need of the infusion, simply assess the child and provide transport to the ED. Dislodged or broken catheters may result in leakage of fluid or blood. In such a case, use sterile technique to clamp off the broken line to minimize risk of infection or air embolus.

On rare occasions, you will be confronted with a child who has a functioning central line but requires emergency IV access for field treatment. Because these permanent lines carry a high risk for infection, look for peripheral access and avoid using the central line whenever possible.

Ventricular Shunts

Ventricular shunts are inserted to drain excessive fluid from the brain, thereby normalizing ICP. A neurosurgeon places the tube and connects it to a one-way, pressure-sensitive valve that runs from the enlarged ventricle subcutaneously into the abdominal peritoneal space **Figure 43-34**. When pressure builds up in the ventricle, the one-way valve opens, and CSF drains into the peritoneum, where it is reabsorbed.

A ventricular shunt obstruction occurs when the drainage of fluid from the brain through the shunt tubing becomes blocked—perhaps due to a break in the tubing, problems with the valve, or buildup of debris in the tubing. Without adequate fluid drainage, the CSF fluid continues to accumulate, resulting in hydrocephalus. A child with a shunt obstruction will show signs of increased ICP, which may range from subtle changes in behavior to impending brain herniation. Typical symptoms include headache, fatigue, vomiting, and even coma.

A ventricular shunt infection results from bacterial contamination during the surgery to place the shunt or from bacteria in the blood adhering to and infecting the hardware. Infections are encountered most frequently within months of shunt surgery. Children with shunt infections are generally extremely sick and have fever and signs of shunt obstruction.

Shunt obstructions and shunt infections are true medical emergencies. The patient should be transported to an appropriate treatment facility where neurosurgical evaluation is available. The child's condition can deteriorate rapidly, so maintain continuous cardiopulmonary monitoring during transport. Shunt obstruction may be recognized by signs and symptoms of increased ICP, including Cushing triad.

▶ Assessment and Management of Children With Special Health Care Needs

Follow the standard pediatric assessment sequence when you are approaching children with special health care needs. Ask questions of the parent or caregiver to establish the child's baseline level of neurologic function and baseline physiologic status. Meet every child at his or her unique developmental level. An otherwise healthy 10-year-old child with a perinatal brain injury may have the developmental skills of a toddler. Conversely, a 6-year-old child with severe cardiopulmonary compromise may be ventilator dependent and have an oxygen saturation percentage in the 80s but be cognitively intact.

Your treatment goal is to restore a child to his or her own physiologic baseline, which will require collaboration with caregivers to determine what is normal for the child and management strategies that have been successful in the past.

Special Populations

Caregivers will be key resources when you are managing a child with special health care needs. Draw on their expertise to assist you in assessing and managing the child.

▶ Transport of Children With Special Health Care Needs

Most children with special health care needs will have a medical home—that is, a hospital, clinic, or private practice where they receive their care. Transporting the child to a facility where the clinical team is familiar with the patient's history and needs will streamline the child's care. If this is not possible, take along any medical records available to assist the team at the receiving facility to sort out the potentially complex issues faced by the patient.

Take any assistive devices as well, including home ventilators and feeding pumps. Most important, take the parent or caregiver of the child! Children with special health care needs rely on their caregivers for much—if not all—of their caretaking needs, so it can be emotionally difficult for the child to be separated from the caregiver.

■ An Ounce of Prevention

Emergency care for children involves a team approach by health care professionals in the community and in the ED. Paramedics are a crucial part of the community responsible for caring for sick and injured children, but their role in prevention is not always highlighted, even though this is an area in which they can have a greater public health impact than possible by running a code or controlling an airway. To be an effective child safety advocate, you must be knowledgeable about local and national prevention programs, such as those conducted through the Emergency Medical Services for Children (EMSC) initiative.

▶ Emergency Medical Services for Children

EMSC is a federally funded program that was created in the 1990s in an effort to reduce child disability and death due to severe illness and injury.[41] EMSC works with local communities and hospitals to improve care for children in and out of the ED. It also works with existing EMS systems to improve the quality of children's emergency care, such as by creating pediatric-specific protocols and procedures. For example, EMSC has helped provide ambulances and EDs with child-appropriate equipment. The program supports training EMTs, paramedics, and other emergency care providers in pediatric-specific emergency care.

▶ Prevention of Injuries

Most injuries are not accidents, but rather are predictable and preventable events. When injury patterns are tracked and tabulated, this knowledge helps emergency care providers target potential areas for intervention and prevention. For example, childhood poisonings can be prevented by effective storage of medications and chemicals. Risk of toddler drowning and submersion in pools can be almost completely eliminated by installation of four-sided pool fencing. The risk of serious injury from a bike crash is lessened by use of a helmet. The morbidity and mortality from motor vehicle crashes is dramatically decreased by the appropriate use of child restraint devices.

As you care for children, you may be frustrated by the illnesses and injuries that you encounter, especially when they are preventable. Take this frustration as a call to action. Get involved in your community. Participate in existing prevention programs or start your own program. Numerous types of pediatric injury can be targeted Table 43-27 ; choose something that interests you, and take a leadership role.

Table 43-27	Examples of Common Injuries and Possible Prevention Strategies	
Injury	**Preventive Measures**
Vehicle trauma	Infant and child restraint seats Seat belts and airbags Pedestrian safety programs Motorcycle helmets
Cycling	Bicycle helmets Bicycle paths separate from vehicle traffic
Recreation	Appropriate safety padding and apparel Cyclist, skateboard, skater, ski, and snowboarder safety programs, helmets, and wrist guards Soft, energy-absorbent playground surfaces
Drowning and submersion	Four-sided locked pool enclosures Pool alarms Immediate adult supervision Caregiver CPR training Swimming lessons Pool and beach safety instruction Personal flotation devices
Poisoning and household injuries	Proper storage of chemicals and medications Child safety packaging
Burns	Proper maintenance and monitoring of electrical appliances and cords Fire and smoke detectors Proper placement of cookware on stove top
Other	Discouragement of infant walker use Gated stairways Babysitter first aid training Child care worker first aid training

Abbreviation: CPR, cardiopulmonary resuscitation

© Jones & Bartlett Learning.

YOU ⟩ are the Paramedic   SUMMARY

1. Using the Pediatric Assessment Triangle (PAT) as a guide, what is your general impression of the child?

By using the PAT, you should be able to determine that the child is sick and requires immediate attention. Further application will help you figure out what may be wrong with him. His initial appearance is abnormal. His work of breathing is normal because he has an adequate respiratory rate and tidal volume and there are no retractions or audible sounds. Circulation is definitely abnormal, with pale skin and some mottling seen on the extremities. The combination of an abnormal appearance, normal respiratory status, and abnormal circulation should guide you toward looking for a circulatory problem.

2. Which information would you like to get from the sister?

It is important to get as much information as possible to help you figure out what the problem might be and what the best approach for treatment is. Information that could provide you with clues would be how long the child has been sick, what he has been complaining of, when he last ate or drank, if he has been urinating regularly, and when he was last awake and talking with his sister.

3. What is the significance of the child's blood pressure?

The child's blood pressure is extremely low. The minimum acceptable systolic blood pressure for a 3-year-old child is 76 mm Hg, calculated as 70 + (2 × age in years). This blood pressure should grab your attention; you need to take action before the child deteriorates further!

4. What should your treatment consist of at this point?

You have the child on high-flow oxygen and identified the cardiac rhythm as sinus tachycardia. Because the child is in decompensated shock, the focus of your treatment should be fluid replacement and checking the glucose level to prevent missing hypoglycemia. Insertion of an IO needle is the ideal way to gain vascular access due to the child's poor hemodynamic status.

5. What are the potential complications of IO needle insertion?

Use caution when you are inserting the IO needle to help minimize the chance for complications. Complications such as compartment syndrome, failed infusion, injury to the growth plate, infection, and fracture have all occurred as a result of IO needle insertion.

6. How should you manage the blood glucose level?

This child is hypoglycemic! Administer glucose at a dose of 0.5 to 1 g/kg to bring the glucose level back to a normal level. Depending on the concentration you have available, you can give 5 to 10 mL/kg of 10% dextrose (D_{10}) solution, 4 to 8 mL/kg of 12.5% dextrose ($D_{12.5}$) solution, or 2 to 4 mL/kg of 25% dextrose (D_{25}) solution. Always remember to recheck the blood glucose level after you have administered IV glucose to ensure the child is not hyperglycemic.

7. What do you think was the cause of shock in this patient?

Hypovolemia and dehydration secondary to prolonged vomiting and diarrhea were the conditions that caused the development of shock in this child.

8. Which additional treatment should be given en route to the hospital?

Now that the child is beginning to respond to treatment and improve, it is your job to keep him warm and perform frequent reassessments.

EMS Patient Care Report (PCR)

Date: 07-06-18	**Incident No.:** 05839		**Nature of Call:** Altered mental status		**Location:** 3920 E. 152 Ave.
Dispatched: 1325	**En Route:** 1327	**At Scene:** 1333	**Transport:** 1350	**At Hospital:** 1359	**In Service:** 1431

Patient Information

Age: 3 **Sex:** M **Weight (in kg [lb]):** 14 kg (30 lb)	**Allergies:** None known **Medications:** None known **Past Medical History:** None known **Chief Complaint:** Altered mental status

Vital Signs

Time: 1338	**BP:** 68/42	**Pulse:** 180	**Respirations:** 22	**Spo₂:** 99%
Time: 1342	**BP:** 74/50	**Pulse:** 180	**Respirations:** 22	**Spo₂:** 99%
Time: 1348	**BP:** 80/54	**Pulse:** 160	**Respirations:** 20	**Spo₂:** 99%

YOU are the Paramedic   SUMMARY (continued)

EMS Treatment (circle all that apply)				
Oxygen @ __12__ L/min via (circle one): **NC** (**NRM**) **Bag-mask device**		**Assisted Ventilation**	**Airway Adjunct**	**CPR**
Defibrillation	**Bleeding Control**	**Bandaging**	**Splinting**	(**Other:** IO insertion)

Narrative
Dispatched to an apartment for a 3-year-old boy with altered mental status. Upon arrival, met at door by 14-year-old sister, who is the only other person on scene. Brought to living room, where the child is observed lying on the couch. Pt is unresponsive to painful stimuli. Skin is noted to be pale, cool, and dry, with mottled extremities. Unable to palpate radial pulse. Carotid pulse is weak. Capillary refill is 5 seconds. Pt placed on O_2 at 12 LPM via nonrebreathing mask. Cardiac monitor applied showing a sinus tachycardia. Lung sounds are clear and equal. Unable to locate peripheral vein for IV access. IO inserted into left tibia. Placement confirmation: needle stands upright on its own, small amount marrow aspirated, fluids flowing easily, and no signs of infiltration. 1,000-mL bag of normal saline hung and initial fluid bolus of 280 mL infused. Blood glucose 28 mg/dL. Administered 28 mL of D_{25}. Reassessment prior to transport shows improving mental status and circulation. Child is waking up as we leave. En route, pt becomes fully awake and alert and radial pulses can be palpated. Contacted Northwest Regional Medical Center, which advised to continue fluid administration. Pt remained stable during transport. Arrived at the ED and care was transferred to Jocelyn, RN. Rescue 20 returned to service at 1431.**End of report**

Prep Kit

▶ Ready for Review

- Children differ anatomically, physiologically, and emotionally from adults.
- Sick or injured children present unique challenges in evaluation and management. Their perceptions of their illness or injury, of their world, and of paramedics differ from the perceptions of adults.
- The majority of children you treat will be accompanied by at least one parent or caregiver. Thus, in many pediatric calls, you will be dealing with more than one patient—even if only the child is ill or injured.
- Serious illness or injury to a child is one of the most stressful situations caregivers can face.

- An assessment tool called the Pediatric Assessment Triangle (PAT) has been developed to help EMS providers form a from-the-doorway general impression of pediatric patients.
- Respiratory problems are among the medical emergencies that you will most frequently encounter in children. Pediatric patients with a respiratory chief complaint will span the spectrum from mildly ill to near death.
- Hypoxia can lead to respiratory failure and arrest, and it precedes the majority of pediatric cardiopulmonary arrests.
- The types of shock that you may encounter are the same in adults and children. Because children typically have strong cardiovascular systems, they are able to compensate for inadequate perfusion more efficiently than adults are.

Prep Kit *(continued)*

- Cardiovascular emergencies are relatively rare in children. When such problems arise, they are often related to volume or infection rather than to a primary cardiac cause, unless the child has congenital heart disease.
- Through the PAT and primary survey, you can quickly identify a cardiovascular emergency, understand the likely pathologic cause, and institute potentially lifesaving treatment.
- Children are particularly difficult to assess neurologically because they can often be uncooperative during the assessment.
- The ingestion of foreign bodies is a common cause of gastrointestinal complaints in pediatrics.
- Children and young adults are much more commonly diagnosed with type 1 diabetes compared to adults; as a result of this endocrine condition, they are susceptible to diabetic ketoacidosis, a life-threatening event.
- Hematologic and immunologic diseases are common in pediatric patients. Because of their altered immunity, many of these children have severe presentations of illness and even shock when EMS is called.
- Toxic exposures account for a significant number of pediatric emergencies; they can take the form of ingestion, inhalation, injection, or application of a substance.
- Behavioral and psychiatric problems relating to pediatric patients may range from out-of-control behavior to a suicide attempt.
- Fever itself is not dangerous, but rather a sign of an underlying process. Most pediatric fevers are caused by viral infections that are often mild and self-limiting. In other cases, fever can be a symptom of a more serious bacterial infection.
- Child abuse or maltreatment comes in many forms: physical abuse, sexual abuse, emotional abuse, and child neglect.
- The sudden death of an apparently healthy baby is devastating to families and the EMS crew responding to the call.
- A brief resolved unexplained event (BRUE; formerly called an apparent life-threatening event [ALTE]) is an episode during which an infant becomes pale or cyanotic; chokes, gags, or has an apneic spell; or loses muscle tone.
- Pediatric trauma is the leading cause of death among children older than 1 year.
  - Motor vehicle crashes cause the most deaths in this age group, followed by falls and submersions.

- Among adolescents, homicide and suicide are major causes of death.
- The initial assessment and management of pediatric burn victims is similar to that of adults, with a few key differences.
  - The higher ratio of skin surface to body mass in children makes them more susceptible to heat and fluid loss.
  - Worrisome patterns of injury or suspicious circumstances should raise concerns of child abuse.
- Children with special health care needs include children with physical, developmental, and learning disabilities.
  - These disabilities have a broad range of causes, including premature birth, traumatic brain injury, congenital anatomic anomalies, and acquired illnesses.
  - Advances in technology and drugs have enabled an increasing number of children with disabilities to receive care in the community, leading to a corresponding increase in the number of EMS calls for this medically complex population.
- Emergency care for children involves a team approach by health care professionals in the community and in the hospital.

▶ Vital Vocabulary

abandonment A type of child maltreatment in which a parent or guardian physically leaves a child without regard to the child's health, safety, or welfare.

absence seizures A type of seizure characterized by a brief lapse of attention during which the patient may stare and not respond; formerly known as a petit mal seizure.

acrocyanosis Cyanosis of the extremities.

bacterial tracheitis An acute bacterial infection of the subglottic area of the upper airway that is complicated by copious thick, pus-filled secretions.

blow-by technique A method of delivering oxygen by holding a face mask or similar device near an infant's or a child's face; used when a nonrebreathing mask is not tolerated.

brief resolved unexplained event (BRUE) An unexpected sudden episode of color change, tone change, or apnea that requires mouth-to-mouth resuscitation or vigorous stimulation; formerly known as apparent life-threatening event (ALTE).

bronchiolitis A condition seen in children younger than 2 years, characterized by dyspnea and wheezing.

Prep Kit (continued)

bronchopulmonary dysplasia A spectrum of lung conditions found in premature neonates who require long periods of high-concentration oxygen and ventilator support, ranging from mild reactive airway to debilitating chronic lung disease.

central venous catheter A catheter inserted into the vena cava to permit intermittent or continuous monitoring of central venous pressure and to facilitate obtaining blood samples for chemical analysis.

child abuse Any improper or excessive action that injures or otherwise harms a child or infant; includes physical abuse, sexual abuse, neglect, and emotional abuse.

child protective services (CPS) The community-based legal organization responsible for protection, rehabilitation, and prevention of child maltreatment and neglect. This agency has the legal authority to temporarily remove children from homes if there is reason to believe they are at risk for injury or neglect and to secure foster placement.

complex febrile seizures An unusual form of seizure that occurs in association with a rapid increase in body temperature.

complex partial seizures A type of seizure characterized by alteration of consciousness with or without complex focal motor activity.

congenital adrenal hyperplasia (CAH) Inadequate production of cortisol and aldosterone by the adrenal gland.

croup A common disease of childhood due to upper airway obstruction and characterized by stridor, hoarseness, and a barking cough.

cystic fibrosis (CF) A genetic disease that primarily affects the respiratory and digestive systems.

dilated cardiomyopathy A condition in which the heart becomes weakened and enlarged, making it less efficient and causing a negative impact to the pulmonary, hepatic, and other systems.

epiglottitis Inflammation of the epiglottis.

gastrostomy tube (G-tube) A tube that is surgically placed directly into the patient's stomach through the skin to provide nutrition or medications.

generalized seizures A type of seizure characterized by manifestations that indicate involvement of both cerebral hemispheres.

grunting A short, low-pitched sound at the end of exhalation, present in children with moderate to severe hypoxia. It reflects poor gas exchange because of fluid in the lower airways and air sacs.

hemophilia A bleeding disorder that is primarily hereditary, in which clotting does not occur or occurs insufficiently.

hydrocephalus The increased accumulation of cerebrospinal fluid within the ventricles of the brain.

hypertrophic cardiomyopathy A condition in which the heart muscle is unusually thick, forcing the heart to pump harder to get blood to leave.

hypopituitarism A condition in which the pituitary gland does not produce normal amounts of some or all of its hormones. It can be congenital; occur secondary to tumors, infection, or stroke; or develop after trauma or radiation therapy.

inborn errors of metabolism (IEMs) A group of congenital conditions that cause either accumulation of toxins or disorders of energy metabolism in the neonate. These conditions are characterized by an infant's failure to thrive and by vague signs such as poor feeding.

intussusception Telescoping of the intestines into themselves.

malrotation with volvulus A condition that occurs when there is a twisting of the bowel around its mesenteric attachment to the abdominal wall.

Meckel diverticulum One of the most common congenital malformations of the small intestines, which presents with painless rectal bleeding.

meningitis Inflammation of the meningeal coverings of the brain and spinal cord; usually caused by a virus or bacterium. The viral type is less severe than the bacterial type; the bacterial type can result in brain damage, hearing loss, learning disability, or death.

mottling A condition of abnormal skin circulation, caused by vasoconstriction or inadequate perfusion.

myocarditis Inflammation of the myocardium.

neglect Refusal or failure on the part of the caregiver to provide life necessities. Compare to emotional abuse, which involves a lack of emotional support by the caregiver.

nuchal rigidity A stiff or painful neck; commonly associated with meningitis.

ossification center An area where cartilage is transformed through calcification into a new area of bone.

panhypopituitarism The inadequate production or absence of the pituitary hormones, including adrenocorticotropic hormone, cortisol, thyroxine, luteinizing hormone, follicle-stimulating hormone, estrogen, testosterone, growth hormone, and antidiuretic hormone.

Prep Kit (continued)

partial seizures A type of seizure that involves only one part of the brain.

Pediatric Assessment Triangle (PAT) An assessment tool that allows rapid formation of a general impression of the type and level of illness or injury in an infant or child without touching him or her; consists of assessing appearance, work of breathing, and circulation to the skin.

pertussis An acute infectious disease characterized by a catarrhal stage, followed by a paroxysmal cough that ends in a whooping inspiration; also called whooping cough.

petechial Characterized by small purple, nonblanching spots on the skin.

pneumonia An inflammation of the lungs caused by bacterial, viral, or fungal infections or infections with other microorganisms.

purpuric Pertaining to bruising of the skin.

pyloric stenosis Hypertrophy (enlargement) of the pyloric sphincter of the stomach; ultimately leads to intestinal obstruction, often in infants.

respiratory arrest The absence of respirations with detectable cardiac activity.

respiratory distress A clinical state characterized by increased respiratory rate, effort, and work of breathing.

respiratory failure A clinical state of inadequate oxygenation, ventilation, or both.

respiratory syncytial virus (RSV) A virus that affects the upper and lower respiratory tracts. Disease—namely, pneumonia and bronchiolitis—is more prevalent in the lower respiratory tract.

retractions A sign of respiratory distress characterized by skin pulling inward between and around the ribs and clavicles during inhalation.

sepsis A pathologic state, usually in a febrile patient, resulting from the presence of invading microorganisms or their poisonous products in the bloodstream.

sickle cell disease A disease that causes red blood cells to be misshapen, resulting in a poor oxygen-carrying capability and potentially resulting in lodging of the red blood cells in blood vessels or the spleen.

simple febrile seizures A brief, self-limited, generalized seizure in a previously healthy child between ages 6 months and 6 years that is associated with the onset of or sudden increase in fever.

simple partial seizures A type of seizure that involves focal motor jerking or sensory abnormality in a patient who remains conscious.

slipped capital femoral epiphysis (SCFE) A dislocation of the epiphyseal end of the femur, usually found in children and adolescents.

sniffing position An upright position in which the patient's head and chin are thrust slightly forward to keep the airway open; the patient appears to be sniffing when in this position.

status epilepticus A seizure that lasts longer than 4 to 5 minutes or consecutive seizures without a return to consciousness between seizures.

stoma In the context of the airway, the resultant orifice of a tracheostomy that connects the trachea to the outside air; located in the midline of the anterior part of the neck.

subglottic space The narrowest part of the pediatric airway.

sudden infant death syndrome (SIDS) The sudden death of an infant younger than 1 year that cannot be explained after a thorough investigation is conducted, including a complete autopsy, examination of the death scene, and a review of the clinical history.

synchronized cardioversion The use of synchronized direct current (DC) electric shock to convert tachydysrhythmias (such as atrial fibrillation) to normal sinus rhythm.

tenting A sign of dehydration in which the skin slowly retracts after being pinched and pulled away slightly from the body.

thrombocytopenia A reduction in the number of platelets in the blood.

thrombosis The development of a blood clot.

tonic-clonic seizures A type of seizure that features rhythmic back-and-forth motion of an extremity and body stiffness.

tripoding An abnormal position that a person assumes to keep the airway open; involves leaning forward onto two arms stretched forward.

ventricular shunt A surgically inserted tube draining cerebrospinal fluid from the cerebral ventricles into a body cavity, often the peritoneal cavity or the right atrium.

von Willebrand disease A bleeding disorder in which the patient is missing the von Willebrand factor (a protein essential for platelet adhesion), preventing the blood from clotting well.

Prep Kit (continued)

▶ References

1. Fleming S, Gill P, Jones C, et al. Validity and reliability of measurement of capillary refill time in children: a systematic review. *Arch Dis Child*. 2015;100(3):239-249.

2. National Association of State EMS Officials. *National Model EMS Clinical Guidelines*. V.11.14. Croup (p. 108). https://nasemso.org/Projects /ModelEMSClinicalGuidelines/documents /National-Model-EMS-Clinical-Guidelines -23Oct2014.pdf. Accessed April 17, 2017.

3. Atkins DL, Berger S, Duff JP, et al. Part 11: pediatric basic life support and cardiopulmonary resuscitation quality: 2015 American Heart Association Guidelines Update for Cardiopulmonary Resuscitation and Emergency Cardiovascular Care. *Circulation*. 2015;132(suppl 2):S519-S525.

4. Hendry PL. The pediatric airway in health and disease. In: Fuchs S, Yamamoto L, eds. *APLS: The Pediatric Emergency Medicine Resource*. 5th ed. Burlington, MA: Jones & Bartlett Learning; 2012:48-95.

5. US Food and Drug Administration. EpiPen and EpiPen Jr. (epinephrine injection) auto-injector. https://www.fda.gov/safety/medwatch /safetyinformation/ucm505913.htm. Published May 2016. Accessed April 17, 2017.

6. CPR to Go Training Center Administration. Update to instructions for use of epinephrine autoinjectors. CPR to Go Training Center website. http://www .cprtogo.org/index.php/2017/02/12/update-to -instructions-for-use-of-epinephrine-autoinjectors/. Published February 12, 2017. Accessed April 17, 2017.

7. Cukor J, Manno M. Pediatric respiratory emergencies: upper airway obstruction and infections. In: Marx JA, Hockberger RS, Walls RM, eds. *Rosen's Emergency Medicine: Concepts and Clinical Practice*. 8th ed. Philadelphia, PA: Saunders; 2014:2016-2116.

8. Choi J, Lee GL. Common pediatric respiratory emergencies. *Emerg Med Clin North Am*. 2012;30(2):529-563.

9. Global Initiative for Asthma. *Global Strategy for Asthma Management and Prevention, 2017*. http://ginasthma.org/2017-gina-report-global -strategy-for-asthma-management-and-prevention/. Updated 2017. Accessed April 17, 2017.

10. National Association of State EMS Officials. *National Model EMS Clinical Guidelines*. V.11.14. Bronchospasm (p. 133). https://nasemso.org /Projects/ModelEMSClinicalGuidelines/documents /National-Model-EMS-Clinical-Guidelines -23Oct2014.pdf. Accessed April 17, 2017.

11. National Association of State EMS Officials. *National Model EMS Clinical Guidelines*. V.11.14. Bronchiolitis (p. 103). https://nasemso.org/Projects /ModelEMSClinicalGuidelines/documents /National-Model-EMS-Clinical-Guidelines -23Oct2014.pdf. Accessed April 17, 2017.

12. American Heart Association. Equipment and procedures for management of respiratory emergencies. In: Chameides L, Samson RA, Schexnayder SM, Hazinski MF, eds. *Pediatric Emergency Assessment, Recognition, and Stabilization Provider Manual*. Dallas, TX: American Heart Association; 2012:51-72.

13. de Caen AR, Berg MD, Chameides L, et al. Web-based integrated guidelines for cardiopulmonary resuscitation and emergency cardiovascular care— part 12: pediatric advanced life support. In: *2015 American Heart Association Guidelines for CPR and ECC*. American Heart Association website. https:// eccguidelines.heart.org/index.php/circulation/cpr -ecc-guidelines-2/. Published October 2015. Accessed April 17, 2017.

14. Berg MD, Nadkarni VM, Gausche-Hill M, Kaji AH, Berg RA. Pediatric resuscitation. In: Marx JA, Hockberger RS, Walls RM, eds. *Rosen's Emergency Medicine: Concepts and Clinical Practice*. 7th ed. Philadelphia, PA: Saunders; 2010:64-76.

15. Perkin RM, de Caen AR, Berg MD, Schexnayder SM, Hazinski MF. Shock, cardiac arrest, and resuscitation. In: Hazinski MF, ed. *Nursing Care of the Critically Ill Child*. 3rd ed. St. Louis, MO: Mosby; 2013:101-154.

16. National Association of State EMS Officials. *National Model EMS Clinical Guidelines*. V.11.14. Shock (p. 72). https://nasemso.org/Projects /ModelEMSClinicalGuidelines/documents /National-Model-EMS-Clinical-Guidelines -23Oct2014.pdf. Accessed April 17, 2017.

17. Doniger SJ, Sharieff GQ. Pediatric dysrhythmias. *Pediatr Clin North Am*. 2006;53(1):85-105.

18. Topjian AA, Berg RA, Nadkarni VM. Advances in recognition, resuscitation, and stabilization of the critically ill child. *Pediatr Clin North Am*. 2013;60(3):605-620.

19. Link MS. Commotio cordis: ventricular fibrillation triggered by chest impact-induced abnormalities in repolarization. *Circulation: Arrhythmia Electrophysiol*. 2012;5(2):425-432.

20. Douglas RJ. Sudden cardiac death following blunt chest trauma: commotio cordis. *World J Emerg Med*. 2011;2(3):234-236.

21. Maron BJ, Haas TS, Ahluwalia A, Garberich RF, Estes NA, Link MS. Increasing survival rate from commotio cordis. *Heart Rhythm*. 2013;10(2):219-223.

22. Schroeder ML, Delaney A, Baker A. The child with cardiovascular dysfunction. In: Hockenberry MJ, Wilson D, eds. *Wong's Nursing Care of Infants and Children*. 10th ed. St. Louis, MO: Mosby; 2015:1251-1321.

Prep Kit *(continued)*

23. Schoen FJ, Mitchell RN. The heart. In: Kumar V, Abbas AK, Aster JC, eds. *Robbins and Cotran Pathologic Basis of Disease*. 9th ed. Philadelphia, PA: Saunders; 2015:523-578.

24. Holmes GL. Febrile seizures. Epilepsy Foundation website. http://www.epilepsy.com/learn/types -seizures/febrile-seizures. Published September 2013. Accessed April 17, 2017.

25. Sencer A, Aras Y, Akcakaya MO, Goker B, Kiris T, Canbolat AT. Posterior fossa epidural hematomas in children: clinical experience with 40 cases. *J Neurosurg Pediatr.* 2012;9(2):139-143.

26. Rodgers CC. The child with cerebral dysfunction. In: Hockenberry MJ, Wilson D, eds. *Wong's Nursing Care of Infants and Children*. 10th ed. St. Louis, MO: Mosby; 2015:1425-1492.

27. Pepper VK, Stanfill AB, Pearl RH. Diagnosis and management of pediatric appendicitis, intussusceptions, and Meckel diverticulum. *Surg Clin North Am.* 2012;92(3):505-526.

28. National Association of State EMS Officials. *National Model EMS Clinical Guidelines*. V.11.14. Hypoglycemia/hyperglycemia (p. 57). https:// nasemso.org/Projects/ModelEMSClinicalGuidelines /documents/National-Model-EMS-Clinical -Guidelines-23Oct2014.pdf. Accessed April 17, 2017.

29. Bryant R. The child with hematologic or immunologic dysfunction. In: Hockenberry MJ, Wilson D, eds. *Wong's Nursing Care of Infants and Children*. 10th ed. St. Louis, MO: Mosby; 2015:1322-1378.

30. Allen JD, Casavant MJ, Spiller HA, Chounthirath T, Hodges NL, Smith GA. Prescription opioid exposures among children and adolescents in the United States: 2000-2015. *Pediatrics.* AAP News and Journals Gateway website. http://pediatrics .aappublications.org/content/early/2017/03/16 /peds.2016-3382. Published March 2017. Accessed April 17, 2017.

31. American Academy of Pediatrics. Ipecac. https:// www.aap.org/en-us/about-the-aap/aap-press-room /aap-press-room-media-center/Pages/Ipecac.aspx. Accessed April 17, 2017.

32. National Association of State EMS Officials. *National Model EMS Clinical Guidelines*. V.11.14. Poisoning/overdose universal care (p. 175). https:// nasemso.org/Projects/ModelEMSClinicalGuidelines /documents/National-Model-EMS-Clinical -Guidelines-23Oct2014.pdf. Accessed April 17, 2017.

33. National Institute of Mental Health. Any disorder among children. https://www.nimh.nih.gov/health /statistics/prevalence/any-disorder-among-children .shtml. Accessed April 17, 2017.

34. Centers for Disease Control and Prevention. Leading causes of death reports, national and regional, 1999–2015. WISQARS. http://webappa.cdc.gov /sasweb/ncipc/leadcaus10_us.html. Updated June 24, 2015. Accessed April 17, 2017.

35. Child abuse statistics and facts. Child Help website. https://www.childhelp.org/child-abuse-statistics/. Accessed April 17, 2017.

36. Pierce MC, Kaczor K, Aldridge S, et al. Bruising characteristics discriminating physical child abuse from accidental trauma. *Pediatrics.* 2010;125:67-74.

37. Galanti G. *Caring for Patients From Different Cultures*. 4th ed. Philadelphia, PA: University of Pennsylvania Press; 2008:197-200.

38. Centers for Disease Control and Prevention. About SUID and SIDS. https://www.cdc.gov/sids /aboutsuidandsids.htm. Updated February 1, 2017. Accessed April 17, 2017.

39. Tieder JS, Bonkowsky JL, Etzel RA, et al; Subcommittee on Apparent Life Threatening Events. Brief resolved unexplained events (formerly apparent life-threatening events) and evaluation of lower-risk infants. *Pediatrics.* 2016;137(5):pii.

40. National Association of State EMS Officials. *National Model EMS Clinical Guidelines*. V.11.14. Head injury (p. 163). https://nasemso.org/Projects /ModelEMSClinicalGuidelines/documents /National-Model-EMS-Clinical-Guidelines -23Oct2014.pdf. Accessed April 17, 2017.

41. Emergency Medical Services for Children. About. https://emscimprovement.center/about/. Accessed April 17, 2017.

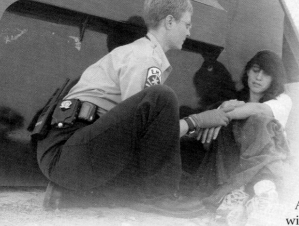

Assessment in Action

You and your partner are dispatched to an elementary school for a 7-year-old child experiencing a seizure. On arrival, you are met by the school principal, who escorts you to the playground. As you enter the area, you observe a young girl next to the swings exhibiting tonic-clonic movement. A teacher approaches and tells you the girl was playing tag with her friends when she stated she "felt funny" and collapsed. According to the teacher, the girl has a history of seizures and has been actively seizing for approximately 15 minutes.

1. Which of the following types of seizures is your patient most likely having?

   A. Absence
   B. Febrile
   C. Generalized
   D. Partial

2. Which type of seizure would be caused by a body temperature increasing rapidly to 101.8°F (38.8°C)?

   A. Generalized
   B. Partial
   C. Simple partial
   D. Febrile

3. Based on the reported length of this seizure active (approximately 15 minutes), what classification would you give this seizure?

   A. Complex
   B. Generalized
   C. Status epilepticus
   D. Partial

4. Which of the following medications may be used as first-line anticonvulsant therapy?

   A. Phenytoin
   B. Morphine
   C. Phenobarbital
   D. Lorazepam

5. What is a major adverse effect associated with the administration of benzodiazepines?

   A. Hypertension
   B. Tachycardia
   C. Respiratory depression
   D. Vomiting

6. If you have chosen to give the anticonvulsant intranasally, what is the maximum amount of volume you can give per nostril?

   A. 1.0 mL
   B. 1.5 mL
   C. 2.0 mL
   D. 2.5 mL

7. Bradycardia that causes severe cardiopulmonary compromise in an infant or child is initially treated with:

   A. administration of atropine.
   B. transcutaneous pacing.
   C. synchronized cardioversion.
   D. effective oxygenation and ventilation.

8. A 9-month-old infant has a history of poor feeding. You note that the infant appears pale and limp in her mother's arms. Intercostal retractions are present. She does not respond when her mother speaks her name. From the information provided, complete the following documentation regarding the PAT.

   Appearance: _____
   Breathing: _____
   Circulation: _____

9. Why are pediatric patients able to maintain their blood pressure longer than adults are when they are in a state of shock?

10. Even though the 7-year-old child in the preceding scenario has a history of seizures, what other clinical exam should you implement to rule out seizure cause or side effect of the seizure activity?

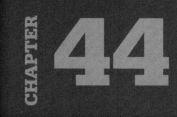

CHAPTER 44

Geriatric Emergencies

National EMS Education Standard Competencies

Special Patient Populations

Integrates assessment findings with principles of pathophysiology and knowledge of psychosocial needs to formulate a field impression and implement a comprehensive treatment/disposition plan for patients with special needs.

Geriatrics

Impact of age-related changes on assessment and care (pp 2214-2219)

Changes associated with aging, psychosocial aspects of aging, and age-related assessment and treatment modifications for the major or common geriatric diseases and/or emergencies
> Cardiovascular diseases (pp 2209-2210, 2221-2223)
> Respiratory diseases (pp 2208-2209, 2219-2221)
> Neurologic diseases (pp 2210-2211, 2223-2226)
> Endocrine diseases (pp 2212, 2230-2231)
> Alzheimer disease (pp 2225-2226)
> Dementia (p 2225)
> Fluid resuscitation in older adults (pp 2212, 2229, 2231, 2235, 2240)

Normal and abnormal changes associated with aging, pharmacokinetic changes, psychosocial and economic aspects of aging, polypharmacy, and age-related assessment and treatment modifications for the major or common geriatric diseases and/or emergencies
> Cardiovascular diseases (pp 2209-2210, 2221-2223)
> Respiratory diseases (pp 2208-2209, 2219-2221)
> Neurologic diseases (pp 2210-2211, 2223-2226)
> Endocrine diseases (pp 2212, 2230-2231)
> Alzheimer disease (pp 2225-2226)
> Dementia (p 2225)
  • Acute confusional state (pp 2223-2225)
> Fluid resuscitation in older adults (pp 2212, 2229, 2231, 2235, 2240)
> Herpes zoster (p 2235)
> Inflammatory arthritis (p 2236)

Patients With Special Challenges

> Recognizing and reporting abuse and neglect (pp 2240-2241 and see Chapter 43, *Pediatric Emergencies*)

Health care implications of
> Abuse (pp 2240-2241 and see Chapter 43, *Pediatric Emergencies*)
> Neglect (pp 2240-2241 and see Chapter 43, *Pediatric Emergencies*)
> Homelessness (see Chapter 45, *Patients With Special Challenges*)
> Poverty (see Chapter 45, *Patients With Special Challenges*)
> Bariatrics (see Chapter 45, *Patients With Special Challenges*)
> Technology dependent (see Chapter 45, *Patients With Special Challenges*)
> Hospice/terminally ill (see Chapter 45, *Patients With Special Challenges*)
> Tracheostomy care/dysfunction (see Chapter 45, *Patients With Special Challenges*)
> Home care (see Chapter 45, *Patients With Special Challenges*)
> Sensory deficit/loss (see Chapter 45, *Patients With Special Challenges*)
> Developmental disability (see Chapter 45, *Patients With Special Challenges*)

Trauma

Integrates assessment findings with principles of epidemiology and pathophysiology to formulate a field impression to implement a comprehensive treatment/disposition plan for an acutely injured patient.

Special Considerations in Trauma

Recognition and management of trauma in the
> Pregnant patient (see Chapter 41, *Obstetrics*)
> Pediatric patient (see Chapter 43, *Pediatric Emergencies*)
> Geriatric patient (pp 2236-2240)

Pathophysiology, assessment, and management of trauma in the
> Pregnant patient (see Chapter 41, *Obstetrics*)
> Pediatric patient (see Chapter 43, *Pediatric Emergencies*)

> Geriatric patient (pp 2236-2240)
> Cognitively impaired patient (see Chapter 45, *Patients With Special Challenges*)

Knowledge Objectives

1. Describe the old-age dependency ratio. (p 2207)
2. Describe the phenomenon known as "the graying of America." (p 2207)
3. Discuss the social, economic, and psychosocial factors affecting the older population. (pp 2207-2208)
4. Identify the physiologic changes that occur in the various body systems as people age. (pp 2208-2214)
5. Identify special considerations when performing patient assessment of a geriatric patient. (pp 2214-2219)
6. Describe the steps in the primary survey for providing emergency care to a geriatric patient, including the elements of the GEMS diamond. (pp 2215-2217)
7. Describe the pathophysiology of geriatric respiratory conditions, the signs and symptoms, and the emergency medical care strategies used in the management of each condition. (pp 2219-2221)
8. Describe the pathophysiology of geriatric cardiovascular conditions, the signs and symptoms, and the emergency medical care strategies used in the management of each condition. (pp 2221-2223)
9. Describe the pathophysiology of geriatric nervous system conditions, the signs and symptoms, and the emergency medical care strategies used in the management of each condition. (pp 2223-2226)
10. Describe the pathophysiology of geriatric gastrointestinal conditions, the signs and symptoms, and the emergency medical care strategies used in the management of each condition. (pp 2226-2228)
11. Describe the pathophysiology of geriatric renal conditions, the signs and symptoms, and the emergency medical care strategies used in the management of each condition. (pp 2228-2230)
12. Describe the pathophysiology of geriatric endocrine conditions, the signs and symptoms,

and the emergency medical care strategies used in the management of each condition. (pp 2230-2231)
13. Describe the pathophysiology of sepsis, the signs and symptoms, and the emergency medical care strategies used in the management of sepsis. (p 2232)
14. Describe the pathophysiology of geriatric toxicology, the signs and symptoms, and the emergency medical care strategies used in the management of adverse drug reactions. (pp 2232-2233)
15. Discuss polypharmacy and medication noncompliance and their effects on patient assessment and management. (p 2232)
16. Describe the pathophysiology of geriatric depression, the signs and symptoms, and the emergency medical care strategies used in the management of depression. (pp 2233-2234)
17. Describe the pathophysiology of geriatric integumentary conditions, the signs and symptoms, and the emergency medical care strategies used in the management of each condition. (p 2235)
18. Describe the pathophysiology of geriatric musculoskeletal conditions, the signs and symptoms, and the emergency medical care strategies used in the management of each condition. (pp 2235-2236)
19. Describe special considerations for a geriatric patient who has experienced trauma, including performing the patient assessment process on a geriatric patient with a traumatic injury. (pp 2236-2240)
20. Discuss elder abuse and neglect, and their implications for assessment and management of the geriatric patient. (pp 2240-2241)
21. Describe the role of hospice as part of end-of-life care. (p 2241)

Skills Objectives

There are no skills objectives for this chapter.

YOU are the Paramedic PART 1

At 0630 hours, your unit is dispatched to 127 Henderson Avenue for an 84-year-old man with altered mental status. The patient's daughter is on scene and called 9-1-1 when her father did not answer the door.

1. What might be the nature of illness you suspect based on the information provided by dispatch?
2. When responding to a geriatric patient, what makes the assessment different from a nongeriatric assessment?

■ Introduction

Geriatrics is the assessment and treatment of disease and/or injury in someone 65 years or older. According to the 2015 US Census estimates, there are more than 44.6 million Americans who are age 65 years and older —a 13.2% increase from the 2010 Census.[1] While people of all ages are now receiving more of their care outside of hospitals, older adults constitute an ever-increasing proportion of patients in the health care system, particularly in the emergency care sector. The older adult population accounts for 15% of all emergency department (ED) visits.[2] The geriatric population also has more contacts with doctors than do people younger than 65 years. As a result, as the number of older Americans increases, the need for physician services will also likely increase.

The **old-age dependency ratio** is used to determine the number of older people in a society as compared with the number of potential workers who are theoretically capable of providing resources to sustain the whole population. This ratio is the number of older people (65 years and older) for every 100 adults (potential caregivers) between the ages 18 and 64 years. It is used by social scientists and researchers to compare the differences in age structure between time periods in a single society or to compare age structures between two different societies. It can be used as an indicator of the aging of a population as a whole.

Many social scientists refer to the phenomenon known as "the graying of America"—a term used to describe the increasing number of older Americans. In 1990, there were 20 older people for every 100 working-age people in the United States. By 2025, however, it is projected that there will be 32 older people for every 100 working-age people.[3] In other words, the supply of people capable of providing resources for the older population is not keeping pace with the growth of the older population. The need for caregivers will certainly increase, and society may have difficulty keeping up with the demand for services as the population continues to age. As the older population grows, emergency medical services (EMS) personnel will be required to offer services that are cost-effective and efficient.

Most of your geriatric patients will not reside in nursing homes. Although nursing home admissions are increasing because of the larger number of older adults in the United States, a countertrend is for older people to maintain independent lives. Many older adults continue to live at home with support from a spouse or family member and a visiting nurse; others live in a more dependent-care environment such as a senior center facility. Still others may reside in an assisted-living facility or a total-care nursing home, which is also known as a skilled nursing facility.

Determining how and where older adults will spend their retirement years is a difficult and complex process involving numerous social and economic issues, such as the person's marital status, financial resources, religious beliefs, ethnicity, gender, and general health. Because such

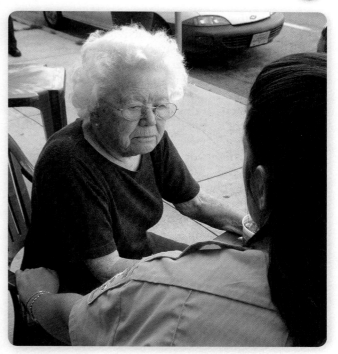

Figure 44-1 EMS professionals should be familiar with the resources available in their community for geriatric care so they can present the options to their patients.
© Jones & Bartlett Learning. Courtesy of MIEMSS.

decisions may place a burden on grown children and other family members, their wishes must be considered by health care providers when making care decisions. Older adults and their families may also seek advice from medical social workers, professional care managers, discharge planners at health care facilities, and a large number of private and public resources. The range of services available includes delivered meals, personal care, housekeeping, adult day care, transportation, caregiver support, respite care, and emergency response systems, including EMS and lifelines **Figure 44-1**.

One factor that frequently affects decisions regarding living conditions and services used by older adults is their financial situation. You cannot assume that all retired people live comfortably. Older adults who report concerns about having enough food to eat each day generally have poorer nutrition, poorer self-reported health, and more limitations in their abilities to care for themselves. Not surprisingly, older people who live in poverty are less likely to feel confident that they will have enough food. They may also have difficulty paying for medical expenses and housing costs and may attempt to save money by skipping doses of medication or using a kerosene heater rather than the central heating unit; these actions may pose serious risks to their health.

Psychosocial factors may influence successful aging. For example, at retirement, some people may no longer feel useful or productive in society and may experience diminished self-esteem. They may also feel frustrated at their inability to do things as easily as they once did, or they may mourn the loss of activities in which they can no longer participate because of complications from medical conditions. Conversely, some people experience feelings of freedom on retirement and accomplishment when looking back on their lives. The psychologist Erik Erikson refers to this stage of development as the crisis of integrity versus despair; at this point in life, a person can experience either integrity because of his or her accomplishments or despair at the idea that he or she may not have enough time to accomplish all of the desired goals. When people are unable to view their lives with integrity, they are significantly more likely to feel depressed, useless, or as though they are a burden on others.

Age may also bring **bereavement**—sadness over the loss of friends and loved ones. As friends and family die, older adults tend to experience increasing loneliness and isolation—factors shown to have negative effects on health. The death of a spouse, in particular, may also increase financial concerns, especially in lower-income families who may not have adequate retirement resources or life insurance coverage. Those people who were previously reliant on their spouse for daily assistance may no longer be able to meet basic needs on their own, requiring more help from their children or from other sources.

The social situations and health problems of older people are quantitatively and qualitatively different from the problems of younger people. As a consequence, you cannot simply transfer the principles of caring for and interacting with the younger population without modification to the older adult population. The special problems of older people require special approaches.

Geriatric Anatomy and Physiology

Human growth and development peak in the late 20s and early 30s, at which point the aging process sets in. Aging is a linear process; that is, the rate at which a person loses functions does not increase with age. A 35-year-old person is aging just as fast as an 85-year-old person, but the older person exhibits the cumulative results of a longer process. Organ and tissue aging may be accelerated by a variety of factors, including genetic qualities, preexisting diseases, diet, exposure to toxins, activity levels, and psychosocial characteristics. It is difficult to make general statements about the rate of aging for all people, as this process can vary dramatically from one person to another. You can most likely recall meeting 60-year-old people who look frail and 80-year-old people who are healthy enough to run a marathon **Figure 44-2**.

The aging process is inevitably accompanied by changes in physiologic function, such as a decline in the function of the liver and kidneys. All tissues in the body undergo aging, albeit not at the same rate. The decrease in the

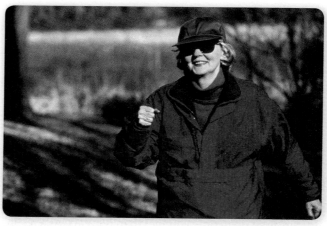

Figure 44-2 Many older people, especially those who have hobbies and activities, are healthy and vital.
Courtesy of the National Cancer Institute.

functional capacity of various organ systems is normal but can affect the way in which a patient responds to illness. Geriatric patients may report signs and symptoms different from those generally experienced by younger people, even when both groups of patients are experiencing the same disease or disorder. In addition, diseases that may generally be short-lived and without detrimental effect can have a much longer course and cause significantly worse effects in older patients.

The aging process and its associated changes can also affect the way health professionals respond to a patient's illness. It is important to differentiate between normal physiologic changes of aging and acute changes that indicate pathologic processes. For example, a health care provider who is unaware of the normal changes of aging may mistake these changes for signs of illness and be tempted to provide treatment when none is necessary. At the other end of the spectrum, the health care provider may attribute genuine disease symptoms to "just getting old" and fail to provide proper treatment. For these reasons, it is particularly important for you to determine the patient's baseline level of function when you are caring for older patients.

The physical changes that occur in older adults are discussed in Chapter 10, *Life Span Development*; the following section identifies additional changes that can occur in the aging adult.

▶ Changes in the Respiratory System

A person's respiratory capacity undergoes significant reductions with age, largely due to decreases in the elasticity of the lungs and in the size and strength of the respiratory muscles. In addition, calcification of costochondral cartilage tends to make the chest wall stiffer. As a result of these changes, the vital capacity (the amount of air that can be exhaled following a maximal inhalation) decreases, and the residual volume (the amount of air left in the lungs at the end of a maximal exhalation) increases. Thus, although the total amount of air in the lungs does not change with age, the proportion of that air usefully used in gas exchange progressively declines. Airflow, which depends largely on airway size and resistance, also deteriorates somewhat with age. Respiratory rates increase to approximately 16 to 25 breaths/min, with breathing also becoming shallower.

Meanwhile, changes in the distribution of blood flow within the lungs result in declining partial pressure of oxygen (PaO_2). The PaO_2 is a measurement of the amount of oxygen in the blood. As the aging process takes place a decline in PaO_2 can have a significant impact on the patient maintaining homeostasis. Furthermore, the respiratory drive becomes dulled as a person ages because of decreased sensitivity to changes in arterial blood gases or decreased central nervous system response to such changes.

Musculoskeletal changes, such as kyphosis (outward curvature of the thoracic spine), may also affect pulmonary function by limiting lung volume and maximal inspiratory pressure. The thoracic cage becomes increasingly stiff, owing to calcification of the costal cartilage. Chest expansion is also limited by decreased pulmonary muscle strength and mass. The decreased mass and strength require an older person to exert a greater amount of energy to perform ventilations.

The respiratory system is physically limited by these changes in its ability to modify either the respiratory rate or tidal volume as a compensatory mechanism. In addition, the lung's defense mechanisms become less effective as a natural consequence of aging. The cough and gag reflexes decrease with age, increasing the risk of aspiration. Furthermore, the ciliary mechanisms that normally help remove bronchial secretions are markedly slowed. Retention of these secretions and mucus produces a breeding ground for bacteria, putting geriatric patients at increased risk of respiratory infection. See Chapter 10, *Life Span Development*, for more information on respiratory changes.

▶ Changes in the Cardiovascular System

As with the respiratory system, a variety of changes occur in the cardiovascular system as a person grows older, with their net effect being to decrease the efficiency of this system. The wall of the left ventricle thickens and elastin in the vessel walls decreases, causing thickening and rigidity, particularly in the coronary arteries.[4] Arteriosclerosis contributes to systolic hypertension in many older patients, which places an extra burden on the heart. This phenomenon may be a consequence of disease states such as diabetes, atherosclerosis and renal compromise, and it is associated with an increased risk of cardiovascular disease, dementia, and death. Compliance of the vascular walls depends on the production of collagen and elastin, proteins that are the primary components of muscle and connective tissue. An increase in blood pressure (normal hypertension seen in aging) leads to overproduction of abnormal collagen and decreased quantities of elastin, both of which contribute to vascular stiffening. The result is a widening pulse pressure, decreased coronary artery perfusion, and changes in cardiac ejection efficiency. Many geriatric patients also exhibit an S_4 heart sound.

Aortic sclerosis occurs when the aortic valve thickens due to fibrosis and calcification. The thickening of the aortic valve obstructs blood flow from the left ventricle. Aortic sclerosis ultimately leads to aortic stenosis, a condition in which the aortic valve does not open fully, decreasing blood flow from the heart. The walls of peripheral vessels also lose elasticity with age, which can result in a higher blood pressure due to less flexibility. The older patient is at a higher risk for the development of peripheral vascular disease, dependent venous pooling, and stasis ulcers.

In addition, the electrical conduction system of the heart undergoes changes over time. For example, the sinoatrial (SA) node, atrioventricular node, and the bundle of His become fibrotic and the number of pacemaker cells in the SA node decreases with age.[4] In many cases, the changes in the conduction system lead to bradycardia, which can in turn contribute to the decline in cardiac output. Other possible changes include the failure of the SA node, which can lead to atrial dysrhythmias, such as atrial fibrillation (AF), which may cause clots to be distributed within the body. Additionally, it is much more difficult for the aging conduction system to produce a faster heart rate as a compensatory mechanism for decreased circulatory volume or increased cellular demand. In older adults, electrocardiography (ECG) may reveal a notched P wave, a prolonged P-R interval, decreased amplitude of the QRS complex, and a notched or slurred T wave.[4]

Some changes in cardiovascular performance are probably not a direct consequence of aging, but rather reflect the deconditioning effect of a sedentary lifestyle. Whether because of other disabilities (such as **arthritis**, inflammation of the joints) or for social, financial, or psychologic reasons, many people tend to decrease their physical activity as they grow older. An older person's heart rate both increases more slowly during physical activity and takes longer to return to the resting rate after becoming elevated. In older adults, cardiac output during exercise may decline by as much as 30% to 40%. Nevertheless, these factors do not ultimately affect the ability to engage in physical activity.

The sum of these changes leaves the cardiovascular system more vulnerable to dysfunction. Because the aging heart is less efficient at its baseline, its ability to compensate for circulatory changes is less than the heart of a younger person. All potential cardiac compromise should be recognized and treated quickly, and you should always be alert for presenting or potential cardiac concerns.

▶ Changes in the Nervous System

Aging produces changes in the nervous system that are reflected in the neurologic exam. In the central nervous system, the brain weight may shrink 10% to 20% by age 80 years.[5] The functional significance of these changes is not clear, however. The human brain has an enormous reserve capacity, and having a smaller and lighter brain does not interfere with the mental capabilities of productive older adults.

Because the brain is responsible for coordinating the other systems of the body, as mental function declines, the specific functions of other body systems may decline as well. Regulation of respiratory rate and depth, pulse rate, blood pressure, hunger, and thirst may all be affected by changes to the central nervous system. Reflexes often slow, resulting in older people not being able to protect themselves in normal ways. For example, older patients with slowed responses to pain may sustain a serious burn if it takes them longer to remove their hand from a hot surface. Changes in both temperature regulation and temperature perception also occur, meaning older people are less capable of recovering from exposure to extreme temperatures and less likely to recognize these exposures.

Sensory Changes

The performance of most of the sense organs declines with increasing age. Decreases in the ability to see and hear are the most common sensory impairments among older adults, along with a decreased ability to discern tastes and decreased tactile sensation. Although these senses may not be as sharp as they once were, you should not assume that all older people are blind or deaf. Use the same communication techniques that you would use with other age groups when you are caring for geriatric patients. If you sense an inability to communicate effectively, gradually modify your technique until you are able to speak with the patient in a comfortable manner.

Visual changes may begin as early as age 40 years. Tear production decreases with age, which can lead to sensations of dry or itchy eyes and increase the chances of mild eye injury (such as corneal abrasion) and infection. Causes of visual impairment in older adults may include diabetes, age-related macular degeneration, and retinal detachment, which may also be associated with diabetes.

The two most common causes of visual disturbances in older adults are cataracts and glaucoma. A cataract is a result of hardening of the lenses over time. The lenses eventually become opaque, preventing light and images from being transmitted to the rear of the eye. Patients with cataracts may report blurred vision, double vision, spots, and ghost images. Surgical treatment may be required to improve vision. By contrast, glaucoma is caused by an increase in intraocular pressure severe enough to damage the optic nerve, potentially resulting in permanent loss of peripheral and central vision. Treatment of glaucoma consists of oral medications and eye drops.

Decreases in visual acuity are common in older people, even without disease processes such as cataracts. Night vision becomes impaired, as does the ability to adjust to rapid changes in lighting conditions, depth perception, and perception of color. Presbyopia, or "far-sightedness," is caused by a loss of elasticity in the lens of the eye. Difficulty differentiating among colors is also more common in older age. Changes in a patient's vision can affect independence, the ability to read, and the ability to drive a vehicle. All of these factors may increase the risk of injury from a vehicle crash or an unintentional overdose of medications.

Although not all older people experience hearing loss, some gradual loss of hearing is not uncommon as people age. A common cause of hearing impairment in geriatric patients is **presbycusis**, a progressive hearing loss, particularly in the high frequencies, along with a lessened ability to discriminate between a particular sound and background noise. Patients who lose the ability to interpret most speech experience a decreased ability to communicate, which may lead to isolation and depression. Even when hearing loss is not severe enough to consistently interfere with conversation, certain activities, such as going to the movies or listening to music, may be less enjoyable. Hearing loss may also threaten safety because many warnings, such as smoke detectors and car horns, are auditory.

Hearing aids are among the most commonly used assistive devices in the United States **Figure 44-3**. These devices generally consist of a microphone and an amplifier, and some models are so small that they fit entirely into the ear canal. Hearing aids are almost always battery operated. If inspection of the ear canal is necessary during EMS care, hearing aids will most likely need to be removed. If the patient is conscious and able to remove them, you should ask the patient to do so because manipulation of hearing aids may cause loud feedback or a squealing

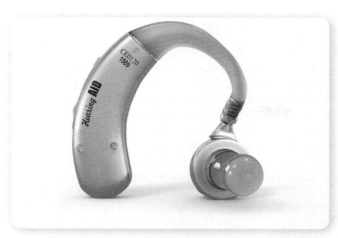

Figure 44-3 Hearing aids are among the most commonly used assistive devices in the United States.
© Maxx-Studio/Shutterstock.

noise. These devices are expensive and not always covered by insurance, so be certain that they are not lost during transport or transfer of patient care.

Another hearing-related impairment noted in the older adult population is Ménière disease. The onset of this disease's symptoms usually occurs in early middle age, with symptoms presenting in cycles that last several months at a time. The typical symptoms include vertigo (a sudden loss of normal balance or equilibrium), hearing loss, tinnitus, and pressure in the ear.

Special Populations

With patients who have some degree of hearing loss, do not yell! Lean closer and speak into the patient's ear using a somewhat low pitch. Remember that patients with limited vision are not necessarily hard of hearing. Also, ensure there is enough light for the patient to see your lips as you speak; lipreading may be how the person compensates for hearing loss.

Changes in appetite in older adults may occur because of a decrease in the number of taste buds, medications, viral infections, and upper respiratory conditions. Although these changes are gradual, the salty and sweet sensation appears to be among the first to diminish.

The sense of touch decreases from aging-related loss of the end nerve fibers. This loss, in conjunction with the slowing of the peripheral nervous system, can result in a delayed reflex reaction in geriatric patients.

The sense of smell is among the last to diminish in older adults. However, factors such as upper respiratory infections (ie, the common cold), to which older persons are more prone, can affect the sense of smell.

For many older people, physiologic changes make it difficult to produce speech that is loud enough, clear, and well spaced. Weakness, paralysis, poor hearing, or brain damage can damage the delicate functions that make these abilities possible. Changes in cognition may also affect speech and conversation, because the person may not be able to recall specific information fast enough to carry on a normal conversation. This may be frustrating to patients, as well as to their conversational partners, so do not rush them for answers to your questions or interrupt them; give them time to put their thoughts together.

Sense of body position (**proprioception**) also becomes impaired with age. Proprioception enables a person to maintain postural stability by using a variety of receptors in the joints and information provided by the eyes. As these mechanisms fail with age, people become less steady on their feet, and the tendency to fall increases markedly. This tendency may be exacerbated by many of the previously described changes in sensory perception.

▶ Changes in the Digestive System

The process of digestion begins in the mouth, which is also where aging-related changes in the digestive system may first be noted. As discussed previously, a decrease in the number of taste buds and changes in olfactory receptors may diminish an older person's senses of taste and smell, which may in turn interfere with the enjoyment of food. The consequent decrease in appetite may lead to malnutrition. Other aging-related changes in the mouth include a reduction in the volume of saliva, with a resulting dryness of the mouth. Dental loss is not a normal result of the aging process, but rather the result of disease of the teeth and gums; nevertheless, dental loss is widespread in the older adult population and contributes to nutritional and digestive problems. Even when dentures are present, ill-fitting dentures may result in pain or discomfort when eating, or they may not allow the wearer to chew effectively, increasing the likelihood of choking, heartburn, and abdominal pain.

Like oral secretions, gastric secretions are reduced as a person ages—although enough acid is still present to produce ulcers under certain conditions. Because of the esophageal sphincter's weakening and decreased ability to hold back stomach contents, the acid present in the stomach may also cause heartburn, indigestion, or acid reflux. Whereas these symptoms tend to be related to diet and eating practices, the possibility exists that the patient may ignore symptoms of cardiac compromise, thinking of them simply as the aftereffects of a spicy or greasy meal. Changes in gastric motility also occur that may lead to slower gastric emptying—a factor of some importance when you are assessing the risk of aspiration, and a factor contributing to uncomfortable (but not life-threatening) heartburn and acid reflux.

The functions of the small and large bowels change little as a consequence of aging, although the incidence of certain diseases involving the bowel (such as diverticulosis) increases as a person grows older. As with other sphincters within the body, rectal sphincter muscles may decrease in size and strength, potentially leading to unintentional bowel release, or fecal incontinence.

Slowing of peristalsis can lead to constipation in older adults. Constipation may also be caused or worsened by certain medications, changes in diet, and decreased physical activity. Collectively, these factors may lead to difficult bowel movements with straining that can cause hemorrhoids. Forceful straining or retching (vagus nerve stimulation) may also lead to syncope or bradycardia. The patient may attempt to treat constipation without the assistance of a physician, often with diet techniques or medications that may or may not be intended to treat constipation. When treated too aggressively, diarrhea may result, sometimes leading to dehydration. For constipation that cannot be resolved with diet and medications, manual removal of stool by a physician or nurse may be necessary.

In the liver, aging brings changes in hepatic enzyme systems, with some systems declining in activity and others increasing. Notably, the activity of the enzyme systems concerned with the detoxification of drugs declines as a person ages. The decrease in hepatic function can complicate drug absorption, resulting in drug toxicity. When patients are prescribed numerous medications, the risk for hepatic damage or drug toxicity increases.

▶ Changes in the Renal System

The kidneys are responsible for maintaining the body's fluid and electrolyte balance; they also have important roles in maintaining the body's long-term acid-base balance and eliminating drugs from the body. The kidneys grow in size and weight until around the age of 40 years old, when the kidneys begin to decline in weight along with a decline in body surface.[6] This decline in weight results from a loss of functioning nephron units, which translates into a smaller effective filtering surface.

Acute illness in geriatric patients is often accompanied by derangements in fluid and electrolyte balance. Aging kidneys, for example, respond sluggishly to sodium deficiency. A geriatric patient may lose a large amount of sodium before the kidneys halt urinary sodium excretion, a problem that is exacerbated by the markedly decreased thirst mechanism in older adults. The net result may be a rapid development of severe dehydration.

Conversely, older adults are at considerable risk of overhydration if they are exposed to large sodium loads (such as from intravenous [IV] saline solutions or heavily salted foods). Because of its lower glomerular filtration rate, the aging kidney is less able to excrete a large sodium load, making the patient vulnerable to acute volume overload.

The same factors that reduce an older person's ability to handle sodium also affect the body's ability to handle potassium. Thus, geriatric patients are prone to hyperkalemia that can reach serious—even lethal—levels if the patient becomes acidotic or if the potassium load is increased from any source.

▶ Changes in the Endocrine System

According to the US Centers for Disease Control and Prevention, 25.9% of US residents, or 11.2 million people, aged 65 years and older had diabetes in 2012.[7] The reason older people are at greater risk for developing type 2 diabetes is multifaceted. As people age, the metabolism of carbohydrates becomes more difficult to process; insulin production and glucose metabolism gradually decrease as the aging organs begin to decrease in functionality. Furthermore, older adults who are diagnosed with diabetes may have a multitude of comorbid disorders and may be prescribed various medications that may affect glucose metabolism.

As people age, an increase in the production of antidiuretic hormone can occur. This change can cause various electrolyte imbalances, particularly hyponatremia, as well as fluid balance issues. Patients may present with pedal or other peripheral edema, although peripheral edema may also be the result of cardiovascular compromise. Again, it is important for you to determine the patient's baseline status in terms of edema; worsening of edema is much more significant than its presence alone.

In women, menopause (or cessation of the reproductive cycles of menstruation and ovulation) results in decreased secretion of hormones, specifically estrogen. Because estrogen plays an important role in the preservation of bone mass, the decline in estrogen levels may lead to decreased bone density and osteoporosis, leading to easily fractured bones in the older adult population. Paired with their increased risk of falls, weakened bones are a significant concern in this population.

▶ Changes in the Immunologic System

Because nearly every function of the immune system is affected by aging, older persons are more prone to infection and secondary complications compared to younger people. Chronic conditions such as diabetes, dementia, malnutrition, and cardiovascular disease place older people at greater risk of serious infection.

Older persons manifest infections differently. Although fever is often present with minor illness in young people, fever in older persons usually indicates a serious infection. However, not all older adults with a serious infection have a fever, due to the decreased ability of the aging immune system to initiate a fever.

▶ Changes in the Integumentary System

Wrinkling and loss of resiliency of the skin are the most visible signs of aging. Wrinkling occurs because the skin becomes thinner, drier, less elastic, and more fragile with age. As subcutaneous fat becomes thinner, bruising becomes more common because subcutaneous fat normally cushions blood vessels from mild blunt forces. Both elastin (the substance that makes the skin pliable) and collagen (the substance that makes the skin strong) levels decrease with age. Thinner skin tears much more easily, and the loss of elasticity allows for more bleeding before hemostasis occurs. Because of the decreased resiliency of the skin, it may also be more prone to tenting when skin turgor is checked, even when dehydration is not present.

As a person ages, the sebaceous glands produce less oil and the skin becomes drier. Sweat gland activity also decreases, hindering the ability to sweat and to regulate heat. Hair follicles produce thinner hair or may stop producing hair. Follicles produce less melanin (the pigment that gives hair color), making the hair color change to gray or white. The number of melanocytes in the epidermis decreases, making the skin appear paler than in younger years and increasing sensitivity to sun exposure. As the number of melanocytes decreases, existing melanocytes grow larger. This process may lead to benign pigmentation changes in sun-exposed areas, such as age spots, or "liver spots."

The blood vessels that supply the skin also are affected by atherosclerosis and provide less oxygenated blood at the cellular level. As a consequence of the skin's lower metabolism, epidermal cells develop more slowly and do not replace outgoing cells as quickly as occurs in younger skin. Fingernails and toenails may change as well, generally becoming thinner and more brittle. More profound changes are noted in these areas when patients have inadequate nutrition from any of a number of causes. Fingernails that are poorly cared for can be a source of infection, particularly for patients with significantly decreased cognitive abilities. Inadequate or incorrect self-care of toenails can result in infection of the soft tissue of the toes, and when combined with peripheral vascular disease or diabetes, the complications from poor toenail care can lead to amputation.

▶ Homeostatic and Other Changes

Homeostasis is the process by which the body maintains a constant internal environment. Many homeostatic mechanisms work on a feedback principle, much like the thermostat in a house; that is, a change in the internal environment feeds back to the control system and induces a corrective response. For example, when the body temperature starts to rise, temperature sensors are activated, which in turn activate compensatory responses: cutaneous blood vessels dilate, and excess heat is transferred from the body to the environment. Similarly, when the concentration of glucose in the blood rises, the pancreas is stimulated to secrete insulin, which leads to uptake of glucose by cells and reduction of the blood glucose level back toward normal.

With aging, there is a progressive loss of these homeostatic capabilities. For that reason, a specific illness or injury in older adults is more likely to result in generalized deterioration compared to the same condition in younger people. For example, the thirst mechanism that ordinarily protects a person from dehydration becomes depressed in older adults. Likewise, temperature-regulating mechanisms tend to become disordered, which when combined with integumentary changes makes older adults much more vulnerable to environmental stresses such as heat exhaustion and accidental hypothermia after relatively minor exposures. A defect in temperature regulation also may account for the absence of a febrile response to illness in some older adults. As discussed previously, infections that would ordinarily produce high fever, such as pneumococcal pneumonia, may produce only a low-grade or no fever in older adults.

Words of Wisdom

A specific illness or injury in an older person is more likely to result in generalized deterioration.

The regulatory system that manages the blood glucose level similarly becomes impaired with increasing age, such that an elevated blood glucose level occurs quite commonly in older patients. Ordinarily, moderate hyperglycemia does no harm, but overly aggressive treatment of this problem may produce damaging hypoglycemia.

▶ Changes in the Musculoskeletal System

Aging brings a widespread decrease in bone mass in men and women, but especially among postmenopausal women. Bones become more brittle and tend to break more easily. Tendons and ligaments begin to lose elasticity, synovial fluids in joints thicken, and the cartilage that ordinarily cushions the joints decreases. Narrowing of the intervertebral disks and compression fractures of the vertebrae contribute to a decrease in height as a person ages, along with changes in posture. Joints lose their flexibility and may be further immobilized by arthritic changes. Muscle mass decreases throughout the body, with an accompanying decrease in muscle strength. Atrophy, or wasting of muscles, occurs when mobility is limited for a prolonged period, such as during bed confinement after surgery or illness.

From the paramedic's perspective, the changes in the musculoskeletal system most often translate into fractures incurred as the result of falls. The aging musculoskeletal system not only makes the geriatric patient more susceptible to fractures when falls occur, but also increases the likelihood of falling, because joint stiffness, loss of elasticity in tendons and ligaments, and weakening of muscles may impair mobility. Aging-related changes may cause patients to have difficulty caring for themselves; this is especially true regarding tasks that require fine motor coordination and strength in the hands and fingers. As a consequence, patients may have difficulty taking medications, self-administering medication, or caring for wounds.

Loss of bone density and muscle mass may be slowed if people remain physically active throughout the life span. People who enter older adulthood with larger muscles and a history of performing physical labor or participating in regular strenuous exercise are the least susceptible to musculoskeletal decline. Older adults may also experience less pain from arthritis when they consistently and gently use arthritic joints.

Geriatric Patient Assessment

Although illness is common among older adults, it is not an inevitable part of aging. All complaints made by older adults cannot be ascribed simply to "getting old." Aging is a continuous process and a normal development sequence that affects people in multiple ways. The normal wear-and-tear concept and genetic makeup are two theories that have been suggested to explain the biologic effects of aging.

> ### Special Populations
>
> Getting old is not a disease, and it does not by itself produce symptoms of disease.

Along the same lines, there is a widespread *misconception* that older adults tend to be hypochondriacs, with many imaginary or minor complaints. In reality, hypochondria is far less common among older patients than among younger patients. Indeed, older patients tend not to complain, even when they have legitimate symptoms. When an older adult calls for an ambulance, he or she usually has a real problem.

Knowing what is and what is not part of the aging process constitutes the first challenge when you are assessing geriatric patients. A second challenge is that signs and symptoms of disease may present differently in this population than in younger patients as a consequence of the aging process. A myocardial infarction may present without chest pain; fever may be minimal in pneumonia; and uncontrolled diabetes may present as hyperglycemic hyperosmolar syndrome (HHS), also called hyperosmolar nonketotic coma (HONK). A variety of acute illnesses—from heart failure to an acute abdomen—may present simply as delirium.

Another challenge relates to the fact that the older the patient, the more likely there will be multiple problems—medical, psychologic, and social. Debilitating health conditions often found in this population include hypertension, arthritic symptoms, heart disease, cancer, diabetes, stroke, and chronic obstructive pulmonary disease (COPD).

The co-occurrence of multiple pathologic conditions has several consequences for patients and health care providers alike. Notably, the symptoms of one disease or disability may alter or hide the symptoms of another condition. The patient with severe leg pain from arthritis, for example, may not pay much attention to new pain caused by thrombophlebitis. In addition, when several organ systems are in borderline condition, a disturbance in function in only one of the systems may have repercussions throughout the body, leading to failure of multiple organs in a domino-like manner. The presence of multiple underlying illnesses also makes it much more difficult for you to sort out which problem is causing which symptom. Furthermore, chronic comorbidities may make it much more difficult to treat the patient's acute problem. For example, the medication a

YOU are the Paramedic   PART 2

On your arrival at the scene, you hear a woman yell, "We're up here!" As you approach the master bedroom, you find the patient lying on the floor, halfway between the bed and the toilet. He appears to have tripped on a rug. You notice a medical alert pendant on the patient's nightstand, along with stacked pillows on the bed. The patient is responsive to painful stimuli and is wearing a nasal cannula that is flowing oxygen at 2 L/min, with tubing stretching from a concentrator in the next room.

Recording Time: 1 Minute	
Appearance	Pale with an altered level of consciousness
Level of consciousness	Responsive to verbal stimuli
Airway	Open and clear
Breathing	Irregular
Circulation	Bounding

3. Could injury prevention methods have been used prior to this incident to help minimize the chances of a fall? If so, which kind?

4. What are your primary responsibilities at this point during the call?

patient needs for a cardiac problem may be contraindicated because of a renal or hepatic problem or, at the least, may require a major modification in the dosage.

Scene Size-up

Begin the patient assessment process by ensuring scene safety, and take standard precautions. Be mindful of clues that may help you determine the mechanism of injury/nature of illness, the environment, and potential for danger. Immediately determine the number of patients who require your assistance, and consider any additional or specialized resources that may need to be called. You also need to be aware of the numerous factors that affect the assessment process in geriatric patients: sensory alterations, verbal communication skills, and mental and physical capabilities. You need to be able to accommodate and comprehend these conditions.

Words of Wisdom

Always assume that a geriatric patient's mental status is normal until you have evidence to the contrary.

Primary Survey

As you approach the patient, you will want to form a general impression that may prove relevant to the case and help you to address life threats. To do so, look for potential clues such as general living conditions; availability of social and family support; activity level; medications; and overall appearance with respect to nutrition, general health, cleanliness, personal hygiene, and attitude and mental well-being.

Many acronyms are used in the prehospital setting to help you remember steps in the assessment and treatment processes. The GEMS diamond was created to help providers recall key themes when caring for geriatric patients Table 44-1 . It was designed to assist the prehospital professional in the assessment and treatment of geriatric patients.

The "G" of the GEMS diamond calls upon you to recognize that the patient is a geriatric patient. In such a case, your thought process needs to be geared toward the possible problems of an aging patient. When you are responding to an emergency involving an older patient, you should consider that older patients are different from younger patients and may present atypically.

The "E" of the GEMS diamond stands for environmental assessment. Assessment of the environment can help give clues to the patient's condition or the cause of the emergency. Is the home too hot or cold? Is the home well kept and secure? Are there hazardous conditions? Preventive care is also important for a geriatric patient, who may not carefully study the environment or may not realize where risks exist.

The "M" of the GEMS diamond stands for medical assessment. Older patients tend to have a variety of medical problems and may be taking numerous prescription, over-the-counter, and herbal medications. Obtaining a thorough history is important in older patients. Keep this point in mind throughout the assessment process.

The "S" stands for social assessment. Older people may have less of a social network because of the death of a spouse, family members, or friends. Older people may also need assistance with activities of daily living (ADLs), such as dressing and eating. Numerous social agencies are readily available to help geriatric patients, and these agencies can share with you and your patients a listing of the services they provide.

The GEMS diamond provides a concise way for you to remember the important issues for older patients. Using this concept will help you make appropriate referrals, and as a result, you will help older patients maintain their quality of life.

Anatomic changes occur as a person ages, predisposing geriatric patients to airway problems. Aging and disease can compromise a patient's ability to protect his or her airway through loss of a gag reflex and normal swallowing mechanisms. Changes in level of consciousness, dementia, and post-stroke weakness or paralysis can cause airway obstruction or aspiration. Ensure that the patient's airway is open and is not obstructed by dentures, vomitus, fluids, or blood. Suction may be necessary.

Anatomic changes with aging may also affect a person's ability to breathe effectively. Increased chest wall stiffness, brittle bones, weakening of the airway musculature, and decreased muscle mass may contribute to breathing problems. Loss of mechanisms that protect the upper airway, such as cough and gag reflexes, may cause a decreased ability to clear secretions. A decrease in the number of cilia that line the bronchial tree may result in the patient's inability to remove material from the lung, which can cause infection. In some patients, the alveoli are damaged, and a lack of elasticity results in a decreased ability to exchange oxygen and carbon dioxide. Superimposed on aging-related physiologic changes in breathing are the chronic respiratory diseases common in older adults that affect their ability to breathe effectively. Airway and breathing issues should be treated with oxygen as soon as possible.

People who normally live with compromised circulation have little in the way of reserves during a circulatory crisis. In addition, aging-related physiologic changes may negatively affect circulation. Less-responsive nerve stimulation may lower the rate and strength of the heart's contractions, so lower heart rates and weaker and irregular pulses are common in older patients. Vascular changes and circulatory compromise might make it difficult to feel a radial pulse on an older patient. If choosing an alternative pulse point like the carotid, press gently. Another option is to listen to the apical pulse right over the heart. The pulse may be irregular because of common heart rhythm problems. Circulation problems in older adults should be treated with oxygen as soon as possible.

Table 44-1	The GEMS Diamond

G   Geriatric Patients

- Present atypically
- Deserve respect
- Experience normal changes with age

E   Environmental Assessment

- Check the physical condition of the patient's home: Is the exterior of the home in need of repair? Is the home secure?
- Check for hazardous conditions that may be present (eg, poor wiring, rotted floors, unventilated gas heaters, clutter that prevents adequate egress).
- Are smoke detectors present and working?
- Is the home too hot or too cold?
- Is there an odor of feces or urine in the home?
- Is bedding soiled or urine soaked?
- Are pets well cared for?
- Is food present in the home? Is it adequate and unspoiled?
- Are liquor bottles present? If so, are they empty?
- Are there burn patterns on the walls, cabinets, or floors?
- Are there unsecured throw rugs that could result in falls?
- If the patient has a disability, are appropriate assistive devices (eg, a wheelchair or walker) present and in adequate condition?
- Does the patient have access to a telephone?
- Are medications prescribed to someone else, expired, unmarked, or from many physicians?
- If living with others, is the patient confined to one part of the home?
- If the patient is residing in a nursing facility, does the care appear to be adequate to meet the patient's needs?

M   Medical Assessment

- Older patients tend to have a variety of medical problems, making their assessment complex. Keep this consideration in mind in all cases—both trauma and medical. A trauma patient may have an underlying medical condition that could have caused or may be exacerbated by the injury.
- Obtaining a medical history is important in older patients, regardless of the chief complaint.
- Perform a primary survey.
- Perform a reassessment.

S   Social Assessment

- Assess activities of daily living (eating, dressing, bathing, toileting).
- Are these activities being provided for the patient? If so, by whom?
- Are there delays in obtaining food, medication, or toileting? The patient may complain of such a delay, or the environment may suggest a problem.
- Does the patient have regular visits from family members, live with family members, or live with a spouse?
- If in an institutional setting, is the patient able to feed himself or herself? If not, is food still sitting on the food tray? Has the patient been lying in his or her own urine or feces for prolonged periods?
- Does the patient have a social network? Does the patient have a mechanism to interact socially with others on a daily basis?

Documentation & Communication

Be patient when you are interviewing older people, recognizing that physical, cognitive, and psychologic barriers may slow or interfere with effective communication.

Your most important tasks during the primary survey are to identify any life-threatening conditions, treat them to the best of your ability, and transport priority patients. Older adults do not have the reserves that younger people have, and they will easily decompensate. Even a general complaint of weakness and dizziness in a geriatric patient can be an indication of something more serious, such as a heart problem. Consider early on in your call whether advanced life support (ALS) treatment and immediate transport are appropriate. If the patient's condition is nonemergent, and the facility is otherwise appropriate based on the patient's condition, consider taking him or her to a facility where the patient has been treated before and his or her medical records are available.

Patient Safety

Remember that some older patients will be on medications that could mask findings that would normally indicate physiologic instability. For example, if the patient is on a beta-blocker, the early sign of tachycardia in a shock patient could be masked.

Documentation & Communication

The following interviewing techniques may enhance communication with geriatric patients:

- Introduce yourself.
- Speak to the patient first rather than to family or bystanders.
- Be aware of your body language.
- Look directly at the patient.
- Speak slowly and distinctly.
- Explain what you are doing.
- Allow time for the patient to answer.
- Show the patient respect, and preserve his or her dignity.
- Do not talk about the patient with others in front of the patient.
- Be patient.
- Locate hearing aids or eyeglasses if needed.
- Turn on lights.

History Taking

Good communication skills will help you gather the information you need during your assessment. Without good communication skills, you could frighten, alienate, insult, anger, or even harm your patients. Your first words should focus on gaining the patient's trust. Introduce yourself. Use respect when you are addressing the patient; use his or her name, if you know it; and do not use terms such as "buddy," "honey," "dear," and "grandma" when addressing an older patient unless the patient asks to be called by that phrase. Speak slowly, distinctly, and respectfully. Do not raise your voice excessively. Attempt to get the patient history from the patient, rather than from family and bystanders, whenever possible. The ability to elicit a thorough patient history reflects education and experience. For example, a thorough knowledge of prescription medications will help in understanding the patient's diagnoses as well as medication compliance.

Communication is not just talking; it involves active listening. When you are asking questions of older patients, wait for their answers. Active listening also involves paying attention to the patient's tone, especially if it conveys fear or confusion.

Nonverbal communication is just as important as verbal communication. Eye contact, hand gestures, body position, facial expressions, and touch communicate a message. When you are speaking with patients, get face to face with them and make sure there is plenty of light. Have patients put in hearing aids (ensure they are turned on) or wear glasses to facilitate better communication, and be sure to take these aids with the patients to the hospital so other health care providers can communicate with these patients using the devices.

Explain everything you plan to do, especially if the patient seems confused. Part of your task in the assessment is to determine whether this confused state is normal, a new manifestation of a preexisting medical problem, or a result of the patient's lack of understanding. Preserve the patient's dignity during exposure and when you are discussing his or her history around others.

A comprehensive patient history includes many elements to investigate—the patient's chief complaint, present illness or injury, pertinent medical history, and current health care status and needs. Keep in mind that pertinent past medical history would include current cardiovascular health (such as palpitations or flutters), exercise tolerance, diet history, medications, smoking and drinking habits, sleep patterns, and other intrinsic and extrinsic factors. Obtaining the chief complaint would seem to be a straightforward procedure, but it may not be simple with some geriatric patients. Older patients tend not to report significant symptoms for several reasons. Many share the misconception that illness and assorted aches and pains are simply part of aging. Others may not mention even legitimate symptoms to avoid being identified as old and a hypochondriac. Some older patients fear that mentioning a symptom will lead to a diagnosis or treatment that will jeopardize their independence. "If I mention those pains in my stomach," the person may reason, "they'll put me in the hospital, and I may never come out of that place again."

Geriatric patients may underreport serious symptoms, and the symptoms they do report may sound trivial. It may be difficult for older patients to report symptoms, particularly in front of their spouse or other family members. Furthermore, they are likely to have several chief complaints, each of which may have a different source.

When a patient's chief complaint seems trivial, it may be necessary to go through a standard list of screening questions to confirm that you are not missing important pieces of information. In such a review of systems, the questions are designed to evaluate the functions of the body's major organ systems. In the field, you do not have sufficient time to conduct a complete review of all systems, but a few well-chosen questions can provide you with a great deal of information about the function of the patient's more important systems:

- Cardiovascular
  - Have you had any pain or discomfort in your chest? When?
  - Have you had any pain in your left arm or jaw?
  - Have you noticed any fluttering in your chest or fast heartbeats?
- Respiratory
  - Do you ever get short of breath? When?
  - Have you had a cough lately? Is it painful and, if productive, what color?
  - What position have you been sleeping in? (Recall that patients with heart failure may find themselves sleeping in an upright position in bed, with pillows behind their back, or in a reclining chair.)
- Neurologic
  - Can you explain the reason for calling 9-1-1?
  - Have you had any dizzy spells? Have you fainted?
  - Have you had any trouble speaking?
  - Have you had headaches recently?
  - Have you noticed any unusual weakness or odd sensations in your arms or legs?
- Gastrointestinal
  - Have there been any changes in your appetite lately?
  - Have you gained or lost any weight?
  - Have there been any changes in your bowel movements?
  - Have you had any nausea or vomiting?
- Genitourinary
  - Do you have any pain or difficulty urinating?
  - Have you noticed any change in the color of your urine?
  - Have you noticed any changes in the frequency of urination?

If any of these screening questions yields a positive answer, follow up with further questions. For example, if the patient states that he or she has been coughing lately, find out whether the patient is bringing up sputum and, if so, what the sputum looks like (eg, is there blood in the sputum?).

Once you have elicited what you believe to be the chief complaint, go through the usual process of assembling the history of the present illness. This history may be complicated if other chronic problems are affecting the acute problem. To sort out which symptoms relate to the current chief complaint and which are chronic difficulties, try asking questions such as "How does this problem differ from what it was like last week?" or "What happened today to make you decide to get help?" Be aware of your tone and body language while asking these questions—you do not want to appear condescending.

Just as it is not practical to go through a comprehensive review of systems in the field, it is not usually feasible to obtain a complete medical history in the prehospital setting. Nevertheless, you should obtain a SAMPLE history to inquire about recent hospitalizations and allergies **Table 44-2** .

Most important, you should obtain the most detailed history possible of the patient's medications, because medications account for a significant percentage of medical

Table 44-2	SAMPLE History Components	
Component	**Features**
Signs and symptoms	Onset and nature of symptoms of pain or fever
Allergies	Known medication reactions or other allergies
Medications	Exact names and doses of ongoing medications (including over-the-counter, prescribed, herbal, and recreational drugs) Timing and amount of last dose Time and dose of analgesics or antipyretics
Past medical history	Previous illnesses or injuries Immunizations Important family history
Last oral intake	Timing of the last food or drink What was ingested and when
Events leading to illness or injury	Key events leading up to the current injury or illness

© Jones & Bartlett Learning.

problems in older adults. A medication history should include all medications, not just prescription drugs, because many people do not think to mention common over-the-counter preparations such as aspirin, antacid tablets, and herbal medicines. Ask the patient to list the medications by name, and determine the dosing and frequency for each one. Also, inquire about medications that are prescribed but not taken (eg, because of cost issues or side effects) and medications that may have been provided by other sources (eg, a spouse's medication). Obtain the patient's permission to take medications to the hospital, and then collect them all—prescription and nonprescription. If the patient cannot tell you where the medicines are stored, check the bathroom medicine cabinet, the bedside table, the kitchen table and counters, and the refrigerator.

Obtaining a history from a geriatric patient requires patience. You must be prepared to listen, often for an extended period. But your listening will be rewarded—not only by helping you discover the patient's problem, but also by allowing you to provide part of the solution to the problem. Listening is a demonstration of caring, and your caring can mean a great deal to a lonely or frightened older person.

Secondary Assessment

During the secondary assessment of a geriatric patient, you may have to adjust your usual examination methods. Poor cooperation and easy fatigability on the part of the patient may require that you keep manipulations to a minimum. In addition, older people are more prone to hypothermia, so be sure to keep the patient warm and maintain body temperature. Inspection and palpation can be hampered by multiple layers of clothing, so remove only the clothing that is necessary to perform an accurate examination. Be sure to cover the patient when you are finished.

Words of Wisdom

Cover the patient with a blanket to protect privacy and keep the patient warm. This action shows respect for the patient and will improve your exam.

Postural changes in blood pressure vary among older adults, but changes increase with increasing frailty and heighten the person's risk for falls. Marked postural changes in blood pressure and pulse rate may indicate hypovolemia or overmedication. As you obtain the vital signs, bear in mind that blood pressure tends to be higher in older adults; thus, an older patient who has a blood pressure in the normal adult range could actually be hypotensive. If possible, determine the patient's baseline blood pressure. When you are obtaining a patient's blood pressure, be aware of the possibility of significant hypertension and

orthostatic changes. Consider obtaining vital signs in both arms and checking pulses proximally and distally in all extremities. This process will allow you to gather information and observe for signs of dependent edema, dehydration, and the patient's circulatory status without raising his or her anxiety level.

Special Populations

Consider the possibility of hypovolemia in any older person whose systolic blood pressure is less than 120 mm Hg.

Pay close attention to the geriatric patient's respiratory rate. Tachypnea can be a sensitive indicator of acute illness in older people—especially pulmonary infection—even when patients show few, if any, other signs. When you are assessing the patient's respirations, listen to lung sounds in all fields, noting adventitious sounds that might aid in the development of a treatment plan. You can also use the stethoscope to listen for carotid bruits; note jugular vein distention.

When you are examining the mouth, make a note of any upper or lower dentures. In the chest exam, keep in mind that older adults may have pulmonary crackles without apparent pathology. Similarly, edema in the legs may be the result of chronic venous insufficiency and not right-sided heart failure.

Reassessment

Reassess the geriatric patient often because the condition of an older adult may deteriorate quickly. Repeat the primary survey. Reassess the vital signs and the patient's complaint. Recheck interventions. Identify and treat changes in the patient's condition.

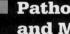

Pathophysiology, Assessment, and Management of Respiratory Conditions

Most patients with COPD, pulmonary edema, and other common respiratory ailments are in the second half of their lives. Geriatric patients also occasionally have pertussis, presumably because their childhood immunization is no longer protective.

▶ Pneumonia

Pneumonia involves an inflammation of the lung, secondary to infection by bacteria, viruses, or other organisms. Although it can affect people at any age, this disease has its biggest impact on very young children and older adults, typically during the colder seasons (winter and early spring). People considered at increased risk for pneumonia include older people; people with underlying health problems such as COPD, diabetes mellitus, and vascular diseases; and any person with a depressed immune system because of acquired immunodeficiency syndrome, cancer therapy, or organ transplantation. Presence of a tracheostomy, ventilator dependence, general immobility, bed confinement (eg, rehabilitation from a fractured hip), and conditions that limit the ability to breathe deeply, such as rib fractures, also increase the risk for pneumonia. Be sure to thoroughly evaluate the patient's medications or medication list for recently prescribed antimicrobial medications, even if the course has been completed. The presence of an infectious process that continues despite proper antimicrobial administration should be noted.

Older patients with pneumonia often do not have the classic presentation of chills, fever, and productive cough, particularly if they take a nonsteroidal anti-inflammatory drug (NSAID) regularly for joint pain or another comorbidity. Instead, these symptoms are often supplanted by acute confusion (delirium), normal temperature, and a minimal to absent cough. Some patients may also report abdominal pain. Rhonchi may be auscultated in the affected lobes, and inflammation of the bronchi may result in wheezing.

Treatment is primarily supportive, consisting of placing the patient in a position of comfort that allows for the best possible ventilation, plus giving fluids, oxygen therapy via a nasal cannula or mask to relieve dyspnea, and analgesics to reduce fever. These patients may benefit from application of continuous positive airway pressure (CPAP). Preventive measures include a *Pneumococcus* vaccine given once, with booster doses after 3 to 5 years (although this will not prevent infection from other bacterial species), along with smoking cessation and respiratory exercises during bed confinement. The receiving facility will determine whether antibiotics are necessary.

▶ Chronic Obstructive Pulmonary Disease

COPD is the name given to a set of diseases, including chronic bronchitis, asthma, and emphysema, all of which are characterized by the presence of bronchial obstruction and airway inflammation. Distinguishing among these diseases can be difficult, so the problem may not be diagnosed or treated correctly. The effects of COPD reflect the age-related loss of elastic tissue in the lungs (senile emphysema) and a decreased ability to defend against infection. These factors may increase the baseline disability of COPD and set up older patients for an increased risk of acute exacerbation, often caused by infection. Patients with COPD may experience dyspnea upon exertion, and when the disease is in its later stages, even minor physical activities such as position changes and walking may become difficult for the patient. Thus,

along with shortness of breath, presenting symptoms in an acute COPD exacerbation may include fatigue and a decreased activity level.

Preventive measures for COPD include smoking cessation, avoidance of certain environmental pollutants, and immunization for influenza and pneumococcal pneumonia. In a patient of any age, treatment goals for COPD are to reduce the symptoms and complications. Long-term oxygen therapy has proved helpful in patients with hypoxemia. In addition, pulmonary rehabilitation may improve functional status and the quality of life for some patients. Patients with COPD frequently use inhaled beta-adrenergic agents and inhaled or oral steroids.

In the field, treatment for acute episodes related to COPD consists of immediate assessment and correction of respiratory difficulties with the application of supplemental oxygen. Use of CPAP has been shown to decrease the morbidity and mortality of patients with COPD.[8] Patients may also receive bronchodilators to decrease the shortness of breath, inhaled or oral steroids to decrease inflammation, and antibiotics to treat infection.

Patients with COPD often express significant anxiety when they have trouble catching their breath despite oxygen or bronchodilator medications. They may be hesitant to go to the hospital because they are fearful of having another intubation, being placed on a ventilator, or dying in the hospital.

> **Patient Safety**
>
> Patients with COPD often have a reduced tidal volume because of their respiratory disease. Keep this in mind if you are using a bag-mask device for ventilatory support. Your normal 500-mL squeeze of the bag may be more than the patient's lungs can handle. Recall when ventilating a patient to squeeze only until you see visible chest rise and/or resistance is met.

▶ Asthma

Asthma is a common disease among older adults. Onset of this disease can occur in old age with presenting symptoms of shortness of breath (especially with effort), chronic or nocturnal cough, and wheezing. Patients with asthma that is worsened by exertion may find that they are more susceptible to asthma attacks as they age.

Management of asthma in the geriatric population is similar to management in other age groups, although when asthma and cardiac disease coexist, the administration of preferred beta-adrenergic agents for asthma may exacerbate cardiac symptoms. Asthma clinical practice guidelines are the same for younger and older patients **Figure 44-4** . On rare occasions, epinephrine may be indicated for a life-threatening asthma exacerbation. See Chapter 16, *Respiratory Emergencies*, for more information about asthma.

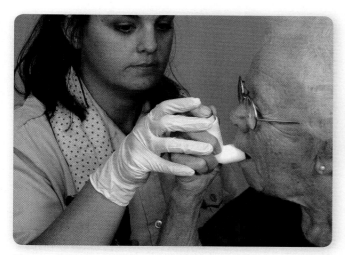

Figure 44-4 A patient having an asthma attack may have a bronchodilator medication in a metered-dose inhaler. An older patient may need assistance with the use of an inhaler.

© Jones & Bartlett Learning.

▶ Pulmonary Embolism

Another condition that can cause respiratory distress is pulmonary embolism. Pulmonary embolism occurs when a blood vessel supplying the lung becomes blocked by a clot. Just as is true with the heart, any obstruction in blood flow to the lung can result in irreversible damage or infarction. An embolus is often released from a vein in a lower extremity, the pelvis, or the abdomen, but could also result from a heart dysrhythmia such as AF. Deep vein thrombosis (DVT) is a common cause of pulmonary embolus in which an embolus may become displaced from the vein in which it formed (generally one of the larger veins in the leg).

Prevention of embolism is based on the patient's risk level—high, moderate, or low. Surgical patients are in the highest risk category for potential emboli, and prophylaxis is generally recommended in such cases, including warfarin (Coumadin) and/or heparin and compression stockings. To ensure that these patients are receiving therapeutic levels of these anticoagulant medications, serum plasma levels and coagulation laboratory tests are regularly performed. The risk of pulmonary embolus increases with age because of older adults' increasing immobility and increased vascular stasis in the lower extremities. Bed confinement during illness or after surgery will further decrease blood flow in the legs and feet, increasing the chance of DVT and pulmonary embolism. In addition, geriatric patients have an increased incidence of diseases associated with a higher risk of pulmonary embolus, such as cancer, heart attack, cardiac dysrhythmias, and clotting disorders.

Many pulmonary emboli are silent or present with tachypnea alone; that is, the classic triad of dyspnea, chest pain, and hemoptysis is often altered or absent. If you suspect a pulmonary embolus, check for swelling, erythema, and warmth or tenderness of the lower leg; all of these are

signs of a DVT. If DVT might be present, handle the leg gently and monitor the patient for respiratory changes. Prehospital treatment is largely supportive after ensuring that the airway and ventilation are adequate.

■ Pathophysiology, Assessment, and Management of Cardiovascular Conditions

Diseases of the heart remain the leading cause of death among older adults in the United States, and coronary artery disease (CAD) is the number one culprit.[9] Heart attack or myocardial infarction is the major cause of morbidity and mortality in people older than 65 years, and its potential for mortality increases significantly after a person reaches 70 years.[9]

▶ Acute Coronary Syndromes

Although chest pain is a common presentation for acute coronary syndromes (ACSs) in older patients, it may be decreased in intensity or present atypically in this age group. In fact, pain may even be absent, with the patient instead reporting dyspnea, syncope, weakness, confusion, nausea, vomiting, or fatigue.

As a result of the wide array of atypical clinical presentations that can occur in patients with an ACS, providers should maintain a high index of suspicion for this condition in older patients who have any complaints between their waist and their nose. Any complaint within this region should be assessed with a prompt 12-lead ECG evaluation.

▶ Heart Failure

People 65 years and older are a high-risk group for heart failure.[10] Risk factors include sex, ethnicity, family history and genetics, long-term alcohol abuse, and multiple medical conditions.[10] As with ACS, prevention is aimed at lifestyle changes: cessation of tobacco use, eating a healthy diet, control of blood glucose (in patients with diabetes), exercise, weight control, and control of hypertension.

Acute exacerbation of heart failure results in pulmonary edema that decreases the ability of the lungs to exchange gases. This condition can often be assessed with the use of end-tidal carbon dioxide ($ETCO_2$) monitoring, which will likely reveal hypercapnic values. It may present with dyspnea or orthopnea. Because of the decreased oxygenation of all of the organ systems, including the brain, mental status changes may also be seen in an acute exacerbation of heart failure, including a sensation of air hunger, or the perception that the person cannot take deep enough breaths to get enough air. Peripheral edema may also indicate worsening heart failure, although in the absence of other more serious symptoms, it may be the result of any number of other circulatory, integumentary, or infectious conditions.

You should pay close attention to the position in which the patient with heart failure is found. When assessing for peripheral edema, the ankles are the logical site for evaluation. Because edema is likely to be formed in the lowest point to the ground on the patient's body, those patients who are confined to bed may present instead with sacral edema, edema that presents around the sacral region of the spinal column.

The presentation of heart failure in an older person can be masked by symptoms and signs symbolic of old age and shared by a number of chronic diseases—for example, dyspnea on exertion, easy fatigability (especially with left-sided heart failure), confusion, crackles on lung exam, orthopnea, dry cough progressing to productive cough, and dependent peripheral edema in right-sided heart failure. Acute exacerbations of heart failure are often related to poor diet (eg, high salt content leading to increased BP and increased afterload, which increases left heart failure), medication noncompliance, onset of dysrhythmias such as AF, or acute myocardial ischemia.

Prehospital treatment is unchanged from that of younger patients, although greater consideration is given to becoming familiar with the patient's medications and their implications for your proposed treatment. ETCO$_2$ should be evaluated immediately and monitored throughout the transport to observe for trends. Additional treatments by prehospital providers should include close monitoring of fluids and avoidance of excessive fluid overload, consideration of the use of CPAP, and potential use of diltiazem (Cardizem) in patients with AF or atrial flutter.

Sometimes heart failure may be exacerbated by fluid imbalances, particularly when overhydration occurs. Because the weakened and less-effective heart is not able to adequately pump normal vascular volumes, an increase in volume within the vascular system may stress the heart further. IV fluids should be administered judiciously in patients with heart failure, as even slight changes can result in significant negative outcomes, and achieving an appropriate balance of fluid and electrolyte administration may be complicated when both dehydration and heart failure are present. If hypoperfusion is present, consider the use of vasopressors in accordance with your local protocols.

▶ Dysrhythmias

Rhythm disturbances (dysrhythmias) of the heart occur when the electrical system controlling the heartbeat experiences an interruption or malfunction. These irregularities cause heartbeats that are too fast, too slow, irregular, or absent. Many people experience an occasional or harmless dysrhythmia that they may describe as a skipping, fluttering, or fast heartbeat. Dysrhythmias in older people are generally a result of age-related changes in the heart, existing cardiac disease, adverse medication effects, or a combination of these factors.

AF, which is the most common dysrhythmia among older people, increases the risk of stroke and heart failure. The fibrillating atria allow for stasis of the blood, thereby encouraging clot formation and increasing the chances that a clot fragment might travel to the brain and cause a stroke.

Bradycardias are also more common in older people. The aging conduction system may produce dysrhythmias such as sick sinus syndrome and atrioventricular blocks. Medications such as beta-blockers or calcium channel blockers can cause excessive slowing of the heart rate. Even seemingly benign conditions, such as constipation, can result in bradycardia, particularly when the patient strains to have a bowel movement. Persistent bradycardic states are often addressed with an internal pacemaker.

▶ Hypertension

More than one-half of all older persons are hypertensive.[11] The majority have isolated systolic hypertension resulting from a loss of arterial elasticity. Controlling systolic and diastolic hypertension in older people helps prevent both stroke and myocardial infarction. Unfortunately, hypertensive emergencies require a controlled decline in blood pressure that often cannot be achieved in the field, and the use of sublingual nitroglycerin for treatment of hypertensive emergencies is generally not accepted because of the risk of rebound hypertension. In case of rapid onset of symptomatic systolic hypertension, treatment aims to gradually reduce the systolic pressure with antihypertensive therapy, which can minimize cardiovascular and cerebrovascular morbidity and mortality. Regardless of which medications are used to treat these emergencies, the patient's head should be placed at a 30° angle to minimize intracranial pressure.

▶ Aneurysms

An aneurysm is a weakness in any artery that produces a balloon defect, weakening the arterial wall. This weakness may be congenital (present at birth) or acquired. In the latter case, hypertension, atherosclerotic disease, and obesity are contributing factors to development of this defect. Life-threatening aneurysms can develop in the brain, chest, or abdomen. The incidence of aneurysm increases with age.

A new headache that the patient describes as "the worst headache of my life" or a change in chronic headache patterns may signal early cerebral bleeding from an aneurysm. All too often, however, the first manifestation of an aneurysm is a sudden and devastating stroke. Use of anticoagulants for the management of cardiac disease increases the negative effects of an aneurysm by increasing the amount of time necessary for bleeding to stop. Preventive measures—proper diet, exercise, smoking cessation, and cholesterol control—aim to control the risk factors associated with hypertension and atherosclerotic diseases.

Thoracic aneurysms generally remain asymptomatic until they become large or rupture. Early symptoms may be related to compression by the aneurysm, such as difficulty swallowing or hoarseness from laryngeal nerve pressure. AAAs present typically with abdominal pain or possibly only with back pain. Asymptomatic thoracic and abdominal aneurysms that do not exceed a certain size and are not expanding are generally treated without surgery but are reassessed on a regular schedule. In an older patient with back pain, examine the chest and abdomen carefully. The treatment of abdominal emergencies is surgical, so early recognition, assessment, stabilization, and rapid transport to an appropriate medical facility are essential.

► Traumatic Aortic Disruption

Traumatic aortic disruption or aortic dissection occurs when the inside wall of the artery becomes torn and allows blood to collect between the arterial wall layers. It may occur with trauma or sustained hypertension, particularly when an abdominal aortic aneurysm (AAA) is present. Dissection weakens the arterial wall, making it prone to rupture. A thoracic dissection, for example, can produce chest pain that is difficult to differentiate from cardiac ischemia. For this reason, it is helpful to obtain blood pressure readings and to palpate a heart rate in both arms in all patients with chest pain. A systolic blood pressure difference of 15 mm Hg or higher suggests a thoracic dissection. Similarly, the presence of palpable pulses in one arm that is greater than the other is suggestive of a thoracic dissection. This blood pressure or heart rate deviation may be either continuous or transient.

► Stroke

Stroke is a significant cause of death and disability in older people. It is the leading cause of long-term disability at any age.[12] Strokes are mainly caused by atherosclerosis. The risk of stroke doubles each decade after 55 years, mirroring the increase in risk factors such as hypertension and AF.[12] Hypertension is the primary risk factor for stroke, but age, family history, smoking, diabetes, high cholesterol, and heart disease also contribute to its incidence. Normal changes of aging, such as loss of vascular elasticity, also place the older patient at an increased risk of hemorrhagic stroke. Prevention is aimed at reduction of risk factors, with emphasis on improving diet, exercising, and lowering cholesterol. Because time is crucial in stroke treatment, many communities have launched public media campaigns aimed at encouraging early recognition of stroke symptoms.

Effective prehospital acute stroke care includes early recognition, discovery of conditions that mimic strokes (such as hypoglycemia or hypoxia), and timely transport to the most appropriate facility. Use a stroke assessment tool as appropriate, taking the patient's history into account when you are assessing the components of the scale. An older person with severe arthritis may not move as well on one side, or damage from a previous stroke may make a patient's speech difficult to assess. Always ask family or caregivers for information that may help you identify deviations from the patient's normal pattern of behavior or activity.

Family members or caregivers can provide valuable input into the patient's baseline cognitive status, personality, and ability to perform ADLs (the skills required for daily self-care). When you are evaluating the patient's cognitive level, evaluate his or her ability to perform basic cognitive functions such as recalling events, learning, and remembering (such as the provider's name) and the ability to follow commands. Caregivers will also have an insight into the patient's normal responses. They will be able to inform the providers if the patient is normally agitated, irritable, or depressed; if the personality change has a recent onset; if the personality change is a symptom of an underlying disorder; or if the change is caused by the presence of unfamiliar people. ADLs include the ability to walk, the ability to dress appropriately for the environment, the ability to maintain reasonable standards for home cleanliness, and the ability to care for basic hygiene needs. Caregivers will be aware of the patient's ability to perform ADLs and can indicate whether this ability has decreased.

Documentation & Communication

A stroke is a traumatic and emotional event for the patient, and a sensitive and compassionate approach is essential. Even though these patients may not be able to communicate with you, they can often understand what you say. Communicate with them as you would any other patient—in a calm and reassuring manner.

► Transient Ischemic Attack

As discussed in more detail in Chapter 18, *Neurologic Emergencies,* any patient experiencing stroke-like symptoms should be treated as though he or she is having a stroke. Furthermore, patients who report a history of previous transient ischemic attacks (TIAs) should be considered at a much higher risk of having a stroke instead of another TIA.

■ Pathophysiology, Assessment, and Management of Neurologic Conditions

Normal age-related cognitive changes have two major features: (1) they are relatively isolated (ie, they are not associated with multiple abnormal neurologic findings that suggest specific disease states), and (2) the onset and progression of these findings are "in time" with the person's aging process (ie, the findings are not sudden or extreme, and they do not extend to other abnormalities).

► Delirium

Delirium (also known as acute brain syndrome or acute confusional state) is a symptom, not a disease. This temporary state is generally a reflection of an underlying disturbance to a person's well-being (usually a treatable physical or mental illness) and is usually reversible.

Delirium is characterized by disorganized thoughts, inattention, memory loss, disorientation, striking changes in personality and affect, hallucinations, delusions, or a decreased level of consciousness. The confusion and disorientation fluctuate with time, and hallucinations may lead to bizarre, uncharacteristic, or confusing behavior. The patient experiences a rapid alteration between mental states, such as lethargy and agitation, serious attention disruption, disorganized thinking, and changes in perception and sensation. Symptoms of delirium may mimic those associated with intoxication, drug abuse, or severe psychologic disorders, such as schizophrenia.

The process of assessing and subsequently managing the numerous causes of delirium is complicated. In such cases, you should assess for recent changes in the patient's level of consciousness or orientation. Specifically, look for an acute onset of anxiety, an inability to think logically or maintain attention, and an inability to focus. Also assess for changes in vital signs, temperature (indicating infection), glucose level, and medications—all frequent causes of delirium.

In older adults, delirium often replaces or confounds the typical presentation caused by a medical problem, an adverse medication effect, or drug or alcohol withdrawal. Causes of delirium may include medications; poisons; electrolyte imbalances; nutritional deficiencies; respiratory, cardiovascular; or nervous system disorders; hyperglycemia or hypoglycemia; environmental emergencies; trauma; and infections such as urinary tract infections (UTI) and pneumonia. Most important, prehospital providers need to consider neurologic causes (such as Alzheimer disease and Parkinson disease) and endocrine changes (such as diabetes).

Use the mnemonic "DELIRIUMS" to identify other causes of delirium:

D Drugs or toxins (including intoxication or withdrawal)
E Emotional (psychiatric)/electrolyte imbalance
L Low PaO_2 (carbon monoxide poisoning, COPD, heart failure, ACS, pneumonia)
I Infection (pneumonia, UTI, sepsis)
R Retention of stool or urine
I Ictal state (seizures)
U Undernutrition (including vitamin deficiencies) or underhydration
M Metabolism (thyroid or endocrine, electrolytes, kidneys)
S Subdural hematoma

With delirium, confusion or disorientation has an abrupt onset—occurring within hours to days—and generally resolves with treatment of the underlying problem. Given this pattern, treatment of delirium focuses on the causative disease or disorder, but establishing this link

---

YOU are the Paramedic   PART 3

While packaging the patient, you ask his daughter, "When was the last time your father seemed normal, and do you know how long he's been here?" You also ask, "How did you know to check on him?" She responds, "I haven't seen him since last night after the 10 o'clock news. I went home and he went to bed. We were supposed to go out for breakfast this morning. I don't know how long he's been there."

Recording Time: 4 Minutes	
Respirations	20 breaths/min and irregular
Pulse	74 beats/min, regular and strong
Skin	Pale and moist
Blood pressure	208/114 mm Hg
Oxygen saturation (Spo$_2$)	88% on 2 L/min by nasal cannula
Pupils	6 mm on the right, 2 mm on the left; minimally reactive

5. In asking the patient's daughter the question, "When was the last time you saw your father appear normal?" what will her response help you to determine, based on the GEMS diamond?

6. Where would you transport this patient?

7. How would you manage this patient's hypoxia?

may be complicated by the patient's inability to provide an accurate medical history and uncooperative behavior while obtaining diagnostic information.

▶ Dementia

Unlike delirium, **dementia** produces irreversible brain failure. Signs and symptoms of dementia take months to years to become apparent. They may include short-term memory loss or shortened attention span, jargon aphasia (talking nonsense), hallucinations, confusion, disorientation, difficulty in learning and retaining new information, and personality changes such as social withdrawal or inappropriate behavior.

Disorders that cause dementia include conditions that impair vascular and neurologic structures within the brain, such as infections, strokes, head injuries, poor nutrition, and medications. The two most common degenerative types of dementia in older people are Alzheimer disease (the fifth leading cause of death in the United States[13]) and multi-infarct or vascular dementia, both of which cause structural damage to the brain. Dementia may also be the result of tumors within the brain, emotional disorders, Parkinson disease, or Huntington chorea.

Risk factors that may predispose a patient to dementia include a low level of education, female sex, and African American ethnicity, although these are more accurately described as correlating factors rather than causes of dementia.

Dementia is typically diagnosed when two or more cognitive and psychomotor functions are impaired, including language, memory, visual perception, emotional behavior and/or personality, and cognitive skills. Patients with dementia experience progressive loss of cognitive function; impairments in long-term or short-term memory, or both; loss of communication skills; inability to perform daily activities; an increased tendency to become lost, even in familiar places; and changes in temperament and affect, especially increasing anger.

Because dementia is a chronic condition, most requests for emergency care will be related to new presentation of dementia-related symptoms or inability to manage behavioral disruptions, such as angry outbursts. There is no treatment for dementia, but acute changes in mental status may be related to underlying medical problems that can be treated. It is important to ascertain from caregivers the patient's baseline behaviors and abilities and to ask specifically about the changes that led them to request emergency services at the point that services are provided. Patients may provide inaccurate or conflicting information about their own conditions, and information provided by patients with advancing dementia should be checked against information provided by caregivers.

Despite the weakened physical condition of patients with dementia, you should be cautious when you are caring for patients with dementia-related complaints. These patients may not be able to rationally evaluate the impact of their behaviors and may attempt to harm you because of confusion or anxiety. Patients with dementia are also at an increased risk of victimization at the hands of caregivers because they are unable to report injury or neglect accurately. Caregiver stress is an additional concern when caring for patients with dementia; referrals to home health agencies, respite care programs, and other community services may be helpful.

▶ Alzheimer Disease

Alzheimer disease is a progressive loss of function that begins with subtle symptoms, such as frequently losing items or having difficulty recalling the names of people. With time, patients lose their ability to think, reason clearly, solve problems, and concentrate. They may forget the identities of close family members, including their spouses and children, and their own past experiences. Symptoms may present as confusion (lack of familiarity with surroundings), changes in personality or judgment, and extreme difficulty with daily activities, such as feeding, bathing, and bowel and bladder control. This progressive disease cannot be cured or reversed by any known treatment or intervention.

Progression of Alzheimer disease is classified into stages. The earliest stage, mild cognitive impairment, is more accurately described as a pre-Alzheimer stage because not all patients who develop mild cognitive impairment will progress to full-blown Alzheimer disease. Mild cognitive impairment is characterized by forgetfulness, especially forgetting earlier conversations or recent events, difficulty when attempting to perform more than one task at once, diminished problem-solving skills, and increases in the amount of time required to perform more difficult tasks.

Early-stage Alzheimer disease involves more cognitive impairment than mild cognitive impairment. It is characterized by language problems, misplacing items, getting lost on familiar routes, personality changes and loss of social skills, loss of interest in previously enjoyed activities, and difficulty performing moderately complex tasks that were once easy, such as balancing a checkbook or preparing food using a recipe.

As Alzheimer disease progresses, symptoms become more profound. Symptoms include forgetting details about current events and components of a person's life history; changes in sleep patterns, sometimes called "sundowning"; difficulty reading and writing; impairment in assessment of danger and risk; disorganized language use and construction of nonsensical sentences; hallucinations and delusions; dangerous or violent behaviors and agitation; and difficulty performing basic tasks such as preparing simple foods, choosing proper clothing, and driving.

Severe or end-stage Alzheimer disease is seen when people forget things learned in the first 2 or 3 years of life. These patients can no longer understand language, recognize even close family members, or perform basic self-care tasks, such as eating, dressing, and bathing. Patients with end-stage Alzheimer disease may no longer interact verbally with family members or caregivers. They may also have medical devices, such as gastric tubes and urinary catheters, placed to facilitate the tasks that they can no longer perform, such as eating and voiding.

Alzheimer disease is not diagnosed by specific tests, but rather through the exclusion of other causes of dementia. The only way to truly confirm the presence of Alzheimer disease is after death, by evaluating the patient's brain tissue. Affected patients develop neurofibrillary tangles, or thickened neurofilaments that encircle and obscure the nuclei of nerve cells. Neurotic plaques also form when neurons die and accumulate into clusters. When dying neurons accumulate around proteins, they develop a product known as senile plaque.

Treatment of Alzheimer disease in the prehospital and interfacility setting will generally revolve around supportive care and treatment of symptoms. Communicate slowly with these patients and consider the possibility of other illnesses. Antipsychotics or benzodiazepines may be used for combative patients who are a danger to themselves or others. Nevertheless, the use of chemical restraints should be considered only after other means of verbal containment have proved ineffective. Daily medication regimens that these patients may be prescribed include antidepressants to assist with depression and cholinesterase inhibitors (eg, donepezil, rivastigmine, and rivastigmine transdermal) to prevent further deterioration and further cognitive decline associated with Alzheimer disease. Medications that have been introduced for patients with Alzheimer disease include memantine, which is an N-methyl-D-aspartate inhibitor, and galantamine, which is an acetylcholinesterase inhibitor.

Experts have not identified a single cause for Alzheimer disease, but most believe it is not a normal part of the aging process. Although age is a significant risk factor for this disease, age is not the sole cause of its development.

▶ Parkinson Disease

Patients with **Parkinson disease**—another age-related neurologic disorder—have two or more of the following symptoms: resting tremor of an extremity, slowness of movement (bradykinesia), rigidity or stiffness of the extremities or trunk, and poor balance. Parkinson disease is discussed in Chapter 18, *Neurologic Emergencies*. Parkinson disease can affect one or both sides of the body and leads to a wide range of functional loss. It may present as dyskinesia (involuntary movements or tremors affecting one or both sides of the body), dementia, depression, autonomic dysfunction (bladder and gastrointestinal [GI] problems), and postural instability (loss of reflexes or inability to "right oneself").

▶ Seizures

The incidence of seizures (including status epilepticus) is increased in the geriatric population, partly because of this age cohort's increase in risk factors such as stroke, dementia, primary or metastatic brain tumors, and acute metabolic disorders (such as hyperglycemia, hyponatremia,

and alcohol withdrawal). Prehospital treatment for seizures is the same for younger and older patients and is discussed in Chapter 18, *Neurologic Emergencies*.

■ Pathophysiology, Assessment, and Management of Gastrointestinal Conditions

Constipation is a frequent and significant problem in older people. Although it can cause acute abdominal pain, it should not be the initial condition suspected when a patient experiences such discomfort. Instead, causes with high mortality, such as bleeding from an acute abdominal aneurysm or dead bowel from mesenteric ischemia, should be investigated first. In your assessment of a gastric emergency, ask the patient about food and fluid intake, history of abdominal complaints, current bowel and bladder habits, and medications and supplements before proceeding with a physical exam.

Symptoms of GI conditions are often vague and manifest only as diffuse abdominal pain with no particular point of origin. Older patients can have a diminished ability to detect pain, and as a result they may not display rigidity or guarding. This absent sign can hamper diagnosis, but more importantly, it can delay access to health care. If an older patient does not feel pain, he or she may not know why a fever has occurred. The patient may try to treat it at home and by the time EMS is activated, the patient is already septic and seriously ill.

Abdominal pain can also be a symptom of a cardiac condition. Imagine how difficult it would be to initially distinguish the source of abdominal pain in a 75-year-old man with a history of gastric ulcers, diverticulitis, and heart disease. Additionally, vascular pathology such as an AAA can cause abdominal pain. Comorbidity creates great difficulties for health care providers, but success can be achieved by obtaining a thorough history and performing a thorough physical exam. Consider obtaining a 12-lead ECG and establishing IV access on patients with abdominal pain who have comorbid factors. Finally, monitor vital signs and be ready for any changes in the patient's status.

Abdominal and gastric complaints often require surgical treatment, so early recognition and rapid transport for definitive hospital care are the best practice.

▶ Bowel Obstruction

Large bowel obstructions in older people are likely to be caused by cancer, impacted stool, or sigmoid volvulus. In addition, small bowel obstruction secondary to gallstones increases significantly with age. With one or more episodes of cholecystitis (inflammation of the gallbladder), the gallbladder adheres to the small bowel and, over time, creates an opening, or fistula. The stone or stones drop into the bowel and produce the obstruction. The large and small intestines are also at risk for obstruction from adhesions due to previous surgery or infection or when a segment of bowel is forced into a fascial defect (hernia) in the abdominal wall. Other causes of bowel obstruction include diet or medication use. Some medications—especially analgesics such as opiates—can lead to constipation and a bowel obstruction.

Gastroesophageal reflux disease (GERD) is prevalent within the geriatric community. These patients may take proton-pump inhibitors, calcium carbonates, or both to manage their GERD. Typically, older patients with this condition have had GERD for several years and are familiar with how to manage it. Thus, a chief complaint of GERD or indigestion should be an immediate red flag for providers; it may be a symptom of a more serious cardiac condition such as myocardial infarction. GERD is typically a diagnosis of exclusion that is made after serial ECGs and cardiac enzyme measurements are performed to rule out a cardiac event. Providers treating patients with GERD symptoms (and potentially cardiac problems) should be sure to perform a 12-lead ECG and transport these patients to a medical facility capable of performing percutaneous coronary intervention.

▶ Biliary Diseases

In addition to presenting in conjunction with small bowel obstructions, biliary diseases—including cirrhosis, hepatitis, and cholecystitis—may occur independently in older patients. Signs and symptoms of biliary disease include jaundice, fever, right upper quadrant pain with possible radiation to the upper back or shoulder, and vomiting or nausea. Jaundice may be more profound in paler patients because less melanin is present to interfere with visibility of bilirubin. Although these diseases cause fever, this response may be muted in older patients. Pain sensation may be altered as well, resulting in unusual referral paths or the absence of abdominal pain.

Pain management may be indicated for patients with acute cholecystitis. Be cautious when administering opiates to older patients, however, because of their decreased ability to compensate for the cardiovascular and respiratory changes that may accompany use of these medications.

▶ Peptic Ulcer Disease

Older patients are more likely than younger ones to have stomach or duodenal ulcers (peptic ulcer disease). The main risk factors for development of peptic ulcer are regular use of NSAIDs and infection with *Helicobacter pylori* (an ulcer-associated bacterium of the stomach), both of which are more common in older patients. Other medications have also been implicated in ulcer formation. Social factors, such as high-stress professions, and certain personality types have been associated with ulcer formation as well. The main symptom of peptic ulcer disease is dyspepsia (gnawing, burning pain in the upper abdomen), which usually improves immediately after eating but returns

several hours later. Other causes of dyspepsia include acid reflux, gastritis, and gastric cancer.

▶ Gastrointestinal Bleeding

GI bleeding also becomes more common with age, and it is almost always the result of either physiologic changes that lead to an increased likelihood of bleeding systemically or pathologic processes that specifically impact the digestive system. A number of normal changes of aging increase the time needed for the geriatric patient's body to achieve hemostasis, including decreased vascular tone and thinning of various epithelial tissues. Decreased rates of peristalsis also increase the likelihood that irritating substances will damage the gastric lining. In addition, older patients are more likely to take medications that alter coagulation, including warfarin, aspirin, and heparin. Pathologic processes within the GI system that are sometimes responsible for bleeding include ulcers and varices; cancers of the stomach, esophagus, colon, and rectum; diverticulitis; cirrhosis; and bowel obstructions.

Although the source of GI bleeding may vary, the signs and symptoms vary more by the location of the bleeding than by its origin. Bleeding from the esophagus is most commonly associated with varices and alcohol abuse; the patient will present with violent vomiting of emesis that contains almost no food and a large quantity of bright red, uncoagulated blood. Bleeding from the stomach may produce either red or darker coffee-ground emesis, and it is most commonly associated with peptic ulcer disease. Bloody stool is usually indicative of bleeding from the lower GI system, although blood from the stomach may be digested and appear as dark, tarry stool. Bright red blood in the stool usually comes from the large intestine or rectum and may be caused by diverticulitis, large bowel obstructions, anal fissures, or hemorrhoids. In general, the darker the blood, the longer it has been in the body and, therefore, the farther the distance between the site of bleeding and the portal of exit.

Upper GI hemorrhage occurs in conjunction with bleeding from the esophagus, stomach, or duodenum **Figure 44-5**. When severe, this condition is a true medical emergency that must be recognized and assessed quickly. Not only are older people more prone to upper GI bleeding, but they are also in need of urgent surgery and at a greater risk of complications and death from this cause.

It is not possible to determine the cause of upper GI bleeding without an endoscopic examination (inspection of the inside of a hollow organ or body cavity) of the esophagus, stomach, and duodenum. Nevertheless, obtaining a thorough history can provide you with clues to the cause. Regular use of NSAIDs or alcohol may result in bleeding from irritation of the lining of the stomach or from ulcers (a hollowing out or disintegration of tissue) in the stomach or duodenum. Forceful vomiting can cause tears in the esophagus that lead to bleeding. Cirrhosis of the liver from long-term alcohol use or chronic infectious

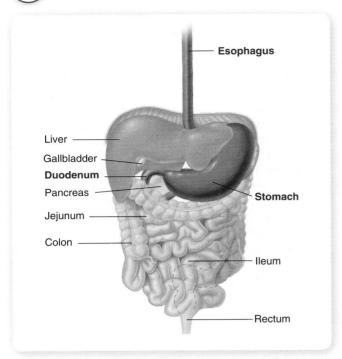

Figure 44-5 Upper gastrointestinal bleeding occurs in the stomach, esophagus, and duodenum.
© Jones & Bartlett Learning.

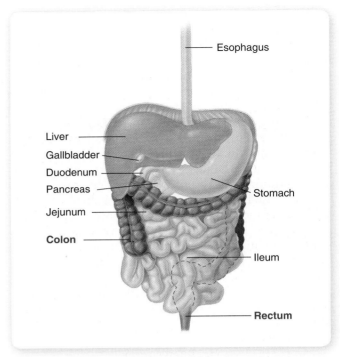

Figure 44-6 Lower gastrointestinal bleeding takes place primarily in the colon and rectum.
© Jones & Bartlett Learning.

hepatitis may cause enlargement of the veins (varices) in the esophagus; these varices can subsequently rupture and result in massive bleeding. Stomach cancer or esophageal cancer can also produce upper GI bleeding. Recent weight loss or difficulty swallowing would raise the suspicion of cancer as the source of bleeding.

Lower GI hemorrhage primarily describes bleeding from the colon and rectum and should never simply be attributed to hemorrhoids **Figure 44-6**. Colon polyps and colon cancer are also possible causes, among others. Minor lower GI bleeding is characterized by small amounts of red blood covering formed brown stools or scant amounts of red blood noticed on the toilet paper. Severe lower GI bleeding is characterized by passing significant amounts of red blood or maroon-colored stools.

Assessment should begin with identifying risk factors such as a history of previous lower GI bleeding, symptoms or signs suggestive of colon cancer, recent constipation or diarrhea, and use of medications such as blood thinners. Treat the patient for shock. Blood administration may be necessary during interfacility transport if the patient's hematocrit and hemoglobin decrease significantly. Severe lower GI bleeding requires immediate transport to the nearest ED.

Some signs and symptoms of GI bleeding are associated with hypovolemia that occurs from the blood loss—namely, agitation, dizziness, syncope, hypotension, and changes in mental status. Others may be associated with the disease processes that caused the bleeding, including jaundice, hepatomegaly, constipation or diarrhea, pain with voiding, nausea, and abdominal pain.

When you arrive at the scene of a patient with GI bleeding, it is more important to assess the severity of the bleeding than to determine the cause of bleeding. Slower bleeding is characterized by emesis with coffee-grounds appearance. With minor bleeding, the pulse rate and systolic blood pressure are normal. Brisk bleeding presents with hematemesis (vomiting red blood) or melena (black, tarlike stools). Note that melena—not pain—is the most common presenting symptom of GI bleeding. Prehospital treatment is supportive, including adequate pain control.

Regardless of the cause of GI bleeding, treatment should focus on recognition and management of hypovolemic shock, along with transport to a facility capable of providing definitive care: many patients with GI bleeding may require surgery to repair the site of injury or disease. Be cautious when administering fluids, and bear in mind that geriatric patients' compensatory mechanisms may be altered because of normal aging processes. Finally, keep in mind that these patients may be on blood-thinning medications (eg, warfarin) that prevent them from forming clots following major injuries.

Pathophysiology, Assessment, and Management of Renal Conditions

Although the kidneys of an older adult may be capable of dealing with the day-to-day demands of the person's body, they may not be able to meet unusual challenges, such as those imposed by illness.

▶ Urinary Tract Infections

UTIs are common in the older adult population.[14] UTIs usually develop in the lower urinary tract (urethra and bladder) when normal flora (the bacteria that naturally populate the skin) enter the urethra and begin to grow there. Although UTIs are usually more common in women due to the relatively short female urethra and its close proximity to the vagina and rectum, after age 50 years, there is an increase in UTIs in men because of obstruction of the urethra by the prostate. Common risk factors for UTIs include diabetes, prostatitis, cystocele (prolapse of the bladder into the vagina), urethrocele (prolapse of the urethra into the vagina), kidney obstruction, and indwelling urinary catheters.

While you are performing a physical assessment of a patient with UTI, you may notice a fever, shortness of breath, GI symptoms, neurologic symptoms, poor urinary output, increased urinary frequency, and hematuria. The patient will typically report painful urination, frequent urges to urinate, and difficulty urinating. You should evaluate the patient's indwelling catheter, if applicable, for sediment, opacity, color, or presence of blood. A strong odor may be present. Later signs and symptoms may include hypotension, tachycardia, diaphoresis, and pale skin.

▶ Renal Failure

Renal failure is a sudden decrease in the rate of filtration through the glomeruli, causing toxins to accumulate in the blood. If the kidneys are no longer able to excrete waste, concentrate urine, and control electrolytes, pH, or blood pressure, then renal failure develops. Risk factors for chronic renal failure include diabetes, cardiac disease, pyelonephritis, hypertension, autoimmune disorders, glomerulonephritis, and polypharmacy. Chronic renal failure may require lifelong hemodialysis or a kidney transplant. Hemodialysis is a process in which the patient is attached to a hemodialysis machine for a period of 3 to 4 hours three times a week so that his or her blood can be filtered through the machine and wastes in it removed.

Whereas dialysis treatments are generally considered a basic life support (BLS) nonemergency transport, if a patient misses a treatment, the situation can evolve into an ALS emergency. Signs and symptoms of such a renal emergency include hypertension, headache, anxiety, fatigue, anorexia, vomiting, increased dark urination, altered mental status, and seizures. A thorough assessment will include obtaining a 12-lead ECG; electrolyte changes may be noted on the ECG. Although all of the patient's vital signs should be monitored regularly, you should not take blood pressures on the same arm that has a fistula. $ETCO_2$ should be monitored throughout the transport, as should breath sounds and bowel sounds. The patient should be transported to a hospital that has hemodialysis capabilities. IV fluids should be administered to assist circulation as necessary. If dysrhythmias are present, they should be treated according to current American Heart Association ACLS guidelines.

If the patient has a urinary catheter in place, urine output should be closely monitored and documented. Also, document the patient's fluid input (in the form of fluid resuscitation) and relay this information upon patient transfer.

▶ Incontinence

Bowel and bladder continence require anatomically correct GI and genitourinary tracts, functioning and intact sphincters, and properly working cognitive and physical functions. Although urinary incontinence (involuntary loss of urine) can have significant social and emotional impacts, relatively few people admit to this problem and even fewer seek treatment for it. Over time, incontinence can lead to skin irritation, skin breakdown, and UTIs.

As people age, both the capacity of the bladder and the strength of the sphincter muscles decrease. Because pressure on the urinary sphincter is responsible for triggering recognition of the need to urinate, a decrease in sphincter tone may keep older people from realizing that their bladder is full until they can no longer wait to urinate. As a consequence, older people may find it difficult to postpone voiding or may have involuntary bladder contractions. Nighttime incontinence may also be problematic for older people because the weakened sensations of the need to urinate are less likely to wake them from sleep. Additionally, incontinence sometimes occurs when older adults recognize the need to urinate and have adequate sphincter control to prevent accidental bladder release, but their physical ability to move to the restroom is limited. In this case, simple modifications, such as placing a toilet chair in the person's bedroom, may eliminate incontinence.

Two major types of incontinence are distinguished: stress and urge. Stress incontinence occurs during activities such as coughing, laughing, sneezing, lifting, and exercise. Urge incontinence is triggered by hot or cold fluids, running water, and sometimes the simple thought of going to the bathroom.

Because incontinence can be embarrassing, always be discreet and nonjudgmental when you are addressing this topic with patients. If you have enough time and the patient's condition allows you to do so, you may want to help the patient gather his or her own incontinence supplies before being transported to the hospital. If the patient experiences a loss of bladder control, you should cover the patient until his or her clothing can be changed. During long transports, you should make an effort to reduce the amount of time that the patient wears urine-soaked clothing or absorbent undergarments; beyond the temporary discomfort and shame associated with incontinence, a patient who must sit in urine for a long time may experience new or worsening skin breakdown.

The opposite of incontinence is urinary retention or difficulty urinating. Patients may have difficulty voiding or absence of voiding as a result of many medical causes. In men, benign enlargement of the prostate (also known as benign prostatic hypertrophy) can place pressure on the urethra, making voiding difficult and frequent. Patients with this condition may experience difficulty sleeping because of the frequent need to urinate with little production. Bladder infections and UTIs can also cause inflammation that results in retention of urine; the pain associated with urination during such infections may lead patients to intentionally avoid urination. The placement and subsequent removal of a urinary catheter can lead to retention as well. Because of the loss of elasticity of the bladder wall, some patients are able to urinate and empty most of the bladder's contents while retaining a small amount of urine; this residual retention may then lead to an increased risk of UTIs.

Temporary urinary retention may lead to pain and abdominal distention. In severe or prolonged cases of urinary retention, patients may have acute or chronic renal failure.

Pathophysiology, Assessment, and Management of Endocrine Conditions

In many older patients, endocrine changes may have occurred earlier in life and been diagnosed before intervention by prehospital providers became necessary. In particular, geriatric patients may have endocrine-related diseases such as Graves disease (hyperthyroidism), Addison disease (hypoadrenalism), Cushing syndrome (hyperadrenalism), osteoporosis, or diabetes.

▶ Diabetic Disorders

In the United States, one out of every four people older than 65 years has diabetes—primarily type 2 diabetes (formerly called adult-onset, or non–insulin-dependent diabetes mellitus).[15] Type 1 diabetes has historically been referred to as insulin-dependent diabetes mellitus or juvenile diabetes, because it generally affects children. Many normal changes of aging contribute to the development of diabetes. The most common risk factor for this disease is having more than one chronic disease, and many older people with diabetes also have hypertension, heart disease, and stroke. Other risk factors for diabetes include a family history of diabetes, genetics, age, diet, obesity, and a sedentary lifestyle. Management of diabetes is complicated when other acute diseases are present, particularly infections; because older adults are more likely to have several comorbid disorders, this concern is especially pertinent for them. In addition, they are often on many medications.

In the emergency setting, diabetes can result in two life-threatening conditions: hypoglycemia and hyperglycemia. Normal blood glucose levels range from approximately 60 to 120 mg/dL. Hypoglycemia occurs when blood glucose levels drop to 45 mg/dL or less, whereas hyperglycemia occurs when the levels of glucose in the blood exceed the normal range.

Geriatric patients with diabetes are at increased risk for hypoglycemia for several reasons: confusion about medication doses or usage, inadequate or irregular dietary intake, inability to recognize the warning signs due to cognitive problems, and blunted warning signs.

YOU are the Paramedic   PART 4

Your partner places the patient on a nonrebreathing mask. The patient's medications include prednisone, furosemide, omeprazole, metoprolol, warfarin, nitroglycerin, and diltiazem.

Recording Time: 8 Minutes	
Respirations	24 breaths/min and irregular
Pulse	78 beats/min, regular and strong
Skin	Pale and moist
Blood pressure	202/106 mm Hg
Oxygen saturation (Spo$_2$)	90% on 15 L/min by NRM
Pupils	Unchanged

8. What do the patient's medications tell you about his current clinical condition?

9. Which type of medical history would you suspect?

In a geriatric patient, delirium may be the only indication of hypoglycemia. Other symptoms may include mental status changes and confusion, diaphoresis, and decreased respiratory effort. New-onset diabetes in geriatric patients often follows a mild progression and produces no symptoms.

As mentioned previously, older people with diabetes and consistently high blood glucose levels are more prone to HHS/HONK, than to diabetic ketoacidosis (DKA). DKA is a life-threatening condition that is associated predominantly with type 1 diabetes (patients who have this condition tend to be young—teenagers and young adults). See Chapter 23, *Endocrine Emergencies*, for more information on this condition.

The most frequent cause of HHS/HONK is infection, but other potential risk factors include hypothermia, hyperthermia, cardiac disease, pancreatitis, and stroke. The patient is likely to present with hyperglycemia (blood glucose level is generally greater than 600 mg/dL) and acute confusion with dehydration, although signs of dehydration may be altered in older adults (Table 44-3). With HHS/HONK, hyperglycemia and hyperosmolarity lead to osmotic diuresis and an osmotic shift of fluid to the intravascular space, resulting in further intracellular dehydration. Signs and symptoms include dizziness, confusion, altered mental status, and polydipsia. Prehospital treatment remains the same as for younger patients, albeit with a cautious approach to fluid resuscitation.

Assessment of hyperglycemia and hypoglycemia is complicated by many of the changes associated with aging. Changes in peripheral vascular function, in particular, make assessment of skin condition for key signs of hypoglycemia much more difficult because many older patients may be paler and cooler at baseline. Diaphoresis may also be less prominent due to changes in regulatory mechanisms and secretory functions of the skin. Moreover, baseline alterations of mentation may be confused with acute mental status changes that are related to either hyperglycemia or hypoglycemia.

In patients with suspected diabetic emergencies, you should assess all vital signs—including blood pressure, blood glucose levels, temperature, and distal pulses—every 15 minutes and monitor them for changes. Obtain

a 12-lead ECG to evaluate the patient for other possible causes of the emergency. Throughout the transport, use capnography to monitor the patient's $ETCO_2$ ventilatory status. SpO_2 is a valuable tool in patients of all ages, but poor perfusion in an older adult may make it more difficult to rely on the SpO_2 values obtained. You may need to look for alternative sites to obtain a reliable reading.

Treatment of diabetic emergencies in geriatric patients is no different than treatment in other populations, although careful attention must be paid to fluid resuscitation and electrolyte balance in older adults.

Prevention of type 2 diabetes focuses on changes in lifestyle that include dietary restrictions, exercise, and controlling obesity. Long-term management may include limiting carbohydrate intake and use of insulin and oral antihyperglycemic agents. Diabetes management also focuses on preventing many of the devastating systemic effects of the disease, including aggressive wound management, frequent screening for impaired renal function, and management of pain associated with neuropathy.

▶ Thyroid Disorders

Thyroid abnormalities increase with aging. Many older patients remain asymptomatic, however, with their disease being diagnosed only when a routine blood test reveals a thyroid problem. Adult hypothyroidism (*myxedema*) is manifested by a general slowing of the body's metabolic processes due to the reduction or absence of thyroid hormone. In patients with hypothyroidism, the signs and symptoms may match those seen with normal aging: cold intolerance, constipation, dry skin, weakness, and weight gain. Prior thyroidectomy is also more common in geriatric patients, who typically take synthetic thyroid hormones to compensate for the body's inability to produce them.

With acute-onset hyperthyroidism (thyrotoxicosis), the presentation can be blunted in older people; although tachycardia is generally present, older patients may experience less tremor, anxiety, or hyperactive reflexes compared to younger patients. AF is more likely to be induced by an overactive thyroid gland in a geriatric patient. A smaller percentage of older patients with hyperthyroidism present with symptoms opposite of those expected: weakness, lethargy, and depression.

Patients with hyperthyroidism or hypothyroidism are likely to require supplemental oxygen. Hypoglycemia may need correction with 50% dextrose (D_{50}). Hypothyroid conditions may lead to diminished respiratory effort that may require positive pressure ventilation.

Continued decrease in the patient's hormone levels may lead to myxedema coma, an extreme manifestation of hypothyroidism that is accompanied by physiologic decompensation. Myxedema coma is more likely in women than in men and occurs primarily in the geriatric population.[16] See Chapter 23, *Endocrine Emergencies*, for more information on these conditions.

Table 44-3	**Signs of Dehydration in Older Adults**

- Dry tongue
- Longitudinal furrows in the tongue
- Dry mucous membranes
- Weak upper body musculature
- Confusion
- Difficulty in speech
- Sunken eyes

Pathophysiology, Assessment, and Management of Immunologic Conditions

Infections in older persons can be severe and dangerous. Sepsis occurs when the patient develops an infection (which may be caused by bacteria, fungi, or viruses) and microorganisms or their toxic products enter the bloodstream. This disease state is a serious problem that you should know how to recognize and treat. Think of sepsis whenever you see a hot, flushed patient who is also tachycardic and tachypneic. Other signs of sepsis include an oral temperature of greater than 100.4°F (38°C) or less than 96.8°F (36°C), a respiratory rate of more than 20 breaths/min or a partial pressure of carbon dioxide in the blood ($PaCO_2$) of less than 32 mm Hg, and a pulse greater than 90 beats/min. If available, consider measuring lactate levels with a point-of-care device. Some systems have the ability to call a sepsis alert based on these criteria or an ETCO_2 of 25 mm Hg or less.

In older patients, the first sign of sepsis may be confusion or otherwise altered mental status. Because of the systemic nature of sepsis, along with the polypharmacy and comorbidities that tend to exist in the geriatric population, elevated temperature and altered vital signs may not always be evident in older patients with this condition. Care is discussed in Chapter 26, *Infectious Diseases*.

Pathophysiology, Assessment, and Management of Toxicologic Conditions

As the number of uses for medications increases, the likelihood of adverse drug reactions and interactions increases in tandem. Older adults are particularly prone to adverse reactions, even when they take drugs at doses that would be safe in younger people. This increased incidence of adverse drug reactions among older people seems to reflect aging-related changes in drug metabolism because of diminished hepatic function; in drug elimination because of diminished renal function; in body composition, including increased body fat and decreased body water, which alters the distribution of drugs through the various body compartments; and in the responsiveness to drugs that affect the central nervous system. A change in any one of these processes can lead to toxic effects in older people.

Other body changes may affect medication use by geriatric patients in a more general way. As vision declines with age, reading small print becomes more difficult. Night vision becomes less acute, so reading labels in dim light can lead to errors. Short-term memory loss may lead to forgetfulness about whether medications have been taken.

▶ Polypharmacy and Medication Noncompliance

Polypharmacy, the use of multiple medications, is common among older adults. Polypharmacy may be therapeutic when multiple drugs are used to manage different medical problems, but it may prove harmful when these medications interact, because their doses have not been adjusted to account for the multiple medications or multiple organs that are affected.[17] Geriatric patients are particularly prone to having multiple chronic diseases, which may lead to a vicious cycle: the presence of multiple disease states leads to the use of multiple medications, which increases the likelihood of adverse reactions, which in turn leads to treatment with more medications. A person's risk of ending up in the hospital because of an adverse reaction to a medication increases with the number of drugs taken—a factor that should be considered when you are assessing the patient's chief complaint. Ultimately, the best dosage of a drug for an older patient is the lowest dosage that will achieve a therapeutic effect.

Another issue that may sometimes arise and compound the patient's medical problems is caregiver theft of medications, which then leaves the patient undermedicated. This risk is not isolated to home caregivers, but can also occur in long-term care facilities. Such a crime should be suspected if patients report immense pain and their vital signs correspond to an undermedicated state.

Medication noncompliance in older patients is also associated with negative effects on health. Many patients—not just older patients—do not follow instructions or advice on the use of their medications. Because older adults take more medications than the rest of the population, noncompliance issues are more likely to arise with these patients. Noncompliance issues include failure to fill a prescription (eg, the patient does not have the money to pay for the medication or does not see the benefits of it), improper administration of medication (eg, the patient decreases the dosage to make the prescription last longer), discontinuation of medication (eg, the patient feels better and decides not to take the medication), and taking inappropriate medications (eg, the patient had medication left over from a previous prescription or shares the medicine with family or friends). Patients may be taking medications prescribed by more than one physician, each of whom dispenses prescriptions without knowledge of the others' orders. Patients may also take over-the-counter medications or medications prescribed for a family member or friend. Compliance can become complicated because of difficult drug regimens that may change based on physician evaluation. Difficult medication regimens may be forgotten by the patient, especially if one has changed recently. Furthermore, patients may not understand the prescribed drug regimen or may have difficulty opening the medication containers.

▶ Pharmacokinetics

Another factor contributing to the toxic effects of drugs in older adults is aging-related alterations in pharmacokinetics—that is, the absorption, distribution, metabolism, and excretion of drugs. Geriatric patients are predisposed to medicine-related reactions owing to the previously mentioned age-related physiologic changes that occur in body systems and body composition. For example, an increase in the proportion of adipose tissue can prolong the half-life of a drug in the body. In particular, medications that affect the central nervous system are the most common source of adverse or unexpected reactions, with barbiturates and benzodiazepines being the drugs most often associated with toxic effects.[18] For this reason, when caring for older patients, you should consider reducing the dosage of medications that affect the central nervous system. For example, consider administering 25 mcg instead of 50 mcg of fentanyl for pain relief. A reduction in the nervous system response—especially the decrease in parasympathetic activity typically seen with the aging process—increases the risk that adverse anticholinergic effects will occur. Reduced beta-adrenergic receptor sensitivity (which is responsible for bronchodilation) makes most bronchodilator medications less effective in older patients. The use of diuretics and antihypertensive medications can cause hypotension and orthostatic changes due to reduced cardiac output and a decrease in total body water. Finally, decreased glucose tolerance may cause medications such as diuretics and corticosteroids to have hyperglycemic effects in older adults.

Pharmacokinetics may also be influenced by diet, smoking, alcohol consumption, and use of other drugs. Drugs such as digoxin that depend on the liver and kidney for metabolism and excretion are particularly likely to accumulate to toxic levels in older patients. With most drugs, little is known about the optimal dosage for older adults, because nearly all clinical trials to establish the safe dosages of drugs are performed in young populations. For the most part, however, dosages for geriatric patients need to be reduced compared with those for younger patients ("start low, go slow").

Although almost any medication can produce toxic effects in an older person, certain medications and their classes are implicated more often than others are. Antibiotics, anticoagulants, digoxin, diuretics, antineoplastic agents, and NSAIDs commonly cause toxic reactions.[19] Typically, toxic effects present with psychiatric symptoms (such as hallucinations, paranoia, delusions, agitation, and psychosis) and cognitive impairment (such as delirium, confusion, disorientation, amnesia, stupor, and coma) **Figure 44-7** .

▶ Drug and Alcohol Abuse

Many geriatric patients see multiple physicians for various disorders that may include pain management or require sedation. Some states have instituted a statewide system to control and monitor scheduled medication distribution,

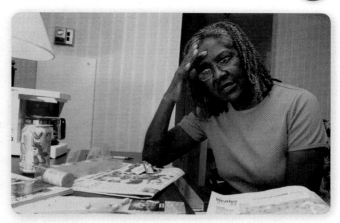

Figure 44-7 The toxic effects of medications may initially manifest in the form of confusion.
© Jones & Bartlett Learning.

which is then used by all pharmacies in the state. These measures help prevent the problem of the same medications being prescribed by multiple physicians.

Substance abuse among older adults is often in response to a life-changing event such as the loss of a spouse, declining health, or low self-esteem. The prevalence of alcohol and drug misuse among older people is also attributable to the multiplicity of medications that are prescribed for them and their heightened vulnerability to abuse owing to the effects of aging. Their decreased body mass and total body water means that alcohol consumption leads to higher concentrations of blood alcohol in older adults compared to consumption of the same amount of alcohol by younger adults; at the same time, the combination of digestive, renal, and hepatic system changes leads to slower elimination of alcohol from the older adult's body.

As the geriatric population continues to grow and members of this age cohort experience even more chronic disabilities, the likelihood of substance abuse–related problems in this group will increase. Recognizing substance abuse in older people can be difficult. If they have engaged in this behavior for a long time, it may be well hidden from—or even accepted by—family and friends. Because substance abuse can complicate your field assessment and treatment, it is important to ask about this issue.

■ Pathophysiology, Assessment, and Management of Psychologic Conditions

As people age, they encounter new experiences and changes to routines they may have established over many years. Some of these experiences may produce physical and psychological changes in the older adult. For example, dementia may result from Alzheimer disease, chronic alcohol abuse, cumulative effects of multiple strokes, or nutritional deficiencies. The loss of loved ones or the moving away of family may cause loneliness. Financial worries, dissatisfaction with living arrangements, or doubts about the significance of one's life accomplishments may become a significant concern as well. Such thoughts often produce psychologic distress and physical pain, which may manifest as abnormal behavior.

All too often, health care providers incorrectly consider anxiety and depression to be a normal part of aging—a belief that can be considered ageism. Ageism is discrimination against older people because of their age. To avoid engaging in ageism and to provide proper care to the geriatric population, particularly those with mental health conditions, you must first identify your own attitudes toward older people and the mentally ill. With this awareness, you will be able to perform a complete physical and psychosocial assessment without bias and will understand the complexity of caring for older people.

Depression is not part of normal aging, but rather a medical disease. Depression can be a normal, short-term reaction to a particular event. When sadness, restlessness, fatigue, and hopelessness persist for weeks, however, this issue becomes a larger concern. Depression in the geriatric population is a major health problem, the incidence of which is growing in tandem with the progressive aging of the population. This trend can be attributed to increases in polypathology, psychosocial stress, and aging-related changes in the brain that collectively lead to greater cognitive impairment, increased medical illness, dependency on health care services, and more suicide attempts **Figure 44-8** . Depression may also occur when a patient takes a variety of medications; such polypharmacy is more likely when the person has multiple medical conditions that result in greater vulnerability to toxic effects.

Depression in geriatric patients can mimic the effects of many other medical problems (such as dementia). Risk factors for depression in older people include a history of depression, chronic disease, and loss (function, independence, or significant others). This condition may be difficult to recognize in older people because many do not want to complain about feeling sad, worthless, or unwanted.

The high suicide rate among the geriatric population can be attributed to a variety of reasons.[20] Many geriatric patients see no other way out when they have a terminal illness or debilitating cardiac or neurologic condition (such as severe heart disease or stroke).

When you are responding to psychologic emergencies with geriatric patients, you need to determine whether the situation is a true behavioral emergency or a behavioral crisis. A behavioral emergency implies a significant risk of serious harm to self or others unless intervention is undertaken immediately. Examples include serious suicidal states, potential violence, and impaired judgment that could leave a person at risk of injury or death. In a behavioral crisis, the patient's ability to cope is insufficient and he or she becomes overwhelmed, sending the patient in search of alternative methods of coping **Figure 44-9** .

When the situation to which you are responding involves a patient with mental illness or a psychotic episode, always remember that a person who is psychotic is out of touch with reality. Many forms of psychotic behavior are possible, including schizophrenic and paranoid behaviors. All symptoms associated with psychotic conditions may not be present when a patient is having an episode, however. Clues to psychotic behavior might include the patient becoming excited or angry for no apparent reason, engaging in antisocial activity or being a loner, and sleeping during the day and staying awake at night. You should consider underlying medical conditions as possible causes of altered behavior. Information about changes in the patient's normal routine may be obtained from family, friends, or caregivers.

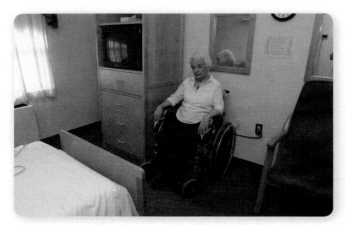

Figure 44-8 Isolation and chronic medical problems are among the factors that contribute to depression in older adults.

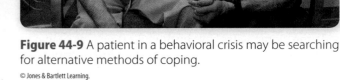

Figure 44-9 A patient in a behavioral crisis may be searching for alternative methods of coping.

Pathophysiology, Assessment, and Management of Integumentary Conditions

Geriatric patients are at high risk for secondary infection after they experience breaks in the skin, skin tumors, and fungal or viral infections of the skin. Many wounds that heal quickly in younger patients take much longer to heal in older patients. Cumulative sun and toxin exposure also increases older adults' likelihood of developing cancerous skin lesions.

▶ Herpes Zoster

Herpes zoster (shingles) is caused by the reactivation of the varicella virus on nerve roots. This condition is more common in the older population, especially if they had chickenpox during the early years of life. Most people with herpes zoster are in good health, but people with cancer or immunosuppression are at higher risk of reactivation of varicella. Shingles can affect any nerve in the body, but the thoracic nerves and the ophthalmic division of the trigeminal nerve are the most common targets. The disease usually starts with pain in the affected area. Subsequently, a cluster of tiny blisters (vesicles) erupts on reddened skin in the same area. The rash is typically unilateral; it rarely crosses the midline.

One of the most common complications of herpes zoster is pain, or postherpetic neuralgia. During the acute phase of the infection, the person may have severe pain and require narcotic pain relievers. Antiviral medications can be used, preferably within 48 hours of the activation of the disease. These medications decrease healing time, new lesion formation, and pain.

▶ Cellulitis

Cellulitis is an acute inflammation in the skin caused by a bacterial infection **Figure 44-10**. This condition usually affects the lower extremities. Symptoms include fever, chills, and general malaise. Cellulitis can cause warmth, swelling, redness, tenderness, and enlarged nodes in the affected area. Blood tests may show elevation of the white blood cell count and the presence of bacteria. Treatments include antibiotic therapy, ensuring adequate fluid intake, and local dressings if there is an open wound.

▶ Pressure Ulcers

Pressure ulcers, also called decubitis ulcers or pressure sores, are a major concern in the care of geriatric patients, particularly those who are bedridden. They occur when pressure is applied to body tissue, resulting in a lack of perfusion and ultimately necrosis. Possible risk factors include brain or spinal cord injury, neuromuscular disorders, and nutritional problems. These ulcers are exacerbated by fecal and urinary incontinence, particularly when the patient is exposed to saturated materials for a prolonged time. Sores are most commonly located on the lower legs, sacrum, greater trochanter, and gluteus maximus.

Pressure ulcers can be classified as follows:

- **Stage 1.** A persistent area of skin redness (without a break in the skin) does not disappear when pressure is relieved.
- **Stage 2.** A partial thickness of skin is lost and may appear as an abrasion, blister, or shallow crater.
- **Stage 3.** A full thickness of skin is lost, exposing the subcutaneous tissues; it presents as a deep crater with or without undermining adjacent tissue.
- **Stage 4.** A full thickness of skin and subcutaneous tissues are lost, exposing muscle or bone.

Prehospital treatment for pressure ulcers is mostly BLS care. However, ulcers that remain untreated can evolve to become a source of significant infection and potentially lead to sepsis. When you observe pressure ulcers that are suggestive of infection in a patient, you should monitor the patient's body temperature and vital signs, administer oxygen if needed, establish an IV line, and consider administration of a fluid bolus.

Pathophysiology, Assessment, and Management of Musculoskeletal Conditions

Changes in physical abilities can affect older adults' confidence in their mobility. Many older adults choose to limit their physical activity due to a fear of falling and sustaining injuries. The muscle system atrophies and weakens with age. Muscle fibers become smaller and fewer in number, motor neurons decline in number, and strength declines. The ligaments and cartilage of the joints lose their elasticity. Cartilage also goes through degenerative changes with aging, contributing to arthritis.

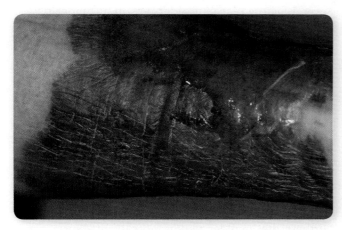

Figure 44-10 Cellulitis is a localized, acute inflammation in the skin caused by bacterial infection.

The stooped posture of older people reflects atrophy of the supporting structures of the body. Many older patients will show some degree of kyphosis (outward curvature of the thoracic spine). Lost height in older adults generally results from compression in the spinal column, first in the disks and then from the process of osteoporosis in the vertebral bodies.

▶ Osteoporosis

Osteoporosis is characterized by a decrease in bone mass leading to reduction in bone strength and greater susceptibility to fracture. The extent of bone loss that a person experiences is influenced by numerous factors, including genetics, smoking, level of activity, diet, hormonal factors, and body weight and structure. Use of anticonvulsant medications, steroids, and alcohol also increases the likelihood of developing osteoporosis. Generally speaking, women are more likely to develop osteoporosis than men are.[21]

Osteoporosis is classified into two categories. The most rapid loss of bone, which typically occurs in women during the years following menopause, is identified as type I osteoporosis. The most common fractures that occur from type I osteoporosis are radius and hip fractures. Type II osteoporosis is seen in both men and women, generally older than 50 years. The most common fractures associated with type II osteoporosis include hip and vertebral fractures. The vertebral fractures may cause the patient to develop dorsal kyphosis.

Although hormone replacement therapy (HRT) was the preferred treatment to prevent or slow osteoporosis in the past, medications that specifically target the bones are now available. These medications, which are classified as bisphosphonates, include alendronate (Fosamax) and ibandronate (Boniva); they generally have lower risks than HRT. The bisphosphonates are also useful in the treatment of bone loss in men, which is generally not true of HRT. Calcium and vitamin D supplementation is another treatment for the condition, and many other medications are available to improve bone strength. Older people should remain active and perform low-impact exercises to maintain bone and muscle strength.

▶ Arthritis

Osteoarthritis is a progressive disease of the joints that destroys cartilage, promotes the formation of bone spurs in joints, and leads to joint stiffness. This type of arthritis is thought to result from "wear and tear" and, in some cases, from repetitive trauma to the joints. Typically, osteoarthritis affects several joints of the body—most commonly those in the hands, knees, hips, and spine. Patients report pain and stiffness that gets worse with exertion; some also report increasing pain with changes in outside temperature or humidity levels. The end result is often substantial disability and disfigurement. Patients are typically treated with anti-inflammatory medications and physical therapy to improve the range of motion. Some patients may use topical lidocaine patches or opiates to manage pain, along with herbal supplements that claim to improve cartilage

health. Although arthritis is not life threatening, patients may seek emergency care for pain management.

Rheumatoid arthritis (RA) is a long-term autoimmune disorder that is characterized by inflammation of the joints and the surrounding tissues. Symptoms are usually bilateral and most commonly affect the hands, feet, wrists, ankles, and knees. Patients may note pain and stiffness at the joints, with smaller joints in the fingers and toes usually being affected long before larger joints, such as the elbows, shoulders, knees, or hips. You may observe deformities that are part of the patient's state as well as a poor range of motion. Care for RA is strictly supportive in the prehospital setting. If RA causes chest pain associated with pleurisy, this symptom should be treated according to pain management protocols.

▮ Management of Medical Emergencies in Older Adults

With the exception of patients who require immediate interventions to maintain a patent airway, adequate and supportive breathing, or circulatory status, most prehospital care of medical emergencies in geriatric patients is supportive and focuses on pain relief and palliative interventions. Additional steps in the patient treatment plan will depend on the patient's specific medical emergency and chief complaint.

Words of Wisdom

Compensatory mechanism changes + aging systems + preexisting conditions = bad outcomes.

▮ Pathophysiology, Assessment, and Management of Geriatric Trauma Emergencies

Several factors place an older person at higher risk of trauma than a younger person—namely, slower reflexes, visual and hearing deficits, equilibrium disorders, and an overall reduction in agility. In particular, changes in the body's homeostatic compensatory mechanisms combined with the effects of aging on body systems and any preexisting conditions usually add up to less favorable outcomes for older adults in trauma situations. Compensation in trauma is successful when an increased pulse rate, increased respirations, and adequate vasoconstriction make up for trauma-related blood loss. Reduced cardiac reserve, decreased respiratory function, impaired renal activity, and ineffective vasoconstriction, by contrast, may lead to unsuccessful recovery from traumatic situations. Furthermore, an older adult is more likely to sustain serious injury in a trauma situation because stiffened blood vessels and fragile tissues tear more readily, and brittle, demineralized bone is more vulnerable to fracture.

Many geriatric trauma cases involve falls or motor vehicle crashes. Although most falls do not produce serious injury, they do result in increased mortality in geriatric patients—a trend that is directly related to the patient's age, preexisting disease processes, and complications related to the trauma. Falls are associated with a higher incidence of anxiety and depression, a loss of confidence, and postfall syndrome. In postfall syndrome, geriatric patients develop a lack of confidence and anxiety about potential falls.

Evidence-Based Medicine

In regard to falls in the geriatric population in the United States, the Centers for Disease Control and Prevention reports the following:[22]

- One in four Americans aged 65+ falls each year.
- Every 11 seconds, an older adult is treated in the emergency room for a fall; every 19 minutes, an older adult dies from a fall.
- Falls are the leading cause of fatal injury and the most common cause of nonfatal trauma-related hospital admissions among older adults.
- Falls result in more than 2.8 million injuries treated in emergency departments annually, including over 800,000 hospitalizations and more than 27,000 deaths.
- In 2014, the total cost of fall injuries was $31 billion.
- The financial toll for older adult falls is expected to increase as the population ages and may reach $67.7 billion by 2020.

Reproduced from National Council on Aging. © 2017 National Council on Aging. www.ncoa.org/news/resources-for-reporters/get-the-facts/falls-prevention-facts/. Accessed August 15, 2017.

Falls among older adults are divided between those resulting from extrinsic (external) causes, such as tripping on a loose rug or slipping on ice, and those resulting from intrinsic (internal) causes, such as a dizzy spell or a syncopal attack Table 44-4 . The risk of falls increases in people with preexisting gait abnormalities (such as from neurologic or musculoskeletal impairment) and cognitive impairment. Older patients with osteoporosis have lower-density bones, so even a sudden, awkward turn may fracture a bone.

When you are treating a patient who has fallen, you need to obtain a careful history. Although the patient may attribute the fall to an accidental cause ("I must have tripped over the rug"), meticulous questioning often reveals a period of dizziness or palpitations just before the fall, suggesting a different cause.

Home safety assessments by EMS—during a routine visit or as part of an outreach program—may reduce fall incidence. Components of this assessment should include clear pathways to and from the bathroom, handrails in bathtubs and on steps, no loose rugs or other objects on the floor, wheelchair ramps with grip tape, and caregivers who are trained to lift and move patients.

After falls, motor vehicle crashes are the second leading cause of accidental death among older adults. An older patient is far more likely than a younger patient to be fatally injured in a motor vehicle crash.[23] Impaired vision, errors in judgment, and underlying medical conditions contribute to the higher risk. Impairments in vision and hearing, along with diminished agility, also contribute to pedestrian deaths involving older adults.

▶ Pathophysiology of Trauma

Changes associated with normal aging and the presence of preexisting conditions impact morbidity and mortality in older adults who experience trauma. Five conditions that appear to influence outcome in trauma patients are

Table 44-4	Causes of Falls in Older Adults
Cause	**Clues to Suggest This Cause**
Extrinsic (accidental)	Obvious environmental hazard at the scene, such as poor lighting, scatter rugs, uneven sidewalk, or ice or other slippery surface
Intrinsic drop attacks	Sudden fall; patient found on the ground somewhat confused, often temporarily paralyzed and unable to get up; no premonitory symptoms
Postural (orthostatic) hypotension	Fall when getting up from a recumbent or sitting position (Check medications the patient is taking, and ask about occult blood loss, such as presence of black stools. Measure blood pressure in recumbent and sitting positions.)
Dizziness or syncope	Marked bradycardia or tachydysrhythmias
Stroke	Other characteristic signs of stroke, such as hemiparesis, hemiplegia, or aphasia
Fracture	Patient report of feeling something snap before falling

cirrhosis, congenital coagulopathy, COPD, ischemic heart disease, and diabetes mellitus. Patients with one or more of these preexisting conditions are twice as likely to die as those without.[24]

Head trauma or injury is a serious problem in this population. The increased fragility of the cerebral blood vessels, enlargement of the subdural space, and a decrease in the supportive tissue of the meninges all combine to make an older adult more vulnerable than a younger person to intracranial bleeding, particularly subdural hematoma. In many cases, the hematoma develops slowly, over a period of days or weeks as a result of the pathophysiologic changes in the brain and skull. By the time the patient becomes symptomatic, the person or his or her caretakers may not remember the initial incident, or the family or caretakers may feel guilty about their own negligence in the incident. As a result, it may be difficult to obtain an accurate history of the initial trauma. The most important early symptom of a subdural hematoma is a headache that may be worse at night. Sometimes the headache occurs on the same side of the head as the blood clot. With increasing intracranial pressure, the state of consciousness becomes depressed and the patient becomes increasingly drowsy.

Older adults are also more vulnerable than their younger counterparts to cervical spinal cord injury and cord compression, even after apparently minor trauma. Degenerative changes in the cervical spine (cervical **spondylosis**) cause arthritic "spurs" and narrowing of the vertebral canal; the nerve roots exiting from the cervical spine gradually become compressed, and pressure on the spinal cord increases. Any injury to the cervical spine, therefore, is much more likely to injure the already compromised spinal cord. Even a sudden movement of the neck may result in spinal cord injury.

Injuries to the chest in older adults are much more likely to produce rib fracture and flail chest, owing to the brittleness of the ribs and overall stiffening of the chest wall as the costochondral cartilage becomes calcified. Abdominal trauma often produces liver injury, perhaps because the liver is less protected by the abdominal musculature.

Hip fracture may occur as a result of relatively minor trauma given the potential precedence of osteoporosis. The most important risk factor for hip fracture is osteoporosis. In older patients, pelvic fractures are more likely to produce hemorrhage than in younger patients, and older patients are nearly four times as likely to require blood transfusions.[25] In addition, patient outcome is significantly worse in older patients with pelvic fractures than in younger patients.[25]

Burns are a significant risk of morbidity and mortality in older adults because of physiologic and pathophysiologic changes related to aging. The risk of mortality is increased when the patient has one or more preexisting medical conditions, defense mechanisms to protect against infection are weakened, and fluid replacement is complicated by renal compromise. When you are assessing a burn patient, you need to monitor the patient's hydration status by assessing current vital signs, mucous membranes, and urine output, which is typically 50 to 60 mL/h or 0.5 to 1.0 mL/kg/h for adults.

Internal temperature regulation is slowed in older adults and continues to slow with increasing age. The body's ability to recognize fluctuations in temperature becomes delayed owing to a slowed endocrine system. Heat gain or loss in response to environmental changes is delayed by atherosclerotic vessels, slowed circulation, and decreased sweat production in the skin. In addition, thermoregulation can be adversely affected by chronic disease, medications, and alcohol use, all of which are more frequent in older adults.

Not surprisingly, given these physiologic characteristics, about half of all deaths from hypothermia occur in older adults, and most indoor hypothermia deaths involve geriatric patients.[26] Although living in an area prone to harsh winters is a risk factor, hypothermia can develop at temperatures above freezing when an older person is exposed for a prolonged period.

Providers should be aware of environmental emergencies during extreme heat and cold, particularly in lower-socioeconomic areas where homes may not have sufficient heat or air conditioning. Managing such events may require public awareness and preplanning. You may have to keep the ambulance's patient compartment at a temperature that is higher than normal, and perhaps uncomfortable for you, to adequately maintain the geriatric patient's temperature.

▶ Assessment and Management of Trauma

Begin the assessment by looking at the mechanism of injury. Always look for signs or symptoms that the patient may have experienced a medical problem before the trauma. A syncopal event while driving, for example, may result in a crash.

The initial management of an injured geriatric patient follows the basic ABCDE (Airway, Breathing, Circulation, Disability, and Exposure) pattern of trauma care, albeit with some special concerns.

When you are securing the airway, check for dentures. If they are intact and in place, leave them where they are; if the dentures are broken or loose in the mouth, remove them and place them in a safe container. Dentures that are properly adhered to a patient's gum line can help achieve a good seal with a bag-mask device. Conversely, patients with loose dentures can easily develop an obstructed airway. Aggressive suctioning of blood or secretions is required because of the older patient's lessened airway and gag reflexes **Figure 44-11** .

When you are assessing breathing, check for rib fracture. If assisted ventilation is required, use a bag-mask device gently, exerting just enough pressure to inflate the lungs so as to lessen the chance of creating a pneumothorax. Administer supplemental oxygen early to assist the patient's body in compensating for early states of trauma.

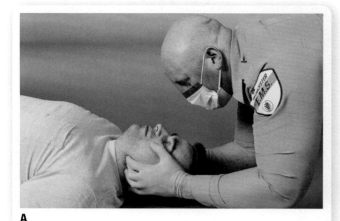

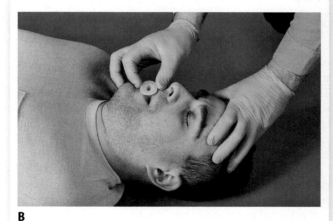

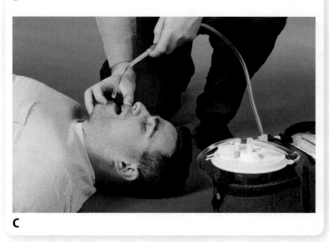

Figure 44-11 The airway should initially be addressed using simple techniques, such as **(A)** the jaw-thrust maneuver, **(B)** placement of an oropharyngeal or nasopharyngeal airway, and **(C)** suctioning.

© Jones & Bartlett Learning.

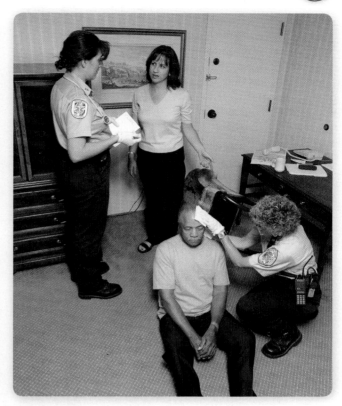

Figure 44-12 History is especially important in older patients who have lost consciousness.

© Jones & Bartlett Learning. Courtesy of MIEMSS.

When you are evaluating circulation, remember that what is a normal blood pressure in a younger person may mean hypotension in an older person. If possible, try to determine the patient's normal baseline blood pressure and circulatory status.

The assessment of disability (neurologic status) should include an evaluation of the patient's pupils and level of consciousness, according to the AVPU (Awake and alert, responsive to Verbal stimuli, responsive to Pain, Unresponsive) scale. Finally, be sure to expose the entire injured area, even if it means peeling away many layers of clothing. Depending on local protocol, hypertonic saline (3% NaCl) can be used to help reduce intracranial pressure in patients with intracranial bleeding, particularly those with asymmetrical pupils and hypertension.

Once the primary survey is complete, try to obtain a complete history of the trauma event from the patient and from anyone who may have witnessed the event **Figure 44-12**. Be aware that the patient may have sustained the trauma several hours or days prior to the ambulance call, with symptoms subsequently developing due to the patient's medication regimens. If the patient fell, from what height? Did the patient have any symptoms beforehand, such as dizziness? If the patient was struck by a car, how fast was the car moving? If the patient was the driver of a car involved in a crash, did he or she feel dizzy or black out before the crash? Did the patient have chest pain? Did witnesses notice the car moving erratically before it crashed?

Obtain a complete list of all medications the patient takes regularly. Inquire in particular about beta-blockers, antihypertensives, and medications for diabetes, because they may affect the patient's response to resuscitation measures and to anesthesia.

Conduct the secondary assessment as usual, paying particular attention to signs of injuries to the head, cervical spine, ribs, abdomen, and long bones. Pain from fractures or peripheral injury may be difficult to assess if the patient has decreased pain perception.

Additional treatment will depend on the patient's specific injuries, although there are a few general principles to keep in mind:

- Use caution when inserting IV catheters and administering isotonic solutions. It is very easy to overload an older person with sodium, and you must balance that risk with the need to maintain adequate perfusion pressure. Use small boluses, and reassess the patient frequently, especially for signs of pulmonary edema.
- Monitor cardiac rhythm throughout care of the patient, and be alert for changes. Previous or continuing cardiac disease predisposes a person to ECG changes.
- Take steps to preserve temperature in geriatric trauma patients. Regulation of temperature is slowed in older adults, and the blood in cold patients does not clot as well.
- Frail geriatric patients may not do well with a traction splint for a femoral fracture. If possible, place the patient on a well-padded backboard and buttress him or her well with pillows secured firmly in place.
- Consider the use of pain medication. Remember that geriatric patients require a lower dosage of pain medications to reach therapeutic levels.
- Immobilize the cervical spine before transporting the patient. Pad the backboard generously, because the skin of an older person may be damaged by the direct trauma of the pressure and the decrease in blood flow. Target areas where the bone is near the surface, from top to bottom: occiput, scapula, spinous processes, elbows, sacrum, and heels. A pressure ulcer can develop in as little as 45 minutes and can complicate the original injury.

Elder Abuse

A category of geriatric trauma that deserves special mention is elder abuse—that is, any form of mistreatment that results in harm or loss to an older person. Five types of abuse are distinguished: physical, sexual, emotional, neglect, and financial. The first four are similar to the forms found in child abuse. Financial abuse involves improper use of an older person's funds, property, or assets. The average victim of elder abuse is 77.9 years old, is female, and has multiple chronic conditions.[27] These conditions

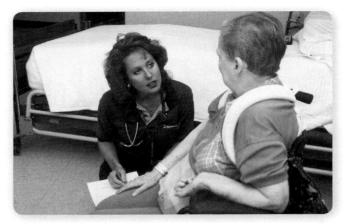

Figure 44-13 Take time to listen patiently to older patients.
© Jones & Bartlett Learning. Courtesy of MIEMSS.

make patients unable to function on their own, leaving them dependent on others for at least part of their care. The abuser is almost always known to the abused and is often a family member (such as adult children or a spouse). Although elder abuse does occur in long-term care facilities, it is more likely to occur at the patient's home or the home of a caregiver.

One clue to elder abuse is unexplained injuries that do not fit the stated cause. Assessment of elder abuse must include not only the physical exam (including the unexplained presence of bruises, burns, and scars, which should be thoroughly documented without speculating about their cause), but also the environmental and social clues. Look at the patient's overall hygiene, and review how he or she interacts with caregivers. Also assess the caregiver's attitudes: Does a caregiver seem unconcerned about the patient's condition, defensive or evasive, or untruthful? Take adequate time to listen patiently to any concerns expressed by older patients about their care (or lack of it) **Figure 44-13** . If the patient is in stable condition but the situation is unsafe, see if the patient will accept transport to the hospital. If the patient refuses transport, see if he or she will accept help from the local **adult protective services (APS)** agency. In some cases, patients may be hesitant to go with EMS personnel because of fear of caregiver retaliation. If the situation is immediately unsafe, notify law enforcement personnel and remain with the patient only if the scene remains safe to do so.

Many states have elder abuse statutes, and the reporting of suspected abuse is mandatory in some jurisdictions. Nevertheless, only 1 out of every 14 cases of elder abuse is ever reported.[24] The way elder abuse is defined varies considerably from state to state, so it is advisable to become familiar with the legislation that applies to your own area. However, regardless of the legislation, if you have any reason to suspect elder abuse in a given case of geriatric injury—for example, if you found evidence of gross patient neglect in the patient's residence—objectively document your observations and report your findings and suspicions to the receiving facility. APS could use these observations as an indicator of whether assistance is required.

End-of-Life Care

You will inevitably be involved with end-of-life care for many patients. Of course, "do not resuscitate" (DNR) does not mean "do not respond to the needs of a terminal patient." You can treat various disorders, administer various medications, and perform other various treatments as long as they do not include providing artificial ventilations or cardiovascular assistance. There is much you can do for patients at the end of life, beginning with demonstrating a caring and concerned attitude and approach. Many of your visits may be "no transport" decisions and may not be perceived as valuable by those who decide on reimbursement, but they are no less valuable to the patient than are more aggressive measures.

Controversies

Is a DNR order from a state other than yours valid? It depends on your state's law. Approximately a dozen states recognize out-of-state DNR orders.

Many communities have a local **hospice**, an organization that provides terminal care for patients and support for their families. If one exists in your community, consider how you or your service might collaborate on providing quality care for a person at the end of life Figure 44-14 .

Hospice is staffed with an array of clinicians who focus on patient comfort and become a valuable resource for the patient's family. Although hospice is commonly associated with patients with terminal cancer, these services are also available to patients with other terminal conditions. For

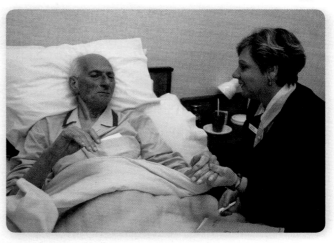

Figure 44-14 Hospice care allows people with terminal illnesses to receive palliative care in their own homes.
© Photofusion Picture Library/Alamy.

example, hospice manages patients with head injuries who have been disconnected from a mechanical ventilator and patients with renal failure who are unable to continue dialysis, among many other patients. The clinicians attempt to administer regular, therapeutically appropriate doses of analgesia to help minimize the amount of patient discomfort. Patients are also generally removed from any life-assistive devices such as a mechanical ventilator, gastric tubes, and cardiac assist devices.

Although many communities have hospice units that operate in their own buildings, in a designated wing of a hospital or in specific health complexes, patients and their families may choose to receive hospice care at their own residence. This arrangement gives the family an opportunity to maximize their time with their loved one, and it gives the patient the comfort of being surrounded by familiar people in a familiar environment in his or her final days. During hospice care in the home, hospice nurses regularly visit patients and their families to provide therapeutic interventions and emotional support.

1. **What might be the mechanism of illness you suspect based on the information provided by dispatch?**

   Based on the nature of the call, there might be a multitude of conditions that could have caused the patients altered level of consciousness. Recall that with any altered level of consciousness patient, you should be evaluating using the mnemonic AEIOUTIPS to help identify the cause or causes.

2. **When responding to a geriatric patient, what makes the assessment different from a nongeriatric assessment?**

   When treating a geriatric patient, it is important to use the GEMS diamond to guide your assessment. The GEMS diamond helps you identify the four categories of geriatric care.

3. **Could injury prevention methods have been used prior to this incident to help minimize the chances of a fall? If so, which kind?**

   An injury prevention home checklist for older patients may have identified the loose rug in the walkway; it may also have encouraged the use of the medic alert button and skid-resistant shoes.

4. **What are your primary responsibilities at this point during the call?**

   After ensuring the safety of the scene, this patient needs supportive care and expeditious transport. ALS interventions should be minimized on scene to ensure timely transport and access to the appropriate specialty services.

5. **In asking the patient's daughter the question, "When was the last time you saw your father appear normal?" what will her response help you to determine, based on the GEMS diamond?**

   Her response will allow you to determine whether the patient is within the appropriate time frame for fibrinolytic

therapy if he was experiencing an ischemic stroke. The response would also help to address the social aspect of your assessment: Is someone checking in on the patient on a normal basis or is he being checked on only occasionally.

6. **Where would you transport this patient?**

   This patient should be transported to the nearest Level I trauma center.

7. **How would you manage this patient's hypoxia?**

   The patient should be placed on a nonrebreathing mask because his oxygen saturation has remained less than 94% despite oxygen delivery by nasal cannula. If the patient's ventilation becomes inadequate, his breathing should be assisted with a bag-mask device.

8. **What do the patient's medications tell you about his current clinical condition?**

   The warfarin indicates that the patient may bleed easily, increasing the likelihood of a subdural hematoma or intracranial hemorrhage. It is also concerning that the patient's blood pressure is so high given that he is already taking a beta-blocker (ie, metoprolol).

9. **Which type of medical history would you suspect?**

   Prednisone indicates a respiratory disorder, furosemide indicates heart failure, omeprazole indicates GERD, metoprolol indicates hypertension, diltiazem indicates AF, warfarin may be clotting prophylaxis due to the AF, and nitroglycerin indicates a history of coronary heart disease.

YOU are the Paramedic **SUMMARY** *(continued)*

EMS Patient Care Report (PCR)

Date: 03-15-18	**Incident No.:** 572819	**Nature of Call:** Altered mental status	**Location:** 127 Henderson Ave

Dispatched: 0630	**En Route:** 0632	**At Scene:** 0640	**Transport:** 0648	**At Hospital:** 0705	**In Service:** 0731

Patient Information

Age: 84 **Sex:** M **Weight (in kg [lb]):** 75 kg (165 lb)	**Allergies:** No known drug allergies **Medications:** Prednisone, furosemide, omeprazole, metoprolol, warfarin, nitroglycerin, diltiazem **Past Medical History:** COPD, HF, AF, ACS, GERD **Chief Complaint:** Altered mental status

Vital Signs

Time: 0644	**BP:** 208/114	**Pulse:** 74	**Respirations:** 20	**Spo$_2$:** 88% NC
Time: 0648	**BP:** 202/106	**Pulse:** 78	**Respirations:** 24	**Spo$_2$:** 90% NRM
Time: 0653	**BP:** 200/104	**Pulse:** 72	**Respirations:** 22	**Spo$_2$:** 90% NRM
Time: 0659	**BP:** 202/108	**Pulse:** 78	**Respirations:** 20	**Spo$_2$:** 94% NRM

EMS Treatment (circle all that apply)

Oxygen @ __15__ L/min via (circle one): NC **(NRM)** Bag-mask device	**Assisted Ventilation**	**Airway Adjunct**	**CPR**
Defibrillation	**Bleeding Control**	**Bandaging**	**Splinting**	**Other:**

Narrative

Dispatched for pt with altered mental status. Arrived to find an 84-year-old male pt on the ground who is responsive to painful stimuli. The pt has been down for an unknown amount of time. Pt was maintaining his own airway, on home O$_2$ by NC at 2 L/min (Spo$_2$ 88%). A 32F NPA was inserted into the R nostril. O$_2$ via NRM @ 15 L/min was applied. Pt is hypertensive, lungs CTA, skin pale/warm/dry to touch, asymmetrical pupils, BG 114 mg/dL. IV of NS was established in L AC with 18g @ TKO (Medic 4). We packaged the pt, with full spinal immobilization with good MSPs before and after and kept the head elevated at 30°, and loaded the pt into the ambulance. Secondary exam was unremarkable. Contacted med control with negative orders. We transported the pt to a Level I trauma center and left in care of ED staff.**End of report**

Prep Kit

▶ Ready for Review

- Older adults constitute an ever-increasing proportion of patients presenting to the health care system, particularly in the emergency care sector.
- The health problems of older people are quantitatively and qualitatively different from those of younger people. The special problems of older people require special approaches.
- The aging process is accompanied by changes in physiologic function. The decrease in the functional capacity of various organ systems can affect the way in which the patient responds to illness.
- A person's respiratory capacity undergoes significant reductions with age due to decreases in the elasticity of the lungs and in the size and strength of the respiratory muscles, calcification of costochrondral cartilage in the chest wall, and musculoskeletal changes.
- A variety of changes occur in the cardiovascular system as a person ages. The wall of the left ventricle thickens and elastin in the vessel walls decreases, causing thickening and rigidity, particularly in the coronary arteries. Arteriosclerosis develops, and the conduction system of the heart deteriorates.
- Changes in the nervous system lead to a decrease in the performance of sense organs, as evidenced by visual changes (glaucoma and cataracts are common) and hearing loss.
- Digestive system changes include a decrease in taste buds and a reduction in saliva and gastric secretions. These changes may interfere with the enjoyment of food, leading to malnutrition in older adults.
- Geriatric patients may experience renal system changes. Although the kidneys of an older person may be capable of handling day-to-day demands, they may not be able to meet unusual challenges, such as those imposed by illness. Therefore, acute illness in geriatric patients is often accompanied by derangements in fluid and electrolyte balance.
- Changes in the endocrine system may lead to diabetes and thyroid abnormalities in older patients.
- Nearly every function of the immune system is affected by aging. Older persons are therefore more prone to infection and secondary complications compared to younger people.
- Age-related changes in the integumentary system include thinner skin and loss of elasticity, allowing skin to be torn easily and more bleeding to occur.
- Aging is accompanied by a progressive loss of homeostatic capabilities. A specific illness or injury in an older person is more likely to result in generalized deterioration. Notably, the regulatory system that manages the blood glucose level becomes impaired with increasing age, such that an elevated blood glucose level occurs quite commonly in older patients.
- Aging brings a widespread decrease in bone mass in men and women, but especially among postmenopausal women. Bones become more brittle and tend to break more easily, especially during falls.
- Knowing what is and what is not part of the aging process constitutes the first challenge when you are assessing geriatric patients. A second challenge is recognizing that signs and symptoms of disease may be altered from their presentation in younger patients as a consequence of aging.
- The GEMS diamond was designed to assist the prehospital professional in the assessment and treatment of geriatric patients. Its elements—recognition that the person is a geriatric patient, environmental assessment, medical assessment, and social assessment—can be integrated into the patient assessment process, helping you to form a general impression of the patient.
- A comprehensive patient history includes many elements to investigate—the patient's chief complaint, present illness or injury, pertinent medical history, and current health care status and needs. A key consideration with geriatric patients is their tendency not to report significant symptoms, which makes it difficult to ascertain the chief complaint.
- Most patients with chronic obstructive pulmonary disease, pulmonary edema, and other common respiratory ailments are in the second half of their lives, and such conditions lead to high mortality in geriatric patients.
- Diseases of the heart remain the leading cause of death among older adults in the United States.
- More than one-half of all older persons are hypertensive, with the majority having isolated systolic hypertension resulting from a loss of arterial elasticity. Controlling systolic and diastolic hypertension in older adults helps prevent both stroke and myocardial infarction.
- Stroke is a significant cause of death and disability in older adults. Hypertension is the primary risk factor for stroke, but age, family history, smoking, diabetes, high cholesterol, and heart disease also contribute to its incidence. Effective prehospital acute stroke care includes early recognition, discovery of conditions that mimic strokes (such as hypoglycemia or hypoxia), and timely transport to the most appropriate facility.
- In geriatric patients, delirium often replaces or confounds the typical presentation caused by a medical problem, an adverse medication effect, or drug withdrawal. Disorders that cause delirium may also include poisons, electrolyte imbalances,

Prep Kit (continued)

nutritional deficiencies, and infections such as urinary tract infections and pneumonia.

- Unlike delirium, dementia is a disease that produces irreversible brain failure. Disorders that cause dementia include conditions that impair vascular and neurologic structures within the brain, such as infections, stroke, head injuries, poor nutrition, and medications.
- The two most common degenerative types of dementia in older people are Alzheimer disease and multi-infarct or vascular dementia, both of which cause structural damage to the brain. Treatment of Alzheimer disease in the prehospital and interfacility setting will generally revolve around supportive care and treatment of symptoms.
- Gastrointestinal problems in older adults include small bowel obstruction due to gallstones, gastroesophageal reflux disease, biliary diseases (cirrhosis, hepatitis, and cholecystitis), stomach or duodenal ulcers (peptic ulcer disease), and gastrointestinal bleeding.
- Renal failure is a sudden decrease in the rate of filtration through the glomeruli, causing toxins to accumulate in the blood. Chronic renal failure may require lifelong hemodialysis or a kidney transplant; missing a dialysis treatment can lead to a renal emergency and a 9-1-1 call.
- A geriatric patient with diabetes is at increased risk for hypoglycemia for several reasons: medications, inadequate or irregular dietary intake, inability to recognize the warning signs due to cognitive problems, and blunted warning signs. Delirium may be the only indication of hypoglycemia in a geriatric patient.
- Older patients with diabetes whose blood glucose levels tend to be high are prone to hyperosmolar hyperglycemic syndrome (HHS), also called hyperosmolar nonketotic coma (HONK). The most frequent cause for HHS/HONK is infection. The patient presentation is likely to consist of acute confusion with dehydration.
- In geriatric patients with hypothyroidism, the signs and symptoms may match those seen with normal aging (eg, cold intolerance, constipation, dry skin, weakness, weight gain); with acute-onset hyperthyroidism (thyrotoxicosis), the presentation can be blunted in geriatric patients.
- In geriatric patients, the first sign of sepsis may be confusion or otherwise altered mental status; elevated temperature and altered vital signs may not always be evident in older patients with this condition.

- Older adults are particularly prone to adverse drug reactions because of changes in the following aspects of functioning: drug metabolism, because of diminished hepatic function; drug elimination, because of diminished renal function; body composition, including increased body fat and decreased body water, which alters the distribution of drugs through the various body compartments; and the central nervous system's responsiveness to drugs.
- Depression in geriatric patients can mimic the effects of many other medical problems (such as dementia). Risk factors for depression in an older person include a history of depression, chronic disease, and loss (function, independence, or significant others).
- Geriatric patients are at higher risk for secondary infection after they experience breaks in the skin, skin tumors, and fungal or viral infections of the skin. Other integumentary conditions that disproportionately affect geriatric patients include herpes zoster (shingles), cellulitis, and pressure ulcers.
- Osteoporosis is characterized by a decrease in bone mass leading to reduction in bone strength and greater susceptibility to fracture. Osteoarthritis is a progressive disease process of the joints that destroys cartilage, promotes the formation of bone spurs in joints, and leads to joint stiffness.
- Several factors put an older adult at higher risk of trauma than a younger person: slower reflexes, visual and hearing deficits, equilibrium disorders, and an overall reduction in agility.
- Elder abuse is any form of mistreatment that results in harm or loss to an older person. Five types of abuse are distinguished: physical, sexual, emotional, neglect, and financial.
- Hospice provides terminal care for patients and support for their families, often allowing patients to receive palliative care in their own homes. You will be involved with end-of-life care for many patients.

▶ Vital Vocabulary

adult protective services (APS) An organization that investigates cases involving abuse and neglect and provides case management services in some cases.

Alzheimer disease A progressive organic condition in which neurons die, causing dementia.

arthritis Inflammation of the joints.

bereavement Sadness from loss; grieving.

cellulitis An acute inflammation in the skin caused by a bacterial infection.

Prep Kit (continued)

delirium An acute confusional state characterized by global impairment of thinking, perception, judgment, and memory.

dementia A chronic deterioration of mental functions.

geriatrics The assessment and treatment of disease in someone 65 years or older.

herpes zoster Shingles; a contagious condition caused by the reactivation of the varicella virus on nerve roots.

homeostasis A tendency toward constancy or stability in the body's internal milieu.

hospice An organization that provides end-of-life care to patients with terminal illnesses and their families.

old-age dependency ratio A formula used to determine the number of older people in a society as compared with the number of potential workers who are theoretically capable of providing resources to sustain the whole population. It is the number of older people (65 years and older) for every 100 adults (potential caregivers) between the ages of 18 and 64 years.

osteoarthritis The degeneration of a joint surface caused by wear and tear that leads to pain and stiffness.

osteoporosis A decrease in bone mass and density.

Parkinson disease A neurologic condition in which the portion of the brain responsible for production of dopamine has been damaged or overused, resulting in tremors.

polypharmacy The use of multiple medications.

presbycusis Progressive hearing loss, particularly in the high frequencies, along with lessened ability to discriminate between a particular sound and background noise.

pressure ulcer An ulcer that occurs when pressure is applied to body tissue, resulting in a lack of perfusion and ultimately necrosis.

proprioception The ability to perceive the position and movement of one's body or limbs.

rheumatoid arthritis (RA) An inflammatory disorder that affects the entire body and leads to degeneration and deformation of joints.

sacral edema Swelling that presents around the sacral region of the spinal column.

sepsis A disease state that results from the presence of microorganisms or their toxic products in the bloodstream.

spondylosis A degenerative condition resulting in decreased mobility of vertebral joints and compression of neural elements.

▶ References

1. Population 65 years and over in the United States: 2011-2015. American community survey 5-year estimates. American Fact Finder, United States Census Bureau website. https://factfinder.census .gov/faces/tableservices/jsf/pages/productview .xhtml?pid=ACS_15_5YR_S0103&prodType=table. Accessed April 7, 2017.

2. National Center for Health Statistics. Emergency department visits. Centers for Disease Control and Prevention website. https://www.cdc.gov/nchs /fastats/emergency-department.htm. Updated March 17, 2017. Accessed April 25, 2017.

3. United States—age dependency ratio. Index Mundi website. http://www.indexmundi.com/facts /united-states/age-dependency-ratio. Accessed April 7, 2017.

4. Upadhyaya RC. Cardiovascular function. In: Meiner SE, ed. *Gerontologic Nursing*. 5th ed. Maryland Heights, MO: Mosby; 2015:388-421.

5. Balter M. The incredible shrinking human brain. Science website. http://www.sciencemag.org /news/2011/07/incredible-shrinking-human-brain. Published July 25, 2011. Accessed April 25, 2017.

6. Weinstein JR, Anderson S. The aging kidney: physiological changes. *Adv Chronic Kidney Dis.* 2010;17(4):302-307.

7. *2014 National Diabetes Statistics Report.* Centers for Disease Control and Prevention website. https://www.cdc.gov/diabetes/data /statistics/2014statisticsreport.html. Updated May 15, 2015. Accessed April 25, 2017.

8. CPAP reduces risk of death in people with COPD and sleep apnea. American Academy of Sleep Medicine website. http://www.aasmnet.org/articles .aspx?id=4107. Published August 14, 2013. Accessed May 4, 2017.

9. National Center for Chronic Disease Prevention and Health Promotion, Division for Heart Disease and Stroke Prevention. Heart disease facts. Centers for Disease Control and Prevention website. https://www.cdc.gov/heartdisease/facts .htm. Updated November 30, 2016. Accessed March 2, 2017.

10. Who Is at Risk for Heart Failure? National Heart, Lung, and Blood Institute website. https://www .nhlbi.nih.gov/health/health-topics/topics/hf/atrisk. Updated June 22, 2015. Accessed May 3, 2017.

11. National Center for Chronic Disease Prevention and Health Promotion, Division for Heart Disease and Stroke Prevention. High blood pressure facts. Centers for Disease Control and Prevention website. https://www.cdc.gov/bloodpressure/facts .htm. Updated November 30, 2016. Accessed March 2, 2017.

Prep Kit (continued)

12. Stroke statistics. The Internet Stroke Center website. http://www.strokecenter.org/patients /about-stroke/stroke-statistics/. Accessed January 2, 2017.

13. National Center for Health Statistics. Deaths and mortality. Centers for Disease Control and Prevention website. http://www.cdc.gov/nchs /fastats/deaths.htm. Updated March 17, 2017. Accessed April 25, 2017.

14. Rowe TA, Mehta MJ. Urinary tract infection in older adults. *Aging Health.* 2013;9(5). https://www.ncbi .nlm.nih.gov/pmc/articles/PMC3878051/. Accessed April 2, 2017.

15. Gupta S. Type 2 diabetes and the elderly. Everyday Health website. http://www.everydayhealth.com /sanjay-gupta/type-2-diabetes-and-the-elderly/. Updated October 10, 2013. Accessed March 2, 2017.

16. Wall CR. Myxedema coma: diagnosis and treatment. *Am Fam Physician.* 2000;62(11):2485-2490.

17. Hajjar ER, Cafiero AC, Hanlon JT. Polypharmacy in elderly patients. *Am J Geriatr Pharmacother.* 2007;5(4):345-351.

18. Wright RM, Roumani YF, Boudreau R, et al. *J Am Geriatr Soc.* 2009;57(2):243-250.

19. Routledge PA, O'Mahony MS, Woodhouse KW. Adverse drug reactions in elderly patients. *Br J Clin Pharmacol.* 2004;57(2):121-126.

20. Conwell Y, Van Orden K, Caine ED. Suicide in older adults. *Psychiatr Clin North Am.* 2012;34(2):451-468.

21. Bennington-Castro J. Everyday guide to osteoporosis: What is osteoporosis? Everyday Health website. http://www.everydayhealth.com /osteoporosis/guide/. Updated October 9, 2015. Accessed April 9, 2017.

22. Falls prevention facts. National Council on Aging website. https://www.ncoa.org/news/resources -for-reporters/get-the-facts/falls-prevention-facts/. Accessed June 13, 2016.

23. Yee WY, Cameron PA, Bailey MJ. Road traffic injuries in the elderly. *Emerg Med J.* 2006;23(1):42-46.

24. Morris JA Jr, MacKenzie EJ, Edelstein SL. The effect of preexisting conditions on mortality in trauma patients. *JAMA.* 1990;263(14):1942-1946.

25. Henry SM, Pollak AN, Jones AL, Boswell S, Scalea TM. Pelvic fracture in geriatric patients: a distinct clinical entity. *J Trauma.* 2002;53(1):15-20.

26. Hypothermia. University of Maryland Medical Center website. http://umm.edu/health/medical /altmed/condition/hypothermia. Reviewed May 26, 2014. Accessed April 3, 2017.

27. National Center on Elder Abuse, Bureau of Justice Statistics. Elderly abuse statistics. Statistic Brain website. http://www.statisticbrain.com/elderly -abuse-statistics/. Research conducted October 30, 2016. Accessed April 7, 2017.

Assessment in Action

It is just after 1000 hours when you are dispatched to a residence for a fall. Upon your arrival at the address, a man meets you at the door and tells you that his mother is "not acting right." He also tells you that she lives alone and apparently fell sometime during the night. He says that she has been confused lately and that the doctor ran tests but found nothing significant. She takes medication for hypertension and has had a stroke and a myocardial infarction in the past. The son says that the doctor thinks his mother may have mild dementia. She also takes "many medications." The son has not seen or talked to his mother since yesterday morning and came over to check on her just prior to calling 9-1-1.

Assessment *in Action* (continued)

You enter the kitchen to find an older woman sitting at the kitchen table looking at you in a bewildered fashion. She has dried blood matted in the back of her white hair, and her son tells you the blood is from her fall. You also note blood on the edge of the countertop that she apparently struck on the way down. She says that she does not remember what happened and cannot tell you her age or what day of the week it is. You note several loose throw rugs on the floor, and her clothes are disheveled and buttoned inappropriately. Her vital signs are within normal limits, pupils are equal and reactive to light, and the blood glucose level is normal. She says she is fine and does not want to go to the hospital.

1. The loose rugs may have contributed to the patient's fall. Which part of the GEMS diamond does this represent?

   A. Geriatric assessment
   B. Environmental assessment
   C. Medical assessment
   D. Social assessment

2. If the rugs are the cause of the fall, this would be considered:

   A. an extrinsic factor.
   B. an intrinsic factor.
   C. proprioception.
   D. a result of spondylosis.

3. The state of the patient's clothing offers important information corresponding to which portion of the GEMS diamond assessment?

   A. Geriatric assessment
   B. Environmental assessment
   C. Medical assessment
   D. Social assessment

4. Changes in the patient's neurologic system due to the aging process and her history of a stroke may indicate which condition as the cause of her confusion?

   A. Delirium
   B. Presbycusis
   C. Dementia
   D. Organic brain syndrome

5. This patient's confusion and instability may be the result of a toxicologic impairment as a result of:

   A. polypharmacy.
   B. alcohol.
   C. noncompliance.
   D. psychiatric conditions.

6. The patient's fall may have resulted from a cardiac dysrhythmia as a result of her aging cardiovascular system. What is the most common dysrhythmia among older adults?

   A. Sinus tachycardia
   B. Sinus bradycardia
   C. Ventricular fibrillation
   D. Atrial fibrillation

7. Confusion in any patient may be the result of endocrine disorders. Older patients, particularly those with a known history of diabetes, are more likely to present with which condition as a result of elevated glucose levels?

   A. Diabetic ketoacidosis
   B. Hyperosmolar hyperglycemic syndrome
   C. Hyperthyroidism
   D. Thyrotoxicosis

8. As a paramedic, it is important for you to assess any geriatric patient for signs of abuse. What should you look for and how should you proceed if abuse is suspected?

9. What is meant by a *review of systems*, and why is it important when you are assessing a geriatric patient?

10. Explain why it is so important to obtain the most detailed history possible of an older patient's medications.

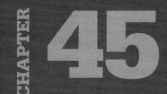
Patients With Special Challenges

National EMS Education Standard Competencies

Special Patient Populations

Integrates assessment findings with principles of pathophysiology and knowledge of psychosocial needs to formulate a field impression and implement a comprehensive treatment/disposition plan for patients with special needs.

Patients With Special Challenges

Recognizing and reporting abuse and neglect (pp 2254-2258)

Health care implications of:

> Abuse (pp 2253-2258 and see Chapter 43, *Pediatric Emergencies*, and Chapter 44, *Geriatric Emergencies*)
> Neglect (pp 2253-2258 and see Chapter 43, *Pediatric Emergencies*, and Chapter 44, *Geriatric Emergencies*)
> Homelessness (pp 2252-2253)
> Poverty (pp 2252-2253)
> Bariatrics (pp 2259-2260)
> Technology dependent (pp 2261-2278)
> Hospice/terminally ill (pp 2258-2259)
> Tracheostomy care/dysfunction (pp 2261-2264)
> Home care (pp 2251-2252)
> Sensory deficit/loss (pp 2278-2285)
> Developmental disability (p 2278)

Trauma

Integrates assessment findings with principles of epidemiology and pathophysiology to formulate a field impression to implement a comprehensive treatment/disposition plan for an acutely injured patient.

Special Considerations in Trauma

Pathophysiology, assessment, and management of trauma in the

> Pregnant patient (see Chapter 41, *Obstetrics*)
> Pediatric patient (see Chapter 43, *Pediatric Emergencies*)
> Geriatric patient (see Chapter 44, *Geriatric Emergencies*)
> Cognitively impaired patient (p 2285)

Knowledge Objectives

1. Discuss how poverty and homelessness adversely impact patient health and EMS system performance. (pp 2252-2253)
2. Identify ways to advocate for patients' rights to health care services. (pp 2252-2253)
3. Recognize signs and symptoms of neglect and various forms of abuse, including physical abuse, neglect, sexual abuse, and emotional abuse. (pp 2253-2255)
4. Identify benign physical findings that may be confused with signs of abuse. (pp 2255-2256)
5. Discuss the unique management and documentation concerns related to suspected cases of abuse or neglect. (p 2257)
6. Describe mandatory reporting and how it relates to cases of suspected abuse. (pp 2257-2258)
7. Describe specific concerns related to patients with a terminal illness, including situations in which hospice may be involved. (pp 2258-2259)
8. Discuss situations in which advance directives and do not resuscitate (DNR) orders may exist, and how the paramedic should proceed in situations where the validity of such a document is in question. (p 2259)
9. Describe specific clinical and management concerns related to bariatric patients. (pp 2259-2260)
10. Discuss operational concerns related to emergency management of bariatric patients. (p 2260)
11. Describe specific concerns related to patients with a communicable disease. (pp 2260-2261)
12. Discuss the purpose of tracheostomy tubes, and how to troubleshoot problems that may occur in a patient with a tracheostomy. (pp 2261-2264)
13. Discuss medical technology and adaptive devices used in the prehospital setting, including long-term ventilators, ventricular assist devices, apnea monitors, long-term vascular access devices, medication infusion pumps, gastric tubes, colostomies, urinary diversion devices, dialysis shunts, surgical drains and devices, and cerebrospinal fluid shunts. (pp 2264-2274)

14. Discuss the types of medical technology that may be used during interfacility transports, including hemodynamic monitoring, intra-aortic balloon pumps, and intracranial pressure monitoring. (pp 2274-2277)

15. Identify strategies for providing care to patients with cognitive impairment, including patients with development delay, Down syndrome, intellectual disability, and autism/autism spectrum disorders. (pp 2278-2280)

16. Identify strategies for providing care to patients with communication impairment, including hearing, vision, and speech impairments. (pp 2280-2284)

17. Identify strategies for providing care to patients with sensory impairment, including paralysis, paraplegia, and quadriplegia. (pp 2284-2285)

18. Discuss concerns related to managing a cognitively impaired patient who experiences trauma. (p 2285)

19. Identify chronic medical conditions likely to be encountered by paramedics, including cancer, cerebral palsy, congenital heart disease, cystic fibrosis, multiple sclerosis, muscular dystrophy, myasthenia gravis, spina bifida, postpolio syndrome, and traumatic brain injury. (pp 2285-2291)

20. Discuss treatment and transport concerns for patients with a chronic illness. (pp 2285-2291)

Skills Objectives

1. Demonstrate how to suction and clean a tracheostomy. (pp 2263-2264, Skill Drill 45-1)

2. Demonstrate how to replace an ostomy device. (pp 2269-2270, Skill Drill 45-2)

3. Demonstrate how to catheterize an adult male patient. (p 2271, Skill Drill 45-3)

4. Demonstrate how to catheterize an adult female patient. (p 2272, Skill Drill 45-4)

YOU are the Paramedic   PART 1

It is approximately 0200 hours when you and your partner respond to a call for a 13-year-old boy with respiratory distress. On arrival, Mrs. Morton, the patient's mother, greets you at the door and shows you to the patient's room. She informs you that your patient, Kyle, was in an all-terrain vehicle crash 18 months ago in which he fractured multiple vertebrae and became paralyzed and partially ventilator dependent. He had a tracheostomy placed at that time because of his need for long-term mechanical ventilation. Mrs. Morton says Kyle woke up about 20 minutes ago coughing and producing a large amount of mucus from his tracheostomy tube. His ventilator is producing a "high-pressure" alarm, and Kyle appears to be anxious and in moderate respiratory distress.

Recording Time: 1 Minute	
Appearance	13-year-old boy in a home hospital bed with head elevated 30°
Level of consciousness	Anxious
Airway	Open, tracheostomy tube in place
Breathing	Partially ventilator dependent, appears to have moderately increased work of breathing
Circulation	Strong radial pulse palpated

1. What other questions would you ask the mother at this time?
2. What is the significance of the high-pressure alarm?

■ Introduction

As a paramedic, you will encounter patients with a wide variety of special challenges. It is often necessary to modify how you communicate with, assess, treat, or transport a patient when that person has a chronic medical condition, sensory impairment, cognitive or emotional disorder, or other anomaly. An understanding of many of the special challenges highlighted in this chapter will help you provide optimal care when emergency medical services (EMS) assistance is required for these patients.

The combined incidence of cognitive, sensory, and communication impairments in the US population is staggering. One to three percent of the population has **intellectual disability**, making it the cognitive impairment that you are most likely to encounter.[1] Slightly more than 1% of children have **autism** or a related condition.[2] Overall, 13% of children have some form of **developmental disability**.[3]

Patients with complicated illnesses and those who require invasive medical devices are no longer confined to acute health care settings (Table 45-1). In 2014, more than 8.7 million patients received medical treatment in long-term care, skilled nursing care, **hospice** care, residential care, adult day care, or home health settings.[4] The largest portion of patients utilizing home health services are doing so as a result of diabetes or its complications.[5] This is in contrast to hospice (at home or in a residential setting) where the majority of patients are enrolled due to a terminal diagnosis of Alzheimer disease or some other form of dementia.[5]

The current data from the CDC indicate that about 15% of home health patients required an emergency department (ED) visit during their enrollment in home health services.[6] Approximately 17% of home health patients required an overnight stay in the hospital during that same time period.[6]

Table 45-1	Home Care Patients in the United States, 2013 and 2014
Age	**Average Percentage of Long-Term Care Services Users**
Under 65	16%
65–74	18%
75–84	29%
85 and over	37%

Data from: Harris-Kojetin L, Sengupta M, Park-Lee E, et al. Long-term care providers and services users in the United States: data from the national study of long-term care providers, 2013–2014. National Center for Health Statistics. *Vital Health Stat.* 2016;3(38):36-37. https://www.cdc.gov/nchs/data/series/sr_03/sr03_038.pdf. Accessed May 4, 2017.

Many life-sustaining therapies such as mechanical ventilation and intravenous (IV) medication administration are continued outside the hospital, often performed by members of the patient's family or by the patients themselves. You should expect to provide care to these patients during EMS response in the community and when these patients require transport between various health care facilities.

Many social and economic factors adversely impact the health of people. Paramedics are frequently requested as a last resort when a patient cannot otherwise access health care services or when attempts to manage an illness, injury, or chronic medical condition without assistance have suddenly failed. This situation can overwhelm EMS and ED resources, placing a heavy burden on paramedics in many EMS systems.

Patient care is further complicated when caregivers abuse or neglect people who are dependent on them. You must learn to recognize signs and cues that suggest abuse or neglect. Abuse and neglect recognition and reporting become essential when children, older adults, and many patients with the special challenges outlined in this chapter are victimized.

▶ General Strategies for Patients With Special Challenges

You should not feel overwhelmed when you are confronted by a patient with special challenges. In many instances, the patient and his or her caregivers have already become experts on a particular condition or impairment. An open mind and willingness to listen are often your greatest assets. You should demonstrate confidence while enlisting the expertise of the patient or other caregiver when you are determining the optimal method to communicate with, assess, treat, and transport a patient. This alliance will help you provide optimal patient care while minimizing the risk of mistakes, complications, or injuries to the patient or others. The collaboration may be as simple as the patient showing you the best place to start an IV line or as complicated as helping you troubleshoot a malfunctioning ventilator or infusion pump.

Patients and caregivers have often received large amounts of education related to a particular condition, device, or technique. It is a mistake for you to claim to have more familiarity with the situation than you actually have. The patient or caregivers are likely to immediately recognize any disparity, and their trust in you will be undermined. Conversely, a well-educated paramedic may be able to explain some important nuance related to the situation, greatly enhancing the understanding by the patient or his or her caregiver.

Resources such as online medical control, electronic medical reference materials, and the experience of coworkers will also prove extremely valuable when you encounter unfamiliar conditions, technology, or situations. A dedicated paramedic will learn from these encounters and become better prepared for similar challenges in the future.

EMS, Health Care, and Poverty

Paramedics, other EMS providers, and EDs are on the frontlines of the economic and health care crisis facing the United States. According to the US Census Bureau report *Income and Poverty in the United States: 2015*, 43.1 million people were in poverty in the United States in 2015.[7] The definition of poverty depends on a calculation that factors how many people are in a household, their ages, and the household's combined total income. For example, two people younger than age 65 years who have two children would be in poverty if their combined annual income was less than $24,257.[8] These trends profoundly impact EMS.

Poverty and the lack of health insurance impact a person's health habits in a variety of ways. As people lose the ability to pay for health care, they stop seeking or receiving many preventive health services. Without preventive measures, the incidence and severity of a disease process can increase significantly. Health care is often delayed until an emergent situation develops.

Chronic medical conditions such as diabetes, hypertension, reactive airway disease, mental disorders, and certain infectious diseases such as tuberculosis and acquired immune deficiency syndrome (AIDS) require ongoing medication to control the disease process. Poverty and the lack of health insurance may prevent patients from receiving needed medications. People may be forced to choose between paying for medications

and paying for other necessities such as food, clothing, or shelter. Interruption of needed medications can lead to catastrophic complications. Exacerbation of chronic illness due to lack of medication may lead to expensive hospitalization and worsening financial woes. Loss of a job or depletion of personal savings during periods of economic hardship can cause a patient to lose access to basic health care services.

Homelessness is a complicated economic and social problem. Homeless people are typically prone to numerous chronic medical conditions, frequently accompanied by mental illness and substance abuse. Medical care for homeless people is made more difficult by problems associated with environmental exposure, crime/violence, malnutrition, and lack of adequate hygiene. Rates of pregnancy, infectious diseases, and mental illness in homeless people far exceed rates in the general population.[9,10] People who are homeless have difficulty accessing preventive health care services and are subject to the same financial barriers to health maintenance as other people who live in poverty.

Patients frequently seek EMS and ED assistance when a chronic medical condition becomes severe or when health care is needed and no other options are available. Federal laws such as the Emergency Medical Treatment and Labor Act (EMTALA, discussed in Chapter 4, *Medical, Legal, and Ethical Issues*) require EDs to stabilize patients experiencing an emergency or active labor, regardless of the patient's ability to pay. This protection allows people with no means to pay for health care services to access health care providers without demand for upfront payment. The stress that this practice places on EDs is significant.

An alarming number of EDs have closed because of financial pressures and changes within the health care industry.[11,12] Many of the EDs that remain are becoming overcrowded. You may be forced to transport patients greater distances to an available ED or experience longer delays when turning patients over to ED staff due to overcrowding.[12]

The situation is further complicated by seemingly frivolous requests for EMS assistance and transportation. Paramedics and other EMS providers are often placed in a precarious position because they may believe a patient does not need to be taken to an ED, but they still feel obligated to transport the patient because of a fear of legal liability or regulations prohibiting patient abandonment. Sometimes, people may request EMS assistance simply as a method to obtain a "free ride" to the hospital or in an attempt to bypass overcrowded ED waiting rooms. Although other health care settings may be more appropriate for the needs of a particular patient, paramedics must be extremely careful to avoid legal liability or charges of patient abandonment. The distinction between an informed patient refusal and abandonment by EMS providers becomes problematic in many situations. Paramedics are in the unique position to assist people in the community by advocating for patient rights and suggesting safe alternatives so patients can receive appropriate medical care. Remember, when patients call for assistance, even when you do not believe such assistance is necessary, the safest thing to do is to provide that assistance. Never refuse to transport a patient if requested unless your EMS system and medical director specifically authorize you to do so.

Various health care organizations and communities have taken creative approaches to providing health care services outside the ED to people without health insurance or those who have limited financial resources. Whereas EDs are well suited to handle a patient in crisis, management of chronic medical conditions is often less than optimal. Such issues as medication monitoring, prescription refills, diagnostic testing, referrals, and coordination among specialists, as well as assistance with social needs, lifestyle modification, or long-term care, are best coordinated by primary health care providers. You may see changes in education and scope of practice as practices in the health care industry place increasing stress on EDs and EMS systems. Some hospital systems increase access to medical care by establishing free-standing EDs in strategic areas to ease overcrowding or facilitate referrals into larger tertiary centers. Creative ideas include having EMS providers offer more primary care services or allowing EMS providers to transport 9-1-1 patients to health care settings other than EDs. Other efforts include establishing formal community paramedicine programs, or placing midlevel personnel on certain EMS vehicles to provide definitive treatment in the patient's home without the need to transport the patient to a health care facility.

Health care resources are available for patients with financial need. Government agencies and private organizations provide health care services to at-risk groups through a variety of community-based health care facilities. These services may target homeless people, children, families, or any person with financial need. Many immunizations are provided at little or no cost by the government in the interest of public health. Hospitals are frequently able to provide financial assistance, payment plans, low-cost health care services, or help enrolling eligible people in government health insurance programs. EMS treatment or transportation should never be discouraged because of a person's perceived financial difficulty.

Care of Patients When Abuse or Neglect Is Suspected

You are likely to provide care to victims of abuse and neglect. However, you will most likely find that caring for these patients is made difficult by a host of emotional, legal, and regulatory concerns. In addition, the care you are trying to provide is frequently complicated by your interactions with the possible perpetrator or perpetrators. You must continue to provide effective care to these patients while taking affirmative steps to protect the potential victim from future harm.

Several groups of people are particularly susceptible to abuse or neglect by caregivers. Children and dependent older adults are at high risk for abuse and neglect, as discussed in Chapter 43, *Pediatric Emergencies*, and Chapter 44, *Geriatric Emergencies*. Adults with medical, cognitive, or emotional impairments may also be subject to abuse or neglect by caregivers. Many adult patients with specific challenges discussed later in this chapter are potential victims of abuse and neglect by family members or caregivers.

▶ Epidemiology of Abuse and Neglect

As discussed in Chapter 43, *Pediatric Emergencies*, and Chapter 44, *Geriatric Emergencies*, millions of children and vulnerable adults are abused or neglected each year in the United States. In most situations, the perpetrator is a family member.[13] Abuse and neglect occur with varied frequency across the spectrum of race and socioeconomic status. Child maltreatment can be committed by any person who has care, custody, or control of the child, including parents, step-parents, foster parents, babysitters, and relatives. Abusive parents frequently receive little enjoyment from parenting and are more isolated from the community than are nonabusive parents. They have unrealistic expectations of their children and try to control their children through negative and authoritarian means. Abusive parents are often afraid of asking for help from sources of support in their communities, or are emotionally unable to ask for help. Most were themselves abused or neglected as children. The determination of abuse and neglect becomes extremely difficult when factors such as poverty, religious beliefs regarding medical treatment, autonomy of mature minors, and potential victims with concomitant emotional or behavioral disorders are present.

▶ Definitions of Abuse and Neglect

Physical Abuse

Abuse and neglect may occur in a variety of ways. The Federal Child Abuse Prevention and Treatment Act, which broadly defines child abuse or neglect as "any recent act or failure to act on the part of a parent or caregiver which results in death, serious physical or emotional harm, **sexual abuse** or exploitation, or an act or failure to act which presents an imminent risk of serious harm."[14] Legal definitions of the different types of abuse and neglect vary significantly from state to state.

Physical abuse is generally defined as an intentional act such as throwing, striking, hitting, kicking, burning, or biting a child (or other vulnerable person) that results in physical impairment or injury. You may encounter victims of physical abuse when you are requested to respond for a dramatic injury, or suspected abuse may be discovered while you are treating and transporting patients with a seemingly unrelated complaint. Physical abuse also occurs if a caregiver places the child or other susceptible person in circumstances that create a substantial risk of harm. When a child is injured because of inadequate supervision or the caregiver's failure to use seat belts or other safety devices, it may or may not be considered physical abuse depending on the specific circumstances or the particular state where the injury occurred.

Neglect

Neglect of vulnerable people is roughly four times more common than is physical abuse, and it results in a higher percentage of child fatalities than does physical abuse.[15,16] Children, certain vulnerable or impaired adults, and dependent older adults require the assistance of caregivers to provide basic necessities such as food, shelter, medical care, supervision, and possibly financial guidance. When caregivers fail to provide such protection and the health or well-being of the vulnerable person is impacted, neglect occurs. Signs of neglect are often subtle, requiring greater awareness on the part of paramedics and other health care providers.

Sexual Abuse and Sexual Exploitation

Vulnerable people may become victims of sexual abuse or **sexual exploitation**. These acts may range from outright sexual contact, to forced prostitution, inappropriate undressing, sexually suggestive photography, or simply forcing the victim to watch sexual acts or pornography. Roughly 8.4% of reported child abuse or neglect cases involve sexual abuse or exploitation, though the actual incidence is unfortunately underreported.[16] Actual elder sexual abuse statistics are not readily available, although one study revealed that 81% of elder sexual abuse incidents involving a female victim were committed by the patient's primary caregiver.[17,18] Certain behavioral cues, genital trauma, and the presence of a sexually transmitted disease are highly suggestive of sexual abuse. In extreme cases, comatose women have become pregnant, leading to criminal charges for caregivers.[19,20]

Emotional Abuse

Emotional abuse impacts children, dependent older adults, and other vulnerable people. This abuse causes a substantial change in the victim's behavior, emotional response, or cognitive function, or it may manifest as a variety of mental illnesses. Emotional abuse may be verbal in the form of ridicule, threats, blaming, or humiliation. It also occurs nonverbally when a caregiver ignores the victim or isolates the victim from others.

Caregiver Substance Abuse

Various states have enacted laws that specifically address substance abuse by the parents or other caregiver. It may be considered abuse or neglect when pregnant women use alcohol, illicit drugs, or other harmful substances,

causing injury to the unborn child. Other state statutes address situations in which a caregiver provides alcohol or drugs to a child, manufactures or sells drugs in the presence of a child, or becomes impaired by alcohol or drugs while caring for a child or other vulnerable person. States may prosecute adults for child abuse when they drive while intoxicated with a child in the car or allow an underage child to become the designated driver for an intoxicated caregiver.

Abandonment

Caregivers may be prosecuted for abandonment in certain states. Abandonment occurs when a child or vulnerable adult suffers harm because the identified caregiver has failed to maintain adequate contact. Leaving a young child home alone and/or allowing the child to wander the streets unsupervised are two examples of possible abandonment.

▶ Recognizing Abuse or Neglect

Paramedics and other health care providers have a legal duty to recognize and report suspected abuse or neglect in children and vulnerable adults. A variety of behavioral cues and physical findings will prompt suspicion of abuse or neglect in these patients.

The demeanor, behaviors, and history provided by the caregiver are often the first clues that abuse or neglect may be present. You should become immediately suspicious if the designated caregiver appears to be under the influence of alcohol or other intoxicating substance. Agitation, slurred speech, bloodshot eyes, speech alteration, unsteady gait, or other unexplained abnormality is suggestive of intoxication.

Caregivers in abuse or neglect situations may interfere with the physical examination of the child or vulnerable adult. Behaviors such as refusing to allow a physical exam, looming over the health care provider during the physical exam, preventing paramedics from removing clothing during the physical exam, or offering unsolicited explanations for abnormal physical findings during the exam may all be suggestive of abuse or neglect. The caregiver may also interrupt or otherwise prevent the patient from answering questions related to the particular illness or injury. Remember, do not confront a suspected perpetrator; rather, simply report to the "hotline" and ED physician. These behaviors should raise your suspicion of abuse or neglect.

You should pay particular attention when a caregiver provides the history of present illness/injury or describes the events that prompted the call for EMS involvement. In many instances, the story provided by the caregiver simply does not make sense in relation to the age, capability, or medical condition of the patient. In other situations, the story provided by the caregiver will frequently change with each subsequent discussion or the explanations provided by the patient and various caregivers will be significantly different.

A caregiver may occasionally self-report facts that are highly suggestive of abuse or neglect. Statements such as "I lost my temper," "I couldn't get her to stop crying," or "I did it to teach him a lesson" should raise immediate concerns regarding abuse or neglect. Other situations, such as a child being injured due to obviously careless actions of an intoxicated caregiver, should trigger your concerns regarding abuse or neglect. More information on child abuse and neglect is discussed in Chapter 43, *Pediatric Emergencies*.

In many instances, there is a legitimate reason for the findings that is related to normal growth and development or a particular medical or mental health condition, not resulting from any maltreatment. You should discuss abnormal behavioral cues or other findings with receiving health care providers when you observe unusual findings during patient assessment.

A variety of physical signs are highly suggestive of the possibility of nonaccidental trauma, particularly in young children and infants. Physical abuse is commonly associated with fractures, burns, and bruises. Bruises on the torso, ears, proximal arms, abdomen, and buttocks are suggestive of abuse **Figure 45-1** . Closed head injury in the absence of a realistic mechanism is also suggestive of abuse. One author reports that 24% to 56% of head injuries in patients younger than age 2 years are a result of physical abuse.[21] Burns, particularly symmetric burns or those without splash marks, and ligature marks suggest abuse **Figure 45-2** . Bruises in patterns resembling finger marks, shoes, or other common items are also extremely concerning for physical abuse. Seizure activity without a prior history in an afebrile child should raise suspicion for the possibility of physical abuse.

▶ Benign Physical Findings

Paramedics and other EMS providers should be aware of notable physical findings that mimic signs of physical abuse. At first glance these findings may appear highly suggestive of nonaccidental trauma, but on further investigation, maltreatment is often ruled out.

As discussed in Chapter 43, *Pediatric Emergencies*, children are prone to bruising or minor injuries as psychomotor skills develop through early childhood. Recall that people sometimes have marks that are not the result of abuse. Examples of these include Mongolian spots, and marks from the practices of coining and cupping **Figure 45-3** . Another example is phytophotodermatitis, which can result from application of citrus or vegetable juices to the patient's skin for healing purposes.

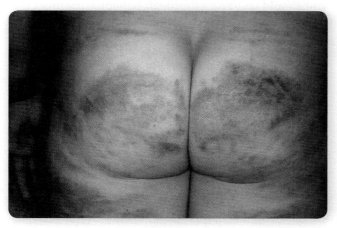

Figure 45-1 Bruises on the buttocks are usually inflicted injuries.

Courtesy of Ronald Dieckmann, M.D.

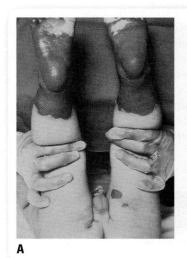
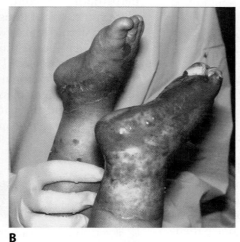
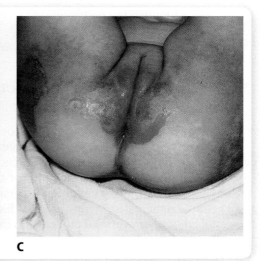

A **B** **C**

Figure 45-2 A. A symmetric scald is a sign of child abuse. **B.** Stocking/glove burns of the feet or hands in an infant or a toddler are almost always inflicted injuries. **C.** A doughnut burn occurs when a child is held in a hot bath and the area in contact with the cooler porcelain is spared.

Courtesy of Ronald Dieckmann, M.D.

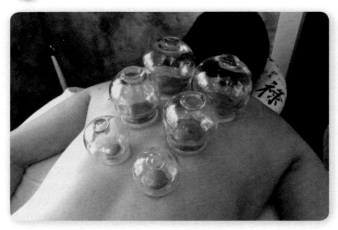

Figure 45-3 Cupping is the cultural practice of placing warm cups on the skin to extract illness from the body. The red, flat, rounded skin lesions are often more intensely red at the borders.

© Cora Reed/Shutterstock.

You may also encounter benign physical findings that are suggestive of sexual abuse. Poor hygiene, masturbating, skin irritation from cleansing products, marks from poorly fitting undergarments, and various infections can all cause physical findings that are suggestive of sexual abuse. You should use caution before labeling manifestations of many of these benign conditions as sexual abuse.

> ## Words of Wisdom
>
> It is a good idea to establish a "code" between you and your partner indicating that the provider should discreetly call for police. This signal can be as simple as "Could you go to the ambulance and get the extra set of latex-free gloves?" This way, you will not aggravate or "tip off" the abuser to your request for police, further riling him or her.

► Management of Suspected Abuse or Neglect

Care of patients who are victims of abuse or neglect may present a considerable challenge for paramedics. Innocent victims suffer devastating injuries at the hands of people who are supposed to be responsible for the patient's well-being. When innocent children, vulnerable adults, or frail geriatric patients are victimized, it is likely to evoke powerful emotions in you and other health care providers. These emotions have the potential to undermine patient care and ultimately worsen the situation for the patient.

Assessment

You should focus on several key priorities when you are caring for a patient with suspected abuse or neglect.

Domestic violence incidents are notorious for placing police, emergency responders, and even innocent bystanders at considerable risk of harm. Law enforcement assistance should be requested whenever the threat of continued violence is present. Scene safety is discussed in greater depth in other areas of this text.

The second priority is for you to provide optimal clinical care to any patient whom you suspect to be the victim of abuse or neglect. This includes patient assessment that is appropriate for the clinical situation. You should not waste time conducting a meticulous head-to-toe examination when immediate threats to a patient's life are present. Life-sustaining interventions and prompt transport are the most appropriate treatment for any patient with a critical illness or injury. Immediate threats to life must be treated aggressively, regardless of whether abuse or neglect is present or suspected. As time permits, you should conduct a thorough patient assessment that includes a history of present illness, head-to-toe exam, and any relevant medical and psychosocial history. The value of full patient exposure must be balanced against privacy needs of the patient and the risks of further traumatizing a victim of suspected abuse or neglect.

It is likely that all the facts of a particular situation will not be fully disclosed when you initially interact with the patient and any caregivers present. You should not make any hasty assumptions regarding the identity of an alleged perpetrator or circumstances surrounding a particular event. It is possible that the caregiver present with the patient is also a victim of abuse, neglect, or violence.

You must use careful judgment when you are deciding whether to allow a particular parent or caregiver to remain or travel with the patient. Separating an ill or injured patient from a trusted caregiver may cause additional stress, especially if this caregiver turns out not to be a perpetrator or in situations when no abuse or neglect has actually occurred. Conversely, the presence of a violent perpetrator may continue to threaten the patient and place you at risk of injury.

You should make every attempt to remain nonjudgmental when you are providing patient care. This is often not easy when powerful emotions are present. You need to remain professional and provide the patient with the best treatment possible. Comments and hostility directed toward the patient's caregiver are unlikely to do anything except complicate the situation, and are unprofessional.

> ## Words of Wisdom
>
> If you and your partner can safely get the patient and the person suspected of abuse away from each other, by all means do so. This separation will help make the scene safer; it also gives you a chance to compare current histories.

Documentation

Careful documentation is essential whenever abuse or neglect is present or suspected. You should expect that any patient care reports (PCRs) and related documentation are going to be reviewed by law enforcement officers, by social service agencies, and in court. Simple documentation errors such as incorrect spelling or grammar and inconsistent times will undermine both the credibility of the documentation and the paramedic responsible for the documentation. Use accurate quotations whenever possible, identifying the source of the information. Carefully document any physical findings or indicate whether assessment of a particular body area was accomplished or deferred. Avoid inaccurate terms such as "normal" or "within normal limits," if a particular area has not been adequately evaluated. Use objective descriptions and measurements whenever possible when you are documenting findings on the physical exam. You should carefully document the timing or time frame of a particular injury or event. Subsequent changes in the reported timing of an event may disclose or substantiate suspicions of abuse or neglect. Avoid labeling a person as a victim or perpetrator. Cite a specific source when you are charting a history of present illness. Avoid photography unless there is a formal policy at the EMS agency that outlines appropriate consent, technique, storage, security, and release of any patient photographs. Special training is often required for forensic photography. It is quite easy for an otherwise well-intentioned paramedic to violate the Health Insurance Portability and Accountability Act (HIPAA) or other patient privacy rules by taking and sharing patient photographs.

Mandatory Reporting and Legal Involvement

Paramedics, EMS providers, and other health professionals are **mandatory reporters** of suspected child abuse and neglect. If you have a reasonable suspicion that child abuse or neglect has occurred, you must report the circumstances to the appropriate child welfare agency for a particular jurisdiction. If you fail to report suspected child abuse or neglect, you may be subject to a variety of civil, criminal, or regulatory penalties. Many states have enacted statutes specifically addressing mandatory reporting of abuse to older and incapacitated adults, though the scope of these statutes may vary significantly from state to state. You should consult your applicable state laws and EMS regulations regarding mandatory reporting of suspected abuse and neglect of older adults and other vulnerable adults.

Suspected abuse and neglect are reported to the state or government social services agency of a particular jurisdiction. Agency titles vary by location but are usually called something similar to Adult Protective Services, Child Protective Services, Department of Youth Services, or Children Youth and Family Division. In most states, central hotline telephone numbers are available for abuse or neglect reports involving children or vulnerable adults. These agencies evaluate the circumstances of a particular report and determine whether an investigation is indicated.

YOU are the Paramedic PART 2

Your partner begins to obtain a set of vital signs as you initiate care for Kyle. His mother says that he has coughing fits like this from time to time and that normally they use their home suction machine, but it suddenly stopped working when this episode began. She has contacted the home health nurse, and he is on his way to the home but will not arrive for another hour. Kyle's condition has affected his quality of life dramatically, but he is not terminally ill. He is not on hospice, and there is no do not resuscitate order on record for him.

Recording Time: 3 Minutes	
Respirations	18 breaths/min; mechanically ventilated with bilateral breath sounds and symmetrical chest rise present, with diminished tidal volume noted
Pulse	114 beats/min, regular, strong peripheral pulses
Skin	Pale, clammy
Oxygen saturations (Spo$_2$)	86% on room air
Pupils	PERRLA

3. In addressing this patient's respiratory status, what strategy could you use to quickly rule out or address the most life-threatening conditions?
4. Given this patient's clinical presentation, what is a likely cause for his respiratory distress?

Unfortunately, not every report of abuse or neglect will automatically trigger an investigation. Rates of investigations of abuse and neglect reports vary significantly from state to state. Circumstances of the case and the severity of the alleged abuse or neglect will determine whether an investigation is initiated or how urgently the social services agency intervenes. Intervention may range from providing support to an at-risk family all the way to immediate removal of the victim from the home or facility.

Law enforcement personnel frequently become involved in cases of suspected abuse or neglect. Law enforcement officers may respond simultaneously with EMS, may discover abuse or neglect while engaged in other law enforcement activities, or may be requested by health care providers, EMS responders, or an investigator from the social services agency. Law enforcement officers have two primary roles when abuse or neglect is suspected. They may intervene when there is an immediate threat to the health or safety of a child or vulnerable adult. Officers are typically empowered to take custody of a child or vulnerable adult for a short duration until the appropriate social services agency can intervene or the immediate threat resolves. In addition, law enforcement officers conduct a simultaneous investigation into potential criminal activity associated with the suspected abuse or neglect. When suspected abuse or neglect results in death, these cases are referred to the medical examiner for autopsy.

Paramedics and other emergency responders may benefit from emotional support following their response to dramatic or heart-wrenching cases of abuse or neglect. Many areas have specially trained crisis intervention personnel who are familiar with the difficult role of EMS and other emergency responders. These personnel can help paramedics and other emergency medical responders recognize and manage the enormous emotional stress associated with these extremely challenging situations.

Care of Patients With Terminal Illness

Despite advances in the science and technology of modern health care, many disease processes simply cannot be reversed. As patients confront the reality of failing health, many choose to forego uncomfortable, invasive, and often marginally effective medical treatment of a particular condition or disease. Paramedics and other EMS providers will encounter patients with a wide variety of terminal illnesses as well as those who decline aggressive medical intervention for otherwise potentially treatable conditions.

Most sources define **terminal illness** as a disease process that is expected to cause death within 6 months, verified by a physician. These conditions may persist for years as the health of the patient either fluctuates or steadily declines. Common terminal conditions include **cancer**, heart failure, pulmonary disease, liver failure, human immunodeficiency virus (HIV), Alzheimer disease, and amyotrophic lateral sclerosis (also known as Lou Gehrig disease). When you are treating these patients, you must be prepared to alter or forego the aggressive, lifesaving interventions that have historically defined the paramedic profession. If you are called to a scene in which death is imminent, the actions you take will have a lasting impact on the family. This is a time when compassion, understanding, and sensitivity are most needed.

Patients with a terminal illness often receive continued medical care. Some continue aggressive medical treatment, hoping for a statistically improbable recovery or attempting to prolong life as much as possible. This approach is known as **curative care**. Other patients may pursue curative care, but refrain from treatment options that are risky, minimally effective, or cause significant discomfort. As the disease process worsens and hopes for recovery fade, patients may transition from curative care to **comfort care**, also known as **palliative care**. When a patient is receiving comfort or palliative care, the focus changes from prolonging life to improving the quality of the time that the patient has left. Medical care continues, but aggressive, invasive, and uncomfortable interventions cease. Patients undergoing comfort care frequently continue to receive analgesic medications, oxygen, IV fluids, treatment of fevers, and possibly antibiotic medications.

Terminally ill patients seen by EMS usually need only supportive care. Therapy is usually aimed at making the patient as comfortable as possible. The patient may have a displaced urinary catheter, need assistance in returning to bed, or need intervention in a pain crisis.

Patients with a terminal illness and their caregivers will often know the best way to manage sudden increases in discomfort. Pain assessment and management are often primary tasks for paramedics treating patients with a terminal illness. Patients should be assessed for pain using a variety of techniques depending on the patient's age, ability to communicate, and cognitive function. You should obtain a history that includes the patient's use of, effectiveness of, and adverse reactions to particular pain medications, especially if you have limited pharmacologic options for pain management. Terminally ill patients may use a complex array of pain medications, transdermal patches, or self-administered pain management devices. You should perform a patient assessment that includes the patient's level of consciousness, vital signs, past medical history, and pain medication history, and then either follow standing protocols or contact medical control to administer analgesic or sedative medications for patient comfort.

Many patients with a verified terminal illness choose to enter hospice treatment. Hospice is a program and philosophy that attempts to help the patient maximize the quality of remaining life. Hospice programs provide social and emotional support, treat discomfort with pharmacologic and nonpharmacologic approaches, and help patients and families cope with the prospect of impending death. Patients may receive hospice treatment at home, in hospitals, or while living at long-term care facilities.

► Advance Directives

Approximately one-quarter of adults in the US have some form of advance directive.[22] These forms are signed by either the patient or the **surrogate decision maker**. A surrogate decision maker is someone who is legally authorized to make health care decisions for that patient when the patient is not capable of making or communicating the decision himself or herself. As discussed in Chapter 4, *Medical, Legal, and Ethical Issues*, the forms instruct health care providers regarding how medical decisions for the patient are to be made when the patient is unable to comprehend or communicate such a decision due to incapacity. Remember, patients with decision-making capacity may revoke a prior advance directive. You should contact online medical control when there is any confusion regarding the documentation or in situations when a patient's surrogate decision maker is contradicting a written advance directive.

Hospice patients, along with many hospital patients and those living at home or in long-term care facilities, have do not resuscitate (DNR) orders in place. EMS providers can be placed in a precarious situation when they are encountering a patient in cardiac or respiratory arrest. State EMS agencies may require a specific DNR form for prehospital providers in the event of a prehospital cardiac or respiratory arrest. These forms may not be readily available when a prehospital resuscitation decision must be made. Other indicators of DNR status include wristbands and bracelets. EMS regulations will specify whether a symbolic indication of DNR status is sufficient for EMS providers to withhold resuscitation efforts. The situation becomes further complicated when conflict exists between DNR paperwork and the stated wishes of a family member or surrogate decision maker for the patient. Consult the EMS regulations for your state for specific requirements related to DNR orders and advance directives.

Patient Safety

In situations where resuscitation efforts may not be helpful (terminal illness, hospice settings, etc), be sure to ask the patient or caregivers if an advance directive or DNR order exists. It is always better to ask these questions before respiratory or cardiac arrest occurs in case any clarification or discussion with online medical control is needed.

■ Care of Bariatric Patients

Caring for patients with **obesity** present challenges for health care providers. Paramedics and other EMS responders must overcome many significant clinical and logistical hurdles when they are treating and transporting patients with profound obesity. As the obesity epidemic worsens, EMS systems may require additional resources to provide optimal care to this at-risk patient population.

Table 45-2	Causes of and Contributing Factors to Obesity
Poor dietary choices	
Excessive food intake	
Lack of exercise	
Hormonal changes	
Inadequate sleep	
Low basal metabolic rate	
Environmental toxins	
Genetic predisposition	
Cessation/reduction of cigarette smoking	
Widespread dependence on air conditioning	

Data from: Dare S, Mackay DF, Pell JP. Relationship between smoking and obesity: a cross-sectional study of 499,504 middle-aged adults in the UK general population. *PLoS One*. 2015;10(4):e0123579. https://www.ncbi.nlm.nih.gov/pmc /articles/PMC4401671/. Accessed May 4, 2017.

The medical specialty of **bariatrics** has emerged in response to the widespread and profound incidence of adult and childhood obesity. Over one-third of American adults are considered to have obesity, defined by a body mass index (BMI) of greater than 30 kilograms per meter squared (kg/m^2).[23] People with a BMI between 40 and 49.9 kg/m^2 are considered to have morbid obesity. A BMI above 50 kg/m^2 is considered extreme obesity. Approximately 20% of children and adolescents have obesity.[24] According to the US Centers for Disease Control and Prevention (CDC), obesity adds more than $147 billion to annual US health care costs.[25,26] Several studies have found that the obesity rates of EMS personnel and firefighters exceed the general population; one such study demonstrated that 75% of firefighter and paramedic recruits in a particular state either were overweight or had obesity.[27]

A wide variety of lifestyle, genetic, metabolic, and environmental causes are responsible for obesity **Table 45-2**.

Obesity causes or worsens a number of serious medical conditions. Heart disease, cerebrovascular accident, diabetes, hypertension, some cancers, and asthma are only some of the diseases linked to obesity. These patients are also prone to physical injury and a variety of musculoskeletal problems.

► Clinical Concerns for the Bariatric Patient

Routine procedures for patients with obesity can become extremely complicated. Airway procedures are made more

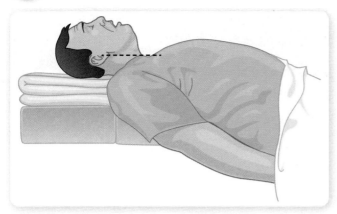

Figure 45-4 The ramped position with the head and shoulders elevated approximately 25° to 30° increases the chance of successful airway management. It is important to confirm that the external auditory meatus is in line with the sternal notch.

Data from: Miller RD, Cohen NH, Erikkson LI, et al. Chapter 55: Airway management in the adult. In: Miller's Anesthesia. 8th ed. Philadelphia, PA: Elsevier; 2015:1666.

difficult by a larger tongue, larger patient head size, and limited neck mobility associated with obesity. Bag-mask ventilation may be ineffective with patients in a supine position. Multiple studies have demonstrated that ramped positioning of the patient with obesity has a positive impact on the chances of successful airway management.[28-33] Ramping of the patient with obesity may be accomplished by utilizing pillows and/or blankets to achieve the desired position or with commercially-manufactured ramping devices **Figure 45-4**. Both methods carry equivalent rates of success and complication.[28-33] Patients with obesity may have a diminished respiratory reserve, decreasing the window to perform airway procedures before the patient becomes hypoxic. These patients often require bag-mask ventilations with positive end-expiratory pressure (PEEP), continuous positive airway pressure (CPAP), or bilevel positive airway pressure (BPAP) as a way to avoid endotracheal intubation or as a bridge until successful intubation can occur. Even bag-mask ventilation can become difficult because of poor mask seal or increased resistance due to excess body tissue on the chest wall and abdomen.

Peripheral IV access is often problematic in patients with obesity. A large neck mass may obscure landmarks for external jugular IV line placement or surgical cricothyrotomy. Many conventional intramuscular (IM) needles will not be able to actually reach the IM space through

Words of Wisdom

When you are transporting a bariatric patient or a patient with obesity, alert the receiving facility in advance if special accommodations, equipment, or other resources may be needed.

excess adipose tissue. Absorption and distribution will be altered for many lipophilic medications, potentially causing dramatic patient response at a given dose. Auscultation of heart, lung, or bowel sounds may be more difficult through extra abdominal and chest wall mass.

▶ Operational Concerns for the Bariatric Patient

EMS treatment and transport of patients with obesity can quickly become complicated. These patients are often too heavy for traditional two-person EMS crews to package and transport safely or effectively. Additional lifting assistance is frequently necessary, although small rooms and narrow staircases limit the utility of additional lifting personnel. As patient weights become extreme, the capacity of EMS equipment such as stretchers, backboards, and stair chairs is quickly exceeded. EMS providers have attempted novel solutions such as using doors, tarps, or plywood for transporting patients with extreme obesity. These improvised devices are not designed to be carried safely and typically have no reliable way to secure the patient. Careful planning and proper body mechanics are essential to avoid injury to emergency responders or the patient.

Paramedics need to advocate for EMS equipment that is capable of safely transporting patients with obesity. Some EMS systems use ambulances with special winches, stretchers, and ramps that allow safe loading of bariatric patients. Even simple items such as larger blood pressure cuffs, longer injection or intraosseous (IO) needles, or special cervical collars may dramatically improve your ability to provide patient care.

The obesity epidemic will likely continue to grow. You should be prepared to encounter these patients with a vast array of illnesses and injuries in any conceivable scene location. Careful planning, a thorough understanding of the challenges involved, and the proper equipment will help you provide the best care possible to this extremely high-risk group.

■ Care of Patients With Communicable Diseases

As discussed in Chapter 26, *Infectious Diseases*, communicable diseases are infectious diseases that can be passed from one person to another by a variety of modes. The severity of these diseases ranges from almost completely undetectable to causing death within several days or weeks. Many patients live for years with a particular communicable disease and the continuous potential to transmit this disease to others. You should expect to encounter patients with communicable disease in every segment of the population and every geographic region. As discussed in Chapter 2, *Workforce Safety and Wellness*, always follow safety protocols and wear proper protective equipment.

Many communicable diseases have significant psychosocial implications. Having a communicable disease can take an emotional toll on the patient, his or her family, and loved ones. Also, certain communicable diseases are commonly associated with particular lifestyle choices that may not be well accepted by others. Communicable diseases often prompt paranoia in people who lack an understanding of the actual risk and mode or modes of transmission. People suspected of having a communicable disease may face discrimination, stigmatization, threats, or hostile treatment in the community. To provide optimal care, paramedics must have the patient's trust, which requires maintaining his or her privacy and treating the patient with respect.

Patient assessment and communication should be conducted with as much privacy as possible. Bystanders, other emergency responders, and even personnel at a receiving facility may have an indirect relationship with the patient. Any unnecessary release of private information could adversely affect the patient. Violation of patient privacy rules can ultimately have harsh legal consequences for you, the paramedic, as well.

You should endeavor to treat patients who have a communicable disease with all the respect and dignity afforded other patients. Patients may acquire a communicable disease through occupational exposure, sexual assault, blood transfusion, close family contact, or other method, without ever participating in any high-risk behaviors. Assumptions based on stereotypes of a particular communicable disease are unlikely to accomplish anything aside from undermining patient care efforts.

Medical Technology in the Prehospital Setting

Patients with complex medical needs are no longer confined to acute health care settings. Many invasive, unusual, or life-sustaining therapies, once reserved for hospitals, are now widely used in patient homes and long-term care facilities. Chronically ill patients are cared for at home by a wide range of caregivers who may include family members, unlicensed caregivers, licensed nonprofessional caregivers, licensed professionals, or a combination of these. As mentioned, many family members who care for chronically ill patients are medically knowledgeable and are often your best source for information and care guidelines. In addition to frail or chronically ill geriatric patients in the home care setting, you may encounter patients, for example, who have recently had a hospital stay, surgery, or a high-risk pregnancy, or a newborn with medical complications. When you encounter medical technology and adaptive devices during an EMS response or an interfacility patient transport, this technology may simplify, complicate, or have no impact whatsoever on your patient care. You may need to troubleshoot these devices when they malfunction or incorporate this technology into traditional prehospital patient care.

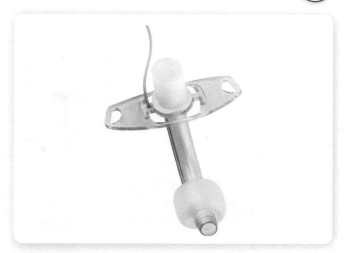

Figure 45-5 Tracheostomy tube.
Portex® Blue Line® Ultra Tracheostomy courtesy of Smiths Medical.

▶ Tracheostomy Tubes

A **tracheostomy tube** `Figure 45-5`, often referred to simply as a *trach* (pronounced "trake") *tube*, functions as a long-term replacement for an endotracheal (ET) tube. These devices are used for patients requiring long-term ventilator support, frequent tracheal suctioning, or airway protection resulting from a long list of possible medical conditions. If a patient experiences an unexpected loss of a tracheostomy tube due to occlusion or an accidental removal, it may or may not create an emergency. Many patients, even those on long-term ventilators, may tolerate interruptions in ventilator support for a period of time. Other patients, including those with cervical spinal cord injuries or serious neuromuscular disease are completely dependent on the ventilator. Loss of a tracheostomy tube may become an immediate threat to life.

Tracheostomy tubes can be placed emergently by health care providers when a profound upper airway obstruction occurs. They may also be placed electively in patients already receiving mechanical ventilation via ET tubes or in patients with a slowly evolving upper airway obstruction or tumor. Tracheostomy tubes may be used by patients in the community, with or without an attached ventilator.

The tracheostomy tube passes directly from an opening in the anterior neck, below the thyroid cartilage, into the trachea. Speech is not possible unless expired air is allowed to pass around the tracheostomy tube and through the larynx (vocal cords). A tracheostomy tube bypasses the nasal passages that filter, warm, and humidify inspired air. Patients with a tracheostomy tube in place will need humidification and heating of inspired air whenever possible. These patients also need frequent deep suctioning with an appropriately sized suction catheter. In health care settings, deep tracheal suctioning is performed with sterile technique. Secretions may accumulate above the

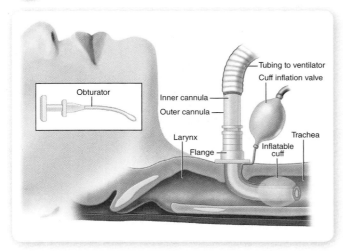

Figure 45-6 A tracheostomy is a surgical procedure in which an opening is placed in the trachea below the cricoid ring. A tracheostomy tube can be inserted into the opening to maintain it. It can also be attached to a ventilator or bag-mask device to assist with ventilations.

© Jones & Bartlett Learning.

tracheostomy tube, requiring oral suctioning in addition to deep tracheal suctioning.

Tracheostomy tubes consist of three main parts with several notable additional features Figure 45-6 . The **outer cannula** is the larger tube that passes from the anterior neck surface, inferior to the thyroid cartilage, into the trachea. Part of the outer cannula is a **flange** that helps stabilize the tracheostomy tube on the skin of the patient's neck and gets secured with ties or a strap around the patient's neck. The outer cannula may or may not have a cuff, similar to an ET tube cuff. If a cuff is present, a short length of tubing with a cuff port (pilot balloon) and Luer valve will be visible. In adults, tracheostomy tube cuffs are necessary for bag-mask or ventilator assistance. Children may or may not require a tracheostomy tube cuff for assisted ventilation.

The second part of the tracheostomy tube is the **inner cannula**. The inner cannula is a tube that runs inside the outer cannula and can typically be removed for cleaning, although not all inner cannulas are capable of being removed. The inner cannula has a 15-mm port that can be attached to a bag-mask or ventilator circuit.

Words of Wisdom

If a tracheostomy tube becomes plugged, the patient may be ventilated by deflating the cuff, covering the nose and mouth with a mask, and using a bag-mask device. If you are unable to ventilate the patient through the tracheostomy tube, plug the tracheostomy stoma and attempt to ventilate the patient in the traditional manner with a bag-mask device.

Special Populations

If you are transporting a child with a tracheostomy tube in a standard car seat, avoid using seats with a tray or shield. The tray or shield could come into contact with the tracheostomy tube and injure the child or block the airway.

The third part of the tracheostomy tube is the removable **obturator**, which is a solid plug with a rounded tip that extends out the bottom (inside) end of the trachea. The obturator is used for initial insertion and reinsertion of the tracheostomy tube (outer cannula) if it becomes dislodged. In the unlikely event that traditional mask-to-mouth ventilations must be performed on a patient with a tracheostomy tube in place, such as cuff failure in a ventilator-dependent patient with no backup outer cannula, the obturator may be inserted to keep air from escaping out the tracheostomy tube.

Tracheostomy tubes may be **fenestrated**, which means that holes or openings are present in the outer cannula or both the inner and the outer cannula. These holes allow the patients to speak, breathe, or clear secretions from the upper airway. Not every tracheostomy tube has fenestrations. These may be used for patients who are being evaluated for tracheostomy tube removal or for patients who require only intermittent ventilator support. It is essential that any cuff be deflated before a fenestrated tube is capped for speaking or clearing of secretions.

Patients and their family members or caregivers are likely to be thoroughly familiar with tracheostomy tube problems. You should not be afraid to accept assistance when you are evaluating, using, or troubleshooting a tracheostomy tube. Any needed equipment is likely to be close by if the patient is at home or in a long-term care facility. Many health care facilities have a policy to keep an extra correctly sized tracheostomy tube at the patient's bedside at all times. Routine care for tracheostomy tubes includes keeping the stoma clean and dry. The outer cannula should be changed as needed. Patients may also require periodic suctioning, depending on their ability to keep the airway clear of secretions or sputum.

Troubleshooting tracheostomy tube problems is similar to troubleshooting ET tube problems. You should follow the DOPE acronym (Dislodged/displaced/disconnected, Obstruction, Pneumothorax, Equipment). First, check for a dislodged, displaced, or disconnected tracheostomy tube. It is possible for a tracheostomy tube to end up in a **false lumen**, outside the trachea, following removal and reinsertion or partial removal. A false lumen can be detected by placing an endotracheal suction catheter into the tracheostomy tube. If the suction catheter meets resistance immediately beyond the expected end of the tracheostomy tube, placement into a false lumen should be considered. If this happens, the tracheostomy outer cannula will need to be removed and then reinserted. Continuous end-tidal capnography monitoring will alert you of any unexpected dislodging, displacement, or disconnect of the tracheostomy tube during transport.

You also need to evaluate for tracheostomy (or ventilator circuit) obstruction. Obstruction of a tracheostomy tube may be cleared by removing the inner cannula and then using a suction catheter to push the mucous plug out. Alternatively, an obstruction may be removed by using a combination of tracheostomy tube suctioning and mechanical ventilation through the tracheostomy tube to loosen and remove a mucous plug.

If the patient's only available tracheostomy tube becomes lost or unusable, you can carefully insert an appropriately sized ET tube into the tracheostomy tube opening (called a stoma). Care must be taken to ensure that the ET tube enters the trachea, not a false lumen under the skin but outside the trachea. Various techniques such as bougie, gloved finger, or hemostat guidance can be used to ensure correct placement. A correctly placed ET tube will appear unusually shallow when placed directly into the trachea. Correct placement is confirmed using a combination of end-tidal carbon dioxide, breath sounds, ventilation compliance, chest rise, and clinical improvement. Finally, pneumothorax and equipment (ventilator or ventilator tubing) failure should be evaluated when you are attempting to troubleshoot a malfunctioning tracheostomy tube.

To suction and clean a tracheostomy tube, follow the steps in **Skill Drill 45-1**.

Skill Drill 45-1 Cleaning a Tracheostomy Tube

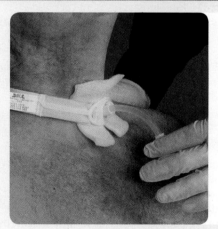

Step 1 Wash your hands and apply a mask, goggles, and clean nonlatex gloves. Suctioning a home care patient is a clean procedure, not a sterile one. Open supplies may be used. For cost reasons, home care patients often reuse their suction catheters. If the catheters do not have visible contamination and have been stored in a clean manner, they are acceptable for use. Remove the inner cannula and check with your patient's caregiver, if available, regarding the appropriate solution for soaking the device, then place the device to soak in the recommended solution. If the caregiver is not available, use a 50/50 mixture of hydrogen peroxide and water. Placing the cannula in plain water is acceptable in short-term situations. With one-piece tracheostomy tubes, this step is unnecessary. If the patient is dependent on a ventilator, have a replacement cannula immediately available.

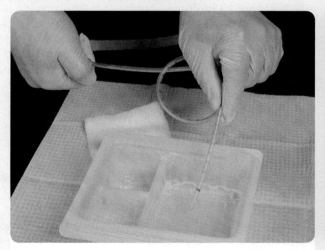

Step 2 Attach the catheter to negative pressure. Check the suction and clear the catheter by drawing up a small amount of saline.

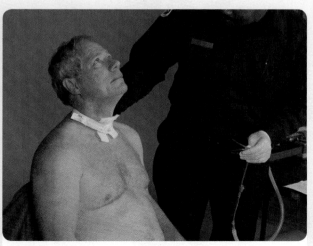

Step 3 Have the patient take a deep breath or preoxygenate the patient using the ventilator.

(continued)

Skill Drill 45-1 Cleaning a Tracheostomy Tube *(continued)*

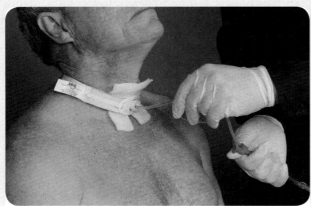

Step 4 Insert the catheter into the trachea without suction. Apply intermittent suction while removing the catheter. Repeat as necessary. Ensure the patient's oxygen saturation remains adequate throughout the procedure.

Step 5 Clean the inner cannula with the tracheostomy brush, rinse, and replace and lock into place. Omit this step for a one-piece tracheostomy tube. Remove your gloves and wash your hands. Document the procedure and assessment on your PCR.

© Jones & Bartlett Learning. Courtesy of MIEMSS.

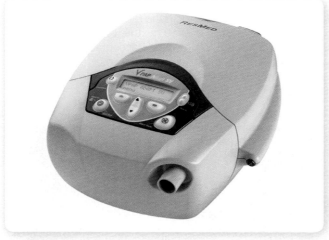

Figure 45-7 A home ventilator.
© ResMed 2012. Used with permission.

Patient Safety

Patients requiring long-term mechanical ventilation are susceptible to the same pathogens as non–ventilator-dependent patients, but they may contract infections with these pathogens more easily. These organisms are typically gram negative and are often resistant to multiple antibiotics.[34] *Pseudomonas aeruginosa* is a common cause of nosocomial and community-acquired pneumonia in patients on long-term mechanical ventilation. Patients may be colonized with bacteria and not have an active infection, yet still be able to infect others when proper personal protection and hand hygiene recommendations are not followed.[35] Ventilator-dependent patients are also susceptible to opportunistic infections that healthy individuals do not routinely contract, due to diminished host defense mechanisms.

▶ Long-Term Ventilators

Patients may be on long-term ventilators at home for a variety of reasons **Figure 45-7**. Spinal cord injury, neuromuscular disease, and lung injury are all conditions associated with long-term ventilator use. It is possible that ventilator use will have nothing at all to do with the reason that EMS was requested for a particular patient.

The primary survey for any patient on a long-term ventilator should include determining whether the ventilator is working effectively for the patient. Patients with a chronic lung disease may have oxygen levels well below what is considered normal for healthy people. You should inquire whether unusual findings such as an elevated respiratory rate or decreased oxygen saturation level are "normal" for this particular patient. Certain serious medical conditions can be made worse by overly aggressive oxygenation and ventilation. If the ventilator appears to be adequate for the patient, it is typically best to leave the ventilator settings unchanged and leave the ventilator connected to the patient.

If the ventilator does not appear to be working effectively for the patient, you have two possible options. It is possible to work with the patient or caregiver to adjust ventilator settings. You should be familiar with the clinical impact of various ventilator changes before attempting to adjust the patient's ventilator. It is possible to severely injure a patient by improperly adjusting his or her ventilator. Additional discussion of ventilator management is in Chapter 15, *Airway Management*.

You always have the option of disconnecting the ventilator completely if the patient is in unstable condition or there is a ventilator malfunction that you are unable to correct. You may choose to disconnect the ventilator during cardiac arrest or other critical illness and initiate ventilation with a bag-mask device or via the patient's tracheostomy tube. PEEP is likely to be needed during bag-mask ventilations for patients who are receiving long-term ventilator support. PEEP valves can be attached to many disposable bag-mask devices.

Patients often have CPAP and BPAP devices in homes and long-term care facilities. These devices offer a noninvasive option for patients who require oxygenation and ventilation support.

Diaphragm and phrenic nerve stimulators (pacemakers) allow certain groups of patients to breathe without the assistance of a ventilator. External electrical impulses cause the diaphragm to contract and then passively relax. This movement creates enough tidal volume for effective respiration, eliminating the need and risks associated with ventilator support. In the event of failure of these devices, you can support ventilation using conventional bag-mask technique. It is possible that asynchrony (a lack of synchronization) may occur between patient breathing and mechanical ventilations if the nerve stimulator device is activated while patients are receiving bag-mask or ventilator assistance. These devices typically consist of a small box connected to wires that are inserted into the anterior lower chest/upper abdominal wall.

▶ Ventricular Assist Devices

As discussed in Chapter 17, *Cardiovascular Emergencies*, ventricular assist devices provide a lifesaving bridge for patients with severe heart failure. In the hospital setting, ventricular assist devices are temporarily placed into a patient's chest cavity during or after heart surgery to augment the performance of a failing heart. Advances in medical technology have allowed these devices to become portable for use by persons with heart failure in the community.

Other than correcting problems with the battery or power supply, there are very few interventions that you can perform on ventricular assist devices in the prehospital setting. In the event of ventricular assist device failure, provide supportive treatment and immediate transport to a facility capable of definitive intervention.

▶ Apnea Monitors

You may occasionally encounter patients using an apnea monitor. Infants who are identified as having a high risk for sudden infant death syndrome or other causes of apnea are provided with apnea monitors along with infant cardiopulmonary resuscitation (CPR) instruction for parents and caregivers. Adults and children may be using apnea monitors for diagnosis and evaluation of sleep apnea.

Sleep apnea monitors will vary depending on purpose. Infant apnea monitors typically record an electrocardiogram

YOU are the Paramedic PART 3

Your partner reports that Kyle's work of breathing is increasing and his oxygen saturation is 86%. You ask Mrs. Morton if she can retrieve a replacement inner cannula and the obturator for Kyle's tracheostomy. You attach a bag-mask device to supplemental oxygen and disconnect Kyle from the ventilator to provide manual positive pressure ventilation and preoxygenate him. Kyle's mother returns to the room and hands you the obturator and a replacement inner cannula. You insert the obturator and remove the inner cannula, noting a large amount of thick secretions.

Recording Time: 5 Minutes	
Respirations	1 breath every 5 to 6 seconds via bag-mask device
Pulse	118 beats/min, strong peripheral pulses
Skin	Capillary refill: approximately 3 seconds
Oxygen saturations (Spo₂)	94% after preoxygenation with 15 L/min oxygen via bag-mask device

5. What is an appropriate course of action to address this patient's deterioration?

(ECG) tracing and record respirations based on transthoracic electrical impedance. Central apnea (usually from neurogenic causes) will be detected, but apnea caused all or partially by airway obstruction may or may not be detected until cardiac arrest occurs.

Many home apnea models do not display numeric values or ECG and respiratory waveforms. It is essential that you use advanced life support (ALS) resuscitation equipment rather than home apnea monitors for any patient requiring EMS assistance. You may or may not need to remove apnea monitor leads and electrodes to perform ALS monitoring or procedures.

Words of Wisdom

False alarms are common with apnea monitors and may be caused by movement, loose lead wires, or improperly placed electrodes. When you are in doubt, follow your local EMS protocols and have the family contact the manufacturer of the device.

▶ Long-Term Vascular Access Devices

In your work as a paramedic, you will encounter patients with a variety of long-term vascular access devices Figure 45-8 . Patients may also present with central venous access devices during interfacility transport. Central and long-term vascular access devices are placed for a variety of reasons including inadequate or impossible peripheral IV access, administration of medications that are irritating to smaller blood vessels, vasopressor medication infusion, chemotherapy, frequent blood draws, long-term antibiotic therapy, or dialysis.

Extreme caution is required when you are considering whether to use a long-term vascular access device. Many of these devices are maintained with the anticoagulant heparin, some in high concentrations. You must obtain additional

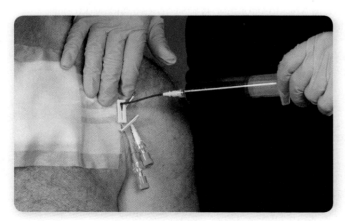

Figure 45-8 You may encounter patients with long-term vascular access devices.
© Jones & Bartlett Learning. Courtesy of MIEMSS.

training and medical director authorization prior to using any long-term vascular access devices.

In emergency situations, the patient's long-term vascular access device may be the only IV access available. You should contact online medical control for guidance in these situations. As a general rule, to remove any heparin, these catheters require up to 10 mL of blood to be removed and discarded before any flush, medication push, or infusion is given. Contamination of these catheters can lead to serious bloodstream infections. Meticulous sterile technique or port cleaning should be used when you are accessing these devices. The following are common long-term vascular access devices that you may encounter:

- **Peripherally inserted central catheter (PICC).** This long IV catheter is usually placed in either arm and follows peripheral veins into the superior vena cava. It may be in place up to 1 year. The smaller diameter and longer catheter length may increase resistance during rapid infusion. A PICC may or may not be flushed with heparin after use.
- **Midline catheter.** This catheter is placed into an upper extremity and is not as long as a PICC, not reaching central circulation. Midline catheters are longer than traditional peripheral IV catheters and are better suited for many irritating medications. These catheters typically contain heparin.
- **Double- or triple-lumen central catheter.** Traditional central lines are placed through the skin in relatively close proximity to a large central vein. The femoral, internal jugular, and subclavian veins are the most common sites. These catheters are placed in an acute care setting but still may be in place for a short time following discharge or transfer to another health care facility. They also contain heparin when not being used for an ongoing infusion.
- **Hickman, Broviac, and Groshong catheters.** These three similar brands of catheters are "tunneled" under the skin and placed into the superior vena cava. These catheters typically contain heparin and look similar to a dialysis catheter, described below. The ports of these catheters may be colored red, blue, or green. Contrary to many other uses in medicine, red does not indicate that this port enters an artery. Do not use any clamps or hemostats on the catheter itself. These catheters contain heparin when not in use.
- **Implanted ports (Port-a-Cath or similar).** These catheters are placed completely under the patient's skin and are tunneled into a central vein, typically the superior vena cava Figure 45-9 . The ports are similar in size and shape to one or two large hazelnuts under the skin. The top of the implanted ports have a flat

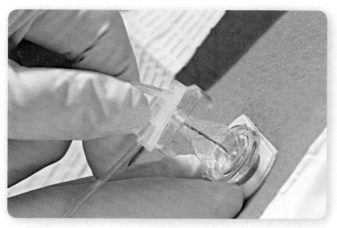

Figure 45-9 A Huber needle is used to access an implanted port.

© 2010 B. Braun Medical Inc., Bethlehem, PA. All Rights Reserved.

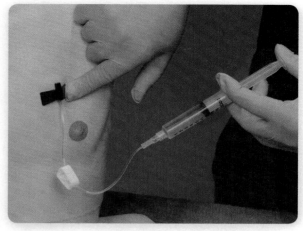

Figure 45-10 Medications are administered through an implantable venous access device through a line flushed with normal saline.

© Jones & Bartlett Learning. Courtesy of MIEMSS.

or slightly rounded top with a clearly palpable edge. These ports are accessed with a needle bent to a 90° angle that has plastic wings for the health care provider to hold while inserting. A metal plate in the base of the port keeps the needle from piercing the bottom. Implanted ports contain heparin when not in use.

- **Dialysis catheter (Vas-Cath/Permcath).** These devices are thick-walled, high-volume catheters, usually placed into a patient's neck or groin for dialysis. Many hospitals require that only dialysis nurses or specially trained registered nurses (RNs) access or use dialysis catheters. These devices are stored with high-dose heparin that can become problematic if adequate blood is not discarded before the catheter is used. The large catheter diameter may allow significant bleeding if the caps and clamps are not used properly.

Accessing an implantable venous access device is out of scope for paramedics in most places. Check with your service's medical director if you are uncertain whether this is in your scope of practice. The general steps for this skill are as follows:

1. Wash your hands and apply a mask, goggles, and nonlatex gloves. Open needed supplies, including the port access kit. Palpate the skin over the device.
2. Cleanse the skin over the device using a cleansing solution (eg, Betadine).
3. Draw up a small amount of saline. Prime the needle tubing and needle with saline. Use a special access needle, called an unbeveled or noncutting needle, to avoid slicing the silicone reservoir wall.
4. While you are stabilizing the device, insert the needle at a 90° angle to the skin until the needle tip reaches the back of the device.
5. Aspirate 5 mL of blood.

6. Block the flow in the line using the crimping device, and then discard the initial aspirate. Obtain additional blood samples as necessary. To avoid air aspiration into the line, never remove the syringe without blocking the flow in the line.
7. Flush the line with normal saline.
8. Block the flow in the device. Administer medications or fluids as directed **Figure 45-10**.
9. Flush the device.
10. Secure the needle with a sterile dressing or remove by pulling straight out of the device. Apply a dressing to the skin over the device if the needle was removed. Identify the tubes of blood by writing the date and time drawn and your name on the side of the tube, and ready them for transport by securing them in a leakproof protected container. Transport tubes to the patient's physician, hospital personnel, or usual lab. Do not shake blood collection tubes, because doing so may cause the blood to hemolyze. Document the procedure and assessment on the PCR. Dispose of contaminated equipment.

▶ Medication Infusion Pumps

Patients receive a wide assortment of IV medications in their homes. Medication categories include inotropic medications for heart failure, IV nutrition, chemotherapy, IV antibiotics, and a variety of other substances. Many of these medications will be administered with infusion pumps, discussed in Chapter 14, *Medication Administration* **Figure 45-11**. If infusion pumps fail while the patient is receiving certain vasoactive medications, a life-threatening emergency may result.

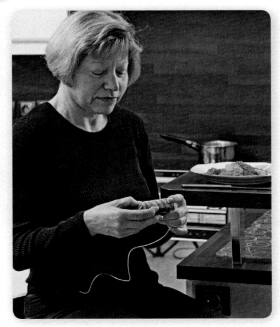

Figure 45-11 Patients may receive intravenous medication at home via a medication infusion pump.

© BELMONTE/age fotostock.

Several problems related to medication infusion pumps will trigger requests for EMS assistance. The underlying medical condition may become exacerbated, despite a properly functioning medication infusion system. In these situations, it is often advisable for you to continue the current medication infusion while contacting medical control for guidance, especially with unfamiliar medications or medical conditions. Most situations will not require titration or manipulation of a patient's medication infusion pump.

It is also possible that problems will occur with a long-term vascular access device. Each device outlined above has a limited life span. These devices can become clogged with blood clots and can harbor infections, and all are subject to either potential mechanical failure or accidental removal. You may need to emergently reestablish alternative vascular access such as a peripheral IV line or IO needle.

You may need to troubleshoot a medication infusion system. Medication infusion pumps require either a battery or a continuous power supply. An electrical outage or battery depletion has the potential to become a life-threatening emergency for the patient. Device malfunction is also a continuous possibility. Sudden, unexpected loss of a medication infusion pump may present you with a considerable challenge.

Simple solutions such as using an ambulance inverter to provide external power after a device battery failure may prove lifesaving. In other instances, another suitable backup device may be available in the patient's home or facility. You should not overlook the timeless practice of calculating the drip rate of IV tubing when a malfunctioning infusion pump cannot be immediately repaired

or replaced. Collaboration with the patient or caregivers and creative solutions for infusion pump malfunction have the potential to save the patient's life.

▶ Tube Feeding

Patients in homes and long-term care facilities may receive some or all nourishment from tube feeding. Flexible catheters can be placed through the mouth or nose, or directly through the skin into the patient's stomach or small intestine. These tubes allow nourishment and water to enter the digestive system directly without the need for chewing or swallowing. These tubes can decrease, but not completely eliminate, the risk of aspiration in patients who lack the ability to swallow effectively or protect his or her airway. It is still possible for a patient to aspirate while being fed through a tube, especially when feeding tubes are placed into the stomach rather than intestine.

Nasogastric and orogastric feeding tubes are placed from the nose and mouth, respectively, into the patient's stomach. Nasoduodenal and nasojejunal feeding tubes are inserted through the nose and end in the duodenum and jejunum, respectively, of the small intestine. Gastrostomy tubes are surgically inserted through the skin into the patient's stomach. Jejunostomy tubes are placed through the patient's skin directly into the jejunum of the small intestine. Percutaneous endoscopic gastrostomy and percutaneous endoscopic jejunostomy tubes are placed into the stomach and jejunum, respectively, using endoscopic surgical technique.

It is unlikely that you will need to troubleshoot or otherwise manipulate feeding tubes during an EMS response. Unless a nasogastric or orogastric tube interferes with the bag-mask seal on a patient's face and cannot be adequately displaced to the side, you will likely not need to remove a feeding tube.

You may need to monitor continuous tube feeding during interfacility transports. An infusion pump is typically used at a rate specific for a particular patient. You should monitor for malfunction of the infusion pump and any signs of the patient vomiting, or aspirating while being fed through a tube. The patient's head should remain elevated during and after completion of tube feeding.

If any complications develop, you should simply stop the tube feeding infusion and possibly flush the catheter with tap water to prevent the tube feed solution from clogging the catheter.

To replace an ostomy device, follow the steps in **Skill Drill 45-2** .

Words of Wisdom

Be careful not to cut an ostomy appliance when you are using trauma shears to cut away clothing. The drainage can contaminate wounds and damage intact skin.

► Colostomy

Patients may receive a **colostomy** following intestinal trauma or surgery. A colostomy is a surgical procedure that directs the large intestine (colon) out through an opening in the anterior abdominal wall called a stoma.

The stoma has a raised, circular mass of tissue that appears moist and vascular. A **colostomy bag** is a plastic bag with a hard, circular opening that is attached around the stoma by an adhesive ring called a wafer **Figure 45-12**. Stool and intestinal liquid are collected in this plastic bag for disposal.

Skill Drill 45-2 — Replacing an Ostomy Device

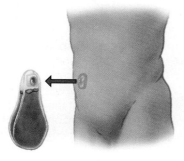

Step 1 Help position the patient in a comfortable area in which to change the appliance and easily dispose of the contaminated articles. Wash your hands and apply a mask, goggles, and clean nonlatex gloves. Open the supplies. Ostomy equipment includes a skin barrier called a wafer and one of several styles of drainage bags. Some bags can be opened along the bottom and emptied at regular intervals; others are sealed around a system similar to a urine drainage bag. Empty/remove the current appliance and dispose of it appropriately.

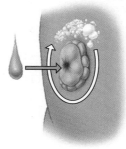

Step 2 Wash the area around the stoma with soap and water. Cleanse the stoma with water only, being careful not to rub or irritate the area.

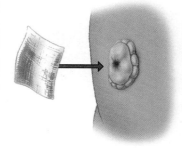

Step 3 Place a clean gauze pad over the stoma to prevent contamination of the clean skin with stool or urine.

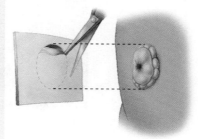

Step 4 Cut the wafer to the correct size using the patient's measurement or tracing. Home care patients usually have the stoma already sized or have a tracing to cut a hole in the wafer large enough for the stoma but keeping exposed skin to a minimum.

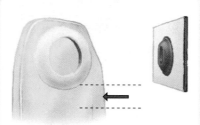

Step 5 Attach the appliance to the wafer. Be sure the distal end is closed.

(continued)

Skill Drill **45-2** **Replacing an Ostomy Device** *(continued)*

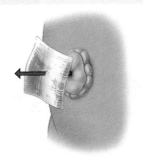

Step 6 Remove the gauze.

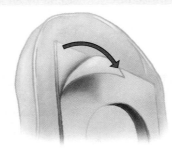

Step 7 Remove the paper backing from the wafer.

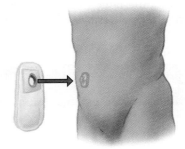

Step 8 Apply the appliance with the stoma centered in the wafer cutout. Remove your gloves and wash your hands. Document the procedure and assessment on the PCR.

© Jones & Bartlett Learning.

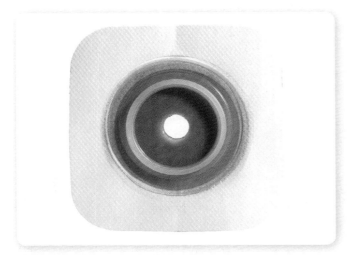

Figure 45-12 An ostomy skin wafer.

Courtesy of ConvaTec. ©/™ indicated a registered trademark of E.R. Squibb & Sons, LLC.

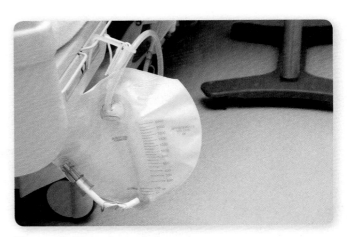

Figure 45-13 A urinary drainage bag.

© Rob Byron/Shutterstock.

You generally do not need to do much in the way of care for a colostomy or colostomy bag. Occasionally the bag will separate from the abdominal wall, requiring replacement or temporary reinforcement with tape. If the colostomy bag becomes full, you may need to assist the patient in emptying the bag. A clamp is located at the bottom of the bag. The clamp is opened and any contents are drained into a suitable collection device. Take care to avoid spilling or splashing the contents of the bag. Abdominal gas may accumulate in the colostomy bag, requiring periodic release during longer transports.

▶ Urostomy and Urinary Diversion

Patients occasionally require urinary diversion for certain medical conditions. Bladder cancer, congenital anomalies, and massive urinary tract obstructions are possible indications for urinary diversion.

Part of the urinary system is diverted through an opening in the anterior abdominal wall, also called a stoma. This procedure is called a **urostomy**. Urine is collected in a plastic bag, similar to the colostomy bag discussed earlier **Figure 45-13**. Interventions by paramedics are similar to those for a colostomy. Occasional emptying and reinforcement or reattachment are likely to be all that you will be required to perform in most EMS settings.

► Urinary Catheterization

Patients who are not able to void (urinate) on their own may need to be catheterized. Catheters may remain in place (ie, indwelling catheters such as Foley catheters) or may be used intermittently (ie, straight catheters). Whereas the principles for catheterization remain the same for either sex, anatomy differences change the process.

Urinary catheterization is not typically in paramedic scope of practice in the prehospital environment. Check with your service's medical director if you are uncertain whether this is in your scope of practice. The steps to catheterize an adult male patient are shown in Skill Drill 45-3.

The steps to catheterize an adult female patient are shown in Skill Drill 45-4.

Skill Drill 45-3 Catheterizing an Adult Male Patient

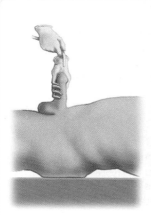

Step 1 Help position the patient supine with the legs slightly spread apart. Maintain privacy as much as possible. Wash your hands and apply a mask, goggles, and sterile nonlatex gloves.

Open the supplies, including the urinary catheter and placement kit. Home care patients may reuse their catheters provided that they have been stored in a clean manner. Place necessary supplies onto a clean area within reach. If placing an indwelling catheter, use sterile technique throughout. Do not allow the catheter that will be inserted to come into contact with anything that is not also sterile. If you are inserting an indwelling catheter, connect a syringe filled with saline to the balloon port. Also, connect the indwelling catheter to the drainage system. There are no connecting ports for either a balloon or a drainage bag on a straight catheter.

Wash the penis with the solution included in the kit. Make sure the foreskin has been retracted. Use great caution throughout to avoid breaks in sterile technique.

Coat the end of the catheter with a water-soluble gel. Hold the penis at a 90° angle to the body and insert the catheter.

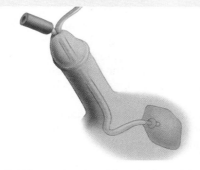

Step 2 When urine is evident in the tubing, insert the catheter until the Y between the drainage port and the balloon port is at the tip of the penis. For a straight catheter, insert approximately 1 inch (2.5 cm) more.

Inflate the balloon and gently pull back on the catheter until you feel resistance, which indicates that the balloon is snug against the neck of the bladder. This step is unnecessary for a straight catheter. Never inflate the balloon if you do not see any urine in the tubing or if you meet resistance to inflation, as doing so may indicate that the balloon is in the urethra instead of the bladder and inflation would therefore cause urethral injury.

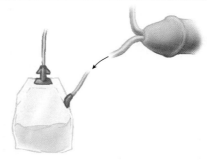

Step 3 Allow urine to drain. Note the amount and color.

To remove a catheter, remove the saline in the balloon port and pull back gently until the catheter is free of the tip of the penis. Never remove an indwelling catheter without using a syringe to remove the saline from the balloon, because it may damage the urinary sphincter. For a straight catheter, simply pull back gently to remove the catheter. Wash according to the home care instructions. Remove your gloves and wash your hands, taking standard precautions.

If the catheter is to remain in place, secure it to the patient's leg according to the home care instructions. Document the procedure and assessment on the PCR.

Skill Drill 45-4 Catheterizing an Adult Female Patient

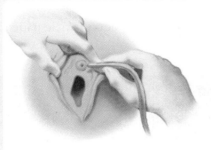

Step 1 Help position the patient supine with the legs spread apart or side lying with the top knee flexed. Maintain privacy as much as possible. Wash your hands and apply nonlatex gloves.

Open supplies including the urinary catheter and placement kit. Home care patients may reuse their catheters provided that they have been stored in a clean manner. Place necessary supplies onto a clean area within reach. If placing an indwelling catheter, use sterile technique throughout. Do not allow the catheter that will be inserted to come into contact with anything that is not also sterile. If you are inserting an indwelling catheter, connect a syringe filled with saline to the balloon port. Also, connect the indwelling catheter to the drainage system. There are no connecting ports for either a balloon or a drainage bag on a straight catheter.

Wash the perineal area with the solution included in the kit. First cleanse the outer area of the perineum, and then spread the labia minora and thoroughly wash the mucosa surrounding the vagina and the urinary meatus. Dry with a clean towel. Coat the end of the catheter with a water-soluble gel. Locate the urinary meatus anterior to the vagina and insert the catheter. Depending on the age of the patient, the integrity of her pelvic musculature, and other factors, locating the urinary meatus can be difficult.

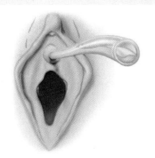

Step 2 When urine is evident in the tubing, insert the catheter another 1 to 3 inches (2.5 to 8 cm).

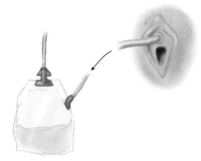

Step 3 Inflate the balloon and gently pull back on the catheter until you feel resistance, which indicates that the balloon is snug against the neck of the bladder. This step is unnecessary for a straight catheter. Allow urine to drain. Note the amount and color.

To remove a catheter, remove the saline in the balloon port and pull back gently until the catheter is free of the tip of the meatus. Never remove an indwelling catheter without using a syringe to remove the saline from the balloon, because it may damage the urinary sphincter. For a straight catheter, simply pull back gently to remove the catheter. If the catheter is to be reused, it should be cleaned. Remove your gloves and wash your hands.

If the catheter is to remain in place, secure it to the patient's leg or abdomen according to the patient's needs. Document the procedure and assessment on the PCR.

© Jones & Bartlett Learning.

▶ Dialysis

As discussed in Chapter 21, *Genitourinary and Renal Emergencies*, patients undergo dialysis as a replacement for failed or failing kidneys. Kidney failure is associated with many chronic conditions. As kidney function declines, fluids, excess electrolytes, and toxins accumulate within the body. If left untreated, these substances will cause death. Coma, cardiac dysrhythmia, and circulatory overload are late signs of kidney failure, requiring prompt intervention to prevent death.

Hemodialysis and peritoneal dialysis may be performed in multiple environments, including the hospital, free-standing dialysis clinics, or even in the patient's home in some cases **Figure 45-14** . As a paramedic, you may be called to assist the dialysis patient in any of these environments.

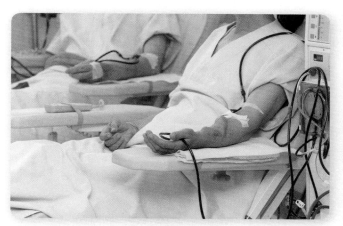

Figure 45-14 Patients may receive hemodialysis and peritoneal dialysis in community-based centers or in their homes.
© Picsfive/Shutterstock.

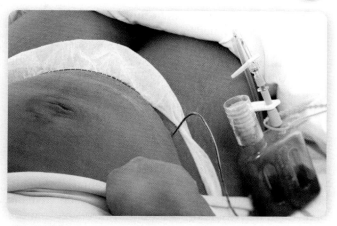

Figure 45-15 A surgical drain is used to monitor and assist wound healing and closure.
© CHASSENET/age fotostock.

A wide variety of complications are possible during or following dialysis treatment. During dialysis, large volumes of fluid are moved into and out of the patient's body. Incorrect calculation during either method of dialysis can create massive abnormalities of fluids and electrolytes that cannot otherwise be compensated for. Both hypovolemia and fluid overload are possible during and after dialysis. Electrolyte abnormalities, including electrolyte depletion, may result from miscalculation. Infection can occur at the site of the dialysis **fistula**—the surgical connection between an artery and a vein, usually in one of the patient's upper extremities—used for hemodialysis. An intra-abdominal infection can occur with peritoneal dialysis.

A severe, life-threatening hemorrhage can occur if the hemodialysis fistula is damaged or the catheter is improperly removed. Other problems with hemodialysis fistulas include thrombosis (blood clot) and stenosis (narrowing).

You need to use caution when you are treating patients who receive dialysis. Modest volumes of IV fluids may cause fluid overload, particularly in otherwise susceptible patients. IV fluids need to be monitored carefully and titrated judiciously to patient response. If too much IV fluid is given, it will be impossible to correct in the prehospital setting.

Patients with renal failure are prone to electrolyte abnormalities, particularly hyperkalemia, and an elevated blood potassium concentration. You need to avoid medications known to increase serum potassium levels such as succinylcholine (Anectine), digoxin, and beta-adrenergic (beta) blockers.

You must also use caution when a hemodialysis fistula is present. Dialysis fistulas are prone to both clots and infection. Avoid blood pressure measurements, blood draws, and IV access on the same arm as the dialysis fistula. Patients with impending dialysis may have already chosen which arm will be used for the fistula. Again, avoid using this arm whenever possible. Both arterial and venous bleeding can occur from the fistula site, especially if improper care was taken during needle removal.

If you are called to respond to an emergency for a patient at a hemodialysis center, it is important to inquire whether the patient had received the dialysis treatment already. It is possible for a significant amount of the patient's blood to be in the dialysis machine during dialysis treatment. You and the dialysis center staff need to carefully coordinate when to remove the patient from the dialysis machine if dialysis is still in progress on your arrival.

Dialysis is both a lifesaving and a life-sustaining therapy for patients in renal failure. Understanding dialysis will dramatically improve your ability to provide care to dialysis patients who become ill or injured.

▶ Surgical Drains and Devices

Patients are often discharged to home or a long-term care facility soon after many surgical procedures. A variety of drains and devices are used following surgery to monitor and assist wound healing or closure **Figure 45-15**. Complications in the postoperative period can trigger requests for EMS assistance. Consequently, you may have to provide care to patients with many different types of surgical drains and devices.

The list of possible surgical drains and devices that you will encounter is extensive. Wound drains prevent pockets of fluid from collecting at the surgical site while allowing health care providers to monitor volume, appearance, and composition of the fluid being drained. Other devices use mechanical forces to stabilize a particular surgical site and promote healing.

It is typically outside the paramedic scope of practice to manipulate many of these items. Improper manipulation or premature removal of a surgical drain or wound device can have significant complications for the patient, including hemorrhage, infection, or the need for additional surgery.

You should contact medical control in the event that additional guidance is needed. In most cases, any needed manipulation of a wound drain or other device will be done by an ED provider or other specialist. If any leakage is present, consider the leaking substance to be potentially highly infective and use appropriate PPE.

Orthotic devices, prosthetic limbs, and braces should also not be manipulated by paramedics. In many instances, these items are fitted and adjusted for the needs of a particular patient. Improper adjustment may reduce the therapeutic benefit or lead to patient injury. Whenever possible, these devices should accompany the patient to the hospital, even if unrelated to the reason for EMS assistance.

▶ Cerebrospinal Fluid Shunts

Hydrocephalus, a condition involving an excess volume of cerebrospinal fluid (CSF) around the brain, can develop either before or after a person is born. CSF is produced in the brain to protect, cushion, provide nourishment, and remove waste products from the brain and spinal cord. If the brain becomes injured, swelling of the brain can be offset by a reduction of CSF volume to maintain a lower intracranial pressure (ICP). Approximately 17 ounces (500 mL) of CSF is produced daily by the choroid plexus of the brain. As CSF is being produced by the brain, it is constantly being reabsorbed by the bloodstream to maintain a balance within the central nervous system. The total volume of CSF is replaced almost four times each day. Excess production or decreased absorption of CSF causes hydrocephalus.

Excess CSF causes increased ICP. Increased ICP leads to signs and symptoms such as headaches, visual disturbances, unsteady gait, nausea and vomiting, seizures, altered mental status, and numerous other effects. Increased ICP will cause the relatively malleable skulls of fetuses, infants, and young children to enlarge, without generally distorting facial features.

Treatment of congenital hydrocephalus (occurring before birth) or acquired hydrocephalus (occurring after birth) involves surgical placement of a **cerebrospinal fluid shunt (CSF shunt)** to drain excess CSF from the central nervous system. The shunt consists of three parts: the inflow (proximal) catheter, the valve, and the outflow (distal) catheter **Figure 45-16**. The inflow catheter is typically placed into the ventricle of the brain of the patient. Occasionally, the inflow catheter is placed in CSF outside the spinal cord. This catheter is connected to a tiny valve. The valve may have fixed opening pressure (pressure required to open the valve) and closing pressure (pressure at which the valve will close), or these may be adjustable. Newer valves can be adjusted by a physician using a magnet that is placed near the valve, outside the patient's body. The outflow catheter is most commonly placed into the patient's peritoneal cavity. This particular placement is known as a ventriculoperitoneal shunt. The outflow catheter can also be placed into the patient's right atrium or pulmonary cavity.

Patients often demonstrate substantial clinical improvement following CSF shunt placement. Improvement can be significant enough to eliminate the need for long-term care when the diagnosis of hydrocephalus is made in older adults and a CSF shunt is placed.

Patients and caregivers need to monitor closely for complications related to shunt malfunction. Many complications develop in the immediate postoperative period,

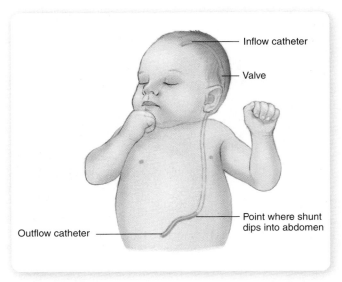

Figure 45-16 A cerebrospinal fluid (CSF) shunt, which drains excess CSF from the central nervous system, consists of the inflow (proximal) catheter, the valve, and the outflow (distal) catheter.

© Jones & Bartlett Learning.

often related to the surgery itself. Shunts need periodic revisions as children grow or bodies change. Infection, shunt valve malfunction, and mechanical damage to either catheter will present with signs suggestive of increased ICP. You should suspect shunt malfunction in any patient with a CSF shunt who presents with a headache, visual disturbances, seizures, or altered mental status.

■ Medical Technology Used During Interfacility Transport

Paramedics perform both 9-1-1 emergency response and interfacility patient transport in many EMS systems and organizations. State EMS regulations and individual service medical directors determine which medications and procedures paramedics are permitted to use and under what circumstances. Medication infusion pumps, ventilators, and cardiac monitors are used routinely by paramedics performing interfacility transport and are discussed in greater detail throughout this text. Paramedics do not generally use the skills and devices outlined next without additional specialized training. The skills and devices discussed next are likely to be encountered as paramedics interact with air medical units and ground critical care transport organizations across the nation. Understanding this technology will help you provide greater assistance when it is encountered in the interfacility transport setting.

▶ Hemodynamic Monitoring

Hemodynamic monitoring is a broad term that describes the movement and various forces applied to blood within the human body. You are actually performing

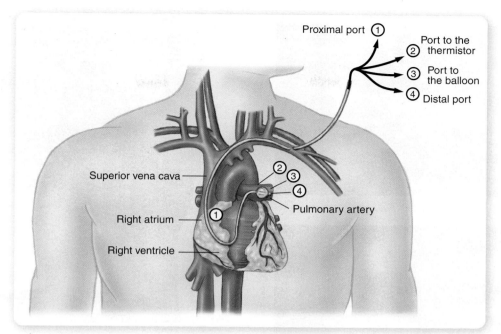

Figure 45-17 An example of catheter placement for hemodynamic monitoring. This example shows pulmonary artery catheter placement.
© Jones & Bartlett Learning.

cursory hemodynamic monitoring by assessing items such as patient blood pressure, pulse rate, pulse strength, urinary output over time, skin temperature, end-tidal carbon dioxide, and mental status. Assessing these items provides you with valuable information regarding the effectiveness of perfusion to a patient's body organs, tissues, and cells.

Patients receive invasive hemodynamic monitoring when health care providers need to evaluate the effectiveness of specific components within the cardiovascular system or carefully guide fluid administration. Monitoring continues as medications are administered and procedures are performed to improve body function or the chances of survival following a critical illness, traumatic injury, or major surgery. Invasive monitoring includes values such as continuous arterial blood pressure, central venous pressure or right atrial pressure, pulmonary artery pressure, direct or indirect measurements of left atrial and left ventricular pressure, systemic vascular resistance, and pulmonary vascular resistance. Interpreting and manipulating these values allows you to optimize cardiovascular function in critically ill patients.

Hemodynamic monitoring technology is constantly evolving. The majority of current hemodynamic monitoring involves placement of different types of catheters into areas within the cardiovascular system, such as arteries, central veins, and various chambers of the heart **Figure 45-17** . The catheter is connected to special tubing, typically filled with normal saline or **heparinized solution** (solution with heparin added to prevent clotting). The solution is kept under constant pressure through the use of a pressure bag or similar device to prevent blood from

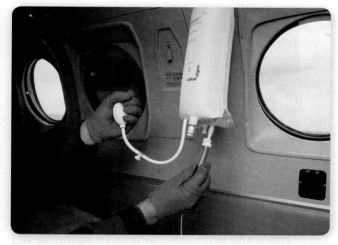

Figure 45-18 An inflated pressure bag used to increase fluid infusion rates.
© Jones & Bartlett Learning. Courtesy of MIEMSS.

being pushed out of the body through the catheter and tubing **Figure 45-18** . This tubing is connected to a **transducer** that converts subtle changes in pressure of this fluid into electrical impulses **Figure 45-19** . These electrical impulses are interpreted by the monitor and displayed as both waveforms and numeric values. Continuous interpretation of the values and waveforms allows providers to precisely titrate many inotropic and vasoactive medications to the desired patient response. Invasive monitoring will identify impending heart failure, guide fluid resuscitation, demonstrate the effectiveness

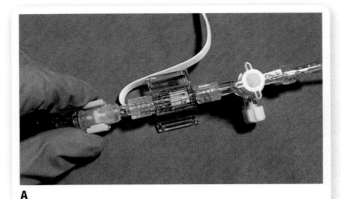

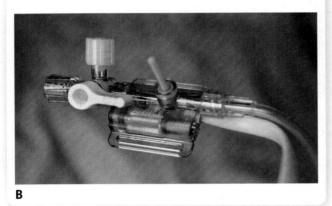

Figure 45-19 The two most common transducer flush system devices. **A.** Squeezable. **B.** Pull-style.

© Jones & Bartlett Learning. Photographed by Andrew Bartkus.

of compressions during CPR, help differentiate various shock states, and provide much potentially useful information in high-risk patients.

Arterial pressure monitoring is a component of hemodynamic monitoring that requires additional consideration. In addition to monitoring blood pressure, arterial lines are used as continuous access when critically ill patients require frequent blood tests or arterial blood gas sampling. Conditions such as sepsis, respiratory failure, diabetic ketoacidosis, or salicylate overdose require frequent testing of blood samples that may be impossible or impractical to obtain from repeated puncture of arteries or veins.

Paramedics may also encounter larger arterial sheaths that have been placed for a cardiac catheterization. These sheaths are placed into a femoral artery and provide a route to cardiac blood vessels. Arterial sheaths are occasionally left in place after a diagnostic cardiac catheterization if the patient needs to be transported to another hospital for further invasive cardiac care or cardiac surgery. Patients should remain supine with legs straight during placement of a femoral arterial sheath, and for a period of time after placement.

Bleeding associated with a displaced arterial catheter or arterial sheath can be immediately life threatening. Anytime a catheter or sheath is in an artery, it must be continuously monitored by a trained health care provider. Patients can quickly exsanguinate from unrecognized

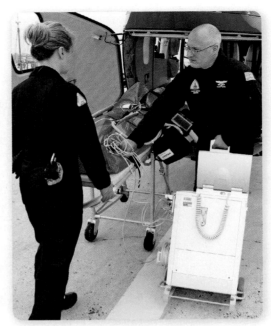

Figure 45-20 A patient being transported with an intra-aortic balloon pump.

© Jones & Bartlett Learning. Courtesy of MIEMSS.

displacement of an arterial catheter. Large quantities of blood can become sequestered in a patient's groin area and stretcher linens before being recognized by transport personnel. Use extreme caution while moving or transporting a patient who has an arterial catheter or arterial sheath in place even if other trained health care personnel are present.

▶ Intra-aortic Balloon Pumps

You may need to assist with transport of patients being treated with an **intra-aortic balloon pump (IABP)**. IABPs are used to decrease cardiac workload and augment perfusion in patients with cardiogenic shock, structural abnormalities in the heart, or myocardial infarction, or following cardiac surgery. It is unlikely that a paramedic will be solely responsible for care of a patient on an IABP. It is quite conceivable, however, that paramedics will accompany a critical care transport team or other health care provider who is responsible for managing the IABP during interfacility transport of a patient.

IABPs consist of a relatively large machine, connecting tubing, monitor cables, and the balloon catheter itself **Figure 45-20**. A cylindrical balloon is inserted through the femoral artery and placed in the aorta, just outside the heart. Tubing connects the balloon catheter to the machine. Monitor leads from the machine are connected to the patient. Movement of both the patient and the IABP machine requires careful planning and coordination among members of the transport team.

The balloon is inflated and actively deflated at precise times during the cardiac cycle. During diastole (relaxation of the heart), the balloon inflates, pushing blood forward

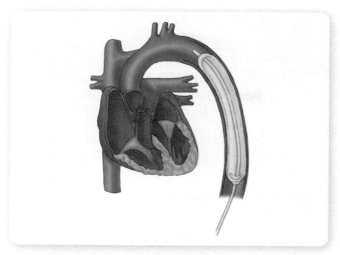

Figure 45-21 Intra-aortic balloon pump inflation.

Illustration from source material by Datascope Corp. and Maquet Cardiovascular. Used with permission.

into systemic circulation **Figure 45-21**. During systole (contraction of the heart), the balloon actively deflates, creating a brief vacuum and reducing cardiac afterload. This process decreases myocardial oxygen demand, reduces cardiac workload, and improves systemic circulation.

The IABP is bulky and often difficult to move and secure in an ambulance. Additional straps need to be used to prevent the machine from injuring the patient or transport team in the event of an ambulance crash. Care needs to be taken when you are handling and securing the connecting tubing between the machine and the balloon catheter. Accidental removal of the balloon catheter often creates a life-threatening emergency for the patient.

▶ Intracranial Pressure Monitor

Patients with intracranial hemorrhage or severe head trauma or who have undergone neurosurgery may have an ICP monitor or drain placed. These devices allow health care providers to monitor ICP, evaluate the appearance of CSF, and allow drainage of CSF to maintain a lower ICP.

It is possible that you will assist other providers with interfacility transport of patients with these devices. Monitoring of ICP is similar to hemodynamic monitoring discussed previously, although newer technology is also in use. The transducer or drainage system is typically aligned at the same height as the patient's ear canal, which may take some creativity to accommodate in the back of an ambulance. Positioning of the drainage system is extremely important. Improper placement of an open drainage system can cause large volumes of CSF to quickly enter or leave the patient's central nervous system.

▶ Doppler Devices

Certain EMS systems and critical care transport programs utilize handheld doppler devices. These devices use ultrasound waves to detect heartbeats and blood flow in situations where palpation and auscultation are not effective. The ultrasound waves are converted into artificial sounds that allow confirmation of underlying movement. Doppler devices are used to detect and calculate fetal heartbeats in pregnant patients, detect pulses

YOU are the Paramedic PART 4

You take a flexible suction catheter, insert it without suction into Kyle's tracheostomy, and apply suction while withdrawing the catheter, removing a large amount of thick secretions. You repeat the suctioning one more time, then reinsert the inner cannula with the obturator and apply the bag-mask device with supplemental oxygen to assist Kyle's ventilations. Kyle's oxygen saturation begins to climb and eventually reaches 99%. His mother informs you that his baseline without supplemental oxygen is 95%.

Recording Time: 7 Minutes	
Respirations	1 breath every 5 to 6 seconds via bag-mask device
Pulse	102 beats/min, regular, strong peripheral pulses
Blood pressure	114/76 mm Hg
Temperature	98.4°F (36.9°C)
Oxygen saturations (Spo$_2$)	99% with 15 L/min oxygen via bag-mask device

6. Is transport always necessary for a patient who is ventilator dependent and has had a deterioration event like the one described in this scenario?

7. Now that the patient's airway is clear, what interventions are appropriate in continuing care?

in compromised extremities, and obtain blood pressure or pulses that are too weak to palpate. To use the device, place a small amount of water-based gel between the probe and the patient's skin over the appropriate area. Move the probe slowly until you detect the underlying flow or movement.

Care of Patients With Cognitive, Sensory, or Communication Impairment

The presence of a cognitive, sensory, or communication impairment can create unique challenges as you assess, treat, and transport a patient. Routine tasks become complicated, requiring creative approaches to provide effective patient care. Patients and their caregivers are often valuable resources for paramedics providing care during EMS response or interfacility transport. The special challenges discussed in this section, with the exceptions of autism and mental/emotional impairment, may appear early in life as a developmental disability or present later due to a medical condition or injury.

▶ Developmental Disability

The CDC defines developmental disability as a diverse group of conditions that are due to physical, learning, language, or behavioral impairments.[36] These impairments appear prior to age 22 years and usually continue throughout the person's lifetime. Communication, movement, the ability to care for oneself, prospects for employment, and a host of other important human attributes are adversely impacted. Profound vision or hearing impairment can disrupt other developmental progression, leading or contributing to a developmental disability. Certain conditions such as autism do not have a readily identifiable cause, although a variety of theories have been proposed. Known causes of other developmental disabilities are listed in Table 45-3 .

▶ Developmental Delay

Developmental delay is a broad term that describes an infant or child's failure to reach a particular developmental milestone by the expected time. Milestones include gross and fine motor skills, such as crawling, walking, and hand-eye coordination; cognitive skills, such as reaching, object permanence, or problem solving; and social skills, such as interacting and forming relationships with others. Language milestones include talking, listening, and comprehending. Signs of problems may be primarily in one developmental area, such as language or social skills, or delays in multiple areas may exist. Developmental delay is linked to many causes of developmental disabilities listed in Table 45-3. **Down syndrome** and autism are associated with potentially significant signs of developmental delay. Depending on the cause, developmental delays may persist into adulthood or resolve as a person's medical or social

Table 45-3	Known Causes of Development Disabilities
Genetic abnormality (for example, phenylketonuria, chromosomal disorder, or fragile X syndrome)	
Hypoxia, malnutrition, or toxic exposure during fetal development (such as to tobacco, alcohol, or other drugs)	
Maternal trauma, hemorrhage, or infection during fetal development	
Premature birth, low birth weight	
Malnutrition	
Abuse or neglect; improper treatment of common childhood illnesses	
Neurologic insult, injury, or infection	
Severe metabolic abnormality	
Toxic exposure (for example to lead, mercury, or another environmental toxin)	
Inadequate stimulation during childhood	
Near drowning	
Hyperthermia	
Trauma or hypoxia during delivery	
Traumatic injuries	

Data from: Facts about developmental disabilities. Centers for Disease Control and Prevention website. https://www.cdc.gov/ncbddd/developmentaldisabilities/facts.html. Updated July 9, 2015. Accessed May 4, 2017; Pivalizza P, Lalani SR. Intellectual disability in children: evaluation for a cause. UpToDate website. http://www.uptodate.com/contents/intellectual-disability-in-children-evaluation-for-a-cause. Updated May 26, 2016. Accessed May 4, 2017; and Privalizza P, Lalani SR. Intellectual disability in children: definition, diagnosis, and assessment of needs. UpToDate website. http://www.uptodate.com/contents/intellectual-disability-in-children-definition-diagnosis-and-assessment-of-needs?source=see_link. Updated August 15, 2016. Accessed May 4, 2017.

situation improves. Early intervention focused on children with developmental delays may allow these children to recover previously missed developmental milestones.

You may encounter children and adults with developmental delays that encompass the entire spectrum of possible severity. Cues from the patient and caregivers will help you determine how best to interact and communicate with a particular patient. Patients can regress to a lower developmental level following a stressful event, illness, or injury. You may find that experience and approaches used while treating younger children are useful when you are interacting with older children and adults with developmental delay. Additional time may be needed when you are assessing these patients, performing procedures, or preparing for transport.

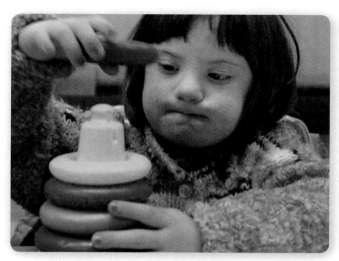

Figure 45-22 A child with Down syndrome.
© PhotoCreate/Shutterstock.

▶ Down Syndrome

Down syndrome is an inherited genetic disorder that is responsible for developmental delay, cognitive impairment, and a pattern of unusual physical features. Patients with Down syndrome can often be identified visually from certain telltale features of the person's head, face, and neck Figure 45-22 . Features include a flattened face and nose, short neck, upward slanting eyes, and often a protruding tongue. Additionally, only a single crease is noted on the palms of the patient's hands.

Down syndrome is also known as trisomy 21. Normal human cells have 23 pairs of chromosomes that create the cell's genetic identity. In Down syndrome, an extra chromosome attaches to the 21st pair, thus, becoming the third chromosome 21, or trisomy 21. The risk of an infant having Down syndrome is greater when a sibling or the mother has Down syndrome. The risk of Down syndrome also increases with older maternal age at the time of conception.

Chromosomal changes associated with Down syndrome may cause structural heart defects, seizures, numerous gastrointestinal problems, speech alterations, hearing loss, and many other abnormalities. Persons with Down syndrome also have a shorter life expectancy. Cognitive deficits with Down syndrome range from barely noticeable to profound impairment. Persons with Down syndrome, depending on their level of mental disability, may function relatively independently or require constant assistance with even basic tasks.

▶ Intellectual Disability

Intellectual disability, formerly called mental retardation, is a primarily cognitive disorder that appears during childhood and is accompanied by lack of "adaptive" behaviors. Adaptive behaviors include the ability to live and function independently or interact successfully with others. Diagnosis of intellectual disability requires that the patient have deficits in the areas of general mental abilities and adaptive functioning, and that the deficits are present before the patient turns 18 years of age.[37]

General mental ability is assessed by a trained clinician through the use of intelligence quotient (IQ) and other cognitive testing in combination with clinical assessment and judgment. In general, an IQ score of 65 to 75 is sufficient to diagnose intellectual disability, so long as the patient also has impairment in everyday adaptive functioning when compared to their peers.[37]

The use of IQ score as the sole determinant of intellectual disability is no longer supported by the American Psychiatric Association in the *Diagnostic and Statistical Manual of Mental Disorders*, Fifth Edition (DSM-5).[37]

Many causes of development delay listed in Table 45-3 will cause intellectual disability. As with Down syndrome and autism, the clinical presentation and severity of symptoms will vary dramatically among people with this type of disorder.

▶ Autism and Autism Spectrum Disorders

Autism and **autism spectrum disorders** are conditions involving developmental delay that are being diagnosed with increased frequency in the United States. These complex disorders of brain development are characterized by difficulties in social interaction, repetitive behaviors, and verbal and nonverbal communications. Increased rates of diagnosis may be due to better awareness and screening or an actual increase in the occurrence of autism in the population.

Patients demonstrate a wide variety of symptoms that often relate to communication, social interaction, sensory processing, the ability to purposefully shift attention, and the ability to play. A large number of people who are autistic will either be completely nonverbal throughout their lifetime or become nonverbal during periods of stress. Developmental regression in absence of another cause in young children should raise concerns for the possibility of autism. Cognitive function can vary significantly among people with autism. Some people with autism may have impaired cognitive function, meeting the criteria for intellectual disability discussed above. Other people with autism may demonstrate highly sophisticated skills with mathematics, puzzles, memory, or art. Some patients will achieve a large degree of independence while others will continue to rely on others for basic needs throughout their lives.

When you are treating patients with autism, you should be extremely mindful of your actions when you are attempting to communicate and initiate physical contact. Commotion and excess stimuli may cause a patient with autism to have bizarre or aggressive behaviors. Any physical contact should be preceded by a careful explanation and go from distal to proximal on the patient. Any questions should be repeated to the patient in a variety of ways to determine whether there is a consistent response. Patients with autism may exhibit minimal reactions to significantly painful injuries or may experience great discomfort with minor physical contact or injuries.

You should be prepared for many possible challenges while providing care to patients with autism. Including the caregivers in assessment, treatment, and transport will often be extremely helpful.

▶ Mental/Emotional Impairment

Mental illness can occur in persons with mental or emotional disability just as it can arise in healthy people. (The care of mentally ill patients is discussed in depth in Chapter 28, *Psychiatric Emergencies*.)

You may be particularly challenged when you encounter patients who demonstrate a **conversion disorder**, previously referred to as hysteria. Certain patients can present with focal neurologic abnormalities as a physical manifestation of an underlying mental illness. Blindness, paralysis, and impaired speech can occur as a response to stress in susceptible people. In this situation, the manifestations such as blindness or paralysis are not voluntary and the patient is not faking the sign or symptom. Diagnosis and treatment of conversion disorders require intervention from an experienced mental health provider and are beyond the scope of your training. When a conversion disorder is suspected, maintain a professional demeanor and continue to assess the patient for other potentially life-threatening causes of the sign or symptom.

▶ Hearing Impairment

Over 37 million adults and children have some degree of hearing loss.[38] Hearing loss inhibits communication, limits social interaction, interferes with infant development, and renders many safety and warning devices ineffective. Patients with profound hearing impairment can pose a considerable challenge to EMS providers.

Hearing impairment may be congenital (present since birth) or acquired. Genetic factors are believed to cause 50% to 60% of congenital hearing loss in children.[39] Twenty-five percent of hearing loss is caused by such environmental factors as maternal infection, Rh incompatibility, hypoxia, maternal diabetes, and pregnancy-induced hypertension.[39] The majority of acquired hearing loss in children and adults is a result of excessive exposure to loud noise. Other causes of acquired hearing loss include various infections, including otitis media (middle ear infection), viral infections, tumors such as acoustic neuroma (a tumor that grows on the eighth cranial nerve), ototoxicity of many kinds of medications, diseases such as Meniere disease (discussed in Chapter 19, *Diseases of the Eyes, Ears, Nose, and Throat*, and Chapter 44, *Geriatric Emergencies*), and degenerative processes associated with aging.

There are two types of hearing loss—**conductive hearing loss**, which is an inability of sound to travel from the outer ear through to the inner ear, and **sensorineural hearing loss**, which is caused by problems with the uptake of sound through tiny hairs within the ear and subsequent conduction of nerve impulses. Patients may have hearing

loss of either type or may have a combination of both conductive and sensorineural hearing loss (mixed hearing loss). It is also possible for patients to have normal hearing physiology but be unable to interpret sounds, particularly speech, due to **central auditory processing disorder (CAPD)**. CAPD is an auditory process deficit that can be characterized by difficulty interpreting speech when other background noises are present. Finally, **auditory neuropathy**, also known as auditory dyssynchrony, is a condition characterized by normal function of the structures of the ear without a corresponding stimulation of auditory centers of the brain. Auditory neuropathy is linked to prematurity, congenital anomalies, and several other neurologic conditions.

Patients with profound or total hearing loss, sometimes called deafness, may be able to communicate using sign language or written and printed words. EMS personnel who regularly provide care to patients who are deaf may find it extremely helpful to learn some sign language, even if that is limited to the words and phrases most relevant to the care they are likely to provide **Figure 45-23**. The California Department of Social Services distributes a medical sign language reference card that is readily available for no charge on the Internet.[40] Writing on simple notepads or on electronic devices will assist you in communicating with patients who are hard of hearing but able to read and write. If patients have minimal or partial hearing loss, slow, deliberate, and sometimes repetitive speech will facilitate communication.

Special Populations

Some patients who are hard of hearing are overly sensitive to loud noises close to their ears. Remember to use a normal tone of voice when you are speaking to them.

When you are caring for a patient who is hard of hearing, one easy solution is to place the earpieces of your stethoscope into the patient's ears while you speak into the bell of the stethoscope.

Hearing Aids

A hearing aid is essentially a device that makes sound louder. Hearing aids cannot restore hearing to normal, but they do improve hearing and listening ability. Several types of hearing aids are available **Figure 45-24**:

- **Behind the ear.** All parts are contained in a plastic case that rests behind the ear.
- **Conventional body.** This older style is generally used by people with profound hearing loss.
- **In the canal and completely in the canal.** These hearing aids are contained in a tiny case that fits partly or completely into the ear canal.
- **In the ear.** All parts are contained in a shell that fits in the outer part of the ear.

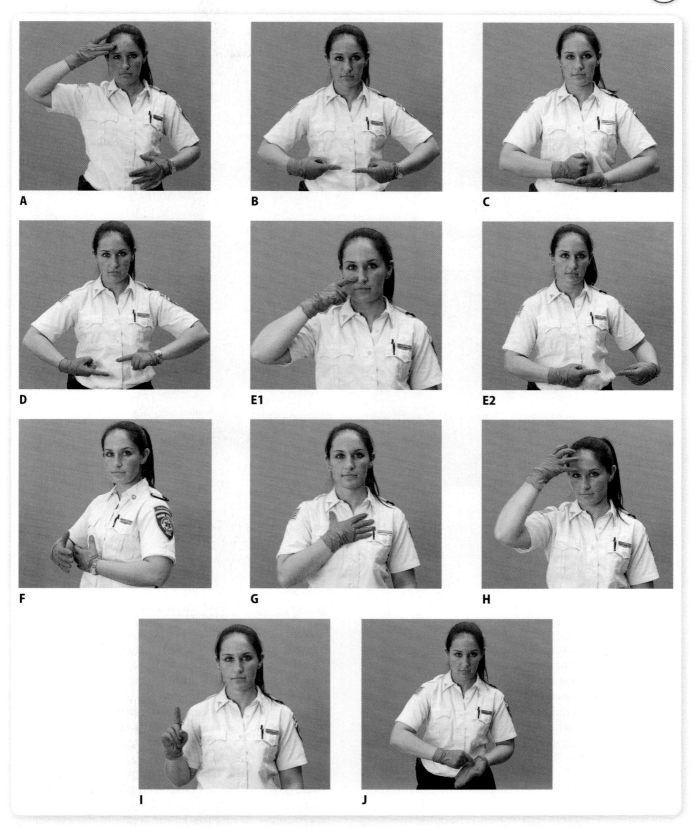

Figure 45-23 Consider learning the American Sign Language signs for common terms related to illness and injury.
A. Sick. **B.** Hurt. **C.** Help. **D.** Ache/pain. **E.** Allergy (the sign is performed in two steps; first the motion shown in **E1**, followed by the motion shown in **E2**). **F.** Breath. **G.** Chest. **H.** Dizziness. **I.** Where. **J.** Write.

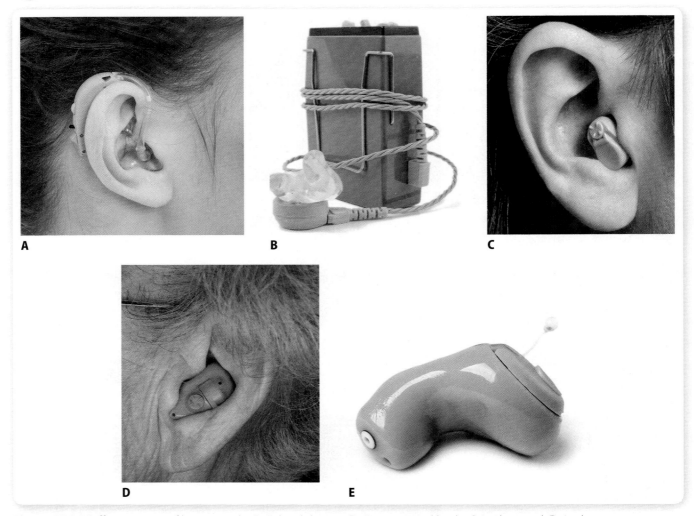

Figure 45-24 Different types of hearing aids. **A.** Behind the ear. **B.** Conventional body. **C.** In the canal. **D.** In the ear. **E.** Completely in the canal.

A: © Piotr Marcinski/Shutterstock; B: Stine Lise Nielsen/Shutterstock; C: Steve Hamblin/Alamy; D: Terry Smith Images/Alamy; E: Jiri Hera/Shutterstock.

Implantable hearing aids are also an option for patients with less profound hearing loss.

To insert a hearing aid, follow the natural shape of the ear. The device needs to fit snugly without being forced. If you hear a whistling sound, the hearing aid may not be in far enough to create a seal or the volume may be too loud. Try repositioning the hearing aid, or remove it and turn down the volume. If you cannot insert the hearing aid after two tries, put it in the box, take it with you, and document the transport and transfer of hearing aids to hospital personnel. Never try to clean hearing aids, and never get them wet.

If a patient's hearing aid is not working, try troubleshooting the problem. First, make sure the hearing aid is turned on. Try a fresh battery, and check the tubing to make sure it is not twisted or bent. Check the switch to make sure it is set on M (microphone), not T (telephone). For a body aid, try a spare cord because the old one may be broken or shorted. Finally, check the ear mold to make sure it is not plugged with wax.

▶ Visual Impairment

An estimated 1.3 million people age 40 years and older in the United States are considered legally blind, with a corrected vision of worse than 20/200.[41,42] If you add to that total the people who cannot effectively perform everyday tasks without the help of eyeglasses, contact lenses, or vision correction, the incidence of visual impairment is staggering.

Visual impairment can be caused by a variety of congenital and acquired conditions. Genetic factors may predispose people to develop vision loss later in life. Congenital causes include fetal exposure to cytomegalovirus, hypoxia during delivery, albinism, hydrocephalus, and retinopathy of prematurity. **Retinopathy** refers to any number of diseases of the retina of the eye that do not involve inflammation. High levels of supplemental oxygen given to infants during the neonatal period have been linked to retinopathy of prematurity. Acquired causes of visual impairment include trauma, cerebrovascular accident, age-related macular degeneration, glaucoma (increased pressure within the eye), cataracts (lens of the eye becomes opaque), uncontrolled hypertension, diabetic retinopathy, or degeneration of the eyeball, optic nerve, or nerve pathway (eg, with aging). Vitamin A deficiency is a significant cause of acquired visual impairment in many developing countries. Patients may have impaired vision due to **optic nerve hypoplasia**, a congenital condition characterized by failure of the optic nerve to completely develop. Over time, it is possible for optic nerve atrophy to occur following a cerebrovascular accident, brain tumor, certain toxic chemical exposures, trauma, and a variety of other causes. Optic nerve atrophy is permanent, but prompt identification and treatment of the underlying cause may slow or stop further vision loss.

Visual impairment can present in several notable patterns. **Table 45-4** outlines common patterns of visual impairment.

Hysterical blindness is an antiquated term for conversion disorder, a mental health condition. Blindness results as the body "converts" an extreme psychologic stressor into a physical manifestation. Diagnosis and treatment of conversion disorders are often quite challenging.

Acute angle-closure glaucoma (AACG) is a true ocular emergency. You should suspect AACG in patients who experience a sudden onset of unilateral eye or periorbital pain accompanied by visual changes. Prompt recognition and patient transport to an ED are imperative.

Other patients with profound visual impairment will benefit from explanation before any physical contact by EMS providers. You should warn your patient in advance if you are going to begin palpation of a body region or perform a procedure such as starting an IV line. A brief discussion with the patient prior to moving or transferring the patient will likely be greatly appreciated.

▶ Speech Impairment

You may encounter patients exhibiting impaired speech. Changes in speech may be associated with neurologic injury, toxicologic exposure, anatomic abnormalities of the face or neck, and numerous other conditions. Speech impairment has the potential to adversely impact the information obtained during assessment and treatment of patients receiving EMS assistance.

Speech impairment may be divided into disorders impacting language, voice production, fluency, and articulation. Articulation disorders essentially involve forming particular words or sounds incorrectly. They may manifest as a lisp or difficulty producing certain sounds. Voice disorders alter the pitch, volume, or tone of the patient's voice. Voices may appear muffled, raspy, or unusually high or low. Fluency disorders affect speech patterns. There may be unusual pauses or patterns to otherwise appropriate speech. Particular words or phrases may be prolonged, repeated, or avoided. Language disorders impair the manner in which ideas, thoughts, and feelings are expressed or understood. A patient may cognitively understand what he or she is trying to say but be unable to decide which words or phrases should be used to express the material. When difficulties with reading, spelling, or writing cause a person to fall behind expectations for a given age, the person has a **language-based learning disability**. Other types of language-based learning disabilities include problems with phonation. **Phonologic process disorders** impact a person's ability to produce sounds that combine into spoken words.

Patients with autism (discussed earlier) and others may present with a **semantic-pragmatic disorder** of speech. This condition is characterized by delayed language developmental milestones, with the person repeatedly using irrelevant phrases out of context, confusing word pairs such as the use of "I" and "you," and having difficulty following the conversations of others. A semantic-pragmatic disorder impacts both reception of communication and the person's ability to express himself or herself.

There are also two types of motor speech disorders that may adversely impact communication. **Dysarthria** is a failure of neurotransmission between the nervous system and muscles of the face and throat that causes impaired speech. Dysarthria is characterized by consistent repetition of the same impairment of speech. **Apraxia** is a neurologic impairment originating in the brain that inconsistently

Table 45-4	**Common Patterns of Visual Impairment**
Type of Impairment	**Characteristics**
Amblyopia	Partial or complete vision loss in one eye
Blindness	Total visual impairment; patients may report the ability to see certain lights or shadows
Cortical visual impairment	Visual impairment caused by a brain abnormality
Hyperopia	Farsightedness; problem with light refraction that makes closer objects appear blurry
Myopia	Nearsightedness; problem with light refraction that makes distant objects appear blurry
Presbyopia	Adult-onset farsightedness; problem with light refraction that makes closer objects blurry
Scotoma	Area missing from the visual field
Strabismus	Misaligned eyes

activates muscles needed to form particular sounds or words. The patient may understand what he or she is trying to say, but the pattern of muscle activation during attempts to form particular words becomes more or less random, resulting in the erratic production of sounds. The differentiation between apraxia and a phonologic process disorder is challenging and will likely require specialist consultation.

Impaired speech can be caused by many conditions other than intoxication. You may need to exercise patience and deliberation when you are communicating with patients who have speech impairment. Enlisting the help of family or caregivers familiar with the unusual speech can prove quite valuable, especially when specific information is needed from the patient.

▶ Paralysis, Paraplegia, and Quadriplegia

Paralysis is simply defined as the inability to move. Muscles in affected areas of the body may become flaccid or fail to move because of continued spasm, known as **spastic paralysis**. Many chronic medical conditions discussed in this chapter can cause paralysis. Head trauma, cerebrovascular accident (stroke), spinal cord injury, malignancy, and other neuromuscular diseases can lead to long-term paralysis. Paralysis affecting the lower extremities but not upper extremities is known as **paraplegia**. If paralysis affects both the upper extremities and the lower extremities, it is known as **quadriplegia**. In many instances, paralysis is accompanied by sensory deficits and loss of bowel or bladder control.

Patients with paralysis often experience serious complications. Paralysis of the respiratory muscles causes patients to be completely dependent on a mechanical ventilator or similar device. Interruption of assisted ventilation for even brief periods may have devastating consequences.

Pressure ulcers, discussed in Chapter 44, *Geriatric Emergencies*, are a constant threat. Patients require frequent mechanical or caregiver assistance to change their position. Tissue perfusion to the coccyx region and over bony prominences becomes compromised when external pressure is applied to these areas for a long period. Anywhere from 25% to 66% of patients with spinal cord injury have pressure ulcers.[43] Infection related to pressure ulcers is a significant cause of mortality in these patients.

Patients who have paralysis related to spinal cord injury are at risk for a life-threatening condition known as autonomic dysreflexia. A stressor within the body, sometimes as simple as a full bladder, constipation, or pain, triggers a large release of catecholamines from the autonomic nervous system. This release causes vasodilation above the level of the spinal cord injury as well as massive arterial vasoconstriction. The patient's blood pressure can become dangerously high.

External devices such as halo rings and vests are used to stabilize structures of the spine following initial management of significant fractures or dislocations

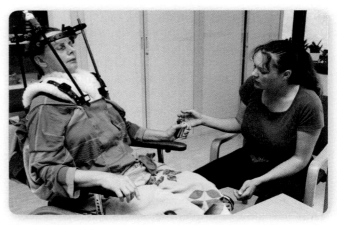

Figure 45-25 A halo ring/vest combination used for spinal stabilization after initial management of significant fracture or dislocation is shown here.

© Henny Allis/Science Source.

Figure 45-25 . These devices require additional consideration and coordination while you are moving these patients. Halo rings and vests have substantial weight. It is necessary to support the halo ring and vest, without applying any force to these devices during patient movement. In the event of cardiac arrest, there is typically an Allen/hex key attached to the anterior chest portion of the vest for removal only to perform external cardiac compressions. Paramedics and other prehospital providers should not attempt to reposition or adjust the halo ring or vest.

Patients with paralysis are particularly susceptible to environmental extremes. It is often impossible for these patients to regulate perfusion to the skin. Fluctuations of the autonomic nervous system place patients at risk for both hypothermia and hyperthermia, particularly hyperthermia.

Paralysis does not always entail a loss of sensation. In some cases, the patient will have normal sensation or hyperesthesia (increased sensitivity) that may cause the patient to interpret touch as pain in the affected area. Conversely, for some patients, pressure that would be experienced by those with normal sensation may not be felt. Some male patients with a severe spinal cord injury will present with priapism, a prolonged penile erection, not at all related to sexual arousal. Depending on the pattern of sensation loss, the priapism may be associated with discomfort for the patient. You should maintain patient privacy and continue to provide interventions related to the patient's presenting complaint.

Scheduled urinary catheterization is required for many patients with paralysis. Urinary infection, urinary reflux, and autonomic dysreflexia are all possible if patients do not have regular bladder emptying.

Total lifting assistance is typically required for many patients with quadriplegia. These patients may or may not need to use a tracheostomy tube, indwelling urinary catheter, colostomy, or ventilator. You may need to request additional lifting assistance or specialty consultation regarding the ventilator or a similar device. Patients with significant paralysis may present serious challenges for EMS providers.

▶ Trauma in Cognitively Impaired Patients

You are likely to encounter children or adults with a developmental disability at the scene, possibly as the victim of a traumatic event. Many of the cognitive, sensory, and communication impairments discussed earlier will become particularly problematic when these patients experience a traumatic injury or become involved in a traumatic event such as a motor vehicle crash. Isolated sensory or communication impairments can cause additional anxiety, confusion, delays, and disruption of patient care or transport. Patients with severe cognitive impairments will have all of the above problems and may present with a variety of abnormal behavioral responses. You may need to significantly modify how communication, assessment, interventions, and patient transport are performed.

Cognitively impaired patients present a number of significant challenges for prehospital providers. These patients may have considerable difficulty communicating under normal circumstances, and when injury, stress, and the excitement of a traumatic event are added in, effective communication can become almost impossible. These patients may not be able to provide a thorough, accurate, or meaningful medical history. If the patient's caregiver is not available, you must rely on physical or behavioral cues when you are providing treatment to these patients. Environmental clues such as the type of business (group home), school (for example, school for the deaf), or lettering on the vehicle may provide you with hints regarding the nature of the disability. Altered or decreased pain sensation, concomitant neurologic disorders, and atypical presentation of physical signs and symptoms are characteristic of many people with profound cognitive impairment. Patients with autism may demonstrate unusual communication patterns or have an exaggerated reaction to physical contact by prehospital providers.

Consent for medical treatment may present some uncertainty. Adults with profound cognitive, sensory, or communication impairment may not have decision-making capacity to consent or refuse medical treatment. You may need to locate a valid surrogate decision maker or initiate treatment under the doctrine of implied consent, particularly in emergency situations.

You will need to modify patient assessment techniques for patients with cognitive impairment. These patients may present with an education level at sixth grade or lower. A second- or third-grade education level is not uncommon. Patients with cognitive impairment may have difficulty understanding or communicating the timing or relationship of particular events. The use of open-ended questions during patient assessment may offer clues regarding the patient's cognitive ability and decision-making capacity. Assess for understanding by having the patient paraphrase or repeat back information conveyed by you or your partner, especially in situations such as obtaining patient consent or refusal.

Caregivers can become valuable resources following a traumatic event with a cognitively impaired patient. Caregivers will be able to relay how that person normally communicates, his or her level of awareness and understanding, physical abilities such as motor skills or activity, and additional information such as sleep patterns and eating habits. Consider allowing the caregiver to remain with the patient during the physical exam or deferring measurement of the vital signs in patients who are outwardly demonstrating sufficient oxygenation, ventilation, and perfusion until the patient is calm and cooperative.

Interventions may require additional time, explanation, and holding assistance. The management of traumatic injuries with fluid resuscitation, airway and ventilation support, bleeding control, and immobilization are generally the same as for patients without cognitive impairment. You should expect many of these patients to have concomitant neurologic disorders such as seizures, delirium, weakness, or muscle spasm. Psychiatric disorders, gastrointestinal abnormalities, and chronic or frequent infections are also common in this patient population. Assess for and treat preexisting injuries, and remain alert for signs or clues of abuse and neglect.

■ Other Notable Chronic Medical Conditions

You should be aware of several notable medical conditions. These conditions may meet the criteria for developmental disability noted earlier but are not primarily associated with sensory, cognitive, or communication impairment. The conditions discussed next are included to provide you with additional understanding of the impact of these chronic conditions when they are encountered in patients during an EMS response or interfacility transport.

Special Populations

You should remain alert when you are treating or transporting patients with arthritis associated with systemic lupus erythematosus (SLE), gout, or RA. In these patients, arthritis discomfort may be accompanied by other potentially significant medical concerns. Symptoms associated with these diseases include chest pain, sensory changes or deficits, and skin changes. Patients with SLE can experience life-threatening cardiac, pulmonary, and neurologic events associated with this debilitating disease process. SLE is discussed in greater detail in Chapter 25, *Immunologic Emergencies*.

▶ Cancer

You are likely to become involved in the medical care or transport of patients with active or successfully treated cancer. *Cancer* is a term applied to various conditions that result from excessive growth and division of abnormal cells within the body. This abnormal cell growth may linger for long periods with minimal clinical impact or progress rapidly, causing death in a relatively short period. Many body systems, tissues, and organs can be targeted and damaged by various types of cancer.

Cancer frequently targets organs and body systems such as the brain, breasts, skin, blood, stomach, liver, immune (lymphatic) system, and colon. Abnormal cells can multiply within a particular organ or body system, causing dysfunction of that organ or system. Cancer cells may also metastasize (spread) to another area of the body that is more susceptible to the effects of abnormal cell growth. In either scenario, critical illness or death may occur.

Signs, symptoms, clinical presentation, and treatment will largely depend on the present location of the cancer or the primary site of origin. Cancer conditions are typically treated by radiation therapy, chemotherapy medications, or some form of surgical removal. These treatment methods may be used alone or in combination, depending on the site or severity of the cancerous condition and other considerations specific to the patient. Treatment for cancer may increase the susceptibility of patients to other unrelated medical conditions.

Chemotherapy medications are notorious for causing nausea and vomiting, loss of appetite, discomfort, and immune system compromise. When patients have a compromised immune system following chemotherapy, otherwise routine infections can become life-threatening emergencies. In many instances, patients will receive chemotherapy, analgesic medications, and blood product replacement through implanted ports and other long-term vascular access devices. These devices reduce patient discomfort and prevent irritation of smaller blood vessels while allowing reliable access for frequently administered medications. Long-term vascular access devices were discussed in greater detail previously in this chapter.

You may need to correct dehydration issues and administer pain or antiemetic medications for patients diagnosed or being treated for cancer. In addition to long-term vascular access devices, patients may use transdermal patches for administration of analgesic or antiemetic medications. You should inquire about or inspect for transdermal medication patches prior to administering medications to these patients. These patients frequently receive hospice treatment (discussed earlier). You should inquire about the patient's wishes regarding resuscitation and obtain copies of advance directives or DNR paperwork when applicable.

▶ Cerebral Palsy

Cerebral palsy (CP) is a potentially devastating, nonprogressive neurologic disorder that results from injury to brain tissue during brain development. Injury to the brain may occur during fetal development, labor and delivery, or the child's first 2 years of life. CP may be caused by genetic defects that alter brain development, maternal infections during fetal development, fetal cerebrovascular accident (stroke), excessive fetal bilirubin (kernicterus) or hemolysis, hypoxia before or during birth, infant infection (eg, postpartum encephalitis, meningitis), or head trauma.

CP generally produces altered skeletal muscle function or contraction. Muscles are poorly controlled; they may be unusually contracted, flaccid, or paralyzed. Severity of this condition may range from almost unnoticeable, with children appearing and acting normal, to profoundly devastating, with paralysis of the arms and legs combined with severe intellectual disability (discussed earlier). Children with mild symptoms may function well in regular school programs. More severely affected patients may present with an exhaustive list of chronic signs and symptoms, including seizure disorders, hearing loss, and a variety of neurologic disorders. It is possible for CP to primarily affect only certain body regions such as hemiplegia (one side of the body) or be more pronounced in either the arms or the legs (paraplegia) **Figure 45-26** . When CP affects all fours limbs, it is known as **spastic tetraplegia**. Movement disorders include tremors, unsteady gait (ataxia), and athetosis (involuntary writhing movement). Severe cases may present with seizures, loss of bladder control, inability to swallow, joint contractures, and impaired respiratory function. Often, severe manifestations of CP will require that the patient receive total assistance from caregivers.

Careful movement and positioning is essential during treatment and transport of the patient. These patients may have significant musculoskeletal changes that make patient assessment and safe movement extremely difficult.

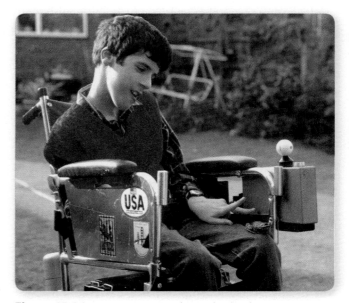

Figure 45-26 A young man with cerebral palsy.
© Sally and Richard Greenhill/Alamy.

Seizures, infection, and respiratory distress, along with many other potential complications, may prompt requests for EMS assistance.

▶ Congenital Heart Disease in Adults

Congenital heart disease (CHD), discussed in depth in Chapter 42, *Neonatal Care*, is a broad term that describes many potential abnormalities of the heart or great blood vessels that develop before birth. The severity of these conditions can range from insignificant to immediately life-threatening. These conditions are often diagnosed shortly after birth, but may also escape detection for many years. In the United States, an estimated 800,000 adults have some form of congenital heart disease.[44]

When treating an adult with a known history of a congenital heart disease condition, your best source of information is often the patient or their family members or caregivers. They will likely have a thorough understanding of the severity and implications of a particular condition, and actively contribute to treatment decisions. Significant physiologic stressors such as pneumonia, pregnancy, sepsis, etc, may unexpectedly complicate an otherwise stable CHD condition. When presented with a patient with an unusual CHD condition, consider seeking assistance from online medical control, particularly when contemplating intravenous fluid boluses, vasoactive medications, or similar interventions.

You should consider the possibility of undiagnosed congenital heart disease when patients present with a heart murmur accompanied by signs and symptoms of heart failure. Certain manifestations of CHD may present with very subtle signs and symptoms, escaping detection until an accidental discovery or abrupt change during adulthood. Patients without access to modern health care resources may survive to adulthood with an undiagnosed and untreated CHD condition that would have otherwise been treated surgically when they were infants or children.

▶ Cystic Fibrosis

Infants and young children may be diagnosed with **cystic fibrosis (CF)** (mucoviscidosis), a genetic disorder that is characterized by increased production of mucus in the lungs and digestive tract. CF is caused by a defective recessive gene, inherited from each parent, that makes it difficult for chloride to move through cells. This causes unusually high sodium loss (resulting in salty skin). Mild cases can go undetected until after a patient reaches adulthood. Sweat glands, reproductive glands, and a variety of body systems may also become adversely affected. The increased mucus impairs respiration, disrupts digestion of food, and may become a life-threatening emergency in severe situations.

CF is suspected in newborn infants who present with meconium or odd-smelling or odd-appearing stool (usually pale, greasy-looking, and foul-smelling). Gastrointestinal symptoms include nausea, anorexia, constipation, pancreatitis, and distended abdomen, as well as bowel obstruction or **ileus** (loss of gastrointestinal motility). CF impairs the release of pancreatic enzymes used to digest and absorb fats in the intestine. Patients with CF are prone to the development of venous thrombosis. Pulmonary manifestations include pneumonia, pneumothorax, persistent cough, respiratory distress, and respiratory failure. Malnutrition and poor growth rate are not uncommon symptoms; in some cases a child with CF may fail to thrive. Other symptoms include infertility, chronic sinus congestion, and bone mineral loss.

Patients with CF receive frequent or continuous treatment with various antibiotics. These antibiotics may be administered intravenously through long-term vascular access devices (discussed earlier). Medical devices promoting lung function and removal of mucus may be used by patients with CF. Patients may be on intermittent or continuous home oxygen. A significant number of patients with CF await or receive lung transplants to prolong and improve their quality of life. It is possible that patients with CF will have a long, complex medical history and a vast array of clinical abnormalities requiring additional time for patient assessment. You may encounter patients with CF who may have minimal to profound respiratory or gastrointestinal compromise from this disorder. You should expect to administer oxygen, provide frequent deep suctioning, and assist ventilation for patients with CF. CF is usually diagnosed in infants and children, but some cases, usually those people with mild or atypical symptoms, are diagnosed in adults. Diagnosis of CF requires specialized testing not available in the prehospital setting. You should alert receiving physicians if a strong suspicion for the possibility of CF exists.

▶ Multiple Sclerosis

As discussed in Chapter 18, *Neurologic Emergencies*, multiple sclerosis (MS) is a severe, incurable degenerative disorder involving the central nervous system (brain and spinal cord). Immune cells within the body attack the myelin sheath of certain nerve fibers, ultimately destroying nerve fibers and preventing nerve transmission to other body tissues **Figure 45-27**. It is not entirely clear what causes MS, although some sources describe a connection between genetic predisposition, environmental factors, and possibly nutrition or exposure to a particular virus. This disease strikes women in their 20s to 40s two to three times more often than it affects men.[45,46] Approximately 400,000 Americans have MS, some with serious disabilities.[46]

Patients typically present with problems related to muscle coordination, muscle tone, altered sensation, and gait disturbances. These patients report periods of varied improvement followed by relapse and progression of the disease. A vast array of signs and symptoms related to neurologic function are possible with MS. Patients may develop problems with the musculoskeletal system such as clumsiness and ataxia, constipation or bladder incontinence, fatigue, decreased sexual performance, extremities

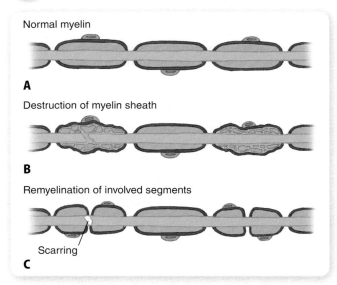

Normal myelin

A

Destruction of myelin sheath

B

Remyelination of involved segments

Scarring

C

Figure 45-27 Progression of multiple sclerosis. **A.** Normal myelin. **B.** Destruction of myelin sheath. **C.** Remyelination of involved segments with scarring.

© Jones & Bartlett Learning.

that feel heavy or weak, altered sensations (dizziness/vertigo), numbness or tingling in parts of the body, cognitive impairment, disruption of speech or swallowing,

and visual impairment. Skin breakdown may result from immobility or poor positioning. Severe manifestations of the disease may render patients bedridden and incontinent.

The patient's life span may be almost normal or markedly decreased depending on the presentation and the severity of the disease. Symptoms can present in many different combinations and last anywhere from several days to months, often interrupted by periods of absent or reduced symptoms. Though life expectancy may be normal, profound symptoms may cause significant disability or impairment, depending on the severity of the disease process.

MS is managed with medications, physical therapy, and counseling. There is no specific EMS treatment for MS. You should allow additional time for assessment due to cognitive or communication barriers. Because of the disease process, the patient may lack sensation, so the physical exam findings may be difficult to interpret. Other supportive measures include IV hydration, analgesic or muscle-relaxing medications, careful patient positioning, and assisted ventilation when indicated.

▶ Muscular Dystrophy

Muscular dystrophy is a broad term that actually describes a category of incurable genetic diseases that cause a slow,

---

YOU ▶ are the Paramedic — PART 5

Your partner reassesses Kyle's breathing and informs you that it is significantly improved, with much better air movement and fewer secretions present. Mrs. Morton calls Kyle's home health nurse, who is still about 30 minutes away, and confirms that he is coming with a new suction machine. Kyle's mother puts his normal settings into the ventilator and reattaches the circuit without difficulty. Kyle's anxiety has significantly improved and he is much more comfortable. Mrs. Morton does not wish to have Kyle transported to the hospital at this time and signs a transport refusal document, fully understanding the risks. You contact your supervisor and medical control, who are in agreement that this refusal is okay provided that you wait for the arrival of the home health nurse. You inform Mrs. Morton that you would like to stay and monitor Kyle until the home health nurse arrives in case he has another episode of respiratory distress. She is greatly appreciative and you monitor Kyle's respiratory status until approximately 0311 when the home health nurse, Brian Ortega, arrives with a new suction machine. You briefly inform him of what happened and the care you provided. You tell the mother to call 9-1-1 again immediately if she has any concerns, and she expresses understanding. You and your partner return to the ambulance so that you may finish your patient care report and clear the scene to return to service.

Recording Time: 15 Minutes	
Respirations	18 breaths/min; mechanically ventilated
Pulse	84 beats/min, regular, strong peripheral pulses
Blood pressure	116/78 mm Hg
Oxygen saturations (Spo$_2$)	97% on room air with mechanical ventilation via home ventilator

8. To what type of infections are patients who require long-term mechanical ventilation susceptible?
9. What actions might a community's emergency medical systems take to improve care for patients such as Kyle who are technology dependent and may have unique needs from the EMS system?

progressive degeneration of the muscle fibers. In many cases, the destroyed fibers are replaced by fat or connective tissue. Specific diseases in this category can be diagnosed by certain genetic markers, age at the time of onset, rate at which the disease progresses, and gender of the patient in certain cases.

Children may present with obvious facial muscle changes, altered gait, delayed psychomotor developmental milestones, and changes in posture. Severe manifestations of certain specific diseases in this group include cardiomyopathy, cognitive impairment, and respiratory compromise. Muscular dystrophy may show obvious signs when an infant is born or have an onset as late as adulthood. Profound symptoms or death from muscular dystrophy may occur in children and teenagers in severe cases. Death typically occurs secondary to cardiac or respiratory dysfunction associated with the disease.

Duchenne muscular dystrophy (DMD), the most common type, is caused by a sex-linked, recessive gene that chiefly affects boys (1 of every 7,250 males aged 5 to 24 years).[47] This disorder is characterized by enlarged heart muscle tissue (dilated cardiomyopathy), heart dysrhythmias, scoliosis (abnormal curvature) of the spine, and gait disturbances. Children with DMD often require the use of a wheelchair by age 15 years.

EMS treatment is primarily limited to careful positioning, supportive treatment, and assisted ventilation in severe cases. Smaller or younger children with muscular dystrophy are typically relatively easy to examine or transport. Larger children or adults may require additional assistance during movement to or from an ambulance.

▶ Myasthenia Gravis

Myasthenia gravis is a rare autoimmune disorder that suddenly or gradually impacts neuromuscular transmission, causing muscles to weaken and tire easily. Although it affects all ethnic groups and sexes, myasthenia gravis is most commonly found in women younger than 40 years (typically between 20 and 30 years) and men older than 60 years.[48] This disease may remain localized to the eyelids and extraocular muscles in a manifestation known as **ocular myasthenia gravis** or become "generalized," affecting respiratory muscles and a variety of skeletal muscles. The skeletal muscles of the face, jaw, neck, and upper extremities are most commonly affected. Patients often demonstrate difficulty speaking, chewing, or swallowing. Respiratory failure due to respiratory muscle fatigue is the most serious manifestation of myasthenia gravis, called a **myasthenic crisis**. A crisis may occur if the patient's respiratory muscles are damaged by infection, stress, side effects of medications, or even menstruation.

Signs and symptoms of this disease will fluctuate over time, either as the impact of the disease varies or in response to immune-based treatment or anticholinergic medication. Classic signs and symptoms include drooping eyelids; double vision; difficulty speaking, chewing, or swallowing; and muscle weakness in the extremities.

You may be requested to transport patients with myasthenia gravis as complications of the disease develop or because patients request EMS assistance for unrelated needs. It is possible that symptoms will resolve completely with rest or during transient remission of the disease process. Treatment is generally supportive and based on patient presentation. Patients having a myasthenic crisis may require airway protection and assisted ventilation. No other specific treatment options are generally available in the prehospital setting.

▶ Myelomeningocele (Spina Bifida)

Myelomeningocele, also known as **spina bifida**, is a birth defect caused by improper development of the fetal neural tube consisting of the brain and spinal cord.

During fetal development, a defect in the vertebral column creates an opening that exposes the spinal cord and meninges. There is also a corresponding defect in the overlying skin that exposes the spinal cord and meninges to the outside environment **Figure 45-28**. Spina bifida may be associated with hydrocephalus or occur as an isolated neurologic abnormality. Spinal cord involvement negatively impacts both bowel and urinary elimination in almost all patients with spina bifida, similar to other patients with spinal cord injury. Scoliosis and other orthopaedic disorders frequently accompany spina bifida. Surgical treatment of spina bifida typically occurs within 1 to 2 days of the patient's birth, although several specialized health care facilities are having significant success with repair of spina bifida while the fetus is still in the mother's uterus.

You may provide care to patients with spina bifida in one of two vastly different scenarios: when delivering a newborn, or when an older adult patient with spina bifida seeks assistance from EMS or requires interfacility

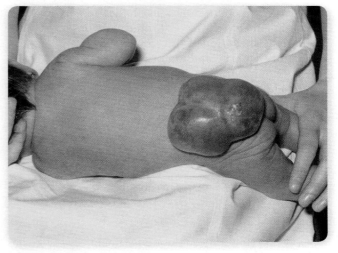

Figure 45-28 Spina bifida is characterized by exposure of part of the spinal cord.
© Biophoto Associates/Photo Researchers, Inc.

transport. It is possible that you may need to perform a prehospital delivery of a fetus with diagnosed or undiagnosed spina bifida. Spina bifida is typically diagnosed by routine prenatal ultrasound. If a patient has not received or followed up with prenatal care, it is conceivable that spina bifida could remain undiagnosed until after delivery. Successful vaginal delivery of a fetus with spina bifida is possible, particularly if hydrocephalus is not also present. Once the fetus is delivered, smaller spinal cord openings should be covered with a moist, sterile dressing. Larger openings should be covered with a sterile occlusive dressing to prevent neonatal hypothermia. The newborn should be placed in a prone or lateral position to keep pressure off of the spinal cord. Prompt transport to a hospital specializing in the care of critical newborns is required.

Modern medicine is able to keep patients with this disorder alive well into adulthood. You may also encounter infants, children, and adults with spina bifida who have already received surgical evaluation and correction of spina bifida. These patients may present with medical issues related to or completely unrelated to this disorder. These patients are likely to require careful positioning, related to the severity of vertebral column and orthopaedic abnormality.

Spina bifida may cause a wide range of clinical manifestations, ranging from minimal to severe. Most patients will present with some degree of bladder dysfunction, known as a neurogenic bladder, requiring frequent urinary catheterization. Scoliosis is also quite common, even after surgical correction of the initial abnormality. Patients may or may not have associated neurologic conditions, such as a seizure disorder, hydrocephalus, CP, or intellectual disability. Patients may also present with complete or partial paralysis of the legs and abnormalities of various bones or joints.

The severity of the spina bifida and presence of other neurologic abnormalities will determine the amount or type of interventions that you will need to provide. It is possible that spina bifida will not significantly impact patient care in certain situations. In the most severe cases, these patients are in need of multiple types of medical technology, including feeding tubes, long-term IV access, ventilatory support, ambulatory assistive devices, and intraventricular shunts to drain excess CSF from the brain's ventricles. To avoid complications, consult with family members and other home health care personnel when attempting to transport the patient.

Remember that latex allergies are common in this population, so carefully consider any medical equipment and supplies you use.

▶ Poliomyelitis/Postpolio Syndrome

Poliomyelitis (polio) is a devastating viral infection that has caused significant morbidity and mortality throughout the world. Since the 1950s, aggressive vaccination campaigns based on the Salk and Sabin vaccines have eradicated the poliovirus in many countries, including the United States. Despite stopping the flow of new cases, more than 640,000 people in the United States live with sometimes-profound consequences of this problematic disease.[49]

Humans are the only known hosts for the poliovirus (poliovirus hominis). Polio initially presents similarly to the common viral syndrome with headache, sore throat, fever, malaise, and vomiting. As the infection progresses, other somewhat generic symptoms present. Patients report back pain, diarrhea, leg pain, continued fever, and muscle discomfort or stiffness. Polio may or may not cause paralysis (paralytic and nonparalytic forms). In nonparalytic forms of polio, recovery is complete. In severe cases, muscle weakness evolves to paralysis of various muscles (most often the legs and lower trunk), muscle spasm, respiratory distress, drooling, difficulty swallowing, and other signs and symptoms. Any weakness or paralysis lasting longer than 12 months after the infection is a sign of permanent damage and disability. Complications include hypertension, respiratory failure, myocarditis, shock, loss of intestinal function, or death.

Those who survive an initial attack from the poliovirus are still at risk for **postpolio syndrome**. This disorder is characterized by progressive or sudden worsening of muscle weakness, previously caused by the poliovirus. Muscle atrophy also occurs. Patients are at renewed risk for developing respiratory insufficiency or respiratory failure, difficulty swallowing, or impaired speech. These adverse changes are frequently accompanied by significant pain or fatigue.

Most cases of polio in children, approximately 72%, are asymptomatic.[50] Polio may cause brief, mild symptoms lasting less than 72 hours in up to 24% of pediatric cases, known as subclinical polio.[50] In either instance, the long-term prognosis is quite favorable. Paralysis occurs in less than 1 percent of pediatric polio cases.[50] However, death occurs in anywhere from 2% to 75% of polio cases associated with paralysis, depending on the patient's age or portion of the CNS and corresponding muscle groups involved.[51]

The treatment for polio and postpolio syndrome remains primarily supportive. Patients with actual or impending respiratory failure require assisted ventilation and oxygenation. Movement and traditional EMS equipment are likely to cause patients significant discomfort. You should be prepared to assist patients with transfer or movement. Careful positioning and padding are essential. Patients with lower body paralysis may require assistance with urinary catheterization due to urinary retention.

▶ Traumatic Brain Injury

Traumatic brain injury (TBI) is a potentially devastating condition associated with many serious short- and long-term complications. You may encounter patients immediately after they experience the injury. Care of these patients in emergency situations is discussed in depth in Chapter 34, *Head and Spine Trauma*. Once the acute crisis has resolved, many of these patients continue to experience serious or life-altering long-term complications.

Patients may demonstrate a wide assortment of cognitive, emotional, behavioral, sensory, and communication disorders. Depending on the location and severity of the TBI, along with other associated injuries, these patients may also present with seizures, impaired movement, gastrointestinal dysfunction, urinary retention, paralysis, and almost any other conceivable problem.

You should be prepared to encounter a patient with a wide range of impairment or complications. The location or severity of the brain injury may cause you great difficulty during patient assessment and transport. In these situations, the caregiver's assistance is often essential as you interact with the patient or attempt to differentiate between new and preexisting signs and symptoms. Patients may not be cooperative or capable of providing a meaningful history or history of present illness. Communication and other common tasks may require additional time and attention while assessing, treating, and transporting patients with a TBI. These patients may not understand or voluntarily allow a physical examination or interventions such as initiating IV access. Patient restraint may be needed when the safety of the patient or prehospital providers is at risk.

YOU are the Paramedic   SUMMARY

1. **What other questions would you ask the mother at this time?**

In many cases, when a patient has a long-term, chronic health problem, the family members become very knowledgeable about the patient's condition. Additional questions to ask to gather important information include the following: Has this happened before? If so, how often, and what do you normally do to handle this situation? Is there a do not resuscitate order in place? Have you contacted your home health care service or hospice service, if applicable?

2. **What is the significance of the high-pressure alarm?**

Ventilator high-pressure alarms can be triggered for many reasons, but two of the most emergent causes are obstruction of the airway or ventilator circuit and tension pneumothorax. It is important to rapidly assess the situation for life-threatening conditions and mitigate those circumstances as soon as possible. The type of alarm that is triggered on the ventilator can be an important clue when correlated with the patient's presentation.

3. **In addressing this patient's respiratory status, what strategy could you use to quickly rule out or address the most life-threatening conditions?**

In patients receiving assisted ventilation who are deteriorating, the DOPE mnemonic (Dislodged/displaced/disconnected, Obstruction, Pneumothorax, Equipment) may be used to quickly address life-threatening issues. Removing the patient from the ventilator and using a bag-mask device with supplemental oxygen can address the *E* for equipment. Auscultating bilateral breath sounds, evaluating the compliance of the chest (Is the patient difficult to ventilate with the bag-mask device, or does the patient ventilate easily?), looking for jugular venous distention (JVD) and tracheal symmetry, and evaluating the symmetry of chest rise can address the *P* for pneumothorax. Clinical history, breath sounds, and patient presentation can aid in determining if an obstruction, the *O* in DOPE, is present. Finally, the *D* for displacement may be ruled in by excluding and addressing the other three items along with correlating the patient's presentation to the physical exam.

4. **Given this patient's clinical presentation, what is a likely cause for his respiratory distress?**

The presence of copious amounts of mucus, a tracheostomy in place, sudden onset of difficulty breathing, and a triggering high-pressure alarm on the ventilator strongly favors obstruction. Another possible cause could be tension pneumothorax, but the symmetrical chest rise and absence of JVD or tracheal deviation (late signs) make tension pneumothorax less likely than obstruction in this case.

5. **What is an appropriate course of action to address this patient's deterioration?**

At a minimum, the patient needs to be removed from the ventilator and have his ventilations assisted with a bag-mask device attached to supplemental oxygen. This step will rule out ventilator equipment problems (the *E* in DOPE) and supply supplemental oxygen if he is not already on it at home. Additionally, you need to prepare to remove the cannula and suction if necessary, as was done in this scenario. It is also important to prepare a backup plan in case suctioning is not successful or you are unable to reinsert the cannula for some reason. This plan can include bag-to-stoma ventilation or occlusion of the stoma and standard bag-mask ventilation over the mouth and nose in appropriate patients.

YOU are the Paramedic SUMMARY (continued)

6. Is transport always necessary for a patient who is ventilator dependent and has had a deterioration event like the one described in this scenario?

In cases where the cause of the problem is easily identified and resolved, transport may not be necessary and can be left to the discretion of the parent or caregiver. In this scenario, in which the patient routinely requires suctioning for his secretions and his home suction equipment malfunctioned, the risk for deterioration and access to replacement equipment should be evaluated. When replacement equipment is accessible and the risk for deterioration is low, the refusal of transport is not inappropriate as long as the risks and benefits are understood and the involved parties understand that they can call 9-1-1 again at any time if they have a concern. If the situation does not have a reversible cause or there is concern about lack of access to care or resources, it is best to encourage transport. In cases where the patient began with an apparently life-threatening condition and has improved after intervention, you should transport the patient; if the patient or family would like to refuse transport, consult with online medical direction.

7. Now that the patient's airway is clear, what interventions are appropriate in continuing care?

The patient has responded well to suctioning and tracheostomy cannula replacement. Because he has recovered to above his normal baseline oxygen saturation, it is appropriate to try to transition him back to his home ventilator. In cases where supplemental oxygen is being used at home, once the patient is stable, it is appropriate to attempt weaning the patient back to his or her original oxygen requirement while closely monitoring for decompensation. In this case, allowing the mother to aid in transitioning the patient back onto his home ventilator is appropriate, as she expresses a comfort level in managing this aspect of caring for the patient. As mentioned earlier, the family and caregivers of technology-dependent patients can be excellent resources to assist in caring for the patient when they are comfortable and express knowledge of the patient's medical devices.

8. To what type of infections are patients who require long-term mechanical ventilation susceptible?

Patients requiring long-term mechanical ventilation are susceptible to the same pathogens as non–ventilator-dependent patients, but they may contract infections with these pathogens more easily. Ventilator-dependent patients are also susceptible to opportunistic infections that healthy people do not routinely contract, due to diminished host defense mechanisms.

9. What actions might a community's emergency medical systems take to improve care for patients such as Kyle who are technology dependent and may have unique needs from the EMS system?

Technology-dependent and chronically ill patients may often call with requests for assistance with common chief complaints that have uncommon complicating factors (eg, difficulty breathing in a patient who is normally on a home ventilator). It is appropriate for the dispatch system to give prearrival information to emergency responders while en route, as long as doing so is consistent with individual department policy and the guidelines of the Health Insurance Portability and Accountability Act. In some cases, such as those involving patients who rely on ventricular assist devices for cardiac support, the home health care service may reach out to the fire department or EMS agency responsible for responding to that patient's address and provide general instructions on caring for a patient with that particular device should complications arise.

EMS Patient Care Report (PCR)

Date: 08-22-18	**Incident No.:** 07453	**Nature of Call:** Respiratory distress		**Location:** 2340 SW 20th Avenue	
Dispatched: 0200	**En Route:** 0203	**At Scene:** 0208	**Transport:** N/A	**At Hospital:** N/A	**In Service:** 0326

Patient Information

Age: 13 **Sex:** M **Weight (in kg [lb]):** 48 kg (106 lb)	**Allergies:** None known **Medications:** Gabapentin **Past Medical History:** Severe trauma with neurologic injury, partially ventilator dependent **Chief Complaint:** Respiratory distress

YOU are the Paramedic SUMMARY (continued)

Vital Signs

Time: 0211	**BP:** Not obtained	**Pulse:** 114	**Respirations:** 18 breaths/min via home ventilator	**Spo$_2$:** 86% on room air via ventilator
Time: 0213	**BP:** Not obtained	**Pulse:** 118	**Respirations:** 10–12 breaths/min via bag-mask device	**Spo$_2$:** 94% on 15 L/min bag-mask device
Time: 0215	**BP:** 114/76	**Pulse:** 102	**Respirations:** 10–12 breaths/min via bag-mask device	**Spo$_2$:** 99% on 15 L/min bag-mask device
Time: 0223	**BP:** 116/78	**Pulse:** 84	**Respirations:** 18	**Spo$_2$:** 97% on room air via ventilator
Time: 0245	**BP:** 114/78	**Pulse:** 79	**Respirations:** 18	**Spo$_2$:** 96% on room air via ventilator
Time: 0310	**BP:** 116/74	**Pulse:** 76	**Respirations:** 18	**Spo$_2$:** 97% on room air via ventilator

EMS Treatment (circle all that apply)

Oxygen @ __15__ L/min via (circle one): NC NRM **(Bag-mask device)**	**(Assisted Ventilation)**	**Airway Adjunct**	**CPR**
Defibrillation	**Bleeding Control**	**Bandaging**	**Splinting**	**(Other:** Tracheal cannula change with suctioning**)**

Narrative

Dispatched to a private residence for a chief complaint of breathing difficulty. Arrived to find partially ventilator-dependent pt with a tracheostomy in place secondary to history of severe traumatic injury and complete neurologic deficit at the level of the upper cervical spinal cord. Pt was in moderate respiratory distress on our arrival and attempting to clear thick mucous secretions. Pt's mother informed the EMS crew that pt routinely requires suctioning to aid in the clearance of his mucous secretions; however, their home suctioning equipment malfunctioned during this episode and was inoperable, which is why she contacted 9-1-1. Pt's respiratory status began to deteriorate and the decision was made to exchange this tracheostomy cannula and provide tracheal suctioning. Pt's mother provided a replacement tracheostomy inner cannula with obturator, and pt was preoxygenated prior to the procedure, achieving an Spo$_2$ of 94%. The old cannula was removed and pt was suctioned without incident. The new cannula was placed and pt was assisted with bag-mask ventilations until oxygen saturation of 99% was achieved (97% after transition back to room air). Pt's respiratory status was significantly improved, as demonstrated by decreased work of breathing and improved vital signs. Pt was weaned from bag-mask ventilation back onto his home ventilator and tolerated the transition well. The mother informed the EMS crew that a home health nurse was en route to the home with a new suction device and would arrive within the hour. She declined further treatment and transport at this time and demonstrated an understanding of the risks and benefits. Contacted supervisor and medical control; both agreed with this refusal provided we wait for arrival of the home health nurse. Brian Ortega, RN, arrived at approximately 0311 with a functioning suction machine. We briefly explained Kyle's status and the care we provided to Mr. Ortega and he was comfortable with Kyle's current condition. The mother was informed that if at any time she changed her decision or required further assistance, she could call 9-1-1. The mother signed a transport refusal form and EMS crew was clear from the scene. Available at 0326.**End of report**

Prep Kit

▶ Ready for Review

- Patients with special challenges and their caregivers have likely become experts on a particular condition or impairment.
- Poverty and patients' lack of health insurance have a direct impact on EMS nationwide. These patients may not receive preventive health services or may not purchase needed medications, thereby increasing the incidence and severity of disease and making an emergency more likely.
- Homeless and low-income patients are prone to numerous chronic medical conditions.
- Federal laws require emergency departments to stabilize patients experiencing an emergency or active labor, regardless of the patient's ability to pay. Become familiar with health care resources for low-income and homeless people.
- Abuse, neglect, and assault occur at all levels of society. Because maltreatment and assault are common reasons for calls to EMS, you must recognize the signs and symptoms of these problems.
- Physical abuse includes any improper or excessive action or force that injures or otherwise harms an individual who is dependent on the care of others, including children, incapacitated adults, and older adults.
- Some benign physical findings may mimic abuse. These include bruising in toddlers due to developing psychomotor skills, injuries from sports or recreation in older children, Mongolian spots in infants of Asian or African origin, or marks from practices such as coining and cupping.
- Your own safety is the number one priority when you are encountering an abusive situation. These situations can evoke powerful emotions; it is imperative that you remain calm and neutral while providing optimal clinical care. As always, treating life threats takes priority over collecting history.
- Careful, objective documentation of potential abuse or neglect is essential. Reporting suspected abuse or neglect is mandatory in most states. Failure to report may lead to a variety of civil, criminal, or regulatory penalties.
- Terminal illnesses are those that cannot be cured. As health care providers, you and your team will sometimes be called on to assist a patient who is facing imminent death. With such a patient, always ask if there is an advance directive or DNR order.
- Bariatric patients and patients with obesity may present significant clinical and logistical hurdles for EMS providers. For example, airway procedures and IV access are physically more difficult to perform. These patients may be too heavy for traditional EMS crews to package and transport safely and effectively. Careful planning and proper body mechanics are essential to avoid injury to emergency responders or the patient, and special equipment may be needed.
- Patients with communicable diseases deserve treatment with the same respect and dignity as any other patient.
- Many patients require physical support and care of chronic illnesses. This care may take place in the home setting. You may need to troubleshoot these devices when they malfunction or incorporate this technology into traditional prehospital patient care.
- Like caregivers of patients with special challenges, family members who care for chronically ill patients are often your best source of information and care guidelines.
- Medical technology likely to be encountered by EMS providers includes tracheostomy tubes, long-term ventilators, apnea monitors, long-term vascular devices, medical infusion pumps, nasogastric or orogastric feeding tubes, colostomy, urostomy, dialysis, surgical drains/devices, and cerebrospinal fluid shunts.
- Patients with tracheostomy tubes may experience emergencies related to occlusion or accidental removal. In some patients, loss of a tracheostomy tube may become an immediate threat to life. Follow the DOPE acronym for troubleshooting tracheostomy tube problems (Dislodged/displaced/disconnected, Obstruction, Pneumothorax, Equipment).
- Patients may be on long-term ventilators at home for a variety of reasons, including spinal cord injury, neuromuscular disease, and lung injury. If you are called to an emergency for a patient who is on a long-term ventilator, ensure that the long-term ventilator is working effectively. It is possible to severely injure a patient by improperly adjusting his or her ventilator. If the ventilator appears to be adequate for the particular patient, it is typically best to leave the ventilator connected to the patient and unchanged.
- Long-term vascular access devices require guidance from medical control before removal, replacement, or flushing.
- Use extreme caution when you are treating patients who receive dialysis; IV fluid administration requires careful monitoring.
- Do not manipulate orthotic devices, prosthetic limbs, or braces; such equipment should always accompany the patient to the hospital.
- When you are assisting with interfacility transport, you may encounter any of the following: hemodynamic

Prep Kit *(continued)*

monitoring, intra-aortic balloon pumps, or intracranial pressure monitors.

- Use extreme caution when you are transporting a patient with an arterial sheath because any associated bleeding may be life threatening.
- Special challenges may include cognitive, sensory, or communication impairment in your patients.
- Developmental delay covers a spectrum of cognitive impairment. Early intervention may allow these children to recover previously missed developmental milestones. With these patients, it may be useful to use the same approaches used for working with young children.
- Autism and autism spectrum disorders are complex disorders of brain development characterized by difficulties in social interaction, repetitive behaviors, and verbal and nonverbal communications. Patients with autism require a mindful approach to communication and physical contact. Limit external stimuli. These patients may have minimal reaction to pain, or exaggerated discomfort to minor physical contact or injuries.
- Learning cursory sign language can help facilitate communication with patients who are hard of hearing.
- Patients who are visually impaired may benefit from more detailed explanation of any physical contact or intervention before it occurs.
- Speech impairment can occur for a number of reasons and may be unrelated to cognitive impairment.
- Paramedics may encounter patients with spastic paralysis, paraplegia, or quadriplegia. Paralysis of respiratory muscles can make the patient dependent on a ventilator. Patients with paralysis are also prone to pressure ulcers. These patients will likely require total lifting assistance.
- When caring for cognitively impaired patients who have experienced trauma, remember that these patients will not necessarily be able to give you a reliable medical history. You may need to locate a valid surrogate decision maker. Interventions may require additional time, explanation, and holding assistance.
- Chronic conditions that EMS providers may encounter include cancer, cerebral palsy, congenital heart disease, cystic fibrosis, multiple sclerosis, muscular dystrophy, myasthenia gravis, poliomyelitis, spina bifida, and traumatic brain injury. Become familiar with these conditions so that you can recognize them and manage emergencies in patients with these conditions.

▶ Vital Vocabulary

acute angle-closure glaucoma (AACG) Increased intraocular pressure that leads to ocular pain and decreased visual acuity. Sudden onset is a medical emergency.

apraxia A neurologic impairment in which the brain is intermittently unable to carry out the command for speech or other tasks.

auditory neuropathy A condition characterized by normal function of the structures of the ear without a corresponding stimulation of auditory centers of the brain; also called auditory dyssynchrony.

autism A developmental disorder characterized by impairments of social interaction; may include severe behavioral problems, repetitive motor activities, and impairment in verbal and nonverbal skills.

autism spectrum disorder A group of complex disorders of brain development, characterized by difficulties in social interaction, repetitive behaviors, and verbal and nonverbal communication.

bariatrics The medical specialty dedicated to prevention and treatment of obesity.

cancer Excessive growth and division of abnormal cells within the body that can occur in many body systems, tissues, and organs and that can progress rapidly and cause death in a relatively short period.

central auditory processing disorder (CAPD) A disorder in which patients have difficulty interpreting speech and differentiating it from other sounds that are present.

cerebral palsy (CP) A developmental condition in which damage is done to the brain. It presents during infancy as a delay in walking or crawling and can take on a spastic form in which muscles are in a nearly constant state of contraction.

cerebrospinal fluid shunt (CSF shunt) A tube placed in the body to relieve pressure by drawing excess cerebrospinal fluid away from the brain or spinal cord.

colostomy The surgical establishment of an opening between the colon and the surface of the body for the purpose of providing drainage of the bowel.

colostomy bag A plastic pouch or bag attached over a colostomy to collect stool.

comfort care Medical treatment aimed at symptom relief and providing comfort for the patient.

conductive hearing loss A type of hearing impairment due to problems with the middle ear bones' ability to conduct sounds from the outer ear to the inner ear.

Prep Kit (continued)

conversion disorder A psychologic condition in which stress or mental conflict is converted into physical complaints.

curative care Medical treatment aimed at curing an illness.

cystic fibrosis (CF) A genetic disorder of the endocrine system that makes it difficult for chloride to move through cells; primarily targets the respiratory and digestive systems.

developmental delay A broad term that describes an infant or child's failure to reach a particular developmental milestone by the expected time.

developmental disability Insufficient development of a portion of the brain, resulting in some level of dysfunction or impairment.

Down syndrome A genetic chromosomal defect that can occur during fetal development and that results in intellectual disability and certain physical characteristics, such as a round head with a flat occiput and slanted, wide-set eyes.

dysarthria A speech disorder caused by neuromuscular disturbance that causes speech to become slow and slurred.

emotional abuse A form of abuse that may be verbal (such as ridicule, threats, blaming, or humiliation) or nonverbal (such as caregiver ignoring the victim or isolating the victim from others). The abuse causes a substantial change in the victim's behavior, emotional response, or cognitive function, or may manifest as a variety of mental illnesses.

false lumen An area that a device was not intended to be inserted into—for example, a tracheostomy tube inserted into an area other than the trachea.

fenestrated Having perforations, holes, or openings.

fistula A surgically created connection between an artery and a vein, usually in the arm, for dialysis access.

flange The part of a tracheostomy tube that is used to stabilize the tube to the patient's neck.

hemodynamic monitoring Monitoring and measurement of blood movement, volume, and pressure.

heparinized solution A saline solution mixed with heparin, an anticoagulant used to prevent blood clots from forming.

hospice An organization that provides end-of-life care to patients with terminal illnesses and their families.

hydrocephalus A medical condition in which there is an abnormal buildup of cerebrospinal fluid in the skull; this can be acquired (occurring after birth) or congenital (developing before birth).

ileus Disruption or loss of normal gastrointestinal motility.

inner cannula The inner tube that is inserted into the outer cannula of a tracheostomy tube.

intellectual disability A primarily cognitive disorder that appears during childhood and is accompanied by lack of adaptive behaviors, such as the ability to live and function independently or interact successfully with others; generally defined as an intelligence quotient below 70; formerly called mental retardation.

intra-aortic balloon pump A balloon that is inserted into the aorta and connected to a pump via a catheter. This therapy helps to increase the blood flow to the coronary arteries during diastole (inflation) and decrease afterload of blood from the left ventricle (deflation).

language-based learning disability A type of disability in which difficulties with reading, spelling, or writing cause a person to fall behind expectations for a given age.

mandatory reporter A category of professional required by some states to report suspicions of child maltreatment. Prehospital professionals may be included.

muscular dystrophy A broad term that describes a category of incurable genetic diseases that cause a slow, progressive degeneration of the muscle fibers.

myasthenia gravis A condition in which the body generates antibodies against its own acetylcholine receptors, causing muscle weakness, often in the face.

myasthenic crisis A complication of myasthenia gravis in which weakened respiratory muscles lead to respiratory failure.

myelomeningocele A developmental anomaly in which a portion of the spinal cord or meninges protrudes outside the spinal column or even outside the body, usually in the area of the lumbar spine (the lower third of the spine); also called spina bifida.

obesity A condition in which a person's body mass index is greater than 30 kilograms per meters squared (kg/m^2).

obturator A solid plug at the end of a tracheostomy tube.

ocular myasthenia gravis An autoimmune disorder in which the extraocular muscles become weakened and are fatigued.

optic nerve hypoplasia A congenital condition characterized by failure of the optic nerve to completely develop, possibly resulting in optic nerve atrophy over time.

Prep Kit *(continued)*

outer cannula The larger (outer) tube of a tracheostomy tube.

palliative care Medical care aimed at relief of pain and suffering in terminally ill patients.

paraplegia Paralysis of the lower extremities.

phonologic process disorders A category of disorders that impact a person's ability to produce sounds that combine into spoken words.

physical abuse A form of abuse that involves an intentional act such as throwing, striking, hitting, kicking, burning, or biting a vulnerable person.

poliomyelitis A viral infection that attacks and destroys motor axons. The disease can cause weakness, paralysis, and respiratory arrest. Because an effective vaccine has been developed, the incidence of the disease is now rare.

postpolio syndrome The death of nerve fibers as a late consequence of polio. The syndrome is characterized by swallowing difficulties, weakness, fatigue, and breathing problems.

quadriplegia Paralysis of the upper and lower extremities.

retinopathy Any eye disorder in which the retina becomes diseased, leading to partial or total vision loss.

semantic-pragmatic disorder A condition characterized by delayed language developmental milestones, resulting in the person repeatedly using irrelevant phrases out of context, confusing word pairs, and having trouble following conversations.

sensorineural hearing loss A permanent lack of hearing caused by a lesion or damage of the inner ear.

sexual abuse A form of abuse that involves a vulnerable person being forced into unwanted sexual acts, or into involvement in sexual activities such as pornography.

sexual exploitation A form of abuse that involves forcing a vulnerable person to perform or be involved in sexual acts, or to be involved in sexual activities such as pornography, in return for something they need or want, such as money, food, or shelter.

spastic paralysis A chronic form of paralysis in which the affected muscles experience continued spasm.

spastic tetraplegia A form of cerebral palsy in which all fours limbs are affected.

spina bifida A developmental anomaly in which a portion of the spinal cord or meninges protrudes outside the spinal column or even outside the body, usually in the area of the lumbar spine (the lower third of the spine); also called myelomeningocele.

surrogate decision maker A person legally authorized to make health care decisions on behalf of a patient who is incapable of making or communicating the decision on his or her own.

terminal illness A disease that a patient cannot be cured of. Death is imminent.

tracheostomy tube A plastic tube placed within the tracheostomy site (stoma).

transducer A device that converts energy or pressure into electrical signals.

urostomy A surgically constructed opening for the urinary system.

▶ References

1. Mental retardation. Centers for Disease Control and Prevention website. https://www.cdc.gov /healthcommunication/toolstemplates /entertainmented/tips/mentalretardation.html. Updated February 22, 2011. Accessed March 19, 2017.

2. Division of Birth Defects, National Center on Birth Defects and Developmental Disabilities, Centers for Disease Control and Prevention. Autism spectrum disorder (ASD). Centers for Disease Control and Prevention website. https://www.cdc.gov/ncbddd /autism/data.html. Updated July 11, 2016. Accessed March 26, 2017.

3. Boyle CA, Buolet S, Schieve LA, et al. Trends in the prevalence of developmental disabilities in US children, 1997-2008. *Pediatrics*. 2011; 127(6):1034-1042.

4. Harris-Kojetin L, Sengupta M, Park-Lee E, et al. Long-term care providers and services users in the United States: data from the national study of long-term care providers, 2013-2014. National Center for Health Statistics. *Vital Health Stat*. 2016;3(38):34. https://www.cdc.gov/nchs /data/series/sr_03/sr03_038.pdf. Accessed March 26, 2017.

5. Harris-Kojetin L, Sengupta M, Park-Lee E, et al. Long-term care providers and services users in the United States: data from the national study of long-term care providers, 2013-2014. National Center for Health Statistics. *Vital Health Stat*. 2016;3(38):40. https://www.cdc.gov/nchs/data/series/sr_03 /sr03_038.pdf. Accessed March 26, 2017.

6. Harris-Kojetin L, Sengupta M, Park-Lee E, et al. Long-term care providers and services users in the United States: data from the national study of long-term care providers, 2013-2014. National Center for Health Statistics. *Vital Health Stat*. 2016;3(38):42. https://www.cdc.gov/nchs/data/series/sr_03 /sr03_038.pdf. Accessed March 26, 2017.

7. Proctor BD, Semega JL, Kollar MA. Income and poverty in the United States: 2015. US Census Bureau. 2016:P60-256. https://www.census.gov /library/publications/2016/demo/p60-256.html.

Prep Kit (continued)

Updated September 26, 2016. Accessed April 27, 2017.

8. How is poverty measured in the United States? Institute for Research on Poverty website. http://www.irp.wisc.edu/faqs/faq2.htm. Accessed March 22, 2017.

9. Maness DL, Khan M. Care of the homeless: an overview. *Am Fam Physician*. 2014;89(8):634-40.

10. Crawford DM, Trotter EC, Hartshorn KJS, Whitbeck LB. Pregnancy and mental health of young homeless eomen. *Am J Orthopsychiatry*. 2011;81(2):173-183.

11. Hsia RY, Kellerman AL, Shen YC. Factors associated with closures of emergency departments in the United States. *JAMA*. 2011;305(19):1978-1985.

12. Liu C, Srebotnjak T, Hsia RY. California emergency department closures are associated with increased inpatient mortality at nearby hospitals. *Health Aff (Project Hope)*. 2014;33(8):1323-1329.

13. What is elder abuse? National Council on Aging website. https://www.ncoa.org/public-policy-action /elder-justice/elder-abuse-facts/. Accessed March 20, 2017.

14. What is child abuse and neglect? Recognizing the signs and symptoms. Child Welfare Information Gateway website. https://www.childwelfare.gov /pubpdfs/whatiscan.pdf. Published 2013. Accessed April 27, 2017.

15. US Department of Health and Human Services, Administration for Children and Families, Administration on Children, Youth and Families Bureau. *Child Maltreatment 2015*. Children's Bureau website. https://www.acf.hhs.gov/cb/resource /child-maltreatment-2015. Published January 19, 2017. Accessed March 27, 2017.

16. National statistics on child abuse. National Children's Alliance website. http://www .nationalchildrensalliance.org/media-room/media -kit/national-statistics-child-abuse. Accessed March 27, 2017.

17. Acierno R, Hernandez-Tejada M, Muzzy W, Steve K. National elder mistreatment study. *NCJ*. 2009.

18. Ramsey-Klawsnik H. Elder sexual abuse within the family. *J Elder Abuse Negl*. 2004;15(1):43-58.

19. Dobbin B. Rapist impregnates comatose woman in nursing home. *Los Angeles Times* website. http://articles.latimes.com/print/1996-02-18/news /mn-37303_1_nursing-home. Published February 18, 1996. Accessed March 19, 2017.

20. Ferdin P. 5-year coma patient gives birth in Mass. *Washington Post* website. https://www .washingtonpost.com/archive/politics/1998 /10/25/5-year-coma-patient-gives-birth-in-mass /9f6b9637-25e9-493e-b3b7-be9a8fe486e7/?utm _term=.340d8e184163. Published October 25, 1998. Accessed March 27, 2017.

21. Verive MJ. Pediatric head trauma. Medscape website. http://emedicine.medscape.com/article/907273 -overview#a5. Updated November 27, 2016. Accessed March 27, 2017.

22. Rao JK, Anderson LA, Lin FC, Laux JP. Completion of advance directives among U.S. consumers. *Am J Prev Med*. 2014;46(1):65-70.

23. Ogden CL, Carroll MD, Fryar CD, Flegal KM. Prevalence of obesity among adults and youth: United States, 2011-2014. Centers for Disease Control and Prevention website. https://www.cdc .gov/nchs/data/databriefs/db219.pdf. Published November 2015. Accessed March 22, 2017.

24. Division of Population Health, National Center for Chronic Disease Prevention and Health Promotion. Childhood obesity facts. Centers for Disease Control and Prevention website. https://www.cdc.gov/healthyschools/obesity /facts.htm. Updated January 25, 2017. Accessed March 27, 2017.

25. Cawley J, Meyerhoefer C. The medical care costs of obesity: an instrumental variables approach. *J Health Econ*. 2012;31(1):219-230.

26. Finkelstein EA, Trogdon JG, Cohen JW, Dietz W. Annual medical spending attributable to obesity: payer- and service-specific estimates. *Health Aff (Millwood)*. 2009;28(5):w822-w831.

27. Tsismenakis AJ, Christophi CA, Buress JW, et al. The obesity epidemic and future emergency responders. *Obesity*. 2009;17(8):1648-1650.

28. Collins JS, Lemmens HJ, Brodsky JB, et al. Laryngoscopy and morbid obesity: a comparison of the "sniff" and "ramped" positions. *Obes Surg*. 2004;14(9):1171-1175.

29. Frappier J, Guenoun T, Journois D, et al. Airway management using the intubating laryngeal mask airway for the morbidly obese patient. *Anesth Analg*. 2003;96(5):1510-1515, table of contents.

30. Lee BJ, Kang JM, Kim DO. Laryngeal exposure during laryngoscopy is better in the 25 degrees back-up position than in the supine position. *Br J Anaesth*. 2007;99(4):581-586.

31. Navarro Martínez MJ, Pindado Martínez ML, Paz Martín D, et al. [Perioperative anesthetic management of 300 morbidly obese patients undergoing laparoscopic bariatric surgery and a brief review of relevant pathophysiology]. *Rev Esp Anestesiol Reanim*. 2011;58(4):211-217.

32. Neligan PJ, Porter S, Max B, et al. Obstructive sleep apnea is not a risk factor for difficult intubation in morbidly obese patients. *Anesth Analg*. 2009;109(4):1182-1186.

33. Rao SL, Kunselman AR, Schuler HG, DesHarnais S. Laryngoscopy and tracheal intubation in the head-elevated position in obese patients: a

Prep Kit (continued)

randomized, controlled, equivalence trial. *Anesth Analg.* 2008;107(6):1912-1918.

34. Noah ZL, Budek CE. Long-term mechanical ventilation. In: Kliegman RM, Stanton BF, St. Geme JW III, Schor NF, eds. *Nelson Textbook of Pediatrics.* 20th ed. Philadelphia, PA: Elsevier; 2016:2153.

35. Noah ZL, Budek CE. Long-term mechanical ventilation. In: Kliegman RM, Stanton BF, St. Geme JW III, Schor NF, eds. *Nelson Textbook of Pediatrics.* 20th ed. Philadelphia, PA: Elsevier; 2016:1414.

36. National Center on Birth Defects and Developmental Disabilities, Centers for Disease Control and Prevention. Developmental disabilities. Centers for Disease Control and Prevention website. https:// www.cdc.gov/ncbddd/developmentaldisabilities /index.html. Updated September 8, 2015. Accessed April 27, 2017.

37. American Psychiatric Association. *Diagnostic and Statistical Manual of Mental Disorders. 5th ed.* Washington, DC: American Psychiatric Association; 2013.

38. Quick statistics about hearing. National Institute on Deafness and Other Communication Disorders (NICDC) website. https://www.nidcd.nih.gov /health/statistics/quick-statistics-hearing. Updated December 15, 2016. Accessed April 27, 2017.

39. Centers for Disease Control and Prevention, National Center on Birth Defects and Developmental Disabilties. Genetics of hearing loss. Centers for Disease Control and Prevention website. https://www.cdc.gov/ncbddd/hearingloss/genetics .html. Updated February 18, 2015. Accessed April 27, 2017.

40. California Department of Social Services Office of Deaf Access. Basic medical sign language. Deaf and Hard of Hearing Service Center website. www.dhhsc .org/resources/pub391.pdf. Published November 2007. Accessed April 27, 2017.

41. Eye health statistics: eye diseases. American Academy of Ophthalmology website. https://www .aao.org/newsroom/eye-health-statistics. Accessed March 27, 2017.

42. Blindness. National Eye Institute website. https:// www.nei.nih.gov/eyedata/blind. Accessed April 27, 2017.

43. Kruger EA, Pires M, Ngann Y, et al. Comprehensive management of pressure ulcers in spinal cord injury: Current concepts and future trends. *J Spinal Cord Med.* 2013;36(6):572-585.

44. Guidelines for treating adults with congenital heart disease. American College of Cardiology website. https://www.cardiosmart.org/heart-conditions /guidelines/achd. Accessed May 2, 2017.

45. Harbo HF, Gold R, Tintoré M. Sex and gender issues in multiple sclerosis. *Ther Adv Neurol Disord.* 2013;6(4):237-248.

46. Hersh CM, Fox RJ. Multiple sclerosis. Cleveland Clinic Center for Continuing Education website. http://www.clevelandclinicmeded.com/medicalpubs /diseasemanagement/neurology/multiple_sclerosis/. Published June 2014. Accessed April 27, 2017.

47. Division of Human Development and Disability, National Center on Birth Defects and Developmental Disabilities, Centers for Disease Control and Prevention. Muscular dystrophy. Centers for Disease Control and Prevention website. https://www.cdc.gov/ncbddd/musculardystrophy /data.html. Updated July 19, 2016. Accessed April 28, 2017.

48. Bird SJ. Clinical manifestations of myasthenia gravis. UpToDate website. https://www.uptodate .com/contents/clinical-manifestations-of -myasthenia-gravis. Updated March 22, 2017. Accessed April 28, 2017.

49. Simionescu L, Jubelt B. Post-polio syndrome. UpToDate website. https://www.uptodate.com /contents/post-polio-syndrome. Updated July 8, 2015. Accessed May 2, 2017.

50. United States Centers for Disease Control and Prevention. Poliomyelitis. Epidemiology and prevention of vaccine-preventable diseases. 13th ed. 2015:298. https://www.cdc.gov/vaccines/pubs /pinkbook/downloads/polio.pdf. Accessed May 4, 2017.

51. United States Centers for Disease Control and Prevention. Poliomyelitis. Epidemiology and prevention of vaccine-preventable diseases. 13th ed. 2015:299. https://www.cdc.gov/vaccines/pubs /pinkbook/downloads/polio.pdf. Accessed May 4, 2017.

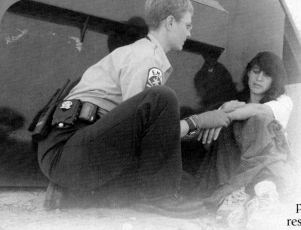

Assessment
in Action

You and your partner are dispatched to a private residence for a 44-year-old patient with difficulty breathing. On arrival, you are directed to the third floor of a "walk-up" (no elevator) apartment building. Upon entering the residence, you observe an approximately 440-pound (200-kg) man sitting partially upright in a recliner. The patient is awake, is in obvious respiratory distress, is speaking in three- to four-word sentences, has pale skin, and appears anxious. He has a nasal cannula in place. As you approach the patient, you observe that he has been incontinent of urine and stool. A neighbor who is present in the apartment informs you that the patient has not been able to get up from the recliner for several days and has now run out of home oxygen.

1. What should be your initial action in this situation?

   A. Place the patient supine and begin bag-mask ventilations.
   B. Attempt IV access to administer an IV fluid bolus.
   C. Administer high-flow oxygen via bag-mask device.
   D. Obtain a full set of vital signs.

2. Based on the information in this scenario, which body system requires the most urgent intervention?

   A. Cardiac
   B. Respiratory
   C. Gastrointestinal
   D. Endocrine

3. If this patient weighs 440 pounds (200 kg) and is 69 inches (176 cm) tall (roughly, the average height in the United States), what is his estimated body mass index?

   A. 54.5 kg/m^2
   B. 64.6 kg/m^2
   C. 69.7 kg/m^2
   D. 70.8 kg/m^2

4. Which of the following methods is most likely to be successful for fluid resuscitation and medication administration if this patient goes into cardiac arrest?

   A. External jugular IV placement
   B. Intraosseous
   C. Peripheral IV placed in proximal finger
   D. Peripheral IV placed in antecubital fossa

5. Which of the following would be the best position to perform bag-mask ventilation on this patient?

   A. Supine
   B. High Fowler
   C. Prone
   D. Ramp position

6. Which extrication device would be most appropriate to transport this patient from his apartment to the ambulance, in his current condition?

   A. Bariatric EMS stretcher
   B. Bariatric transfer sheet
   C. Bariatric extrication chair
   D. Bariatric backboard

7. If this patient were to require intubation and mechanical ventilation, which ventilation adjunct would you expect?

   A. Prone positioning
   B. Bifurcated (double-lumen) ET tube
   C. Inverse-ratio ventilation
   D. Positive end-expiratory pressure

8. What equipment is needed to safely and effectively provide emergency medical care to bariatric patients?

9. How should you safely and effectively manage patients in the prehospital setting with unfamiliar medical devices?

10. How can you offer optimal care to patients with unusual chronic medical conditions?

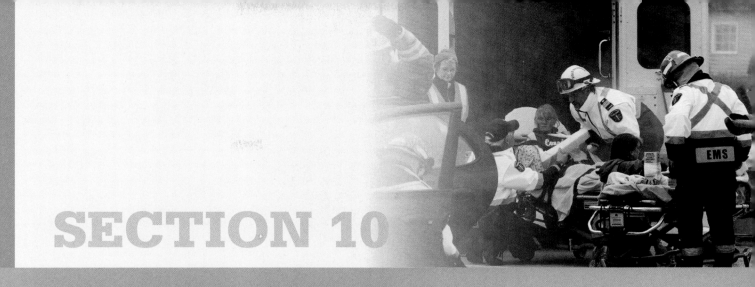

SECTION 10

Operations

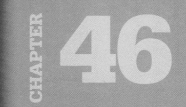
Transport Operations

National EMS Education Standard Competencies

EMS Operations

Knowledge of operational roles and responsibilities to ensure patient, public, and personnel safety.

Principles of Safely Operating a Ground Emergency Vehicle

> Risks and responsibilities of emergency response (pp 2306-2307, 2310-2313, 2317-2319)
> Risks and responsibilities of transport (pp 2310-2313, 2317-2319)

Air Medical

> Safe air medical operations (pp 2322-2326)
> Criteria for utilizing air medical response (pp 2321-2322)
> Medical risks/needs/advantages (pp 2320-2321)

Medicine

Integrates assessment findings with principles of epidemiology and pathophysiology to formulate a field impression and implement a comprehensive treatment/disposition plan for a patient with a medical complaint.

Infectious Diseases

Awareness of
> A patient who may have an infectious disease (p 2311)
> How to decontaminate equipment after treating a patient (pp 2311-2312)

Assessment and management of
> A patient who may have an infectious disease (see Chapter 26, *Infectious Diseases*)
> How to decontaminate the emergency vehicle and equipment after treating a patient (pp 2311-2312)
> A patient who may be infected with a bloodborne pathogen (see Chapter 26, *Infectious Diseases*)
  • Human immunodeficiency virus (HIV) (see Chapter 26, *Infectious Diseases*)
  • Hepatitis infections (see Chapter 26, *Infectious Diseases*)
> Antibiotic-resistant infections (see Chapter 26, *Infectious Diseases*)

> Current or new emergent infectious diseases prevalent in the community (see Chapter 26, *Infectious Diseases*)

Knowledge Objectives

1. Summarize the medical equipment, safety equipment, and operations equipment carried on an emergency medical vehicle. (pp 2304-2306)
2. Discuss the importance of performing regular vehicle inspections, and list the specific parts of an emergency vehicle that should be inspected daily. (pp 2306-2308)
3. Provide examples of some high-risk situations and hazards that may affect the safety of the emergency vehicle and its passengers during both pretransport and transport. (pp 2309-2310)
4. Discuss specific considerations that are required for ensuring scene safety, including personal safety, patient safety, and traffic control. (pp 2310-2311)
5. Define the terms cleaning, disinfection, high-level disinfection, and sterilization, and explain how they differ. (p 2311)
6. Identify the dangers to consider when operating an emergency vehicle in the emergency mode. (pp 2312-2316)
7. Discuss the guidelines for driving an emergency vehicle safely and defensively, and identify key steps emergency medical services (EMS) personnel can take to improve safety while en route to the scene, the hospital, and the station. (pp 2313-2316)
8. Describe the elements that dictate the use of lights and siren to the scene and to the hospital and the factors required to perform a risk-benefit analysis regarding their use. (pp 2313-2314, 2318-2319)
9. Give examples of the specific, limited privileges that are provided to emergency vehicle drivers by most state laws and regulations. (p 2318)
10. Explain why using police escorts and crossing intersections pose additional risks to EMS personnel during transport, and discuss special considerations related to each. (p 2319)
11. Describe the capabilities, protocols, and methods for accessing air medical transport. (pp 2319-2322)

12. List the safety concerns when operating a landing zone for helicopter transport. (pp 2322-2326)
13. Describe key scene safety considerations when preparing for a helicopter medevac, including establishing a landing zone, securing loose objects, mitigating on-site hazards, and approaching the aircraft. (pp 2322-2326)

Skills Objectives

1. Demonstrate how to perform a daily inspection of an emergency vehicle. (pp 2306-2307)
2. Demonstrate how to clean and disinfect the emergency vehicle and equipment during the postrun phase. (pp 2311-2312)

■ Introduction

Today's emergency vehicles are equipped with state-of-the-art technology, including defibrillators and monitors that can transmit information directly to the emergency department (ED) or catheterization laboratory, blood and oxygen testing equipment, automatic transport ventilators, CPR adjuncts to circulation devices, global positioning systems (GPS), and mobile data terminals. Even when all safety guidelines are being followed, the emphasis on rapid response places you and your crew members in great danger while driving to calls.

Driving an emergency vehicle is a tremendous responsibility. Not only do you have to be aware of the safety of your crew and passengers, but you are also responsible for the safe passage of other vehicles and pedestrians you encounter on the road. Activating the lights and siren does not ensure that you will be heard or understood by other drivers. More importantly, the use of lights and siren is usually only a request for the right-of-way.

This chapter discusses emergency vehicle design and how to equip and maintain an emergency vehicle. It also focuses on the techniques and judgment that you will need to learn to safely operate an emergency vehicle, which includes parking considerations, emergency vehicle control and operation, the effects of weather on driving, and common hazards that are encountered in driving an emergency vehicle. Finally, it describes how to work safely with patient transport aircraft.

■ Emergency Vehicle Design

Current specifications for emergency medical transport vehicles were originally developed by the US General Services Administration (GSA) in the early 1970s. Design and manufacturing specifications are outlined in the **DOT KKK 1822** federal guidelines for the purchasing of emergency vehicles.[1] These guidelines were reviewed and updated every 5 years based on recommendations from manufacturers and operators of the vehicles. Many states adopted the GSA guidelines for emergency vehicles in their area because the guidelines allow for more eligibility in government grant funding. When the GSA announced that the KKK 1822 specifications would be discontinued, the National Fire Prevention Agency (NFPA) began working on a replacement standard and published their first specifications for emergency transport vehicles in the NFPA 1917 guidelines in 2013.[2] The Commission on Accreditation of Ambulance Services has also developed a set of guidelines for emergency vehicle specifications in GVS-2015. Both of these specifications are being considered as replacements for the GSA KKK 1822 guidelines.[3] As of the start of 2017, the KKK 1822 standards are still in use and will be extended until alternative standards are developed and approved by the GSA for the purchasing of government vehicles.

The original guidelines required that all emergency medical vehicles be painted Omaha orange and white, allowing them to be easily recognized by other drivers.

YOU ▶ are the Paramedic   PART 1

You and your partner are getting ready to order lunch at your favorite lunch spot when you are dispatched for a multi-vehicle crash on the interstate nearby. It has been raining all day, so you are not surprised a collision has occurred. You exit the parking lot and turn to get to the closest interstate on-ramp.

1. Explain the concept of "due regard."
2. What considerations should you make concerning your route to the interstate?

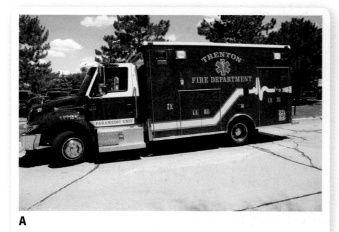

A

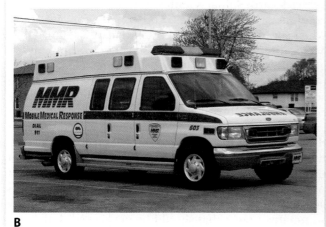

B

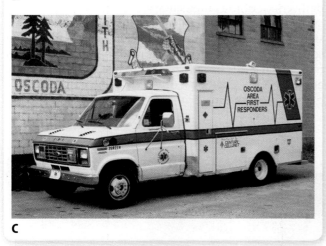

C

Figure 46-1 Basic emergency medical vehicle designs.
A. Type I (a heavy-duty type I is shown here; a standard type I
is shown in Figure 46-5). **B.** Type II. **C.** Type III.

A: © Tom Carter/PhotoEdit, Inc; B and C: Courtesy of Captain David Jackson, Saginaw Township Fire Department.

More recently, standards have been relaxed to allow for
a variety of personalized paint schemes. The KKK 1822
standards also established three major emergency medical
vehicle designs **Figure 46-1** and **Table 46-1** .[4]

Improvements made to emergency vehicles over the
years have made them not only safer for emergency medical

Table 46-1	Basic Emergency Medical Vehicle Designs
Type I emergency medical vehicle	Conventional, truck-cab chassis with a modular body that can be transferred to a newer chassis as needed
Type II emergency medical vehicle	Standard van, forward-control integral cab-body
Type III emergency medical vehicle	Specialty van, forward-control integral cab-body that can be transferred to a newer chassis as needed
Heavy-duty emergency medical vehicle	Extra heavy-duty vehicle

© Jones & Bartlett Learning.

services (EMS) personnel, but also more comfortable.
One of the most significant developments in emergency
vehicle design has been the enlargement of the patient
compartment. The inclusion of padded cabinet corners
as well as safety nets on the squad bench have made it
easier to perform patient care activities with less risk of
injury. In many emergency vehicles, not everyone in the
vehicle is restrained in a five-point harness and wearing
a helmet. Recent studies on vehicle safety for emergency
vehicles have resulted in the addition of newer vehicle
safety designs based on recommendations from SAE
(Society of Automotive Engineers) International. These
include changes in how the patient stretcher is secured in
the rear compartment and equipment securing devices.
These recommendations have been incorporated into the
new emergency medical vehicle standards.[5,6] However,
there is still room for improvement.

■ Emergency Vehicle Equipment

In the patient compartment of an emergency vehicle,
every inch of space is dedicated to storing or securing the
equipment it takes to do the job well. Much like a jigsaw
puzzle, everything must fit tightly together to prevent
injury, yet be easily accessible.

Many organizations have influenced the development
of the supplies and equipment carried on today's units.
The Occupational Safety and Health Administration
(OSHA) makes recommendations regarding infection
control practices to include all areas of personnel protective
equipment, sharps containers, and disinfecting equipment.
The American College of Surgeons (ACS) developed the

first standardized list of equipment to be carried on an emergency vehicle in 1970. The list is now published in a cooperative effort between the ACS, the American College of Emergency Physicians, and the National Association of EMS Physicians, as well as state EMS lead agencies and is continually updated as technologic advances are made in the field.[7]

Checking the Emergency Vehicle

Getting ready to respond to a call is just as important as providing patient care. The crew must ensure that the unit is capable of responding safely and efficiently to calls.

At the beginning of each shift, crew members must check the emergency vehicle to ensure the proper equipment is available and in good working order. Many local or regional regulatory agencies have equipment regulations specifying the minimal equipment or supplies that must be carried on every emergency vehicle. Each time supplies and equipment are used, they should be properly cleaned or replaced and returned to service for the next call. Medication expiration dates must be checked regularly to confirm that they have not expired. In addition, diagnostic equipment, such as defibrillators, pulse oximeters, and glucometers are tested each shift and are calibrated on a regular basis by appropriate preventive maintenance personnel.

Documentation & Communication

Because the mechanical aspects of emergency work, such as driving and moving patients, have an impact on your safety and the safety of others, your service should have specific procedures for daily inspections. Following these procedures protects you physically, and documenting your compliance is an important legal protection. Procedures should call for dating and either signing or initialing the check sheets. Software is available to check your vehicle and record data directly onto a digital device. Store all documentation where it can be found later if needed to support a legal challenge.

The emergency vehicle inspection should include the following:

- Fuel levels
- Oil levels
- Transmission fluid levels
- Engine cooling system and fluid levels
- Batteries
- Brake fluid
- Engine belts
- Wheels and tires, including the spare, if there is one. Check inflation pressure and look for signs of unusual or uneven wear.

- All interior and exterior lights
- Windshield wipers and fluid
- Horn
- Siren
- Air conditioners and heaters
- Ventilating system
- Doors. Make sure they open, close, latch, and lock properly.
- Communication systems, both on-vehicle and portable
- All windows and mirrors. Check for cleanliness and position.

All compartments in the emergency vehicles should be checked regularly, both inside and out. Most emergency vehicles carry spinal stabilization and patient moving equipment in the outside compartments for easy access when speed may be an important factor **Figure 46-2**. Medications and temperature-sensitive equipment are generally stored in the patient compartment area. It is important to maintain temperature control for medications; some emergency vehicles have a medication temperature control unit on-board **Figure 46-3**.

An emergency vehicle needs to be able to do four things 100% of the time: start, steer, stop, and stay running. Any threat to one of the "four Ss" should prompt the operator to put the vehicle out of service immediately. A standard daily checklist is essential to ensure the emergency vehicle is in good operating order. **Table 46-2** summarizes tasks that should be performed during the daily check of the emergency vehicle.

It is also important for you to be cognizant of warning signs of impending problems. **Belt noise** is a chirping or squealing sound, synchronous with engine speed (not road speed). It is usually related to a load on one of the appliances operated by a drive belt—the power steering pump, the water pump, the vacuum pump (in a diesel),

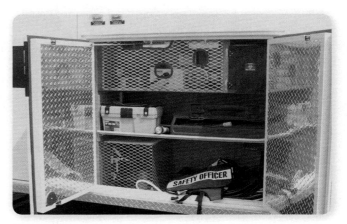

Figure 46-2 The emergency vehicle should have a weatherproof compartment that can be reached from outside the patient compartment. It should hold equipment for safeguarding patients and crew, controlling traffic, and illuminating work areas.

© Jones & Bartlett Learning. Courtesy of MIEMSS.

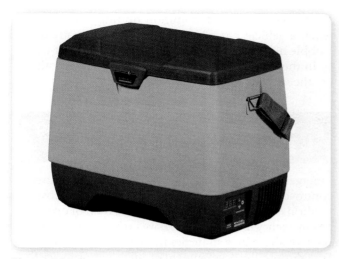

Figure 46-3 Some emergency vehicles have a medication temperature control unit on-board.
Courtesy of Engel USA.

or the alternator. Belt noise is always significant and will eventually keep an emergency vehicle from operating. It does not necessarily warrant taking a unit out of service immediately.

Brake fade is a sensation that an emergency vehicle has lost its power brakes. Its most common causes are overheating of brake surfaces, loss of vacuum, loss of brake fluid, wet or greasy brake drums/disks, or a failed master cylinder. Even a single instance of brake fade warrants taking your vehicle out of service immediately.

Generally, you should not hear, smell, or feel a vehicle's brakes, with occasional exceptions. Cold brakes may squeak intermittently in wet weather. Some kinds of brake pads are equipped with "telltale tabs"—small aluminum projections that are designed to rub on the disk surfaces and squeak, warning an operator when the pads are nearing the end of their useful life. Otherwise, a consistent squeaking or grinding sound warrants immediate attention by a mechanic.

Table 46-2	Daily Emergency Vehicle Inspection Tasks
Tasks	**Tips**
Walk around the emergency vehicle.	Identify unreported body damage, major leaks, inoperative lighting, or damaged tires. Checking brake and backup lights requires assistance of a second person.
Check fuel levels.	Some emergency vehicles carry two fuel tanks; check both.
Check the motor oil.	Do this prior to starting the engine. Check for level and quality. Should be yellow or amber in a gasoline engine, or gray or black in a diesel engine. Should never smell like fuel.
Check transmission fluid.	Often checked with motor running and the gear selector in "park." Should be pink or yellow. Should not smell like charcoal.
Check steering fluid.	Should be pink or yellow. Should not smell like charcoal.
Check lubricants.	Should feel slippery between the fingers. Should appear clean. Should smell like fresh oil.
Check brake fluid.	Should be clear or yellow when fresh; could be amber after a few years of service. Do not uncap brake fluid reservoir; fluid absorbs moisture from the atmosphere.
Check coolant.	May be either red or bright yellow-green. Do not uncap coolant reservoir; it is pressurized and can expand rapidly, causing burns. Check levels at the overflow reservoir and add coolant as needed.
Check the battery.	Should be clean. Top surfaces of battery should be dry and the terminals corrosion-free. System voltage should be 12 to 12.5 volts at rest, 13.5 to 14.5 volts when engine is running. Should not be higher than 15. Should not smell like sewer gas; if so, take out of service immediately, leave hood closed, and do not start the engine.

Brake pull is a sensation that when you depress the brake pedal, someone is trying to jerk the steering wheel to the left or right. It can indicate brake fluid or grease on a brake pad, or it can result from a serious mechanical malfunction. Remove the vehicle from service immediately.

Drift is a finding that when you let go of the steering wheel, the vehicle consistently wanders left or right. Any vehicle may normally drift slightly to the right, because most roads are built with a crown in the center (so water drains toward the gutters). A vehicle should not consistently drift to the left, however.

Steering pull is a persistent tug on the steering wheel that you can feel as the emergency vehicle "drifts" to one side or the other. Its most common cause is uneven tire pressures (possibly a flat tire). Steering pull can also be caused by one or more misaligned wheels or another mechanical problem. It can cause loss of control in the event of a sudden stop. A vehicle's steering geometry is complex. To allow for its adjustment, the entire front suspension system is held together by clamps. Misalignment can occur when a vehicle hits a curb and dislodges one or more of these clamps. The result may be control problems as well as tire damage in short order.

A pulsating brake pedal—an up-and-down motion of the brake pedal during deceleration—is an abnormal condition, especially at low speeds. A pulsating brake pedal usually indicates warped brake rotors or drums but can also suggest a bent wheel. This motion can be severe when the brakes are hot. This condition always warrants service. If your vehicle is equipped with antilock brakes, it is a normal occurrence to feel your brakes pulsate when on wet pavement. This automatic activation of the brakes is to prevent your wheel or wheels from slipping or locking up.

Normally, little effort is required to steer an emergency vehicle. Excessive effort to steer is, therefore, a serious finding and can be caused by inadequate steering fluid or a failed power steering pump or drive belt.

Steering play is a sensation of looseness or sloppiness in a vehicle's steering. This finding is important when accompanied by clunking or banging noises during steering, and it should never be noticeable in a new vehicle. This problem is typically caused by wear, but it can also result from underinflated tires. This situation warrants immediate inspection of the emergency vehicle.

Tire squeal is a singing sound that occurs when you turn the vehicle, especially at parking speeds. Squealing is normal on smooth concrete, but not on asphalt. The most common cause is underinflated tires, but it can also result from misaligned wheels, especially in the presence of other signs. This situation warrants a mechanic's attention as soon as possible.

Wheel bounce is a vibration, synchronous with road speed, that you can feel in the steering wheel (suggesting a front wheel) or driver's seat (rear wheel). Wheel bounce is usually detectable at freeway speeds of over 45 miles per hour (mph). It suggests a defective shock absorber, a bubble in a tire, or an improperly balanced wheel.

Wheel wobble is a common finding at low speeds when a vehicle has a bent wheel. You normally detect wobble in the steering wheel if it involves a front wheel, or in the driver's seat if it is in the rear wheel. Potholes are the most common cause.

Emergency Vehicle Staffing and Development

Emergency vehicle staffing has been a major source of controversy over the few past decades. Escalating costs for medical care, fuel, and the financial burden of operating an emergency medical service have prompted the development of alternative strategies for managing EMS systems. For example, the development of "high-performance EMS systems" represents an effort to maximize personnel productivity and minimize response times. The key factors that are analyzed in an effective, cost-efficient service are summarized as follows.

- **Response times.** High-performance systems typically use a response time standard in which a significant fraction (usually 90%) of all responses must be achieved in an established time—for example, 8 minutes or less in an urban area.[8] These standards are based on the recommendations of the Commission on Accreditation of Ambulance Services.
- **Productivity.** The EMS provider measures how many patient transports per hour each emergency vehicle accomplishes (known as "unit-hour utilization").
- **Unit costs.** Determined by the cost to respond to each call as well as the actual number of hours the units were actively operating, these costs include the paramedics' salaries and benefits, plus the operational cost of vehicles and equipment (gas, routine maintenance, and repairs).
- **Taxpayer subsidies.** The local government may make a financial commitment to help lower user fees. Some services also offer annual subscription fees in return for free services during the year.

▶ Emergency Vehicles and EMS Systems

In the United States, many first-response emergency medical services are delivered by fire department personnel who are cross-trained in EMS. Some emergency medical responders are trained in basic life support (BLS); others have advanced life support (ALS) training. These responders may be paid or volunteer, and they typically respond from fire stations located throughout the community. Many fire services also operate the emergency medical transport services.

In other communities, the emergency medical service is provided by a private, for-profit enterprise. In some areas, a public agency (not part of the fire department) delivers emergency transport services; this system is known as the third service delivery model. Another type of model involves a public-private partnership or a nonprofit corporation.

Staffing of emergency vehicles may be variable between and within EMS systems. Some systems have two or even three paramedics on each emergency vehicle. Others staff the emergency vehicle with basic emergency medical technicians (EMTs). Some systems employ a tiered response system that attempts to assign ALS personnel only where they are needed.

► System Status Management

System status management (SSM) is a concept that was developed by Jack Stout in 1983.[9] The goals of SSM are to maximize efficiency and reduce response time. In SSM, historic data are compiled and used to determine emergency service demands, and SSM then takes into consideration fluctuations in demand to better organize service. For example, an increased demand for service may be noted during certain hours of the day or in certain geographic locations. These demands are termed **peak loads**. In an urban area, the demand for EMS may be higher during the daytime but lighter during the night. SSM attempts to arrange **strategic deployment** of emergency vehicle resources to minimize response times. The strategic deployment of an emergency vehicle to a location, known as **posting**, can take advantage of developments in satellite vehicle location and GPS technologies.[10]

Another component of SSM is the capability to help organize peak demand staffing. Shift schedules are designed to provide a sufficient number of emergency vehicles during peak load hours. For example, more emergency vehicles might be staffed between noon and 1800 hours than between midnight and 0600 hours. One potentially negative aspect of SSM is the toll that it can take on personnel, who have less time to get out of the vehicle and relax in the duty station between calls.

► Emergency Vehicle Stationing

The goals for establishing emergency duty stations are to maximize efficiency and to minimize response times. In most urban and suburban areas, the distance factor may not be as important as the call volume. In a rural setting, both availability of first responders and distance may be equally important. Also, the district may have special facilities that create increased emergency medical demands on long-term care facilities. Other considerations in the design of emergency duty stations include the need for maintenance and cleaning of vehicles and equipment, storage, disinfection facilities, classrooms for training and meetings, and sleeping quarters for personnel who spend the night.

■ Mitigating Hazards Throughout the Call

► En Route to the Scene

In many ways, the en route or response phase of the call is potentially very dangerous[11] for you. Collisions between passenger vehicles and emergency vehicles cause many serious injuries to EMS personnel. Techniques to make

YOU ▶ are the Paramedic | PART 2

You arrive on scene and are directed to a vehicle where a woman is sitting in the driver's seat. There is minimal damage to the vehicle, which appears to have rear-ended the vehicle in front of it. The patient states that she is fine but her knee hurts where it hit the bottom of the dashboard. As you attend to the patient, your partner assesses the driver of the other vehicle and determines he is uninjured.

Recording Time: 1 Minute	
Appearance	Awake
Level of consciousness	Alert (oriented to person, place, time, and event)
Airway	Open
Breathing	Adequate
Circulation	Adequate

3. What equipment and supplies are typically taken from the emergency vehicle to the patient's side?
4. What factors should be considered when you are operating an emergency vehicle in inclement weather?

vehicle operation safer will be discussed later in this chapter. As you and your partner prepare to respond to the scene, make sure you always fasten your seat belts and shoulder harnesses *before* you move the emergency vehicle. At this point, you should inform dispatch that your unit is responding and confirm the nature and location of the call. This is also an excellent time to ask for any other available information about the location.

While en route, you and your team should prepare to assess and care for the patient. Review dispatch information about the nature of the call and the location of the patient. Assign specific initial duties and scene management tasks to each team member, and decide what type of equipment to take initially. Depending on your operation procedures, you may also decide which stretcher to bring to the patient. Communications with dispatch and any use of GPS should be conducted by the officer, not the vehicle operator, since these are distractions to driving.

▶ Securing Equipment

It is important to make sure all equipment (in the cab, patient compartment, and storage compartments) is secured before placing a vehicle in motion. Driving rapidly through heavy traffic will cause objects to shift in the rear compartment. Placing an item such as an open drug or equipment box on the squad bench for easy access may be convenient, but if a quick change in direction occurs, the contents will end up scattered all over the floor, or worse, broken. A piece of diagnostic equipment or a portable oxygen cylinder can become a lethal projectile if not secured correctly.

▶ Arrival at the Scene

On arrival at the incident, you will perform a scene size-up. After you complete your size-up, report to dispatch the nature of the incident if this is part of your local protocol. Also report any unexpected situations, such as the need for backup units, a heavy rescue unit, or a hazardous materials team. Do not enter the scene if there are any hazards to you. If there are dangerous hazards at the scene, the patient should be moved before you begin care. The patient may have to be moved by others if you are not appropriately equipped or trained. Immediately size up the scene by using the following guidelines:

- Look for safety hazards.
- Evaluate the need for additional units or other assistance.
- Determine the mechanism of injury in trauma patients or the nature of the illness in medical patients.
- Evaluate the need for any specialized equipment or additional response vehicles (ie, police department, fire department, rescue, power company, hazardous materials).
- Make sure you take standard precautions. The type of care that you expect to give will dictate what personal protective equipment you should wear.

If you are the first EMS provider at a scene with multiple patients, quickly estimate the number of patients. Inform dispatch if additional units are needed at the scene. Such incidents may qualify as mass-casualty incidents, which involve complex organization of personnel under the incident command system (see Chapter 47, *Incident Management and Mass-Casualty Incidents*). In this system, individual EMS providers may be assigned roles to do such things as beginning the triage and tagging process, assist in treating patients, and load patients for transport to a hospital.

Patient Safety

In March of 2014, the American College of Emergency Physicians and the National Association of EMS Physicians issued a policy statement stating that safety must become a foundational component of every EMS system. Providing high-quality EMS requires that we understand risk and embrace practices to prevent harm to patients, EMS personnel, and members of our community. It is the EMS physician's role to develop and support a culture of safety in EMS systems.

▶ Traffic Control

After ensuring your own safety and that of your crew, your first responsibility at a crash scene is to care for the patients. Only when all the patients have been treated and the emergency situation is under control should you be concerned with restoring the flow of traffic. If the police do not arrive quickly at the scene, you might then need to take action.

The purpose of traffic control is to ensure an orderly traffic flow and to prevent another crash. Under ordinary circumstances, traffic control is difficult. A crash or disaster scene presents serious additional problems. Passing motorists often slow down and stare, paying little attention to the roadway in front of them. Some curiosity seekers may park down the road and return on foot, creating still other hazards. Emergency workers are required to wear reflective vests in both daytime and nighttime operations on federal-aid highways. The vests should meet the performance standards of class 2 or 3 of the ANSI/ISEA 107-2015 publication.[12]

As soon as possible, place appropriate warning devices, such as reflectors, on both sides of the crash. Remember, the main objectives in directing traffic are to warn other drivers, to prevent additional crashes, and to keep vehicles moving in an orderly fashion so that care of injured patients is not interrupted.

▶ Safe Patient Transport

Many patients have said that one of the most frightening parts of being suddenly ill or injured is the emergency vehicle ride to the hospital. Already anxious, a patient may experience increased anxiety during a fast, bumpy ride with a siren blaring. Such a ride is not likely to be lifesaving. In most cases, excessive speed is unnecessary and dangerous and reckless. What is necessary is safe transport of the patient to an appropriate medical care facility in the shortest practical time. Realizing this objective takes common sense and defensive driving techniques. Speed is no substitute for these qualities. In almost every case, you will provide lifesaving care right where you find the patient, before moving the patient to the emergency vehicle. You may then begin less urgent measures, such as bandaging, splinting, and reassessment. Next, you must package the patient for transport, securing him or her to a device such as a backboard, a scoop stretcher, or the wheeled patient stretcher. Then move to the emergency vehicle, and properly lift the patient into the patient compartment.

No matter how careful the driver may be, a patient who is riding to the hospital while lying on his or her back on a stretcher can experience discomfort and possibly even danger. Secure the patient according to the manufacturer's recommendations, which typically includes the use of shoulder straps and at least three straps across the body. Use deceleration or stopping straps over the shoulders to prevent the patient from continuing to move forward in the event the emergency vehicle suddenly slows or stops. Always follow your service's standard operating procedures on strapping the patient, and also the recommendations of the stretcher manufacturer.

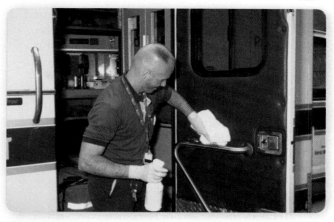

Figure 46-4 Be sure to clean and disinfect the emergency vehicle and equipment at the station if you did not do so at the hospital.

© Jones & Bartlett Learning. Courtesy of MIEMSS.

routine inspections. Use a written or electronic checklist to document needed repairs or replacement of equipment and supplies.

It is also important to **decontaminate** the emergency vehicle after the call. Terms related to decontamination include *cleaning, disinfection, high-level disinfection,* and *sterilization.* The definitions are as follows:

- **Cleaning.** The process of removing dirt, dust, blood, or other visible contaminants from a surface.
- **Disinfection.** The killing of pathogenic agents by directly applying a chemical made for that purpose to a surface.
- **High-level disinfection.** The killing of pathogenic agents by the use of potent means of disinfection.
- **Sterilization.** A process, such as the use of heat, that removes all microbial contamination. The use of ultraviolet lighting to decontaminate an emergency vehicle is becoming a practice in areas around the country.[13]

You must ensure that the following steps are taken after each trip:

1. Strip used linens from the stretcher immediately after use, and place them in a plastic bag or in the designated receptacle in the ED.
2. In an appropriate receptacle, discard all disposable equipment used for care of the patient that meets your state's definition of medical waste. Most items will be considered general trash.
3. Wash all contaminated areas with soap and water. Scrub blood, vomitus, and other substances from the floors, walls, and ceilings with soap and water. For disinfection to be effective, cleaning must be done first.

Special Populations

The National Association of EMS State Officials (NASEMSO) is working with other agencies on the development of evidence-based standards for the safe transport of children by ambulance. Until such standards are in place, NASEMSO suggests that EMS officials work to establish interim steps, such as encouraging EMS transport agencies to implement cost effective means to lessen risk while transporting children and working with other state EMS officials to determine uniform approaches and policy language, including information relating to ambulance crash-related injuries.

► Postrun Activities: Restocking, Cleaning, and Disinfection

As soon as you are back at the station, you should do the following:

- Clean and disinfect the emergency vehicle and any equipment that was used per your service's exposure control plan, if you did not do so before leaving the hospital **Figure 46-4** .
- Restock any supplies you did not get at the hospital.

To maintain the emergency vehicle so that it is safe and available on a moment's notice, you should perform

4. Disinfect all nondisposable equipment used in the care of the patient. For example, the blood pressure cuff should be cleaned after each patient use as recommended by the manufacturer.

5. Clean the stretcher with an Environmental Protection Agency–registered germicidal/virucidal solution or with bleach and water at 1:100 dilution.

6. If any spillage or other contamination occurred in the emergency vehicle, clean it up with the same germicidal/virucidal or bleach/water solution.

7. Clean the outside of the emergency vehicle as needed.

8. Replace or repair broken or damaged equipment without delay.

9. Replace any other equipment or supplies that were used.

10. Refuel the vehicle if the fuel tank is below required reserves. The oil level should be checked each time the vehicle is refueled or as your service's standard operating procedure requires.

Restock any supplies you did not get at the hospital. Finally, have a written policy/procedure for cleaning each piece of equipment. Refer to the manufacturer's recommendations as a guide.

Defensive Emergency Vehicle Driving Techniques

Every year there are more than 6,000 emergency medical vehicles involved in crashes, some of them fatal. Between 1992 and 2011, the National Highway Traffic Safety Administration reported that there was an average of 4,500 motor vehicle crashes per year involving an emergency medical transport vehicle **Figure 46-5**.

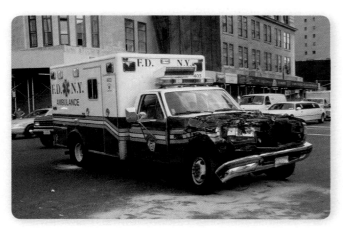

Figure 46-5 A wrecked emergency medical vehicle (type I style).
© Robert Brenner/PhotoEdit, Inc.

Approximately 65% of crashes per year (totaling 2,925 crashes) resulted in property damage only; 34% (1,530) of crashes per year resulted in an injury to individuals in all vehicles involved in the crash. There was an average of 29 crashes involving fatalities annually. More than half of those fatal crashes occurred while the emergency vehicle was in the emergency mode. Even more troubling is the fact that 42% of the fatal crashes involved the emergency medical vehicle in the *nonemergency* mode.[14]

Learning how to properly operate your vehicle is just as important as learning how to care for patients when you arrive on the scene. An emergency vehicle that is involved in a crash delays patient care, at a minimum, and, at the worst, may take the lives of the EMS providers, other motorists, or pedestrians. The following section introduces you to safe driving techniques; however, you cannot become a proficient and safe operator of an emergency vehicle without specialized training and practice. You are strongly encouraged to participate in an emergency driving program, such as the NAEMT EMS Vehicle Operator Safety (EVOS) course, designed for the EMS vehicle operator, and offered through your EMS organization, before attempting to operate an emergency vehicle. It is the responsibility of every emergency medical service to ensure that personnel are not only safe drivers *before* they begin employment, but are given emergency vehicle operation courses *after* they are hired, and training in the service's policies, procedures, and state laws appropriate to operating an emergency vehicle.

▶ Driver Characteristics

Not everyone who drives an automobile is qualified to drive an emergency vehicle. In some states, such as Florida, Iowa, and Minnesota, you must successfully complete an approved emergency vehicle operations course before you are allowed to drive the emergency vehicle on emergency calls. In any state, diligence and caution are important characteristics, as are a positive attitude about your ability and tolerance of other drivers.

One basic requirement is physical fitness. Many crashes occur as a result of physical impairment of the driver. You should not be driving if you are taking medications that may cause drowsiness or slow your reaction times. These medications include cold remedies, analgesics, or tranquilizers. And, of course, never drive or provide medical care after drinking alcohol. Fatigue can also play a prominent role in crashes, so it is imperative to get as much rest as possible during downtimes. Driving alone may also be a factor on long transports.

Another requirement is emotional fitness. Emotions should not be taken lightly. A person's personality can change once he or she is behind a steering wheel. Emotional maturity and stability are closely related to the ability to operate under stress. In addition to knowing exactly what to do, you must be able to do it under difficult conditions.

Having the proper attitude is important for the emergency vehicle operator. Never get behind the wheel of an emergency vehicle thinking that you can drive in any manner that pleases you. Great responsibility is placed on the driver of an emergency vehicle.

In addition to training and experience, the good judgment and knowledge that you need to drive an emergency vehicle require practice. Remember, even the best drivers can benefit from practice.

▶ Safe Driving Practices

Route Planning and Navigation

When you are dispatched to an emergency, you must decide which route will be used to arrive at the scene safely. Make sure you have detailed street and area maps in the driver's compartment of the emergency vehicle, along with directions to key locations, such as local hospitals. Even if you have access to and routinely rely on a GPS-enabled computer navigational system for directions, you should still have access to traditional maps in the event that the navigational system becomes disabled.

Become familiar with the roads and traffic patterns in your town or city so that you can plan alternative routes to common destinations. Avoid areas of heavy traffic if possible. Pay particular attention to ways around frequently opened drawbridges, congested traffic, or blocked railroad crossings. Often, switching to an alternative route will save more time than driving faster. School zones are especially dangerous at the beginning or ending of classes and should be avoided if possible. Be aware of construction zones in your area as well as railroad crossings. Also become familiar with special facilities and locations within your regional operating area, such as other medical facilities, airports, arenas and stadiums, and chemical or research facilities that might pose unusual problems (staging areas may be predefined for emergency operations).

Fatigue

Fatigue has many causes, such as stress, working the night shift, and lack of quality sleep in accordance with your body's circadian rhythms. As a result of these causes of fatigue, operating a large vehicle, such as an emergency vehicle, creates a large risk. You must be able to recognize when you are fatigued. Do not be ashamed to admit it to yourself, your partner, or your supervisor. If you are feeling fatigued, you should be placed out of service for the remainder of the shift or until the fatigue has passed and you feel capable of operating the vehicle safely.

Distractions

With the availability of digital and electronic devices, there are many things that may distract the driver of an emergency vehicle from focusing on his or her driving. En route to a call, it should not be the driver's responsibility to talk on the radio or operate the emergency vehicle's audible devices. Personnel riding on the passenger side of the vehicle (officer's seat) are not just there to read the road map and guide the driver to the destination.

They serve as another set of eyes and ears to help arrive at a location safely.

GPS is a vital piece of equipment found on most vehicles today, but it can be a hazard if the driver is focused on its directions and not on the roadway. Do not totally rely on a device to lead you to every call, but use it as a supplement to your own territory knowledge base. Study your areas well before getting behind the wheel of an emergency vehicle. Some emergency vehicles come equipped with mobile data terminals (MDT). A driver should *never* attempt to type on the computer while driving the emergency vehicle.

Driving is also not the time to be texting others or operating personal data devices. Many vehicle manufacturers are placing stereos or radios in the emergency vehicle's cab. Such features are nice when you are not committed to an emergency medical call, but you should not listen to music when you are also listening to the service radio.

Eating or drinking in the emergency vehicle may be convenient after a long transfer when personnel are being pressured to get back into service, but it is important for you to take the time to stop and recharge before jumping back into the emergency mode again. Eating in the ambulance may also be against OSHA guidelines. Driving alone while your partner is caring for a patient in the rear compartment is also a challenge, especially if it is in the middle of the night.

Use of Safety Restraints

Standard operating procedures should mandate that everyone in the emergency vehicle, not just the patient, use seat belts. Unless crucial for patient care, all passengers including EMS personnel in the patient compartment should use the vehicle's restraint devices. For example, it is not acceptable or safe to allow parents to hold children in their laps even if both are on the emergency vehicle stretcher. Children should not be transported on the stretcher unless properly restrained. It is not advisable to use adult seat belts for children. Most states now have policies in place that require that all pediatric patients be secured with age-appropriate restraints. Of course, when you are driving the emergency vehicle, you should *always* use a seat belt.

Speed

Do not allow the type of call to affect how you respond to it. When you hear that the call involves children or a severe trauma potential, you may have the urge to drive with less caution, feeling that speed is more important than is safety. You may have the urge to speed up when you receive a call that involves another public safety worker. As a professional, you must not let the nature of the call affect your judgment—always drive with caution.

Siren Risk-Benefit Analysis

Despite improvements in the sophistication of 9-1-1 answering systems and in the accuracy of telephone triage protocols, most emergency medical vehicles use their lights and siren most of the time when responding to emergency calls. However, once a patient is loaded, a conscious decision should be made whether to use the emergency vehicle warning devices en route to the patient destination or drive with the normal flow of traffic. Lights and siren should *never* be used to transport a nonemergency patient. You should drive in an emergency mode only when the patient's condition warrants it. The paramedic riding in the rear compartment of the emergency vehicle with the patient should be the person to make the decision to drive in an emergency mode to the patient destination. Great care must be taken in making that decision, and it should be guided by the stability of the patient and not by the surrounding traffic or closeness to the end of your shift.

Driver Anticipation

The one thing that is predictable about driving an emergency vehicle in the emergency mode is that all other drivers are unpredictable. Do not expect them to pull to the right to allow your vehicle to pass on the left the way public safety vehicles are instructed to do. Expect other vehicles to pull to the left *or* right. Some drivers do not realize an emergency vehicle is behind them because of loud music or inattentive behavior. Drivers may stop suddenly in front of you out of panic. You should always maintain a safe travel distance behind other vehicles. If your emergency vehicle is following too close behind, drivers may not know which lane is safe to move into because their vision is blocked by your unit. Also watch out for the aggressive actions of other drivers. Not everyone respects the passage of an emergency vehicle; some may refuse to grant the right-of-way. Do not respond aggressively in return, but wait until it is safe to pass before doing so.

A wise emergency vehicle driver will not accelerate through all intersections, even if he or she has the right-of-way, but will slow down or even stop in high-traffic areas. It is important to make sure all other drivers are aware of your presence. Make eye contact, especially with the lead vehicles, and be ready to apply your brake until it appears that everyone is clear on your intentions. The emergency vehicle driver should use the vehicle's turn signals the same way other drivers are expected to do. Never force a vehicle into oncoming traffic in an effort to get around; doing so creates a dangerous situation.

The Cushion of Safety

To operate an emergency vehicle safely, you must maintain a safe following distance from the vehicles in front of you and try to avoid being tailgated from behind. You must leave enough space between your vehicle and the one in front when stopped at an intersection so that the emergency vehicle can be safely manipulated around other vehicles when you are responding.

You must also ensure that the **blind spots** in your vehicle's mirrors do not prevent you from seeing vehicles or pedestrians on either side of the emergency vehicle. Keeping a safe distance between your vehicle and the one in front of you, checking for tailgaters behind your emergency vehicle, and keeping aware of vehicles potentially hiding in your mirror's blind spots are considered maintaining a **cushion of safety**. To ensure that you have enough reaction time and stopping distance from the vehicle in front of you, follow at a safe distance, allowing the motorist enough time to move over to the right. If the motorist does not move, you will need to allow for enough time to evade the vehicle. This entails driving about 4 or 5 seconds behind a vehicle traveling at an average speed in good weather conditions.

When you are operating in emergency mode, tailgaters may follow your vehicle dangerously close in congested areas simply to use your emergency vehicle to get through traffic. If the emergency vehicle stops suddenly to avoid a crash, the tailgating vehicle could crash into the rear of the emergency vehicle, possibly causing you to lose control and strike other vehicles or pedestrians. Always scan your rearview camera and side view mirrors for cars that are following too closely.

If you are being tailgated, never speed up to create more distance. The tailgater may, in turn, increase his or her speed to continue to follow you through traffic. Slamming on your brakes to scare the other driver usually does not work either and may cause a crash. You can have your dispatcher contact the local police to let them know that someone is driving recklessly behind you.

Never, under any circumstance, get out of the emergency vehicle to confront a driver. This will only delay your response to or transport of the patient and can lead to a dangerous situation.

Finally, there are three blind spots around the emergency vehicle that you cannot see with the mirrors:

- The mirror itself creates a blind spot, obstructing the view ahead and preventing the driver from seeing objects such as a pedestrian or vehicle. To eliminate this blind spot, you should lean forward in your seat so that the mirror does not obstruct the view, especially when making turns at intersections.
- The rear of the vehicle cannot be seen fully through the mirror and is therefore a blind spot. Because of the configuration of today's emergency vehicle and the relative height of the vehicle, the rearview mirror generally gives the driver a view of the patient compartment, not the vehicle behind the emergency vehicle. Because of this blind spot, many crashes occur when the emergency vehicle is backing up. Follow your service's standard operating procedure on the use of spotters when backing the vehicle.
- The side of the vehicle often cannot be seen through the driver and passenger mirrors at a certain angle. Entire cars may not be seen in the

mirror, even though they are right next to the emergency vehicle. To eliminate this problem, emergency medical vehicular standards require the use of a convex mirror to assist you in visualizing this blind spot. However, even with the use of your mirrors, you need to lean forward or backward in the seat to help eliminate the blind spot. This is an especially important technique to use when changing lanes or making turns. Some of the newer vehicles have blind spot sensors that signal if a vehicle is in your blind spot. Vehicle warning devices are helpful, but they do not take the place of operator awareness and a spotter when available.

You should always scan your mirrors frequently for any new hazards. Remember that your mirrors can give you a false sense of security and may hide people or vehicles.

Vehicle Size and Distance Judgment

Vehicle length and width are critical factors when you are maneuvering, driving, and parking an emergency vehicle. They are especially important with types I and III vehicles, which are wider than they look from behind the steering wheel. To brake and pass effectively, you must know the width and length of your vehicle. Crashes often occur when the vehicle is backing up. Vehicle size and weight will greatly influence braking and stopping distances. Good peripheral vision and depth perception will help you to judge distances, but they are no substitute for intensive training, experience, and frequent evaluation of the vehicle.

Backing Up the Emergency Vehicle

Most EMS systems have established a policy about emergency vehicle backup. Backing up a vehicle is the most common source of vehicle damage and may result in costly repairs. If possible, avoid situations in which the emergency vehicle will have to be backed up. If it must be done, follow these rules:

- Use a **spotter** to guide you **Figure 46-6**.
- Agree with the spotter *before* you place the vehicle in reverse. You may be attempting to back to the left while your spotter is trying to direct you to the right.
- Keep your spotter in view at all times. If you lose sight of the spotter, stop until he or she is back in your line of sight.
- Agree on hand signals with your spotter before moving. For example, some people have different ideas of which gesture means "Stop."
- Keep your window cracked or rolled down when in motion. This may allow you to hear people warning you of unseen dangers.

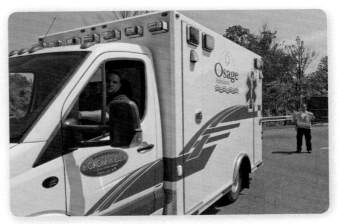

Figure 46-6 Always use a spotter when backing up the emergency vehicle.
© Jones & Bartlett Learning. Photographed by Glen E. Ellman.

- Do a walk-around before getting behind the wheel, and look up as well as down. Objects may not be visible once you start backing up.
- Use audible warning devices whenever the emergency vehicle is in motion.
- Some vehicles have a backup camera, which is helpful, but do not rely totally on the camera.

Parking at an Emergency Scene

When you are parking the emergency vehicle, pick a position that will allow for efficient traffic control and flow around a crash scene. Do not park alongside the scene because you may block the movement of other emergency vehicles. Instead, park about 100 feet (30 m) past the scene on the same side of the road. It is best to park uphill and/or upwind of the scene if smoke or hazardous materials are present. If you must park on the back side of a hill or curve, leave your warning lights or devices on. Do the same when you are parking at night. Always park so as to provide a cushion of space between your vehicle and operations at the scene. This can help prevent personnel from being struck if someone crashes into your vehicle on the scene. Maintain concern for others who are not involved in the incident. For example, if you are parking in an apartment complex, try not to block parked vehicles because the owners of those vehicles may need to leave while you are inside.

Stay away from any fires, explosive hazards, downed wires, or structures that might collapse. Be sure to set the parking brake. If your vehicle is blocking part of the roadway, leave on the emergency warning lights. If your vehicle has them, leave on only the flashing yellow lights. Other drivers tend to drive toward emergency vehicles with flashing red or red and white lights. Within these safety guidelines, you should try to park your emergency vehicle as close to the scene as possible to facilitate emergency medical care. If necessary, you can temporarily block traffic to unload equipment and to load patients quickly and safely. If you must do this, try to do it quickly so that traffic is not blocked any longer than is absolutely necessary. Also, park in a location that will not hamper your departure from the scene.

When you are parking off the side of the road, you must be aware of the terrain. In dry weather, the heat from underneath the vehicle could start a grass fire. In wet weather, the weight of the emergency vehicle makes it susceptible to sinking into mud and getting stuck.

Parking on a roadway at night is especially dangerous **Figure 46-7** . Some drivers may have their attention distracted by the scene, and they may drift toward and collide with a parked emergency vehicle. Sometimes it may be safer to use your emergency flashers instead of all the overhead flashers. Likewise, to avoid blinding oncoming traffic, it may be better to turn off the emergency vehicle's headlights when parked, especially if you are on a two-lane road.

Always wear visible protective clothing when you get out of the vehicle on roadways. Reflective vests are lightweight and have the added benefit of increasing visibility during the day as well as at night. Heavy protective clothing should also be considered when you are responding to crashes where extrication is being performed.

▶ Emergency Vehicle Control

As the driver of an emergency vehicle, you have only two ways to control the vehicle: by changing its direction and

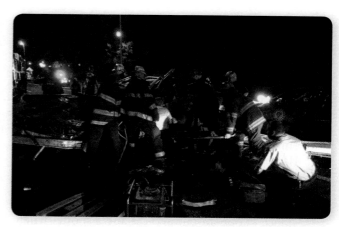

Figure 46-7 Parking on a roadway at night can be extremely hazardous.
© Mark C. Ide.

by changing its speed. Either maneuver requires a continuous rolling contact between the surface of the tires and the surface of the road.

The tire's grip on the road may vary widely on different parts of the same road, depending on the condition of the road's surface, the age of the road, and the weather. Unpaved roadways may present a challenge, especially in inclement weather. Tire grip also varies according to the tire's tread design and wear. As a driver, you must constantly evaluate the road surface: at a given speed,

---

YOU ▸ are the Paramedic   PART 3

Your patient confirms that she was the driver of this vehicle. She is able to recall all events preceding the crash. Her primary survey and secondary assessment are unremarkable except for her right knee, which struck the base of the dash. You assess the knee and find it to be tender on palpation. There are good pulses in the lower leg and foot. The patient has limited range of motion. You allow the patient to self-extricate from the vehicle per local protocol and apply a splint to the knee for comfort. You load the patient in your emergency vehicle for transport.

Recording Time: 5 Minutes	
Respirations	14 breaths/min
Pulse	80 beats/min
Skin	Warm, dry, pink
Blood pressure	126/82 mm Hg
Oxygen saturation (Spo$_2$)	99% on room air
Pupils	PERRLA

5. Should lights and the siren be used while you are transporting this patient? Why or why not?

6. What other actions should be taken before you depart the scene?

how much frictional force can the tires apply before the emergency vehicle becomes unstable? Grip is especially important in cornering, when additional centrifugal force is acting on the vehicle.

Road Positioning and Cornering

Road position refers to the position of the vehicle on the roadway relative to the inside or outside edge of the paved surface. To corner efficiently, you must know the vehicle's present position and its projected path. The aim is to take the corner at the speed that will put you in the proper road position as you exit the curve **Figure 46-8**. The apex of the turn through a curve is the point at which the vehicle is closest to the inside edge of the curve. If you reach the apex early in the curve, the vehicle will be forced toward the outside of the roadway as it exits the curve. If you reach the apex late in the curve, the vehicle will tend to stay on the inside of the roadway; this helps you to keep the vehicle in the proper lane and allows room for error if you enter the turn too fast.

▶ Braking

Getting a feel for the proper brake pressure comes with experience and practice. Each vehicle has a different braking action. For example, the brakes on types I and III vehicles have a heavier feel than the brakes on a type II vehicle. Certain heavy vehicles use air brakes that have yet another feel. You should get to know each vehicle you drive, and be sure you understand its braking characteristics and the best downshifting techniques.

▶ Controlled Braking

Controlled braking is the use of the brakes to control the vehicle. Brakes not only control the movement of

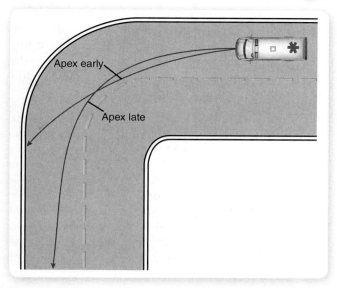

Figure 46-8 To keep the emergency vehicle in the proper lane on a curve, you must know the vehicle's present position and projected path and take the corner at the correct speed.

© Jones & Bartlett Learning.

the vehicle, causing it to slow or stop, but also help to control its direction. Braking while the vehicle is traveling in a straight line is the safest, most efficient method. Braking in a turn causes a loss of efficiency. You might not notice this at a low speed, but it becomes more apparent at higher speeds. Applying the brakes while cornering is not an effective way to slow the vehicle and may actually cause a skid or spin.

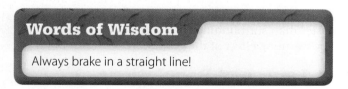

Words of Wisdom

Always brake in a straight line!

Weather and Road Conditions

Because of their higher center of gravity, most emergency vehicles have the tendency to tip over if curves or turns are taken at too great of a speed. On rainy days, there is an even greater danger for this to occur. Water can get trapped between the tires of vehicles with dual tires in the rear and cause the emergency vehicle to start hydroplaning. You should use extreme caution and slow down in inclement weather to take the weight distributions of the vehicle into consideration. Remember that you will need more room to come to a complete stop when compared with driving a regular passenger vehicle. Also, remember that your line of sight is limited to what you can see in the side mirrors; make it a habit to use them frequently when you are driving both the emergency vehicle and your own personal vehicle.

Hydroplaning. On a wet road, at speeds of greater than 30 mph, the tire may be lifted off the road as water "piles up" under it, causing the vehicle to feel as if it is floating. This situation is known as **hydroplaning**. At higher speeds on wet roadways, the front wheels may actually be riding on a sheet of water, robbing the driver of control of the vehicle. If hydroplaning occurs, you should gradually slow down without jamming on the brakes.

Water on the Roadway. Wet brakes will increase the stopping time of the vehicle and pull it to one side or the other. If at all possible, avoid driving through large pools of standing water; often, you cannot tell how deep the water is. If you must drive through standing water, make sure to slow down and turn on the windshield wipers. After driving out of the pool, lightly tap the brakes several times until they are dry. If the vehicle is equipped with antilock brakes, apply a steady, light pressure to dry the brakes. Finally, driving through moving water should be avoided at all times.

Decreased Visibility. In areas where there is fog, smog, snow, or heavy rain, common sense tells you to slow down. At night, use only low headlight beams for maximum visibility without reflection. You should always use headlights during the day to increase your visibility to other drivers. Also, watch carefully for stopped or slow-moving vehicles.

Ice and Slippery Surfaces. A light mist on an oily, dusty road can be just as slippery as a patch of ice. Good all-weather tires and an appropriate speed will significantly reduce traction problems. If you are in an area that often has snowy or icy conditions, consider using studded snow tires, if they are permitted by law. You should be especially careful on bridges and overpasses when temperatures are close to freezing. These road surfaces will freeze much faster than surrounding road surfaces because they lack the warming effect of the ground underneath.

▶ Laws and Regulations

Regulations regarding vehicle operations vary from state to state and from city to city, but some things are the same everywhere. Drivers of emergency vehicles have certain limited privileges in every state; however, these privileges do not lessen their liability in a crash. In fact, in most cases, the driver is presumed to be liable if a crash occurs while the emergency vehicle is operating with warning lights and siren. Motor vehicle crashes are the single largest source of lawsuits against EMS personnel and agencies.

When you are on an emergency call, emergency vehicles typically are exempt from some of the usual vehicle rules. If you are on an emergency call and are using your warning lights and siren, you may be allowed to do the following:

- Park or stand in an otherwise illegal location
- Proceed through a red traffic light or stop sign *after* stopping
- Drive faster than the posted speed limit (note that some states have maximum speeds)
- Drive against the flow of traffic on a one-way street or make a turn that is normally not allowed
- Travel left of center to make an otherwise illegal pass (note that some states have maximum speeds for this maneuver)

Even if you are given specific exemptions to some traffic laws in an emergency, this privilege must be used sparingly. Emergency vehicles are not allowed to pass a stopped school bus with the red light flashing until the school bus operator makes sure the children are safe and turns off the red blinkers.

Right-of-Way Privileges

A right-of-way privilege is just that: a privilege. State motor vehicle statutes or codes often grant an emergency vehicle the right to disregard the rules of the road when responding to an emergency. However, in doing so, the operator of an emergency vehicle must not endanger people or property under any circumstances. Remember that use of lights and siren does not give you the right-of-way; it only requests the right-of-way.

Right-of-way privileges for emergency vehicles vary from state to state. Some states allow you to proceed through a red light or stop sign after you stop and make sure it is safe to proceed. Other states allow you to proceed through a controlled intersection "with **due regard**," using flashing lights and the siren. Due regard means you may proceed only if you consider the safety of all people who are using the roadway. If a crash occurs, your service might be sued even if you were operating the vehicle with due regard. If you are found to be at fault, you may personally have to pay punitive damages or face both civil and criminal sanctions.

Get to know your local right-of-way privileges. Exercise them only when it is absolutely necessary for the patient's well-being. The use of lights and audible warning devices is a matter of local protocol or state law.

Use of Warning Lights and Siren

Three basic principles govern the use of warning lights and siren on an emergency vehicle:

1. The unit must be on a true emergency call to the best of your knowledge.
2. Both audible and visual warning devices must be used simultaneously when taking exemptions to traffic laws.
3. The unit must be operated with due regard for the safety of all others, on and off the roadway.

The siren is probably the most overused piece of equipment on an emergency vehicle. In general, the siren does not help you as you drive; nor does it really help other motorists. Motorists who are driving at the speed limit with the windows up, the radio on, and the air conditioner or heater set on high may not hear the siren until the emergency vehicle is very close. If the radio is particularly loud, they may not hear the siren at all.

If you do have to use the siren, be sure to warn the patient before you turn it on. Be especially mindful not to increase the speed of the emergency vehicle just because the siren is in use. Always travel at a speed that will allow you to stop safely at all times, especially so that you are prepared for drivers who do not give you the right-of-way. Never assume that warning lights and siren will allow you to drive through a congested area without stopping or slowing down. Slow down to ensure that all drivers are stopping as you approach an intersection, and then proceed with due caution.

Use of Escorts

It is typically *not* a good idea to follow another emergency vehicle, such as a police car, through traffic as an escort. Many drivers will see only the first set of lights and sirens and assume that the way is clear once that vehicle has passed. If you are following another emergency vehicle, leave enough space between the vehicles so that other drivers (and you) have enough time to react and safely stop should someone pull in front of you unexpectedly. To alert motorists that a second unit is approaching, use a siren tone that is different from that of the first vehicle.

Another potential danger occurs when family members follow closely behind you on the way to the hospital. Both the emergency vehicle and other drivers may have difficulty seeing the vehicles that are following. If you need to stop suddenly, there may be no time to react and the vehicle could crash into the emergency vehicle. Instruct family members before you leave the scene that they cannot drive closely behind you, and make sure they are aware of how to get to the hospital at a slower speed.

Sometimes family members will not heed your warning about following the emergency vehicle to the hospital. If the patient's family members or another motorist begins to follow you when you are operating your emergency vehicle using lights and siren, consider turning off your lights and siren and slowing down to normal speed, in an effort to prevent a collision.

Intersection Hazards

Intersection crashes are the most common (approximately 72%) and usually the most serious type of crash in which emergency vehicles are involved.[15] Always be alert and careful when you are approaching an intersection. If you are on an urgent call and cannot wait for traffic lights to change, you should still come to a momentary stop at the light; look around for other motorists and pedestrians before proceeding into the intersection.

Motorists who "time the traffic lights" present a serious hazard. You may arrive at an intersection while the light is green. At the same time, a motorist who is timing the lights on the cross street arrives at the intersection. The motorist has a red light but knows that it is about to turn green and is expecting to go through. The stage is now set for a serious crash.

Unpaved Roadways and Rural Settings

When you are required to drive the emergency vehicle on an unpaved roadway, special care must be taken. Unpaved roads may be encountered when the patient's residence is far off the road and may be inaccessible by the emergency vehicle. When you are responding on this type of roadway, you must operate the vehicle at a lower speed and maintain a firm grip on the steering wheel in an effort to maintain complete control of the emergency vehicle at all times. Unpaved roadways often have uneven surfaces and large potholes and may be impassable in rain. Do not drive a heavy emergency vehicle onto unpaved or grassy areas when the ground has been saturated with rain unless you are sure the unit will not get bogged down and stuck.

Rural EMS systems usually have agreements with other agencies, such as the Forestry Service, to help them reach the remote locations. Watch out for animals entering the roadway, especially in the evenings when visibility is decreased. Large deer, moose, and even livestock can migrate onto the roadways, requiring the driver to be extra alert to avoid running into animals.

School Buses

An emergency vehicle is *never* allowed to pass a school bus that has stopped to load or unload children and is displaying its flashing red lights or extended "stop arm." If you approach a school bus that has its lights flashing, you should stop before reaching the bus and wait for the driver to make sure the children are safe, close the bus door, and turn off the warning lights. Only then may you carefully proceed past the stopped school bus.

School Zones

When you respond through a school zone with your emergency lights activated, it is important to remember that lights and siren tend to attract children to the roadway and create a potential hazard. In many states, it is unlawful for an emergency vehicle to exceed the speed limit in school zones regardless of the condition of the patient.

Funeral Processions

There is also no exemption in most states when you are approaching a funeral procession while in the emergency mode. Some escorts will pull the procession over, but others may not. Out of respect, most emergency drivers will maintain the activation of the emergency lights, but turn off the audible devices and slowly pass the procession on the left, using due regard for other approaching drivers.

■ Air Medical Transport

Air medical transport—especially the use of helicopters—has done much to speed up the transfer of patients from the trauma scene to definitive care. This mode of transport presents certain risks, however, and it is appropriate only in certain circumstances. Several factors must be considered before calling for an **aircraft transport**: Does the patient's condition warrant the risk of using air medical transport? Will use of the aircraft truly save the patient time in getting to definitive care once all other factors are considered?

▶ Rotor-Wing Versus Fixed-Wing Aircraft

Rotor-wing aircraft (helicopters) have become a standard of care for the transport of critically injured patients from the scene to a regional trauma center Figure 46-9 . Fixed-winged aircraft are used mainly for the transport of patients over long distances. EMS personnel are frequently called to transport these patients from the airfield to definitive care facilities Figure 46-10 .

▶ Advantages of Using Aircraft Transport

Aircraft transport has an advantage over ground transport in that it reduces transport time if the transport distance is extreme and may help the patient receive definitive treatment within the Golden Hour, also called the Golden Period. The decision to use rotor-wing transport (helicopter) should be made as early in the call as possible. If, after patient assessment, it is determined that the helicopter

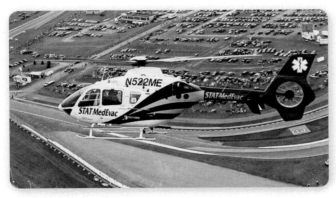

Figure 46-9 Rotor-wing air aircraft.
Courtesy of Brian Denlinger and STAT MedEvac.

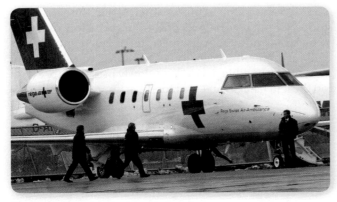

Figure 46-10 Fixed-winged aircraft.
© Hermann J. Knippertz/AP Photo.

Patient Safety

The air transport crew has an even more arduous task than the ground transport crew to ensure safety. Given the noisy and limited space and the low-light operating environment in most rotor-wing aircraft, identifying adverse events is even more difficult. The air transport crew needs to minimize risk by optimizing the patient's condition prior to flight and ensuring adequate monitoring equipment is in place. Additionally, using excellent crew resource management skills and making appropriate go/no-go decisions is crucial to the safety of the patient and the crew.

is not needed, it can always be returned to service. Some districts have "automatic send helicopter" procedures written into their protocols.

You should weigh all the factors that involve time when you are deciding whether the helicopter is appropriate. The machine must be started, personnel and gear loaded, and sometimes great distances covered. Once the helicopter is at the scene, time must be allotted to land the aircraft and transfer the patient to the air crew. Packaging the patient for air transport and loading the patient into the helicopter also require time. Especially in metropolitan areas, it can be difficult to justify use of the helicopter. Severe traffic congestion or prolonged extrication times may sometimes make the use of a helicopter appropriate in urban areas.

Use of aircraft transport may be warranted if the patient has a spinal injury and the terrain over which the patient must be carried is rough. Even though the patient is stabilized, ground transport in a vehicle that is bouncing on the road could further injure the patient. The paramedic on scene is the best judge of the patient's transport needs. Table 46-3 summarizes the advantages of using emergency aircraft for patient transport.

▶ Disadvantages of Using Aircraft Transport

Patients in cardiac arrest or those with peri-arrest conditions, should be transported by ground. Treating a patient in cardiac arrest in the helicopter is difficult due to space limitations.

Table 46-3	**Advantages of Using Helicopter Transport**

- Reduced transport time
- Ability to access patients in remote areas
- Availability of medical crew with advanced skills and equipment

© Jones & Bartlett Learning.

Table 46-4 — Disadvantages of Using Helicopter Transport

- Weather- or environment-related challenges
- Altitude limitations
- Airspeed limitations
- Aircraft cabin size limitations
- Terrain that poses landing challenges
- Cost
- Patient's condition that is not suited to helicopter transport
- Restrictions on the number of responders
- Potential for crash

© Jones & Bartlett Learning.

In addition, to ensure safety, helicopters do not fly when there is poor visibility. The terrain may also make it difficult to land the helicopter safely. Uneven ground and loose objects such as rocks or debris should be taken into account before attempting to land the aircraft. Table 46-4 lists disadvantages of using the aircraft for patient transport.

▶ Helicopter Medical Evacuation Operations

A medical or trauma air evacuation is commonly known as a **medevac** and is generally performed exclusively by helicopters. Most rural and suburban EMS jurisdictions and many urban systems have the capability to perform helicopter medevacs or have a mutual aid agreement with another agency such as a police or hospital-based medevac service to provide such services. You should become familiar with the medevac capabilities, protocols, and procedures of your particular EMS agency because they vary from service to service.

Calling for a Medevac

Every agency has specific criteria for the type of patient who may receive medical evacuation and how and when to call for a medevac. The following basic guidelines will help you to understand the process better:

- **Why call for a medevac?** Medevac may be needed if the transport time to the hospital by a ground emergency vehicle is too long considering the patient's condition. It may also be needed when road, traffic, or environmental conditions limit or completely prohibit the use of a ground transport. Medevac may offer advanced care that you are unable to provide, such as administering pain medications or other specialized medications and inserting advanced airways. When there are multiple patients, it may be necessary to transport the most critical patients to another facility so that the local EDs are not overwhelmed with patients.

YOU are the Paramedic   PART 4

You are transporting your patient to the hospital and the rain has increased to a downpour. Your driver advises that she is slowing down due to weather conditions. You reassess your patient and find her to be resting comfortably with no change in condition.

Recording Time: 10 Minutes	
Respirations	14 breaths/min
Pulse	80 beats/min
Skin	Warm, pink, dry
Blood pressure	124/80 mm Hg
Oxygen saturation (Spo$_2$)	99% on room air
Pupils	PERRLA

7. What should the emergency vehicle operator do if the patient's family is following the emergency vehicle?
8. If the driver of your emergency vehicle approaches a school bus that has activated its warning lights and "stop" sign, what will be the proper way to respond?

- **Who receives a medevac?** Medical evacuations should be used for patients with time-dependent injuries or illnesses. They are widely used for patients suspected of having a stroke, heart attack, or serious spinal cord injury. Serious conditions that may require the use of helicopter medevacs may be found in remote areas and involve scuba diving accidents, submersions, or skiing and wilderness incidents. Other patients who may warrant the use of medical evacuation are trauma patients and candidates for limb replantation (for amputations), a burn center, a hyperbaric chamber, or a venomous bite center. Because specific criteria differ between services, you must be familiar with your local jurisdiction's criteria used to call for this lifesaving service.
- **Whom do you call?** Generally, your dispatcher must be notified first. The request for medevac should include the chief complaint and the patient's weight, as many medevac helicopters have weight limits. (You should be aware the limitations of your local medevac service.) In some regions, after the medevac has been initiated, the ground EMS crew may be able to access the flight crew on a specially designated radio frequency for one-on-one communications. If available, it is important to keep this frequency clear of chatter and long, drawn-out communications. You may be asked to give a brief presentation or update on the patient's condition. In this case, you should gather your thoughts and speak clearly and concisely, avoiding information that is not immediately pertinent. Another important topic of communication between the ground and flight EMS crews will be where to land the helicopter.

Medevac Issues

While you are making the decision to request medevac, several important factors need to be taken into consideration. These factors are weather, the environment/terrain, altitude, airspeed limitations, cabin size, and cost. Typically, helicopters are unable to operate in severe weather such as thunderstorms, blizzards, and heavy rain. The environment may pose a risk as well. In mountainous or desert terrain, there may be too many hazards in the immediate vicinity to safely land the helicopter in the desired location.

Depending on availability and circumstances, a military helicopter might be available to transport critically ill or injured victims. It may be a requirement that an attempt has been made to contact a local helicopter transport service before calling for aid from the military.

The airships used by the military may be too large to land on some of the civilian hospitals' landing zones. Your service should have protocols in place for requesting military assistance.

As the elevation increases, the air thins, making it more difficult for pilots and patients to breathe. Because of this danger, helicopters have a maximum limit on flight elevations.[16] Most helicopter services are limited to flying at 10,000 feet (3,050 m) above sea level. This limit could create a problem if your patient is located at 13,500 feet (4,100 m) above sea level. It is important to remember that medevac helicopters are not jets, and it takes time for them to arrive on the scene because of limitations in airspeed. Typically, medevac helicopters fly between 120 and 150 mph.

Because of the helicopter cabin's confined space, helicopters are limited in the number of patients that can be safely transported and by the size of the patient whom they can safely transport. Although a helicopter may be able to safely lift off with a 500-pound (227-kg) patient, because of his or her size and girth, it may be impossible to safely fit and secure the patient into the cabin area.

▶ Establishing a Landing Zone

Although a helicopter can fly straight up and down, such movement is the most dangerous mode of operation. The safest and most effective way to land and take off is similar to that used by fixed-wing aircraft. Landing at a slight angle allows for safer operations. Takeoff combines a gradual lift and forward motion to travel up and out on a slight angle.

An important part of conducting a medevac is choosing the best location. Establishing a **landing zone** is the responsibility of the ground EMS crew. It involves more than simply looking for a clear space. You must be prepared to take action to make certain that the flight crew is able to land and take off safely. Actions to take and considerations to make when you are selecting and establishing a landing zone include the following:

- The area should be a hard or cropped grassy level surface that measures 100 feet × 100 feet (recommended; 30 m × 30 m) and no less than 60 feet × 60 feet (18 m × 18 m).[17] If the site is not level, the flight crew must be notified of the steepness and direction of the slope.
- The area must be cleared of any loose debris that could become airborne and strike the helicopter or the patient and crew. Such hazards include branches, trash bins, flares, accident tape, and medical equipment and supplies.
- You must survey the immediate area for any overhead or tall hazards such as power lines or telephone cables, antennas, and tall or

leaning trees. The presence of these must be relayed immediately to the flight crew because an alternative landing site may be required. The flight crew may request that the hazard be marked or illuminated by weighted cones or by positioning an emergency vehicle with its lights turned on next to or under the potential hazard.

- To mark the landing site, use weighted cones or position emergency vehicles at the corners of the landing zone with headlights facing inward to form an X. This procedure is essential during night landings as well. Never use accident tape or people to mark the site. The use of flares is also not recommended; not only can they become airborne, but they also have the potential to start a fire or cause an explosion.
- Make sure all nonessential persons and vehicles are moved to a safe distance outside of the landing zone.
- If the wind is strong, radio the direction of the wind to the flight crew. They may request that you improvise some form of wind directional device to aid their approach. A bed sheet tightly secured to a tree or pole may be used to help the crew determine wind direction and strength. Never use tape.
- Many aircraft are now being equipped with night vision goggles for the crew and large landing lights mounted on the underside of the aircraft. Use of such equipment might require turning off any flashing emergency lights on any vehicles at the landing zone once the pilot is aware of the landing area's exact location.

▶ Landing Zone Safety and Patient Transfer

You should be familiar with the capabilities, protocols, and methods for accessing helicopters in your area. Helicopter services provide training for EMS personnel in ground operations and safety. Interactions with flight personnel should be comprehensive. Patients should be packaged prior to arrival of the aircraft and an extensive report given to the flight crew for transfer care. The following discussion is an introduction to safe operations; it is not intended to be substituted for the more extensive courses available locally.

Helicopter safety is nothing more than good common sense, along with a constant awareness of the need for personal safety. The types of helicopters that are used for medical operations vary, but the dangers are the same. If you are familiar with the way helicopters work and follow the pilot's instructions, you will minimize these dangers. You should be sure to do nothing near the helicopter and go only where the pilot or crew directs you.

Keep the pilot in view at all times, and approach and depart the aircraft from the front, then move to the side as directed by the air crew.

The most important rule is to keep a safe distance from the aircraft whenever it is on the ground and "hot," which means the tail rotor is spinning. Most of the time, the rotor blades will remain running because the flight crew does not generally expect to remain on the ground for a long time. This means that every EMS provider should stay outside the landing zone perimeter unless directed by the pilot or a member of the flight crew that he or she is to approach the aircraft. Usually, the flight crew will come to the crew carrying their own equipment and not require any assistance inside the landing zone. If you are asked to enter the landing zone, stay away from the tail rotor; the tips of its blades move so rapidly that they appear invisible. Never approach the helicopter from the rear, even if it is not running. If you must move from one side of the helicopter to another, go around the front. Never duck under the body, the tail boom, or the rear section of the helicopter; the pilot cannot see you in these areas. The proper approach area is between the nine-o'clock and the three-o'clock positions as the pilot faces forward **Figure 46-11**.

Another area of concern is the height of the main rotor blade. On many aircrafts, it is flexible and may dip as low as 4 feet (1.2 m) off the ground **Figure 46-12**. When you approach the aircraft, walk in a crouched position. Wind gusts can alter the blade height without warning, so be sure to protect equipment as you carry it near the blades. Air turbulence created by the rotor blades can blow off hats and loose equipment. These, in turn, can become a danger to the aircraft and personnel in the area. Never carry anything above your head, and make sure someone is always in charge of each piece of equipment when around the aircraft. Stretchers can easily roll into the tail rotors if no one is physically holding onto the cot after the patient is loaded into the helicopter.[18]

When you are accompanying a flight crew member, you must follow directions exactly. Never try to open any aircraft door or move equipment unless a crew member tells you to. When you are told to approach the aircraft, use extreme caution and pay constant attention to hazards.

Keep the following guidelines in mind when you are operating at a landing zone:

- Pay close attention to direction by the flight crew when you are approaching the aircraft.
- Become familiar with helicopter hand signals used within your jurisdiction **Figure 46-13**.
- Do not approach the helicopter unless instructed and accompanied by flight crew.
- Make certain that all patient care equipment is properly secured to the stretcher and that the patient is fastened as well. Equipment includes oxygen tanks, cervical collars, and head immobilizers. Remove sheets from the stretcher

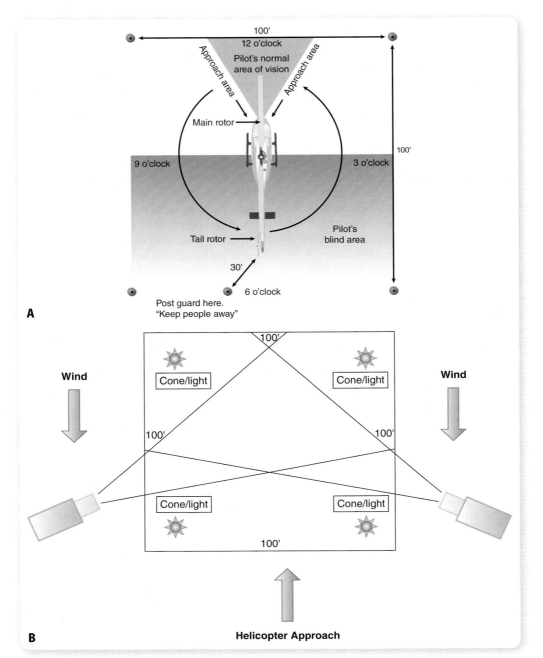

Figure 46-11 A. Approach a helicopter between the nine-o'clock and the three-o'clock positions as the pilot faces forward. **B.** Wind direction and helicopter approach are shown here. Nighttime operations can use emergency vehicle headlights to light the area as shown.
© Jones & Bartlett Learning.

prior to the patient being loaded so that the linen is not drawn up into the rotor blades once the patient has been transferred into the aircraft. Any loose articles or belongings such as hats, coats, or bags that belong to the patient or crew should not be brought into the landing zone and will likely need to be transported to the hospital by ground.

■ Be mindful that some helicopters may load patients from the side, whereas others have rear-loading doors. Regardless of where the patient is being loaded, always approach the aircraft from the front unless otherwise instructed by the flight crew. Always take the same path when you are moving away from the helicopter, transporting the patient headfirst.

■ Smoking, open lights or flames, and flares are prohibited within 50 feet (15 m) of the aircraft at all times.

Communicating With Other Agencies

When you are interacting with other agencies, there is always the possibility of communication issues. Medevacs are no exception. Whereas the typical EMS system has its specific and well-defined jurisdiction, medevacs respond to service requests throughout a large, multijurisdictional area. Because of this large area with numerous jurisdictions, the medevac interacts with many services on a multitude of different radio frequencies.

To prevent any miscommunication, when the request is made for a medevac response, the request should include a ground contact radio channel (typically a preestablished mutual aid channel) and a call sign of the unit with which the medevac should make contact.

Special Considerations

Night Landings

Nighttime operations are considerably more hazardous than daytime operations are because of the darkness. The pilot may fly over the area with the helicopter's lights on to spot obstacles and the shadows of overhead wires, which can be hard to see. Do not shine spotlights, flashlights, or any other lights in the air to help the pilot; they may temporarily blind the pilot. Instead, direct light beams toward the ground at the landing site. Even after the helicopter has landed, you should not aim lights anywhere near it. Of course, smoking, open lights or flames, and flares are prohibited within 50 feet (15 m) of the aircraft at all times.

Landing on Uneven Ground

If the helicopter must land on a grade, extra caution is advised. The main rotor blade will be closer to the ground on the uphill side. In this situation, approach the aircraft from the downhill side only **Figure 46-14**. Do not move the patient to the helicopter until the crew has signaled that they are ready to receive you. A flight crew member will direct and assist you in loading the patient.

Medevacs at Hazardous Materials Incidents

The flight crew must be notified immediately of the presence of hazardous materials at the scene. The

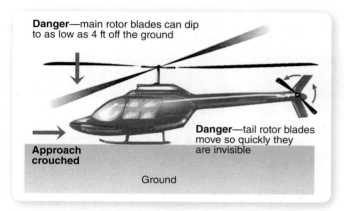

Figure 46-12 The main rotor blade of the helicopter is flexible and may dip as low as 4 feet (1.2 m) off the ground.
© Jones & Bartlett Learning.

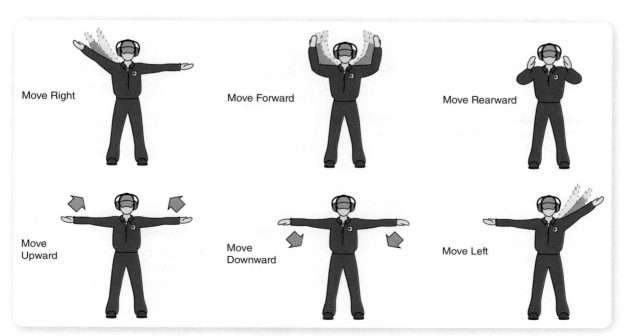

Figure 46-13 Some examples of helicopter hand signals. Be familiar with those used within your jurisdiction.
© Jones & Bartlett Learning.

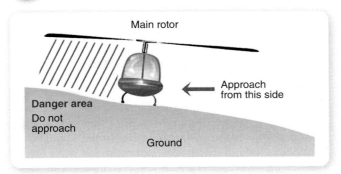

Main rotor

Approach from this side

Danger area
Do not approach

Ground

Figure 46-14 Approach a helicopter on a grade from the downhill side only.

© Jones & Bartlett Learning.

aircraft generates tremendous wind and may easily spread any hazardous vapors present. Always consult the flight crew and incident commander about the best approach and distance from the scene for a medevac. The landing zone should be established upwind and uphill from the hazardous materials scene. Any patients who have been exposed to a hazardous material must be properly decontaminated before they can be loaded into the aircraft. For incident management procedures at hazardous materials incidents, refer to Chapter 47, *Incident Management and Mass-Casualty Incidents*; see Chapter 49, *Hazardous Materials*, for a discussion of decontamination.

YOU ▸ are the Paramedic   SUMMARY

1. **Explain the concept of "due regard."**

   Every state has laws regarding the use of lights and siren when operating an emergency vehicle. The concept of due regard is an important part of those laws. The driver is given a lot of responsibility and exemptions within the law but must take full responsibility for the safety of all others, thus, setting a higher standard than what is expected of the other motorists.

2. **What considerations should you make concerning your route to the interstate?**

   Avoid areas of heavy traffic if possible. School zones are especially dangerous at the beginning or ending of classes and should be avoided if possible. Be aware of construction zones in your area and railroad crossings. Know the best routes in your district before you head out.

3. **What equipment and supplies are typically taken from the emergency vehicle to the patient's side?**

   Many provider agencies have a policy concerning what equipment is taken to the patient on every call. Usually required equipment includes an airway kit, oxygen assembly, and a response bag that contains a minimum of supplies and medications to stabilize a patient prior to transport. In the case of trauma patients, this equipment will also include spinal precaution equipment.

4. **What factors should be considered when you are operating an emergency vehicle in inclement weather?**

   Because of their higher center of gravity, most emergency vehicles have a tendency to tip over if curves or turns are taken at too great of a speed. On rainy days, there is an even greater danger for this to occur. Water can get trapped between the tires of vehicles with dual tires in the rear and cause the emergency vehicle to hydroplane. Use great caution in inclement weather to take the weight distributions of the vehicle into consideration. Remember that you will need more room to come to a complete stop, compared with a regular passenger vehicle.

5. **Should lights and the siren be used while you are transporting this patient? Why or why not?**

   Lights and siren should never be used to transport a nonemergency patient. The paramedic providing patient care in the rear compartment of the emergency vehicle should be the one to decide whether to drive in an emergency mode to the patient destination.

6. **What other actions should be taken before you depart the scene?**

   If your vehicle needs to be backed up, follow your agency's policy. At a minimum, walk around your vehicle to make sure cabinets are secured, and look at the scene behind

YOU are the Paramedic   SUMMARY *(continued)*

your vehicle. If you are on a busy roadway such as an interstate, have a law enforcement officer help you by providing a break in the traffic flow so you can safely exit.

7. What should the emergency vehicle operator do if the patient's family is following the emergency vehicle?

Both the emergency vehicle operator and other drivers may have difficulty seeing vehicles that are following. If you need to stop suddenly, there may be no time to react and the following vehicle could crash into the emergency

vehicle. Instruct family members before you leave the scene that they cannot drive closely behind you.

8. If the driver of your emergency vehicle approaches a school bus that has activated its warning lights and "stop" sign, what will be the proper way to respond?

No specific exemption is allowed when you are approaching a school bus that has its warning devices activated. The emergency vehicle is required to stop and wait for the driver of the school bus to drop the stop signs and lights on the bus before proceeding forward.

EMS Patient Care Report (PCR)

Date: 02-02-18	**Incident No.:** 73542		**Nature of Call:** MVC		**Location:** 224 W/B I-80
Dispatched: 1315	**En Route:** 1316	**At Scene:** 1321	**Transport:** 1328	**At Hospital:** 1342	**In Service:** 1400

Patient Information

Age: 25 **Sex:** F **Weight (in kg [lb]):** 50 kg (110 lb)	**Allergies:** No known drug allergies **Medications:** Pt denies **Past Medical History:** Pt denies **Chief Complaint:** Right knee pain

Vital Signs

Time: 1326	**BP:** 126/82	**Pulse:** 80	**Respirations:** 14	**Spo$_2$:** 99% on room air
Time: 1331	**BP:** 124/80	**Pulse:** 80	**Respirations:** 14	**Spo$_2$:** 99% on room air
Time:	**BP:**	**Pulse:**	**Respirations:**	**Spo$_2$:**

EMS Treatment (circle all that apply)

Oxygen @ _____ L/min via (circle one): NC NRM **Bag-mask device**	**Assisted Ventilation**	**Airway Adjunct**	**CPR**
Defibrillation	**Bleeding Control**	**Bandaging**	**(Splinting:** Knee splint**)**	**(Other:** Spinal precautions**)**

Narrative

Arrived to find 25-year-old female driver of a midsize vehicle that rear-ended a vehicle at low speed. The pt states she was wearing her seat belt. Pt denies any injury except for right knee pain. Pt believes her knee struck the lower dash on impact with the front vehicle. Airbags did not deploy. Primary and secondary assessments are within normal limits with the exception of the right knee. The pt has limited ROM but strong pulses in the lower leg and foot. Pt self-extricated per local protocol from vehicle. Knee splint applied for comfort. Right leg assessed after splinting and no change noted. Pt transported to regional hospital without incident. Report to RN Sullivan upon arrival.**End of report**

Prep Kit

▶ Ready for Review

- Federal Regulation DOT KKK 1822 sets the standards for emergency medical vehicle design and manufacturing specifications.
- Three body style types are identified:
  - Type I: Conventional, truck-cab chassis with a modular body that can be transferred to a new chassis as needed
  - Type II: Standard van, forward-control integral cab-body emergency vehicle
  - Type III: Specialty van, forward-control integral cab-body emergency vehicle
- Check the emergency vehicle, including medical equipment and supplies, at the beginning of every shift to ensure that all equipment is available and in good working order.
- Preventive maintenance is just as important as operating skills. Looking for problems before the unit is in motion may prevent breakdowns while you are en route to calls.
- After the call, be sure to clean, disinfect, and restock. Perform a routine inspection to ensure that the emergency vehicle is ready to respond to the next call.
- Learning how to properly operate your vehicle is just as important as learning how to care for patients when you arrive on the scene. The first rule of safe driving in an emergency vehicle is that speed does not save lives; good care does.
- Drivers must know and follow safe driving practices, including wearing a seat belt, using an appropriate speed, using sirens appropriately, and maintaining a cushion of safety.
- All drivers and passengers should use appropriate safety restraints while a vehicle is in motion. Pediatric patients should be secured in devices designed for them.
- Make sure all equipment is secured before leaving the scene.
- Lights and siren should be used when you are responding to emergencies but used sparingly when transporting a patient to the hospital.
- Avoid backing up the vehicle if possible. If it is necessary, use a spotter to assist in the procedure. Make sure everyone is clear on where the unit is to be placed and that hand signals used are agreed upon.
- Use extreme caution when you are driving in heavy traffic areas or in rural areas where the roadways themselves may not be suitable for travel with a heavy emergency vehicle. Watch out for other dangers such as animals running onto the roadway.
- Slow down in inclement weather, being aware that the emergency vehicle requires greater travel time and distance to stop properly.
- Any specific exemption from traffic laws does not negate your responsibility to proceed with due regard to prevent vehicular crashes.
- Escorts should not be used due to the danger of motorists not seeing both the emergency medical vehicle and the escort.
- Aircraft transport is used to evacuate medical and trauma patients.
- A medical or trauma evacuation is commonly known as a medevac and is generally performed exclusively by helicopters.
- You must follow certain safety rules when you are working around landing zones and helicopters. Be sure that you are familiar with these rules before working any call involving air transport.

▶ Vital Vocabulary

aircraft transport Fixed-wing aircraft and helicopters that have been modified for medical care; used to evacuate and transport patients with life-threatening injuries to treatment facilities.

belt noise A chirping or squealing sound, synchronous with engine speed.

blind spot An area of the road that is blocked from your sight by your own vehicle or mirrors.

brake fade A sensation that an emergency vehicle has lost its power brakes.

brake pull A sensation that when an operator depresses the brake pedal, the steering wheel is being pulled to the left or the right.

cleaning The process of removing dirt, dust, blood, or other visible contaminants from a surface.

cushion of safety A safe distance maintained between your vehicle and other vehicles on any side of you.

decontaminate To remove or neutralize radiation, chemical, or other hazardous material from clothing, equipment, vehicles, and personnel.

Prep Kit (continued)

disinfection The killing of pathogenic agents by direct application of chemicals.

DOT KKK 1822 Federal standards that regulate the design and manufacturing guidelines of emergency medical vehicles.

drift A finding that when the operator lets go of the steering wheel, a vehicle consistently wanders left or right.

due regard Driving with awareness and responsibility for other drivers on the roadways when you are operating an emergency vehicle in the emergency mode, and making sure that other drivers are aware of your approach.

heavy-duty emergency vehicle An extra heavy-duty transport vehicle.

high-level disinfection The killing of pathogenic agents by using potent means of disinfection.

hydroplaning A condition in which the tires of a vehicle may be lifted off the road surface as water "piles up" under them, making the vehicle feel as though it is floating.

landing zone A designated location for the landing of aircraft.

medevac Medical or trauma evacuation of a patient by helicopter.

peak load A time of day or day or week in which the call volume is at its highest.

posting The placement of an emergency vehicle at a specific geographic location to cover larger areas of territory and reduce response times.

spotter A person who assists a driver in backing up an emergency vehicle to compensate for blind spots at the back of the vehicle.

steering play A sensation of looseness or sloppiness in a vehicle's steering.

steering pull A drift that is persistent enough that an operator can feel a tug on the steering wheel.

sterilization A process, such as heating, that removes microbial contamination.

strategic deployment The staging of emergency vehicles to strategic locations within a service area to allow for coverage of emergency calls.

type I emergency medical vehicle Conventional, truck-cab chassis with a modular body that can be transferred to a new chassis as needed.

type II emergency medical vehicle Standard van, forward-control integral cab-body.

type III emergency medical vehicle Specialty van, forward-control integral cab-body.

wheel bounce A vibration, synchronous with road speed, that can be felt in the steering wheel.

wheel wobble A common finding at low speeds when a vehicle has a bent wheel.

▶ References

1. Busch J. Addressing ambulance standards. EMSWorld website. http://www.emsworld.com/article/12051684/ambulance-design-and-safety-standards. Published March 29, 2015. Accessed April 3, 2017.

2. Avsec R. Understanding NFPA's new ambulance rule. FireRescue1 website. https://www.firerescue1.com/fire-products/vehicles/ambulances/articles/2023939-Understanding-NFPAs-new-ambulance-rule/. Published November 18, 2014. Accessed April 3, 2017.

3. JEMS Staff. Ambulance standards update. *Journal of Emergency Medical Services* website. http://www.jems.com/articles/2016/02/ambulance-standards-updated.html. Published February 11, 2016. Accessed April 3, 2017.

4. Ambulance types: what is an ambulance? EMT-Resources website. http://www.emt-resources.com/Ambulance-types.html. Accessed April 3, 2017.

5. Vanarnam M. AEV-AEV briefing on current status of ambulance standards projects. National Association of Emergency Medical Technicians website. https://www.naemt.org/docs/default-source/ems-health-and-safety-documents/health-and-safety-documents/status-of-ambulance-standards-projects-30mar2015.pdf?sfvrsn=2. Published March 30, 2015. Accessed April 3, 2017.

6. Renga S. SAE standards for ambulance safety. EMS1 website. https://www.ems1.com/ems-products/patient-handling/articles/76710048-SAE-Standards-for-ambulance-safety/. Published March 30, 2016. Accessed April 3, 2017.

Prep Kit (continued)

7. Equipment for ambulances. American College of Surgeons website. https://www.facs.org/~/media /files/quality%20programs/trauma/publications /ambulance.ashx. Updated April 2009. Accessed April 3, 2017.

8. Gunderson M, Hatley T. EMS system design. EMS1 website. https://www.ems1.com/ems-management /articles/873958-Understanding-response-interval -statistics/. Published September 2, 2010. Accessed April 3, 2017.

9. Bledsoe B. EMS myth #7: status system management lowers response time and enhances patient care. EMSWorld website. http://www.emsworld.com /article/10325076/ems-myth-7-system-status -management-lowers-response-times-and -enhances-patient-care. December 1, 2003. Accessed April 3, 2017.

10. Dynamic system status management. High Performance EMS website. https://hpems .wordpress.com/2011/08/08/dynamic-system -status-management/. Published August 8, 2011. Accessed April 3, 2017.

11. Prehospital and disaster medicine, April-June 1994, Vol. 9, No. 2. International Academies of Emergency Dispatch website. https://www.emergencydispatch .org/articles/useoflights1.htm. Accessed April 3, 2017.

12. ANSI/ISEA 107-2015. International Safety Equipment Association website. https://safetyequipment.org /ansiisea-107-2015/. Accessed March 12, 2017.

13. McCallion T. How clean is your ambulance? *Journal of Emergency Medical Services* website. http://www .jems.com/articles/2012/04/how-clean-your -ambulance.html. Published April 30, 2012. Accessed March 12, 2017.

14. National Highway Traffic Safety Administration and ground ambulance crashes. National Association of Emergency Medical Technicians website. https://www.naemt.org/Files/HealthSafety /2014%20NHTSA%20Ground%20Amublance%20 Crash%20Data.pdf. Published April 2014. Accessed April 3, 2017.

15. Ballam E. Ambulance crash roundup. EMSWorld website. http://www.emsworld.com /article/10225399/ambulance-crashes. Published February 9, 2011. Accessed April 3, 2017.

16. Brotak E. Into thin air. Flight Safety Foundation website. https://flightsafety.org/asw-article/into -thin-air/. Published November 1, 2013. Accessed April 7, 2017.

17. Penny T. Helicopter field medical landing zones— do you know the risks and controls? Linkedin website. https://www.linkedin.com/pulse /helicopter-field-medical-landing-zones-do-you -know-risks-terry-penney. Published March 29, 2016. Accessed April 3, 2017.

18. Rash CE. Ground safety: walking into trouble. https://flightsafety.org/asw/aug06/asw_aug06 _p28-34.pdf. Published August 2006. Accessed December 31, 2016.

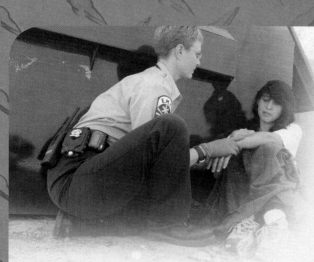

Assessment in Action

You are on scene with a critical trauma patient and are considering whether to transport the patient by ground or by air. You are 20 miles (32 km) away from the closest trauma center, it is nighttime, and the weather is clear.

1. What is the most important factor in determining whether air transport is warranted?

   A. Weather conditions
   B. Whether the difference in time will make a difference in patient outcome
   C. Where the air transport vehicle will be starting from
   D. Whether the air crew can effectively care for the patient in small quarters

2. All of the following are potential reasons to call for air transport on your critically injured patient, EXCEPT:

   A. injuries that may present with airway problems.
   B. multisystem trauma.
   C. pending cardiac arrest.
   D. presentation of shock.

3. Another important consideration when debating the use of medevac transport would be:

   A. your patient's mechanism of injury.
   B. the ability of the aircraft to land at night.
   C. the surrounding terrain.
   D. the aircraft crew's ability to find a receiving facility.

4. You have decided to transport your patient by air. When establishing a landing zone, what is the recommended size of a standard helicopter landing zone?

   A. 25 ft × 25 ft (8 m × 8 m)
   B. 50 ft × 50 ft (15 m × 15 m)
   C. 100 ft × 100 ft (30 m × 30 m)
   D. 150 ft × 150 ft (46 m × 46 m)

5. What is the recommended method of marking a landing zone at night?

   A. Place a vehicle with emergency lights on at each corner of the zone.
   B. Place a single strobe light in the center of the zone.
   C. Have personnel wearing reflective gear stand at each corner of the zone.
   D. Place one flare at each corner of the zone.

6. When is it safe to approach the helicopter?

   A. When the patient care team exits the aircraft
   B. As soon as the helicopter lands
   C. When the rotor blades stop turning
   D. When the pilot signals you to approach

7. What is an important consideration when transporting your patient to the aircraft for loading?

   A. Make sure all loose articles of clothing and equipment are secured.
   B. Approach the aircraft as soon as they have landed to expedite transport time.
   C. Always approach from the rear so as not to blind the pilot with any portable lighting.
   D. Don't approach the aircraft until the crew has approved your immobilization technique.

8. You are advised that the local aircraft is unable to respond due to a mechanical problem. The patient remains in an unstable condition, and you and your partner decide that it would be in the patient's best interest to run lights and siren to the trauma center. What are some potential dangers when transporting a patient with lights and siren?

Assessment *in Action* (continued)

9. You have been dispatched to assist a BLS unit on the scene of a crash approximately 15 miles (24 km) outside of town. The BLS crew reports that they have a 45-year-old man involved in a single-vehicle crash. They advise that the patient is normotensive and reporting abdominal pain. Upon arrival, you find that the patient is a bit worse off than they had conveyed. His blood pressure is 80/50 mm Hg, heart rate is 110 beats/min, and respirations are 16 breaths/min. You believe he has an unstable pelvis. You are 20 minutes by ground from a level 1 trauma center. That center does have a helicopter that will come to the scene. What is your best action?

10. You are en route to an emergency scene. As you approach a busy intersection, you slow down to watch for traffic entering the intersection from all lanes. Your forward lane is presenting with a red traffic light. You see no other approaching traffic, so you proceed forward. Halfway into the intersection, a car suddenly appears from your right and you are unable to avoid a collision. Based on the concept of due regard, can you be charged for the crash if you had approached the intersection appropriately and had looked for approaching vehicles before entering the potential danger area? Why or why not?

Incident Management and Mass-Casualty Incidents

National EMS Education Standard Competencies

EMS Operations

Knowledge of operational roles and responsibilities to ensure patient, public, and personnel safety.

Incident Management

Establish and work within the incident management system. (pp 2335-2344)

Multiple Casualty Incidents

Triage principles (pp 2345-2347)
Resource management (pp 2335-2340)
Triage (pp 2345-2351)
> Performing (pp 2347-2350)
> Retriage (p 2346)
> Destination decisions (p 2351)
> Posttraumatic and cumulative stress (p 2351)

Knowledge Objectives

1. Explain the federal requirements for the minimum entry-level certifications of paramedics and other emergency personnel in incident command system (ICS) training. (p 2334)
2. Describe the National Incident Management System (NIMS) and its major components. (pp 2334-2335)
3. Describe the purpose of the ICS and its organizational structure, and the role of emergency medical services (EMS) response within it. (pp 2335-2339)
4. Describe how the ICS ensures the safety of responders, people injured or threatened by the incident, volunteers assisting at the incident, and the media and general public who are at the scene. (pp 2339-2340)
5. Describe the role of the paramedic in establishing command under the ICS. (pp 2340-2341)
6. Explain the purpose of EMS operations within incident management. (pp 2341-2344)
7. Describe the specific conditions that would define a situation as a mass-casualty incident (MCI), including some examples. (p 2344)
8. Describe what occurs during primary and secondary triage, how the four triage categories are assigned to patients on the scene, and how destination decisions regarding triaged patients are made. (pp 2345-2348, 2351)
9. Explain the need for retriaging of patients during MCIs. (p 2346)
10. Describe how the START and JumpSTART triage methods are performed. (pp 2348-2350)
11. Describe the purpose of critical incident stress management. (p 2351)

Skills Objectives

1. Demonstrate how to perform triage based on a fictitious scenario that involves an MCI. (pp 2345-2351)

Introduction

The most challenging situations you can be called to are disasters and **mass-casualty incidents (MCIs)**. A **disaster** is declared by a locale, county, state, or by the federal government for purposes of providing additional resources and funds to those in need.

A **multiple-casualty incident** refers to any situation with more than one patient, but which will not overwhelm available resources. There is no set numerical cutoff at which a *multiple*-casualty incident becomes a *mass*-casualty incident. Rather, a mass-casualty incident (MCI) is declared when the number of patients and severity of injuries presenting at a given time or place suggest that available community resources could be overwhelmed, therefore requiring assistance per mutual aid response, discussed later in this chapter. For the purposes of this text, the term mass-casualty incident (MCI) is used throughout.

You may be the first responding unit to a scene that can quickly overwhelm your available resources. Even seasoned veterans can lose their ability to control the scene when there is a large number of patients, a lack of resources, or a lack of a structured response. One of the most efficient ways to deal with large-scale events is to adhere to a framework that allows you to structure the emergency response and maintain the flexibility to respond based on the unique needs of the scene. The framework is designed so that emergency responders, regardless of geographic location, can rapidly deploy the system if presented with an MCI.

To promote more efficient coordination of emergency incidents at the local, regional, state, and national levels, the **National Incident Management System (NIMS)** was developed. This system was designed in an effort to improve efficiency in the management of incidents, regardless of size or complexity. NIMS courses may offer certifications that can be prerequisites, corequisites, or part of an entry-level course.

Finally, by learning to use the principles of the **incident command system (ICS)**, you will be better prepared to provide a coordinated effort during an incident. As a paramedic, you will typically be assigned to work within the emergency medical services (EMS)/medical group under an ICS, but you also may be asked to function in other areas (discussed later in this chapter).

■ The NIMS

Although most incidents are handled at the local level, the president of the United States directed the Secretary of Homeland Security to implement the NIMS in February 2003 (Table 47-1). Major incidents require the involvement and coordination of multiple jurisdictions, functional agencies, and emergency response disciplines. The NIMS provides a consistent nationwide template to enable federal, state, regional, and local governments, as well as private sector and nongovernmental organizations, to work together effectively and efficiently. The NIMS is used to prepare for, prevent, respond to, and recover from

Table 47-1	Development of the NIMS
Year	**Development**
1973	First FIRESCOPE technical team is established by the US Forest Service and other major California fire departments.
1982	Modifications are made to the FIRESCOPE management style, and the National Interagency Incident Management System is developed.
1987	NFPA develops *NFPA 1561*—Standard on Fire Department Incident Management System.
1990	National Fire Service Incident Management System Consortium is created.
2003	Homeland Security Presidential Directive (HSPD-5) mandates development of an incident management system for national incidents.
2008	NIMS updated with changes to organization to stress importance of preparedness.

Abbreviations: FIRESCOPE, Firefighting Resources of California Organized for Potential Emergencies; NFPA, National Fire Protection Association; NIMS, National Incident Management System
© Jones & Bartlett Learning.

domestic incidents, regardless of cause, size, or complexity, including acts of catastrophic terrorism and hazardous materials (hazmat) incidents.

Two important features of NIMS are standardization and flexibility. Using common terminology helps define organizational functions, incident facilities, resource descriptions, and position titles. Standardization of ICS organization and associated terms does not limit the flexibility of the system. The organizational structure must

YOU are the Paramedic   PART 1

You have been dispatched to the scene of a motor vehicle crash outside of a church. At 2101, you are the first responding EMS unit to arrive on the scene where a vehicle has left the highway and crashed into a group of people attending a funeral. The crash occurred on a two-lane road, and the scene is located approximately 30 yards (27 m) from the roadway. From inside your ambulance, you can see approximately 12 people lying on the ground around the car and two people lying on top of the car. There are many people crowded around the area. There are no identifiable hazards.

1. When does an event become an MCI?
2. How can you prepare yourself for an MCI?
3. What is the goal of the ICS?

be flexible enough to be rapidly adapted for use in any situation. The ICS organization may be expanded easily from a small size for routine operations to a larger organization capable of handling catastrophic events. Flexibility is acceptable within standard ICS organizational structure.

Another important feature of the NIMS is the concept of *interoperability*, in which a common incident communications plan is developed and facilitates interoperable communications. When responding to a catastrophic event, it is important to remember that additional resources may be responding from other jurisdictions, as well as other states. Everyone must be able to work using a similar framework to efficiently manage the event.

The ICS, which is the focus of this chapter, is one component of the NIMS. The major NIMS components are as follows:

- **Command and management.** The NIMS standardizes incident management for all hazards and across all levels of government. The NIMS standard incident command structures are based on three key constructs: ICS, multiagency coordination systems, and public information systems.
- **Preparedness.** The NIMS establishes measures for all responders to incorporate into their training so that they are prepared to respond to any event.
- **Resource management.** The NIMS sets up mechanisms to identify requirements, order and acquire, mobilize, track and report, recover and demobilize, and reimburse and inventory resources before, during, and after an incident. The NIMS also defines standard procedures to recover equipment used during the incident.
- **Communications and information management.** Effective communications, information management, and sharing are critical aspects of domestic incident management. The NIMS communications and information systems simplify the essential functions needed to provide interoperability.
- **Ongoing management and maintenance.** The US Department of Homeland Security will establish a multijurisdictional, multidisciplinary NIMS Integration Center. This center will provide strategic direction for and oversight of the NIMS, supporting routine maintenance and continuous improvement of the system in the long term.

The Incident Command System

A basic understanding of the core structure and components of the ICS allows you to effectively assist in the management of any incident, regardless of whether you are the first responding unit or the incident commander. Communication is of the utmost importance when managing an emergency response. Common terminology and the use of "clear text" communications help responders from multiple agencies work efficiently together.

When you use the ICS, the basic framework of your response is already laid out. The specific needs of managing a particular event can be modified based on a change in the number of resources available or a change in the size or complexity of the event. The goal of the ICS is to efficiently utilize available resources to manage the event and care for the sick or injured. Make certain to follow your local SOPs for establishing the ICS. The ICS is designed to control duplication of effort and **freelancing**, in which individual units or different organizations make independent and often inefficient decisions about the next appropriate action. These personnel are often not needed. Personnel should respond only when requested or dispatched by an appropriate authority. To understand freelancing, think of a small ambulance company driving their only two ambulances to another state to assist with recovery efforts after a hurricane. If they do not coordinate their response with local authorities, their actions may be a duplication of effort and could even hamper the recovery efforts being coordinated through the ICS.

One of the organizing principles of the ICS is limiting the **span of control**, the number of resources for which a supervisor is responsible, usually expressed as the ratio of supervisors to responders (the optimal span of control is 1:5). To maintain effective communication and management of resources, you should limit the number of subordinates to three to seven people. Factors that may influence the span of control include the size of the event, safety hazards, and physical distance between resources. Tactical operations that pose a significant risk to responders, such as extrication of patients from a building collapse, may call for a smaller span of control, such as three people per supervisor. Lower risk operations, like restocking supplies at an aid station, may allow for a larger span of control of up to seven people per supervisor. As you can imagine, if you go beyond the recommended span of control, the risk of ineffective communication and loss of control of your resources rises significantly.

Organizational structures may include sections, branches, divisions and groups, and resources **Figure 47-1**. In some regions, emergency operations centers may exist. City, state, or federal governments usually operate the centers. They are often designed to serve as a base of operations or command center for representatives from every agency and entity involved in a response. These centers are usually activated during natural disasters, catastrophic events with a large number of patients, or any event that may exceed the available resources.

Your role will normally lie outside of the emergency operations center; however, you should know that some centers utilize the ICS. You should find out from your service if one exists, who is in charge, how it is activated, and what your expected role would be in the event of an MCI.

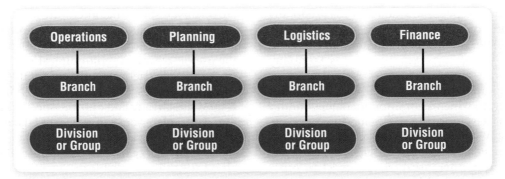

Figure 47-1 Organizational structures may include sections, branches, divisions, and groups.
© Jones & Bartlett Learning.

▶ Incident Command System Roles and Responsibilities

There are many roles defined in the ICS. The general staff includes operations, finance, logistics, and planning roles. These roles have specific responsibilities. It is important that you have a basic understanding of each of these roles so that you can assist if needed.

Command

The **incident commander (IC)** has overall command responsibility for the ICS. The IC oversees the incident, establishes the strategic objectives and priorities, and develops a response plan to manage the incident **Figure 47-2**. The **command** functions include the public information officer (PIO), safety officer, and liaison officer. The number of duties the IC takes on often varies by the size of the incident. As the incident increases in size or complexity, the IC will often delegate duties to other personnel. For example, at a motor vehicle crash with five patients, the IC may choose to assume all of the command functions. In a mass shooting with dozens of patients, the IC may choose to delegate to a PIO, safety officer, and liaison officer. This allows the IC to focus on the most critical tasks in managing the response.

Large MCIs, such as an overturned tanker causing a hazmat incident in a populated area, require a multi-agency or multijurisdictional response and use of a **unified command system**. In this case, plans are drawn up in advance by all cooperating agencies that assume a shared responsibility for decision making and cooperation. The response plan should designate the lead and support agencies in several kinds of MCIs. (The hazmat team will take the lead in a chemical leak, for example. However, the medical team might have a leadership role in a multivehicle car crash.) One of the most important keys to an effective unified command system is frequent training to allow for seamless deployment of the system when a real incident occurs.

A **single command system** has one person in charge and is generally used with small incidents that involve only one responding agency or one jurisdiction. Ideally,

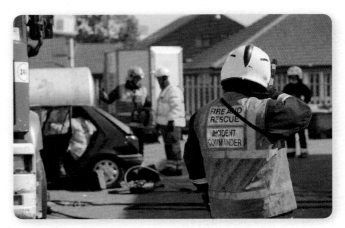

Figure 47-2 The person in command at an MCI oversees the incident and develops a plan for response.
© FirePhoto/Alamy.

it is used for short-duration, limited incidents that require the services of a single agency.

For small-scale incidents that are not anticipated to increase in complexity, the IC may be located somewhere on the fringes of a scene that is clearly identifiable. It is important to know who the IC is, where the command post is located, and how to communicate with the IC. To maintain an effective span of control, you may be reporting to a supervisor who can communicate any needs or vital information to the IC.

For large-scale incidents or incidents with several injured responders, it may be reasonable for the IC to be located a short distance from the scene. To understand this reasoning, remember that the goal of ICS is to effectively manage complex events that are often emotionally charged. If your IC is distracted by seeing injured responders or even becomes focused on providing care for a patient, he or she will no longer have control of the scene. Vital information being relayed to the IC may be missed and fatal errors can be made. Always consider the possibility of secondary devices that may target responders who are establishing command at the original scene of a terrorist attack.

Regardless of physical location, always make sure that the IC is aware of all tactical operations and major plans before they are initiated. This communication is particularly important if a **transfer of command** takes place. Because an MCI can be ever changing and ever increasing in scope, an IC may turn over command to someone with more experience in a critical area. In large-scale events, the transfer of command may occur simply because of the duration of the event. A recovery from a natural disaster could have several transfers of command. The transfer of command should occur in a face-to-face exchange to minimize any errors in communication of essential information. In extreme situations, it could be done by phone, radio, or email. Your agency should have standard operating procedures (SOPs) that govern the transfer of command. Make certain to follow those SOPs. When an incident draws to a close, there should be a **termination of command**. Your agency should have **demobilization** procedures to implement as the situation de-escalates or comes to an end. This allows responders to return to their facilities when the event has ended or their shift is over.

Operations

At a large incident, the **operations section** is responsible for managing the tactical operations, including standard triage, treatment, and transport of patients. Most of what you will be tasked with as a paramedic will be centered in the operations section. While on a smaller scene, there may not be a designated operations section as the IC may be able to effectively manage the tactical operations. In complex scenarios, the IC should appoint an operations section chief. This helps to maintain a proper span of control. The operations section chief supervises the people working at the scene of the incident; these people are assigned to branches, divisions, and groups. The operations section chief is also responsible for reporting back to the IC throughout the event.

Finance

The **finance section chief** is responsible for documenting all expenditures at an incident for reimbursement. A financial person is not usually needed at smaller incidents, but larger incidents demand keeping track of personnel hours and expenditures for materials and supplies and reporting at meetings of the general staff. Responding agencies and organizations may be eligible for some types of reimbursement after the incident, and an efficient finance section chief will help your agency to succeed in the reimbursement process. Finance personnel should be trained in the process of assessing expenditures with an eye to reimbursement long before an actual event.

The various functions within the finance section are the time unit, the procurement unit, the compensation/claims unit, and the cost unit. The time unit is responsible for ensuring the daily recording of personnel time and equipment use. The procurement unit deals with all matters concerning vendor contracts. The compensation and claims unit has two major purposes: dealing with claims as a result of the incident and injury compensation. Finally, the cost unit is responsible for collecting, analyzing, and reporting the costs related to an incident.

Logistics

The **logistics section** or logistics section chief has responsibility for communications equipment, facilities, food and water, fuel, lighting, and medical equipment and

YOU are the Paramedic　PART 2

At 2102 hours, a quick response vehicle with an EMS supervisor arrives on scene within 1 minute of your arrival. Once incident command has been transferred to a supervisor, you are assigned the role of triage supervisor. Patient 1 is an unresponsive older female who has a depressed skull fracture, a closed femur fracture, and a closed humerus fracture.

Recording Time: 1 Minute	
Appearance	Pale, cool, moist skin
Level of consciousness	U (Unresponsive to verbal or painful stimuli)
Airway	Open
Breathing	Adequate
Circulation	Pulse rapid, weak, and regular

4. What are the four general triage categories?
5. How should you triage this patient?
6. What treatment should you initiate for this patient?

Table 47-2	MCI Equipment and Supplies
Airway control	PPE (gloves, face shield, HEPA or N95 mask) Oral airways, nasal airways Suction units (manual units) Rigid tip Yankauer and flexible suction catheters Laryngeal mask airway, i-gel or King LT airway, ET tubes[a] Laryngoscope and blades[a] Commercial tube holder, tape, syringes, stylet[a] ETCO$_2$ device
Breathing	Pocket mask and one-way valve Bag-mask devices (adult and child), spare masks Oxygen delivery devices (nonrebreathing mask, cannula, extension tubing) Oxygen tank, regulator Occlusive dressings Large-bore IV catheter for thoracic decompression[a]
Circulation	Dressings, bandages, tape Sphygmomanometer, stethoscope Burn dressings, burn sheets, sterile water for irrigation One-handed commercial tourniquets Hemolytic dressings 1,000-mL bags of normal saline, IV start kits, catheters[a]
Disability	Rigid collars (universal size) Head beds, wide tape, backboard straps Flashlights, spare batteries
Exposure	Space blanket to cover patients Scissors
Logistic/Command	Sector vests (triage, treatment, transport, staging, command, rescue) Pads of paper, pencils, pens, markers Triage tags or kits used by your regional system Assessment cards Tarps: red, yellow, green, black

[a] These items could be packaged in an ALS kit.

Abbreviations: ALS, advanced life support; ET, endotracheal; ETCO$_2$, end-tidal carbon dioxide; HEPA, high-efficiency particulate air; IV, intravenous; MCI, mass-casualty incident; PPE, personal protective equipment

© Jones & Bartlett Learning.

supplies for patients and emergency responders. Local SOPs will list the medical equipment needed for the incident, depending on the type of incident. Table 47-2 lists common MCI equipment and supplies. Logistics personnel are trained to find food, shelter, and health care for you and the other responders at the scene of an MCI. In a large incident, it is often necessary for many people to handle logistics, even though only one person will report to the IC.

Planning

The **planning section** solves problems as they arise during the MCI. There are typically four units associated with the planning section: resources, situation, demobilization, and

documentation. Each unit has specific responsibilities, but planners usually obtain data about the problem, analyze the previous incident plan, and predict what or who is needed to make the new plan work. They need to work closely with the operations, finance, and, especially, logistics sections. Planners can and should call on technical experts to help with the planning process.

Another function of the planning section is the development of an **incident action plan (IAP)**, which is the central tool for planning during a response to a disaster emergency. The planning section chief prepares the IAP with input from the appropriate sections and units of the incident management team. It should be written at the outset of the response and revised continually throughout the response. In an initial response for an incident that is readily controlled, a written plan may not be necessary. Larger, more complex incidents will require an IAP to coordinate activities. The level of detail required in an incident action plan will vary according to the size and complexity of the response.

Command Staff

Three important positions that help the general staff (all staff described previously) and the IC are the safety officer, the PIO, and the liaison officer. The **safety officer** monitors the scene for conditions or operations that may present a hazard to responders and patients. The safety officer may need to work with environmental health and hazmat specialists. The importance of the safety officer cannot be underestimated—he or she has the authority to stop an emergency operation whenever a rescuer is in danger. While this is an important designation, you must remember that everyone on the scene should be aware of safety hazards. A safety officer should remove hazards to paramedics and patients before the hazards cause injury.

The **public information officer (PIO)** provides the public and media with clear and understandable information. A wise PIO positions his or her headquarters well away from the incident command post and, most important, away from the incident, to minimize distractions. Also, the PIO must keep the media safe and from becoming part of the incident. The designated PIO may work in cooperation with PIOs from other agencies in a **joint information center (JIC)**. In some circumstances, the PIO/JIC may be responsible for disseminating a message designed to help a situation, prevent panic, and provide evacuation directions.

The **liaison officer (LNO)** relays information and concerns among command, the general staff, and other agencies. If an agency is not represented in the command structure, questions and input should be given through the LNO.

▶ Communications and Information Management

Communication has historically been the weak point at most major incidents. To minimize the effects of communications problems, it is recommended that communications be integrated. This means that all agencies involved should be able to communicate quickly and effortlessly via radios. Communications allow for accountability throughout the incident, as well as instant communication between recipients. As always, and more so during a large incident, it is important to maintain professionalism on all radio communications, remembering to communicate clearly, concisely, and using clear text (no codes). Imagine the confusion caused by multiple agencies from different jurisdictions shouting that someone is "10-10." Half of the responders may think the code means "out to lunch" while the other half know it as "fight in progress." Plain language communication is paramount during any MCI.

▶ Mobilization and Deployment

When an incident has been declared and the need for additional resources has been identified, a request is made for additional resources. Once a request is made, these resources are mobilized and deployed to a designated location or staging area. It is important to wait until the request is made, to minimize the potential for freelancing.

Check-in at the Incident

You may be used to checking in with the IC upon arrival at a small-scale incident. On arrival at a large-scale incident or MCI, you should check in with the resource unit, a subsection of the planning section. Checking in accomplishes many different functions. It allows you to be assigned to a supervisor for job tasking and allows for personnel tracking throughout the incident. Checking in also ensures that costs, pay, and reimbursement can be calculated accurately. This is a crucial task—it provides accountability regarding who is present at the incident should something go wrong. Historically, there have been large-scale incidents where a secondary event (like a building collapse) occurred, and the IC was unable to determine exactly how many people he or she had to account for because not all personnel checked in at the incident.

Initial Incident Briefing

After the check-in process is complete, report to your supervisor for an initial briefing that will allow you to get information regarding the incident, as well as specific job functions and responsibilities.

Incident Record Keeping

Record keeping is important for financial reasons and for documentation purposes. If a large piece of equipment becomes inoperable, it may be possible for replacement costs to come from the incident. Record keeping also allows for tracking of time spent on the actual incident for reimbursement purposes.

Accountability

Because of the large number of responders at a large incident, accountability is essential. You may have an identification badge or card for when you check in to an incident. Accountability also means keeping your supervisor advised of your location, actions, and completed tasks. It also includes advising your supervisor of the tasks that you have been unable to complete and what tools you need to complete them.

Incident Demobilization

Once the incident has been stabilized and all of the hazards mitigated, the IC will determine which resources are needed or not needed and when to begin demobilization. This process allows for an expeditious return of resources to their parent organizations to be placed back in service.

■ EMS Response Within the Incident Command System

▶ Preparedness

Preparedness involves the decisions made and basic planning done before an incident occurs. Every area can experience natural disasters, such as hurricanes, tornadoes, earthquakes, or wildfires. Therefore, preparedness in a given area would involve decisions and planning about the most likely natural disasters for the area, among other disasters. While it may not be possible to plan for every conceivable incident, most preparedness plans allow for some flexibility should there be unique circumstances when the event occurs.

Each EMS agency generally has a written disaster plan with which you will be expected to assist in the event of a large-scale incident. These plans are generally located at each EMS station, as well as on each EMS vehicle. In preparation for a disaster, you may have a checklist of supplies that need to be at your station. Supplies may include water, batteries, cots, and other items for the personnel who will be staffing the station. You may also have a list of medical supplies that you must have on hand in sufficient quantities prior to an incident.

Of course, you should have a personal disaster plan for your family. Families need to be prepared and know what to expect should you be required to be a disaster responder. Your EMS agency may have an assistance program for families of EMS responders. It is reasonable to expect that you will be more focused on helping to mitigate a disaster if you know that your family is in a safe place. You should be up-to-date on immunizations for influenza, hepatitis A and B, and tetanus.

One of the most crucial components of preparedness involves training. Mock scenarios requiring multiple agencies to work together should be practiced monthly. This may seem excessive, but frequent training leads to higher performance and increased efficiency during a real MCI. One of the biggest pitfalls of preparedness lies in an organization that has not updated its plans for several years or has not implemented frequent training to evaluate the strengths and weaknesses of the plan. Practice like you're going to play. Continuous, realistic training will improve your performance during an actual emergency response.

▶ Scene Size-up

Remember that sizing up a scene starts with dispatch. If dispatch information indicates a possible unsafe scene, stay away from the scene or get only close enough to make an assessment without putting yourself in harm's way. Dispatch information for an MCI may indicate a large number of patients, or it may sound like a normal dispatch for an unknown problem. As you receive more information indicating a possible MCI, do not hesitate to request more resources early on. This could save precious minutes in a response time. It is much easier to cancel resources that are responding to the scene than it is to wait for them, knowing you could have called for them earlier.

When you arrive first on the scene of an MCI, you will establish command and then perform a size-up and make some preliminary decisions. On many scenes, this initial size-up can be completed from inside the vehicle. The size-up will be driven by two basic questions that responders must ask themselves:

- What do I have?
- What resources do I need?

Never make things more difficult than they have to be. Keep it simple by asking yourself these two questions. If you continually reassess these two questions, you will make it a long way through the initial management of an MCI. Make sure to include others, and work as team when you answer these questions because overlooking a single safety issue early on can start a chain of problems.

What Do I Have?

Start with scene safety. First, assess for hazards. Warn all other responders about hazardous materials, fuel spills, electrical hazards, or other safety concerns as soon as possible. Confirm the incident location. Estimate the number of casualties. Your immediate report to dispatch would be: "Medic One arriving on scene, multiple vehicles involved, all lanes of traffic are shut down, no apparent hazards at this time. Medic One is assuming medical command."

What Do I Need?

Decide what resources are needed. Once you have an accurate count of the number of patients, report this information to dispatch, and confirm that you have enough resources responding to the scene. You may need more EMS responders, ambulances, or other forms of transportation. If extrication is required, a rescue unit and fire department response may be needed. If there are hazmat issues, get a hazmat team immediately. Your second report to dispatch would be "Command to dispatch, there are 12 patients with multiple entrapments. Please start five additional ambulances, the fire department, and heavy rescue to the scene." Many large EMS systems deploy specialized MCI units or mobile emergency department vehicles that are able to treat dozens of patients on the scene **Figure 47-3** .

▶ Establishing Command

Command must be established early, preferably by the most experienced public safety official to arrive first on the scene. These officials may include police, fire, or EMS personnel. A command system ensures that resources are effectively and efficiently coordinated. Make sure that you have evaluated the entire scene. You should quickly walk a circle around the scene to make sure you have not missed any injured people or safety hazards. After doing

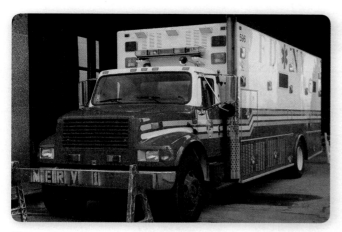

Figure 47-3 Emergency medical technicians, paramedics, nurses, and physicians staff this mobile emergency room. They are able to provide advanced life support to multiple patients simultaneously on the scene of an MCI.

© Jones & Bartlett Learning. Courtesy of MIEMSS.

so, return to your designated command post, which is most likely your ambulance or a quick response vehicle.

If you have assumed the role of IC, do your best to retain the mindset that you are there to serve as command. It is not possible to effectively maintain command of a scene if you are initiating treatment on a critical patient. You can lose situational awareness quickly. You cannot focus on directing arriving resources to where they are needed if you are busy applying a tourniquet or opening a patient's airway. As a paramedic, this may be a difficult concept to grasp because your focus usually lies on providing patient care. However, the success of managing an

MCI relies on you concentrating on your duties as the IC. Additional arriving units may present the opportunity to transfer command to a more qualified individual. Until you transfer command to another person, avoid performing other tasks at the scene.

▶ Communications

Communications is often a key problem at an MCI or a disaster. The infrastructure can be damaged or communications capabilities can be overwhelmed. You may need to move all radio operations for the event to a dedicated channel to minimize radio talk from other calls. Your communications center should have protocols in place that designate specific radio channels for use during an MCI and what resources will be dedicated to those channels. If possible, use face-to-face communications to limit radio traffic. If you communicate via radio, do not use codes or signals. It is imperative that the communication equipment is reliable, durable, and field tested. You should also be aware of what backups are available if the primary communications system does not work. Some regions have mobile self-contained communications centers, whereas others use local radio groups such as HAM radio operators to assist with communications. Most important, your plan should include a "Plan B" in case of communications failure.

■ Medical Incident Command

What has traditionally been referred to as **medical incident command** is also known as the medical (or EMS) group of the ICS **Figure 47-4** . At incidents that have a significant

YOU ▶ are the Paramedic   PART 3

A teenage girl is sitting upright next to the rear bumper of the car. She is awake and responds appropriately to questions. She has a deformity to her right ankle with some abrasions noted around her lower legs. You observe minimal bleeding from the patient's legs.

Recording Time: 4 Minutes	
Appearance	Pink, warm, dry skin
Level of consciousness	Alert (oriented to person, place, time, and event)
Airway	Open
Breathing	Normal, adequate depth, nonlabored
Circulation	Radial pulse is normal, strong, and regular

7. How should you triage this patient?

8. What is the difference between primary and secondary triage?

9. How many ambulances would you request to transport 14 patients?

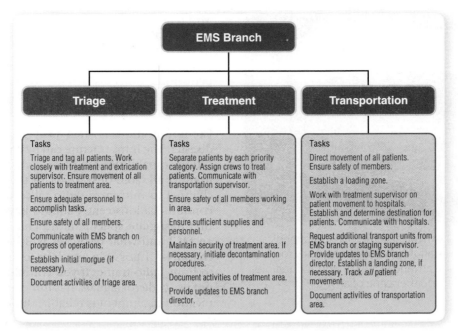

Figure 47-4 Components of the EMS Branch within the incident management system.
© Jones & Bartlett Learning.

Words of Wisdom

Participating in a simulated tabletop MCI can help you better understand how command is established, how the scene is assessed, how scene objectives are determined, how an incident plan is created, how resources are requested, when ICS needs to expand, how communication is coordinated, and how EMS works with other agencies during a large emergency.

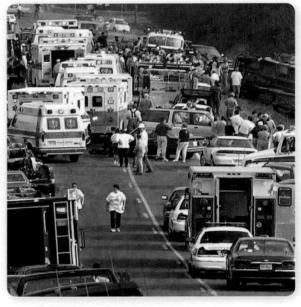

Figure 47-5 MCIs require triage.
© David Crigger, *Bristol Herald Courier*/AP Photo.

medical factor, the IC should appoint someone as the medical group supervisor. This person will supervise the primary roles of the medical group—triage, treatment, and transport of the injured. The medical branch director should help ensure that EMS units responding to the scene are working within the ICS, each medical unit receives a clear assignment before beginning work at the scene, and personnel remain with their vehicle in the staging area until they are assigned their duties. Depending on the scale of the incident, EMS may be a group or may fall under the logistics section as a unit.

▶ Triage Unit Leader

The **triage unit leader** is ultimately in charge of counting and prioritizing patients. During large incidents, a number of triage personnel may be needed **Figure 47-5**. The primary duty of the triage unit is to ensure that every patient receives initial assessment of his or her condition. Paramedics doing triage will help move patients to the appropriate treatment sector. One of the most difficult parts of being

a triage unit leader is that you must not begin standard treatment until all patients are triaged, or you will compromise your triage efforts. Triage is discussed in detail later in this chapter.

▶ Treatment Unit Leader

The **treatment unit leader** will locate and set up the treatment area with a tier for each priority of patient. Treatment unit leaders ensure that secondary triage of patients is performed and that adequate patient care is given as resources allow. Treatment unit leaders also have a responsibility to assist with moving patients to the transportation area. As treatment unit leaders supervise the responders, they must communicate with the medical group leaders to request sufficient quantities of supplies, including bandages, burn supplies, airway and respiratory supplies, and patient packaging equipment.

▶ Transportation Unit Leader

The **transportation unit leader** coordinates the transportation and distribution of patients to appropriate receiving hospitals. Transportation requires coordination with incident command to help ensure that enough personnel and ambulances are in staging or have been requested. A key role of the transportation unit leader is to communicate with the area hospitals to help determine where to transport the patients. One of the first actions of the transportation unit leader should be to contact local hospitals to establish how many patients they can accommodate. Your dispatch communication specialists may be able to help with obtaining that information. Some regions may have planned for a designated hospital within a region to perform the coordination between hospitals on destination decisions. An MCI typically disrupts the everyday functioning of the region's trauma system, so good coordination is needed. If you have only one available trauma center, the transportation unit leader may be tasked with finding other local hospitals where patients can be stabilized before being transferred to an appropriate trauma center. The transportation unit leader documents and tracks the number of vehicles transporting, patients transported, and the facility destination of each vehicle and patient. You must be familiar with and utilize whatever system your EMS agency uses to identify patients. Numbered triage tags can be beneficial for tracking which patients were transported to what facility, because a patient's identity may be unknown. Tags that incorporate bar codes to assist with tracking patients may be available at your local service.

▶ Staging Area Manager

A **staging area manager** should be assigned when MCIs or scenes require response by numerous emergency vehicles or agencies. The vehicles cannot and should not drive into the scene of the MCI without direction from the staging area manager. The staging area should be established away from the scene because the parked vehicles can be in the way. In addition, the potential for staged units to come under attack should be taken into account if the event was a deliberate attack. Make sure that units are staged in a safe area, away from the incident. The staging area manager locates an area to stage equipment and responders, tracks unit arrivals, and sends out vehicles as needed. This position plans for efficient access and exit from the disaster site and prevents traffic congestion among responding vehicles.

The staging area manager releases vehicles and supplies when ordered by command.

▶ Physicians on Scene

In an MCI, some areas have plans in place for physicians on scene. Sometimes, even without a plan, the enormity of the situation may require that physicians be sent to the scene. They provide secondary triage decisions in the treatment unit, deciding which priority patients are to be transported first. Physicians can provide on-scene medical direction for paramedics, and they can provide care in the treatment sector as appropriate. If trained to do so, physicians may be able to assist with difficult triage situations in the treatment sector when the patient is retriaged.

▶ Rehabilitation Group Leader

In disasters or situations that will last for extended periods, a rehabilitation group for the responders should be established. The **rehabilitation group leader** should establish an area that provides protection for responders from the elements and the situation. The rehabilitation area should be located away from exhaust fumes and crowds (especially members of the media) and out of view of the scene itself. Rehabilitation is where a responder's needs for rest, fluids, food, and protection from the elements are met. The rehabilitation group leader must also monitor responders for signs of stress. These signs may include fatigue, altered thinking patterns, and complete collapse. Your service might consider having a defusing or debriefing team in this area. Responders should be encouraged to take advantage of these services but should never be forced to participate.

▶ Extrication and Special Rescue

Some disasters require search and rescue or extrication of patients **Figure 47-6**. An **extrication task force leader** or **rescue task force leader** may need to be appointed. These supervisors determine the type of equipment and

---

Words of Wisdom

MCIs and disasters take a physical and emotional toll on emergency responders. Make certain that you are evaluated medically if you have been injured, come into contact with any hazardous substance, or inhale any dust, fumes, or smoke. Often, the health effects of such exposures do not manifest for years and are difficult to link to a particular event. Also, be aware of signs of stress in yourself and in your coworkers. Consider using the opportunity for stress debriefing after an incident.

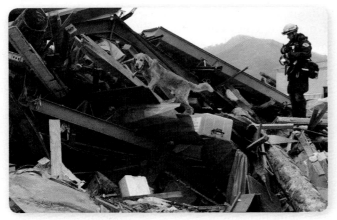

Figure 47-6 Some disasters will involve search and rescue or extrication.

© Courtesy Everett Col/age fotostock.

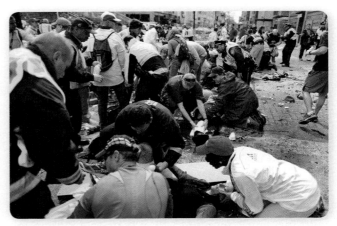

Figure 47-7 In large MCIs, aid may be necessary from a large number of additional jurisdictions.

© John Tlumacki/*The Boston Globe*/Getty.

resources needed for the situation. In some incidents, victims may need to be extricated or rescued before they can be triaged and treated. Because extrication and rescue are medically complex, the supervisors will usually function as a specialty group under the operations group of the ICS. The extrication and rescue supervisors identify the special equipment and personnel needed for the rescue. Extrication and rescue can be dangerous, so crew safety is of utmost importance.

▶ Morgue Unit Leader

In some disasters, there will be many dead patients. The **morgue unit leader** will work with area medical examiners, coroners, disaster mortuary assistance teams, and law enforcement agencies to coordinate removal of the bodies. The morgue supervisor should attempt to leave the dead victims in the location found, if possible, until a removal and storage plan can be determined. The location of victims may help in the identification of the dead victims in multiple-fatality situations, or there may be crime scene considerations. If it is determined that a morgue area is needed, the morgue supervisor should ensure that the morgue is out of view of the living patients and other responders because the psychologic impact could worsen the situation.

■ Mass-Casualty Incidents

As stated earlier, in this text, an MCI refers to an emergency situation that can place great demand on the equipment or personnel of the EMS system or that has the potential to overwhelm available resources. An MCI may also be any incident in which the system would require a **mutual aid response**, an agreement between neighboring EMS systems to respond to MCIs or disasters in each other's region when local resources are insufficient to handle the response **Figure 47-7**. Bus

or train crashes and earthquakes are obvious examples of MCIs. **Figure 47-8** is a diagrammed example of a residential building fire confined to one apartment that may produce only one patient but that has the potential to generate dozens of patients from among the rescuers and residents. Loss of power to a hospital or nursing home with ventilator-dependent and nonambulatory patients could be considered an MCI, although no one is injured.

Your response to MCIs will differ depending on the location and how spread out your patients are. You should be able to recognize an MCI as an open (uncontained) incident or a closed (contained) incident. An **open incident** has a number of casualties not yet located when you answer the initial call. Rescuers may have to search for patients and then triage or treat them in multiple locations. There also may be an ongoing situation that produces more patients while you are at the scene—for example, school shootings, tornadoes, or a hazmat release at an industrial plant.

A **closed incident** is a contained incident in which patients are found in one focal location, and the situation is not expected to produce more patients than initially present. The patients can be triaged and treated as they are removed. Although a closed incident is often easier to handle, a closed incident may suddenly become an open incident. An example of a closed incident would be a bus that was in a rollover crash.

Organizations and emergency services may establish different standards for what constitutes an MCI or for when to implement the ICS, but experience with previous MCIs is helpful in making the determination as well. Agencies and jurisdictions that regularly use the ICS will gain valuable experience and will be better prepared to respond to an MCI or a disaster. By using the ICS and the NIMS and understanding the various roles and responsibilities of each position, the responders and/or IC can manage the incident in a smooth, organized manner.

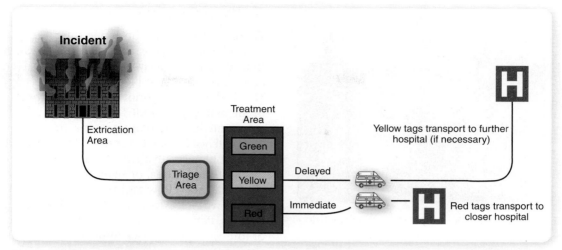

Figure 47-8 Diagram of an MCI. The incident command system established at the scene of a building fire may look similar to this diagram.

© Jones & Bartlett Learning. Courtesy of MIEMSS.

When you are responding to an incident, ask yourself the following questions when you are considering whether the call is an MCI:

- How many injured or ill patients are on scene?
- What are my available resources?
- How long will it take for additional help to arrive?
- Where should these patients be transported? Trauma center? Burn center?

What if you are faced with two critical patients and four patients with seemingly minor injuries and have over 15 minutes until the next ambulance arrives? What should you do? Never initiate transport of patients in your ambulance if there are unattended patients present who are sick or wounded. This would leave patients at the scene without medical care and can be considered abandonment. If there are multiple patients and not enough resources to handle them without abandoning victims, request additional resources and initiate the ICS and triage procedures (described later) **Figure 47-9**. If possible,

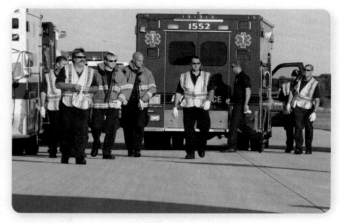

Figure 47-9 MCIs require additional ambulances and emergency medical services providers from the immediate region.

© Nancy G Fire Photography, Nancy Greifenhagen/Alamy Images.

consider relocating the patients into a smaller area that will allow you to initiate treatment on the critical patients while continuing to observe those who are less injured. Do not be afraid to use your resources and delegate tasks to your partner or responders from other agencies, like police officers. Always follow your local protocols.

Triage

Triage means to sort patients based on the severity of their conditions and prioritize them for care accordingly **Figure 47-10**. The goal of doing the greatest good for the greatest number of patients means that the triage assessment is brief and the patient condition categories are basic. **Primary triage** is a type of patient sorting used to rapidly categorize patients; the focus is on speed as you work on locating all patients and determining an

Words of Wisdom

If you are faced with treating a small number of critical patients while awaiting the arrival of additional resources, consider moving the patients to a centralized location, such as to the rear of your ambulance. If necessary, secure patients on long backboards to assist with moving them. Work swiftly to triage all patients and prioritize your interventions. Perform the necessary interventions as you wait for additional help to arrive. Do not hesitate to ask bystanders or other nonmedical responders to assist with simple tasks like bleeding control.

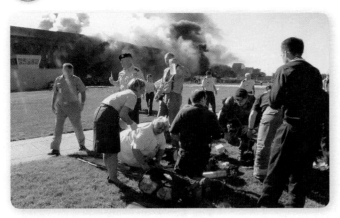

Figure 47-10 Triage is the process of sorting and prioritizing patients based on severity of conditions.
Courtesy of Journalist 1st Class Mark D. Faram/U.S. Navy.

initial priority as their condition warrants. The patients will be identified in some way, such as a triage tag. The main information needed on the triage tag is a unique number and triage category. Effective, rapid triage can help bring structure and calm to the chaos of an MCI. After the primary triage, the team leader should communicate the following information to the medical branch director:

- The total number of patients
- The number of patients in each of the triage categories
- Recommendations for extrication and movement of patients to the treatment area
- Resources needed to complete triage and begin movement of patients

When the initial triage has been completed, **secondary triage** can occur. Secondary triage is a type of patient sorting used in the treatment group that involves retriage of the patients. Patient condition may change rapidly and with little warning; what may have appeared to be a delayed category initially could change to an immediate need, or even an expectant level, before transportation can be arranged. Frequent reevaluations of your triaged patients can help you identify these changes. Depending on your resources and available personnel, retriaging of patients should be performed as frequently as possible. In smaller MCI events, this step may not be necessary if adequate resources have arrived on the scene at this point.

When performing triage, avoid spending too much time assessing a single patient. In a true MCI, there may be dozens of patients to triage quickly. A complete triage assessment should take no more than 30 seconds. Just think how long it would take a single provider to triage 50 patients if the provider repeatedly spent more time assessing the patient than was absolutely necessary. It could take an hour before the provider got to the last patient. That is too long! Lives may depend on your ability to perform triage rapidly and accurately.

▶ Triage Categories

There are four common triage categories. They can be remembered using the mnemonic IDME, which stands for Immediate (red), Delayed (yellow), Minimal (green; hold), and Expectant (black; likely to die or dead) **Table 47-3** . This is the order of priority for treatment and transport of the patients at an MCI.

Immediate (red-tag) patients are your first priority. They will need immediate care and transport. They usually have problems with airway, breathing, or circulation (the ABCs), head trauma, or signs and symptoms of shock.

Delayed (yellow-tag) patients are the second priority and will need treatment and transport, but it can be delayed. Patients usually have multiple injuries to bones or joints, including back injuries with or without spinal cord injury.

Minimal (green-tag) patients are the third priority. Patients may require no field or only "minimal" treatment. In some parts of the world, this is the hold category. These patients are the "walking wounded" at the scene. If they have any apparent injuries, they are usually soft-tissue injuries such as contusions, abrasions, and lacerations.

The last priority is the expectant (black-tag) patients, who are dead or whose injuries are so severe that they have, at best, a minimal chance of survival despite maximal efforts. This category may include patients who are in cardiac arrest or who have an open head injury, for example. If you have limited resources, this category may also include patients in respiratory arrest. Patients in this category receive treatment and transport only after patients in the other three categories have received care.

Patient Safety

Many triage tape kits and triage tags will offer a quick reference guide for identifying the triage categories and the steps to triage a patient (ie, the START algorithm). Using this guide may be reasonable if you need prompting during the first few patients that you triage in a mass-casualty incident. Provide the most accurate triage possible to provide the greatest good to the greatest number of patients.

An interesting development is the possible addition of a new, fifth triage category—the orange-tag category. This category represents an intermediate category between the critical (red-tag) and noncritical, nonambulatory (yellow-tag) categories of patients. During a true MCI, there may be ambulatory patients who require prompt evaluation and treatment for symptoms that are the result of medical comorbidities and not the acute traumatic injuries associated with the initial event. Consider patients who are having nontraumatic chest pain or shortness of breath following the event. In the past, these patients may have been undertriaged as stable, requiring little or no treatment,

Table 47-3	Triage Priorities	
Triage Category	**Patient Description**	**Typical Injuries**
Red Tag: First Priority (immediate)	Patients, including injured rescuers, who need immediate care and transport. Treat these patients first, and transport as soon as possible.	▪ Airway and breathing difficulties ▪ Uncontrolled or severe bleeding ▪ Severe medical conditions ▪ Decreased mental status ▪ Signs of shock (hypoperfusion) ▪ Severe burns ▪ Open chest or abdominal injuries
Yellow Tag: Second Priority (delayed)	Patients whose treatment and transport can be temporarily delayed.	▪ Burns without airway problems ▪ Major or multiple bone or joint injuries ▪ Back injuries with or without spinal cord damage
Green Tag: Third Priority (walking wounded)	Patients who require minimal or no treatment and transportation can be delayed until last.	▪ Minor fractures ▪ Minor soft-tissue injuries
Black Tag: Fourth Priority (expectant; some areas call this Priority Zero)	Patients who are already dead or have little chance for survival. Treat salvageable patients before treating these patients.	▪ Obvious death ▪ Obviously nonsurvivable injury, such as major open brain trauma ▪ Respiratory arrest (if limited resources) ▪ Cardiac arrest

© Jones & Bartlett Learning.

simply because they were ambulatory. A patient placed in this intermediate category could be more appropriately prioritized for treatment and transport if his or her condition required a specific destination that was not a trauma center (ie, cardiac catheterization center or hyperbaric chamber).[1] The New York City Simple Triage And Rapid Treatment (FDNY-START) system now incorporates the orange-tag category, and there may be ongoing developments as other systems adopt similar classifications.

▶ Triage Tags

Whatever triage system is used, it is vital that every patient has a tag or some type of identifying label. Tagging patients early assists in tracking them and can help keep an accurate record of their condition. Triage tags should be weatherproof and easily read **Figure 47-11**. The patient tags or tape should be color coded and should clearly show the category of the patients. The combined use of symbols

YOU are the Paramedic   PART 4

A man reports not being able to feel or move his legs. He is currently pinned under the front of the vehicle.

Recording Time: 7 Minutes	
Appearance	Pale, clammy skin
Level of consciousness	Alert (oriented to person, place, time, and event)
Airway	Open
Breathing	Rapid and deep
Circulation	Radial pulses are slow and regular

10. How should you triage this patient?
11. Would you consider this to be an open or a closed incident?

and colors to indicate the triage categories is important for rescuers who are color-blind.

The tags become part of the patient's medical record. Most have a tear-off receipt with a number correlating with the number on the tag. When torn off by the transportation

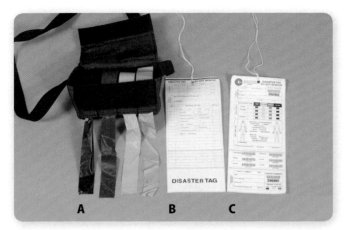

Figure 47-11 Triage tags (from left to right). **A.** Waterproof weapons of mass destruction tags. **B.** Back. **C.** Front.
© Jones & Bartlett Learning.

supervisor, it assists him or her in tracking the patient. If the patient is unresponsive and cannot be identified at the scene, the tag will serve as an identifier for tracking purposes. Some areas use digital photography of patients to assist in later identification. The photo is catalogued with the patient's tag number, and the patient's location is tracked with this. When family members are brought to crisis centers to help locate loved ones, the pictures may be of assistance.

Another method of tracking patients is to use bar-code scanners and triage tags that have bar codes. With adequate training, this method allows for real-time tracking of patients from the initial triage to the destination hospital. Whatever labeling system is used, it is imperative for the transportation supervisor to be able to identify which patient went by which unit and to which destination, as well as the priority of the patient's condition.

▶ START Triage

START triage is one of the easiest methods of triage **Figure 47-12** . The staff members at Hoag Memorial Hospital, Newport Beach, CA, are responsible for developing

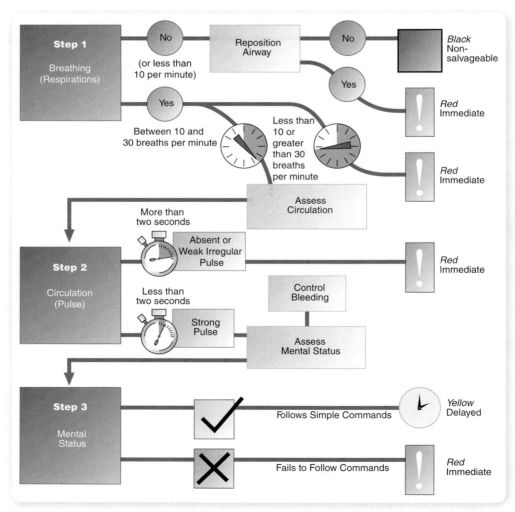

Figure 47-12 The Simple Triage And Rapid Treatment (START) triage system.
© Lou Romig MD, 2002.

this method of triage. It is easily mastered with practice and will give you the ability to rapidly categorize patients at an MCI. START triage uses a limited assessment of the patient's ability to walk, respiratory status, hemodynamic status, and neurologic status.

The first step of the START triage system is performed on arrival at the scene by calling out to the disaster site, "If you can hear my voice and are able to walk to . . . " and then directing patients to an easily identifiable landmark. The injured persons in this group are the "walking wounded" and are considered minimal priority, or third-priority patients.

The second step in the START process is directed toward nonambulatory patients. You move to the first nonambulatory patient and assess the respiratory status. If the patient is not breathing, open the airway by using a simple manual maneuver. A patient who still does not begin to breathe is triaged as expectant (black). If the patient begins to breathe, tag him or her as immediate (red) and place in the recovery position and move on to the next patient.

Words of Wisdom

You do not want to become overwhelmed by the "walking wounded." When you arrive on the scene of an MCI, people who can walk will generally begin walking toward you so that you can help them. Consider picking an identifiable landmark in a safe area (and away from your ambulance) to which you can direct them.

If the patient is breathing, a quick estimation of the respiratory rate should be made. A patient who is breathing faster than 30 breaths/min is triaged as an immediate priority (red). If the patient is breathing fewer than 30 breaths/min, move to the next step of the assessment.

The next step is to assess the hemodynamic status of the patient by checking for a radial pulse. An absent radial pulse implies the patient may be hypotensive and should be triaged as an immediate priority. If the radial pulse is present, go to the next assessment.

The final assessment in START triage is to assess the patient's neurologic status, which simply means to assess the patient's ability to follow simple commands such as, "show me three fingers." This assessment establishes that the patient can understand and follow commands. A patient who is unresponsive or cannot follow simple commands is an immediate priority patient. A patient who complies with a simple command should be triaged in the delayed category.

Remember, as the number of injured increases, so should the speed of your assessment. Make sure you have additional resources on the way to the scene to help with

triage. Triage is meant to do the greatest good for the greatest number of people. The goal of your assessment is to take no more than 30 seconds before moving on to the next patient.

Words of Wisdom

When using START triage, you may hear discussion about RPMs. This acronym refers to checking Respirations, Perfusion, and Mental status.

▶ JumpSTART Triage for Pediatric Patients

Lou Romig, MD, recognized that the START triage system does not take into account the physiologic and developmental differences of pediatric patients Figure 47-13. She developed the JumpSTART triage system for pediatric patients. JumpSTART is intended for use in children younger than 8 years or who appear to weigh less than 100 pounds (45 kg). As in START, the JumpSTART system begins by identifying the walking wounded. Infants or children not developed enough to walk or follow commands (including children with special needs) should be taken as soon as possible to the treatment group for immediate secondary triage. This action assists in getting children who cannot take care of their own basic needs into a caregiver's hands.

There are several differences within the respiratory status assessment compared with that in START. First, if you find that a pediatric patient is not breathing, immediately check the pulse. If there is no pulse, label the patient as expectant. If the patient is not breathing but has a pulse, open the airway with a manual maneuver. If the patient does not begin to breathe, give five rescue breaths and check respirations again. A child who does not begin to breathe should be labeled expectant. The primary reason for this difference is that the most common cause of cardiac arrest in children is respiratory arrest.

The next step of the JumpSTART process is to assess the approximate rate of respirations. A patient who is breathing fewer than 15 breaths/min or more than 45 breaths/min is tagged as immediate priority and you move on to the next patient. If the respirations are within the range of 15 to 45 breaths/min, the patient is assessed further.

The next assessment in JumpSTART triage is also the hemodynamic status of the patient. Just like in START, you are simply checking for a distal pulse. This does not need to be the brachial pulse; assess the pulse that you feel the most competent and comfortable checking. If there is an absence of a distal pulse, label the child as an immediate priority and move to the next patient. If the child has a distal pulse, move on to the next assessment.

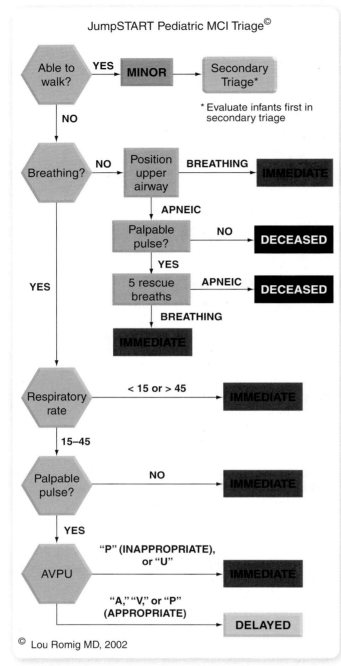

Figure 47-13 The JumpSTART triage system.
© Lou Romig MD, 2002.

The final assessment is for neurologic status. Because of the developmental differences in children, their responses will vary. For JumpSTART, a modified AVPU (Awake and alert, responsive to Verbal stimuli, responsive to Pain, Unresponsive) score is used. A child who is unresponsive or responds to pain by posturing or with incomprehensible sounds or is unable to localize pain is tagged as immediate priority. A child who responds to pain by localizing it or withdrawing from it or is alert is considered a delayed priority patient.

▶ SALT Triage

Another triage method is the Sort, Assess, Lifesaving interventions, and Treatment and/or Transport (SALT) triage system. This triage system begins by using a global sorting of patients. This first step identifies the patients who are ambulatory and can follow commands to walk to a designated area. You will assess these patients last. Patients who are unable to walk should be observed for purposeful movement or the ability to follow verbal commands. They will be given the second priority for assessment. Those patients who lie still or have obvious life-threatening injuries should be assessed first as these patients are the most likely to benefit from the lifesaving interventions allowed in the SALT triage algorithm.[2]

As you begin your assessment on each patient, the SALT method allows for limited rapid interventions. These steps include bleeding control, opening the airway (including two rescue breaths for children), needle decompression for tension pneumothorax, and auto-injector antidotes. As you progress through the assessment, you will assess the airway, mental status, perfusion, respiratory status, and whether or not bleeding has been controlled.

The SALT method is also unique in that there are five patient categories. Black tags are assigned to patients who are dead and should not be moved from the point of injury. Gray tags are assigned to patients who are not expected to survive given the available resources. However, you may consider returning to these patients after patients in the immediate category have been appropriately treated. The other three categories are similar to most triage schemes with immediate, delayed, and minimal categories.

▶ Triage Special Considerations

There are a few special situations in triage. Patients who are hysterical and disruptive to rescue efforts may need to be made an immediate priority and transported out of the disaster site, even if they are not seriously injured. Panic breeds panic, and this type of behavior could have a detrimental impact on other patients and on the rescuers.

Do not hesitate to have the "walking wounded" assist you with simple tasks. If you have identified a patient in the immediate category who requires a jaw thrust to maintain an open airway, it may be reasonable to have someone who is classified as a "green tag," with only minor injuries, help maintain that patient's airway. When resources are scarce, delegating someone to hold pressure on an arterial bleed or hold someone's airway open could help save a life.

A rescuer who becomes sick or injured during the rescue effort should be handled as an immediate priority and be transported off the site as soon as possible to avoid a negative impact to the morale of remaining rescuers. If the rescuer can be treated quickly and return to assist with operations, this also may be beneficial.

Hazardous materials and weapons of mass destruction incidents force the hazmat team to identify patients as contaminated or decontaminated before the regular triage process. Contamination by chemicals or biologic weapons in a treatment area, a hospital, or a trauma center could obstruct all systems and organizations coping with the MCI. Bear in mind that some incidents may require multiple triage areas or teams because the victims are located far apart.

▶ Destination Decisions

Recall the 2011 American College of Surgeons Committee on Trauma field triage decision scheme shown in Chapter 29, *Trauma Systems and Mechanism of Injury*. The decision scheme outlines criteria for referral to a trauma center, including physiologic criteria, anatomic criteria, mechanism of injury criteria, and special considerations such as age or underlying health conditions. These guidelines help prehospital care providers recognize injured patients who are likely to benefit from transport to a trauma center, and are intended for individual patients. You may use this scheme in evaluating individual patients at large-scale incidents.

Another important consideration when you are choosing an appropriate facility for your patients will be the capabilities of local or even distant hospitals. The transportation officer generally will be responsible for obtaining the details about what local hospitals can accommodate in terms of number of patients and acuity. Whereas some hospitals can handle dozens of patients with enough warning, others can be rapidly overwhelmed with only a few critical situations. In the event that a hospital is inundated with a large number of patients, most facilities have a **hospital surge capacity** plan in place to accommodate the overload. This may include rapidly deployed mobile units such as portable tents that can be put in place on site.

When you have an incident that involves hundreds of patients, you must anticipate that not all of the critical trauma patients will go straight to a single trauma center. In extreme circumstances, patients may be transported to a hospital that is not ordinarily capable of accepting a trauma patient. However, the physicians at that hospital can work to stabilize the patient before arranging transfer of the patient to an appropriate facility. In other cases, it may be necessary to transport some patients to specialty centers such as burn units or pediatric facilities that are more capable of handling the particular patient situation.

All patients triaged as immediate (red) or delayed (yellow) should preferably be transported by ambulance or air ambulance, if available. In extremely large situations, a bus may transport the walking wounded. If a bus is used for minimal priority patients, it is strongly suggested that they be transported to a hospital or clinic distant from the MCI or disaster site to avoid overwhelming the local area hospital resources. It is advisable when using a bus to plan for at least one EMT or paramedic to ride on the bus and to have an ambulance follow the bus. If a patient's condition worsens, the patient could be moved to the ambulance and transported to a closer facility. The EMT or paramedic can stay with the patients triaged as needing minimal care until they arrive at the designated hospital. Any worsening of a patient's condition must be relayed to the receiving hospital as soon as possible in whatever manner the incident dictates.

Immediate priority patients should be transported two at a time until all are transported from the site. Then patients in the delayed category can be transported two or three at a time until all are at a hospital. Finally, the slightly injured are transported. Expectant patients who are still alive would receive treatment and transport at this time. Dead victims are handled or transported according to the SOP for the area.

■ Critical Incident Stress Management

Dealing with an MCI places an incredible amount of stress on the responder. There are few things more emotionally wrenching than discussing triage and management of an MCI. Thinking about how you may come upon patients that might be salvageable under normal circumstances and knowing that you have to leave them as they struggle to breathe because you must triage another dozen patients is difficult. What if the patient that you had to leave behind is a child? Fortunately, struggling to deal with the aftermath of an MCI is no longer considered a sign of weakness. Even so, there has been an alarming increase in the number of suicides among EMS workers, firefighters, and police officers. This trend must stop. Debriefing with others who responded to the event may be beneficial. Debriefing with family or others who did not respond to the event can be unhelpful and may create additional issues as they struggle to cope with the horrors that you describe. If you believe a colleague is struggling with the emotional toll of an incident, reach out to that person and offer to help him or her find a way to deal with the stress.

The debriefing or defusing of emergency workers before, during, and after a major MCI should be an available resource in your departmental disaster plan; however, the use of debriefing is considered controversial and will depend on your service director's and medical director's views of its usefulness. **Critical incident stress management (CISM)** should be available to responders but its benefits are not evidence-based.[3] Stress management should not be forced. Forcing stress management can do more harm than good to the psychologic well-being of rescuers.

Everyone should also have access to coping mechanisms after the incident, whether through a service's Employee Assistance Program, mental health professionals, or peer counselors trained in CISM debriefing. This assistance should be available without regard for a specific time frame. Some effects may not be seen until months after the incident and may present as drastic changes in daily routines, physical illnesses, mental illnesses, or even alienation from family members. The impact of the incident on all responders should be included as part of the post-incident evaluation.

▶ After-Action Reviews

After any incident, an after-action review should be done. All agencies involved in the response should participate in the effort to improve future reactions to disasters. If something worked well in the plan, keep it. If something did not work at all, remove it or fix it. Just remember that it is important to be constructive in your criticism of the response. If you highlight an area for improvement, make sure that you are able to suggest a solution to the problem.

No response is ever perfect, but it is up to all participants to keep perfecting their training, equipment, plans, and skills. Leaders in EMS suggest that all observations should be noted, in writing if possible, to allow future review. All MCIs are different; the way you react to each of them will be different, too. By keeping the basic goal of "doing the most good for the most patients" in the forefront, developing plans, using the ICS, and applying a systematic approach to triage, an MCI can be handled effectively. Practice plans often and they will become instinctive.

YOU are the Paramedic   SUMMARY

1. When does an event become an MCI?

An event becomes an MCI once the available resources could become overwhelmed. This may vary in different areas based on location, the size of the department, and immediate resources. What may be easy for a large metropolitan department to handle may completely overwhelm a small rural system.

2. How can you prepare yourself for an MCI?

A good place to start is your agency's policy and procedure manual. Familiarize yourself with the expectations for the roles you may be assigned. Then get involved! Participate in disaster planning drills, tabletop MCI exercises, and other training opportunities. Advocate for frequent training to help identify strengths and weaknesses of the response. Use feedback to help improve future responses. Consider becoming a member of a professional organization that focuses on disaster management.

3. What is the goal of the ICS?

The goal of the ICS is to efficiently utilize available resources to manage the event and care for the sick or injured.

4. What are the four general triage categories?

The four triage categories used most frequently are immediate (red), delayed (yellow), minimal or "walking wounded" (green), and expectant (black).

5. How should you triage this patient?

The patient is unresponsive with signs of shock. The patient should be triaged in the immediate (red) category. This patient should be one of the top priorities once all patients have been triaged and moved into the treatment area.

6. What treatment should you initiate for this patient?

During your initial triage of the scene, you should not provide any immediate care for this patient. Your instinct may be to administer oxygen, initiate intravenous access, and begin treating for shock; however, you must remember that no treatment should be initiated when using the START triage algorithm.

7. How should you triage this patient?

She is sitting upright, alert and oriented. There are no threats to her cardiovascular or respiratory status. Her injuries may require treatment but are minor upon initial assessment. She should be categorized in the minimal (green) category.

8. What is the difference between primary and secondary triage?

For the purpose of this chapter, primary triage is the initial triage performed at the scene. Secondary triage takes place later as the patient is brought to the treatment area. Other sources you read may refer to secondary triage as the assessment of a patient on arrival to the emergency department.

9. How many ambulances would you request to transport 14 patients?

Using a general rule that you could transport two patients in each ambulance, the initial request should be for at least eight additional transport ambulances. Unique circumstances may dictate whether this is an easy or an impossible request. Think outside the box. Should you call for multiple helicopters? Maybe there should be an ambulance that takes several patients to the hospital and then returns to the scene to retrieve more patients.

YOU are the Paramedic **SUMMARY** *(continued)*

10. How should you triage this patient?

This patient is seriously injured. You may have concerns for spinal and thoracic trauma. The patient's tachypnea and respiratory distress is a key physical finding that you should pick up on in your triage assessment. This patient should be categorized in the immediate (red) category. Make sure that you have called for the resources needed to free this patient from under the car.

11. Would you consider this to be an open or a closed incident?

Although scenes involving automotive crashes and roadways always have the potential to destabilize (secondary collision or car catches fire), it would be reasonable to consider this scene to be a closed incident. You are unlikely to have a drastic change in the number of patients or need for available resources in this particular situation.

Patient No. 1
Triage Tag
No. 4862387

Move the Walking Wounded	MINIMAL
No respirations after head tilt	EXPECTANT
☐ Respirations—over 30 or less than 10	IMMEDIATE
☐ Perfusion—capillary refill over 2 seconds	IMMEDIATE
☒ Mental status—unable to follow simple commands	IMMEDIATE
Otherwise	DELAYED

MAJOR INJURIES: Unresponsive, multiple long bone fractures, skull fracture
HOSPITAL DESTINATION: Scotts North
ORIENTED × ☐   DISORIENTED ☐   UNRESPONSIVE ☒

TIME	PULSE	B/P	RESPIRATION
2102	Rapid, weak, and regular	N/A	Adequate
N/A	N/A	N/A	N/A

PERSONAL INFORMATION:
NAME: Unknown
MALE ☐ FEMALE ☒ AGE: EST. 70 WEIGHT: EST. 135 lb (61 kg)
MEDICAL COMPLAINTS/HISTORY
Auto-pedestrian. Unresponsive, long bone fractures, skull fracture

EXPECTANT	No	4862387

IMMEDIATE	No	4862387

Patient No. 2
Triage Tag
No. 4862388

Move the Walking Wounded	MINIMAL
No respirations after head tilt	EXPECTANT
☐ Respirations—over 30 or less than 10	IMMEDIATE
☐ Perfusion—capillary refill over 2 seconds	IMMEDIATE
☐ Mental status—unable to follow simple commands	IMMEDIATE
Otherwise	DELAYED

MAJOR INJURIES: None
HOSPITAL DESTINATION: St. Francis
ORIENTED × ☒4   DISORIENTED ☐   UNRESPONSIVE ☐

TIME	PULSE	B/P	RESPIRATION
2105	Radial pulse is normal, strong, and regular	N/A	Normal, adequate depth, nonlabored
N/A	N/A	N/A	N/A

PERSONAL INFORMATION:
NAME: Jessica Kraft
MALE ☐ FEMALE ☒ AGE: 16 WEIGHT: EST. 100 lb (45 kg)
MEDICAL COMPLAINTS/HISTORY
Dislocated ankle/possible fracture, lower leg abrasions

EXPECTANT	No	4862388

IMMEDIATE	No	4862388

DELAYED	No	4862388

MINIMAL	No	4862388

YOU are the Paramedic   SUMMARY (continued)

Patient No. 3

Triage Tag
No. 4862389

Move the Walking Wounded	MINIMAL
No respirations after head tilt	EXPECTANT
☒ Respirations—over 30 or less than 10	IMMEDIATE
☐ Perfusion—capillary refill over 2 seconds	IMMEDIATE
☐ Mental status—unable to follow simple commands	IMMEDIATE
Otherwise	DELAYED

MAJOR INJURIES: Spinal injury, legs pinned under car

HOSPITAL DESTINATION: Scotts North

ORIENTED × 4   DISORIENTED ☐   UNRESPONSIVE ☐

TIME	PULSE	B/P	RESPIRATION
2108	Radial pulses are slow	N/A	Rapid and deep
N/A	N/A	N/A	N/A

PERSONAL INFORMATION:

NAME: Scott Melbourne

MALE ☒   FEMALE ☐   AGE: 33   WEIGHT: EST. 200 lb (90 kg)

MEDICAL COMPLAINTS/HISTORY

Spinal trauma, legs pinned under car

EXPECTANT   No   4862389

IMMEDIATE   No   4862389

Prep Kit

▶ Ready for Review

- Major incidents require the involvement and coordination of multiple jurisdictions, functional agencies, and emergency response disciplines.
- The National Incident Management System (NIMS) provides a consistent nationwide template to enable federal, state, and local governments, as well as private sector and nongovernmental organizations, to work together effectively and efficiently. The NIMS is used to prepare for, prevent, respond to, and recover from domestic incidents, regardless of cause, size, or complexity, including acts of catastrophic terrorism and hazardous materials (hazmat) incidents.
- The major NIMS components are command and management, preparedness, resource management, communications and information management, and ongoing management and maintenance.
- The purpose of the incident command system (ICS) is to ensure responder and public safety, achieve incident management goals, and ensure the efficient use of resources.
- Using the ICS gives you a modular organizational structure that is built on the size and complexity of the incident.
- Preparedness involves the decisions made and basic planning done before an incident occurs.
- Your agency should have written disaster plans that you are regularly trained to carry out.
- General ICS staff roles include operations, finance, logistics, and planning.
- At incidents that have a significant medical factor, the incident commander should appoint someone as the medical group supervisor who will supervise triage, treatment, and transport of injured patients.
- A mass-casualty incident refers to any situation that places such a great demand on available equipment or personnel that the system would require a mutual aid response, or any incident that has a potential to create one of the previously mentioned situations.
- The goal of triage is to do the greatest good for the greatest number of patients. This means that the triage assessment is brief and patient condition categories are basic.
- The four common triage categories are immediate (red), delayed (yellow), minimal (green; hold), and expectant (black; likely to die or dead).
- It is vital to tag each patient during triage to help keep an accurate record of his or her condition. Triage tags become part of the patient's medical record.
- START triage (Simple Triage And Rapid Treatment) uses a limited assessment of the patient's ability to walk, respiratory status, hemodynamic status, and neurologic status to quickly and efficiently triage patients.
- JumpSTART triage modifies the START triage system to take into account the physiologic and developmental differences of pediatric patients. It is intended for use in children younger than age 8 years or who appear to weigh less than 100 pounds (45 kg).
- The Sort, Assess, Lifesaving interventions, and Treatment and/or Transport triage system uses a global sorting approach to help determine who should be triaged first, second, and third. It also allows for rapid life-saving interventions to be performed during the initial triage assessment.
- Consider critical incident stress management before, during, or after an event. It is normal to sometimes feel overwhelmed. Recognize the need for assistance for yourself as well as for others.

▶ Vital Vocabulary

closed incident A contained incident in which patients are found in one focal location and the situation is not expected to produce more patients than are initially present.

command In incident command, the position that oversees the incident, establishes the objectives and priorities, and from there develops a response plan.

critical incident stress management (CISM) A process that confronts responses to critical incidents and defuses them.

demobilization The process of directing responders to return to their facilities when work at a disaster or mass-casualty incident has finished, at least for the particular responders.

disaster A situation declared by a locale, county, state, or by the federal government for the purposes of providing additional resources and funds to those in need.

extrication task force leader In incident command, the person appointed to determine the type of equipment and resources needed for a situation involving extrication or special rescue; also called the rescue task force leader.

finance section chief In incident command, the position in an incident responsible for accounting of all expenditures.

freelancing When individual units or different organizations make independent and often inefficient decisions about the next appropriate action.

hospital surge capacity The capabilities of a receiving hospital to handle a large number of unexpected emergency patients, such as those seen in a mass-casualty incident.

Prep Kit (continued)

incident action plan (IAP) An oral or written plan stating general objectives reflecting the overall strategy for managing an incident.

incident commander (IC) The overall leader of the incident command system to whom commanders or leaders of the incident command system divisions report.

incident command system (ICS) A system implemented to manage disasters and mass-casualty incidents in which section chiefs, including operations, finance, logistics, and planning, report to the incident commander.

joint information center (JIC) An area designated by the incident commander, or a designee, in which public information officers from multiple agencies disseminate information about the incident.

JumpSTART triage A sorting system for pediatric patients younger than 8 years or weighing less than 100 pounds (45 kg). There is a minor adaptation for infants and children (including those with special needs) who cannot ambulate on their own.

liaison officer (LNO) In incident command, the person who relays information, concerns, and requests among responding agencies.

logistics section In incident command, the section that helps procure and stockpile equipment and supplies during an incident.

mass-casualty incident (MCI) An emergency situation that can place great demand on the equipment or personnel of the EMS system or has the potential to overwhelm available resources.

medical incident command A group of operations in a unified command system, whose three designated sector positions are triage, treatment, and transport.

morgue unit leader In incident command, the person who works with area medical examiners, coroners, and law enforcement agencies to coordinate the disposition of dead victims.

multiple-casualty incident Any situation with more than one patient, but which will not overwhelm available resources.

mutual aid response An agreement between neighboring EMS systems to respond to mass-casualty incidents or disasters in each other's region when local resources are insufficient to handle the response.

National Incident Management System (NIMS) A Department of Homeland Security system designed to enable federal, state, and local governments and private sector and nongovernmental organizations to effectively and efficiently prepare for, prevent, respond to, and recover from domestic incidents, regardless of cause, size, or complexity, including acts of catastrophic terrorism.

open incident An ongoing or uncontained incident in which rescuers will have to search for patients and then triage or treat them. The situation may produce more patients. Examples include school shootings, tornadoes, a hazardous materials release, and rising floodwaters.

operations section In incident command, the section that is responsible for managing the tactical operations, including standard triage, treatment, and transport of patients.

planning section In incident command, the component that ultimately produces a plan to resolve any incident.

primary triage A type of patient sorting used to rapidly categorize patients; the focus is on speed in locating all patients and determining an initial priority as their condition warrants.

public information officer (PIO) In incident command, the person who keeps the public informed and relates any information to the press.

rehabilitation group leader In incident command, the person who establishes an area that provides protection for responders from the elements and the situation.

rescue task force leader In incident command, the person appointed to determine the type of equipment and resources needed for a situation involving extrication or special rescue; also called the extrication task force leader.

safety officer In incident command, the person who gives the "go ahead" to a plan or who may stop an operation when rescuer safety is an issue.

secondary triage A type of patient sorting used in the treatment sector that involves retriage of patients.

single command system A command system in which one person is in charge, generally used with small incidents that involve only one responding agency or one jurisdiction.

span of control In incident command, the subordinate positions under the commander's direction to which the workload is distributed; the supervisor-to-worker ratio.

staging area manager In incident command, the person who locates an area to stage equipment and personnel and tracks unit arrival and deployment from the staging area.

START triage Simple Triage And Rapid Treatment; a patient sorting process that uses a limited assessment

Prep Kit (continued)

of the patient's ability to walk, respiratory status, hemodynamic status, and neurologic status.

termination of command The end of the incident command structure when an incident draws to a close.

transfer of command In incident command, when an incident commander turns over command to someone with more experience in a critical area.

transportation unit leader In incident command, the person who coordinates transportation and distribution of patients to appropriate receiving hospitals.

treatment unit leader In incident command, the person responsible for locating, setting up, and supervising the treatment area.

triage To sort patients based on the severity of their conditions and prioritize them for care accordingly.

triage unit leader The person in charge of prioritizing patients, whose primary duty is to ensure that every patient receives initial triage.

unified command system A command system used in larger incidents in which there is a multiagency or multijurisdictional response to coordinate decision making and cooperation among the agencies.

▶ References

1. Arshad FH, Williams A, Asaeda G, et al. A modified simple triage and rapid treatment algorithm from the New York City (USA) Fire Department. *Prehosp Disaster Med.* 2015;30(2):199-204. https://www .ncbi.nlm.nih.gov/pubmed/25687598. Published February 17, 2015. Accessed February 23, 2017.
2. SALT Mass Casualty Triage Algorithm (Sort, Assess, Lifesaving Interventions, Treatment/Transport)— adapted for a very large radiation emergency. Radiation Emergency Medical Management website. https://www.remm.nlm.gov/salttriage.htm. Published February 22, 2017. Accessed April 13, 2017.
3. Jacobs J, Horne-Moyer HL, Jones R. The effectiveness of critical incident stress debriefing with primary and secondary trauma victims. *Int J Emerg Ment Health.* 2004;6(1):5-14. https://www.ncbi.nlm.nih .gov/pubmed/15131998. Published Winter 2004. Accessed April 14, 2017.

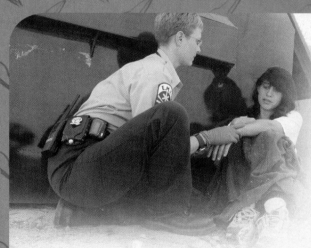

Assessment in Action

You are responding to a local marina for reports of a boat that collided into the dock. As you arrive at the marina, you can see a large speedboat sticking out of the side of a larger yacht at the end of the dock. Bystanders and other boaters are pulling people out of the water and onto a section of the dock.

1. As the first arriving emergency responder, what should be one of your first actions?

   A. Assume incident command and call for additional resources.
   B. Shout on the public address system for people to get out of the water.
   C. Exit the vehicle and immediately count the number of people.
   D. Turn off all emergency lights and sirens so the crowd does not run toward you.

2. What type of command structure would you expect to use during this type of event?

   A. Single command
   B. Unified command
   C. Divisive command
   D. Multiagency command

Assessment *in Action* (continued)

3. What type of incident would you expect this to be classified as?

    A. Closed
    B. Open
    C. Linear
    D. Complex

4. As you continue to triage the scene, you see that two additional transport units have arrived on scene. Because you were the only ambulance on scene, what two roles should these receiving crews seek to establish immediately?

    A. Triage and transport
    B. Triage and treatment
    C. Transport and treatment
    D. Morgue and transport

5. Which triage method uses a limited assessment of the patient's ability to walk, respiratory status, hemodynamic status, and neurologic status?

    A. JumpStart
    B. START
    C. SALT
    D. SMART

6. You are assessing a patient who has been struck by a propeller of a boat. She is breathing spontaneously approximately 40 breaths per minute and has weak radial pulses. You notice that she is bleeding profusely from a large laceration on her leg. What triage category should she be placed in?

    A. Expectant
    B. Delayed
    C. Minimal
    D. Immediate

7. What information should be communicated to the medical branch director following primary triage?

    A. Number of patients in each triage category
    B. Resources required to account for expectant patients
    C. Transportation assignment of each patient
    D. Presence of media reporters at the site

8. Why is the concept of an accurate primary and secondary triage so important?

9. What is the importance of after-action reviews?

10. If you notice a coworker who seems irritated or depressed following an MCI, what should you do? Could this be a sign of emotional stress related to the response?

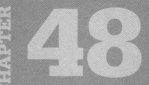
Vehicle Extrication and Special Rescue

National EMS Education Standard Competencies

EMS Operations

Knowledge of operational roles and responsibilities to ensure patient, public, and personnel safety.

Vehicle Extrication

> Safe vehicle extrication (pp 2370-2372, 2374-2376)
> Use of simple hand tools (pp 2370-2371, 2374-2377)

Knowledge Objectives

1. Explain the three levels of training in technical rescue incidents in the context of NFPA 1006, *Standards for Technical Rescue Personnel Professional Qualifications.* (p 2361)
2. Discuss guidelines for assisting special rescue teams in the context of NFPA 1670, *Standard on Operations and Training for Technical Search and Rescue Incidents.* (pp 2361-2362)
3. Discuss the steps in special rescue, including preparation, response, arrival and scene size-up, scene stabilization, access, disentanglement, removal, and transport in the context of NFPA 1670. (pp 2362-2367)
4. Discuss specific hazards that may be encountered during the arrival and scene size-up of a technical rescue incident. (pp 2363-2365)
5. Discuss how to ensure situational safety at the site of a vehicle extrication, including controlling traffic flow, performing a 360° assessment, stabilizing the vehicle, dealing with unique hazards, and evaluating the need for additional resources. (pp 2363-2365)
6. Discuss how to ensure safety at the scene of a rescue incident, including scene size-up and the selection of the proper personal protective equipment and additional necessary gear. (pp 2363-2366)
7. Explain the importance of the incident management system during technical rescue incidents. (p 2364)
8. Explain the simple methods used to access the patient during an incident that requires extrication. (pp 2366, 2372-2375)

9. Discuss disentanglement methods and considerations, including airbag safety, displacing the seat, removing the windshield, removing the roof, and displacing the dash. (pp 2366, 2374-2377)
10. Outline the standard terminology used to describe the anatomy of a vehicle. (pp 2368-2369)
11. Describe the specific hazards associated with alternative power vehicles. (pp 2369-2370)
12. Identify the hazards posed by specific types of hazardous materials. (p 2370)
13. Recall how hand tools for striking, prying, cutting, and lifting are used in rescue operations. (pp 2370-2371)
14. Identify various types of cribbing used for vehicle stabilization. (pp 2371-2372)
15. Outline the ways in which a patient can be accessed, from simple to complex. (pp 2372-2374)
16. Recognize the hazards to providers' and patients' safety during disentanglement, including undeployed airbags. (pp 2374-2376)
17. Give examples of situations that would require special technical rescue teams, and describe the paramedic's role in these situations. (pp 2378-2387)
18. Summarize the special hazards and challenges posed by entrapment in and rescue from a confined space. (pp 2378-2379)
19. Describe why collapse is a key safety concern in trench rescue and how this threat can be managed. (pp 2379-2380)
20. Compare the variables of depth, temperature, and current in surface water rescue, cold water submersion, and rescue from floodwaters. (p 2380)
21. Differentiate the equipment and techniques used in high- and low-angle rope rescue. (pp 2382, 2384)
22. Define and contrast wilderness search and rescue with lost person search and rescue. (pp 2384-2385)
23. Describe the steps in making a safe approach to a structure fire. (p 2385)
24. Cite the similarities between agricultural and industrial rescue. (pp 2385-2386)
25. Explain the special considerations applicable to tactical response scenarios. (pp 2386-2387)

26. Sequence the metabolic cascade that occurs in a patient with crush syndrome. (p 2388)

27. Articulate the patient care considerations involved in providing prehospital pain management. (p 2388)

28. Using a basket stretcher as an example, explain the importance of proper equipment selection in patient packaging. (pp 2388-2390)

Skills Objectives

1. Describe how to remove or cut battery cables in traditionally fueled, electric, and hybrid vehicles. (p 2369)

2. Demonstrate how to stabilize a vehicle. (pp 2371-2373)

3. Demonstrate how to gain access to the patient by opening the door. (pp 2372-2373)

4. Demonstrate how to gain access to the patient and provide initial medical care. (pp 2372-2375)

5. Demonstrate how to gain access to the patient by breaking tempered glass using a spring-loaded center punch. (pp 2373-2375, Skill Drill 48-1)

6. Outline techniques for patient extrication: seat displacement, windshield removal, roof removal, and dash displacement. (pp 2376-2377)

7. Demonstrate use of a throw bag in a *reach-throw-go* water rescue. (pp 2381-2382)

8. Demonstrate how to stabilize a suspected spinal injury in the water. (pp 2382-2383, Skill Drill 48-2)

■ Introduction

Most emergency medical services (EMS) departments respond to a variety of special rescue situations Figure 48-1 , including vehicle extrication, collapse, confined space, trench, water, hazmat, agricultural, and wilderness rescue.

Often, the first emergency responders to arrive at a rescue incident are EMS providers. The initial actions paramedics take may secure the safety not only of patients, but also of bystanders, other emergency responders, and the paramedics themselves. Their actions in these first few moments may determine how efficiently the rescue is carried out.

YOU are the Paramedic — PART 1

At 2130 hours, you are dispatched to a motor vehicle crash at 642 Banberry Road. While en route, the dispatcher informs you the police and fire/rescue are also responding, as bystanders report occupants trapped inside a vehicle. Upon arrival, you find a late-model sport-utility vehicle (SUV) that has driven off the road and become wedged between a large tree on the passenger's side and a stone wall on the driver's side. You approach the vehicle to find a 65-year-old woman inside. She is obviously anxious and is crying out for someone to get her out of the vehicle.

Recording Time: 1 Minute	
Appearance	65-year-old woman in obvious distress. Anxious and distraught.
Level of consciousness	Alert (oriented to person, place, time, and event)
Airway	Open
Breathing	Chest rise appears adequate
Circulation	Strong carotid pulse, slightly increased

1. What is a technical rescue incident?

2. What level of rescue training and education is required to operate specialized rescue tools and coordinate patient extrication from a motor vehicle crash?

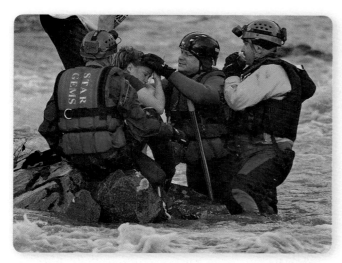

Figure 48-1 Most EMS departments respond to a variety of special rescue situations.

Robert Lasher, *The Charlotte Observer*/AP Photo.

"Rescue" means to deliver from danger or confinement. As an EMS provider, you will find yourself working to deliver patients from some level of danger or confinement on virtually every call, but certain calls will require a higher level of expertise. Imagine you arrive at an extrication incident at which a vehicle has crashed into a metal light pole, and the pole has collapsed onto the vehicle, crushing the windshield, deforming the doors, and trapping the driver inside. Your assessment shows that the patient is in stable condition. The patient care appears routine, but the rescue itself requires great expertise. This patient will need to be extricated.

This chapter discusses general rescue operation guidelines and procedures, using vehicle extrication as the primary example. The chapter includes an overview of other special rescue situations, such as confined space, trench, water, and agricultural rescue.

As a paramedic, you may not be responsible for special rescue and extrication. Nevertheless, you must be prepared for it and be aware of the associated hazards.

Words of Wisdom

Rescue awareness and operations education help you avoid rescue situations that you are not trained to handle.

■ Rescue Training

All EMS providers must have some formalized education or training in basic rescue techniques. Most such training is aimed at awareness, enabling providers to identify hazards, activate the appropriate additional resources,

and secure the scene to prevent additional people from becoming patients.

Your function as a paramedic in rescue operations depends on the type and level of specialized rescue education you have attained and your role at the incident. Some specially trained EMS providers are not in a position to provide rescue services at a given scene because they don't have the appropriate resources or have not been assigned to a rescue role. Your primary concern is always safety, and your primary role is always to provide emergency medical care and prevent further injury to the patient. All providers must wear proper personal protective equipment (PPE) to allow them to access patients and safely administer treatment throughout the incident.

A **technical rescue incident (TRI)** is a complex rescue incident involving vehicle extrication; rescue from water, ice, or confined spaces; rescue following trench, structural, or other collapse; high-angle rescue; response to hazardous materials incidents; or wilderness search and rescue in which specially trained personnel and special equipment and support are required. This chapter describes *how to assist* such rescue personnel in carrying out these tasks, but it will not make you an expert in the skills that require specialized training.

Just as in patient care, the first priority in rescue is rescuer safety. As with hazardous materials and other EMS operations, in rescue (sometimes referred to as "technical rescue"), various circumstances call for different levels of training, skill, and ability. Training in technical rescue areas is conducted at three levels. These levels are defined in NFPA 1006, *Standard for Technical Rescue Personnel Professional Qualifications*, and NFPA 1670, *Standard on Operations and Training for Technical Search and Rescue Incidents*:

1. **Awareness.** This training level is an introduction to the topic, with an emphasis on recognizing hazards, securing the scene, and calling for appropriate assistance. There is no implementation of actual rescue skills at the awareness level. This is the minimum level of capability of a responder who will be providing care.
2. **Operations.** Geared toward working in the "warm zone" of an incident (the area directly around the hazard area), operations training allows you to assist directly in the rescue operation and take a limited part in rescue incidents.
3. **Technician.** At this level, you are directly involved in the rescue operation itself. Training includes the use of specialized equipment, care of patients during the rescue, and management of the incident and of all personnel at the scene. Rescue technicians can provide the highest level of response, employing advanced techniques to identify hazards, use equipment, and coordinate, perform, and supervise TRIs.

Guidelines for Rescue Operations

Follow these guidelines when assisting rescue team members:

- **Be equipped, prepared, and ready to meet the expectations of your role.** For example, if you will be expected to access a patient who is in a hazardous environment, ensure you have the proper protective gear, equipment, and training, and ensure you coordinate with other rescuers and EMS providers. If you are not equipped, prepared, and ready or it is not your role to do so, do not put yourself or others in unsafe situations. All emergency responders have a strong desire to act in times of need, but a rescuer who is not equipped, prepared, ready, and coordinated with the overall rescue effort can distract from or derail the entire rescue.
- **Maintain situational awareness.** Whether directing others or being directed, remain aware of your situation and the conditions under which you are working. Determine whether situation or conditions pose an immediate or eventual threat to you or others. If you notice such a threat, report it to the appropriate person in the chain of command. You must constantly assess and reassess the scene. If you think your assigned task may be unsafe, bring your concern to the incident commander's (IC) or safety officer's attention. You cannot ignore what is happening around you simply because someone else is in charge.
- **Work as a team.** Rescue efforts often require many people to complete a wide range of tasks. Personnel trained in specific operations, such as vehicle extrication, cannot do their jobs without the support of others. Rescue is a team effort, and your role is essential.
- **Follow the golden rule of public service.** As you carry out a rescue effort, it's easy to concentrate only on the technical aspects of the rescue, forgetting about the patient. He or she needs your emotional support and encouragement. It's helpful to have a rescuer stay with the patient whenever possible, updating him or her on which actions will be performed next.

Documentation & Communication

If you do not understand what is expected of you, *ask*. Have the orders clarified so you'll be able to safely complete your assigned task.

Words of Wisdom

As a paramedic, your primary responsibility at the scene of a technical rescue is patient care.

Steps in Special Rescue

Your role can change as a special rescue operation progresses. Rescue and removal of patients involves several steps. You must access the patient and then quickly assess him or her for medical or trauma complications. Treatment in such situations is often hampered by the circumstances surrounding the event. Once you initiate lifesaving treatment, the patient must be released or removed from any **entrapment**. Medical care must nevertheless continue throughout the incident. The toughest part of any rescue is neither the rescue itself nor the treatment, but the coordination and balance of the two.

Although special rescue situations take many different forms, all rescuers should perform the following steps to ensure safety and efficiency:

1. Preparation
2. Response
3. Arrival and scene size-up
4. Stabilization of the scene
5. Access
6. Disentanglement
7. Removal
8. Transport

▶ Preparation

You can prepare for emergency rescue incidents by training with fire departments and special rescue teams in your area. This process will prepare you to respond to a mutual aid call by teaching you about the expertise of the personnel in other departments or agencies and the rescue equipment to which they have access. Knowing the field terminology will also improve communication with other rescuers. However, specialized training and, in some regions, certification are required before you are qualified to fully participate.

Before any technical rescue call, your department must consider the following issues:

- Does the department have the personnel and equipment needed to handle a TRI from start to finish?
- Which equipment and personnel will be first on scene on a TRI call? What resources will be available on a call?
- Do members of the department know the hazards in their response area? Have they visited those areas with local representatives?

► Response

A dispatch protocol should be established for TRIs. If your department has its own **technical rescue team**, it may respond with a rescue squad, ambulance, fire engine company, and chief officer. In some EMS departments, the rescue squad will come from an outside agency. In others, the EMS department itself provides the primary technical rescue services. Many TRIs involving electricity necessitate heavy equipment or require specialized knowledge or other resources. Thus, it's often necessary to notify utility companies, the department of public works, or other outside agencies during a TRI.

► Arrival and Scene Size-up

Starting with the initial dispatch, you should begin compiling information. Scene size-up begins with the facts supplied by the person reporting the incident and continues on the scene with reports from bystanders. This information may reveal the following:

- Location and nature of the incident
- Each patient's condition and position
- Number of patients trapped or injured
- Nature and estimated severity of specific injuries
- Hazards at the scene

As you approach the scene of a TRI, however, you may not know what kind of scene you are entering. Remember, it's the responsibility of each responder to perform his or her own scene size-up. The scene size-up includes *initial evaluation* of the variables, including the following:

- Scope and magnitude of the incident
- Nature of the incident
- Potential number and severity of patients
- Hazards
- Access to and egress from the scene
- Environmental factors
- Operating and immediately available resources
- Additional resources needed

While it can be overwhelming to consider all these items and more, a simple, commonly used format can both focus your awareness and simplify how you communicate important size-up information. Consider using the UCAN (Unit, Conditions, Actions, Needs) format to guide both your size-up process and your size-up communication:

- **Unit.** Consider not just your unit identification, but also your role at the incident. Your role may change as the incident progresses. Clarify this role in your mind and identify or announce it as necessary.
- **Conditions.** What do you see as you approach the scene? While a great deal may be going on, focus on the crucial points related to your role, such as nature and scope of the incident, hazards, and routes of entry and egress.
- **Actions.** Clarify your next immediate actions so you can focus on operating effectively and coordinating well with other rescuers.
- **Needs.** Identify additional resources with which you will need to coordinate immediately, and identify any materials you will need to perform your role. Request those resources as appropriate.

Hazards

At a TRI, you may be tempted to immediately approach the patient or the accident area. However, as a paramedic, your own safety is paramount, and you must also protect your partner and the public. It is crucial that you slow down and properly evaluate the situation. Consider the hazards, such as utilities and environmental conditions, that may be **immediately dangerous to life and health (IDLH)**. If such hazards are identified, call for specialized resources. Do not rush into the incident scene until you have completely assessed the situation. You must stop and think about the dangers that may be present. Do not make yourself part of the problem.

Traffic Incident Management

Perhaps the most common and dangerous hazard encountered on rescue scenes, especially scenes of motor vehicle extrication, is ongoing traffic. **Traffic incident management (TIM)** is the method of controlling the flow of motor vehicle traffic to enhance safety and allow for efficient rescue operations.

While full TIM training is beyond the scope of this chapter, all emergency responders, including paramedics, should know the crucial components of TIM to identify when it is needed and whether it is being managed correctly:[1]

- Paramedics, other emergency responders, patients, and bystanders are at risk of being injured or even killed due to crashes that may occur as traffic flows through and around rescue scenes.
- Rescue operations can operate more efficiently when traffic flow in the area is properly managed.
- When possible, rescue operations should be moved away from flowing traffic.
- Traffic flow sometimes must be halted completely in the area of a rescue incident; however, complete cessation of traffic may have a significant economic impact on the area and is often not the safest traffic management strategy.
- Traffic should typically be diverted around the rescue work zone.
- Flares, cones, flags, and signs should be used to warn oncoming drivers to slow down as they approach the emergency scene.
- All rescuers operating in the area of flowing traffic should wear compliant reflective high-visibility garments.

- Flashing lights, vehicle headlights, or scene lighting aimed in the direction of oncoming traffic is likely to confuse, blind, or even attract drivers.
- If rescue operations must occur close to flowing traffic, a large vehicle such as a fire engine or highway maintenance truck should be positioned to protect the rescue work area.

▶ Scene Stabilization

Once additional resources are on the way, it's time to stabilize the incident. Look around and observe the geographic area, identify the routes of access and exit, note weather and wind conditions, and consider evacuation issues and transport distances. Remember, you may be the first to arrive on the scene. Therefore, you may find yourself temporarily in command until an officer arrives.

The first arriving responder will immediately assume command and initiate the incident command system (ICS). The ICS is the foundation of effective TRI mitigation. Many TRIs become complex situations requiring many assisting units. The National Incident Management System (NIMS) is discussed more fully in Chapter 47, *Incident Management and Mass-Casualty Incidents*. Without the ICS in place, it will be difficult—if not impossible—to ensure rescuers' safety. At any TRI, follow the IC's orders. Your ultimate goal is to protect the team and patients. No matter what type of rescue scene you enter, keep the following three guidelines in mind:

1. Approach the scene cautiously.
2. Position apparatus properly.
3. Assist specialized team members as needed.

Emergency Vehicles

Determine where to locate your emergency vehicle, taking into account the safety of emergency workers, patients, and other motorists. Don't unnecessarily disrupt traffic. Traffic flow is a hazard associated with any operation, especially one located on a highway. Don't hesitate to ask that the road be closed if necessary. Provide a safe ambulance loading zone. Establish staging areas away from the scene.

Use large emergency vehicles to provide a barrier against motorists who fail to heed emergency warning lights. Many departments place apparatus at an angle to the crash. This position ensures that if the apparatus is struck from behind, it will be pushed to the side. You can also place traffic cones or flares to direct motorists away from the crash site. Make sure no obvious fire hazard is present.

You need to be visible, but too many lights tend to distract or confuse drivers. Turn on your headlights and consider using amber lighting at the scene. Use only essential warning lights, but do not assume that motorists will heed them. Let law enforcement personnel coordinate traffic control. Before exiting the ambulance at an emergency scene, be alert for vehicles.

Outer and Inner Circle Surveys

As you approach the rescue area, begin with the outer circle survey. This survey involves evaluating the area surrounding the TRI. For example, at a two-vehicle motor vehicle collision, the outer circle survey would involve evaluating the area surrounding the vehicles and beyond, looking for items such as patients thrown from the vehicles, ingress areas for rescuers and egress areas for patients, and hazards in the area approaching the vehicles. Completing a thorough outer circle survey can be a challenge because bystanders and even other rescuers may be directing you immediately to the center of the incident. Still, this survey is important in identifying any life-threatening hazards and taking measures to avoid or mitigate them, if you are trained to do so. Determine whether the situation is a search, rescue, or recovery. If you need additional resources, they should be requested by the IC, who will establish strategic objectives and unify command with other involved agencies.

Once you have completed an outer circle survey, perform an inner circle survey on the heart of the TRI. If at all possible, do a 360° evaluation around the center of the incident—in this example, the damaged vehicles. Check over and under, continuing to identify patients, hazards, access points, and opportunities to facilitate care and rescue. An inner circle survey might help responders notice downed wires on top of a vehicle or additional victims beneath it.

Control Zones

The IC should coordinate with law enforcement personnel to help secure a perimeter surrounding the scene. In addition, the fire department should implement a strict accountability system to control access to the site. As part of the scene stabilization effort, three controlled zones are established, either formally (with visible markers and barriers) or informally (designated simply by the operations contained within the zones):

- **Hot zone.** This area is only for entry teams and rescue teams. This zone immediately surrounds the site or incident (eg, hazardous materials release or motor vehicle crash (MVC), and its size is proportional to its hazards. Entry into this zone is restricted to properly equipped and prepared essential personnel.
- **Warm zone.** The warm zone is only for properly trained and equipped personnel. This is the area in which personnel and equipment decontamination and hot zone support take place.
- **Cold zone.** The cold zone is the outer perimeter in which vehicles and equipment are staged and the command post is located. The public and the media should be kept clear of the cold zone at all times.

Police or fire line tape or barriers are often used to demarcate these controlled zones. Red tape is typically used for the hot zone, orange tape for the warm zone, and yellow tape for the cold zone. Of course, someone must ensure the zones of the emergency scene are enforced. Scene control activities are sometimes assigned to law enforcement personnel.

Specific Hazards

During scene stabilization, the environment should be monitored for IDLH threats to rescuers or patients. The US Department of Transportation (DOT) publishes an *Emergency Response Guidebook* (*ERG*) that may help TRI rescuers decide which preliminary actions to take. The guide provides information on about 4,000 of the most common chemicals that may be encountered at a highway scene. Expertise should be called in and they will likely bring a computer database to assist as a resource about the specific chemicals involved in the incident.

Motor Vehicle Stabilization. Any motor vehicle involved in a crash must be stabilized before you gain access to the patient. The fire department is usually responsible for vehicle stabilization. If the fire department is not on scene, however, you may be able to perform this task if protocol allows. Simple ways of stabilizing a motor vehicle after a crash include engaging the parking brake, placing the vehicle in park (if it has an automatic transmission), and shutting off the engine. We will discuss motor vehicle stabilization in more detail later in the chapter.

Utility Hazards. Electrical and other utility hazards require the assistance of trained personnel. For electrical hazards, such as downed lines, park at least one full telephone pole span (approximately 50 feet [15 m]) away, and do not park beneath damaged or downed power lines Figure 48-2 . Treat all downed wires, power lines, or other sources of electricity as if they were charged (live), and don't touch or go near them until they've been deenergized by a power company representative. Even if the lights are out along the street where the wires are down, never assume that the wires are dead. Be especially alert for downed wires after a storm that has blown down trees or tree limbs.

It's not just the wires that are hazardous; any metal or conductive material they touch may also be energized. Metal fences or guardrails, for example, can become energized along their entire length. Running or standing water is also an excellent conductor of electricity.

Natural gas and liquefied petroleum gas are flammable. If a call involves leaking gas, call the gas company immediately. Follow your local protocol. The IC must ensure the proper procedures are followed to shut off the utilities in the rescue area.

Words of Wisdom

Remember, utility hazards can be above or below ground, or even overhead, and the rescue situation will dictate which ones need to be addressed first. Ground and aerial ladders must stay at least 10 feet (3 m) away from electrical lines, so that the ladder does not come in contact with the power line and become energized. This is especially true as air humidity or the voltage in the line increases.

Protective Equipment

The IC and the technical rescue team will determine what protective equipment you need while assisting at a rescue scene. Most specialized teams carry unique items, such as harnesses and jumpsuits, which are easier to move in than turnout gear. This specialized equipment must meet certain standards to ensure it is appropriate for the intended rescue environment. Other gear must be specialized as well:

- Your PPE must be bright to help ensure your visibility during daylight hours. Any PPE used at night must be equipped with reflective material to increase your visibility in the darkness.
- For certain rescue situations, PPE must be flame- or flash-protective.
- Footwear is designed and certified for specific rescue environments. It must be highly visible and offer ankle support, traction, and chemical or thermal protection (hot or cold). Some footwear has insoles equipped with puncture barriers. Likewise, puncture- or cut-resistant gloves may be necessary in some rescue situations.
- Protective head gear is designed to be smaller and lighter for specific rescue situations (eg, climbing helmets, firefighter helmets).
- Providers may need to wear safety glasses or goggles approved by the American National Standards Institute (ANSI).

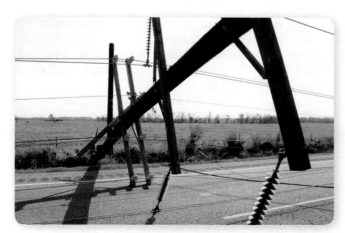

Figure 48-2 Downed electrical wires present a hazard for responding crews.

Courtesy of Robert Kaufmann/FEMA.

■ Chalk or spray paint for marking searched areas, a compass, a first aid kit, a whistle, a handheld global positioning system (GPS) device, cyalume-type light sticks, and binoculars are easy-to-carry items that can be useful in certain types of rescue.

Accountability

The **accountability system** is an important process to ensure rescuers' safety at all emergencies. It allows the IC to manage resources, delegate tasks, track the personnel on the scene (including their identities, assignments, and locations), and restricts scene access to rescuers with specific assignments.

Patient Contact

Technical rescue situations often last for hours, with the patient being left alone for long periods. At any rescue scene, you must try to communicate with the patient, whether by radio, cell phone, or even shouting. Reassure the patient that everything possible is being done to ensure his or her safety.

If you make contact, it's important to maintain communication. Ideally, someone should be assigned to talk to the patient while other personnel focus on the rescue. The patient could be sick or injured and is probably frightened. If you remain calm, your demeanor will in turn calm the patient.

▶ Access

The actions of EMS personnel must be effectively coordinated with ongoing operations during a rescue incident. Your main functions are to treat and monitor all patients throughout the rescue, which may span many hours, and to stand by in case a rescue team member needs medical assistance.

With the scene stabilized, you must now gain access to the patient. How is he or she trapped? Will accessing the patient require simple or complex tasks? For example, in a vehicle extrication, will the doors unlock and open, or will you need to use tools and equipment to gain access? **Simple access** may require hand tools, such as a sledge hammer, spring-loaded center punch, glass saw, Halligan bar, or pry bar. **Complex access** may require special tools, such as a reciprocating saw, hydraulic ram, spreader, or cutter. Using such tools requires specialized training and frequent practice. You can take a vehicle extrication course that covers the selection and use of such tools in a variety of TRI scenarios.

Remember, communication with patients during the rescue is essential to ensure they are not injured further by the rescue operation. Even if they are uninjured, they need to be reassured that the team is working as quickly as possible to free them.

Gaining access to the patient will depend on the type of incident. For example, in an incident involving a motor vehicle, you must consider its location and position, the type of damage to the vehicle, the patient's position, and the nature and severity of the patient's injuries. You may decide to use a different means of access during the course of the rescue as the patient's injuries become apparent, particularly if his or her condition begins to deteriorate.

Keep in mind that you might not be able to gain full access to the patient right away. Initial access may be limited because of safety hazards or physical restrictions. As a result, assessment and treatment might be limited as well. If you need priority access to part of a patient to provide crucial assessment or treatment, inform the appropriate person in the ICS chain of command.

▶ Disentanglement

Initiate emergency medical care as soon as you have access to the patient. Some fire, EMS, and law enforcement agencies have technical rescue paramedics who can not only establish intravenous (IV) lines and treat medical conditions, but also handle special equipment and participate in advanced procedures.

A team member should remain with the patient to direct the rescuers who are performing the disentanglement. Unless there is an immediate threat, such as a possibility of fire or explosion, you should perform a primary assessment and any necessary crucial interventions before disentanglement begins. Such interventions may include immobilizing the cervical spine, securing the airway, administering oxygen, providing ventilation, or controlling significant bleeding. Once life threats have been treated, disentanglement can begin.

Disentanglement involves freeing patients from the area or object in which they are trapped. For example, in vehicle extrication, disentanglement would involve using rescue tools and various other methods to cut the vehicle (or machinery) away from trapped or injured patients.

▶ Removal

Once patients have been disentangled and life threats treated, the effort shifts to removing the patients from the hazard area. In some instances, this may simply amount to having someone help a patient out of the hazard area; in other situations, spinal immobilization may be necessary before the patient can be removed. A wide variety of stretchers, scoops, and backboards may be used **Figure 48-3** .

To prepare the patient for removal, you must control all life-threatening conditions, dress wounds as appropriate, and stabilize suspected fractures and spinal injuries. It can be tricky to use standard splints in confined areas, but splinting the patient's arms to his or her trunk and strapping the legs to each other will often suffice until the patient can be positioned on a backboard or scoop, which will serve as the ultimate splint for the whole body. A short backboard, such as the Kendrick Extrication Device (KED), is typically used to stabilize a sitting patient. Some specialized rescue and extrication devices can serve these functions as well.

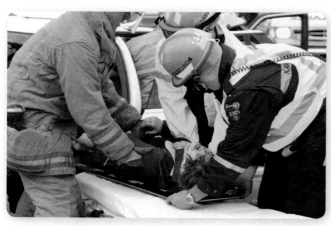

Figure 48-3 Patient removal.
© Murray Wilson/Fotolia.

The patient should be moved prior to completion of initial care, assessment, stabilization, and treatment only when the patient's or emergency responder's life is in immediate danger. Sometimes the patient's general condition is deteriorating and time does not permit meticulous splinting and dressing procedures. Quick removal may also be necessary if hazards are present, such as a gas leak.

Packaging is preparing the patient for movement as a unit by means of a backboard or similar device. Backboards can be helpful for moving patients with suspected or actual spine injuries.

Using a Basket Stretcher

A basket stretcher, often called a Stokes litter or Stokes basket, facilitates moving patients to a place of safety and can be used in a variety of situations. The manner in which a patient is packaged in a basket stretcher depends on his or her medical condition, the environment, and the manner in which the patient will be evacuated. Basket stretchers can be lifted by rope, carried by vehicles, or, most commonly, hand-carried by rescuers. In case of vertical evacuation, pack excess gear around the patient to prevent undue movement. While you are handling the patient, ensure you communicate and keep him or her apprised of the situation and your progress.

Carrying a standard basket stretcher typically involves a team of six to eight rescuers distributed around the stretcher, three or four to a side. Normally, the person at the front of the left side is in charge. This method is fast because little teamwork is required, and it usually gives the patient a comfortable ride. However, this carrying method is tiring for the handlers because it puts constant strain on certain muscles. In addition, ground vision is compromised, especially at night; a handler can easily trip over a rock and drop the stretcher.

More than one team will be needed if the stretcher must be carried over a distance farther than the team can cover in about 15 to 20 minutes. A good method to use on long evacuations is team *leapfrogging*, in which one team takes the litter for a given distance while the other team goes ahead to rest and plan the next stretch.

When footing is highly unstable, an obstacle prevents the team from progressing, or falling becomes a hazard, the so-called caterpillar or lap pass is a useful option. When the stretcher reaches the obstacle, the team pauses while every extra person lines up on the route ahead of the perilous terrain or obstacle. The rescuers form two adjacent lines facing each other, about the width of the stretcher apart and alternate (in other words, they are not all opposite each other). They usually sit down to make themselves as stable as possible. When everyone is set, rescuers pass the stretcher down between the two lines. As the stretcher passes a person, he or she gets up and carefully but quickly moves around the line in the direction of travel, and gets set to pass the stretcher again. Done correctly, this technique provides a stable and secure passage of the stretcher.

Words of Wisdom

If you will be assisting a technical rescue team, training with the team is probably the most important step you can take to prepare for a TRI. Training gives you a feel for how the team members operate; likewise, it gives them an opportunity to gauge your level of expertise. The more knowledge you have, the more you can participate.

▶ Transport

Once the patient has been removed from the hazard area, EMS will transport him or her to an appropriate medical facility. The type of transport depends on the severity of the patient's injuries and the distance to the medical facility. For example, if a patient is critically injured or if the rescue is taking place some distance from the medical facility, air transport may be more appropriate than an ambulance.

■ Vehicle Extrication

According to the National Highway Transportation Safety Administration, in 2014, an estimated 2,338,000 injuries and 32,675 fatalities occurred as a result of MVCs.[2]

Words of Wisdom

All new vehicles and pickup trucks have driver-side and passenger-side airbags. Many vehicles have **supplemental restraint systems** in other places as well. If these airbags do not activate during a crash, they may deploy unexpectedly during rescue operations. They must be deactivated to prevent injury to rescuers.

Although the number of injuries and fatalities has slowly declined since 1974, MVCs remain a significant cause of morbidity and mortality in the United States.

▶ Vehicle Anatomy and Structural Components

Standardized Vehicle Terminology

Using standardized terminology to refer to specific parts of a vehicle will reduce confusion and mistakes at vehicle extrication scenes. For example, the front of a vehicle is the portion that normally travels down the road first. The hood is on the front of the vehicle, and the trunk is in the rear.

The left side of a vehicle is on the driver's left as he or she sits in it. In the United States and Canada, the driver's seat is on the left. The passenger's seat is on the right. Always refer to left and right as they relate to the vehicle—not as they refer to your own left and right. You can also refer to the left and right sides of the vehicle as the driver and passenger sides, respectively.

Roof posts (or pillars) add vertical support to the roof of a vehicle. The posts are generally designated by letters (A, B, C, and D) **Figure 48-4**:

- The A posts are located closest to the front of the vehicle; they form the sides of the windshield.

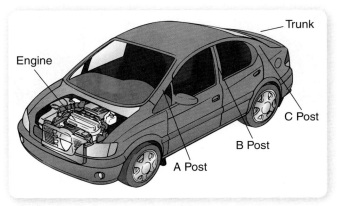

Figure 48-4 The anatomy of a vehicle.

© Jones & Bartlett Learning.

YOU ▶ are the Paramedic   PART 2

While you wait for the fire department rescue crew to secure the vehicle, you and your partner don extrication PPE jumpsuits so that you can work in the hot zone of the TRI. About 5 minutes later, the crew gains access to the patient from a rear door. As you and your partner make entry, the rescue crew continues to work to remove the roof of the vehicle to free the patient. During your initial contact with the patient, you calm her and explain what's going to happen as you, your partner, and the fire department work to rescue her. One of the firefighters has been maintaining manual spinal immobilization. You ask him to continue to assist while you perform your primary survey.

The patient tells you it's hard for her to "catch her breath" and repeatedly asks you what happened. She says that as she was driving, she felt a tire leave the roadway. She tried to steer the vehicle back onto the road, but the vehicle crossed over to the other side and stopped suddenly when it became wedged between the tree and the rock wall. The next thing she knew, she was yelling for help and heard sirens. She's not sure whether she lost consciousness. The patient has a history of type 1 diabetes, for which she takes metformin and insulin.

Recording Time: 5 Minutes	
Respirations	26 breaths/min
Pulse	Carotid pulse, 108 beats/min, regular and strong
Skin	Pale, cool, and diaphoretic
Blood pressure	Unable to obtain due to access problems
Oxygen saturation (Spo$_2$)	Unable to obtain due to access problems
Pupils	PERRLA

3. What are the three control zones that will be established while the scene is being stabilized?

4. Why is it important to use the ICS during a TRI?

- In four-door vehicles, the B posts are located between the front and the rear doors; in some vehicles, they do not reach all of the way to the roof.
- In four-door vehicles, the C posts, if present, are located behind the rear doors.
- D posts can be found on larger vehicles, such as SUVs, station wagons, and vans, that have windows behind the rear doors.
- On large vans, buses, and other vehicles with numerous windows, the lettering process continues from front to back, with posts E, F, G, and so forth.

The hood covers the engine compartment. The bulkhead divides the engine compartment from the passenger compartment. An insulating metal piece known as the firewall temporarily protects the passengers in the event of an engine fire. The passenger compartment, or cab, includes the front and back seats, including the driver's seat. This part of a vehicle is sometimes called the occupant cage or occupant compartment.

Structural Integrity

Most modern vehicles have **unibody construction**, in which the body and frame of the vehicle are fused into a single component **Figure 48-5** . Although such a vehicle can split apart during a severe crash, unibody design is safer than older frame types. Unibody construction directs energy away from the passenger compartment during a crash by incorporating crumple zones into the front and sometimes the rear of the vehicle. The crumple zones collapse on impact, absorbing and diverting the force or energy of the crash and preventing intrusion into the cab of the vehicle. To fully comprehend this process, you must understand the law of conservation of energy, particularly the forces of mechanical energy unleashed during a MVC. For more information, refer to Chapter 29, *Trauma Systems and Mechanism of Injury*.

▶ Alternative Power Vehicles

Many vehicles worldwide are now powered by something other than a traditional petroleum-based fuel (gasoline or diesel fuel). The term **alternative power vehicles** encompasses vehicles powered by electricity (supplied by batteries), liquefied petroleum gas, ethanol, biodiesel fuels, and other, less common alternative power sources.

Sources of Alternative Power

Electric and Hybrid Power. Electric vehicles are powered by hydrogen fuel cells, all-electric batteries, or a combination (hybrid) of gasoline and electric power. These are the most common types of alternative power vehicles rescuers are likely to encounter. In any vehicle that contains a battery or batteries, trained rescue personnel can secure the electrical system by disconnecting the batteries. Electric and hybrid vehicles contain large banks of batteries and high-voltage wires in various locations throughout. While the high-voltage wires, which are covered in orange insulation for easy identification, present a hazard, the high-voltage systems in hybrid and electric vehicles do shut down when the vehicle is powered down. The systems can be completely disabled by disconnecting the standard 12-volt car battery. The decision to do so and the disconnection procedure itself are typically the responsibility of the IC or rescue crew, who are aware of special considerations that may apply. For example, in alternative power vehicles, the standard car battery is often not found in its traditional location under the hood.

The less commonly encountered but more serious hazard is leakage of chemicals from damaged battery packs, releasing toxic gels, liquids, or gases. These chemicals should be handled in the same way as other hazardous materials.

Liquefied Petroleum Gas (LPG). Vehicles fueled by LPG are similar to traditionally fueled vehicles but use compressed propane gas (CPG) or a mixture of propane and butane, sometimes referred to as Autogas. Fuel sources similar to LPG include liquefied natural gas (LNG) and compressed natural gas (CNG). These fuels are most commonly used to power fleet vehicles, such as school buses, service or delivery trucks, or municipal vehicles, including some police vehicles.

Vehicles powered by hydrogen fuel cells, LPG, or other compressed gases present a hazard after a crash if large amounts of highly flammable or reactive gases leak from breached containers in or around the vehicle.

Ethanol and Flex Fuel. Vehicles powered by ethanol and flex fuel (a blend of up to 85% ethanol with gasoline, referred to as E85) are almost identical to traditional gasoline-powered vehicles in appearance and operation.

Biodiesel and Dimethyl Ether. These fuels for diesel engines are almost identical to their traditional diesel counterparts in appearance and operation.

Flex fuel, biodiesel, and other alternative fuels for gasoline or diesel engines may present various health, reactivity, and flammability hazards. They should be handled using the same procedures followed for leaking gasoline, diesel fuel, or other hazardous liquids.

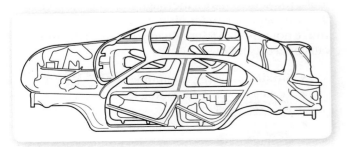

Figure 48-5 Unibody design.
© Jones & Bartlett Learning.

Words of Wisdom

A fire fueled by ethanol or methanol burns bright blue, and gives off little or no smoke, so it can be hard to see on a clear day.

Safety

While these vehicles present a range of safety concerns and special challenges to responding personnel, most basic safety procedures are the same at the scene of a MVC regardless of the vehicle. Evaluate the hazards presented by alternative power vehicles in the same careful way in which you would evaluate initial and evolving hazards at the scene of any other extrication or rescue incident. Follow these tips for managing alternative power vehicle hazards:

- Look for markings specific to alternative power vehicles, and call early for assistance **Figure 48-6** .
- Do not use flares to mark off the incident scene; use nonsparking markers, such as cones or reflective triangles.
- Stabilize the vehicle by engaging the brakes, setting the parking brake, putting the transmission in park (or neutral), turning off the ignition, and stabilizing the scene if applicable.
- A quiet hybrid or electric vehicle is not necessarily turned off or powered down.
- Be aware of the possibility of toxic vapors, gases, or fumes even if no fire is present. Also, remember, daylight may conceal the flames of a methanol- or ethanol-fueled fire.
- Avoid contact with any fluids leaking from the vehicle.
- Call for a hazardous materials team as soon as possible, and set up a safety zone around the perimeter.

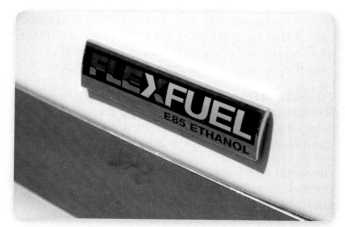

Figure 48-6 A flex fuel identification badge. Flex fuel vehicles are capable of running on either gasoline alone or a blend of up to 85% ethanol and 15% gasoline (referred to as E85).
© GIPhotoStock Z/Alamy.

▶ Hazardous Materials

Depending on the complexity of the incident, a vehicle extrication could require a specialized team to manage hazardous materials. For example, an accident involving a tanker or semitruck containing a known or unknown hazardous product would require hazardous materials personnel or a hazardous materials team to respond. Before approaching a wreck, consider additional hazards that may be posed by the vehicle or vehicles involved, such as fire hazards, electrical hazards, fuel sources, or liquid runoff. Keep in mind that the vehicle may be transporting hazardous materials that are not part of the vehicle itself.

In incidents involving hazardous materials, rescuers must follow a proper size-up and evaluation process. All too often in such incidents, rescue personnel are unnecessarily exposed to dangerous agents because they rush into the site before they've gathered vital information pertaining to the material or agent. Although responders trained at the awareness level have only limited participation in such scenarios, they can certainly assist operations- and technician-level responders by, for instance, looking through a set of binoculars to identify placards, product labels, numbers, and other information. They can also assist by sealing the site perimeter and referring to the DOT's *ERG* to identify the product, its flammability and incompatibilities, evacuation distances, and other pertinent data.

Words of Wisdom

Hazards can emerge at any time during an incident. Performing an individual scene size-up is crucial, but so is maintaining situational awareness. Report any immediate threats or evolving hazards to the appropriate person in the ICS.

▶ Hand Tools

A **hand tool** is any piece of equipment operated by human power. Hand tools are the basis of all working tools. In some instances, hand tools are more efficient than power tools. You should have a thorough working knowledge of the basic, simple hand tools used during any TRI even if you're not expected to use them yourself. Hand tools are categorized as follows:

- Striking tools (eg, a hammer) **Figure 48-7**
- Leverage/prying/spreading tools (eg, a pry bar) **Figure 48-8**
- Cutting tools (eg, trauma shears, glass handsaw) **Figure 48-9**
- Lifting/pushing/pulling tools (eg, hooks, pike poles) **Figure 48-10**

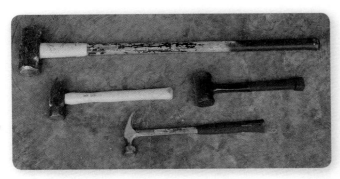

Figure 48-7 Striking tools.
© Jones & Bartlett Learning.

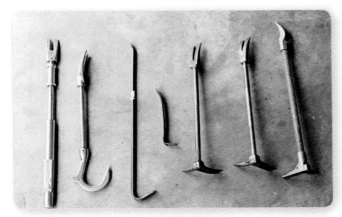

Figure 48-8 Leverage/prying/spreading tools.
© 2003 Berta A. Daniels.

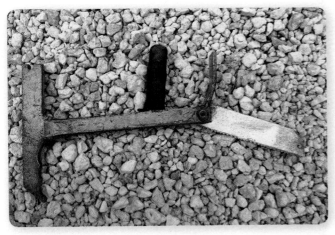

Figure 48-9 A cutting tool such as the Glass Master can be used to cut out a windshield.
Courtesy of David Sweet.

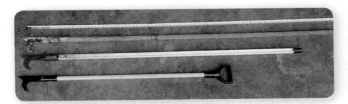

Figure 48-10 Lifting/pushing/pulling tools.
© Jones & Bartlett Learning.

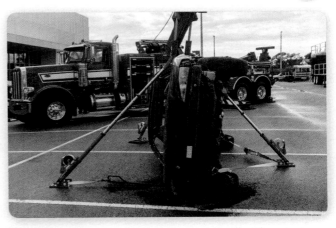

Figure 48-11 This vehicle is being stabilized with a strut.
© Lynn Palmer/Alamy.

▶ Vehicle Stabilization

Objects and vehicles that are unstable pose a threat because they may shift, slide, or fall, injuring victims, rescuers, or bystanders. These objects—most often, the damaged vehicles—need to be properly stabilized before your approach. Stabilization provides a solid foundation from which to work, ensuring safety for patients and rescuers. Specialized tools are sometimes required to stabilize a vehicle Figure 48-11 .

Alternative power vehicles are often identified by markings on the vehicle. Take basic actions to ensure the vehicle is stabilized: set the parking brake; operate any electric features of the vehicle to facilitate access or extrication, such as rolling down windows and adjusting seats; remove the ignition key; and put the vehicle in park.

Words of Wisdom

Even if it's not your job to use specialized equipment to stabilize a vehicle, as with any hazard, it will always be your job to identify the hazard and either correct it yourself or call for another resource to correct it.

Cribbing

The most basic physical support used for vehicle stabilization is **cribbing**. Cribbing is usually made of wood, plastic, composite material, or steel. Several cribbing designs, such as step chocks, wedges, shims, and box cribs, are used for extrication Figure 48-12 . **Step chocks** are specialized cribbing blocks made of wood, plastic, or composite material arranged in a step configuration. **Wedges** are tapered shafts of wood or other material used to snug loose cribbing under a load or fill a void. A **box crib** is a pallet-like framework that can be placed beneath a heavy load. **Shims** are similar to wedges but with a slimmer profile.

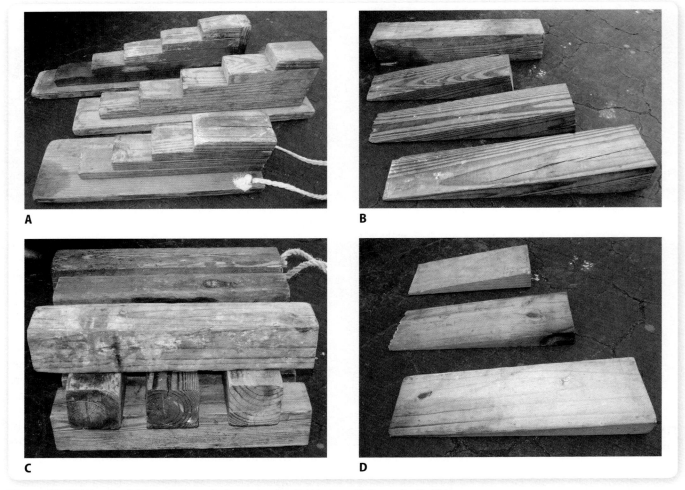

Figure 48-12 Wood cribbing designs. **A.** Step chocks. **B.** Wedges. **C.** Box crib. **D.** Shims.

Courtesy of David Sweet.

After cribbing has been placed, a vehicle may still move because of the give in the suspension system. The five directional movements are horizontal, vertical, roll, bounce, and yaw **Figure 48-13**. Such motion can occur as rescuers enter the vehicle or as patients are extricated from it, causing further injury.

After the vehicle is completely stabilized, set the parking brake, put the vehicle in park (or neutral), and turn off the engine.

▶ Gaining Access to the Patient

This section discusses simple vehicle access techniques.

Opening the Door

After stabilizing the vehicle, the simplest way to access a patient is to open a door. Doing so will allow you to

reach most patients, even those in upside-down vehicles. If the door nearest the patient doesn't work, try all of the others—even if they appear to be badly damaged. It's a waste of time and energy to open a jammed door with heavy rescue equipment when another door can be opened with no special equipment. Make sure the doors aren't locked. If all the doors are locked, consider breaking a window (using the techniques described in

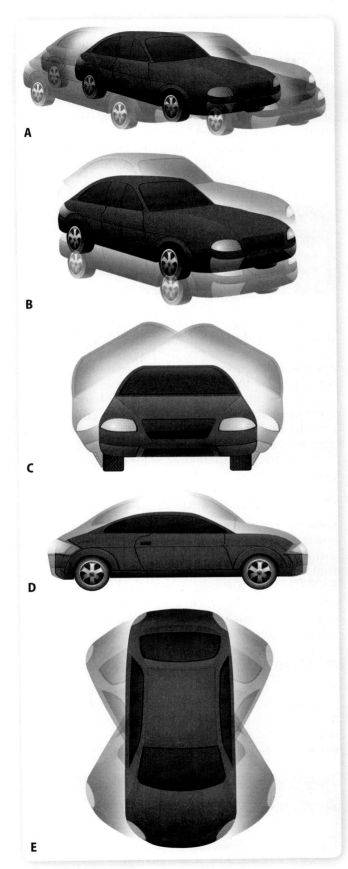

Figure 48-13 Five directional movements. **A.** Horizontal. **B.** Vertical. **C.** Roll. **D.** Bounce. **E.** Yaw.

this chapter), and then attempt to manually unlock the doors. The golden rule of forcible entry and extrication is "Try before your pry!"

> **Words of Wisdom**
>
> Energy-absorbing bumpers can explode when subjected to heat and can spring out when loaded.

Breaking Tempered Glass

If a patient's medical condition is serious enough to require immediate care and you cannot enter the vehicle through a door, consider breaking a window. Auto glass is either tempered or laminated **Figure 48-14** . Side and rear windows are typically made of **tempered glass**, which is designed to break easily into small pieces and shatters easily when hit with a pointed object, such as a spring-loaded center punch or other sharp hand tool **Figure 48-15** . Because these windows don't pose as great a safety threat, they can be your primary access route.

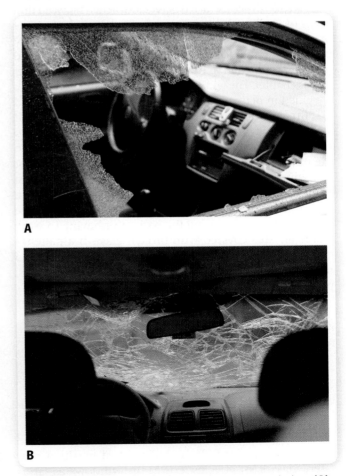

Figure 48-14 Types of glass in vehicles: tempered glass **(A)** and laminated windshield glass **(B)**.

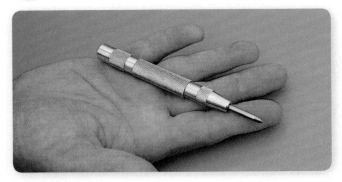

Figure 48-15 For tempered glass, a spring-loaded center punch is the most basic and common of all glass removal tools.

© Jones & Bartlett Learning. Courtesy of MIEMSS.

Some newer vehicles have windows and sunroofs or moonroofs constructed of polycarbonate, which is stronger, lighter, and much harder to break than tempered glass. Avoid obtaining access through a window that feels like plastic.

Do not try to break and enter through the windshield, because it is probably made of laminated glass, which cannot be broken with a spring-loaded center punch. **Laminated glass** is specially constructed glass sandwiched between thin layers of flexible plastic. When it's struck by a sharp stone or center punch, a weblike crack appears, but the structure of the glass remains intact. For this reason, the windshield must be removed in one large piece, as we will discuss later in this chapter. The windshields of most passenger vehicles are glued in place with a strong plastic adhesive.

Breaking the rear window or a side window will sometimes create an opening large enough for you to reach the patient if there is no rapid way to gain access to the passenger compartment. If you must break a side or rear window to gain access, choose the window farthest from the patient or patients, and hit it in the corner, rather than in the center. This approach will minimize the likelihood of injuring the patient or having to work inside an area covered with broken glass. If a patient's condition warrants your immediate entry, however, do not hesitate to break the closest window. If access allows, place a blanket over the patient first.

Words of Wisdom

Always warn trapped passengers that you are going to break the glass!

During this step of the rescue, all rescuers should be wearing proper PPE, including dust mask, gloves, safety glasses, or goggles. Lower the windows as far as possible before breaking the glass. If the window cannot be lowered, place tape on the outside of the window in a "star of life" pattern to help minimize shattering and make it easier to remove broken glass before entry. If you are using something other than a spring-loaded center punch, such as an axe or screwdriver, always aim for a low corner; the window frame will help prevent the tool from entering the vehicle and striking the person inside. Give other EMS personnel a verbal warning, "Breaking glass!" unless a stop/freeze call is made. After breaking the window, use a hand tool to clean out the remaining glass in the window frame so it does not fall onto passengers or injure rescuers. Place the debris in an area where it won't pose a hazard.

Words of Wisdom

Do not use a sledgehammer to crack a walnut. Use the right tool!

To break tempered glass using a spring-loaded center punch, follow the steps in Skill Drill 48-1 .

Once you've removed the remaining fragments of tempered glass from the frame, try again to unlock the door. Release the locking mechanism, and then use both the inside and the outside door handles at the same time. This action may force open a jammed lock, even in a door that is badly damaged. If you cannot gain access to the vehicle using any of these methods, heavier extrication tools must be brought in and trained personnel summoned.

Providing Initial Medical Care

Once you've entered the vehicle and accessed the patient, you must begin to provide emergency medical care. This includes assessment and management of the ABCDEs. Patient care should occur simultaneously with extrication Figure 48-16 . Although it may be necessary to delay some elements of care for short periods, your goal is to stabilize the patient and remove him or her from the vehicle as quickly and safely as possible.

▶ Disentangling the Patient

The next step in the vehicle extrication sequence is disentangling the patient, the process of removing the parts of the vehicle in which he or she is ensnared. The goal is to remove the sheet metal and plastic from around the patient—not to "cut the patient out of the vehicle."

Words of Wisdom

A good extrication is a safe extrication.

Before attempting disentanglement, study the situation. What is trapping the patient in the vehicle? Is he or she wearing a seat belt? Have all airbags been deployed?

Skill Drill 48-1 Breaking Tempered Glass Using a Spring-Loaded Center Punch

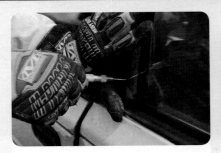 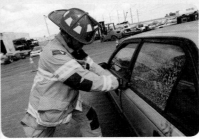 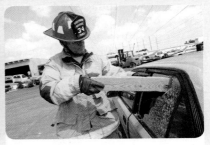

Step 1 Take standard precautions and don the appropriate PPE. Ensure the scene is safe and the vehicle stable. Using the window farthest from the patient, place the palm of your hand facedown against the lower corner of the window and frame, with your index finger and thumb facing upward. Position and rest the body of the spring-loaded center punch in the ridge section of your palm (the V-section of your hand) between your index finger and thumb.

Step 2 Ensure the patient is protected from flying glass. Verbally warn personnel, "Breaking glass!" With the tip of the tool directly on the glass, apply pressure until the spring is activated and the glass breaks.

Step 3 Use a piece of cribbing to remove the remaining fragments of tempered glass from around the window frame.

© Jones & Bartlett Learning. Photographed by Glen E. Ellman.

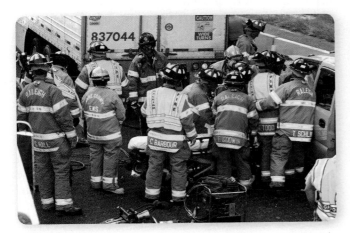

Figure 48-16 Patient care should occur simultaneously with extrication.
© Mike Legeros. Used with permission.

Perform only the disentanglement procedures necessary to remove the patient safely from the vehicle. The order in which you perform them will be dictated by the specific conditions at the incident. Many times it will be necessary to perform one procedure before you can access the parts of the vehicle needed to perform another. For example, you must find and disable undeployed airbags before removing the patient.

Before the patient is disentangled, he or she should be covered with a blanket or protected by using a backboard. Ensure the patient understands what you're doing; the noise of the extrication procedure can be frightening for patients.

To develop expertise in disentangling a patient, you must take an approved extrication course. The following sections provide an overview of the procedures most commonly performed.

Airbag Safety

In modern vehicles, most of the passenger compartment is protected by a variety of airbag systems. Airbag systems are marked with symbols or badges containing abbreviations such as SRS (supplemental restraint system) and HPS (head protection system). These markings are generally located close to the airbag inflator.

No modern airbag system is mechanically deployed. Each system is controlled by a computer that measures forces applied during a MVC and makes an instantaneous determination of which systems should be triggered and whether a passenger is currently occupying the seat position to be protected. Although the computer may retain power for 10 to 30 minutes after the vehicle's power is cut, unless the airbag system is itself damaged during the rescue operation, undamaged and undeployed airbag systems are designed not to self-deploy after a crash. Still, it is prudent to avoid operating unnecessarily in the deployment area of an airbag system immediately after the crash.

Words of Wisdom

A seat belt pre-tensioning system is designed to tighten automatically, eliminating slack when a crash is detected. Such systems are sometimes activated simultaneously with the airbags and sometimes act independently.

Remember the following when you are dealing with airbag systems:

- An airbag that has deployed during a crash presents no safety hazard for rescuers.
- If the airbags did not deploy, disconnect the battery and allow the airbag capacitor to discharge. The time required to discharge the capacitor varies from one model of airbag to another.
- Do not place a hard object, such as a backboard, between the patient and an undeployed airbag.
- Do not attempt to cut a steering wheel if the steering column contains an undeployed airbag.
- For your safety, avoid working in the deployment area of airbags and restraint systems.

Displacing the Seat

In a frontal or rear-end collision, the vehicle may be compressed. The front of the vehicle is pushed back, restricting space between the steering wheel and the seat. Displacing the seat, then, can relieve pressure on the driver and give rescuers more room for removal.

To displace a seat backward, begin with the simplest steps. Many times you can gain some room by moving the seat backward on its track, especially with short drivers who had been driving with the seat forward. Before you move the seat back, first be sure to immobilize the spine. With manually operated seats, you need only release the seat-adjusting lever and carefully slide the seat back as far as it will go. If the seat is electrically operated, check that the vehicle has power, and engage the lever to slide the seat backward. If these methods are unsuccessful, you may need to perform a seat displacement.

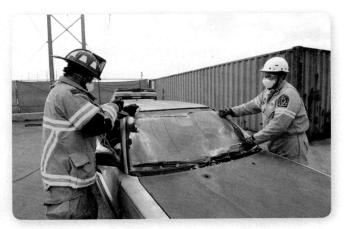

Figure 48-17 A technical rescuer removing the windshield with a glass handsaw.
© Jones & Bartlett Learning. Photographed by Glen E. Ellman.

Removing the Windshield

A second technique that's often necessary for disentanglement is glass removal. Removing the rear window, side glass, or windshield improves communication between rescue personnel inside and outside the vehicle. Sometimes all you need to do is roll down a window. Open windows allow you to pass medical supplies to the personnel inside.

When the roof must be taken off, all of the glass in the vehicle must first be removed. The windshield of a damaged vehicle may be removed by a trained technical rescuer using a glass handsaw **Figure 48-17** .

Removing the Roof

Removing the roof of a vehicle provides additional space, giving EMS better access to the patient and alleviating the patient's feeling of panic caused by being confined inside a wrecked vehicle. Equipment can be more easily passed into the vehicle, and rescuers have better visibility and more space to perform disentanglement. Both the provider and the patient will benefit from the improved air circulation too. Furthermore, removing the roof creates a large exit route for the patient.

A key consideration in displacing the roof is the safety of the rescuers and patient inside the vehicle. In particular, as you cut the roof posts, you must support the roof to keep it from falling on those inside the vehicle. Roof removal may be performed by a trained technical rescuer **Figure 48-18** .

Displacing the Dash

During a frontal collision, the vehicle's dash may be pushed down or backward. When a patient is trapped by the dash, it must be moved using a technique called the dash roll **Figure 48-19** . Its objective is to lift the dash up and move it forward. The process requires pushing or rolling the entire front end of the vehicle—the dashboard, steering wheel, and steering column—off of the entrapped

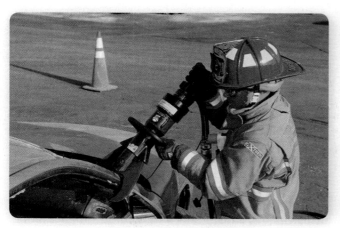

Figure 48-18 A technical rescuer removing the roof.
© Jones & Bartlett Learning. Photographed by Glen E. Ellman.

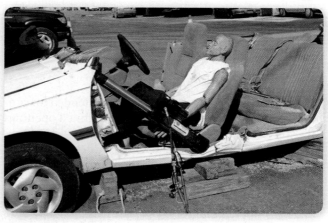

Figure 48-19 The dash roll technique.
© Jones & Bartlett Learning. Photographed by Glen E. Ellman.

occupant. The roof can be removed before a dash roll can be performed. Alternatively, a dash roll can be performed by cutting both A posts segmentally: each A post is cut as low as possible and again, at the level the windshield, it is cut transversely.

The dash roll technique, which may be performed only by a trained technical rescuer, requires a hydraulic cutter. A tool such as the hydraulic ram then pushes the dash forward. The opening made with these tools is maintained with cribbing.

YOU ▶ are the Paramedic   PART 3

You gain entry to the vehicle, make contact with the patient, and immediately notice that the dashboard and left side door have been pushed in and down, partially trapping the patient's lower extremities. You advise the rescue crew that you have limited ability to assess the patient, who now begins to report pain in her left leg. She continues to be concerned and anxious about having been in a crash. You calmly reassure her that all efforts are being made to get her out of the vehicle safely.

After working for about 15 minutes, the rescue crew has displaced the dashboard enough to allow for a full assessment, which reveals tenderness in both sides of the rib cage, with diminished breath sounds bilaterally and symmetric chest rise. The abdomen is soft and tender to palpation of the lower quadrants. The lower portion of the abdomen is bruised beneath the umbilicus. You note a 3-inch (8-cm) laceration of the left thigh, with venous bleeding. You ask your partner, who is outside the vehicle, to obtain IV access with a 18-gauge catheter in the left antecubital space and to initiate a normal saline drip using a 10-drop set running at 10 drops per minute. In the meantime, you focus on controlling bleeding from the leg laceration. Your partner also performs a finger stick to obtain the patient's blood glucose level; the result is 183 mg/dL.

Recording Time: 30 Minutes	
Respirations	22 breaths/min
Pulse	Radial pulse, 126 beats/min, regular and strong
Skin	Pale, warm, diaphoretic
Blood pressure	104/62 mm Hg
Oxygen saturation (Spo₂)	96% on 15 L/min nonrebreathing mask
Pupils	PERRLA

5. Patients requiring extrication often become anxious. What can you do to help calm the patient?
6. In what ways, if any, is this patient at risk of developing crush syndrome?

Additional Specialized Rescue Situations

▶ Confined Spaces

A **confined space** is a structure that is not intended for continuous occupancy and that usually has limited openings for entry and exit. Confined spaces can be found in farm, commercial, and industrial settings. Structures ranging from automobile trunks to grain silos, industrial pits, and below-ground shafts are all considered confined spaces. Confined spaces found in many residential settings include cisterns, well casings, and septic tanks **Figure 48-20** .

Confined spaces present a special hazard because ventilation may be too limited to facilitate adequate air circulation and exchange. The result is an oxygen-deficient atmosphere that may contain poisonous gases. Technical rescue teams must use air sampling monitors to check the atmosphere before making entry. Entering a confined space without doing so and without the proper breathing apparatus can be a fatal mistake.

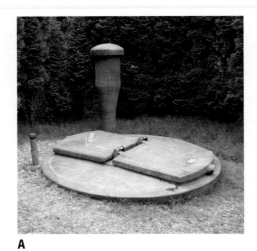

A

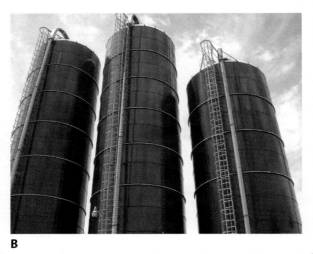

B

Figure 48-20 Confined spaces. **A.** Below ground. **B.** Silo.

A: © Tyler Boyes/Shutterstock; B: © Joan Stabnaw/Shutterstock.

Confined spaces present other risks too. Inadequate ventilation may trap flammable mixtures, presenting a threat of fire or explosion. The contents of a grain silo or trench can suddenly engulf a rescuer like quicksand. Large pieces of machinery often contain confined spaces studded with augers or screws. Any piece of equipment, even if turned off or disconnected from a power source, may contain stored electrical energy, posing a threat of electrocution. Rescuers must never attempt a rescue without proper training.

Do not be overwhelmed by the urgency to begin treating patients; scene safety must always be considered first. Keep in mind that a confined-space call is sometimes dispatched as a heart attack or medical illness call, because the caller assumes that the person who entered the confined space became unresponsive because of a heart attack or medical illness.

> ## Words of Wisdom
>
> Confined spaces such as manholes can be deceptive. They may look survivable, but they can contain unseen hazards, such as inadequate oxygen or toxic, invisible gases.

Oxygen Deficiency and Poisonous Gases

Gases can range from colored to clear and be odorless or have a characteristic smell. Specific situations lend themselves to potential gas presence. Part of scene size-up should be to keep potential gas hazards in mind.

Hydrogen sulfide (H_2S) is a colorless, toxic, flammable gas released as bacteria break down organic matter in the absence of oxygen. It can be found in swamps, standing water, sewers, volcanic gases, natural gas, and in some wells. Hydrogen sulfide is heavier than air and has a pungent odor at first, but quickly deadens a person's sense of smell.

Carbon monoxide (CO) is a colorless, odorless, tasteless gas that cannot be detected by a person's normal senses. Inhaling carbon monoxide gas can result in severe poisoning, because the carbon monoxide molecule binds to the hemoglobin molecule in red blood cells, displacing the oxygen molecules to which the cells would normally bind. A small quantity of carbon monoxide can thereby monopolize the red blood cells and prevent them from transporting oxygen to the body. The signs and symptoms of carbon monoxide poisoning include headache, nausea, disorientation, and unconsciousness.

Carbon dioxide (CO_2) is a colorless gas associated with asphyxiation. It's used to make dry ice and is found in fire extinguishers. It produces a sour taste in the mouth and a stinging sensation in the nose and mouth.

Methane (CH_4)—the principal component of natural gas—is not toxic but will cause burns if ignited. Flammable or explosive mixtures of methane form at lower concentrations than those required for asphyxiation. Methane is used as a fuel from natural gas fields but can also be generated from fermentation of organic matter (eg, manure, waste water, sludge, or municipal solid waste).

Ammonia (NH_3) is a toxic, corrosive chemical with a characteristic pungent odor. Because ammonia gas is lighter than air, it rises to the top of any confined space in which it is trapped. It's typically found in rural areas and is used extensively in agriculture as a crop fertilizer.

Nitrogen dioxide (NO_2) is a red-brown gas with a characteristic sharp, biting odor. It's a primary component of polluted air and is toxic when inhaled.

Safe Approach

As you approach a confined-space rescue scene, look for bystanders who might have witnessed the emergency. Gathering information before the technical rescue team arrives will save valuable time later. Do not assume that a person in a pit, for example, has experienced a medical emergency, such as a heart attack; instead, assume there is an IDLH atmosphere at any confined-space call. An IDLH atmosphere is one that can immediately incapacitate anyone who enters the space without breathing protection. Inevitably, it will take some time for qualified rescuers to arrive on the scene and prepare for safe entry. The person at the original incident may have died before your arrival; do not become part of the problem and make an entry prior to atmospheric monitoring.

Assisting Other Rescuers

You can prevent a confined-space incident from becoming worse by recognizing it, securing the scene, and ensuring that no one enters the space until additional rescue resources arrive.

As trained and equipped personnel arrive, you can help by giving a situation report. Then compare observed conditions with reported conditions and determine if they've changed. Whether an incident appears to be stable or has changed significantly since the first report will affect the operation strategy for the rescue. This scene size-up should be relayed to the specialized rescue team members when they arrive at the scene. Include in your situation report a description of any rescue attempts that have been made, exposures, hazards, extinguishment of fires, the facts and probabilities of the scene, the status and resources of the fire company, an identification of any hazardous materials present, and a progress evaluation.

Confined-space rescues can be complex and lengthy. You may be asked to assist by bringing rescue equipment to the scene, maintaining a charged hose line, or handling crowd control. By understanding the hazards of confined spaces, you will be better prepared to help a specialized team deal with a confined-space emergency.

▶ Trenches

When earth is removed for placement of a utility line or for other construction, the sides of the excavation can

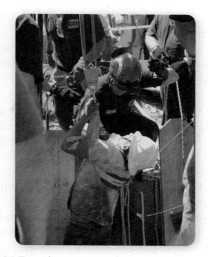

Figure 48-21 Trench rescue.
Courtesy of Captain David Jackson, Saginaw Township Fire Department.

collapse, trapping a worker **Figure 48-21**. Entrapment may also occur when a child plays around a pile of sand or earth that collapses. Unfortunately, many entrapments occur because required safety precautions were not taken.

After a collapse, the collapsed product is unstable and prone to further collapse. In addition, earth and sand are heavy, and a person who is partly entrapped can't simply be pulled out. Instead, he or she must be carefully dug out after **shoring** has stabilized the sides of the excavation. Rescuers should make entry only after shoring has been put in place.

Generating vibrations or placing additional weight on top of displaced earth will increase the probability of **secondary collapse**. A secondary collapse is one that occurs after the initial collapse; it can be caused by equipment vibrations, personnel standing at the edge of the trench, or water washing away the soil. Soil that has been removed from the excavation and placed in a pile is called the **spoil pile**. Avoid disturbing this material; it's unstable and may collapse if placed too close to the excavation.

Safe removal of a trapped person requires a special rescue team trained and equipped to erect shoring that will protect the rescuers and the entrapped person from secondary collapse.

Words of Wisdom

Most trench collapses occur in trenches measuring less than 12 feet (3.7 m) deep and 6 feet (1.8 m) wide. In a collapse, a person is suddenly covered with heavy soil, resulting in asphyxiation.

Safe Approach

Safety is of paramount importance as you approach a trench or excavation collapse. To avoid triggering a secondary collapse, stay away from the edge of the site and keep all workers and bystanders away. In addition, vibrations generated by equipment and machinery can touch off a secondary collapse, so shut down all heavy equipment. Even vibrations caused by nearby traffic can cause collapse, so it may be necessary to stop or divert the flow of traffic.

Make verbal contact with the trapped person if you can do so without placing yourself in danger. Let the trapped person know that a trained rescue team is on the way. If you approach the trench, do so from the narrow end, where the soil is more stable. However, it's best *not* to approach the trench unless absolutely necessary; EMS providers should stay out of a trench unless they've been properly trained in confined-space rescue.

By keeping people away from the edges of the excavation, shutting down machinery, and establishing contact with the patient, you start the rescue process. You can also size up the scene, looking for evidence of where the trapped workers may be located. Hand tools and hard hats are one such indicator. Questioning other workers may also help EMS providers determine where the trapped people were last seen.

▶ Water

Almost all EMS departments must perform water rescue in sites ranging from small streams and swimming pools to rivers, lakes, reservoirs, and oceans. A static body of water, such as a lake, may have no current and is considered flat or slow-moving water. In contrast, a whitewater stream or flooded river may have a swift current. During a flood, even a dry wash in the desert can quickly become a site of raging water.

You may suddenly find yourself immersed during a water rescue, so you should be aware of self-rescue techniques. If you are suddenly pulled into a swift current, you should adopt the **self-rescue position**. The first step is to roll into a faceup, arched position. To avoid contact with objects below the surface, keep your lower back higher than your feet. Keep your feet together and facing in the direction of travel—in other words, float feetfirst—with your arms at your sides, your head down, and your chin tucked in. Keeping toes above surface of water can help prevent feet from getting snagged by objects unseen under the water surface. Use your hands to change direction as needed to avoid objects and to divert your path out of the raging current.

Cold Water Rescue

Water temperature varies widely by season and by geographic area. Even on warm days, the water temperature

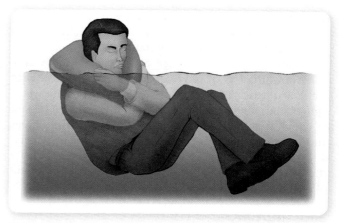

Figure 48-22 The heat-escape-lessening position.
© Jones & Bartlett Learning.

can be low. Water causes heat loss 25 times greater than ambient air temperature. Indeed, any water temperature of less than 98.6°F (37°C) will cause hypothermia; patients who become hypothermic lose the ability to self-rescue. Maintaining body heat is crucial because hypothermia poses an immediate threat, quickly progressing to unconsciousness and death. In extremely cold water (35°F [2°C]), a person is likely to die after 15 to 20 minutes of submersion.

If you find yourself in cold water, make every effort to keep your face above the water, protect your head, minimize movement, and assume the heat-escape-lessening position (HELP) **Figure 48-22**, which helps keep heat in the core of your body. HELP requires a personal flotation device and consists of drawing the knees close to the chest, pressing the arms close to the sides of the body, and keeping the head and neck out of the water. In a group, victims should huddle together to share body warmth.

A person immersed in water colder than 70°F (21°C) may benefit from a phenomenon known as the **cold-protective response**. Essentially, when the body is submerged in cold water, heat is conducted from the body to the water. The resulting hypothermia can protect vital organs from the lack of oxygen. In addition, exposure to cold water will occasionally activate certain primitive reflexes that may preserve bodily functions for prolonged periods. In one case, for example, a 2½-year-old girl recovered fully after being submerged in cold water for at least 66 minutes. For this reason, you should continue to provide full resuscitative efforts for a person who has been submerged in cold water until he or she either responds or is pronounced dead by a physician. See Chapter 38,

Environmental Emergencies, for a more detailed discussion of hypothermia.

Whenever a person dives or jumps into cold water, the diving reflex—the slowing of the heart rate caused by submersion in cold water—may cause immediate bradycardia. Although loss of consciousness may follow, the person may be able to survive for an extended time under water because of a lowered metabolic rate and decreased oxygen demand and consumption associated with hypothermia.

> ### Words of Wisdom
> Remember, hypothermic patients are often dehydrated due to "cold diuresis" and should be removed from the water in a horizontal position to avoid sudden orthostatic changes. In addition, hypothermia makes the heart prone to arrhythmias that can be induced by sudden exertion, so minimize patient activity as you extract them from the water.

Other Water Rescue Situations

In North America, the most common swift water rescue scenario involves people who have attempted to drive through floodwaters. The vehicle stalls in the high water, leaving the occupants stranded in a rising stream or creek with a swift current. If the water rises high enough, the vehicle can be swept away. These incidents are especially dangerous for rescue personnel because it can be hard to determine the depth of the water around the vehicle.

In surface water rescue, rescuers must consider hazards such as the dangerous hydraulics created by moving water. In addition, so-called strainers—floating objects such as trees, branches, debris, or wire mesh—can pose a serious risk for rescuers. Dams and hydroelectric sites are treacherous for even the most skilled rescuer. The height of a dam has no bearing on the severity of the threat to rescuers. Intakes at the base of a dam can act like drains, sucking rescuers down into them. Low-head dams are often associated with dangerous recirculating currents (sometimes referred to as a "boil") **Figure 48-23** . These currents can trap victims and unwary rescuers alike, dragging them underwater, away from the dam, and back to the surface, where the cycle repeats itself. For this reason, low-head dams are often referred to in the field as "drowning machines." Never underestimate the power or intensity of moving water.

> ### Words of Wisdom
> The hydraulics of moving water change with variables such as depth, velocity, and obstruction of flow.

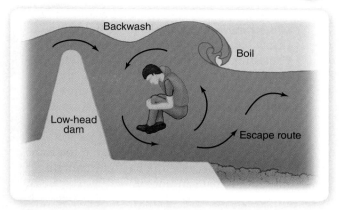

Figure 48-23 Recirculating current at a low-head dam.
© Jones & Bartlett Learning.

Safe Approach

When you respond to a water rescue incident, your safety and that of other rescuers is your primary concern. Your standard EMS gear is not designed for water rescue activities. For anyone working within 10 feet (3 m) of the water or with someone performing a water rescue, the minimum PPE includes a properly sized and certified type III **personal flotation device (PFD)**. You must be familiar with the manufacturer's procedures for donning and removing the PFD. All straps should be tightened, with hanging straps secured to prevent entanglement. Any rescuer directly involved must also have thermal protection, a helmet appropriate for water rescue, a cutting device, a whistle, contamination protection (if necessary), and foot protection, such as wetsuit-type booties. If you're working near but not in the water, shoes that provide solid traction when wet are preferable to standard hard-soled work boots.

If you are a part of the first arriving ambulance crew at the scene of a water rescue, try to communicate with the person in the water, who may be in a vehicle or holding on to a tree or other solid object. Let the person know that more help is on the way.

Do not exceed your level of training and resources. If you can't swim, working around or near water is not recommended. Even someone trained as a lifeguard for still water is not prepared to enter flowing water with a strong current, such as that of a river, stream, or the ocean. Make sure bystanders do not try to rescue the patient and place themselves in a situation from which they too must be rescued.

When you see a person struggling in the water, your first impulse may be to jump in to help. Doing so, however, endangers your life and may not result in a successful rescue. The model most commonly used in water rescue is *reach-throw-row-go*:

- **Reach.** First attempt to *reach* out to the threatened person, using any readily available object. If the person is close to shore, a branch, pole, oar, or paddle may be long enough.

- **Throw.** If you can't reach the person, *throw* something—for example, a life buoy or a throw bag. A throw bag is rescue device consisting of a small sack that contains two ropes and a piece of foam. In an emergency, a rescuer opens the bag, pulls out enough rope to grasp firmly (some rescuers prefer to wrap the rope around their backs), and then throws the bag to the threatened person. He or she is then instructed to grab the rope, not the bag, because the bag may contain more rope that can uncoil.
- **Row.** If you can't reach the drowning person by throwing something that floats, you may be able to *row* out to the person in a small boat or canoe if one is available. Do so only if you know how to propel and steer the craft. Protect yourself by wearing an approved PFD.
- **Go.** As a last resort, *go* into the water to save the threatened person. Enter the water only if you are a capable swimmer trained to the level of swift water rescue.

Words of Wisdom

Personal flotation devices must be worn by all personnel operating near the water.

Many departments in cold geographic regions have developed specialized equipment to assist in ice rescue. Throwing a rope or flotation device may initially be helpful. Ladders can be used to distribute the weight of the rescuer on ice-covered water. You can create a flotation buoy using specially designed hose lines that have end caps and an air line. You can wear a specialized rescue suit designed to prevent hypothermia and supply flotation. If your department is involved in ice rescue, you should receive training in these specialized procedures.

Recovery Situations

On occasion, you may be called to the scene of a drowning at which the patient is not floating or visible in the water. An organized rescue effort in these circumstances calls for personnel who are experienced in a range of recovery techniques and who know how to use specialized equipment, including snorkels, masks, and scuba gear. As a last resort, when standard recovery procedures are unsuccessful, you may have to use a grappling hook or other large hook to drag the river bottom, for example, where the patient is thought to have gone under. Although the hook could seriously wound a submerged person, it may be the only effective way to bring him or her to the surface for resuscitative efforts.

▶ Spinal Injuries in Submersion Incidents

Submersion incidents may be complicated by spinal fractures or other spinal cord injuries. When spinal injury is suspected, the neck must be protected from further injury. Refer to the spinal motion restriction assessment guidelines in Chapter 34, *Head and Spine Trauma*. Follow the steps in Skill Drill 48-2 .

▶ Rope Rescue

Rope rescue is the most versatile and widely used technical rescue skill. Sometimes rope rescue can remove a person from a perilous position.

Types of Rope Rescue

Rope rescue incidents are divided into low-angle and high-angle operations. **Low-angle operations** are situations in which the slope of the ground over which the rescuers are working is less than a 45° angle. In such cases, rescuers depend on the ground for their primary support, and the rope system serves as a secondary means of support. For example, a rope stretched from the top of an embankment can be used for support by rescuers who are carrying a patient up an incline.

A low-angle operation is used when ropes are needed to pull or haul up a patient or rescuer, such as when lifelines are placed during ice or water rescue. Such an operation is typically necessary when the footing is inadequate or slippery—on a dirt or rock embankment, for instance. In such an incident, a rope is tied to your harness and you climb the embankment by yourself, using the rope to keep from falling.

Ropes can also be used to help raise or lower a basket stretcher. This technique frees you from having to carry all of the weight over rough terrain. Rescuers at the top of the embankment can use a rope system to help pull up or lower the basket.

Words of Wisdom

There should be a minimum of six rescuers on basket stretchers, and extra teams of six should be rotated when the patient needs to be carried a long distance.

When rescue personnel are using any rope system to assist in rescue operations, a safety measure is to **belay** the rope. In climbing, belaying is a technique in which you control the rope as it is fed out to the climbers to protect them in the event of a fall. A vital part of the climbing system, belaying can be accomplished with a self-belay or with a secondary lifeline. One possible complication is that belays depend on the angle of operations; as a

Skill Drill 48-2 Stabilizing a Suspected Spinal Injury in the Water

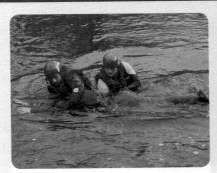

Step 1 Turn the patient supine by rotating the entire upper half of the patient's body as a single unit. Twisting only the head, for example, may aggravate any injury to the cervical spine. Two rescuers are usually required to turn the patient safely, although one may suffice.

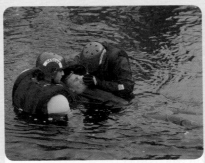

Step 2 As soon as the patient is turned, have the other rescuer support the head and trunk as a unit while you open the airway and begin artificial ventilation using the mouth-to-mouth method or a pocket mask. Immediate ventilation is the primary treatment of all submersion patients as soon as the patient is faceup in the water.

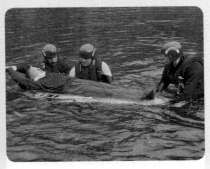

Step 3 Float a buoyant backboard under the patient as you continue ventilation.

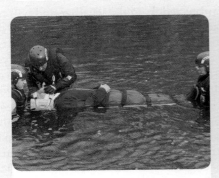

Step 4 Secure the trunk and head of the patient to the backboard to eliminate motion of the cervical spine. Do not remove the patient from the water until this is done.

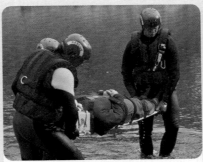

Step 5 Remove the patient from the water, on the backboard.

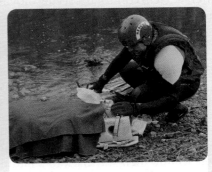

Step 6 Remove the patient's wet clothes and cover him or her with a blanket. Administer supplemental oxygen if the patient is breathing adequately; give positive-pressure ventilation if he or she is apneic or breathing inadequately. Begin cardiopulmonary resuscitation if breathing and pulse are absent.

consequence, the entire load may be transferred to the belay line. This could prove dangerous, depending on the load and the length of the rope.

Another aspect of climbing or rescue situations is the descent. In some descents, the angle is so severe that rescuers must use a technique known as rappelling. To **rappel** is to descend on a fixed rope. **Scrambling**, a method used to ascend rocky faces and ridges, can be described as a cross between hill climbing and rock climbing. These are technical rescue skills that require additional training and resources beyond your paramedic course.

High-angle operations are situations in which the slope of the ground is greater than a 45° angle and rescuers or patients depend on a life safety rope, not a fixed surface of support such as the ground. High-angle rescue techniques are used to raise or lower a person when other means of doing so are not readily available. Such rescues are extremely demanding and dangerous and should be attempted only by expertly trained personnel.

Safe Approach

If you respond to an incident requiring rope rescue, consider both your safety and that of those around you. A rope rescue is among the most time-consuming calls you'll encounter. Extensive setup is necessary, and a considerable amount of equipment must be assembled before you initiate the rescue. Protect your safety by staying clear of the area below the patient and avoiding any loose material that might fall. Help control the scene, moving bystanders to an area where they cannot be injured.

▶ Wilderness Search and Rescue

Wilderness **search and rescue (SAR)** missions, conducted by a limited number of departments, consist of two parts: search (looking for a lost or overdue person) and rescue (removing a person from a hostile environment).

Several types of situations may prompt initiation of an SAR mission. Small children may wander off and be unable to find their way back to a familiar place. Older adults with dementia may forget where they're going and become lost. People who are hiking, hunting, or participating in other wilderness activities may get lost if they lack the right training or equipment. SAR missions may also be initiated if people are caught unaware by unexpected weather changes or if they become sick or injured.

Safe Approach

The term "wilderness" can cover many different environments, such as forests, mountains, deserts, parks, animal refuges, and rain forests. Depending on the terrain and environmental factors, the wilderness can be as little as a few feet off the roadway or several hours' trek into the backcountry. Even with a short access time, the scene could require an extensive evacuation and, thus, qualify as a wilderness incident. Terrain hazards include cliffs, steep slopes, caves, wells, mines, avalanches, rivers, streams, valleys, beaches, and rock slides.

When you participate in an SAR mission, prepare for the weather conditions by bringing drinking water, food, suitable clothing, and the correct PPE for the mission. A handheld strobe light may help paramedics keep track of each other in a crowd or in rural or wilderness locations. Strobe lights are lightweight, durable, and readily visible at night at a distance of approximately 1 mile (1.6 km).

Make sure you don't exceed your physical limitations and don't become embroiled in a situation beyond your ability to handle. Call for a special wilderness rescue team, depending on the situation and your local protocols.

▶ Lost Person Search and Rescue

When a person gets lost in the outdoors and a search effort is initiated, an ambulance is usually summoned to the search base. Each search team is then organized to include a member of EMS. This provider carries the essential equipment to provide simple immediate care. Your role is to stand by at the search base until the lost person or people have been found.

As soon as you arrive at the scene and have been briefed on the situation, you should isolate and prepare the equipment you'll need to carry into the patient's location so that no time is lost when you find the person, or if a member of the search team becomes injured during the search. The prepared carry-in equipment, including a backboard and other equipment you will need to immobilize the patient, should be left in the back of the ambulance. There it will be protected from the weather and will not need to be reloaded (and possibly be left behind) if the ambulance needs to be relocated. You'll usually be given a portable radio tuned to the search frequency so that you can monitor the progress of the search and communicate with and be contacted by those in charge of the operation.

Sometimes you may be asked to stay at the scene with relatives of the lost person. Find out from them whether the lost person has any pertinent medical history, and pass this information along to those in charge of the search. Unless you've been instructed otherwise, only incident command should communicate any news or progress of the search to the family. For this reason, you must be sure that your radio is set to a discreet volume.

Safe Approach

Once the lost person has been found, you'll be guided by search personnel to that location or to a prearranged intersection to which the patient will be carried to decrease the amount of time you need to reach the patient and begin treatment. You should be sure that the carry-in equipment is evenly distributed among personnel and that you proceed at a pace that allows all personnel to stay together easily. Sometimes the time and effort necessary to reach and carry out the patient can be decreased by relocating the ambulance or, if available, by using a four-wheel drive or all-terrain vehicle. As with other technical rescues, although the ambulance crew will assume responsibility for patient care once it reaches the patient's side, cooperation between EMS and the search team is necessary to safely carry the patient to the base and load him or her into the waiting ambulance.

▶ Structure Fires

In most areas, an ambulance is dispatched with the fire department apparatus to any structure fire, regardless of whether injuries are reported. A fire in a house, apartment building, office, school, plant, warehouse, or other building is considered a structure fire. When you respond to a fire scene, you should determine whether any special route will be necessary because of the fire. Once you arrive at the scene, you must park the ambulance far enough away to be safe from the fire itself and from the collapsing building, if building collapse should occur. You must also ensure the ambulance will not impede other arriving equipment or become hemmed in by equipment or hoses. However, the ambulance must be close enough to be visible to rescuers and accessible for arriving patients. Finally, park where you will have unobstructed egress in the event you must initiate emergency transport of an injured patient. The IC will determine this location. In some instances, EMS personnel will also set up a rehabilitation sector for the fire crew.

Words of Wisdom

Threats such as fire, infectious disease, and electricity are not the only safety hazards during an emergency response. Some calls involve violence against rescuers. These calls may evolve into formal tactical situations, or they may be "simple" assaults in which, for example, alcohol or drug abuse has escalated a domestic dispute into a violent outburst. Your training, your attitude when responding to calls, and your daily EMS protocols should help you minimize the likelihood of such incidents and mitigate the outcome when they cannot be prevented.

Your next step is to determine whether there are injured patients at the scene or you've been called to stand by. A number of ambulances may be dispatched to a serious fire to ensure one or more units will remain available at the scene if others must leave to transport injured patients.

Safe Approach

As with other technical rescue situations, SAR in a burning building requires special training and equipment. SAR is performed by teams of firefighters wearing full turnout gear and self-contained breathing apparatus (SCBA) and carrying tools and fully charged hose lines. These teams will bring patients out of the burning building to the area where the ambulance is standing by. Therefore, unless otherwise ordered, you should always stay with the ambulance. You should remain there even after the fire has been extinguished, in the event a firefighter becomes

injured during salvage and overhaul. The ambulance should leave the scene only if you must transport a patient or if the IC has released you.

▶ Agricultural and Industrial Rescue

According to the National Agricultural Safety Database (NASD), about 50% of farm fatalities involve tractors, and 14% are machine related. Tractors and machines have a great deal of power. Thus, in the agricultural or industrial setting, operators, workers, and family members are exposed to extraordinary hazards. Rescue personnel should visit local farms and industrial plants to learn as much as possible about the equipment that's used, how it operates, and how an operator can become entrapped in or confined by the equipment.

Typical machine hazards involve pinch points, wrap points, shear points, crush points, and pull-in points. A particular hazard on farms is the tractor power take off (PTO) shaft that can become entangled on clothing, hair, or straps and cause severe even fatal injuries. Each of these areas is typically protected with a shield or a guard; however, over time, guards may be removed or damaged and not subsequently replaced. To identify such hazards, factory machinery is routinely inspected by the Occupational Safety and Health Administration (OSHA) and other regulating agencies. However, most farms in the United States are not covered under OSHA regulations and are therefore not subject to inspections or other mandates. This is an important consideration if you are in a farming community.

Safe Approach

A crucial skill for rescue personnel is effective cribbing to stabilize a vehicle or other agricultural or industrial equipment. During such a rescue, because of uneven ground, large spaces, and the necessity of supporting heavy loads, using the proper technique is essential for everyone's safety. Tractor rescue operations, in particular, require many cribbing blocks because large voids must be shored up and a suitable lifting platform provided.

Machinery is made of steel or other strong cast metals that will challenge most rescue tools designed for vehicle extrication. If the right tools are available, it's often easier to dismantle farm machinery than to cut it apart. Depending on the situation and your local protocol, it may be prudent to call for a special agricultural rescue team.

Once you're able to get close to the patient, carefully evaluate how he or she is trapped. Rescue personnel must secure the machine on either side of the entrapped patient to prevent any movement during disentanglement and extrication. At this point, the extent of the patient's injuries has not been determined. To isolate the injury site, as it's called, you must focus on the part of the machine in which the patient is trapped. Then study the machine to determine alternative methods of disentangling the patient. You should always have alternative plans of attack.

One approach may be slow and methodical while another is an aggressive plan to be implemented if the patient's condition warrants rapid disentanglement and extrication.

As rescue plans proceed, you must assess the patient and determine your index of suspicion based on the mechanism of injury and length of entrapment. A crucial difference between entrapment involving farm machinery and entrapment involving any other industrial machinery is the length of time of the entrapment. In a manufacturing setting, if an operator becomes entrapped in a machine, a coworker is usually right there to shut off the power to that machine and call for help while coworkers and maintenance staff begin dismantling the machine and managing the stored energy. In many cases, they actually extricate the patient before rescue personnel arrive. In contrast, a farmer may become entrapped out in a field while working alone. This patient may experience an extended delay between injury and medical treatment because there is no witness to initiate an emergency response. Many agricultural workers carry cell phones, but a farmer may not be able to reach the phone or may be too badly injured to use it. Once the patient has been assessed, technical rescuers, the EMS team, and the IC must decide which approach—methodical, aggressive, or something in between—is wisest.

▶ Tactical Emergency Medical Support

EMS and law enforcement personnel often work together on the scene at which a violent crime has taken place. A paramedic in an urban environment, for example, may work closely with law enforcement personnel almost daily. However, if an incident develops into a **tactical situation** (eg, a high-risk warrant, a hostage situation, or a barricaded suspect), the law enforcement agency may deploy a specialized tactical unit called a **special weapons and tactics (SWAT) team**.

Many SWAT teams now include specially trained EMS providers working in partnership with law enforcement. A paramedic on the tactical team undergoes extensive training in tactical strategies and practices regularly as a functioning member of the team. The tactical paramedic must also be proficient at rendering medical care in tense, perilous situations. Advanced tactical EMS training courses focus on assessing patients under conditions of limited visibility; maintaining concealment and cover; and rapidly extricating patients. The tactical paramedic is trained to enter the hot zone with law enforcement personnel and is equipped with the same PPE body armor, ballistics helmet, and eye protection, at a minimum. The tactical paramedic must also carry a medical kit that meets the needs of the incident but is compact enough not to impede movement. Most of the medical equipment is designed to handle traumatic injuries, bleeding control, airway management, and fluid replacement. A complete set of advanced life support gear is usually cached in the warm zone.

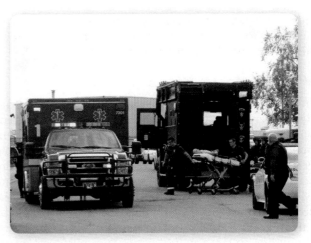

Figure 48-24 Tactical EMS providers move an injured suspect. Only the most basic medical care is provided in an unsecured area.
© Rachel D'Oro/AP Photo.

The tactical paramedic's main duty is to provide immediate medical care to those who are injured during a SWAT team operation. The injured person may be a team member, a civilian, or the suspect **Figure 48-24**. In most situations, the tactical paramedic will begin providing medical care before the scene is declared safe for other EMS personnel to enter.

Evidence-Based Medicine

The Hartford Consensus

In 2013, in response to the Sandy Hook Elementary School shooting of 2012, representatives of fire, rescue, EMS, law enforcement, and emergency care associations gathered in Hartford, Connecticut, to produce a consensus document to enhance survivability from mass-casualty shooting events.[3] With a new focus on early hemorrhage control, rather than the previous common practice of waiting until casualties could be moved to EMS personnel operating in a "safe zone" for care, the Hartford Consensus recommended the following prioritized actions using the THREAT mnemonic:

- **T**hreat suppression
- **H**emorrhage control
- **R**apid **E**xtrication to safety
- **A**ssessment by medical providers
- **T**ransport to definitive care

The Hartford Consensus concluded with the recommendation that care of victims is a shared responsibility between law enforcement, fire/rescue, and EMS and that operations during active shooter events should be guided by jointly developed protocols practiced by all agencies in a coordinated and collaborative manner.

Documentation & Communication

When not responding to an emergency incident, the tactical paramedic is responsible for maintaining medical records for each team member, conducting basic rescue training for the team, and providing suggestions for training evolutions. For planned tactical operations such as high risk search warrants, the tactical paramedic performs a medical threat assessment ahead of time to identify medical resources, environmental threats, and potential special medical needs.

If you are not part of a specially trained tactical EMS team, follow these tips when responding to a tactical situation:

- Turn off lights and sirens as you approach the scene.
- Request direction from the IC when you arrive at the outer perimeter.
- A law enforcement officer will guide you to a shielded area.
- As you exit the ambulance, stay low and remain near the side of the vehicle unless you're directed to another place of safety.

- Do not turn on the vehicle's outside speakers. Turn down the volume of any radios you're carrying.
- Don't look around the sides or over the top of any building or structure that may be shielding you.
- Stand by at the staging area to treat and package injured patients after the SWAT team or other law enforcement officers have evacuated them.
- When you're ready to transport a patient, ask a law enforcement officer to notify the IC. Leave only after the IC has verified that it's safe for the ambulance to move.
- As you exit the scene, follow the specific route indicated by the IC or law enforcement officer assigned to guide you.

■ Patient Care

Virtually any medical or traumatic condition a paramedic might encounter during his or her normal duties may also occur during a rescue call. Some conditions may be significantly aggravated by the situation that necessitated the rescue or even by the rescue process itself. Some medical or traumatic conditions, however, are unique to rescue situations. In patients rescued

YOU ▶ are the Paramedic   PART 4

The rescue crew finishes removing the vehicle's roof. With their help, you and your partner package the patient on a long backboard, lift her out of the vehicle, and transfer her safely to the stretcher. As you are making your way back to the ambulance, the patient begins to report abdominal pain. A quick reassessment shows abdominal distention, with pain in all quadrants on palpation. The patient's skin is now pale, cool, and diaphoretic, and you are no longer able to feel a radial pulse. A carotid pulse is present but weak. Respirations remain slightly rapid but improving, with diminished breath sounds bilaterally. You administer a 250-mL fluid challenge. Ten minutes later, you've secured the patient inside the ambulance, and you reassess her. She still reports severe abdominal pain and is asking for something to ease her discomfort.

Recording Time: 45 Minutes	
Respirations	22 breaths/min
Pulse	Carotid pulse, 136 beats/min, regular and weak
Skin	Pale, cool, and diaphoretic
Blood pressure	86/58 mm Hg
Oxygen saturation (Spo₂)	94% on 15 L/min nonrebreathing mask
Pupils	PERRLA

7. Why must pain medication be administered with caution, if at all, in the prehospital setting?
8. How should you manage your patient during transport?

from confined spaces, especially those rescued from a cave-in or trench, you must consider the possibility of crush injuries and crush syndrome. Crush syndrome occurs when the chest, the abdomen, or a lower limb or other extremity is compressed for 4 to 6 hours, elevating pressure and thereby reducing blood flow. The resulting oxygen deprivation in the area, in turn, necessitates anaerobic metabolism within the tissues. Lactic acid and other metabolic wastes build up, especially in muscle tissue. Consequently, crush syndrome is considered a hypoperfusion injury.

Over a prolonged period, pressure can also break down cell walls, allowing a leakage of metabolic waste and intracellular fluid and electrolytes that would normally be contained within the cell. As long as the area remains under pressure, bleeding is typically controlled and the leakage of cellular materials remains localized. When the patient is extricated and pressure is released, however, not only does blood pressure often plummet and bleeding often resume, but toxic materials that had been contained within localized tissues are released into the bloodstream. Myoglobin from muscle tissue, for example, can impair kidney function, as can phosphorus and uric acid, which are also released. Potassium, no longer regulated because the cellular sodium-potassium pumps are malfunctioning, can affect heart rhythm and may produce pronounced peaked T-waves on an electrocardiogram (ECG). Treatment with positive-pressure ventilation, along with administration of sodium bicarbonate, calcium chloride, and a fluid bolus, can help to reverse the effects of respiratory and metabolic acidosis.

▶ Pain Management

In many rescue situations, patients will be in pain as a result of injuries received during the incident. Paramedics may use both pharmacologic and nonpharmacologic methods to manage pain in injured patients. Nonpharmacologic methods include placing a patient in a position of comfort, splinting and padding to improve stabilization, ensuring gentle handling during treatment and transport, and talking with patients to help keep their minds off of discomfort. EMS providers should also keep patients warm, because shivering can heighten pain.

Providing pharmacologic treatment of pain in the prehospital setting is an important function of paramedic providers. Pain control may be the difference between a patient who endures a rescue scenario relatively easily, with tolerable pain, and an uncooperative patient in substantially more metabolic distress because of significant pain.[4,5] As with any other pharmacologic intervention, pain control should be considered according to the medication's indications, relative and absolute contraindications, and possible side effects.

▶ Medical Supplies

Table 48-1 lists the basic medical supplies you should carry in an off-road medical pack.

Table 48-1 Supplies for an Off-Road Medical Pack

- Vinyl or latex disposable exam gloves
- Face masks
- Hand sanitizer
- Mouth-to-mask resuscitation device
- 1 triangular bandage (cravat)
- Universal trauma dressings
- 4-inch × 4-inch (10-cm × 10-cm) and 5-inch × 9-inch (13-cm × 23-cm) sterile dressings
- Roller gauze bandage
- Gauze-adhesive strips
- Occlusive dressing for sealing chest wounds
- Adhesive tape
- Blankets
- Cold packs
- Alcohol pads
- One 12-mL or larger syringe for wound irrigation
- 2 glucose or energy gel packets
- Heat packs
- Abdominal dressings
- Survival blanket
- Scissors
- Irrigation fluid or wound cleansing soap
- Goggles
- SAM (structural aluminum malleable) splint
- Butterfly bandages
- Cervical collars
- Blood pressure cuff
- Rapid immobilization straps
- Pocket flashlight
- Commercially available tourniquet (CAT or SOF-T)
- Batteries

© Jones & Bartlett Learning.

▶ Patient Packaging

A number of special patient packaging tools are available to help you extricate, move, lift, and load patients. The basket stretcher, or Stokes basket, for example, is a rigid framed structure into which the patient is set and then secured. It comes in two general types Figure 48-25. The most common type is a rigid structure composed of a chicken-wire mesh supported by a metal (aluminum, steel, or titanium) frame and ribs. The other style is a rigid plastic or fiberglass basket supported by a steel or aluminum frame. Both types of baskets are available as either one- or two-piece units. The two-piece units can be latched or joined together for easier packing into the rescue scene.

The wire basket is more suitable for water rescue and helicopter hoists because the wire mesh lets water and moving air (eg, a helicopter's rotor downwash) pass through it easily. Given that water weighs 8.37 pounds (3.79 kg) per gallon, this consideration can be important. Air or water that fails to drain or pass through the

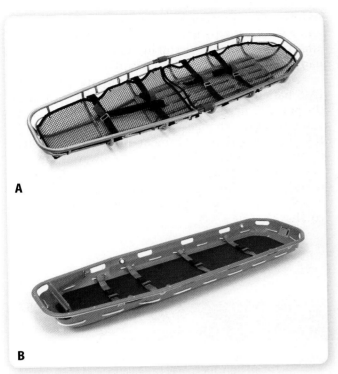

Figure 48-25 A basket stretcher used for secure patient packaging is made in two basic styles. **A.** Wire mesh. **B.** Rigid plastic or fiberglass.

© Ferno-Washington, Inc. Used with permission.

basket can make the basket spin or drag in response to the air or hydraulic forces exerted on it. Unfortunately, a wire basket snags every bit of debris and becomes ensnared on almost any obstruction or obstacle. Thus, for most other types of evacuations, a plastic or fiberglass basket is the superior choice. It slides more easily across heaps of debris, down ladders, and over snow and other surfaces.

Both types of baskets have a wheel device attached to the bottom to facilitate movement over trails and low-level debris. The devices have few or no belts or straps to secure the patient into the basket. Instead, a number of patient packaging systems can be used, including those featuring 5- to 6-mm cord or 1-inch (2.5-cm) tubular webbing. Each packaging system relies on the same basic principle: securing the patient's pelvis, which is the fulcrum of the body, into the basket. Separate techniques are then deployed to secure the patient's legs and/or chest, or to lash or lace the patient's entire body into the basket.

When packaging a patient with a fractured pelvis, the patient's distress may become a hindrance, because these techniques can provoke agonizing pain. Indeed, any sort of patient packaging that involves first anchoring the pelvis causes great discomfort. One highly effective workaround is to secure the patient in a full-body vacuum mattress. Once the patient has been adequately splinted and secured in this device, the mattress is fastened inside

the basket stretcher. As a result, the main attachment/focal point is the entire vacuum splint, not the patient's broken pelvis.

Another frequently encountered necessity is the transport of a spine-immobilized patient in a basket stretcher. Some devices have a leg divider for the lower extremities that precludes use of a backboard. Also, most backboards are too wide, and their rectangular shape won't readily fit inside a basket.

There are two alternative solutions. The first is to place the patient in a Kendrick Extrication Device (KED), rather than on a backboard, and then strap him or her into the basket. The second is to hold the cervical spine, surround the patient with enough rescuers to lift the patient while maintaining spinal immobilization, slide the basket beneath the patient, and then lower him or her back down into it. The patient can then be secured, with the basket serving as the spinal immobilization device.

Once the patient has been safely extricated or evacuated, you can reverse the process and lower/secure the patient to a backboard in preparation for transport. This consideration is especially important in a multiple-patient rescue, because most services have multiple backboards but only one basket stretcher. Don't let the ambulance crew drive off with your basket stretcher unless you have a replacement. The loss of a specialized litter can put a rescue team out of service or necessitate improvisation with alternative packaging.

When you package a patient into a basket stretcher, you must consider all of his or her needs. If you've placed the patient on supplemental oxygen, the portable oxygen tank (preferably an aluminum one) must be secured in the stretcher as well. Likewise, the tubing for the mask or cannula must be secured, because it could catch on a piece of debris or inadvertently become entangled in the raising or lowering mechanism. In addition, personnel must monitor the amount of oxygen in the cylinder. It could be dangerous for the patient if the oxygen supply runs out, especially while he or she is on a mask.

The same holds true for IV lines. Avoid using a gravity-fed system if possible. The IV tubing can get snagged and might even get pulled out of your patient. If the patient requires an IV line, use a pressure infuser and secure the line and tubing along with the patient before extrication and transport.

Basket stretchers are poor insulators. Thus, when you package a patient into one, you must protect him or her from the elements. Keep any IV lines warm as well.

If falling debris, such as rocks, ice, or building materials, is a possible hazard, package your patient with head and eye protection. This protection may be as simple as placing a rock helmet and goggles or other protective eyeglasses on him or her, or as comprehensive as using a shield to protect the patient's head and neck.

Some tight or confined spaces are so narrow that they can't accommodate a basket stretcher. Your patient, however, may require spinal immobilization. In such a case, use a KED or KED-SKED combination. A KED is a spinal immobilization device that captures the three planes of the spinal column (ie, the head, shoulders, and pelvis). This narrow-profile device was originally designed by an EMT for extrication of Formula One race car drivers. Apply the KED to the patient and then rig it for raising or lowering as you would for an uninjured person—namely, by using a seat harness and applying a chest harness around the patient and the KED. Devices similar to the KED have also been approved as vertical lifting harnesses.

Another option is to place the patient in a KED and then secure both in a SKED device. A SKED litter is a flexible, wrap-around litter—essentially a drag sheet made of heavy-duty polyethylene plastic that wraps around and cocoons the patient, with prerigged securing and attachment points. It's useful in sliding patients through narrow passages and over rough surfaces.

Adaptability and improvisation are essential in EMS patient care practices. In rescue and extrication, the patient's needs, your resources, and the techniques you rely on can change as the rescue process develops. If you lack the right equipment, use your ingenuity to create the necessary tools. You can always splint one body part to another, by attaching the upper extremities to the torso and the lower legs to each other. This kind of splinting can be surprisingly effective when it's all you have.

YOU are the Paramedic SUMMARY

1. What is a technical rescue incident?

A technical rescue incident (TRI) is a challenging, complex rescue situation that requires the expertise of specially trained people equipped with special resources. This distinction is important, as paramedics and other responders may have specialized and appropriate training but lack the specialized resources needed to handle a specific incident. Examples of TRIs include vehicle extrication, trench collapse, confined spaces, wilderness rescue, and water rescue.

2. What level of rescue training and education is required to operate specialized rescue tools and coordinate patient extrication from a motor vehicle crash?

Of the three levels of training, education, and capability in technical rescue, the first level, awareness, allows rescuers only to identify a TRI and summon additional resources. The middle level, operational training, allows rescuers to do all that awareness-level providers can, plus assist as directed in the rescue operation. At the technician level, rescuers can operate specialized tools and coordinate the strategic and tactical extrication of a patient from a motor vehicle crash.

3. What are the three control zones that will be established while the scene is being stabilized?

Control zones are necessary to ensure the safety of all parties. Three areas, or zones, must be established, as follows:

- **Hot zone.** This area is for entry teams and rescue teams only. The hot zone is the area in which immediate hazards are present; for example, rescue tools may be in operation, fuels may be leaking, and there may be the possibility of material collapse.
- **Warm zone.** Only properly trained and equipped personnel are permitted access to the warm zone. This is the site at which personnel and equipment decontamination takes place. This area is also used to support the hot zone.
- **Cold zone.** The purpose of the cold zone is to stage vehicles and equipment and establish a command post.

4. Why is it important for the ICS to be used during a technical rescue incident?

TRIs often are complex, requiring the coordination of many resources. Using the ICS keeps the scene organized and ensures the safety of those involved by clarifying the roles of each responder, their lines of communication, and the control zones in which they operate.

5. Patients requiring extrication often become anxious. What can you do to help calm the patient?

The most important thing you can do is to maintain communication with your patient in a calm and collected manner.

6. In what ways, if any, is this patient at risk of developing crush syndrome?

The patient was trapped under the dashboard for a considerable amount of time, but not the 4 to 6 hours that it would take for significant crush syndrome to develop. If she had been unable to call for help for several more hours, the areas of her body that were not able to receive oxygenated blood to feed the tissues would have switched to anaerobic metabolism for energy. As a result,

YOU are the Paramedic   SUMMARY (continued)

lactic acids and other waste products would have formed and accumulated in the tissues. Once the pressure was released, the waste products would be carried throughout her body by the bloodstream, creating a situation that could be lethal.

7. Why must pain medication be administered with caution, if at all, in the prehospital setting?

The patient is demonstrating signs and symptoms of shock. Although the patient is experiencing significant amounts of pain, the administration of pain medications may contribute to a further decrease in blood pressure.

8. How should you manage your patient during transport?

As mentioned, the patient is exhibiting signs and symptoms of shock. Your priority should be to support and maintain the ABCs. This may entail providing assisted ventilations, intubating, and administering medications to raise the blood pressure. Remember to also keep the patient warm. Multisystem trauma patients as well as patients in shock can lose significant amounts of body heat, which can worsen their condition.

EMS Patient Care Report (PCR)

Date: 03-06-18	**Incident No.:** 22487		**Nature of Call:** Motor vehicle crash		**Location:** 642 Banberry Rd.

Dispatched: 2130	**En Route:** 2131	**At Scene:** 2139	**Transport:** 2224	**At Hospital:** 2257	**In Service:** 2315

Patient Information

Age: 65 **Sex:** F **Weight (in kg [lb]):** 75 kg (165 lb)	**Allergies:** None **Medications:** Metformin, insulin **Past Medical History:** Diabetes **Chief Complaint:** Shortness of breath and abdominal pain

Vital Signs

Time: 2144	**BP:** N/A	**Pulse:** 108	**Respirations:** 26	**Spo$_2$:** N/A
Time: 2209	**BP:** 104/62	**Pulse:** 126	**Respirations:** 22	**Spo$_2$:** 96%
Time: 2224	**BP:** 86/58	**Pulse:** 136	**Respirations:** 22	**Spo$_2$:** 94%
Time: 2239	**BP:** 90/60	**Pulse:** 132	**Respirations:** 22	**Spo$_2$:** 96%
Time: 2254	**BP:** 94/60	**Pulse:** 130	**Respirations:** 20	**Spo$_2$:** 96%

EMS Treatment (circle all that apply)

Oxygen @ ___15___ L/min via (circle one): NC **(NRM)** Bag-mask device	**Assisted Ventilation**	**Airway Adjunct**	**CPR**
Defibrillation	**(Bleeding Control)**	**(Bandaging)**	**(Splinting)**	Other:

YOU are the Paramedic   SUMMARY (continued)

Narrative

Dispatched to motor vehicle crash with possible entrapment. En route informed that law enforcement and fire crew on-scene advising a single vehicle off the road with a single patient trapped inside. Technical response team en route. Upon arrival IC advises that our pt is a 65-year-old woman who is trapped from the lower portion of her chest down by the dashboard with several inches of passenger compartment intrusion. Initial information provided by firefighter Holland: Pt is currently awake, alert, and oriented to person, place, time, and event. Airway is patent, and chest rise appears adequate. Carotid pulses are regular, strong, and elevated. The pt is complaining of difficulty breathing and is concerned about the location of her grandson. Initial pt contact was made at approximately 2140. Pt remains awake and alert and states "she can't catch her breath." Manual spinal immobilization held by firefighter Holland. Pt states that she was driving down the road when, for an unknown reason, her vehicle left the roadway. Vehicle became wedged between a large tree and a stone wall, precluding simple extrication. Pt is unsure whether she lost consciousness. Pt states that she has a history of diabetes, takes metformin and insulin, and has no known drug allergies. Debris removed at approximately 2208 allowing for full assessment. Assessment reveals bilateral chest rise with tenderness to both sides of the rib cage. Breath sounds are diminished bilaterally. Abdomen is soft and tender to both lower quadrants. Bruising is noted to both lower quadrants beneath the umbilicus. A laceration approximately 3 inches (8 cm) in length was noted on the left thigh. Venous blood steadily coming from the wound. Bleeding controlled with direct pressure and bandage. Oxygen applied via nonrebreathing mask at 15 L/min. IV started in the left antecubital space with 18-gauge Angiocath. Normal saline 1,000 mL hung with 10 gtt set and ran at 10 gtt/min. Blood glucose is 183 mg/dL, which is normal for pt. Pt had c-collar placed. No noted pain to the neck prior to collar. Back reveals no trauma or pain to palpation. The pt is packaged with a vacuum splint and basket stretcher. While the pt is being moved to the truck, she begins to report severe abdominal pain. Reassessment reveals abdomen is distended and tender to palpation to all quadrants. Skin is pale, cool, and diaphoretic. Radial pulses are absent. Carotid pulses present and weak at a rate of 136 beats/min. Administered 250-mL fluid challenge. Pt moved to stretcher and secured inside the ambulance. Pt still reports severe abdominal pain and requests pain medication. Explained to pt that she is unable to have any due to her condition. En route to Baptist Medical Center at 2224. Head-to-toe assessment: Pupils equal and reactive. No noted trauma to the head or face. No fluids coming from the nose, mouth, or ears. No tracheal deviation or JVD noted. Bilateral breath sounds diminished bilaterally with pain upon palpation to the chest. Bruising now noted to the chest walls bilaterally. Abdomen distended and becoming rigid. Tender to palpation of all quadrants. Lower extremities have multiple abrasions. Bleeding from laceration on the left thigh has stopped. Upper extremities have multiple abrasions; no other trauma noted. PMS present in all four extremities. No further changes noted during transport. Arrived at Baptist Medical Center at 2257. Report given and pt care turned over to RN Jenkins.**End of report**

Prep Kit

▶ Ready for Review

- "Rescue" means to deliver from danger or confinement.
- A technical rescue incident (TRI) is a complex rescue incident involving vehicle extrication; rescue from water, ice, or confined spaces; rescue following trench, structural, or other collapse; high-angle rescue; response to hazardous materials incidents; or wilderness search and rescue (SAR) that requires specially trained personnel and special equipment.
- Technical rescue training occurs on three levels: awareness, operations, and technician. Most of the training and education EMS providers receive is aimed at the awareness level, enabling them to identify the hazards and secure the scene to prevent additional people from becoming patients. Additional levels of response require additional training and preparation.

Prep Kit (continued)

- As you assist the rescue team, be safe, follow orders, maintain situational awareness, work as a team, and always remember the patient.
- The hardest part of any rescue is neither the rescue itself nor the treatment, but coordination and balance of the two.
- Although special rescue situations may take many different forms, most involve the following steps: preparation, response, arrival and scene size-up, scene stabilization, access to the patient, disentanglement, removal, and transport.
- At a TRI, it is crucial to take time to properly evaluate the situation. Consider the possible general hazards of live utilities, confined spaces, and environmental conditions, as well as hazards that are immediately dangerous to life and health.
- The first arriving officer at a rescue scene should immediately assume command and start using the incident command system. This step is crucial because many TRIs eventually become complex, requiring a large number of assisting units.
- Whenever possible, park emergency vehicles in a manner that promotes safety and doesn't unnecessarily disrupt traffic. Traffic flow is the largest single hazard associated with any highway operation.
- Accountability should be practiced at all emergencies, no matter how small.
- Many vehicle extrication techniques require the use of specialized skills and training, as well as hydraulic or pneumatic tools.
- Basket stretchers facilitate movement of patients to a place of safety and can be used in a variety of situations. The way in which a patient is packaged in a basket stretcher depends on his or her medical condition, the environment, and the plan for his or her evacuation.
- Simple vehicle extrication techniques include unlocking and opening the door and breaking tempered glass. Once you've entered the vehicle and accessed the patient, you will provide initial medical care.
- Use of standardized terminology reduces confusion at vehicle extrication scenes: A posts are those closest to the front of the vehicle; B posts are located between the front and rear doors; C posts, if present, are located behind the rear doors; D posts can be found on larger vehicles, such as SUVs and vans, that have windows behind the rear doors. On large vehicles, the lettering process continues from front to back, with posts E, F, G, and so forth.
- Vehicles may be powered by electricity, by hybrid systems that use both electricity and gasoline, or by fuels such as propane, natural gas, methanol, or hydrogen. There are many hazards associated

with alternative power vehicles, but the general approach to safety is the same.
- You should have a thorough working knowledge of the basic, simple hand tools. Hand tools can be categorized as striking tools, leverage/prying/spreading tools, cutting tools, and lifting/pushing/pulling tools.
- Vehicle extrication could require a specialized team to manage hazardous materials. These materials might be part of the vehicle, or the vehicle might be transporting dangerous chemicals or other agents.
- Vehicle movement after stabilization is caused by give in the suspension system. The five directional movements are horizontal, vertical, roll, bounce, and yaw.
- The most basic physical tool used for vehicle stabilization is cribbing.
- During disentanglement, responders need to be mindful of undeployed airbags.
- A confined space is a location surrounded by a structure that is not designed for continuous occupancy and that usually has limited openings for entry and exit.
- Confined spaces present a special hazard because they may have limited ventilation to provide for air circulation and exchange, which can make them an oxygen-deficient atmosphere, or they may contain poisonous gases.
- Trench rescue may become necessary when earth is removed for placement of a utility line or for other construction and the sides of the excavation collapse, trapping a worker.
- Because almost any EMS provider may respond to a water rescue situation, you should know how to use a personal flotation device correctly and how to employ self-rescue positions.
- To immobilize the spine while a patient is still in the water, turn the patient supine, attend to the airway and ventilation, place the patient on a buoyant backboard, secure the trunk and head, remove the patient from the water, remove his or her wet clothes, and cover him or her with a blanket.
- Rope rescue incidents are divided into low-angle and high-angle operations.
  - In low-angle operations, the slope of the ground over which the rescuers are working is less than 45°. Low-angle operations are used when the scene requires ropes to be used only as assistance to pull or haul up a patient or rescuer.
  - In high-angle operations, the slope of the ground is greater than 45°, and rescuers or patients are dependent on a life safety rope, not a fixed surface of support such as the ground.

Prep Kit (continued)

- Wilderness SAR missions consist of two parts: search (looking for a lost or overdue person) and rescue (removing a patient from a hostile environment).
- During lost person SAR, your role is to stand by at the search base until the lost person or people have been found.
- You should always stay with your ambulance during a structure fire. SAR during a fire is performed by trained personnel.
- Machines in factories and on farms have pinch points, wrap points, shear points, crush points, and pull-in points that can cause injury.
- Dismantling a piece of farm or factory equipment may be more effective than cutting it apart when extricating a patient, because rescue tools designed for the vehicle extrication cannot cut through the steel or other cast metals of which the industrial or agricultural equipment is made.
- If an incident develops into a tactical situation, law enforcement agencies may deploy a specialized law enforcement tactical unit called a special weapons and tactics (SWAT) team.
- Many SWAT teams now include a specially trained paramedic skilled in rendering medical care during tense tactical situations.
- Pain control in rescue situations should take the form of nonpharmacologic methods, such as splinting to minimize movement and gentle handling.
- A number of special patient packaging tools are available to help extricate patients from their situation and move them up, down, or out to the ambulance. The basket stretcher is an example of a packaging tool.
- You should carry an off-road medical pack containing medical supplies, such as dressings and disposable exam gloves, and gear, such as a survival blanket and flashlight.

▶ Vital Vocabulary

accountability system A method of accounting for all personnel at an emergency incident and ensuring only those with specific assignments are permitted to work within the various zones.

alternative power vehicle A vehicle powered by energy other than petroleum-based fuel, or a vehicle that relies on a combination of petroleum and another fuel or energy source for power.

awareness The first level of rescue training provided to all responders; emphasizes recognizing hazards, securing the scene, and calling for appropriate assistance. There is no use of actual rescue skills.

belay A technique used to control a rope as it is fed out to climbers.

box crib A pallet-like framework used to shore up a heavy load.

cold-protective response A phenomenon associated with cold-water immersion in which the body reflexively lowers its metabolic rate in an effort to preserve basic bodily functions.

cold zone A safe area for agencies involved in a rescue operation; the incident commander, command post, EMS providers, and other necessary support functions should be located in the cold zone.

complex access Complicated entry requiring special tools, advanced training, and the use of force, such as breaking windows.

confined space A space that is not meant for continuous occupancy and to which access is limited or restricted, such as a manhole, well, or tank.

cribbing A type of basic physical support, such as blocks or short lengths of wood, used to stabilize a vehicle during a rescue operation.

disentanglement Use of specialized tools and advanced techniques to free a patient from the area or object in which he or she is trapped.

entrapment A circumstance in which a patient is unable to extricate himself or herself from an impediment, such as debris or soil.

hand tool Any tool or piece of equipment operated by human power.

high-angle operation A rope rescue operation in which the angle of the slope is greater than 45°. Rescuers depend on life safety rope rather than working from a fixed support surface, such as the ground.

hot zone The area that directly surrounds an incident site and is considered immediately dangerous to life and health. All personnel working in the hot zone must wear all appropriate protective clothing and equipment. Entry requires approval by the IC or a designated sector officer. Complete backup, rescue, and decontamination teams must be in place at the perimeter before operations begin.

immediately dangerous to life and health (IDLH) An atmospheric concentration of any toxic, corrosive, or asphyxiant substance that poses an immediate threat to life or could cause irreversible or delayed adverse health effects. There are three general IDLH atmospheres: toxic, flammable, and oxygen-deficient.

laminated glass A type of window glazing that incorporates a sheeting material to keep the glass from breaking into shards. This kind of glass, often used for windshields, resists even deliberate breakage.

low-angle operation A rope rescue operation carried out on a mildly sloping surface (less than 45°) or on level ground. The ground is the rescuer's

Prep Kit (continued)

primary means of support, and the rope system is the secondary means of support.

operations The technical rescue training level geared toward working in the warm zone of an incident. Training at this level allows responders to directly assist those conducting the rescue operation and to use certain rescue skills and procedures.

packaging The act of preparing a patient for movement as a unit by means of a backboard or similar stabilization device.

personal flotation device (PFD) Also known as a life vest, a water rescue device that allows the body to float.

rappelling The act of descending from a height on a fixed rope.

scrambling A cross between hill climbing and rock climbing used to ascend rocky surfaces and ridges.

search and rescue (SAR) The process of locating a lost or overdue person and removing him or her from a hostile environment.

secondary collapse A collapse that occurs after the primary trench, excavation, or structural collapse.

self-rescue position A position used by a swift-water rescuer to avoid objects below the surface; the rescuer rolls into a faceup arched position, with the lower back higher than the feet (which are held together and face in the direction of travel—that is, feet first) and the arms at the sides.

shim A slim, low-profile, wedgelike object used to snug loose cribbing under a load or to fill a void.

shoring A hydraulic, pneumatic, or wood system to support a trench wall or reinforce building components such as walls, floors, or ceilings to prevent collapse.

simple access Access easily achieved with the use of simple hand tools or application of force.

special weapons and tactics (SWAT) team A specialized law enforcement tactical unit.

spoil pile The pile of dirt unearthed from an excavation. The pile may be unstable and prone to collapse.

step chock A specialized cribbing assembly of wood or plastic blocks arranged in a step configuration.

supplemental restraint system A system of specialized devices, such as airbags and seat belt pre-tensioners, used to restrain a driver or passenger in the protected passenger compartment of a motor vehicle during a crash.

tactical situation A high-risk situation involving the potential for physical violence or armed combat typically involving law enforcement teams interacting with potentially dangerous criminal suspects.

technical rescue incident (TRI) A complex rescue requiring specially trained personnel and sophisticated equipment and involving vehicle extrication; rescue from water, ice, or confined spaces; rescue following trench, structural, or other collapse; high-angle rescue; response to hazardous materials incidents; or wilderness search and rescue.

technical rescue team A group of rescuers expertly trained in the various disciplines of technical rescue.

technician The level of training necessary for a rescuer directly involved in a rescue operation; indicates a high level of competency in technical or hazardous materials rescue.

tempered glass A type of glass that is heat-treated so that it breaks into small, relatively dull pieces.

traffic incident management (TIM) The process of coordinating different partner agencies to detect, respond to, and clear traffic incidents as quickly as possible to reduce the impacts of incidents on safety and congestion, while protecting the safety of on-scene responders and the traveling public.

unibody construction A vehicle design with no formal frame structure. The body and frame are one piece, which is considered to be the structural integrity of the vehicle.

warm zone The area located between the hot and cold zones at an incident. Decontamination stations are located in the warm zone.

wedge A tapered shaft of wood or other material used to snug loose cribbing.

► References

1. US Fire Administration, Federal Emergency Management Agency. *Traffic Incident Management Systems.* https://www.usfa.fema.gov/downloads/pdf/publications/fa_330.pdf. Published March 2012. Accessed March 20, 2017.

2. U.S. Department of Transportation. National Highway Traffic Safety Administration. *Traffic Safety Facts: 2014 Motor Vehicle Crashes: Overview.* https://crashstats.nhtsa.dot.gov/Api/Public/ViewPublication/812246. Published March 2016. Accessed March 24, 2017.

3. Jacobs LM, McSwain NE, Rotondo MF, et al. Improving survival from active shooter events: the Hartford Consensus. *Bull Am Coll Surg.* 2013;98(6):14-16.

4. Alonso-Serra HM, Wesley K, National Association of EMS Physicians Standards and Clinical Practices Committee. Prehospital pain management [National Association of EMS Physicians position paper]. *Prehosp Emerg Care.* 2003;7(4):482-488.

5. Dailey MW, Burton J, Day L, DeMartino W. Prehospital analgesic protocols in the United States: a national survey [abstract]. *Acad Emerg Med.* 2009;16(suppl 4):S197.

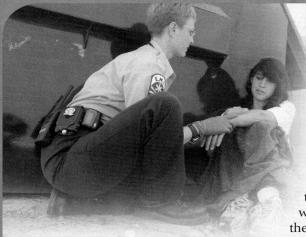

Assessment *in Action*

It is 0800 hours, and the morning rush-hour commute is underway. The weather is cool, with a light rain reducing visibility on the road and slowing traffic to a stop-and-go crawl in some places. You and your partner are dispatched to the scene of a motor vehicle collision on the highway in which a hybrid SUV has rear-ended a box truck. Apparently, the SUV struck the rear bumper of the box truck, and the engine compartment of the hybrid SUV is now partially wedged under the back of the truck. The driver of the truck is out of the vehicle and claims to be uninjured. The driver of the SUV appears to be unconscious and is trapped inside her vehicle.

1. Which of the following pose significant scene hazards?

    A. The driver of the box truck
    B. The driver of the SUV
    C. Environmental conditions
    D. Leaking gasoline from the box truck

2. What is the most significant hazard associated with any highway operation?

    A. Visibility
    B. Traffic flow
    C. Access to the scene
    D. Bystanders and media

3. Which of the following are capable of stabilizing a vehicle?

    A. Steel-reinforced cables
    B. Stairs
    C. Airbags
    D. Cribbing

4. Which tool should be used to break tempered glass?

    A. Sledgehammer
    B. Spring-loaded center punch
    C. Axe
    D. Pike pole

5. What actions should be taken by emergency responders to secure a hybrid SUV involved in a motor vehicle collision?

    A. Leave the key in the ignition.
    B. Secure the registration information
    C. Crib the front and back of the vehicle
    D. Disconnect the 12-volt battery.

6. At what point during the rescue operation should initial medical care be rendered?

    A. Immediately on arrival at the scene
    B. After the patient has been disentangled from the vehicle
    C. Once the patient is in the ambulance
    D. Upon first patient contact

7. To be directly involved with the rescue operation itself, what level of training must you have completed?

    A. Master
    B. Technician
    C. Awareness
    D. Operations

8. In a mass-shooting scenario, who might provide hemorrhage control prior to the patient being delivered to EMS waiting in a safe area or cold zone?

9. If you are trained in special rescue operations, is it appropriate for you to act in that capacity whenever necessary?

10. Who is responsible for performing a size-up upon arrival at an emergency scene?

Hazardous Materials

National EMS Education Standard Competencies

EMS Operations

Knowledge of operational roles and responsibilities to ensure patient, public, and personnel safety.

Hazardous Materials Awareness

Risks and responsibilities of operating in a cold zone at a hazardous materials or other special incident. (pp 2410-2414)

Knowledge Objectives

1. Define the term hazardous material. (p 2398)
2. Describe the OSHA HAZWOPER regulation and the entry-level training or experience requirements identified by the HAZWOPER regulation for a paramedic to respond to a hazardous materials incident. (pp 2398-2399)
3. Describe the hazard classification system used by the National Fire Protection Association (NFPA). (p 2399)
4. Explain the role of paramedics during a hazardous materials incident both before and after the hazardous materials team arrives, including precautions required to ensure the safety of civilians and public service personnel. (pp 2399-2401)
5. Discuss the specific types of information and reference resources a paramedic can use to recognize a hazardous materials incident. (pp 2401-2402)
6. Describe some of the containers and vehicles used to transport hazardous materials on the roadway. (pp 2403-2404, 2406-2410)
7. Explain how the three safety zones are established at a hazardous materials incident, and discuss the characteristics of each zone, including the personnel who work within each one. (pp 2410-2412)
8. Describe the four levels of personal protective equipment (PPE) that may be required at a hazardous materials incident to protect personnel from injury by or contamination from a particular substance. (pp 2411, 2413-2414)
9. Describe how the route of the exposure, the dose and concentration of the hazard, and the length of time the hazard is in contact with the body affect the body. (pp 2414-2415)
10. Provide examples of how understanding the chemical and physical properties of a substance may give you some valuable insight when it comes to providing care. (pp 2415-2417)
11. Describe decontamination techniques, including emergency decontamination, mass decontamination, and technical decontamination. (pp 2418-2420)
12. Describe patient care at a hazardous materials incident and explain special requirements for specific exposures. (pp 2420-2422)

Skills Objectives

1. Identify Department of Transportation labels, placards, and markings that are used to designate hazardous materials. (pp 2401-2405)
2. Demonstrate the ability to use a variety of reference materials to identify a hazardous material. (pp 2401-2405)

Introduction

One of the inevitable consequences of living in an industrialized world is the proliferation of hazardous materials. A **hazardous material**, as defined by the Department of Transportation (DOT), is any substance or material that is capable of posing an unreasonable risk to human health, safety, or the environment when transported in commerce, used incorrectly, or not properly contained or stored. The products of our civilization require the manufacture, transport, storage, use, and disposal of tens of thousands of potentially toxic substances. Thousands of hazardous materials releases occur each year, with the great majority of these being highway transportation incidents.

This chapter will take a broad look at some of the unique aspects you should consider when you are responding to hazardous materials incidents. The information provided here is **not** intended to: (1) be comprehensive coverage of hazardous materials incident response procedures, (2) certify you to any recognized level of hazardous materials response, or (3) turn you into a hazardous materials expert. The material provided is intended to help you understand a hazardous materials incident, the consequences of exposure to those substances, and your role in responding to a hazardous materials incident. Operating at a hazardous materials scene presents many challenges that are not encountered during a normal emergency medical services (EMS) response. These challenges include avoiding exposure to a toxic substance, so that you don't turn into a victim like those patients already exposed, and handling exposures properly and with confidence.

Regulations and Standards

The primary regulations for hazardous materials response are put forth by the Occupational Safety and Health Administration (OSHA) and the Environmental Protection Agency (EPA). The OSHA document containing the hazardous materials response competencies is commonly referred to as **HAZWOPER (HAZardous Waste OPerations and Emergency Response)**. The complete HAZWOPER regulation can be found in Title 29 of the Code of Federal Regulations (CFR), standard 1910.120(q)(6)(i). The training levels found in the OSHA regulation are identified as awareness, operations, technician, specialist, and incident commander. According to OSHA, "First responders at the awareness level are people who are likely to witness or discover a hazardous substance release and who have been trained to initiate an emergency response sequence by notifying the proper authorities of the release. They would take no further action beyond notifying the authorities of the release." Based on the OSHA HAZWOPER regulation, first responders at the awareness level should have sufficient training or experience to objectively demonstrate competency in the following areas:

- An understanding of what hazardous substances are and the risks associated with them

YOU are the Paramedic PART 1

You and your partner are en route to an anhydrous ammonia leak at a food processing plant. Initial reports state that approximately 20 people were in the immediate vicinity of the leak. The hazardous materials team is on scene setting up safety zones, and the incident command system has been established. On your arrival, the incident commander assigns your unit to the medical treatment group. When you arrive at the designated area in the cold zone after decontamination of all victims, the medical group leader indicates there is one person requiring medical attention and provides you with the safety data sheet for anhydrous ammonia. You are escorted to the patient, a 50-year-old man complaining of burning eyes and respiratory distress.

Recording Time: 1 Minute	
Appearance	Anxious and restless
Level of consciousness	Alert (oriented to person, place, time, and event)
Airway	Open
Breathing	30 breaths/min; shallow; increased work of breathing with accessory muscle use and audible expiratory wheezes
Circulation	Strong radial pulse, tachycardic

1. Are the signs and symptoms of an anhydrous ammonia exposure consistent with what you observe during the rapid full-body scan?
2. What chemical reference sources could assist you with the treatment of your patient?
3. Explain what actions you might take if you feel the scene is not safe.

- An understanding of the potential outcomes of an incident
- The ability to recognize the presence of hazardous substances
- The ability to identify the hazardous substances, if possible
- An understanding of the role of the first responder awareness individual in the emergency response plan
- The ability to determine the need for additional resources and to notify the communication center

Consensus-based standards such as the National Fire Protection Association (NFPA) 472 standard, *Standard for Competence of Responders to Hazardous/Materials/Weapons of Mass Destruction Incidents*, are also available to guide responders. Additionally, NFPA 473, *Standard for Competencies for EMS Personnel Responding to Hazardous Materials/ Weapons of Mass Destruction Incidents*, is a good resource to offer guidance to those EMS responders rendering medical care at hazardous materials incidents. OSHA and the EPA have established mandatory safety procedures for personnel who deal with problems involving hazardous materials. OSHA's HAZWOPER standard (CFR 1910.120 (q)) provides for the safety of personnel who work on hazardous waste cleanup sites or hazardous waste treatment storage and disposal sites or who respond to hazardous materials emergencies. The EPA also has a parallel HAZWOPER standard (40 CFR 311) that extends coverage to governmental employees and volunteers who would not normally be covered under OSHA standards.

Words of Wisdom

According to the NFPA, the authority having jurisdiction (AHJ) is an organization, office, or person responsible for enforcing the requirements of a code or standard, or for approving equipment, materials, an installation, or a procedure.[1]

All EMS personnel should receive appropriate hazardous materials response training, based on the needs and requirements of the **authority having jurisdiction (AHJ)** and the local EMS agency. In many cases, the AHJ may decide that the awareness level of training may be appropriate. In other instances, the AHJ may choose to train EMS responders to a higher level, such as the operations or technician level. Whatever the case, it is up to the AHJ to decide how much hazardous materials response training will be required of EMS responders. The level of training will dictate when and where you might use your EMS skills. Training in hazardous materials is conducted at three levels:

- **Awareness.** Responders who encounter a hazardous materials incident are trained to recognize hazardous materials, isolate the area, and call for appropriate assistance. Although the awareness level has no set training hour requirement, OSHA has defined, specific objectives that must be met in this training. In contrast, NFPA 472 does not consider awareness-level personnel to be *responders* in the typical sense of the word. Paramedics must realize the awareness level is designed for the recognition of hazardous materials incidents. Responders trained to this level may not be initially dispatched to a scene that is known to involve hazardous materials.
- **Operations.** Personnel who respond to protect nearby people, property, and the environment from the effects of a hazardous materials incident are trained to operate in a defensive manner and not make direct, intentional contact with the hazardous substance. Because of the limitations imposed on responders trained at the awareness level, many EMS agencies provide this level of training for paramedics. Paramedics are commonly trained to the operations level if they may be called to the scene of a hazardous materials incident for stand-by or need to treat patients outside of the hot zone.
- **Technician.** At this level, you may be directly involved in a contaminated atmosphere or be part of the hazardous materials response operation itself. Responders who are usually members of a hazardous materials team make direct, intentional contact with a spilled material to mitigate the problem. Training includes the use of specialized equipment, care of patients during the rescue, and management of the incident and of all personnel at the scene.

Keep in mind that federal, state, and local regulations and standards govern the use, storage, and transport of hazardous materials. These regulations and standards are designed to improve the public's ability to know and to help protect workers and emergency responders as they try to protect the public. Become familiar with the laws of the state and locality in which you serve. To determine what level of hazardous materials training you may need, consult experts in the field from your local jurisdiction.

Paramedics and Hazardous Materials Incidents

A good guess is not enough to identify potential hazardous materials scenes and determine how to safely operate if you are first on scene or called to provide medical support at a hazardous materials incident; you must also rely on training and reference sources. You should know how and when to access specific toxicologic information (reference sources, poison control center, medical control) and/or a hazardous materials team when the situation calls for it. You should understand how a hazardous materials scene is organized from a command and control perspective, including how you fit into the command structure and operational plan. You also need to be familiar with the different types of personal protective equipment (PPE) used at a hazardous materials scene, how the hazardous materials team or other responders will decontaminate patients, and how to assess and treat exposures. In addition, you may be called on to support hazardous materials teams through on-scene medical monitoring and/or provide treatment in the event responders are exposed.

Hazardous materials incidents may include but are not limited to the following:

- A highway or railroad incident in which a substance is leaking from a cargo tank or railroad tank car
- A leak, fire, or other emergency at an industrial plant, refinery, or other fixed facility where chemicals or explosives are produced, used, or stored
- A leak or rupture of an underground natural gas pipe
- Incidents in an agricultural setting in which insecticides may be in use or accidentally released
- Buildup of methane or other by-products of waste decomposition in sewers, sewage processing plants, or landfills
- An incident with criminal intent in which a suspected hazardous materials agent is intentionally released

Scene Size-up

When you first arrive at any scene and recognize the presence or potential presence of a hazardous material release, your most important job is to ensure your own safety. Unfortunately, identifying the hazard might not be possible, which could complicate your ability to rapidly understand the threat and initiate protective actions. In some cases, the presence of a hazardous material can be recognized from warning signs such as victim/patient signs and symptoms, placards, labels, or other clues found at the scene. Placards or labels may be found in the following locations:

- On buildings or in areas where hazardous materials are produced, used, or stored
- On trucks and railroad cars that transport certain types/amounts of a hazardous material
- On drums or other storage vessels that contain a hazardous waste or hazardous material

Sometimes, transporters do not label containers or vessels appropriately, and the labeling of packages and transport vehicles can be misleading.

Always maintain a high index of suspicion as you perform your scene size-up. Even the most mundane looking scene could present significant dangers. Intentional ingestion of chemicals and activities occurring at illicit labs or potential terrorist activities may have no obvious warning signs. You could be well into the call before you have a

firm grasp of what is really happening. In some cases, you may be able to identify leaks or spills by the following:

- A visible cloud or unusual-looking smoke or vapor resulting from the escaping substance
- A leak or spill from a tank, container, truck, or railroad car with or without hazardous materials placards or labels
- An unusual, strong, noxious, acrid odor in the area

Some chemicals are odorized to indicate the presence of normally odorless gases (eg, propane and methane). However, there are a number of dangerous substances that are odorless and can be detected only by air monitoring instruments (eg, carbon monoxide). To that end, never rely solely on your sense of smell to identify the presence of a hazardous material; if you smell it, you are exposed! Remember, a large number of people, including you, could be exposed before the presence of a hazardous materials incident is identified.

If you approach a scene where more than one person has collapsed or is unconscious or in respiratory distress, especially at a mass gathering event such as a political convention or sporting event, you should suspect the presence of a hazardous materials agent.

If you do not follow the proper safety measures when you are faced with a hazardous materials incident, you and many others could end up needlessly exposed or injured. The safety of you and your team, the other responders, and the public must be your most important concern. There will be times when your ambulance crew is the first set of responders to arrive at the scene. If, as you approach, any signs suggest that a hazardous materials incident has occurred, you should stop at a safe distance, upwind and uphill from the scene. After rapidly sizing up the scene, isolate the hazardous area to the best of your ability; deny entry to the affected area and call for additional resources. These resources may include law enforcement officers, firefighters, hazardous materials responders, or additional EMS responders.

Once your safety is ensured, you may begin the process of identifying victims and beginning patient care if appropriate. There are, however, many factors that could impact your ability to provide care. More on this topic will be explored throughout the rest of the chapter. If you do not recognize the danger until you are too close, immediately leave the danger zone. Once you have reached a safe place, reassess the situation and provide as much information as possible when you are calling for additional resources. Examples of items to report include the following:

- Your exact location
- Atmospheric conditions, if appropriate
- Size and shape of containers or cargo tankers
- The exact name of the substance, if known
- The chemical ID number or symbols if visible
- The number of victims, including signs and symptoms, if observed
- The type and number of additional resources requested

- Location of safe staging areas for incoming resources
- Location of incident command post

Do not reenter the scene or leave the area until you have been cleared by the hazardous materials team, or you may contribute to the situation by spreading hazardous materials.

> ### Words of Wisdom
>
> Do not rush into a hazardous materials scene. Stop and assess the situation first.

▶ Identification of Hazardous Materials

Information is one of the most valuable commodities at a hazardous materials incident. This information can come to you in the form of your own observations, reports from bystanders, signs and symptoms of victims, and other sources, including labels and placards, shipping papers, or safety data sheets. In some cases, labels and placards will provide you with basic information about the materials involved in the release. Remember, take no risks, but when applicable, try to read the marking and placards required at hazardous materials storage sites and on vehicles.

The most recent edition of the *Emergency Response Guidebook* (*ERG*) should be carried on every emergency response vehicle **Figure 49-1**. The *ERG* is a guidebook for first responders during the initial phase of a dangerous goods/hazardous materials transportation incident. It is available in a mobile version and a free smartphone application is available for download.[2] The *ERG* provides information on specific properties and hazards of

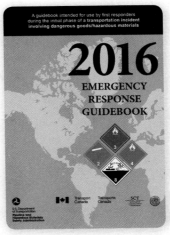

Figure 49-1 The *Emergency Response Guidebook* is a reference used as a base for your initial actions at a hazardous materials incident. These are the most common chemicals found in transportation but only a small percentage of all the chemicals that exist.
Courtesy of U.S. Department of Transportation.

substances, what is shown on placards, and recommended isolation distances. There is also a section on using the *ERG* that will walk you through the "how to" of using it as a reference source.

To use the *ERG*, follow the steps in **Skill Drill 49-1** (NFPA 472, 4.1.2.2, 4.2.3, 4.4.1, 5.2.3):

The nine DOT chemical families recognized in the *ERG* are as follows:

- **DOT Class 1:** Explosives
- **DOT Class 2:** Gases
- **DOT Class 3:** Flammable/combustible liquids
- **DOT Class 4:** Flammable solids, spontaneously combustible materials, and dangerous-when-wet materials or water-reactive substances

Skill Drill 49-1 Using the *ERG* to Research Materials

Step 1 Identify the chemical name and/or the chemical ID number for the suspect placard or label.

Step 2 Look up the material name in the appropriate section. Use the yellow section to obtain information based on the chemical ID number. Use the blue section to obtain information based on the alphabetical chemical name. *Note any listing that has been highlighted as this should lead you to the evacuation distance section of the ERG.*

Step 3 Determine the correct emergency action guide to use for the chemical identified.

Step 4 Identify the potential fire and explosion and/or health hazards of the chemical identified.

Step 5 Identify the isolation distance and the protective actions required for the chemical identified.

Step 6 Identify the emergency response actions of the chemical identified.

Table of Placards and Initial Response Guide To use on Scene
Use this table only if materials cannot be specifically
Identified by using the shipping document, numbered placard,
or orange panel number

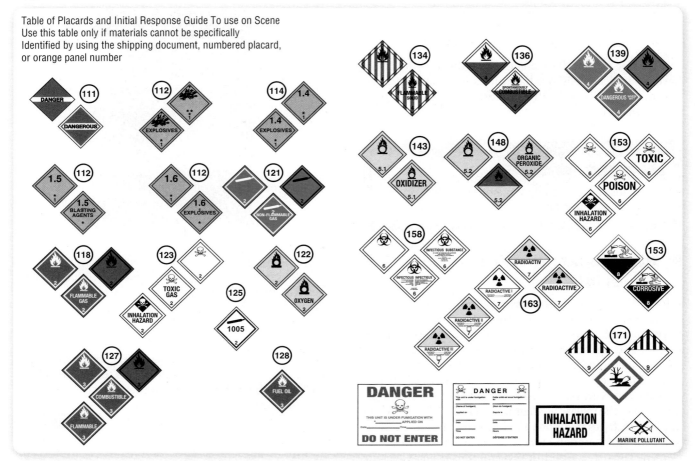

Figure 49-2 The DOT uses labels, placards, and markings (such as these found in the *ERG*) to give responders a general idea of the hazard inside a particular container or cargo tank.

Courtesy of U.S. Department of Transportation.

- **DOT Class 5:** Oxidizing substances and organic peroxides
- **DOT Class 6:** Toxic substances and infectious substances (The word *poison* or *poisonous* is considered synonymous with *toxin* or *toxic*.)
- **DOT Class 7:** Radioactive materials
- **DOT Class 8:** Corrosive substances
- **DOT Class 9:** Miscellaneous hazardous materials/products, substances, or organisms

You can download a free copy of the *ERG* by visiting the US DOT Pipeline and Hazardous Materials Safety Administration website.

Transportation Marking System

The DOT marking system is an identification system characterized by labels, placards, and markings **Figure 49-2**. This marking system is used when materials are being transported from one location to another in the United States. The same marking system is used in Canada by Transport Canada.

Placards are diamond-shaped indicators (at least 10.8 inches [27 cm] on each side) that are placed on all four sides of highway transport vehicles, railroad tank

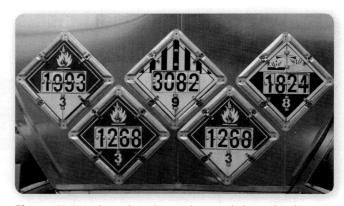

Figure 49-3 A placard is a large, diamond-shaped indicator that is placed on all sides of transport vehicles that carry hazardous materials. The numbers identify the specific material being transported.

© Mark Winfrey/Shutterstock.

cars, and other forms of transportation carrying hazardous materials **Figure 49-3**. Placards identify the broad hazard class (flammable, poison, corrosive) to which the material inside belongs. The most common placards show four-digit numbers that are part of the United Nations/North American coding system for identification of hazardous materials. This number identifies the specific material being transported and corresponds with information in the *ERG*. In addition to the numbers, different symbols are used to help identify different classes of hazardous materials.

Labels are smaller versions (at least 3.9 inches [9.9 cm] on each side) of placards; they are placed on the four sides of individual boxes and smaller packages being transported. A label on a box inside a delivery truck relates only to the potential hazard inside that particular package.

Placards, labels, and markings are intended to give responders a general idea of the hazard inside a particular container or cargo tank. However, the DOT system does not require that all chemical shipments be marked with placards or labels. In most cases, the package or cargo tank must contain a certain amount of hazardous material before a placard is required. Conversely, some chemicals are so hazardous that shipping any amount requires placards or labels.

Other good sources of information for identifying hazardous materials in transport include the **bill of lading**, or freight bill, which should be carried by the truck driver in the cab, and the **waybill**, or "consist," which is carried by the conductor of a train. Additionally, dispatchers may assist in collecting further information from organizations such as **CHEMTREC (Chemical Transportation Emergency Center)**, which operates a telephone line (1-800-262-8200) and has an extensive database to assist emergency responders. CHEMTREC has the ability to provide responders with technical chemical information via the telephone, fax, or other electronic media. Calls can be translated in over 180 languages. There is also a phone conferencing service that will put a responder in touch with thousands of shippers, subject matter experts, and chemical manufacturers. When you call CHEMTREC (a free service), be sure to have the following basic information ready:

- Name of the chemical or chemicals involved
- Name of the caller and callback telephone number
- Location of the actual incident or problem
- Shipper or manufacturer of chemical (if known)
- Container type
- Rail car or vehicle markings or numbers
- Shipping carrier's name
- Recipient of material
- Local conditions and exact description of the situation

The Canadian equivalent of CHEMTREC is known as CANUTEC (Canadian Transport Emergency Centre). This organization serves Canadian responders in much the same way CHEMTREC serves responders in the United States. The Mexican equivalent of CHEMTREC and CANUTEC is SETIQ. Phone numbers for all of these agencies, including the phone number for the National Response Center (NRC) and other important resources, can be found in the *ERG*. The NRC is operated by the US Coast Guard and serves as a central notification point,

Words of Wisdom

There are many legitimate reference sources available to EMS responders when it comes to hazardous materials response. It is up to you to be familiar with what is available within your AHJ.

rather than a guidance center. Once the NRC is notified, it will alert appropriate state and federal agencies.

Fixed-Facility Marking System

The NFPA has developed its own system for identifying hazardous materials. NFPA 704, *Standard System for the Identification of the Hazards of Materials for Emergency Response*, outlines a marking system characterized by a set of diamonds that are found on the outside of buildings, on doorways to chemical storage areas, and on fixed storage tanks. This marking system is designed for fixed-facility use. The NFPA 704 hazard identification system uses a diamond-shaped symbol of any size, which is itself broken into four smaller diamonds, each representing a particular property or characteristic **Figure 49-4**. The placards are colored and indicate specific hazards (red = fire hazard, blue = health hazard, white = special information, and yellow = reactivity hazard). Each small diamond is rated on a scale of 0 (no hazard) to 4 (severe risk).

If you are at a permanent manufacturing or storage facility, you should be able to obtain a **safety data sheet (SDS)** for in-depth information about the hazardous materials present **Figure 49-5**. An SDS provides basic information about the chemical makeup of a substance, the potential hazards it presents, appropriate first aid in the event of an exposure, and other pertinent data for safe handling of the material. Obtaining this information may expedite treatment in the hospital and may be potentially lifesaving.

▶ Containers

In basic terms, a **container** is any vessel or receptacle that holds a material. Often the container type, size, and

Words of Wisdom

To ensure efficiency and safety when you are responding to a potential hazardous materials incident, you should learn the concepts and principles of the National Incident Management System (NIMS) and the incident command system (ICS) discussed in Chapter 47, *Incident Management and Mass-Casualty Incidents*. Hazardous materials incident management may seem laborious, slow, or cumbersome to you, but the potentially extreme hazards and the need to protect rescuers, other health care personnel, and the public from harm mandate a cautious approach.

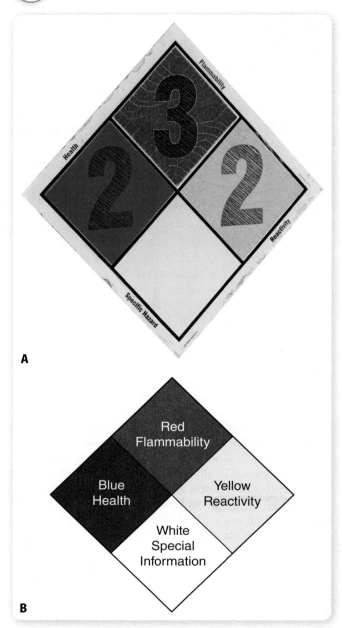

A

B

Figure 49-4 A. Example of a placard using the NFPA 704 hazard identification system. **B.** Each color used in the diamond represents a particular property or characteristic.

© Jones & Bartlett Learning.

material of construction provide important clues about the nature of the substance inside. Nevertheless, you should not rely solely on the type of container when you are making a determination about hazardous materials.

Chemical waste from an illicit laboratory, for example, might be found in an unmarked plastic container of any size. In this case, there may be no legitimate markings to alert you to the possible contents. Gasoline or waste solvents may be stored in 55-gallon (208-L) steel drums. Sulfuric acid, at 97% concentration, could be found in a polyethylene drum that might be colored black, red, white, or blue. In most cases, there is no correlation between the color of the drum and the possible contents.

The same sulfuric acid might also be found in a 1-gallon (4-L) amber glass container. Steel or polyethylene drums, bags, high-pressure gas cylinders, railroad tank cars, plastic buckets, aboveground and underground storage tanks, cargo tanks, and pipelines are all representative examples of how hazardous materials are packaged, stored, and shipped **Figure 49-6** .

Some recognizable chemical containers, such as 55-gallon (208-L) drums and compressed gas cylinders, can be found in almost every type of manufacturing facility. Materials stored in a cardboard drum are usually in solid form. Stainless steel containers hold particularly dangerous chemicals, and cold liquids are kept in containers designed to maintain the appropriate temperature **Figure 49-7** .

One way to distinguish containers is to divide them into two categories based on their capacity: bulk and nonbulk storage containers.

Bulk Storage Vessels

Bulk storage containers include fixed tanks, highway cargo tanks, rail tank cars, totes, and intermodal tanks. In general, bulk storage containers are found in buildings that rely on and need to store large quantities of a particular chemical. Most manufacturing facilities have at least one type of bulk storage container. Often these bulk storage containers are surrounded by a supplementary containment system to help control an accidental release. **Secondary containment** is an engineered method to control spilled or released product if the main containment vessel fails. A 5,000-gallon (18,900-L) vertical storage tank, for example, may be surrounded by a series of short walls that form a catch basin around the tank.

Words of Wisdom

When you consider locations for possible hazardous materials incidents, do not limit your thinking. You may be surprised by how many different kinds of containers you may find in unexpected places.

Large-volume horizontal tanks are also common. When stored aboveground, these tanks are referred to as aboveground storage tanks; if they are placed underground, they are known as underground storage tanks. These tanks can hold a few hundred gallons to several million gallons of product and are usually made of aluminum, steel, or plastic.

Another commonly encountered bulk storage vessel is the tote, also referred to as an intermediate bulk container. Totes have capacities ranging from 119 to 703 gallons (450 to 2,660 L). These portable plastic tanks are surrounded by a stainless steel web that adds both structural stability and protection to the container. They can contain any type of chemical, including flammable liquids, corrosives, food-grade liquids, or oxidizers **Figure 49-8** .

Nitrogen, refrigerated liquid
Safety Data Sheet P-4630
This SDS conforms to U.S. Code of Federal Regulations 29 CFR 1910.1200, Hazard Communication.

Date of issue : 01/01/1979   Revision date : 10/21/2016   Supersedes : 10/03/2014

SECTION: 1. Product and company identification

1.1.   Product identifier

Product form	:	Substance
Name	:	Nitrogen, refrigerated liquid
CAS No	:	7727-37-9
Formula	:	N2
Other means of identification	:	Nitrogen (cryogenic liquid), Nitrogen, Medipure Liquid Nitrogen

1.2.   Relevant identified uses of the substance or mixture and uses advised against

Use of the substance/mixture	:	Medical applications
		Industrial use
		Food applications

1.3.   Details of the supplier of the safety data sheet

XYZ Chemical, Inc.
10 Main Street
Anytown, NY 01234-5678 - USA
T 1-800-555-4321
www.xyzchemical.com

1.4.   Emergency telephone number

Emergency number   : Onsite Emergency: 1-800-555-0011

CHEMTREC, 24hr/day 7days/week
— Within USA: 1-800-424-9300, Outside USA: 001-703-527-3887
(collect calls accepted, Contract 17729)

SECTION 2: Hazard identification

2.1.   Classification of the substance or mixture

GHS-US classification

Refrigerated liquefied gas   H281

2.2.   Label elements

GHS-US labeling

Hazard pictograms (GHS-US)   :

GHS04

Signal word (GHS-US)	:	WARNING
Hazard statements (GHS-US)	:	H281 - CONTAINS REFRIGERATED GAS; MAY CAUSE CRYOGENIC BURNS OR INJURY
		OSHA-H01 - MAY DISPLACE OXYGEN AND CAUSE RAPID SUFFOCATION
Precautionary statements (GHS-US)	:	P202 - Do not handle until all safety precautions have been read and understood
		P271+P403 - Use and store only outdoors or in a well-ventilated place
		P282 - Wear cold insulating gloves/face shield/eye protection.
		CGA-PG05 - Use a back flow preventive device in the piping
		CGA-PG24 - DO NOT change or force fit connections
		CGA-PG06 - Close valve after each use and when empty
		CGA-PG23 - Always keep container in upright position

2.3.   Other hazards

Other hazards not contributing to the classification	:	Asphyxiant in high concentrations
		Contact with liquid may cause cold burns/frostbite

EN (English US)   SDS ID : P-4630   1/9

Figure 49-5 An example of a safety data sheet for liquid nitrogen.

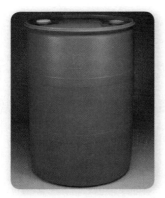

Figure 49-6 Drums may be constructed of many different types of materials, including cardboard, polyethylene, and stainless steel. The drum shown here is a polyethylene drum.

Courtesy of EMD Chemicals, Inc.

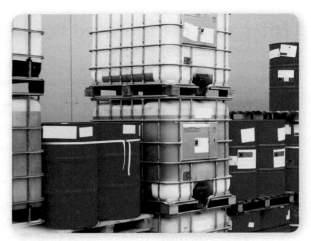

Figure 49-7 A series of chemical storage containers.

© Ulrich Mueller/Shutterstock.

Shipping and storage totes can be hazardous. These containers often are stacked atop one another and moved with a forklift, such that a mishap with the loading or moving process can compromise the tote. Because totes have no secondary containment system, any leak has the potential to create a large puddle. In addition, the steel webbing around the tote makes it difficult to access and patch leaks.

Intermodal tanks are both shipping and storage vessels. They hold between 5,000 and 6,000 gallons (18,900 to 22,700 L) of product and can be pressurized or nonpressurized. Intermodal tanks can also be used to ship and store gaseous substances that have been chilled until they liquefy, such as liquid nitrogen. In most cases, an intermodal tank is shipped to a facility, where it is stored and used and then returned to the shipper for refilling. Intermodal tanks can be shipped by all methods of transportation—air, sea, and land **Figure 49-9** .

Nonbulk Storage Vessels

Essentially, **nonbulk storage vessels** are all types of containers other than bulk containers. Nonbulk storage vessels can hold a few ounces to 119 gallons (450 L) of product

---

YOU are the Paramedic   PART 2

As you begin your assessment, you observe that the patient is seated leaning forward in a tripod position. It is clear that he is in respiratory distress. He has shallow, rapid respirations with intercostal and subcostal retractions. Audible expiratory wheezes are present. You ask your partner to assist the patient's ventilations with a bag-mask device. You place the patient on the cardiac monitor and observe a sinus tachycardia. A coworker is able to tell you that the patient was trapped in the room where the anhydrous ammonia leak occurred for approximately 5 minutes. The patient has a past medical history of hypertension and asthma.

Recording Time: 5 Minutes	
Respirations	30 breaths/min; shallow
Pulse	Radial pulse, 127 beats/min; regular and strong
Skin	Pale, warm, and diaphoretic
Blood pressure	156/84 mm Hg
Oxygen saturation (Spo$_2$)	88% on room air; 93% when assisted with a bag-mask device at 15 L/min
Pupils	PERRLA

4. What should your initial treatment consist of?
5. Based on the SDS for anhydrous ammonia, how would you determine a treatment plan for this patient?
6. Are there any other treatment options at this point?

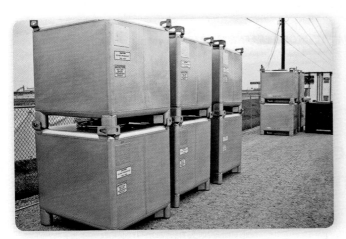

Figure 49-8 A tote is a commonly encountered bulk storage vessel.
Courtesy of Tank Service, Inc.

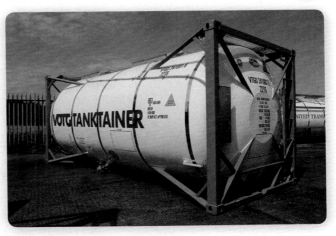

Figure 49-9 An intermodal tank.
Courtesy of UBH International, Ltd.

and include vessels such as drums, bags, compressed gas cylinders, cryogenic containers, and more. Nonbulk storage vessels hold commonly used commercial and industrial chemicals such as solvents, industrial cleaners, and compounds. This section describes the most commonly encountered types of nonbulk storage vessels.

Drums. **Drums** are easily recognizable, barrel-like containers. They are used to store a wide variety of substances, including food-grade materials, corrosives, flammable liquids, and grease. Drums may be constructed of low-carbon steel, polyethylene, cardboard, stainless steel, nickel, or other materials. Generally, the nature of the chemical dictates the construction of the storage drum. Steel utility drums, for example, hold flammable liquids, cleaning fluids, oil, and other noncorrosive chemicals. Polyethylene drums are used for corrosives such as acids, bases, oxidizers, and other materials that cannot be stored in steel containers. Cardboard drums hold solid materials such as soap flakes, sodium hydroxide pellets, and food-grade materials. Stainless steel or other heavy-duty drums generally hold materials too aggressive (ie, too reactive) for either plain steel or polyethylene.

Bags. Bags are commonly used to store solids and powders such as cement powder, sand, pesticides, soda ash, and slaked lime. Storage bags may be constructed of plastic, paper, or plastic-lined paper. Bags come in different sizes and weights, depending on their contents.

Pesticide bags must be labeled with specific information **Figure 49-10** . You can learn a great deal from the label, including the following details:

- Name of the product
- Active ingredients
- Hazard statement
- Total amount of product in the container
- Manufacturer's name and address
- EPA registration number, which provides proof that the product was registered with the EPA

- EPA establishment number, which shows where the product was manufactured
- Signal words to indicate the relative toxicity of the material:
  - Danger—Poison: Highly toxic by all routes of entry
  - Danger: Severe eye damage or skin irritation
  - Warning: Moderately toxic
  - Caution: Minor toxicity and minor eye damage or skin irritation
- Practical first aid treatment description
- Directions for use
- Agricultural use requirements
- Precautionary statements such as mixing directions or potential environmental hazards
- Storage and disposal information
- Classification statement on who may use the product

In addition, every pesticide label must carry the statement, "Keep out of reach of children."

Carboys. Some corrosives and other types of chemicals are transported and stored in vessels called **carboys** **Figure 49-11** . A carboy is a glass, plastic, or steel container that holds 5 to 15 gallons (19 to 600 L) of product. Glass carboys are often placed in a protective wood, foam, fiberglass, or steel box to help prevent breakage. For example, nitric acid, sulfuric acid, and other strong acids are often transported and stored in thick glass carboys protected by a wooden or polystyrene (Styrofoam) crate to shield the glass container from damage during shipping.

Cylinders. Several types of **cylinders** are used to hold liquids and gases. Uninsulated compressed gas cylinders are used to store substances such as nitrogen, argon, helium, and oxygen. They come in a range of sizes. As a paramedic, you are familiar with the shape of a compressed gas cylinder; it holds the oxygen for your patients.

A BIOCHEMICAL FOR MATING DISRUPTION OF OMNIVOROUS LEAFROLLER (Platynota stultana)

ACTIVE INGREDIENTS:
(E) - 11 - Tetradecen-1-yl acetate . . . . 20.57 %
(Z) - 11 - Tetradecen-1-yl acetate . . . . .3.19 %
OTHER INGREDIENTS . . . . 76.24 %
TOTAL . . . . 100.00 %

KEEP OUT OF REACH OF CHILDREN

CAUTION

PRECAUTIONARY STATEMENTS
HAZARDS TO HUMANS AND DOMESTIC ANIMALS

Harmful if absorbed through the skin. Causes moderate eye irritation. Avoid contact with skin, eyes, or clothing. Harmful if inhaled. Avoid breathing vapor or spray mist.

User Safety Requirements: Applicators and other handlers must wear long-sleeved shirt and long pants, waterproof gloves, and shoes plus socks. For overhead exposure wear chemical resistant headgear. Follow manufacturer's instructions for cleaning and maintaining PPE. If no such instructions for washables, use detergent and hot water. Keep and wash PPE separately from other laundry.

FIRST AID STATEMENT

IF SWALLOWED: Call a Poison Control Center or doctor immediately for treatment advice. Have person sip a glass of water if able to swallow. Do not induce vomiting unless told to do so by a Poison Control Center or doctor. Do not give anything by mouth to an unconscious person.

IF ON SKIN OR CLOTHING: Take off contaminated clothing. Rinse skin immediately with plenty of water for 15-20 minutes. Call a Poison Control Center or doctor for treatment advice.

IF INHALED: Move person to fresh air. If person is not breathing, call 9-1-1 or an ambulance, then give artificial respiration, preferably mouth-to-mouth, if possible. Call a Poison Control Center or doctor for further treatment advice.

IF IN EYES: Hold eye open and rinse slowly and gently with water for 15-20 minutes. Remove contact lenses, if present, after the first 5 minutes, then continue rinsing eye. Call a Poison Control Center or doctor for treatment advice.

DIRECTIONS FOR USE

IT IS A VIOLATION OF FEDERAL LAW TO USE THIS PRODUCT IN A MANNER INCONSISTENT WITH ITS LABELING.

Do not apply this product in a way that will contact workers or other persons, either directly or through drift. Only protected handlers may be in the area during application. For requirements specific to your state or Tribe, consult the agency responsible for pesticide regulation.

AGRICULTURAL USE REQUIREMENTS - Use this product only in accordance with its labeling and with the Worker Protection Standard, 40 CFR part 170. This Standard contains requirements for the protection of agricultural workers on farms, forests, nurseries, and greenhouses, and handlers of agricultural pesticides. It contains requirements for training, decontamination, notification, and emergency assistance. It also contains specific instructions and exceptions pertaining to the statements on this label about personal protective equipment (PPE). The requirements in this box apply to uses of this product that are covered by the Worker Protection Standard. Do not enter or allow worker entry into treated areas during application of this product. A restricted entry interval of 0 hours has been established.

Figure 49-10 A pesticide bag must be labeled with the appropriate information.
© Jones & Bartlett Learning.

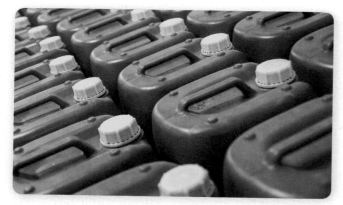

Figure 49-11 A carboy is used to transport and store corrosive chemicals.
© Radu Bercan/Alamy.

▶ Roadway Transport of Hazardous Materials

The most common method of hazardous materials transport is over land, by roadway transportation vehicles. According to the CFR, 49 CFR 171.8(2), or local jurisdictional regulations (for example, Transport Canada), a **cargo tank** is bulk packaging that is permanently attached to or forms a part of a motor vehicle, or is not permanently attached to any motor vehicle and that, because of its size, construction, or attachment to a motor vehicle, is loaded or unloaded without being removed from the motor vehicle. The DOT does not view tube trailers (which consist of several individual cylinders banded together and affixed to a trailer) as cargo tanks.

One of the most common and reliable transportation vessels is the **MC-306/DOT 406 flammable liquid tanker** **Figure 49-12** . These tanks frequently carry liquid food-grade products, gasoline, or other flammable and combustible liquids. The oval-shaped tank is pulled by a diesel tractor and can carry between 6,000 and 10,000 gallons (22,700 to 37,900 L) of product. The MC-306/DOT 406 is nonpressurized (its working pressure is between 2.65 and 4 pounds per square inch [psi], or 18 to 26 kilopascals [kPa]), usually made of aluminum or stainless steel, and offloaded through valves at the bottom of the tank. These cargo tanks have several safety features, including full rollover protection and remote emergency shut-off valves.

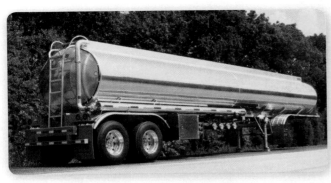

Figure 49-12 The MC-306/DOT 406 flammable liquid tanker typically hauls flammable and combustible liquid.
Courtesy of Polar Tank Trailer, L.L.C.

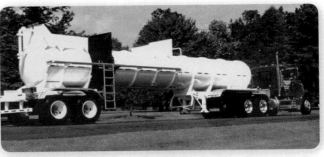

Figure 49-14 The MC-312/DOT 412 corrosive tanker is commonly used to carry corrosives such as concentrated sulfuric acid, phosphoric acid, and sodium hydroxide.
Courtesy of National Tank Truck Carriers Association.

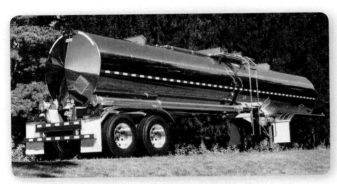

Figure 49-13 The MC-307/DOT 407 chemical hauler carries flammable liquids, mild corrosives, and poisons.
Courtesy of Polar Tank Trailer, L.L.C.

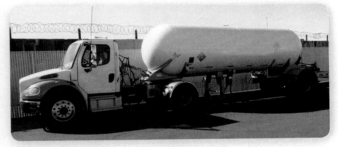

Figure 49-15 The MC-331 pressure cargo tanker carries materials such as ammonia, propane, Freon, and butane.
Courtesy of Rob Schnepp.

A vehicle that is similar to the MC-306/DOT 406 is the **MC-307/DOT 407 chemical hauler**. It has a round or horseshoe-shaped tank and is capable of holding 6,000 to 7,000 gallons (22,700 to 26,500 L) of liquid `Figure 49-13`. The MC-307/DOT 407, which is also a tractor-drawn tank, is used to transport flammable liquids, mild corrosives, and poisons. This type of cargo tank may be insulated (horseshoe) or uninsulated (round) and may have a higher internal working pressure than does the MC-306/DOT 406—in some cases up to 35 psi (240 kPa). Cargo tanks that transport corrosives may have a rubber lining to prevent corrosion of the tank structure.

The **MC-312/DOT 412 corrosive tanker** is commonly used to carry corrosives such as concentrated sulfuric acid, phosphoric acid, and sodium hydroxide `Figure 49-14`. This cargo tank has a smaller diameter than either the MC-306/DOT 406 or the MC-307/DOT 407 and is often identifiable by the presence of several heavy-duty reinforcing rings around the tank. The rings provide structural stability during transport and in the event of a rollover. The inside of an MC-312/DOT 412 tanker operates at approximately 15 to 25 psi (100 to 170 kPa) and holds approximately 6,000 gallons (22,700 L). These cargo tanks have substantial rollover protection to reduce the potential for damage to the top-mounted valves.

The **MC-331 pressure cargo tanker** carries materials such as ammonia, propane, Freon, and butane `Figure 49-15`. The liquid volume inside the tank varies, ranging from the 1,000-gallon (3,800-L) delivery truck to the full-size 11,000-gallon (41,600-L) cargo tank. The MC-331 cargo tank has rounded ends, typical of a pressurized vessel, and is commonly constructed of steel or stainless steel with a single tank compartment. The MC-331 operates at approximately 300 psi (2,100 kPa), with typical internal working pressures being in the vicinity of 250 psi (1,700 kPa). These cargo tanks are equipped with spring-loaded relief valves that traditionally operate at 110% of the designated maximum working pressure. A significant explosion hazard arises if an MC-331 cargo tank is impinged on by fire, however. Because of the nature of most materials carried in MC-331 tanks, a threat of explosion exists because of the inability of the relief valve to keep up with the rapidly building internal pressure. Responders must use great care when they are dealing with this type of transportation emergency.

The **MC-338 cryogenic tanker** is a low-pressure tanker that relies on tank insulation to maintain the low temperatures required for the cryogens it carries `Figure 49-16`. A boxlike structure containing the tank control valves is typically attached to the rear of the tanker. Special training is required to operate valves on this and any other tanker. An untrained person who attempts to operate the valves may disrupt the normal operation of the tank, thereby compromising its ability to keep the liquefied gas cold and creating a potential explosion hazard. Cryogenic tankers have a relief valve near the valve control box. From time to time, small puffs of white vapor will be vented

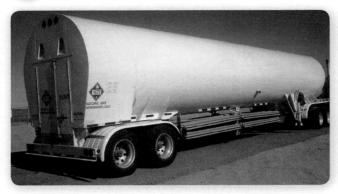

Figure 49-16 The MC-338 cryogenic tanker maintains the low temperatures required for the cryogens it carries.
Courtesy of Jack B. Kelley, Inc.

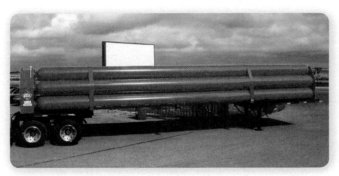

Figure 49-17 Tube trailers carry compressed gases such as hydrogen, oxygen, helium, and methane.
Courtesy of Jack B. Kelley, Inc.

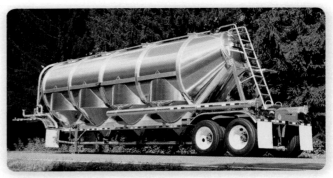

Figure 49-18 A dry bulk cargo tank carries dry goods such as powders, pellets, fertilizers, and grain.
Courtesy of Polar Tank Trailer, L.L.C.

from this valve. Responders should understand that this is a normal occurrence; the valve is working to maintain the proper internal pressure. In most cases, this vapor is not indicative of an emergency situation. Problems can occur however in hot weather if these trucks crash and the freezer unit is damaged.

Tube trailers carry compressed gases such as hydrogen, oxygen, helium, and methane **Figure 49-17** . Essentially, they are high-volume transport vehicles that are made up of several individual cylinders banded together and affixed to a trailer. The individual cylinders on the tube trailer are much like the smaller compressed gas cylinders discussed earlier in this chapter. These large-volume cylinders operate at working pressures of 3,000 to 5,000 psi (20,700 to 34,500 kPa). One trailer may carry several different gases in individual tubes. Typically, a valve control box is found toward the rear of the trailer, and each individual cylinder has its own relief valve. These trailers can frequently be seen at construction sites or at facilities that use large quantities of compressed gases.

Dry bulk cargo tanks are commonly seen on the road; they carry dry bulk goods such as powders, pellets, fertilizers, or grain **Figure 49-18** . These tanks are not pressurized but may use pressure to offload the product. Dry bulk cargo tanks are generally V-shaped with rounded sides that funnel the contents to the bottom-mounted valves.

▶ Establishing Safety Zones

Until the hazardous materials technical team arrives to determine the hazard zone, you should be aware of the safety perimeters that are necessary for hazardous materials that are toxic (poisonous) and those that pose a danger of fire or explosion. If you are dispatched to a hazardous materials incident, take the following precautions:

- Protect yourself first!
- Isolate the incident as much as possible to avoid the risk of further harm to other people—laypeople, EMS staff, firefighters, and law enforcement responders. No one should risk his or her life or health at a hazardous materials incident. The *ERG*, which you should carry in your vehicle, can help determine initial isolation distances.
- Notify your dispatcher and any other EMS, fire, or law enforcement responders that a hazardous materials incident is in progress.
- Inform incoming responders of what you observe about wind direction, terrain features, and a safe response route.

As the hazardous materials incident progresses, hazardous materials specialists will establish the hot, warm, and cold zones. The hot zone is the contamination zone where only properly trained rescuers wearing appropriate PPE are allowed. The warm zone surrounds the hot zone. Typically, the decontamination corridor is located in the warm zone. This zone should be entered only by trained hazardous materials specialists wearing appropriate PPE. The cold zone provides a further buffer from the hazards present in the hot and warm zones. Paramedics normally perform triage and patient treatment in the cold zone **Figure 49-19** .

Initial Isolation and Protection Distance

There may be times when a decision must be made to shelter in place, evacuate, or rescue people in danger. In those instances, responders may need to consult printed and electronic reference sources for guidance on evacuation

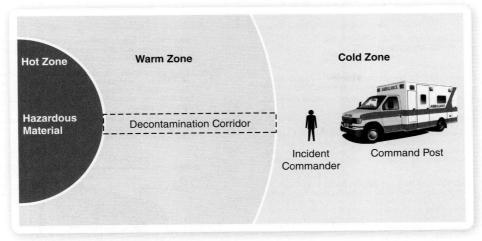

Figure 49-19 Hot, warm, and cold zones.
© Jones & Bartlett Learning.

distances and other safety information. The most accessible resource for evacuation distances is the green section of the *ERG* (Figure 49-20). This reference book identifies and outlines predetermined evacuation distances and basic action plans for chemicals highlighted in the yellow or blue sections of the book, based on spill size estimates.

Hazardous materials teams also use air-monitoring equipment to help determine explosive limits, oxygen levels, and the concentration of hydrogen sulfide and carbon monoxide. They will also be able to determine the pH of spills and may have capability for specific agent testing using colorimetric devices.

There are also a number of computer programs such as Computer-Aided Management of Emergency Operations (**CAMEO**) to help predict downwind concentrations of hazardous materials based on the input of environmental factors into a computer model. When used properly, these computer programs can be a valuable source of information for predicting the size and direction of gas or vapor clouds. This type of program is typically used by hazardous materials responders but may also be available to EMS personnel.

▶ Personal Protective Equipment

You should be familiar with the PPE used at hazardous materials scenes even if you are not expected to use it. In most cases, the hazardous materials team or other trained responders will determine the appropriate PPE needed for a specific task or mission. Your job as an EMS provider is to recognize certain levels or combinations of PPE and understand the potential hazards encountered by the people inside the garments. Various sections of NFPA 472 provide guidance on the selection, use, and components of chemical protective equipment. It could be that the highest hazard is not posed by the released substance! EMS providers should consider the effects of heat and

cold stress on the people inside the PPE in addition to the chemical threats posed by the hazardous materials agent. The astute EMS provider will evaluate the environmental conditions present at the scene, formulate a plan to deal with responders experiencing heat- or cold-related issues, determine the potential health risks that could be posed by an exposure, and determine how that exposure should be treated along with the appropriate transport decision. A proactive EMS provider, operating at the scene of a hazardous materials incident, already has a basic plan in place to treat civilians and responders alike.

Hazardous materials responders classify chemical protective clothing by level A through level D (Figure 49-21). Most paramedic ambulances do not carry this equipment, but again, you should be familiar enough with it to understand what the wearer of the garment is experiencing.

Words of Wisdom

The NFPA publishes protective clothing standards to provide guidance on the performance of certain types of chemical-protective garments. NFPA 1991, for example, is the *Standard on Vapor-Protective Ensembles for Hazardous Materials Emergencies.* NFPA 1992, *Standard on Liquid Splash-Protective Ensembles and Clothing for Hazardous Materials Emergencies*, covers a different type of chemical-protective garment. The NFPA also acknowledges the importance of chemical-protective garments as they relate to weapons of mass destruction response. To obtain guidance in this area, responders may reference NFPA 1994, *Standard on Protective Ensembles for First Responders to CBRN Terrorism Incidents* (CBRN stands for chemical, biologic, radiologic, and nuclear).

HOW TO USE TABLE 1 - INITIAL ISOLATION AND PROTECTIVE ACTION DISTANCES

(1) The responder should already have:

- Identified the material by its ID Number and Name; (if an ID Number cannot be found, use the Name of Material index in the blue-bordered pages to locate that number.)
- Found the three-digit guide for that material in order to consult the emergency actions recommended jointly with this table;
- **Noted the wind direction.**

(2) Look in Table 1 (the green-bordered pages) for the ID Number and Name of the Material involved in the incident. Some ID Numbers have more than one shipping name listed - look for the specific name of the material. (If the shipping name is not known and Table 1 lists more than one name for the same ID Number, use the entry with the largest protective action distances.)

(3) Determine if the incident involves a SMALL or LARGE spill and if DAY or NIGHT. A SMALL SPILL consists of a release of less than 208 liters (55 US gallons). This generally corresponds to a spill from a single small package (e.g. a drum), a small cylinder, or a small leak from a large package. A LARGE SPILL consists of a release of more than 208 liters (55 US gallons). This usually involves a spill from a large package, or multiple spills from many small packages. DAY is any time after sunrise and before sunset. NIGHT is any time between sunset and sunrise.

(4) Look up the INITIAL ISOLATION DISTANCE. This distance defines the radius of a zone (Initial Isolation Zone) surrounding the spill in ALL DIRECTIONS. Within this zone, all public should be evacuated (protective clothing and respiratory protection is required in this zone). Persons should be directed to move out of the zone in a direction perpendicular to wind direction (crosswind), and away from the spill, to a minimum distance as prescribed by the Initial Isolation Distance.

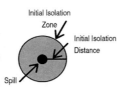

(5) Look up the initial PROTECTIVE ACTION DISTANCE. For a given material, spill size, and whether day or night, Table 1 gives the downwind distance—in kilometers and miles—from the spill/leak source for which protective actions should be considered. For practical purposes, the Protective Action Zone (i.e., the area in which people are at risk of harmful exposure) is a square, whose length and width are the same as the downwind distance shown in Table 1. Protective actions are those steps taken to preserve the health and safety of emergency responders and the public. People in this area should be evacuated and/or sheltered-in-place.

(6) Initiate Protective Actions to the extent possible, beginning with those closest to the spill site and working away from the site in the downwind direction. When a water-reactive TIH (PIH in the US) producing material is spilled into a river or stream, the source of the toxic gas may move with the current or stretch from the spill point downstream for a substantial distance.

The shape of the area in which protective actions should be taken (the Protective Action Zone) is shown in this figure. The spill is located at the center of the small circle. The larger circle represents the INITIAL ISOLATION zone around the spill.

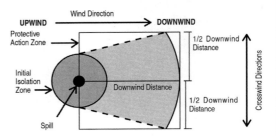

NOTE 1: See "Introduction To Green Tables - Initial Isolation And Protective Action Distances" under "Factors That May Change the Protective Action Distances" (page 289)

NOTE 2: When a product in Table 1 has the mention "(when spilled in water)", refer to Table 2 – Water-Reactive Materials which Produce Toxic Gases for the list of gases produced when these materials are spilled in water.

Call the emergency response telephone number listed on the shipping paper or the appropriate response agency as soon as possible for additional information on the material, safety precautions and mitigation procedures.

Page 294

Page 295

Page 296

TABLE 1 - INITIAL ISOLATION AND PROTECTIVE ACTION DISTANCES

ID No.	Guide	NAME OF MATERIAL	SMALL SPILLS (From a small package or small leak from a large package) First ISOLATE in all Directions Meters (Feet)	SMALL SPILLS Then PROTECT persons Downwind during DAY Kilometers (Miles)	SMALL SPILLS Then PROTECT persons Downwind during NIGHT Kilometers (Miles)	LARGE SPILLS (From a large package or from many small packages) First ISOLATE in all Directions Meters (Feet)	LARGE SPILLS Then PROTECT persons Downwind during DAY Kilometers (Miles)	LARGE SPILLS Then PROTECT persons Downwind during NIGHT Kilometers (Miles)
1005 1005	125 125	Ammonia, anhydrous Anhydrous ammonia	30 m (100 ft)	0.1 km (0.1 mi)	0.2 km (0.1 mi)	Refer to table 3		
1008 1008	125 125	Boron trifluoride Boron trifluoride, compressed	30 m (100 ft)	0.1 km (0.1 mi)	0.7 km (0.4 mi)	400 m (1250 ft)	2.2 km (1.4 mi)	4.8 km (3.0 mi)
1016 1016	119 119	Carbon monoxide Carbon monoxide, compressed	30 m (100 ft)	0.1 km (0.1 mi)	0.2 km (0.1 mi)	200 m (600 ft)	1.2 km (0.7 mi)	4.4 km (2.8 mi)
1017	124	Chlorine	60 m (200 ft)	0.3 km (0.2 mi)	1.1 km (0.7 mi)	Refer to table 3		
1026	119	Cyanogen	30 m (100 ft)	0.1 km (0.1 mi)	0.4 km (0.3 mi)	60 m (200 ft)	0.3 km (0.2 mi)	1.1 km (0.7 mi)
1040 1040	119P 119P	Ethylene oxide Ethylene oxide with Nitrogen	30 m (100 ft)	0.1 km (0.1 mi)	0.2 km (0.1 mi)	Refer to table 3		
1045 1045	124 124	Fluorine Fluorine, compressed	30 m (100 ft)	0.1 km (0.1 mi)	0.2 km (0.1 mi)	100 m (300 ft)	0.5 km (0.3 mi)	2.2 km (1.4 mi)
1048	125	Hydrogen bromide, anhydrous	30 m (100 ft)	0.1 km (0.1 mi)	0.2 km (0.2 mi)	150 m (500 ft)	0.9 km (0.6 mi)	2.6 km (1.6 mi)
1050	125	Hydrogen chloride, anhydrous	30 m (100 ft)	0.1 km (0.1 mi)	0.3 km (0.2 mi)	Refer to table 3		
1051	117	AC (when used as a weapon)	60 m (200 ft)	0.3 km (0.2 mi)	1.0 km (0.6 mi)	1000 m (3000 ft)	3.7 km (2.3 mi)	8.4 km (5.3 mi)
1051 1051 1051	117 117 117	Hydrocyanic acid, aqueous solutions, with more than 20% Hydrogen cyanide Hydrogen cyanide, anhydrous, stabilized Hydrogen cyanide, stabilized	60 m (200 ft)	0.2 km (0.2 mi)	0.9 km (0.6 mi)	300 m (1000 ft)	1.1 km (0.7 mi)	2.4 km (1.5 mi)

Figure 49-20 Instructions and example pages from the Initial Isolation and Protective Action Distances table found in the *ERG*.

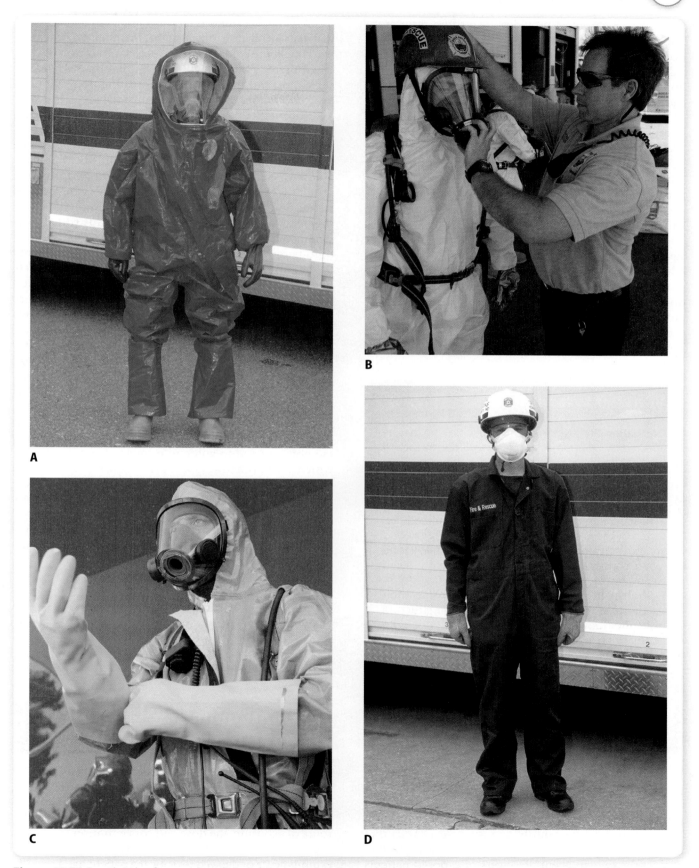

Figure 49-21 Four levels of protection. **A.** Level A protection. **B.** Level B protection. **C.** Level C protection. **D.** Level D protection.

A **level A ensemble** provides the greatest respiratory and skin protection from exposure to hazardous substances because it is "fully encapsulating." These garments fully cover the body and the self-contained breathing apparatus (SCBA) or other supplied air system worn by the responder. The suits are rigorously tested by manufacturers to determine resistance to many chemicals. Because they are considered to be "gastight," and completely cover the wearer, you may be asked to monitor or evaluate the technicians for heat stress. Additionally, you should familiarize yourself with the procedures for getting into and out of these types of garments in the event a responder has an in-suit emergency and you are called on to provide patient care.

A **level B ensemble** is called for when the responder needs a high level of respiratory protection, but the released substance does not pose a lethal threat via skin absorption. It is not fully encapsulating like level A, and it is worn with SCBA, or supplied air on the outside of the suit. Level B protection is often worn by hazardous materials responders who are performing decontamination.

Words of Wisdom

Evacuation: Removing/relocating people who may be affected by an approaching release. If the threat will be sustained over a long period, it may be advisable to evacuate people from a predicted or anticipated hazard area, making sure to evacuate those in higher danger first.

Rescue: Removing/relocating people already affected by the release. If you are wearing PPE while you are moving people from one place to another, it is no longer considered to be an evacuation; it is considered to be a rescue.

Shelter-in-place: Keeping people inside their residence, commercial building, or other structure instead of moving them away from the path of an approaching release. In some cases, usually in the case of a transitory problem such as a mobile vapor cloud, it is advisable to use the shelter-in-place method. This method is desirable only when the population being protected in place can care for themselves and control air-handling equipment, and the structure can be sealed.

A **level C ensemble** is designed to protect against a known substance. The equipment provides minimal splash protection and is worn with an air-purifying respirator (APR) or powered air-purifying respirator (PAPR) that must have filters specifically chosen to provide protection against the known agent. Receivers of exposed patients in the emergency department (ED) and law enforcement officers providing perimeter protection at a scene would be good candidates for wearing level C protection.

A **level D ensemble** is typically not worn in hazardous materials incidents by anyone other than support personnel working in the cold zone. This level of protection is worn when there is little or no threat posed by the released substance, and the responder is wearing no respiratory protection other than perhaps a dust mask.

The NFPA does not "certify" any garments. This is a common misperception in the hazardous materials and weapons of mass destruction response industry. Instead, the intent of the NFPA clothing standards is to provide guidance on manufacturing quality and performance standards. A third-party testing laboratory carries out the testing and "certifies" the garment in question. In short, the NFPA publishes performance standards (durability, flammability, chemical resistance, and cold temperature); third-party laboratories then test manufacturers' garments to determine if they meet the NFPA standards. Much like other NFPA committees, the Technical Committee for Chemical Protective Clothing consists of end users (responders), manufacturers, government representatives, and other recognized experts in the field.

When it comes to the selection and use of PPE, responders must understand how standards and regulations influence their decisions made in the field. The NFPA protective clothing standards do not tell you when, or under which conditions, to wear a particular level of chemical protection. Rather, these standards are performance documents for the garments only; they are not intended to guide responders. For guidance on which level of chemical protection to use under specific conditions, you may consult the OSHA HAZWOPER regulation, 29 CFR 1910.120; Appendix B of the OSHA HAZWOPER regulation offers guidance on which components should be worn for certain levels of protection, and under which conditions the various levels of protection should be chosen.

Words of Wisdom

If you are not dressed for the game, stay on the sidelines.

Contamination and Toxicology

The health hazards that hazardous materials present depend on the ability of the hazardous material to get into the body and interfere with the body's processes. The harm caused by a hazardous material is affected by the route of exposure, the dose and concentration, how long the toxin was in contact with the body, and whether it exhibits acute or delayed toxicity. If a patient has a chronic preexisting condition, like a respiratory ailment, then a minor anhydrous ammonia exposure could prove to be more dangerous than would be expected.

► Primary and Secondary Contamination

There are two basic types of contamination—primary and secondary. **Primary contamination** is the direct exposure of a patient to a hazardous material. **Secondary contamination** takes place when a hazardous material is transferred to a person from another person or from contaminated objects.

► Routes of Exposure

The physical properties of hazardous materials and the physical surroundings at the hazardous materials incident can expose your patient in different ways. As described in Chapter 27, *Toxicology*, the four primary methods of entry are ingestion, inhalation, injection, and absorption. However, other factors will affect your treatment priorities, including air temperature, the concentration of the hazard, and the amount of time that a patient is exposed.

A **local effect** may be described as reddening of the skin, localized pain, or the formation of blisters. Some chemical substances may have a **systemic effect** on your patient. Carbon monoxide, for example, could be inhaled without causing any damage to the airway, but ultimately render your patient unconscious, or in respiratory or cardiac arrest. These types of exposures are difficult to handle because the damage is occurring inside the body. Your job may entail identifying the exposure scenario and the substance involved and providing supportive care during transport. In some patients, if it is within your scope of practice, you might be able to deliver an antidote to reverse the systemic effects of an exposure.

Some hazardous materials can have a significant adverse effect on the neurologic, renal, or hepatic systems. These toxic effects may be seen immediately in the field or may be delayed for hours or even years, eventually presenting in the form of cancer. When the reaction shows up hours or even days after your initial treatment, your careful documentation becomes invaluable to patients. Your records should include, among other elements required by the AHJ or your medical director, a description of the scene, anything the hazardous materials team told you about the substance, how your patient looked initially, the treatments rendered, and the positive or negative changes since initial contact.

Regardless of the route or type of exposure, the **dose effect** principle applies: the greater the length of time or the greater the concentration of the material, the greater the effect probably will be on the human body. For example, people who have a substance briefly splashed on their skin will be exposed to a much lower dose than if they were lying in a puddle of that same substance for 30 minutes. The cycle of poison action includes absorption into the body, delivery to target organs, and binding to the organs. The cycle continues with biotransformation and elimination of the toxin through the gastrointestinal, kidney, or respiratory systems. These concepts should be considered as decontamination decisions are made with the hazardous materials team.

► Chemical Terms

When you are providing care and/or medical support at a hazardous materials incident, it is important to understand the terms and definitions used by the responders and how those terms and definitions relate to the released material. Additionally, understanding the chemical and physical properties of a substance may give you some valuable insight when it comes to providing care. For example, if your patient was rescued from a below-grade entrapment and propane was released during the event, would you expect the vapors to collect in low-lying areas (where your patient might have been trapped) or rise up and away from the below-grade situation? Propane is heavier than air and does in fact collect in low-lying areas, so you might have an additional issue to deal with from a patient care perspective.

For the purpose of this chapter, the definition of **vapor pressure** will pertain to liquids held inside any type of closed container. When liquids are held in a closed 55-gallon (208-L) drum or a 4-liter glass bottle, for example, some amount of pressure (in the headspace above the liquid) will develop inside. All liquids, even water, will develop a certain amount of pressure in the airspace between the top of the liquid and the container.

The key point to understanding vapor pressure is this: the vapors released from the surface of any liquid must be contained for them to exert pressure. What happens if the container is opened or spilled onto the ground to form a puddle? The liquid still has a vapor pressure, but it is no longer confined to a container. In this case, you can conclude that liquids with high vapor pressures will evaporate much more quickly than liquids with low vapor pressures. Vapor pressure directly correlates to the speed at which a material will evaporate once it is released from its container.

For example, motor oil has a low vapor pressure. When it is released, it will stay on the ground for a long time at normal temperature. Chemicals such as isopropyl alcohol or diethyl ether have the opposite reaction. When either of these materials is released and collects on the ground, it will evaporate rapidly. If the ambient air temperature or pavement temperature is elevated, the evaporation rate will increase. Wind speed, shade, humidity, and the surface area of the spill also influence how fast the chemical will evaporate.

Vapor density is another concept for figuring out where a gas or vapor might go once released from its container. Vapor density compares the hazardous material gas to air (air has a vapor density of 1). If the gas is heavier than air, the gas will sink into little valleys and ditches. Gases such as propane, butane, and carbon dioxide are heavier than air. But, if the vapor rises and dissipates as it travels with the wind, then the vapor density is less than that of the air. Gases like anhydrous ammonia, acetylene, methane, and hydrogen are lighter than air. This is why you are taught to approach a scene from upwind and uphill!

Of course, the situation changes dramatically if a fire is involved. **Flash point** is an expression of the temperature at which a liquid fuel gives off sufficient vapors that, when an ignition source is present, will result in a flash fire. The flash fire involves only the vapor phase of the liquid and will go out once the vapor fuel is consumed.

For example, the flash point of gasoline is minus 45°F (minus 43°C). When the temperature of gasoline reaches minus 45°F (minus 43°C), either from an external source or from the surrounding environment, it gives off sufficient flammable vapors to support combustion. Diesel fuel, on the other hand, has a much higher flash point than gasoline, approximately 100°F to 160°F (38°C to 71°C) depending on the fuel grade. In either case, once the temperature of the liquid surpasses its flash point, the fuel will give off sufficient flammable vapors to support combustion. Because of this, responders should always be mindful of ignition sources at flammable/combustible liquid incidents. Low flash point liquids typically have high vapor pressures. Subsequently, low flash point liquids can be expected to produce a significant amount of flammable vapors at all but the lowest ambient temperatures.

Ignition temperature is the next important combustion landmark after flash point. When a liquid fuel is heated beyond its ignition temperature, it will ignite without an external ignition source. For example, think of a pan full of cooking oil being heated on the stove. For illustration purposes, assume that the ignition temperature of the oil is 300°F (149°C). What will happen if the burner is set on high, left unattended, and the oil is heated past 300°F (149°C)? Once the temperature of the oil exceeds its ignition temperature, it will ignite; there is no need for an external ignition source. This is a common cause of stove fires.

Flammable range is another important term for you to understand. In broad terms, **flammable range** is an expression of a fuel-air mixture, defined by upper and lower limits, that reflects an amount of flammable vapor mixed with a given volume of air. Gasoline again can serve as the example. The flammable range for gasoline vapors is 1.4% to 7.6%. The two percentages, called the **lower flammable limit (LFL)** (1.4%) and the **upper flammable limit (UFL)** (7.6%), define the boundaries of a fuel-air mixture necessary for gasoline to burn properly. If a given gasoline-air mixture falls between the upper and lower flammable limits, and that mixture reaches an ignition source, there will be a flash fire.

Hazardous materials teams can, in many cases, cool down the heat or dissipate the concentration of vapors by pouring on streams of cool water. However, before any water is applied, the hazardous materials team will make crucial decisions about whether the material may be **water reactive** or **water soluble**. If they are going to use water, they will also determine the hazardous material's **specific gravity**—whether the hazardous material will sink or float in water.

▶ Toxicology Terms

Chemistry experts and medical providers should communicate with each other using agreed-upon terms to describe the health hazards any incident might present. You will be a better provider and incident historian if you can master these terms.

The **threshold limit value (TLV)** is the maximum concentration of a toxin that someone can be exposed to for a 40-hour workweek over a typical 30-year career. This value is established by the American Conference of Governmental Industrial Hygienists. The corresponding value, established by OSHA, is called the **permissible exposure limit (PEL)**.

YOU are the Paramedic   PART 3

The patient reports increased difficulty breathing. A nebulizer is attached to the bag-mask device and your partner administers 2.5 mg of albuterol and 0.5 mg of ipratropium (Atrovent) while you establish an 18-gauge intravenous line in the patient's right antecubital space and draw up 125 mg of methylprednisolone (Solu-Medrol).

Recording Time: 10 Minutes	
Respirations	Assisted with a bag-mask device
Pulse	Radial pulse, 134 beats/min; regular and strong
Skin	Pale, warm, and diaphoretic
Blood pressure	152/84 mm Hg
Oxygen saturation (Spo$_2$)	93% via bag-mask device at 15 L/min
Pupils	PERRLA

7. Explain the difference between primary and secondary contamination.
8. Explain why a water-based decontamination would be appropriate for an anhydrous ammonia exposure.

If you see both of these values listed in a reference source, you can assume the definitions are the same even if the values are different. OSHA is the law, but from an operational perspective, you should also pay attention to the more conservative of the two values if there is a conflict. The **threshold limit value/short-term exposure limit (TLV-STEL)** is the concentration that a person can be exposed to for a limited number of brief periods (eg, four 15-minute exposures per day). The **threshold limit value/ceiling (TLV-C)** is the concentration that a person should never be exposed to. Keep in mind this value is established for workplace environments and hazardous materials responders often will be operating in emergency environments that are many times greater than these values.

Lastly, the **threshold limit value/skin** indicates that direct or airborne contact with a material could result in possible and significant exposure from absorption through the skin, mucous membranes, and eyes.

Sometimes you will hear the experts refer to the lethal dose or lethal concentration value. The **lethal dose (LD)** of a material is a single dose that causes the death of a specified number of the group of test animals exposed by any route other than inhalation. The **lethal concentration (LC)** is the concentration of the material in air that, on the basis of laboratory tests (inhalation route), is expected to kill a specified number of the group of test animals when administered over a specified period. You can use these values as rough guidelines in the field when you are gauging the amount of toxicity of a particular substance. From a toxicity standpoint, you should be more concerned with substances that can be harmful at low levels. The following information will give you an idea of how to gauge toxicity in the field if an LD or LC value is known.

Toxic, as defined by OSHA 29 CFR 1910.1200, is a chemical that falls in any of the following three categories:

- A chemical that has an **LD_{50}** (a dose that would be lethal to 50% of the test population) of more than 50 milligrams per kilogram but not more than 500 milligrams per kilogram of body weight when administered orally to albino rats weighing between 200 and 300 grams each
- A chemical that has an LD_{50} of more than 200 milligrams per kilogram but not more than 1,000 milligrams per kilogram of body weight when administered by continuous contact for 24 hours (or less if death occurs within 24 hours) with the bare skin of albino rabbits weighing between 2 and 3 kilograms each
- A chemical that has an LC_{50} in air of more than 200 parts per million but not more than 2,000 parts per million by volume of gas or vapor, or more than 2 milligrams per liter but not more than 20 milligrams per liter of mist, fume, or dust, when administered by continuous inhalation for 1 hour (or less if death occurs within 1 hour) to albino rats weighing between 200 and 300 grams each

Highly toxic is defined by OSHA 29 CFR 1910.1200 as follows:

- A chemical that has an LD_{50} of 50 milligrams or less per kilogram of body weight when administered orally to albino rats weighing between 200 and 300 grams each
- A chemical that has an LD_{50} of 200 milligrams or less per kilogram of body weight when administered by continuous contact for 24 hours (or less if death occurs within 24 hours) with the bare skin of albino rabbits weighing between 2 and 3 kilograms each
- A chemical that has an LC_{50} in air of 200 parts per million by volume or less of gas or vapor, or 2 milligrams per liter or less of mist, fume, or dust, when administered by continuous inhalation for 1 hour (or less if death occurs within 1 hour) to albino rats weighing between 200 and 300 grams each

You might also hear the industrial hygienists or other hazardous materials responders use the term **immediately dangerous to life and health (IDLH)**, which means the atmospheric concentration of any toxic, corrosive, or asphyxiant substance will pose an immediate threat to life, irreversible or delayed adverse effects, or serious interference for a team member's attempt to escape from the dangerous atmosphere. From a response perspective, this is the value you will be most concerned with and the value that is likely to be the cause of an exposure that requires some form of clinical intervention. Along with these toxicologic terms, when reference sources are available, you should also attempt to identify the expected signs and symptoms of exposure. This may help you make a differential diagnosis in the field or better correlate the patient's response to the exposure.

Decontamination and Treatment

Treating patients who have been exposed to hazardous materials can be a difficult and emotionally challenging experience. Remember, your safety comes first. If you are first on the scene, you cannot immediately begin care until you fully understand the situation. Even if a patient is visible and requires rescue, you must resist the temptation to enter the scene unless you have the appropriate training, knowledge, equipment, and personnel. Staying safe is a tough decision that requires discipline and emotional coolness. You must work as part of the team to prevent more casualties. When the substance presents an unacceptable risk to the responders, decontamination must be given the highest priority and you must wait until your patient or patients have been decontaminated. Then you can apply your knowledge and skills, in the cold or support zone, to treat the patient safely.

► Decontamination

Decontamination methods will depend on the type of hazardous material involved, the stability of the scene, and the number, condition, and location of patients. In some cases, decontamination can be a form of treatment to reduce the dose of hazardous material in contact with the patient and decrease the risk of secondary contamination to others (including rescuers and ED personnel). Protection of the environment during decontamination is important and in most cases, plans should be made for containment of runoff. When lives are at stake, however, containing runoff is secondary.

There are four types of common decontamination methods you will see in the field—dilution, absorption, neutralization, and disposal. **Dilution** is the most common method and the easiest to perform in the field. Dilution typically relies on the use of copious amounts of water to flush the contaminant from the skin or eyes. This action decreases the dose effect of the hazardous material on the patient. Sometimes a simple soap, such as tincture of green soap, is used in the decontamination process. Other decontamination agents are rarely used, although vegetable or mineral oil is sometimes used if the contaminant is a water-reactive substance. Be cautious when you are using brushes; abrasion of a patient's skin increases the potential for hazardous material absorption. Pay special attention when your patient has been exposed to a solvent. Solvents are especially difficult to remove from the skin with water only; the patient may still have a solvent odor for quite some time after decontamination has been performed. Be aware of this during transport, or you may fall victim yourself to the off-gassing of solvents!

Absorption is accomplished with large pads that the hazardous materials team carries to soak up liquid and remove it from the patient. Towels can also be used in the same way. Absorption is not the most effective way to remove contamination from the skin as a rule, but it is a method. **Neutralization** involves the use of a chemical to change the hazardous material into less harmful substances. Neutralization on the skin is almost never used when a person has been in contact with hazardous substances because of the dangers of uncontrolled exothermic reactions. When acids are used on bases, or vice versa, heat is generated as a by-product of the reaction. Such reactions could be detrimental to the patient, making neutralization an action that is almost always contraindicated. **Disposal** is not so much of a decontamination strategy as it is a result of the process. EMS responders should be mindful of removing as much of the patient's clothing as possible (in some cases, this is all of it) to reduce the amount of contamination that contacts the body. Simply removing the clothing of a person exposed to chemicals can reduce the level of contamination by as much as 80% to 90%.[3]

Emergency Decontamination in "Fast-Breaking" Situations

In some of the most difficult situations, you may be faced with the need to make an immediate decision about whether to treat patients despite the fact that they are contaminated. In this case, you may be responsible for deciding whether to proceed with rapid emergency decontamination. In all cases, you must ensure you have the appropriate protection to protect yourself against the threat and stay clear of the product. Do not make physical contact with it.

Emergency decontamination is the process of removing the bulk of contaminants from a person as quickly and completely as possible. Once you are properly protected, you should instruct the person to disrobe and remove as much of the hazardous materials from his or her body as possible; be prepared to provide assistance if necessary. If available, give the person bags in which personal belongings and clothing can be placed. If the hazardous material is a powder, it should be brushed away first. If the hazardous material is water reactive, water should not be used for decontamination. A quick check of the *ERG* may assist you with identifying any reactivity issues prior to decontamination. Most often, however, water from whatever source is available (garden hose, fire hose, safety showers) is considered to be the universal decontamination solution. Again, when lives are at stake, controlling the runoff is secondary to getting the contaminant off the person. The goal is to get the victim clean enough to allow you the opportunity to render care; this is the point at which the victim becomes a patient!

► Mass Decontamination

In many cases, hose streams can be set up by firefighters to douse a large number of patients with copious amounts of water, thereby effecting **mass decontamination**. Many agencies have commercial mass-casualty decontamination systems as well. It is up to you to know which approach is used in your jurisdiction. In either case, the principle is the same: do the best possible for the most people in the shortest amount of time possible.

An example of such a setup is the creation of an emergency decontamination corridor. A **decontamination corridor** is a controlled area within the warm zone where decontamination takes place. It is not a life safety action; it is the "normal course of business" decontamination that responders do as part of their mitigation efforts. A decontamination corridor may be formed by parking two fire engines parallel to each other and approximately 10 to 20 feet (3 to 6 m) apart **Figure 49-22**. Nozzles can be attached to the side discharge ports of the engines and set to create a fine-particle fog-stream decontamination shower. Patients should disrobe on one end and enter the shower in single file. From a remote location, patients can be advised on how to decontaminate and directed to pay

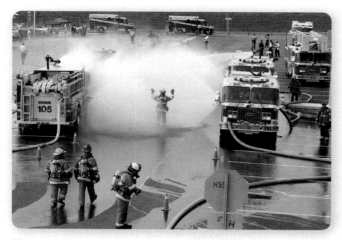

Figure 49-22 A decontamination corridor is established in the warm zone.

Courtesy of Master Sgt. Jim Varhegy/U.S. Air Force.

special attention to the areas of the body that are difficult to rinse such as the axillae, between fingers and toes, around the groin, the scalp, and between the buttocks. Soap and soft brushes should be made available. At the other end of the shower corridor, towels, blankets, and temporary garments should be available. Hypothermia may be a concern for some patient populations, such as young children and older adults, after decontamination. It is at the *end* of this corridor that you would make initial contact with the patients and begin the triage process. Ideally, the runoff water from decontamination should be contained. At a minimum, the runoff should not be allowed to become a source of secondary contamination.

▶ Technical Decontamination

Technical decontamination is the process used by the responders to clean PPE, tools, and equipment. It is a thorough cleaning process, often involving cleaning solutions and scrub brushes and a decontamination corridor. Keep in mind that the process and setup of technical decontamination may differ from jurisdiction to jurisdiction. There is not a single "right" way to do it; it is constructed primarily to accomplish the means, rendering the PPE, tools, and equipment free of contamination.

The following steps are intended to give you an idea of the technical decontamination process and to enhance your awareness of the dangers associated with hazardous materials and the constant need for proper decontamination techniques. The process described is not intended to make you proficient in accomplishing decontamination yourself. You may receive additional training in hazardous materials response that will give you a better understanding of the task.

1. Responders exit the hot zone and approach the decontamination corridor.
2. Contaminated tools and equipment should be left behind at the hot zone end of the decontamination corridor.
3. Hazardous materials personnel are showered and washed using water, brushes, soap, or other appropriate decontamination agents to remove all surface contaminants. This is done with the assistance of other hazardous materials personnel (the decontamination team), who should wear not more than one step lower

YOU ▶ are the Paramedic   PART 4

As you prepare the patient for transport, you note the patient's work of breathing is decreased and he is less anxious. Your partner places the patient on a nonrebreathing mask and the patient is packaged for transport.

Recording Time: 15 Minutes	
Respirations	22 breaths/min; adequate depth and volume
Pulse	Radial pulse, 114 beats/min; regular and strong
Skin	Pale, warm, and dry
Blood pressure	146/80 mm Hg
Oxygen saturation (Spo$_2$)	96% on nonrebreathing mask
Pupils	PERRLA

9. Which areas of the body are difficult to clean and rinse when a patient is being decontaminated?
10. Depending on the type of exposure, the use of invasive procedures should be minimized if possible. Why is this important?

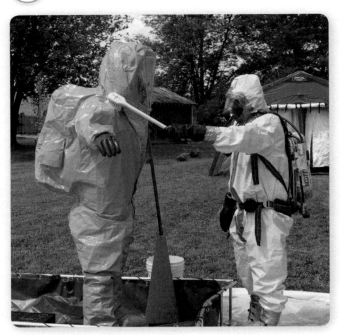

Figure 49-23 Technical decontamination is a thorough cleaning process to clean personal protective equipment, tools, and equipment.

© Jones & Bartlett Learning. Courtesy of MIEMSS.

PPE than the entry team. Because technical decontamination is not aimed at life safety, it is done in a manner that will contain the runoff. Often this is accomplished inside a small wading pool or other disposable basin **Figure 49-23** .

4. Paramedics should stay alert for signs of an ongoing primary or potential secondary contamination problem.

5. The team members move into an area of the decontamination corridor where they are helped out of their PPE by another member of the decontamination team. Contaminated protective clothing and equipment are placed into a bag or receptacle for later decontamination or disposal.

6. Respirators and/or SCBA masks and undergloves are removed last and placed in plastic bags or in other forms of containment.

7. Ideally, the responders should proceed to a location where they can take a personal shower to further reduce the potential for contamination. This is not always possible, but is the best course of action when possible.

8. Entry team personnel undergo medical monitoring.

▶ Treatment of Patients Exposed to Hazardous Materials

In general, patients who are contaminated can be treated using the concepts learned in Chapter 27, *Toxicology*, and Chapter 32, *Burns*. Remember to apply the basics of patient

care. However, there are some special considerations for hazardous materials patients. One of these is that invasive procedures should be minimized if possible. If you know from the hazardous materials team that your patient is contaminated, the process of endotracheal intubation may expose the patient to airway contamination. Placement of an intravenous (IV) or intraosseous (IO) line may allow contamination to bypass the skin barrier. You will need to weigh the risks of invasive procedures against their benefits.

You should be familiar with references and how to access technical expertise when you are deciding how to treat patients during a hazardous materials incident. Some assistance may be obtained from the *ERG* and CHEMTREC. In addition, you may consult with poison control centers, the Agency for Toxic Substances and Disease Registry, and local medical control. The hazardous materials team may have comprehensive reference textbooks that can guide you in treatment decisions and also be of assistance to ED physicians. Never forget that you are the physician's eyes and ears in the field. Share the knowledge you have gained from the hazardous materials team for your patient's sake.

The following categories of exposures are intended to serve as introductory information and should not be viewed as definitive treatment protocols or complete clinical interventions. They are intended to stimulate thinking and prompt you to learn more about the finer points of treating patients with chemical exposures.

Corrosives: Acids and Bases

Corrosives are chemicals that include both acids and bases. Some examples are toilet bowl cleaner, lye, and hydrochloric acid. Acids have a low pH (from 0 to 7), whereas bases have a high pH (7 to 14). Substances with either high or low pH can cause severe burns to the skin, eyes, and mucous membranes. Signs and symptoms include skin irritation, reddening or other discoloration, and blistering. Exposure of the mucous membranes to fumes can also cause burns, including severe life-threatening airway and lung burns.

Once the patient is decontaminated appropriately, treatment is generally supportive: ensure a patent airway, oxygenate the patient, treat for pain if indicated, and treat burns appropriately. Consider transport to a burn center if necessary. Patients showing signs of pulmonary edema secondary to an inhalation exposure may need to be treated for this with diuretics; however, you should always consult medical control to determine the proper course of action when you are treating patients with chemical exposures.

Solvents

Solvents may be liquids, solids, or gases. Common solvents include paint thinner and nail polish remover. **Solvents** are substances that are capable of dissolving other substances. Many solvents give off potent vapors that can be inhaled and can also be absorbed through the skin. Respiratory exposure in particular can cause immediate pulmonary symptoms such as pulmonary edema. Prolonged dermal exposure can cause symptoms as well, including cardiac dysrhythmias and seizures.

Solvent exposures may require extensive decontamination, almost to the point that it may be considered a form of treatment. Some solvents present additional hazards in that they can be metabolized into other toxic substances once absorbed by the body. Acetonitrile, for example, can be metabolized into a form of cyanide. It is important for you to research the substance the patient has been exposed to in order to understand what the substance is doing to the body and what the body may be doing to the substance. In general, solvent exposures require much of the same basic patient care as with any other exposure. Pay special attention to the potential for vomiting if a solvent has been ingested. Vomiting may complicate the patient's airway and be a cause for chemical pneumonitis.

Pesticides

Exposure to organophosphate and carbamate pesticides can produce severe signs and symptoms by interfering with the enzyme acetylcholinesterase, which promotes uptake of the neurotransmitter acetylcholine. In essence, these substances can cause runaway nervous system stimulation that produces a collection of signs known by the mnemonic **DUMBELS**. DUMBELS stands for Diarrhea, Urination, Miosis (constriction of the pupils)/Muscle weakness, Bradycardia/Bronchospasm/Bronchorrhea (discharge of mucus from the lungs), Emesis (vomiting), Lacrimation (excessive tearing of the eyes), Seizures/Salivation/Sweating. The mechanism of action of pesticides is similar to what you would find with most nerve agent exposures. It is recommended that you become more familiar with the mechanism of action of this unique group of chemical substances to fully understand the potential patient presentation. In addition to the DUMBELS symptomology described, exposures can produce tachycardia or bradycardia, twitching muscles (unlike tonic-clonic seizures), and excessive pulmonary secretions. As always, you should protect yourself from secondary contamination, including that from emesis when the exposure has been gastrointestinal.

Treatment of pesticide poisoning includes aggressive decontamination, protection of the airway with intubation and frequent suctioning when necessary, high-flow oxygen, and the use of atropine to block the overstimulation of muscarinic receptors of the parasympathetic nervous system. Pralidoxime may also be recommended to restore the ability of acetylcholinesterase to break down acetylcholine, which reverses the root cause of the exposure. This is a complicated set of chemical interactions, and the full explanation is beyond the scope of this textbook. It is recommended that you fully educate yourself about the mechanism of action of organophosphates and carbamates and the recommended clinical interventions.

Chemical Asphyxiants

Any gas that displaces oxygen from the atmosphere is termed an **asphyxiant**. Colorless, odorless gases (eg, carbon monoxide and hydrogen sulfide) that are confined to an area may represent a deadly trap when would-be rescuers rush in to help a collapsed victim. Substances known as **chemical asphyxiants** interfere with the use of oxygen at the cellular level; **cyanide** is a common example of such an agent. Hydrogen cyanide is used in many industrial processes. The release of cyanide in Bhopal, India, was a major hazardous materials incident that caused thousands of fatalities. Cyanide poisoning can also occur during exposure to the by-products of combustion at structure fires, which is the most common exposure scenario for hydrogen cyanide.

Treatment of cyanide exposure (for patients whose exposure was not due to smoke inhalation) begins with the use of amyl nitrite ampules, which the patient should inhale for 15 seconds of every minute. This step is followed by the IV administration of 300 mg of sodium nitrite, followed by 12.5 g of sodium thiosulfate. Follow the instructions found in the cyanide antidote kit for definitive treatment guidelines.

A treatment option for smoke inhalation cyanide poisoning is the antidote hydroxocobalamin, marketed in the United States and around the world as Cyanokit. Cyanokit is an FDA-approved antidote for known or suspected smoke inhalation exposures. The drug is a precursor to vitamin B_{12} and is safe to use in the field to treat the cyanide component of a smoke exposure. Refer to the manufacturer's guidelines for use. NFPA 473 also provides guidance on the treatment of smoke inhalation.

Another common exposure that results in a chemical asphyxiation is **carbon monoxide**. This gas ties up hemoglobin to the extent that oxygen in the blood becomes inaccessible to the cells. Treatment includes removal of the patient from the source and administration of 100% supplemental oxygen. Consider transport to an ED with hyperbaric oxygen capability.

Toxic Products of Combustion

Toxic products of combustion are the hazardous chemical compounds released when a material decomposes under heat. Remember the process of combustion is a chemical reaction and, like other reactions, will generate a given amount of by-products. You are well aware of the smoke produced by a structure fire, but have you really thought about what the smoke is made of or thought about the toxic gases that are liberated during a residential structure fire?

An easy way to think about the toxic products of combustion is to apply a long-standing phrase: "garbage in, garbage out." This phrase reflects the idea that whatever objects are involved in the fire (eg, chairs, tables, and sofas) will break down in the heat and create a host of chemical by-products in the smoke. In short, the toxic gases and other chemical substances found in the smoke will be determined by what is burning. To that end, smoke is not "just smoke"; it is unique, to some degree, in each and every fire.

Burning wood may seem like simple combustion, but consider this: a burning piece of a common wood used in residential construction, Douglas fir, gives off more than 70 harmful chemical compounds. Other substances found in most fire smoke include soot, carbon monoxide, carbon dioxide, water vapor, formaldehyde, cyanide compounds, and many oxides of nitrogen. Each of these substances is unique in its chemical makeup, and most are toxic to humans, even in small doses.

For example, carbon monoxide affects the ability of the human body to transport oxygen. The red blood cells cannot get oxygen to the cells and, subsequently, a person will die from tissue asphyxiation. Cyanide compounds also affect oxygen uptake in the body and are found to be a prevalent cause of civilian death in structure fires. Formaldehyde is found in many plastics and resins, and is one of the many components of smoke that causes eye and lung irritation. The oxides of nitrogen, including nitric oxide, nitrous oxide, and nitrogen dioxide, are deep lung irritants that may cause a serious medical condition called pulmonary edema, which is fluid buildup in the lungs.

The textbook *Hazardous Materials: Awareness and Operations, Second Edition*, is an excellent source of information on the by-products of combustion and treatment of smoke inhalation.

▶ Transport Considerations

The ideal transport scenario at a hazardous materials incident would be to have a team of paramedics who were not involved with decontamination or cold zone patient treatment standing by to transport patients to the ED. However, if the incident is a large one, the cold zone paramedics may need to both treat and transport patients.

You should remember that patients received after field decontamination should not be assumed to be completely decontaminated. Accordingly, you should take certain precautions to prepare yourself and your equipment for assuming care of the patient from the hazardous materials team and for getting the patient to the ED. First, you should wear appropriate PPE if indicated and be trained to wear the level required. The hazardous materials team may be able to supply some of the PPE if you do not have access to a splash-protective garment, for example. In addition, you should be given a complete report on what hazardous materials have been involved, the patient's source of exposure, and what has been done to decontaminate and/or treat the patient, if appropriate. In no event should you transport a patient if decontamination has not been sufficient. An example of insufficient decontamination would be when a hazardous material on the patient continues to produce toxic gases, such as after a smoke exposure or a liquid splash exposure.

Before receiving and transporting a patient exposed to hazardous materials, you can do several things in preparation. One principle is to reduce the amount of supplies and equipment that the patient will come in contact with. You could remove the mattress from the stretcher because the patient will probably be carried on a backboard; removing the mattress will make decontamination easier later. In general, use as much disposable equipment as possible. Supplies and equipment inside the ambulance should be removed and set aside in a clean, safe place for later retrieval.

It is impractical and time-consuming to line the inside of the ambulance with plastic. Instead, plan to isolate the patient by wrapping him or her in a sheet or other available covering to reduce the potential for secondary contamination. A double-wrap procedure is preferable. In this procedure, the patient is first wrapped in a cloth or plastic sheet, preferably one that helps protect the patient from hypothermia. Then the patient is placed on a backboard and the backboard placed on the stretcher. You should know which EDs in your area have facilities for receiving patients with possible hazardous materials contamination. The ED should be given plenty of notice prior to the transport so that they can assemble the appropriately trained personnel and prepare equipment. Often EDs will have a separate or dedicated treatment and decontamination room for these situations.

■ Medical Monitoring and Rehabilitation

You may be asked to assist with **medical monitoring** of the hazardous materials team. Wearing PPE often causes heat stress, and of course the toxins the team is working with can cause serious health effects. Factors that influence hazardous materials team members' health include level of physical fitness, activity, level of PPE, and environmental factors such as temperature.

Medical monitoring should include documentation of the incident factors including the hazardous materials involved, their toxic effects, what PPE was worn, its resistance to permeability with the hazardous materials, and what type of decontamination was used. You should have a plan for treatment, transport, and potential availability of antidotes in the event that a hazardous materials team member needs medical assistance.

You might be asked to assess hazardous materials team members before they suit up for entry into the hot zone and then again after they come out. Your assessment should include a complete set of vital signs, electrocardiogram, temperature, and body weight. Team members should be encouraged to hydrate with water or a sports drink prior to entering the hot zone. Working inside a level A suit is like being inside a sauna, with no way to lose heat through evaporation, conduction, convection, or radiation. A useful fact that can help you with your assessment is that some hazardous materials teams keep a file of their members' baseline medical status. Be sure to ask for this information.

Before being allowed to reenter the hot zone, the hazardous materials team should be evaluated by paramedics in the rehabilitation area (located in the cold zone) for hydration status, vital signs, and any potential symptoms of exposure to the toxic agent the incident involves. Team members should remove their protective clothing and be given a chance to rest. Reassess vital signs and perform a neurologic assessment (eg, orientation to time, place, and events) as well as an assessment of fine motor skills. Team members with elevated temperatures should be monitored closely for possible heatstroke. The loss of body weight is a direct correlation to the loss of fluids and the risk of dehydration and hypovolemia. Members should be encouraged to rehydrate by drinking water or other appropriate fluids. If there are abnormalities in vital signs or if team members have signs or symptoms, they should not be allowed to return to work until their physical status returns to normal. Setting arbitrary numbers for pulse rate and/or blood pressure may not be an accurate way to determine if a responder is showing adverse signs and symptoms. As an astute paramedic, you must take the entire presentation of signs and symptoms into account when evaluating a responder who has just spent time in PPE. An example of a hazardous materials team rehabilitation log that can assist you in the hazardous materials rehabilitation sector is shown in **Figure 49-24**.

HazMat Medical Monitoring Worksheet

Date:_____   Entry Person:_____

Incident #_____   Medical Monitor:_____

Important: HazMat team members shall not be allowed to don PPE if any of the following conditions are present: systolic BP <100 or >160, diastolic BP >100, pulse rate >120, oral temperature >99.8°F, Respirations >24. Medical monitors must read and be familiar with the "Medical Monitoring Guidelines" before beginning medical evaluations.

Pre-entry Evaluation
Before donning PPE, take and record baseline vital signs.

Time_____ BP_____ Pulse Rate_____ Resp._____ Oral Temp._____°F

Post-entry Evaluation
Immediately after doffing PPE, take vital signs and assess for hyperthermia.

Time_____ BP_____ Pulse Rate_____ Resp._____ Oral Temp._____°F

Reentry Evaluation
Before redonning PPE, take vital signs and reassess for hyperthermia.
Entry person must remain in rehab for a minimum of 30 minutes between entries.

Time_____ BP_____ Pulse Rate_____ Resp._____ Oral Temp._____°F

HazMat Exposure Suspected?
Immediately contact the HazMat Team Leader and see "HazMat Exposure Protocols."

Figure 49-24 Rehabilitation log.
© Jones & Bartlett Learning.

YOU are the Paramedic   SUMMARY

1. Are the signs and symptoms of an anhydrous ammonia exposure consistent with what you observe during the rapid full-body scan?

When you arrive on the scene, you receive a briefing and an SDS for anhydrous ammonia. While you may have never seen a true anhydrous ammonia exposure in your career, it would be reasonable to quickly scan the document to review for any major assessment or treatment recommendations. Do your homework quickly so that you know what to look for and what to do. The SDS tells you that anhydrous ammonia is a respiratory irritant. Your findings are consistent with an anhydrous ammonia exposure.

2. What chemical reference sources could assist you with the treatment of your patient?

The SDS contains valuable information regarding all aspects of the chemical, from ingredients, physical data, and fire/explosion data to health hazard data. Reading the health hazard section will provide you with the signs and symptoms of exposure, which then helps guide patient management. An *ERG* may also have some information that could be beneficial.

3. Explain what actions you might take if you feel the scene is not safe.

If you ever have the feeling the scene is not safe on a hazardous materials incident, you should immediately retreat to a safe location. Ensure you notify the incident commander and any personnel who are near your location. You may not have a significant amount of time from the time you realize the scene is not safe to the time you become ill or incapacitated.

4. What should your initial treatment consist of?

Your patient is suffering from respiratory distress with acute bronchospasm. You know from the SDS that anhydrous ammonia is a respiratory irritant. Based on the knowledge gathered from the SDS and the patient's presentation, initial treatment should include assisted ventilation with a bag-mask device, bronchodilators, and IV access.

5. Based on the SDS for anhydrous ammonia, how would you determine a treatment plan for this patient?

You know anhydrous ammonia is a respiratory irritant. The plan for this inhalation exposure will focus around airway protection and oxygenation. Ensure the patient has a patent airway and is ventilating appropriately. Be aware that swelling of the larynx can cause upper airway obstruction so be prepared to intubate if stridor or other evidence of impending upper airway obstruction develop.

6. Are there any other treatment options at this point?

Because you respond to these situations so rarely, you should consider contacting medical control early in the management of this patient, because you may not be thinking well beyond the first 5 minutes of the initial management.

7. Explain the difference between primary and secondary contamination.

Primary contamination occurs when the patient has been contaminated by the direct source. In this case, the patient was contaminated when the tank leaked out the anhydrous ammonia and he inhaled the gas. Secondary contamination can occur when a responder comes into contact with a substance while assessing or treating the patient. Proper protective equipment and proper decontamination will help minimize the risk of secondary contamination. In this situation, there is minimal risk of secondary contamination.

8. Explain why a water-based decontamination would be appropriate for an anhydrous ammonia exposure.

Anhydrous ammonia does not react with water. Methods for decontamination will call for a solution of detergent/soap, water, and a brush. This approach to decontamination will be used on the patient and any responders who require decontamination after treating the patients.

9. Which areas of the body are difficult to clean and rinse when a patient is being decontaminated?

Several small areas on the body can be quite difficult to clean and rinse. These include the axillae, the area between the fingers and toes, around the groin, the scalp, and between the buttocks. If you are assigned to help with decontamination, ensure you pay close attention to these areas.

10. Depending on the type of exposure, the use of invasive procedures should be minimized if possible. Why is this important?

Protecting the patient from further contamination is an important component of treatment. Any procedure such as endotracheal intubation or insertion of an IV line bypasses normal protective barriers of the body such as the skin and mucous membranes. This is not to say that these procedures should not be performed at all. Just remember to weigh the risks against the benefits of any procedure in that situation.

EMS Patient Care Report (PCR)

Date: 01-15-18	**Incident No.:** 285972		**Nature of Call:** Hazardous materials		**Location:** 674 Chestnut Drive

Dispatched: 1417	**En Route:** 1418	**At Scene:** 1426	**Transport:** 1517	**At Hospital:** N/A	**In Service:** N/A

Patient Information

Age: 50 **Sex:** M **Weight (in kg [lb]):** 59 kg (130 lb)	**Allergies:** None **Medications:** Lisinopril, albuterol **Past Medical History:** Asthma, hypertension **Chief Complaint:** Shortness of breath

Vital Signs

Time: 1501	**BP:** N/A	**Pulse:** Tachycardic	**Respirations:** 30	**Spo$_2$:** N/A
Time: 1505	**BP:** 156/84	**Pulse:** 127	**Respirations:** 30	**Spo$_2$:** 88% RA; 93% bag-mask
Time: 1510	**BP:** 152/84	**Pulse:** 134	**Respirations:** 22	**Spo$_2$:** 93% bag-mask
Time: 1515	**BP:** 146/80	**Pulse:** 114	**Respirations:** 22	**Spo$_2$:** 96% NRM

EMS Treatment (circle all that apply)

Oxygen @ __15__ L/min via (circle one):

NC (NRM) (Bag-mask device)

(**Assisted Ventilation**)	**Airway Adjunct**	**CPR**

Defibrillation	**Bleeding Control**	**Bandaging**	**Splinting**	**Other:** Nebulizer via bag-mask: 2.5 mg albuterol, 0.5 mg Atrovent. Solu-Medrol 125 mg IV.

Narrative

Dispatched to water treatment plant for anhydrous ammonia leak with multiple pts. Upon arrival, unit assigned to medical group by incident command. Provided SDS from group leader and assigned pt. Initial pt contact was made at 1500. Pt appeared in acute respiratory distress as evidenced by intercostal and subcostal retraction and audible expiratory wheezes. Pt was seated on tarp assuming tripod position with difficulty completing sentences. According to coworker, the pt was in the immediate area when the leak occurred and was trapped for approximately 5 minutes. Initial assessment reveals patent airway, rapid and shallow respirations, audible expiratory wheezes, and a regular, rapid radial pulse. Assisted pt ventilations with bag-mask at 15 L/min. At 1508 pt reported increased difficulty breathing. 2.5 mg albuterol and 0.5 mg ipratropium (Atrovent) administered via nebulizer with bag-mask. IV established with 18-gauge catheter in the right antecubital space. 125 mg methylprednisolone (Solu-Medrol) given IV. Pt assessment prior to transport revealed: Pt A&O x 4. PERRLA. No JVD or tracheal deviation noted. Symmetric chest rise with adequate respiratory depth and volume. Abdomen soft and nontender on palpation. PMS present in all extremities. Pt packaged for transport and care was turned over to medic O'Riley at 1517 for transport to Southport Regional Medical Center.**End of report**

Prep Kit

► Ready for Review

- Thousands of hazardous materials incidents occur (and are reported) each year.
- Handling hazardous materials emergencies requires specialized training and equipment.
- You should never enter a hazardous materials scene without understanding the nature of the problem.
- According to the Occupational Safety and Health Administration (OSHA) and the National Fire Protection Association, the levels of hazardous materials response training are awareness, operations, technician, and specialist (OSHA only).
- The great majority of hazardous materials emergencies are transportation incidents, predominantly occurring on roadways.
- When you are approaching an incident, you should be alert for signs of hazardous materials. Signs of hazardous materials include vapor clouds, strange odors, spilled liquids, and multiple victims.
- Sources of information about hazardous materials include labels and placards, transport documents, safety data sheets, and the *ERG*.
- Hazardous materials incident management follows principles of the National Incident Management System and the incident command system.
- Hazardous materials incidents involve hot, warm, and cold zones.
- Without proper personal protective equipment (PPE) and training, you should not enter the hot and warm zones.
- The four levels of hazardous materials PPE are level A, level B, level C, and level D.
- Primary hazardous materials contamination comes from direct contact with the toxin.
- Secondary contamination is spread by people (patients, the hazardous materials team, or EMS providers), clothing, or objects.
- Effects from hazardous materials exposure may be local on the body or systemic.
- Routes of exposure include inhalation, ingestion, absorption, and injection.
- Rescue and decontamination of victims is secondary to rescuer and public protection.
- Decontamination should be undertaken as a methodical process based on the nature of the contaminant.
- Treatment of hazardous materials victims is usually symptomatic and supportive of the ABCs. In some cases, antidotes are indicated and must be approved by the authority having jurisdiction.
- Invasive procedures should be carefully administered to avoid the risk of introducing contamination.
- Paramedics may be directed to support a hazardous materials operation with medical monitoring of the hazardous materials personnel.

► Vital Vocabulary

absorption A type of decontamination that is done with large pads that the hazardous materials team uses to soak up liquid and remove it from the patient.

asphyxiant Any gas that displaces oxygen from the atmosphere; can be deadly if exposure occurs in a confined space.

authority having jurisdiction (AHJ) An organization, office, or person responsible for enforcing the requirements of a code or standard, or for approving equipment, materials, an installation, or a procedure.

bill of lading A document carried by drivers of commercial vehicles that should provide specific information about what is carried on the vehicle.

CAMEO Computer-Aided Management of Emergency Operations; a tool to help predict downwind concentrations of hazardous materials based on the input of environmental factors into a computer model.

carbon monoxide A chemical asphyxiant that results in a cellular respiratory failure; this gas ties up hemoglobin to the extent that oxygen in the blood becomes inaccessible to the cells.

carboy A glass, plastic, or steel nonbulk storage container, ranging in volume from 5 to 15 gallons (19 to 600 L).

cargo tank Bulk packaging that is permanently attached to or forms a part of a motor vehicle, or is not permanently attached to any motor vehicle, and that, because of its size, construction, or attachment to a motor vehicle, is loaded or unloaded without being removed from the motor vehicle.

chemical asphyxiant A substance that interferes with the use of oxygen at the cellular level.

CHEMTREC (Chemical Transportation Emergency Center) A resource available to emergency responders via telephone on a 24-hour basis.

container Any vessel or receptacle that holds material, including storage vessels, pipelines, and packaging.

corrosives A class of chemicals with either high or low pH levels. Exposure can cause severe soft-tissue damage.

cyanide A chemical asphyxiant used in many industrial processes; exposure can occur from by-products of combustion at structure fires.

cylinder A portable, nonbulk, compressed gas container used to hold liquids and gases. Uninsulated

Prep Kit (continued)

compressed gas cylinders are used to store substances such as nitrogen, argon, helium, and oxygen. They have a range of sizes and internal pressures.

decontamination corridor A controlled area within the warm zone where decontamination takes place.

dilution A type of decontamination method that uses copious amounts of water to flush the contaminant from the skin or eyes.

disposal A type of decontamination in which as much clothing and equipment as possible is disposed of to reduce the magnitude of the problem.

dose effect The principle that the longer a hazardous material is in contact with the body or the greater the concentration, the greater the effect will most likely be.

drum A barrel-like nonbulk storage vessel used to store a wide variety of substances, including food-grade materials, corrosives, flammable liquids, and grease. Drums may be constructed of low-carbon steel, polyethylene, cardboard, stainless steel, nickel, or other materials.

dry bulk cargo tank A tank designed to carry dry bulk goods such as powders, pellets, fertilizers, or grain. Such tanks are generally V-shaped with rounded sides that funnel toward the bottom.

DUMBELS A mnemonic that stands for diarrhea, urination, miosis/muscle weakness, bradycardia/bronchospasm/bronchorrhea, emesis, lacrimation, seizures/salivation/sweating, which are the signs and symptoms that can be produced by exposure to organophosphate and carbamate pesticides or other nerve-stimulating agents.

emergency decontamination The process of removing the bulk of contaminants from a person without regard for containment. It is used in potentially life-threatening situations, without the formal establishment of a decontamination corridor.

evacuation The removal or relocation of people who may be affected by an approaching release of a hazardous material.

flammable range An expression of a fuel-air mixture, defined by upper and lower limits, that reflects an amount of flammable vapor mixed with a given volume of air.

flash point The minimum temperature at which a liquid or a solid releases sufficient vapor to form an ignitable mixture with air.

hazardous material Any substance that is toxic, poisonous, radioactive, flammable, or explosive and causes injury or death with exposure.

HAZWOPER (HAZardous Waste OPerations and Emergency Response) The federal OSHA regulation that governs hazardous materials waste site and response training. Specifics can be found in Title 29, standard number 1910.120. Subsection (q) is specific to emergency response.

ignition temperature The minimum temperature at which a fuel, when heated, will ignite in air and continue to burn; also called the autoignition temperature.

immediately dangerous to life and health (IDLH) An atmospheric concentration of any toxic, corrosive, or asphyxiant substance that poses an immediate threat to life, or could cause irreversible or delayed adverse health effects, or serious interference for a team member attempting to escape from the dangerous atmosphere. A respirator is mandatory when working in such an environment.

intermodal tank A bulk container that serves as both a shipping and a storage vessel. Such tanks hold between 5,000 and 6,000 gallons (18,900 to 22,700 L) of product and can be pressurized or nonpressurized. Intermodal tanks may be shipped by all modes of transportation.

label A type of signage at least 3.9 inches (9.9 cm) on each side that is often required on all four sides of individual packages and boxes that are being transported.

LD_{50} A dose that would be lethal to 50% of the test population.

lethal concentration (LC) The concentration of a material in air that, on the basis of laboratory tests (inhalation route), is expected to kill a specified number of the group of test animals when administered over a specified period.

lethal dose (LD) A single dose that causes the death of a specified number of the group of test animals exposed by any route other than inhalation.

level A ensemble The highest level of protective suit worn by hazardous materials personnel; may also be referred to as fully encapsulating because the suit covers everything, including the breathing apparatus.

level B ensemble Personal protective equipment that is one step less protective than level A, but provides for a high level of respiratory protection.

level C ensemble A level of personal protective equipment that provides splash protection.

level D ensemble The level of protection that firefighter turnout gear provides.

local effect An effect of a hazardous material on the body that is limited to the area of contact.

Prep Kit *(continued)*

lower flammable limit (LFL) The minimum amount of gaseous fuel that must be present in the air for the air-fuel mixture to be flammable or explosive.

mass decontamination The physical process of reducing or removing surface contaminants from large numbers of victims in potentially life-threatening situations in the fastest time possible.

MC-306/DOT 406 flammable liquid tanker A vehicle that typically carries between 6,000 and 10,000 gallons (22,700 to 37,900 L) of a product such as gasoline or other flammable and combustible materials. The tank is nonpressurized.

MC-307/DOT 407 chemical hauler A tanker with a rounded or horseshoe-shaped tank capable of holding 6,000 to 7,000 gallons (22,700 to 26,500 L) of flammable liquid, mild corrosives, and poisons. The tank has a high internal working pressure.

MC-312/DOT 412 corrosive tanker A tanker that often carries aggressive (highly reactive) acids such as concentrated sulfuric and nitric acid. It is characterized by several heavy-duty reinforcing rings around the tank and holds approximately 6,000 gallons (22,700 L) of product.

MC-331 pressure cargo tanker A tanker that carries materials such as ammonia, propane, Freon, and butane. This type of tank is commonly constructed of steel and has rounded ends and a single open compartment inside. The liquid volume inside the tank varies, ranging from the 1,000-gallon (3,800-L) delivery truck to the full-size 11,000-gallon (41,600-L) cargo tank.

MC-338 cryogenic tanker A low-pressure tanker designed to maintain the low temperature required by the cryogens it carries. A boxlike structure containing the tank control valves is typically attached to the rear of the tanker.

medical monitoring The process of assessing the health status of hazardous materials team members before and after entry to a hazardous materials incident site.

neutralization A type of decontamination that uses one chemical to change the hazardous material into two less harmful substances; rarely used by hazardous materials teams.

nonbulk storage vessel Any container other than a bulk storage container, such as drums, bags, compressed gas cylinders, and cryogenic containers. Nonbulk storage vessels hold commonly used commercial and industrial chemicals such as solvents, cleaners, and compounds.

permissible exposure limit (PEL) The maximum concentration of a chemical that a person may be exposed to under OSHA regulations.

placard A type of signage at least 10.8 inches (27 cm) on each side that is often required to be on all four sides of transport vehicles identifying the hazardous contents of the vehicle.

primary contamination An exposure that occurs with direct contact with the hazardous material.

safety data sheet (SDS) A document that provides a detailed product description and that is kept on site at workplaces for every potentially hazardous chemical at the workplace.

secondary containment An engineered method to control spilled or released product if the main containment vessel fails.

secondary contamination Exposure to a hazardous material by contact with a contaminated person or object.

shelter-in-place A method of safeguarding oneself or others' position during an emergency or event; in the context of a hazardous material, for example by remaining in a safe atmosphere, usually inside structures.

solvent A substance that is capable of dissolving other substances.

specific gravity The measure that indicates whether a hazardous material will sink or float in water.

systemic effect A physiologic effect on the entire body or one of the body's systems.

technical decontamination A multistep process of carefully scrubbing and washing contaminants from a person or object, collecting runoff water, and collecting and properly handling all items.

threshold limit value (TLV) The concentration of a substance that is supposed to be safe for exposure no more than 8 hours per day and 40 hours per week.

threshold limit value/ceiling (TLV/C) The maximum concentration of hazardous material to which a worker should not be exposed, even for an instant.

threshold limit value/short-term exposure limit (TLV-STEL) The concentration of a substance that a worker can be exposed to for up to 15 minutes but no more than four times per day with at least 1 hour between each exposure.

threshold limit value/skin The concentration at which direct or airborne contact with a material could result in possible and significant exposure from absorption through the skin, mucous membranes, and eyes.

toxic products of combustion Hazardous chemical compounds that are released when a material decomposes under heat.

tube trailer A high-volume transportation device made up of several individual compressed gas cylinders

Prep Kit *(continued)*

banded together and affixed to a trailer. Tube trailers carry compressed gases such as hydrogen, oxygen, helium, and methane. One trailer may carry several different gases in individual tubes.

upper flammable limit (UFL) The maximum amount of gaseous fuel that can be present in the air if the air-fuel mixture is to be flammable or explosive.

vapor density The weight of an airborne concentration (vapor or gas) as compared with an equal volume of dry air.

vapor pressure For the purpose of this chapter, the pressure associated with liquids held inside any type of closed container.

water reactive A property that indicates that a material will undergo a chemical reaction (for example, explosion) when mixed with water.

water soluble A property that indicates a material can be dissolved in water.

waybill A cargo document kept by the conductor of a train; also referred to as a consist.

▶ References

1. National Fire Protection Association. Codes & Standards. NFPA 1710. http://www.nfpa.org /codes-and-standards/archived/safer-act-grant /nfpa-1710. Accessed April 14, 2017.
2. Friese G. *How to download and use the* Emergency Response Guide *app.* EMS1 website. https://www .ems1.com/ems-products/education/articles /1403906-How-to-download-and-use-the -Emergency-Response-Guide-app/. Accessed April 14, 2017.
3. Decontamination procedures. Chemical Hazards Emergency Medical Management, US National Library of Medicine website. https://chemm .nlm.nih.gov/decontamination.htm. Published November 14, 2014. Accessed March 18, 2017.

Assessment in Action

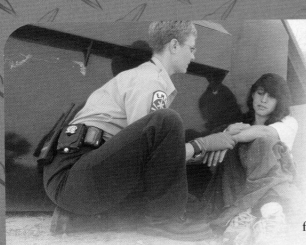

You are employed by a rural EMS system and are dispatched to the scene of an airplane crash with a possible hazardous materials exposure. A crop duster crashed into the terminal of the regional airport, releasing an unknown chemical into the area. Prior to arrival, you are asked to stage 1 mile (1.6 km) from the scene.

1. As you approach the scene, what would be the primary concern given the possible release of a chemical into the air in regard to the location where you are staging?

   A. Number of patients
   B. Amount of chemical stored in the area
   C. Chemical reaction with water
   D. Wind direction

2. After staging, you receive an update that multiple patients have been seen stumbling away from the hangar and onto the tarmac. A thick cloud of smoke is coming from the hangar. Given this information, what type of exposures do you expect to see from the patients?

   A. Absorption
   B. Inhalation
   C. Ingestion
   D. Injection

Assessment *in Action* (continued)

3. What special resources should you make sure you have immediately available while en route to the scene?

   A. Hazardous materials team
   B. Coroner
   C. Transport safety crew
   D. Field amputation team from hospital

4. The local fire department and hazardous materials team have arrived on scene and established command. They report the need to perform emergency decontamination on four patients. Based on your understanding of hazardous materials awareness, when is emergency decontamination appropriate?

   A. When patients are ambulatory and can walk away from the scene
   B. When patients have an immediate life threat due to exposure
   C. When patients are anxious about being near the incident
   D. When first responders have been contaminated upon arrival

5. While the emergency decontamination is taking place, your dispatch center reports the incident commander has requested you to respond to another forward staging area to receive patients who are being removed from the scene after decontamination. What level of PPE should you wear as a minimum given this scenario?

   A. Level A
   B. Level B
   C. Level C
   D. Level D

6. Wearing proper PPE for this incident will help to prevent what type of exposure?

   A. Primary contamination
   B. Secondary contamination
   C. Emergency decontamination
   D. Critical contamination

7. After you have transported one patient to the hospital, you have been asked to respond to the scene to assist with evaluations on the hazardous materials crew. You know this process as:

   A. medical monitoring.
   B. entry evaluation.
   C. exit evaluation.
   D. forecasting.

8. What is a common method used to decontaminate patients during a mass-casualty incident?

9. Why is the identification of the agents involved in a hazardous materials incident so crucial before performing primary decontamination?

10. How is the role of air medical transport affected in transporting patients who were involved in a hazardous materials incident?

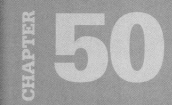

CHAPTER 50

Terrorism Response

National EMS Education Standard Competencies

EMS Operations

Knowledge of operational roles and responsibilities to ensure patient, public, and personnel safety.

Mass-Casualty Incidents Due to Terrorism and Disaster

› Risks and responsibilities of operating on the scene of a natural or human-made disaster. (pp 2433, 2437-2441)

Knowledge Objectives

1. List key questions to consider when responding to a terrorist event. (p 2433)
2. Define international and domestic terrorism. (pp 2434-2435)
3. Define and specify the types of terrorist groups. (p 2436)
4. List various examples of terrorist motivations. (pp 2436-2437)
5. Discuss the color-coded advisory system's replacement with the National Terrorism Advisory System. (p 2437)
6. Explain how to identify potential terrorist targets to which you may respond. (pp 2437-2438)
7. Discuss what actions paramedics should take during the course of their work to heighten their ability to respond to and survive a terrorist attack. (pp 2438-2439)
8. Discuss factors to consider when responding to a potential weapon of mass destruction incident, including preincident indicators, the type of location, the type of call, the number of patients, and victims' statements. (p 2438)
9. Discuss key response actions to take at the scene of a terrorist event. (pp 2438-2441)
10. Define secondary device and the importance of continually reassessing scene safety. (p 2441)
11. List the five main categories of weapons of mass destruction. (p 2441)
12. Define the terms persistency, volatility, contact hazard, and vapor hazard. (p 2442)
13. Describe specific vesicant agents. (p 2442)
14. Explain the signs, symptoms, and emergency medical treatment of a patient with vesicant exposure. (pp 2442-2443)
15. Describe specific pulmonary agents. (p 2443)
16. Explain the signs, symptoms, and emergency medical treatment of a patient with pulmonary agent exposure. (p 2443)
17. Describe specific nerve agents. (pp 2443-2444, 2446)
18. Explain the signs, symptoms, and emergency medical treatment of a patient with nerve agent exposure. (pp 2444-2446)
19. Describe specific industrial chemicals and insecticides. (p 2446)
20. Explain the signs, symptoms, and emergency medical treatment of a patient with cyanide agent exposure. (pp 2446-2447)
21. Define the terms dissemination, disease vector, communicability, and incubation. (p 2447)
22. Explain the signs, symptoms, and emergency medical treatment of a patient with smallpox. (pp 2448-2449)
23. Explain the signs, symptoms, and emergency medical treatment of a patient with viral hemorrhagic fever. (pp 2449-2450)
24. Explain the signs, symptoms, and emergency medical treatment of a patient with inhalation and cutaneous anthrax. (pp 2450-2451)
25. Explain the signs, symptoms, and emergency medical treatment of a patient with plague. (pp 2451-2452)
26. Explain the signs, symptoms, and emergency medical treatment of a patient with botulinum toxin exposure. (p 2452)
27. Explain the signs, symptoms, and emergency medical treatment of a patient with ricin exposure. (pp 2452-2453)
28. Define syndromic surveillance and its importance during a potential terrorist event. (p 2453)
29. Define radiation and the difference between alpha, beta, gamma, and neutron radiation. (p 2455)

30. Describe what a radiologic dispersal device, or dirty bomb, is and how it is used for terrorism. (p 2455)

31. Explain the emergency medical management of a patient who was potentially exposed to radiation. (p 2456)

32. List protective measures to take when responding to a radiologic event. (p 2456)

33. Discuss specific types of explosive devices used by terrorists. (pp 2457-2458)

Skills Objectives

1. Demonstrate how to use a nerve agent antidote kit. (pp 2445-2446)

YOU are the Paramedic | PART 1

You and your partner are dispatched along with multiple other units to an explosion at a political rally outside of a local church. The dispatcher informs you the communications center is receiving multiple reports of people injured called in by police who were already in the area. Prior to arrival, you are asked to stage three blocks north of the church until the scene is declared safe. Initial reports indicate there was a sudden explosion during the height of the rally. First responders report, on arrival, they were finding patients with severe difficulty breathing and bleeding injuries. Fire department and hazardous materials teams are already en route, along with additional law enforcement and emergency medical services (EMS) resources.

Just as you pull into the staging area, the fire department notifies you that you are safe to proceed to the scene. The incident command system has already been established, and a mass-casualty incident has been declared. The hazardous materials team is setting up a decontamination corridor for patients because there has been a report of possible chemical dispersal from the explosion that is causing difficulty breathing. Your unit is assigned to the treatment area. As you arrive, you see that the explosion took place near the front steps of the church. Incident command has been set up across the street from the church. Hazardous materials personnel are performing initial triage in the hot zone. You see a large number of people, many of them obviously injured, being directed by fire department and hazardous materials personnel through the decontamination corridor to the treatment area located in the parking lot behind the church.

There are approximately 15 people entering the treatment area when you arrive. Some have bleeding and respiratory symptoms. There are reports that patients and initial responders were complaining of a strong odor that smelled like bleach. Approximately 15 minutes into the call, you receive your first patient.

Recording Time: 1 Minute	
Appearance	Man in his mid 20s, in respiratory distress. Patient appears confused.
Level of consciousness	Verbal (knows his name, but does not know where he is or how he got there)
Airway	Irritated, but open, maintained by patient
Breathing	Increased work of breathing with accessory muscle use and audible expiratory wheezes
Circulation	Strong radial pulse, decreased; no obvious significant bleeding

1. What are some clues that might help you treat your patient?

2. Chemical agents may be obtained easily and combined with other weapons such as explosives. What types of chemical agents may be likely to cause this patient's signs and symptoms?

Introduction

Preparing for response to acts of terror has become a reality for EMS workers in the United States and around the world. Domestic terrorist groups as well as international terrorists have increased their targeting of civilian populations with acts of terror. The question is not will terrorists strike again, but rather when and where will they strike? You must be mentally and physically prepared for the possibility of a terrorist event.

Your health and safety are primary concerns when you are called to respond to terrorist attacks. The threat that terrorism poses to the health and safety of paramedics was realized even before the September 11, 2001, attacks. The sarin attacks in Tokyo in 1996 sickened approximately 100 emergency medical care providers who rushed to the scene, because they lacked proper personal protective equipment (PPE).[1] The attacks on September 11, 2001, brought the issue of emergency responder health and safety to the forefront because 411 emergency responders were killed on that day.[2] Many more paramedics and emergency medical technicians (EMTs) were injured, developed chronic disorders, or experienced depression and physiologic problems as a result of their response.[2]

Chapter 51, *Disaster Response*, discusses concerns related to disasters in general, but there are some issues specific to terrorist attacks that must be considered. Although it can be difficult to anticipate and plan a response to terrorist incidents, there are several key principles that apply to every response. This chapter describes how you can prepare to respond to these events by discussing types of terrorist events and patient management. You will also learn the signs, symptoms, and treatment of patients who have been exposed to chemical, biologic, radiologic, nuclear, and explosive (CBRNE) agents or injured by explosive attacks. Lastly, issues of responder health and safety at the scene of a terrorist attack will be discussed in detail. At the end of this chapter, you will be able to answer the following key questions:

- What are the most frequent sites for a terrorist attack?
- What are your initial actions when faced with a terrorist event?
- Who should you notify, and what should you tell them?
- What types of additional resources might you require?
- How do you ensure your own safety, your partner's safety, and the safety of victims?
- How should you proceed to address the needs of the victims?
- What is the clinical presentation of a patient exposed to a weapon of mass destruction (WMD)?
- How are WMD patients to be assessed and treated?
- How do you avoid becoming contaminated or cross-contaminated with a WMD agent?
- How do you ensure your health after your response to the incident has concluded?

EMS providers are encouraged to seek additional training and participate in drills and exercises to hone the skills needed to respond safely to a terrorist event.

Terrorism

Although the definition of **terrorism** varies widely, it can be broadly defined as an act or threatened act of violence against innocent people for political purposes. Although by this definition, terrorist acts have surely been around for nearly as long as there have been organized societies, the term *terrorism* was first used in reference to the French government's Reign of Terror in 1793-1794 during the French Revolution.[3]

Terrorism can strike anywhere around the world. In Colombia and oil-rich regions in Africa and the Middle East, political terrorist groups target oil resources (refineries, pipelines, and infrastructure) as a means to instill fear in multinational corporations and governments. To achieve their goals, terrorists do not discriminate when selecting their targets. In one attack in 2004, over 30 heavily armed male and female terrorists and suicide bombers overran a school in Beslan, Russia, and held children as hostages over the course of 3 days. When the siege was over, 334 hostages were killed, many of them children, who were too weak after 3 days of starvation to escape the massacre **Figure 50-1**. In an attack in 2011 in Norway, a

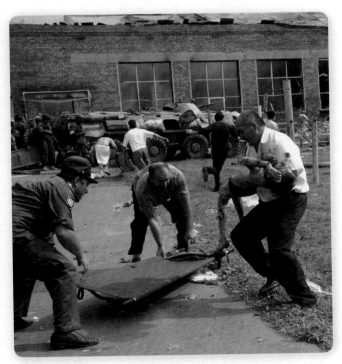

Figure 50-1 In 2004, a terrorist attack at a school in Beslan, Russia, resulted in hundreds of deaths.
© ZUMA Wire Service/Alamy.

lone terrorist exploded a car bomb in Oslo and then targeted a summer camp, opening fire and killing 69 people.

► International Terrorism

The US Federal Bureau of Investigation (FBI) defines two types of terrorism: international terrorism and domestic terrorism. **International terrorism**, also known as cross-border terrorism, is defined as acts of terror committed by foreign agents.[3]

Events such as the attacks on New York City's World Trade Center in 1993 and again on September 11, 2001 (often called "9/11" for short) have changed the way Americans live and travel **Figures 50-2 and 50-3**. In Mumbai, India, international terrorists stormed two landmark hotels popular with Western tourists in a coordinated attack that occurred at 11 sites (including a women and children's hospital and a train station) over the course of 3 days in November of 2008. These highly organized terror attacks killed over 160 people and injured more than 300. In November 2015 in Paris, France, terrorists launched a coordinated series of mass shootings and suicide bombings at cafés, restaurants, and theaters, killing 130 people and injuring more than 350 people.

Although most incidents of international terrorism occur in densely populated areas and mass gatherings, sites of significance to the terrorist might include emergency services in the surrounding areas, to which victims may flee for assistance.

► Domestic Terrorism

Although terrorist attacks planned by foreigners often dominate discussion and planning for large-scale emergency

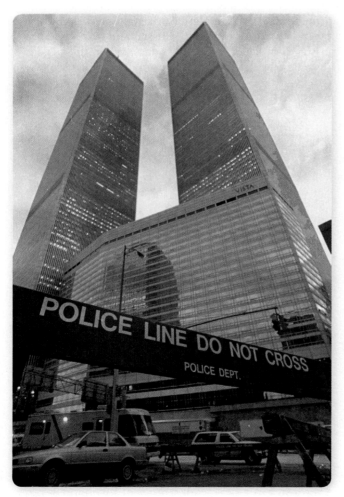

Figure 50-2 The terrorist attack on the World Trade Center in 1993.
© Greg Gibson/AP Photo.

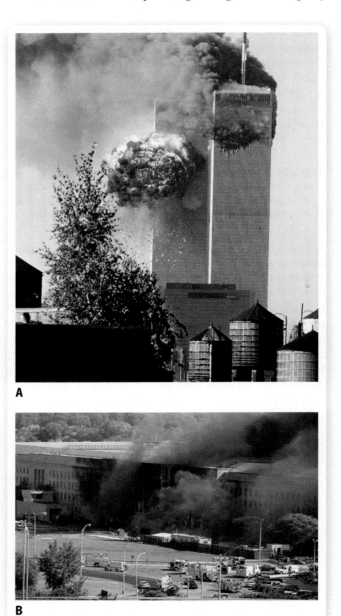

A

B

Figure 50-3 The September 11, 2001, attack on the World Trade Center accounted for the majority of the deaths caused by terrorists in 2001. **A.** The World Trade Center attack. **B.** The Pentagon attack.
© Tom Horan/AP Photo.

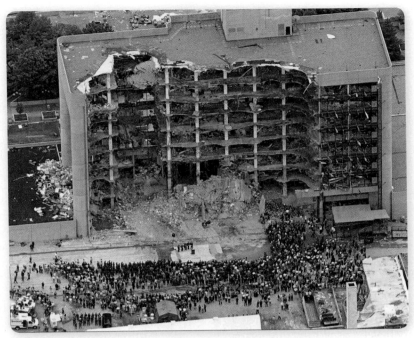

Figure 50-4 The destruction of the Alfred P. Murrah Federal Building in Oklahoma City in 1995 took the lives of 168 people, including 19 children.
© Bill Waugh/AP Photo.

response, **domestic terrorism** is also a fact of life. Domestic terrorism is defined as a terrorist plot or operation originating within the borders of the target country. The United States has a long history of domestic terrorism, including both successful and failed incidents. In recent years, domestic terrorist events number around 12 per year.[4] A partial list includes the following:

- 1984, The Dalles, OR: Salmonella was used as a biologic weapon targeting government officials and the general populace.
- 1995, Oklahoma City, OK: A truck bomb was detonated in front of the Alfred P. Murrah Federal Building, killing 168 and causing the partial collapse of the building **Figure 50-4** .
- 2001, New York, NY, Washington, DC, West Palm Beach, FL: Letters containing anthrax spores killed 5 people and infected 17 other people.
- 2002, Chicago, IL: A US citizen was arrested for plotting to construct a radiologic (dirty) bomb.
- 2013, Boston, MA: Multiple bombs positioned near the finish line of the Boston Marathon exploded, killing 3 and injuring more than 250 people.
- 2013, Washington, DC: Postal letters laced with highly toxic ricin addressed to prominent politicians were intercepted at the US Capitol mail facility.
- 2016, Orlando, FL: A gunman claiming terrorist allegiance opened fire in the Pulse nightclub, killing 49 people **Figure 50-5** .

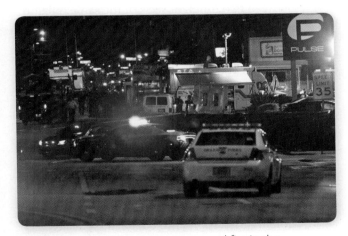

Figure 50-5 In 2016, a gunman opened fire in the Pulse nightclub in Orlando, Florida, claiming the lives of 49 people.
© MANDEL NGAN/AFP/Getty.

- 2016, Seaside Park, NJ, New York, NY: Pipe bombs exploded, injuring 31 civilians. Additional bombs were found and defused.

Unfortunately, this list presents just a small sample of the domestic terror attacks and plots that have involved US citizens or legal residents. Also, though its planning did not originate within the borders of the US, the 2001 attack in which hijacked airplanes flew into the World Trade Center complex in New York, NY, and the Pentagon building in Washington, DC is another incident that occurred domestically.

▶ Motivations of Terrorists

Terrorists can generally be described by their motivations, which fall into one or more of the following categories:

- **State terrorists.** The first formal documented terrorism, state terrorism is the systematic use of terror by an established government to control all or part of its populace. This form of terrorism should not be confused with state-sponsored terrorism, where a government gives direction and resources to a nongovernmental terrorist organization.

- **Religious extremists.** These terrorists hold extreme views within mainstream religions or are members of religious groups that hold extreme views that motivate violent activities. Such groups can be especially dangerous because they may seek **apocalyptic violence** or mass murder as a means to their ends. The fanaticism and suicidal ideologies that accompany such extreme religious viewpoints may see other religions or "nonbelievers" as worthy targets for death, and part of their apocalyptic doctrine is to eradicate or cleanse a region (or the entire earth) of those who do not practice their faith. This ideology fuels intrareligious terrorism between two different sects of the same religion (such as Shiite versus Sunni Muslims). Religious terrorist groups include organizations such as Aum Shinrikyo, who carried out sarin chemical attacks in Tokyo between 1994 and 1995.

- **Issue-oriented groups.** These groups often represent the violent fringe or a splinter group of a legitimate nonviolent group or movement that seeks to effect change through legal and socially acceptable means. If such nonviolent methods are seen as ineffective or time-consuming, or if there is a disagreement in methodology or philosophy between factions in the group, a smaller group may break off and look toward violence for a more immediate and effective response to their demands. Examples include antiabortion groups and eco-terrorists.

- **Right-wing extremists.** The aim of these groups is to limit government, preserve what they perceive to be traditional social orders, and combat left-wing groups. Right-wing groups may be formed as militias or gangs and are often motivated to suppress other racial or cultural groups. According to the FBI, right-wing extremist groups are growing as a domestic terrorist threat.

- **Left-wing extremists.** The aim of these groups is to limit corporations and businesses, overturn what they perceive to be traditional establishment, and combat right-wing groups. Left-wing groups may be formed as loose groups or cells and are often motivated to do away with class and cultural divides. Once the most prominent form of domestic extremist factions, left-wing groups have greatly declined since the 1980s.

- **Separatists.** Terrorists seek political, economic, or social freedom. They may also seek to kill or evict foreigners, migrants, or those with different ethnic, racial, sociologic (poor or lower class), or cultural backgrounds from their own. They often use terror to influence economic or immigration politics and the drawing or redrawing of geopolitical borders to claim or reclaim land. These groups may seek to establish a new country, establish a new individual state or region within a country, or rejoin a country from which their group has been separated.

- **Narcoterrorists.** Narcoterrorism is the use of terror to take control of a region, its politics, or government with the goal of manufacturing, distributing, and selling (trafficking) drugs. They often target military, police, and antidrug politicians or government officials (and their families), as well as innocent civilians, in an effort to gain control over an entire region, usurping the power of the local authority. As a result of the revenue of the drugs that they manufacture and/or distribute, these groups are generally more heavily armed, organized, and funded than are the local authorities. As such, they exert disproportionate and massive amounts of regional control. Other terrorist groups, such as extremist political or violent religious organizations, often use the drug trade to fund their terrorist activities. However, strictly speaking this behavior would not be classified as narcoterrorism, because they are not using terror for the furtherance of drug distribution.

- **Pathologic terrorists.** Terrorists with no motivation beyond their own desire to control and terrorize others. These people do not often conspire with more than two or three other people regarding their terrorist operations. Although "lone wolf" terrorists sometimes fall into this category, pathologic terrorists often do not have a set political or ideologic motivation. This characteristic can cause some confusion, as some lone wolf terrorists are people who are officially or ideologically aligned in their motivations with another category of terrorists.

The hallmark of many of these groups is violent, simultaneous, coordinated attacks. This is primarily meant to confuse, spread thin, and overwhelm emergency response to the incidents, but also to boast the level of sophistication and planning that they have put into committing the acts. These groups exhibit trends toward apocalyptic violence to effect a combination of political, geopolitical, and religious goals.

Terrorist organizations often thrive in areas with little governmental organization. This is an ideal environment for them to train terrorist recruits, store equipment, and plan and operate effectively. As such, many of these groups look to establish training camps and bases of operation in remote, austere locations where they can function with impunity and protect themselves using **guerilla warfare** tactics.

Most terrorist attacks involve coordination between multiple terrorists, or "actors," working together. Recruiters identify willing actors and bring them into the organization, where they are trained, financed, and provided equipment and intelligence on their target or targets, as well as transportation and often lodging. Twenty terrorists worked together to commit the worst act of terror in US history on September 11, 2001, but there were dozens more people directly and indirectly involved in planning and helping to execute the attacks.[5] Four terrorists worked together to carry out the London subway bombings on July 7, 2005, but many more were involved in their training, financing, and planning.[6]

In many cases, such as the Columbine, CO; Newtown, CT; and Orlando, FL mass shootings; and the bombings of the 1996 Summer Olympics, the 2013 Boston Marathon, and the Alfred P. Murrah Federal Building; no more than a few terrorists, and sometimes only a single terrorist, planned and carried out the event. Such lone wolf attacks can be difficult to predict and may occur at mass gatherings, at symbolic sites or events, or in simple, small-town locations.

■ Paramedic Response to Terrorism

▶ Recognizing a Terrorist Event (Indicators)

A hallmark of terrorist events is the planning and preparation leading up to the incident is kept **covert** by the terrorist agents. However, emergency medical responders can prepare themselves for response to terrorist incidents by maintaining good situational awareness as a habit on every call. Responders should raise their level of situational awareness even more when operating at or responding to locations and events that terrorists may see as high-value targets.

Examples of potential high-value targets for terrorists include the following:

- Major sporting events, concerts, ceremonies, and parades where large crowds are gathered
- Locations where damage or destruction will provoke extreme fear, such as nuclear power plants and research facilities, chemical factories, biologic laboratories, and petroleum distillation and storage facilities

- Locations where attacks will provoke extreme emotional reactions, such as day care centers, schools, health care facilities, abortion clinics, and churches
- Locations that are crucial to transportation, such as airports, subway or train stations, tunnels, and bridges
- Critical industry and infrastructure, such as power plants, water treatment plants, manufacturing facilities, shipping facilities, dams and reservoirs, power lines, and natural gas lines
- Locations of symbolic significance, such as local, state, and government buildings, financial buildings, corporate headquarters, military installations, monuments, and national parks
- Locations vital to emergency response, including police stations, fire stations, dispatch centers, command centers, EMS facilities, and hospitals

It is important to understand the **National Terrorism Advisory System (NTAS)**, instituted in 2011 to replace the color-coded Homeland Security Advisory System that had been used since 2002 by the Department of Homeland Security (DHS). NTAS alerts apply to threats to the United States and its territories. The NTAS alerts responders to the potential for an attack, and, as far as practicable, will give specifics of the current threat. If the information is available, the NTAS alert will provide specific details related to who will be potentially affected, such as the geographic area, transportation concerns, and the nature of the threat. It will also include steps that people or communities can take to protect themselves in response to the threat. The advisory will specify whether the threat is **elevated** (there is no specific information about the timing or location) or **imminent** (the threat is believed to be impending or expected to occur soon). The alert will be publicly announced via posting at DHS.gov/alerts and releasing the alert to the news media. DHS will also distribute alerts via social media such as Facebook and Twitter. Updated NTAS alerts are issued if information related to the threat changes; updated alerts are distributed in the same manner as initial alerts. Alerts are automatically canceled on a designated expiration date.[7]

The DHS has not issued specific recommendations for EMS personnel to follow in response to the alert system. Follow your local protocols, policies, and procedures. It is your responsibility to ensure you know the threat level at the start of your workday. Some EMS organizations display the NTAS on communication. On the basis of the current information available, take appropriate actions and precautions while continuing to perform daily duties and responding to calls.

Understanding and being aware of the current threat is only the beginning of responding safely to calls. Once you are on duty, you must be able to make appropriate decisions regarding the potential for a terrorist event.

In determining the potential for a terrorist attack, on every call you should observe the following:

- **Preincident indicators.** Has the NTAS posted a threat warning? Has there been a recent increase in violent political activism? Are you aware of any credible threats made against the location, gathering, or occasion?
- **Type of location.** Is the location a monument, infrastructure, government building, or a specific type of location such as a temple? Is there a large gathering such as a parade or political demonstration? Is there a special event taking place such as a college football game?
- **Type of call.** Is there a report of an explosion or suspicious device nearby? Did the call come into dispatch as a large number of people having unexplained coughing and difficulty breathing? Are there reports of people fleeing the scene?
- **Number of patients.** Are there multiple patients with similar signs and symptoms? This is probably the single most important clue that a terrorist attack or an incident involving a WMD has occurred.
- **Victims' statements.** This is probably the second best indication of a terrorist or WMD event. Are the patients fleeing the scene giving statements such as, "Everyone is passing out," "There was a loud explosion," or "There are a lot of people shaking on the ground." If so, something is occurring that you do not want to rush into, even if it is determined not to be a terrorist event.

Words of Wisdom

Maintaining good situational awareness during all emergency medical calls and understanding when to raise your awareness based on clues and cues on scene will help you remain safe and ready to respond to nearly any incident, terrorist or otherwise. Although some cues to a terrorist incident may be apparent, the confusion caused by large-scale and high-impact incidents may make it difficult to determine whether the incident was caused intentionally or by accident. All high-impact incidents call for high levels of situational awareness. Your EMS operations training, including preparation for disasters, mass-casualty incidents, hazardous materials incidents, and terrorist incidents, will guide you, regardless of the trigger of the event. In any of these situations, you must use good judgment and resist the urge to rush in and help, especially when there are multiple victims from an unknown cause.

▶ Response Actions

Once you suspect that a terrorist event has occurred or a WMD has been used, there are certain actions to take to ensure that you will be safe and be in the proper position to help the community:

- Ensure scene safety and personal safety
- Notify your dispatch and/or supervisor of the incident
- Request additional/specialized resources
- Establish or coordinate with command
- Initiate mass-casualty incident procedures

Scene Safety

If you have any concerns regarding scene safety, do not immediately enter. The best location for staging is upwind and uphill from the incident. As with any other scene that is not safe, wait for assistance from those who are trained in assessing and managing the hazards. Remember, while not every responder is trained to neutralize hazards, every responder has the responsibility to notice suspicious people, objects, and circumstances and report them as appropriate. Remember the following:

- Failure to park your vehicle at a safe location can place you and your partner in danger **Figure 50-6** .
- If your vehicle is blocked in by other emergency vehicles or damaged by a secondary device (or event), you will be unable to provide patients with transport or simply to escape **Figure 50-7** .

Responder Safety (Personal Protection)

Emergency response, by its nature, is a dangerous profession. It is associated with exposure to a multitude of occupational hazards, from ergonomics (lifting and carrying), to workplace violence, hazardous materials, and vehicle crashes, to name just a few. Each day paramedics operate on the scene of hazardous and potentially life-threatening scenes, often without significant injuries or loss of life. However, when emergency workers respond to the scene of a terrorist incident, research shows that responder health and safety suffer greatly. The uniqueness and uncertainty of terrorist and WMD incidents can cloud the decision-making process, and paramedics can develop

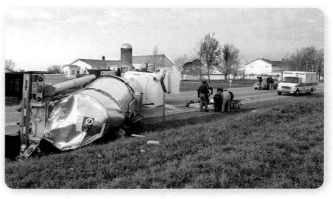

Figure 50-6 Park your vehicle at a safe location and distance.
© Ilene MacDonald/Alamy.

- Previous knowledge, fit-testing, experience, and comfort using multiple types and brands of PPE
- The proper PPE
- Self-enforcement of all protective measures

The best form of protection from a WMD agent is preventing yourself from coming into contact with the agent. Among the greatest threats facing you in a WMD attack are contamination and **cross-contamination**. Contamination with an agent occurs when you have direct contact with the WMD or are exposed to it. Cross-contamination (also known as secondary contamination) occurs when you come into contact with a contaminated person who has not yet been decontaminated. Decontamination of patients is an important part of medical management of patients who have been exposed to or contaminated with a CBRNE agent. Decontamination is covered in Chapter 49, *Hazardous Materials*. If EMS personnel have been appropriately trained in decontamination and have the appropriate PPE, they may be involved in decontamination per their protocols.

Notification Procedure/Resource Requests

When you suspect a terrorist or WMD event has taken place, notify the dispatcher or the incident commander, or both. Vital information needs to be communicated effectively if you are to receive the appropriate assistance. Inform them of the nature of the event, any additional resources that may be required, the estimated number of patients, and the upwind route of approach or optimal route of approach.

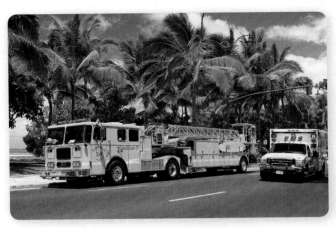

Figure 50-7 Ensure your vehicle is not blocked in by other emergency vehicles.
© pbpgalleries/Alamy.

tunnel vision—a situation in which a person does not see the overall picture, but focuses on only one aspect of it. In short, paramedics can lose their situational awareness.

At large-scale events, you may arrive well before environmental health personnel or trained health and safety professionals arrive. For this reason, you need the following key resources when responding to potentially hazardous scenes:

- Awareness of measures to take for self-preservation
- A culture of safety within your organization

YOU are the Paramedic   PART 2

The patient appears to be in respiratory distress. Your partner obtains vital signs and applies a nonrebreathing mask at 15 L/min as an initial measure while you begin your assessment. The patient reports burning in his chest and shortness of breath along with irritation in his eyes, nose, and throat. His eyes are watering, his nose is running, and he is drooling. You observe intercostal and supraclavicular retractions. Breath sounds are diminished but clear. The patient denies any past medical history or allergies to medications and is repeatedly asking you what happened.

Recording Time: 5 Minutes	
Respirations	24 breaths/min
Pulse	Radial pulse, 112 beats/min, regular and strong
Skin	Pink, warm, and dry with minor abrasions
Blood pressure	138/82 mm Hg
Oxygen saturation (Spo$_2$)	84% on 15 L/min nonrebreathing mask
Pupils	PERRLA, slightly bloodshot

3. On the basis of the information you have, to what agent do you think your patient was exposed?
4. What should be the focus of your initial treatment?

It is extremely important to establish a safe staging area where other units will converge. Be mindful of access and exit routes when you direct units to respond to a location. It is unwise to have units respond to the front entrance of a hotel or apartment building that has had an explosion, because perpetrators may plant secondary devices at entrances, expecting responders to enter there. Finally, trained responders in the proper protective equipment are the only people equipped to handle the WMD incident. These specialized units, traditionally hazardous materials teams, must be requested as early as possible due to the time required to assemble and dispatch the team and their equipment. Many jurisdictions share hazardous materials teams, and the team may have to travel a long distance to reach the location of the event. It is always better to be safe than sorry; call the team early and the outcome of the call will be more favorable. Remember, there may be more than one type of device or agent present.

Command

If the incident command system (ICS) is already in place, then you should immediately seek out the medical staging supervisor to receive your assignment.[8]

The first arriving provider on the scene must begin to sort out the chaos and define his or her responsibilities under the ICS. As the first person on scene, the paramedic may need to establish incident command until additional personnel arrive. Depending on the circumstances, you and other paramedics may function as medical branch supervisors, triage supervisors, treatment supervisors, transportation or logistic supervisors, or staff. Generally, the most senior paramedic on the scene acts as the medical branch director until relieved by a supervisor or EMS physician.

Initial tasks that the first arriving paramedic must perform are as follows:

- Report to incident command post (in unified command).
- Establish a medical branch under the operations section.
- Determine the scope and scale of the incident:
  - Type of incident
  - Hazards to responders and victims
  - Number of patients/deceased
  - Safe access, egress, and staging locations

- Gather information on decontamination area or areas and hot, warm, and cold zones.
- Regularly gather and disseminate information to dispatch.
- Establish and assign a supervisor for the following areas:
  - Decontamination (if established)
  - Triage
    - Minor/walking wounded (green tag)
    - Delayed (yellow tag)
    - Urgent (orange tag, used in some areas)
    - Immediate (red tag)
    - Deceased (black tag)
  - Treatment
  - Transportation (departing units)
  - Staging (arriving personnel and units)
  - Rehabilitation (assessment, monitoring, and treatment for first responders only)
- Report all EMS activities to the operations section chief.

If the ICS is already in place, then you should immediately seek out the EMS staging supervisor to receive your assignment. The ICS and its components are discussed in further detail in Chapter 47, *Incident Management and Mass-Casualty Incidents*.

Paramedics should expect a heavy police presence at each EMS sector (treatment, triage, transportation). Law enforcement is present for several reasons, including the following:

1. To provide site security so the media and onlookers do not mingle with the wounded and interfere with their care
2. To monitor all victims in the event the perpetrator or an accomplice (such as a lookout or secondary attacker) may be among the injured
3. To canvas witnesses who may have valuable information

Paramedics should fully comply with all law enforcement requests. These requests may be safety-related or may be intended to thwart additional planned attacks. Investigators may interview patients during triage or

Patient Safety

Although some incidents may require EMS responders to treat patients as they are found and to "protect in place," at many incidents, it is crucial for the safety of the patient and the responders for patients to be moved away from the **patient generator**, the source that is causing people to become sick or injured. This effort may involve EMS or other responders helping to move patients to a **patient collection point**, also known as a casualty collection point. Responders and patients may still need to follow the instructions of law enforcement, hazardous materials technicians, or other specialists. Patients and responders may require special decontamination or other special screening and treatment as they are moved to safety.

Words of Wisdom

You are of no help to the public if you become a patient. More importantly, once you become a victim of the event, you place an additional burden on your fellow responders, who must treat you. Do not develop tunnel vision. Assess the scene and resist the urge to run in and help; otherwise, you may place yourself and your partner in danger.

treatment, or ride along with them to the hospital to gather information on what they saw or know.

Secondary Device or Event (Reassessing Scene Safety)

Terrorists have been known to plant additional explosives that are set to explode after the initial bomb. This type of **secondary device** is intended primarily to injure responders and to secure media coverage, because the media generally arrives on scene just after the initial response. Do not rely on others to secure your safety. It is every paramedic's responsibility to constantly assess and reassess the scene for safety. It is easy to overlook a suspicious package lying on the floor while you are treating casualties. Stay alert. Something as subtle as a change in the wind direction during a gas attack or an increase in the number of contaminated patients can place you in danger. Never become so involved with the tasks that you are performing that you do not look around and ensure the scene remains safe.

Weapons of Mass Destruction

A **weapon of mass destruction (WMD)** is anything used as a weapon designed to bring about mass death, casualties, and/or massive damage to property and infrastructure

(bridges, tunnels, airports, and seaports). WMDs can be grouped into five major categories: chemical, biologic, radiologic, nuclear, and explosive, known collectively as CBRNE. To date, the preferred WMD for terrorists has been explosive devices. Terrorist groups have favored tactics that use truck or car bombs or pedestrian suicide bombers. Previous terrorist attempts to use either chemical or biologic weapons to their full capacity have been unsuccessful. Nonetheless, as a paramedic, you should understand the destructive potential of these weapons and be aware of the clinical symptomology with which patients who have been exposed or infected with them may present.

As discussed earlier, the motives and tactics of new-age terrorist groups have begun to change. As with doomsday cults, many terrorist groups participate in apocalyptic, indiscriminate killing. This doctrine of total carnage would make the use of WMDs highly desirable. WMDs are easy to obtain or create and are specifically geared toward killing large numbers of people. Had the proper techniques been used during the 1995 attack on the Tokyo subway, there may have been tens of thousands of casualties. With the fall of the former Soviet Union, the technology and expertise to produce WMDs may be available to terrorist groups with sufficient funding. Moreover, the technical recipes for making nuclear, biologic, and chemical weapons and explosive devices can be found readily on the Internet; in fact, they have even been published on terrorist group websites.

The following sections describe the categories of WMDs that EMS personnel and their agencies should prepare to encounter in the field.

Chemical Agents

Chemical agents are human-made substances that can have devastating effects on living organisms. They can be produced in liquid, powder, or vapor form, depending on the desired route of exposure and dissemination technique, and are dispersed to kill or injure. First developed during World War I, these agents have been implicated in thousands of deaths since being introduced on the battlefield; more recently, they have been used to terrorize civilian populations. These agents, categorized based on how they work and the signs and symptoms they produce, are classified as follows:

- Vesicants or blister agents (eg, mustard gas and lewisite)
- Respiratory or choking agents (eg, phosgene or chlorine)
- Nerve agents (eg, sarin, soman, tabun, or VX nerve agent)
- Metabolic or blood agents (eg, hydrogen cyanide, cyanogen chloride)
- Irritating agents (eg, mace, chloropicrin, tear gas, capsicum/pepper spray, and dibenzoxazepine)

Chemical weapons can be liquid, gas, or solid materials. **Persistency** and **volatility** are terms used to describe how long the agent will stay on a surface before it evaporates. Persistent or nonvolatile agents can remain on a surface for long periods, usually longer than 24 hours. Nonpersistent or volatile agents evaporate relatively fast when left on a surface in the optimal temperature range. An agent that is described as highly persistent (such as the VX nerve agent) can remain in the environment for weeks to months, whereas an agent that is highly volatile (such as sarin, also a nerve agent) will turn from liquid to gas (evaporate) within minutes to seconds.

Route of exposure is a term used to describe how the agent most effectively enters the body. Chemical agents can have either a vapor or a **contact hazard**. Agents with a **vapor hazard** enter the body through the respiratory tract in the form of vapors. Agents with a contact hazard (or skin hazard) give off little vapor or no vapors and enter the body through the skin.

▶ Vesicants (Blister Agents)

The primary route of exposure of blister agents, or **vesicants**, is the skin (contact); however, if vesicants are left on the skin or clothing long enough, they produce vapors that can enter the respiratory tract. Vesicants cause burn-like blisters to form on the patient's skin as well as in the respiratory tract. The vesicant agents consist of sulfur mustard, lewisite, and phosgene oxime. The vesicants usually cause the most damage to damp or moist areas of the body, such as the armpits, groin, and respiratory tract. Signs of vesicant exposure on the skin include the following:

- Skin irritation, burning, and reddening
- Immediate intense skin pain (with lewisite and phosgene oxime)
- Formation of large blisters
- Gray discoloration of skin (a sign of permanent damage seen with lewisite and phosgene oxime)
- Swollen and closed or irritated eyes
- Permanent eye injury (including blindness)

If vapors were inhaled, the patient may experience the following:

- Hoarseness and stridor
- Severe cough
- Hemoptysis (coughing up of blood)
- Severe dyspnea

Sulfur mustard, often referred to by the military abbreviation H, is an oily, yellow-brown substance that is generally considered persistent. When released, sulfur mustard has the distinct smell of garlic or mustard and is quickly absorbed into the skin and/or mucous membranes. As the agent is absorbed into the skin, it begins an irreversible process of damage to the cells. Absorption through the skin or mucous membranes usually occurs within seconds, and damage to the underlying cells takes place within 1 to 2 minutes **Figure 50-8**.

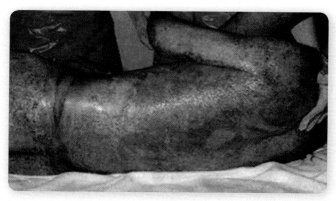

Figure 50-8 Skin damage resulting from exposure to sulfur mustard.

Courtesy of Dr. Saeed Keshavarz/RCCI, Research Center of Chemical Injuries/IRAN.

The patient will experience a progressive reddening of the affected area, which will gradually develop into large blisters. These blisters are similar in shape and appearance to those associated with thermal second-degree burns. The fluid within the blisters does not contain any of the agent; however, the skin covering the area is considered to be contaminated until decontamination by trained personnel has been performed.

If the patient does survive the initial direct injury from the agent, the depletion of the white blood cells leaves the patient with a decreased resistance to infections. Although sulfur mustard is regarded as persistent, it does release enough vapors when dispersed to be inhaled. Inhalation creates upper and lower airway compromise. The result is damage and swelling of the airways. The airway compromise makes the patient's condition far more serious.

Lewisite, often referred to by the military abbreviation L, and **phosgene oxime**, often referred to by the military abbreviation CX, produce blister wounds similar to those of sulfur mustard. They are highly volatile and have a rapid onset of symptoms, as opposed to the delayed onset seen with sulfur mustard. These agents produce immediate intense pain and discomfort when contact is made. The patient may have a gray discoloration at the contaminated site. While tissue damage also occurs with exposure to these agents, they do not cause the secondary cellular injury that is associated with sulfur mustard.

Vesicant Agent Treatment

There are no antidotes for sulfur mustard or phosgene oxime exposure. British anti-lewisite (BAL) is the antidote for lewisite; however, it is typically carried only by specialty military response units. You must ensure the patient has been decontaminated (usually by soap and copious amounts of water) before assessment of ABCDEs (Airway, Breathing, Circulation, Disability, and Exposure) is initiated. The patient may require prompt airway support if any agent has been inhaled, but this should not occur until after decontamination. Initiate transport and gain intravenous (IV) access as soon as possible. Generally, burn centers are best equipped to handle the wounds and subsequent infections produced by vesicants. Follow your local protocols when you are deciding what facility to transport the patient to.

▶ Pulmonary Agents (Choking Agents)

Also known as toxic inhalation hazards, pulmonary agents are gases that cause immediate harm to people exposed to them. The primary route of exposure for these agents is through the respiratory tract, which makes them an inhalation or vapor hazard. Once inside the lungs, they damage the lung tissue and fluid leaks into the lungs. Pulmonary edema develops in the patient, resulting in difficulty breathing due to the inability for air exchange. These agents produce respiratory-related symptoms such as dyspnea, tachypnea, and pulmonary edema. This class of chemical agents consists of **chlorine** (military abbreviation CL) and **phosgene** (military abbreviation CG).

Chlorine was the first chemical agent ever used in warfare. It has a distinct odor of bleach and can create a green haze when released as a gas. Initially it produces upper airway irritation and a choking sensation. The patient may later experience the following signs and symptoms:

- Shortness of breath
- Burning and tightness in the chest
- Hoarseness and stridor due to upper airway constriction
- Gasping and coughing
- Watery eyes and drooling

With serious exposures, patients may experience pulmonary edema, complete airway constriction, and death. The fumes from a mixture of household bleach (chlorine) and ammonia create an acid gas that produces similar effects. Each year, such mixtures overcome hundreds of people when they mix household cleaners.

Another pulmonary agent, phosgene, is not found only in the context of chemical warfare; it is a product of combustion and might be found at a fire at a textile factory or house or at the site of metalwork or burning Freon (a liquid chemical used in refrigeration). Therefore, you may encounter a patient who was exposed to this gas during the course of a normal call or at a fire scene. Phosgene is a potent agent. Its symptoms are usually delayed for hours. Unlike chlorine, when phosgene enters the body, it generally does not produce severe irritation that might cause the patient to leave the area or hold his or her breath. In fact, the odor produced by the chemical is similar to that of freshly mown grass or hay. The result is that much more of the gas is allowed to enter the body unnoticed.

The initial signs and symptoms of a mild exposure may include the following:

- Nausea
- Chest tightness
- Severe cough
- Dyspnea on exertion

The patient with a severe exposure may present with dyspnea at rest and excessive pulmonary edema. The patient will actually expel large amounts of fluid from his or her lungs. The pulmonary edema that is seen with a severe exposure produces such large amounts of fluid from the lungs that the patient may become hypovolemic and subsequently hypotensive.

Pulmonary Agent Treatment

The best initial treatment for any pulmonary agent is to remove the patient from the contaminated atmosphere. Patient removal should be done by trained personnel using the proper PPE. Aggressive management of the ABCs should be initiated, paying attention to oxygenation, ventilation, and suctioning if required. Do not allow the patient to be active because this will worsen his or her condition much faster. There are no antidotes to counteract the pulmonary agents. Managing the ABCs, gaining IV access, allowing the patient to rest in a position of comfort with the head elevated, and initiating rapid transport are the primary goals for care provided in the prehospital setting. Pharmacotherapy of this patient may include the standard treatment for bronchospasm, pulmonary edema, potential corticosteroid use (per local medical direction), and positive pressure ventilation with supplementary oxygen.

▶ Nerve Agents

The **nerve agents** are among the deadliest chemicals developed. Designed to kill large numbers of people with small quantities, nerve agents can cause cardiac arrest within seconds to minutes of exposure. Nerve agents, discovered while in search of a superior pesticide, are a class of chemical called **organophosphates**, which are found in household bug sprays, agricultural pesticides, and some industrial chemicals, at far lower strengths than in nerve agents.

These pesticides kill insects by disrupting their brains and nervous systems. Unfortunately, these same chemicals can also harm the nervous systems of animals and humans. These chemicals block the essential enzyme cholinesterase from working, causing the body's organs to become overstimulated.

G agents came from the early nerve agents, the G series, which were developed by German scientists (hence the G) in the period after World War I and into World War II. The following G agents are listed from high volatility to low volatility:

- **Sarin, military abbreviation GB.** Sarin is a highly volatile colorless and odorless liquid that turns from liquid to gas within seconds to minutes at room temperature. It is highly lethal, with an LD_{50} of 1,700 mg/70 kg (about 1 drop, depending on the purity). The **LD_{50}** is the amount that will kill 50% of people who are exposed to this level. Sarin is primarily a vapor hazard, with the respiratory tract as the main route of entry. This agent is especially dangerous in enclosed environments such as office buildings, shopping malls, or subway cars. When this agent comes into contact with skin, it is quickly absorbed and evaporates. When sarin is on clothing, it has the effect of **off-gassing**, which means that the vapors are continuously released over a period of time (like perfume), effectively following contaminated victims wherever they go.

- **Soman, military abbreviation GD.** Twice as persistent as sarin and five times as lethal, soman is both a contact and an inhalation hazard that can enter the body through skin absorption and through the respiratory tract.
- **Tabun, military abbreviation GA.** Tabun is approximately half as lethal as sarin and 36 times more persistent; under the proper conditions, it will remain for several days. The components used to manufacture tabun are easy to acquire, and the agent is easy to manufacture, which make it unique. Tabun is both a contact and an inhalation hazard that can enter the body through skin absorption and through the respiratory tract.
- **VX nerve agent.** VX is a clear, oily agent that has no odor and looks like baby oil. It is over 100 times more lethal than sarin and is extremely persistent Figure 50-9 . In fact, VX is so persistent that given the proper conditions, it will remain relatively unchanged for weeks to months. These properties make VX primarily

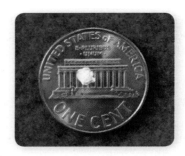

Figure 50-9 VX nerve agent is the most toxic chemical ever produced. The dot on the penny demonstrates the amount needed to achieve the lethal dose.
© Jones & Bartlett Learning. Photographed by Kimberly Potvin.

a contact hazard because it lets off little vapor. It is easily absorbed into the skin, and the oily residue that remains on the skin's surface is extremely difficult to decontaminate.

Nerve agents all produce similar symptoms but have varying routes of entry. Once the agent has entered the body through skin contact or through the respiratory system, the patient will begin to exhibit a pattern of predictable symptoms. Like all chemical agents, the severity of the symptoms will depend on the route of exposure and the amount of agent to which the patient was exposed. The resulting symptoms of nerve agent exposure are described by the mnemonics SLUDGEM and the "killer Bs," as shown in Table 50-1 . The killer Bs mnemonic is more useful to you because it lists the more dangerous symptoms associated with exposure to nerve agents.

YOU are the Paramedic | PART 3

While you are performing your primary survey, the sector leader informs you the hazardous materials team has identified the chemical dispersed along with the explosion as chlorine. A few people from outside the church described the odor as "bleach-like." You obtain IV access in the right antecubital space with an 18-gauge IV catheter with a saline lock. As you do so, the patient's difficulty breathing worsens and you begin to assist ventilations.

Recording Time: 10 Minutes	
Respirations	28 breaths/min, shallow; then ventilated at 12 breaths/min
Pulse	Radial pulse, 112 beats/min, regular and strong
Skin	Pale, warm, dry
Blood pressure	138/82 mm Hg
Oxygen saturation (Spo₂)	86% immediately prior to ventilation
Pupils	PERRLA, bloodshot

5. What smells or colors can you expect to always be present with a chlorine exposure?

Table 50-1	Symptoms of People Exposed to Nerve Agents
Mnemonic: SLUDGEM	
S	Salivation
L	Lacrimation
U	Urination
D	Defecation
G	Gastrointestinal distress
E	Emesis
M	Miosis
Mnemonic: Killer Bs	
B	Bradycardia
B	Bronchorrhea
B	Bronchospasm

© Jones & Bartlett Learning.

There is only a handful of medical conditions that are associated with the bilateral pinpoint constricted pupils (**miosis**) seen with nerve agent exposure. Conditions such as a suspected stroke, basilar skull fracture, direct light to both eyes, and an opiate drug overdose all can cause bilateral constricted pupils. Therefore, assess the patient for all of the SLUDGEM and killer B signs and symptoms to determine whether the patient has been exposed to a nerve agent.

Miosis is the most common symptom of nerve agent exposure and can remain for days to weeks. This symptom, along with the others listed in Table 50-1, will help you recognize exposure to a nerve agent early. The seizures that are associated with nerve agent exposure are unlike those found in patients with a history of seizure. The patient will continue to seize until death or until treatment is given with a nerve agent antidote kit (NAAK), such as the **DuoDote** or **MARK 1** kit.

Nerve Agent Treatment

Fatalities from severe exposure occur as a result of respiratory complications, which lead to respiratory arrest. As with any chemical exposure, EMS personnel should wear appropriate PPE, and the patients should be decontaminated prior to treatment. Common initial findings in nerve agent and organophosphate poisoning include patients who are seizing, vomiting, and expelling a large volume of secretions. As with all emergencies, managing the ABCs is the best and most important treatment that

you can provide. The patient's airway, respirations, and circulation should be rapidly assessed. Be prepared to provide immediate airway control, oxygenation, and ventilatory support. When possible, IV access should be obtained and a cardiac monitor applied. Often these patients will require administration of a NAAK to further support the ABCs by drying secretions and allowing the heart rate to normalize.

The DuoDote antidote kit contains a single injection of both atropine (2 mg) and 2-PAM chloride (pralidoxime chloride; 600 mg). The atropine helps resolve the symptoms while the 2-PAM chloride works to reverse the binding of cholinesterase inhibitors with acetylcholinesterase. While additional doses of atropine may be necessary to continue to manage symptoms, no more DuoDote kits (in particular, the 2-PAM chloride) should be administered. You may also have access to a MARK 1 kit, but these kits are no longer made. The MARK 1 kit contains the same medications that are in the DuoDote antidote kit (atropine and 2-PAM chloride), but they are administered with two separate auto-injectors. In some regions, paramedics may carry a DuoDote or MARK 1 kit on the unit and will be called on to administer it. These medications are delivered using the same technique as the EpiPen auto-injector; however, multiple doses may need to be administered. Also, a benzodiazepine may need to be administered due to the concurrent seizure activity.

Atropine is used to block the nerve agent's overstimulation of the body. However, because the nerve agent may remain in the body for long periods, 2-PAM chloride is used to eliminate the agent from the body. The 2-PAM antidote is effective at relieving the respiratory muscle paralysis and twitching caused by the nerve agent. Many of the symptoms described in the SLUDGEM and killer Bs mnemonic will be reversed with the use of atropine; however, doses of 2 to 6 mg IV or intramuscularly every 5 minutes may need to be administered to see these results. Like virtually all medications, these are most effective if administered before circulation begins to fail. If your service carries a NAAK, refer to your medical director and local protocols for specific dosage and usage information. The standard procedures for using a DuoDote are as follows:

1. Remove the DuoDote kit from its protective pouch. Hold the unit by its body in your dominant hand.
2. Keep the green tip pointed downward. This is the needle end of the auto-injector.
3. Remove the gray safety cap. If the safety cap is in place, the auto-injector will not fire.
4. Choose the location to inject. It should be a large muscle mass. The outer thigh is the most common site. Remove any wallets, pocket guides, or other potential obstructions. The DuoDote is able to deploy through light clothing.
5. Grasp the unit and position the green tip of the auto-injector on the victim's outer thigh at approximately a 90° angle.

6. Push firmly until the auto-injector fires.
7. Hold the auto-injector in place for 10 seconds to ensure the atropine has been properly delivered.
8. Remove the DuoDote auto-injector and inspect for the (now visible) needle extending from the green tip. If the needle is not visible, the auto-injector has not fired. Ensure the gray safety cap is removed and repeat the process.
9. Once the auto-injector has fired, place the unit in an appropriate sharps container.
10. Complete evacuation and decontamination procedures.
11. Reevaluate the patient for need of further intervention.

Table 50-2 offers a quick reference and comparison of the nerve agents.

Words of Wisdom

On March 20, 1995, members of a Japanese cult released sarin in the Tokyo subway. The first arriving medical responders were met with chaos as hundreds and then thousands of people fled the subway system. Many were contaminated and showing signs and symptoms of nerve agent exposure. In the end, more than 6,000 people sought medical care for exposure to sarin, and 13 people died.[9] None of the EMS personnel wore protective clothing and most became cross-contaminated from contact with contaminated patients. Remember, you can avoid becoming exposed. Do not become a victim yourself!

▶ Industrial Chemicals/Insecticides

As previously mentioned, the basic chemical ingredient in nerve agents is organophosphate. This is a common chemical that is used in lesser concentrations for insecticides. Whereas industrial chemicals do not possess sufficient lethality to be effective WMDs, they are easy to acquire, are inexpensive, and would have similar effects as the nerve agents. Crop-duster planes could be used to disseminate these chemicals. You should be cautious when you are responding to calls where insecticide equipment is stored and used, such as a farm or supply store that sells these products. The symptoms and medical management of patients poisoned by organophosphate insecticide are identical to those of the nerve agents.

Metabolic Agents (Cyanides)

Hydrogen cyanide (military abbreviation AC) and cyanogen chloride (military abbreviation CK) are both agents that affect the body's ability to use oxygen. **Cyanide** is a colorless gas that has an odor similar to almonds. The effects of the cyanides begin on the cellular level and are rapidly seen at the organ system level. Beside the nerve agents, metabolic agents are the only chemical weapons known to kill within seconds to minutes. Unlike nerve agents, however, these deadly gases are commonly found in many industrial settings. Cyanides are produced in massive quantities throughout the United States every year for industrial uses such as gold and silver mining, photography, lethal injections, and plastics processing. They are often present in fires associated with textile or plastic factories. In fact, cyanide is naturally found in the pits of many fruits in low doses. There is little difference

Table 50-2	**Nerve Agents**					
Name	**Military Abbreviation**	**Odor**	**Special Features**	**Onset of Symptoms**	**Volatility**	**Route of Exposure**
Tabun	GA	Fruity	Easy to manufacture	Immediate	Low	Contact with skin and vapor hazard
Sarin	GB	None (if pure) or strong	Will off-gas while on victim's clothing	Immediate	High	Primarily respiratory vapor hazard; contact with skin is extremely lethal
Soman	GD	Fruity	Ages rapidly, making it difficult to treat	Immediate	Moderate	Contact with skin; minimal vapor hazard
VX nerve agent	VX	None	Most lethal chemical agent; difficult to decontaminate	Immediate	Very low	Contact with skin; no vapor hazard (unless aerosolized)

in the symptoms found between hydrogen cyanide and cyanogen chloride. In low doses, these chemicals are associated with dizziness, light-headedness, headache, and vomiting. Higher doses will produce symptoms that include the following:

- Shortness of breath and gasping respirations
- Tachypnea
- Flushed skin color
- Tachycardia
- Altered mental status
- Seizures
- Coma
- Apnea
- Cardiac arrest

Words of Wisdom

Always ensure your patients have been thoroughly decontaminated by trained personnel before you come into contact with them. Chemical agents are primarily a vapor hazard, and all of the patient's clothing must be removed to prevent off-gassing. Never perform mouth-to-mouth or mouth-to-mask ventilation on a victim of a chemical agent. Many of the vapors may linger in the patient's airway, and cross-contamination may occur.

The symptoms associated with the inhalation of a large amount of cyanide will all appear within several minutes. Death is likely unless the patient is treated promptly.

Cyanide Agent Treatment. Cyanide binds with the body's cells, preventing oxygen from being used. Several medications act as antidotes, but many services do not carry them. Once trained personnel wearing the proper PPE have removed the patient from the source of exposure, even if there is no liquid contamination, all of the patient's clothes must be removed to prevent off-gassing in the ambulance. Trained and protected personnel must decontaminate any patients who may have been exposed to liquid contamination before you can initiate treatment. Then you should support the patient's ABCs and gain IV access.

Mild effects of cyanide exposure will generally resolve by simply removing the victim from the source of contamination and administering supplementary oxygen. Severe exposure, however, will require aggressive oxygenation and perhaps ventilation with supplementary oxygen, as well as the administration of IV hydroxocobalamin, distributed using the commercial name of Cyanokit. Sodium nitrate and sodium thiosulfate may also be used. Typically, such kits are not carried by EMS agencies, but they may be available from major hospitals since they are more commonly used for victims of commercial chemical exposure and smoke inhalation. Always use a

bag-mask device or oxygen-powered ventilator device to ventilate a patient exposed to a metabolic agent. The agent can easily be passed on from the patient to you through mouth-to-mouth or mouth-to-mask ventilations. If no antidote is available, initiate transport immediately.

Table 50-3 summarizes the chemical agents. The odors of the particular chemicals are provided for informational purposes only. The sense of smell is a poor tool to use to determine whether there is a chemical agent present. Many people are unable to smell the agents, and the odor could be derived from another source. The information in the table is useful to you if you receive reports from victims claiming to smell bleach or garlic, for example. You should never enter a potentially hazardous area and "smell" to determine whether a chemical agent is present.

Biologic Agents

Biologic agents are organisms or products of organisms that are cultivated, synthesized, and mutated in a laboratory to cause disease or death. The **weaponization** of biologic agents is performed to artificially maximize the target population's exposure to the germ, thereby exposing the greatest number of people and achieving the desired result.

The primary types of biologic agents that you may come into contact with during a biologic event include the following:

- Viruses
- Bacteria
- Neurotoxins

Biologic agents pose many difficult issues when used as a WMD. They can be almost completely undetectable. Also, most of the diseases caused by these agents will be similar to other minor illnesses commonly seen by paramedics.

Biologic agents may be spread in various ways. **Dissemination** is the means by which a terrorist will spread the agent—for example, poisoning the water supply or aerosolizing the agent into the air or ventilation system of a building. A **disease vector** is an animal that spreads disease, once infected, to another animal. For example, the plague can be spread by infected rats, smallpox by infected people, and West Nile virus by infected mosquitoes. How easily the disease is able to spread from one human to another human is called **communicability**. When communicability is high, such as with smallpox, the person is considered **contagious**. Typically, standard precautions for blood and airborne pathogens are enough to prevent contamination and transmission. The same core concepts apply to virtually all levels of infection control.

Incubation describes the period between the person's exposure to the agent and the onset of symptoms. The incubation period is especially important for you to understand. Although your patient may not exhibit signs or symptoms, he or she may be contagious.

Table 50-3	Chemical Agents					
Class	Names and Military Abbreviations	Odor	Lethality	Onset of Symptoms	Volatility	Primary Route of Exposure
Vesicants	Mustard (H) Lewisite (L) Phosgene oxime (CX)	Garlic (H) Geranium (L)	Causes large blisters to form on victims; may severely damage upper airway if vapors are inhaled; severe intense pain and gray skin discoloration (L, CX)	Delayed (H) Immediate (L, CX)	Very low (H, L) Moderate (CX)	Primarily skin contact; with some vapor hazard
Pulmonary agents	Chlorine (CL) Phosgene (CG)	Bleach (CL) Cut grass (CG)	Causes irritation; choking (CL); severe pulmonary edema (CG)	Immediate (CL) Delayed (CG)	Very high	Vapor hazard
Nerve agents	Tabun (GA) Sarin (GB) Soman (GD) VX nerve agent (VX)	Fruity or none	Most lethal chemical agents can kill within minutes; effects are reversible with antidotes	Immediate	Moderate (GA, GD) Very high (GB) Low (VX)	Vapor hazard (GB) Vapor and skin contact hazard (GA, GD) Skin contact hazard (VX)
Cyanide agents	Hydrogen cyanide (AC) Cyanogen chloride (CK)	Almonds (AC) Irritating (CK)	Highly lethal chemical gases; can kill within minutes; effects are reversible with antidotes	Immediate	Very high	Vapor hazard

© Jones & Bartlett Learning.

You need to be aware of when you should suspect the use of biologic agents. If the agent is in the form of a powder, such as in the October 2001 incidents involving anthrax powder mailed in letters, the call must be handled by hazardous materials specialists. Patients who have come into direct contact with the agent need to be decontaminated before any EMS contact or treatment is initiated.

▶ Viruses

Viruses are germs that require a living host to multiply and survive. A virus is a simple organism and cannot thrive outside of a host (living body). Once in the body, the virus will invade healthy cells and replicate itself to spread through the host. As the virus spreads, so does the disease that it carries. A virus survives by moving from one host to another by using its transport system—vectors.

Viral agents that may be used during a biologic terrorist release pose an extraordinary problem for health care providers, especially those in EMS. Although some viral agents do have vaccines, there is no treatment for a viral infection other than antivirals for some agents. Because of this characteristic, the following viruses have been used as terrorist agents.

Smallpox

Smallpox is a highly contagious disease. Standard precautions must be used to prevent cross-contamination to health care providers. Simply by wearing examination gloves, a HEPA-filtered respirator, and eye protection, you will greatly reduce your risk of contamination. The last natural case of smallpox in the world was seen in 1977. Before the rash and blisters show, the illness will start with a high fever and body aches and headaches. The patient's body temperature is usually in the range of 101°F to 104°F (38°C to 40°C).

An easy, quick way to differentiate the smallpox rash from other skin disorders is to observe the size, shape, and location of the lesions. In smallpox, all the lesions are identical in their development. In other skin disorders, the lesions will be in various stages of healing and development.

Smallpox blisters also begin on the face and extremities and eventually move toward the chest and abdomen. The disease is in its most contagious phase when the blisters begin to form **Figure 50-10**. Unprotected contact with these blisters will promote transmission of the disease. There is a vaccine to prevent smallpox; however, it has been linked to medical complications and, in rare cases, death **Table 50-4**. Vaccination against the disease is part of a national strategy to respond to a terrorist threat. Because

the vaccine does have some risk, only first responders have been offered the vaccine. If an outbreak occurred, the vaccine would be offered to people at risk.

Viral Hemorrhagic Fevers

Viral hemorrhagic fevers (VHFs) consist of a group of diseases that include the Ebola, Rift Valley, and yellow fever viruses, among others. This group of viruses causes the blood in the body to seep out from the tissues and blood vessels **Figure 50-11**. Initially, the patient will have flulike symptoms, progressing to more serious symptoms such as internal and external hemorrhaging. Outbreaks are common in Africa and South America. Outbreaks in the United States, however, are extremely rare. All standard precautions must be taken when you are treating these illnesses. Mortality rates can range from 5% to 90%, depending on the strain of virus, the patient's age and health condition, and the availability of a modern health care system **Table 50-5**.[10]

► Bacteria

Unlike viruses, **bacteria** do not require a host to multiply and live. Bacteria are much more complex and larger than viruses are and can grow up to 100 times larger than the largest virus. Bacteria contain all the cellular structures of a normal cell and are completely self-sufficient. Most importantly, bacterial infections can be fought with antibiotics.

Like any other types of infections, including viral, bacterial infections must be protected against by avoiding cross-contamination. Proper PPE and effective disinfection and decontamination are the best tools available to protect responders in biologic weapon scenarios, just as proper blood and airborne pathogen protocols protect paramedics every day.

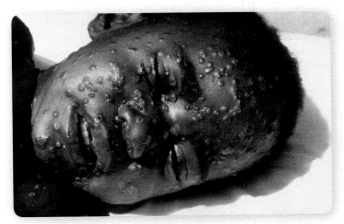

Figure 50-10 In smallpox, all the lesions are identical in their development. In other skin disorders, the lesions will be in various stages of healing and development.

Courtesy of Centers for Disease Control and Prevention.

Table 50-4	Characteristics of Smallpox
Signs and symptoms	Severe fever, malaise, body aches, headaches, small blisters on the skin, bleeding of the skin and mucous membranes. Incubation period is 10 to 12 days, and the duration of the illness is approximately 4 weeks.
Route of entry	Inhalation of coughed droplets or direct skin contact with blisters.
Communicability	High from infected people or items (such as blankets used by infected patients). Person-to-person transmission is possible.
Medical management	Standard precautions. There is no specific treatment for smallpox victims. Patients should be provided with supportive care (management of ABCs).
Dissemination	Aerosolized for warfare or terrorist uses.

© Jones & Bartlett Learning.

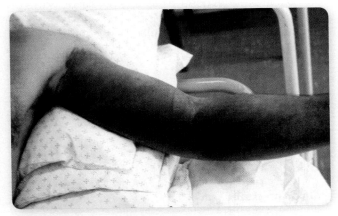

Figure 50-11 Viral hemorrhagic fevers cause the blood vessels and tissues to seep blood. The end result is ecchymosis, hemoptysis, and blood in the patient's stool. Notice the severe discoloration in this patient with Crimean Congo hemorrhagic fever, indicating internal bleeding.

Courtesy of Professor Robert Swanepoel/National Institute for Communicable Disease, South Africa.

Table 50-5	Characteristics of Viral Hemorrhagic Fevers
Signs and symptoms	Sudden onset of fever, weakness, muscle pain, headache, and sore throat. All of these symptoms are followed by vomiting and, as the virus runs its course, internal and external bleeding.
Route of entry	Direct contact with an infected person's body fluids.
Communicability	Moderate from person to person or from contaminated items.
Medical management	Standard precautions. There is no specific treatment for viral hemorrhagic fever. Patients should be provided supportive care (management of ABCs) and treatment for shock and hypotension, if present.
Dissemination	Direct contact with an infected person's body fluids. It can also be aerosolized for use in an attack.

© Jones & Bartlett Learning.

Most bacterial infections will generally begin with flulike symptoms, which make it quite difficult to identify whether the cause is a biologic attack or a natural epidemic. Biologic agents have been developed and used for centuries during times of war.

Inhalation and Cutaneous Anthrax (*Bacillus anthracis*)

Anthrax is a deadly bacterium that lies dormant in a spore (protective shell). When exposed to the optimal temperature and moisture, the pathogen is released from the spore. The routes of entry for anthrax are inhalation, cutaneous, or gastrointestinal (from consuming food that contains spores) **Figure 50-12**. Anthrax spores can be found naturally in soil. As such, cutaneous anthrax is not

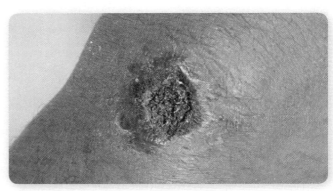

Figure 50-12 Cutaneous anthrax.
Courtesy of James H. Steele/CDC.

YOU ▶ are the Paramedic   PART 4

Your partner provides positive pressure ventilation with a bag-mask device attached to 100% oxygen while you prepare to intubate. The patient's airway is secured with a 7.5-mm endotracheal tube. Tube placement is confirmed with waveform capnography, and the patient is manually ventilated by your partner.

Recording Time: 15 Minutes	
Respirations	12 breaths/min, adequate depth and volume, manual ventilation. Bilateral wheezing is heard.
Pulse	Radial pulse, 108 beats/min, regular and strong
Skin	Pale, warm, and dry
Blood pressure	132/80 mm Hg
Oxygen saturation (Spo₂)	92% on 100% oxygen via bag-mask
Pupils	Dilated, equal, and slow to respond. Bloodshot.

6. What is the treatment of choice for a patient with chlorine gas exposure?

Table 50-6	Characteristics of Anthrax
Signs and symptoms	Flulike symptoms, fever, respiratory distress with tachycardia, shock, pulmonary edema, and respiratory failure after 3 to 5 days of flulike symptoms
Route of entry	Inhalation of spore or skin contact with spore or direct contact with skin wound (cutaneous)
Communicability	Only in the cutaneous form (rare)
Medical management	Pulmonary/inhalation: Standard precautions, supplemental oxygen, ventilatory support for pulmonary edema or respiratory failure, and transport Cutaneous: Standard precautions, application of dry sterile dressings to prevent accidental contact with wound and fluids
Dissemination	Aerosol

© Jones & Bartlett Learning.

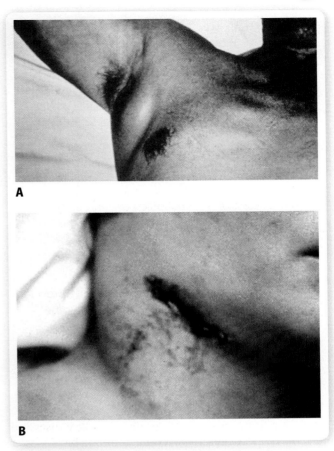

Figure 50-13 A. Plague bubo at lymph node under arm. **B.** Plague bubo at lymph node on neck.

Courtesy of Centers for Disease Control and Prevention.

uncommon among farmers and people who work with soil. The inhalational form, pulmonary anthrax, is the deadliest and often presents as a severe cold. Pulmonary anthrax infections are associated with a 82% death rate if untreated.[11] Antibiotics can be used to treat anthrax successfully. There is also a vaccine to prevent anthrax infections **Table 50-6**.

Plague—Bubonic/Pneumonic

Of all the infectious diseases known to humans, none has killed as many as the plague. The 14th century plague that ravaged Asia, the Middle East, and finally Europe (the Black Death) killed an estimated 33 to 42 million people. Later on, in the early 19th century, almost 20 million people in India and China perished due to the plague. The plague's natural vectors are infected rodents and fleas. When a person is either bitten by an infected flea or comes into contact with an infected rodent (or the waste of the rodent), that person can contract bubonic plague.

Bubonic plague infects the **lymphatic system**—a passive circulatory system in the body that bathes the tissues in lymph and works with the immune system. When this infection occurs, the patient's **lymph nodes**

(area of the lymphatic system where infection-fighting cells are housed) become infected and grow. The glands of the nodes will grow large (up to the size of a tennis ball) and round, forming **buboes** **Figure 50-13**. If the infection is left untreated, it may spread through the body, leading to sepsis and possibly death. This form of plague is not contagious and is not likely to be seen in a bioterrorist incident.

Pneumonic plague is a lung infection, also known as plague pneumonia that results from inhalation of plague bacteria. This form of the disease is contagious and has a much higher death rate than the bubonic form has. This form of plague therefore would be easier to disseminate (aerosolized), has a higher mortality rate, and is contagious **Table 50-7**.

▶ Neurotoxins

Neurotoxins are the deadliest substances known to humans. The strongest neurotoxin is 15,000 times more lethal than VX and 100,000 times more lethal than sarin. These toxins are produced from plants, marine animals, molds, and bacteria. The route of entry for these toxins is ingestion,

Table 50-7	**Characteristics of Plague**
Signs and symptoms	Fever, headache, muscle pain and tenderness, pneumonia, shortness of breath, extreme lymph node pain and enlargement (bubonic)
Route of entry	Ingestion, inhalation, or cutaneous
Communicability	Bubonic: Low, only from contact with fluid in bubo Pneumonic: High, from person to person
Medical management	Standard precautions, management of ABCs, provide supplemental oxygen, and transport
Dissemination	Aerosol

© Jones & Bartlett Learning.

Table 50-8	**Characteristics of Botulinum Toxin**
Signs and symptoms	Dry mouth, intestinal obstruction, urinary retention, constipation, nausea and vomiting, abnormal pupil dilation, blurred vision, double vision, drooping eyelids, difficulty swallowing, difficulty speaking, and respiratory failure due to paralysis
Route of entry	Ingestion or gastrointestinal
Communicability	None
Medical management	Management of ABCs, provide supplemental oxygen, and transport. Ventilatory support may be needed due to paralysis of the respiratory muscles. A vaccine is available.
Dissemination	Aerosol or food supply sabotage or injection

© Jones & Bartlett Learning.

inhalation from aerosols, or injection. Unlike viruses and bacteria, neurotoxins are not contagious and have a faster onset of symptoms. Although these biologic toxins have immense destructive potential, they have not been used successfully as a WMD.

Botulinum Toxin

The most potent neurotoxin is **botulinum**, which is produced by bacteria. When introduced into the body, this neurotoxin affects the nervous system's ability to function. Voluntary muscle control diminishes as the toxin spreads. Eventually the toxin causes muscle paralysis that begins at the head and face and travels downward throughout the body. The patient's accessory muscles and diaphragm becomes paralyzed, and the patient goes into respiratory arrest   Table 50-8 .

Ricin

Although not as deadly as botulinum, **ricin** is still five times more lethal than VX. This toxin is derived from mash that is left from the castor bean   Figure 50-14 . When introduced into the body, ricin causes pulmonary edema and respiratory and circulatory failure, leading to death   Table 50-9 .

The clinical picture depends on the route of exposure. The toxin is quite stable and extremely toxic by many routes of exposure, including inhalation. Perhaps 1 to 3 mg of ricin can kill an adult, and the ingestion of one seed can probably kill a child.

Although all parts of the castor bean are actually poisonous, it is the seeds that are the most toxic. Castor

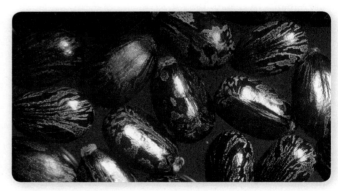

Figure 50-14 These seemingly harmless castor beans contain the key ingredient for ricin, one of the most potent toxins known to humans.
Courtesy of Brian Prechtel/USDA.

bean ingestion causes a rapid onset of nausea, vomiting, abdominal cramps, and severe diarrhea, followed by vascular collapse. Death usually occurs on the third day in the absence of appropriate medical intervention.

Ricin is least toxic by the oral route. This is probably a result of poor absorption in the gastrointestinal tract, some digestion in the gut, and, possibly, some expulsion of the agent as caused by the rapid onset of vomiting. Ingestion causes local hemorrhage and necrosis of the liver, spleen, kidneys, and gastrointestinal tract. Signs and

Table 50-9	Characteristics of Ricin
Signs and symptoms	Inhaled: Cough, difficulty breathing, chest tightness, nausea, muscle aches, pulmonary edema, and hypoxia Ingested: Nausea and vomiting, internal bleeding, and death Injection: No signs except swelling at the injection site and death
Route of entry	Inhalation, ingestion, injection
Communicability	None
Medical management	Management of ABCs. No treatment or vaccine exists.
Dissemination	Aerosol or contamination of a food or water supply by sabotage

© Jones & Bartlett Learning.

symptoms appear 4 to 8 hours after exposure. Signs and symptoms of ricin ingestion are as follows:

- Fever
- Chills
- Headache
- Muscle aches
- Nausea
- Vomiting
- Diarrhea
- Severe abdominal cramping
- Dehydration
- Gastrointestinal bleeding
- Necrosis of the liver, spleen, kidneys, and gastrointestinal tract

Inhalation of ricin causes nonspecific weakness, cough, fever, hypothermia, and hypotension. Symptoms occur about 4 to 8 hours after inhalation, depending on the inhaled dose. The onset of profuse sweating some hours later signifies the termination of the symptoms. Signs and symptoms of ricin inhalation are as follows:

- Fever
- Chills
- Nausea
- Local irritation of eyes, nose, and throat
- Profuse sweating
- Headache
- Muscle aches
- Nonproductive cough
- Chest pain

- Dyspnea
- Pulmonary edema
- Severe lung inflammation
- Cyanosis
- Convulsions
- Respiratory failure

Treatment is supportive and includes both respiratory support and cardiovascular support as needed. Early intubation, ventilation, and positive end-expiratory pressure, combined with treatment of pulmonary edema, are appropriate. IV fluids and electrolyte replacement are useful for treating the dehydration caused by profound vomiting and diarrhea. Table 50-10 summarizes the biologic agents.

▶ Other Paramedic Roles During a Biologic Event

The Worried Well

The term worried well refers to generally healthy people who seek medical treatment because they are concerned they are exhibiting symptoms associated with a particular illness or incident they recently learned about. During a terrorist incident or other type of emergency, these worried well can overwhelm EMS and health care systems that are already managing actual victims in addition to the typical response volume. Do not refuse care of a person whom you suspect to be among the worried well; your role is first to properly assess each patient according to his or her complaint and the nature of the incident.

Paramedics will often be called on to help calm the fears of the worried well and the general public. Depending on the local emergency and public health system, in addition to standard EMS responses to worried well calls, paramedics may be called to assist overwhelmed emergency departments or to help staff public health centers and mobile field hospitals.

Syndromic Surveillance

Syndromic surveillance is the monitoring, usually by local or state health departments, of patients presenting to emergency departments and alternative care facilities, and the recording of EMS call volume and the use of over-the-counter medications. Patients with signs and symptoms that resemble influenza are particularly important. Local and state health departments monitor for an unusual influx of patients with these symptoms in hopes of discovering an outbreak early. The EMS role in syndromic surveillance is a small one, yet valuable in the overall tracking of a biologic terrorist event or infectious disease outbreak. Quality assurance and dispatch operations need to be aware of an unusual number of calls from patients with "unexplainable flu" coming from a particular region or community.

Points of Distribution

Points of distribution (PODs) (Strategic National Stockpile) are strategically placed facilities that have been

Table 50-10	Biologic Agents			
Disease	**Transmission Person to Person**	**Incubation Period**	**Duration of Illness**	**Lethality (approximate case fatality rates)**
Anthrax (inhalation)[a]	No	1 to 6 d	3 to 5 d	High (usually fatal if untreated)
Botulinum[b]	No	1 to 5 d	Death in 24 to 72 h; lasts months if patient does not die	High without respiratory support
Pneumonic plague[c]	High	2 to 3 d	1 to 6 d (usually fatal)	High unless treated within 12 to 24 h
Ricin[d]	No	12 to 24 h; can be as early as 4-6 h	Days; death within 36 h; 12 d depending on dose and route of exposure	High
Smallpox[e]	High	7 to 19 d (average 10 to 14 d)	4 wk	Moderate in most populations; high in the very young, the very old, and those with existing medical conditions
Viral hemorrhagic fevers[f]	Moderate	4 to 21 d	Death between 7 to 16 d	High to moderate, depending on type of fever

Data from: Anthrax. Centers for Disease Control and Prevention website. https://www.cdc.gov/anthrax/basics/. Updated September 1, 2015. Accessed April 8, 2017; Kinds of botulism. Centers for Disease Control and Prevention website. https://www.cdc.gov/botulism /definition.html. Updated May 8, 2017. Accessed May 18, 2017; Plague (*Yersinia pestis*). Centers for Disease Control and Prevention website. https://emergency.cdc.gov/agent/plague/faq.asp. Updated November 18, 2015. Accessed April 8, 2017; Ricin toxin from *Ricinus communis* (castor beans). Centers for Disease Control and Prevention website. https://emergency.cdc.gov/agent/ricin/facts.asp. Updated November 18, 2015. Accessed April 8, 2017; Smallpox. Centers for Disease Control and Prevention website. https://www.cdc.gov /smallpox/index.html. Updated September 26, 2016. Accessed April 8, 2017; Management of patients with suspected viral hemorrhagic fever. *MMWR*. 1988;37(S-3);1-16. https://www.cdc.gov/mmwr/preview/mmwrhtml/00037085.htm. Accessed April 8, 2017.

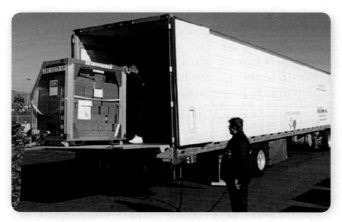

Figure 50-15 The Centers for Disease Control and Prevention Strategic National Stockpile can deliver one of many push packs to any location in the country within 12 hours of an emergency.
Courtesy of the Strategic National Stockpile/CDC.

preestablished for the mass distribution of antibiotics, antidotes, vaccinations, and other medications and supplies. These medications may be delivered in large containers known as "push packs" by the Centers for Disease Control and Prevention **Figure 50-15** . These containers have a targeted delivery time of within 12 hours anywhere in the country and contain antibiotics, chemical antidotes, antitoxins, life-support medications, IV administration, airway maintenance supplies, and medical/surgical items. In some regions, local and state municipalities have started to stockpile their own supplies to reduce the time delay.

Paramedics may be called on to assist in the delivery of the medications to the public (depending on local emergency management planning). The paramedic's role may include triage, treatment of seriously ill patients, and patient transport to the hospital. Most plans for PODs include at least one ambulance on standby for the transport of seriously ill patients.

■ Radiologic or Nuclear Devices

Other than in research and testing, there have been only two publicly known incidents involving the use of a nuclear device. During World War II, Hiroshima and Nagasaki were devastated when they were targeted with nuclear bombs. It has been estimated that a death toll of 214,000 people occurred due to the two bombs and their associated effects. The awesome destructive power demonstrated by the attack ended World War II and has since served as a deterrent to nuclear war.

There are nations that hold close ties with terrorist groups (state-sponsored terrorism) and have obtained some degree of nuclear capability. As an alternative to developing a sophisticated nuclear weapon, it is possible for a terrorist to secure radioactive materials or waste to perpetrate an act of terror. Such materials are far easier for the determined terrorist to acquire and require less expertise to use. The difficulties in developing a nuclear weapon are well documented. Radioactive materials, however, such as those in radiologic dispersal devices (discussed later), can cause widespread panic and civil disturbances.

▶ Radiation

Ionizing radiation is energy that can be emitted in the form of rays, or particles. This energy can be found in **radioactive material**, such as rocks and metals. This material is unstable, and it attempts to stabilize itself in a natural process called **decay**. As the substance decays, it gives off radiation until it stabilizes. The process of radioactive decay can take from as little as minutes to billions of years; meanwhile, the substance remains radioactive.

The energy that is emitted from a strong radiologic source is categorized as **alpha radiation**, **beta radiation**, **gamma radiation** (x-rays), or **neutron radiation** Figure 50-16 . Alpha is the least harmful penetrating type of radiation and cannot travel fast or through most objects. In fact, a sheet of paper or the body's skin easily stops it. Beta radiation is slightly more penetrating than alpha and requires a layer of clothing to stop it. Gamma rays, which share key characteristics with x-rays, are far faster and stronger than alpha and beta rays. These rays easily penetrate the human body and require either several inches of lead or concrete to prevent penetration. Neutron energy is the fastest moving and most powerful form of radiation. Neutrons easily penetrate lead and require several feet of concrete to stop them.

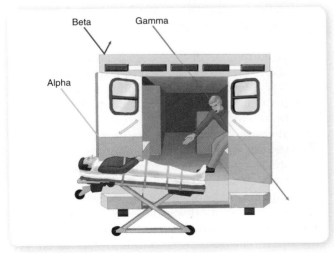

Figure 50-16 Alpha, beta, and gamma radiation.
© Jones & Bartlett Learning.

▶ Sources of Radiologic Material

There are thousands of radioactive materials found on the Earth. These materials are generally used for purposes that benefit humankind, such as medicine, killing of germs in food (irradiation), and construction work. Once radiologic material has been used for its purpose, the material remaining is called radiologic waste. Radiologic waste remains radioactive but has no more usefulness. These materials can be found at the following locations:

- Hospitals
- Colleges and universities
- Chemical and industrial sites
- Power plants

Not all radioactive material is tightly guarded, and the waste is often not guarded. This attainability makes use of radioactive material and substances appealing to terrorists.

▶ Radiologic Dispersal Devices

A **radiologic dispersal device (RDD)** is any container that is designed to disperse radioactive material. This would generally require the use of a bomb, hence the nickname **dirty bomb**. A dirty bomb carries the potential to injure victims with not only the radioactive material but also the explosive material used to deliver it. Just the thought of an RDD creates fear in a population, and so the ultimate goal of the terrorist—fear—is accomplished. In reality, however, the destructive capability of a dirty bomb is limited to the explosives that are attached to it. Therefore, if the explosive is sufficient to kill 10 people without radioactive material, it will also kill 10 people with the radioactive material added. There may be long-term injuries and illness associated with the use of an RDD, yet not much more than the bomb by itself would create. In short, the dirty bomb is an ineffective WMD in terms of physical damage, but can be psychologically potent in terms of the fear it can create.

Nuclear Energy

Nuclear energy is artificially released by altering (splitting) radioactive atoms. The result is an immense amount of energy that usually takes the form of heat. Nuclear material is used in medicine, weapons, naval vessels, and power plants. Nuclear material gives off all forms of radiation, including neutrons (the deadliest type). Like radioactive material, when nuclear material is no longer useful, it becomes waste that is still radioactive.

Nuclear Weapons

The destructive energy of a nuclear explosion is unlike that of any other weapon in the world. That is why nuclear weapons are kept only in secure facilities throughout the world. There are nations that have ties to terrorists and that have actively attempted to build nuclear weapons. However, the ability of these nations to deliver a nuclear weapon, such as a missile or bomb, is, as of yet, incomplete. There is also the deterrent of complete mutual annihilation. Therefore, the likelihood of a nuclear attack is remote.

Unfortunately, due to the collapse of the former Soviet Union, the whereabouts of many small nuclear devices is unknown. These small suitcase-sized nuclear weapons are called **special atomic demolition munitions (SADMs)**. The SADM, or "suitcase nuke," was designed to destroy individual targets, such as important buildings, bridges, tunnels, or large ships. The estimate is that perhaps as many as 80 are missing as of 1998. No other information or updates on the whereabouts of these devices have been made public.

How Radiation Affects the Body

The effects of radiation exposure will vary depending on the amount of radiation that a person receives and the route of entry. There are three levels of radiation exposure:

- **Radioactive exposure.** Exposure to radioactive material occurred, but the body is not necessarily contaminated.
- **External contamination.** The skin was contaminated with radioactive material, but the inside of the body is not necessarily contaminated yet.
- **Internal contamination.** The inside of the body is contaminated.

Radiation can be introduced into the body by all routes of entry, including directly through the body's exterior. The patient can inhale radioactive dust from nuclear fallout or from a dirty bomb, or have radioactive liquid absorbed into the body through the skin. Once in the body, the radiation source will irradiate the person from within rather than from an external source (such

Words of Wisdom

The inverse square law is derived from physics and describes how radiation travels from its source. If you double your distance from a radiologic source, you will decrease the amount of radiation that you are exposed to by a factor of four. For example, if the radiation dose at 2 feet (0.6 m) from the source is 20 rad, at 4 feet (1 m) it will decrease to 5 rad, and at 6 feet (2 m) away it will be 1.25 rad. Therefore, the farther away you get from a radioactive source, the better, but moving even a small distance away greatly reduces your exposure. Remember to use time, distance, and shielding to protect yourself.

as x-ray equipment). Some common signs of acute radiation sickness are dizziness, nausea, vomiting, internal and external bleeding, petechiae, diarrhea, and altered mental status. Unless the radiation exposure is very severe, most, if not all, of these symptoms will be delayed hours to days to weeks. Most patients will be initially asymptomatic.

Medical Management

Being exposed to a radiation source does not make a patient contaminated or radioactive. However, when patients have a radioactive source on their body (such as debris from a dirty bomb), they are contaminated and must be initially cared for by a hazardous materials responder. Once the patient is decontaminated and there is no threat to you, you may begin assessment and treatment of the ABCs and treat the patient for any burns or trauma.

Protective Measures

There are no suits or protective gear designed to completely shield you from radiation. Those people who work in high-risk areas do wear some protection gear (lead-lined suits); however, this equipment is not available to the paramedic. The best ways to protect yourself from the effects of radiation are to use time and distance and to shield yourself in level C protection from the source (protection levels are discussed in Chapter 49, *Hazardous Materials*).

- **Time.** Radiation has a cumulative effect on the body. The less time that you are exposed to the source, the less the effects will be. If you realize the patient is near a radiation source, leave the area immediately.
- **Distance.** Radiation is limited in how far it can travel. Depending on the type of radiation, often moving only a few feet is enough to remove you from immediate danger (inverse square law). You should take this into account when you are responding to a nuclear or radiologic incident and make certain that responders are stationed far enough from the incident.
- **Shielding.** As discussed earlier, the path of all radiation can be stopped by a specific object. It will be impossible for you to recognize the type of radiation being emitted, or even from which direction it is coming. Therefore, always assume you are dealing with the strongest form of radiation and use concrete shielding (such as buildings or walls) between yourself and the incident. The importance of shielding cannot be overemphasized. In one atomic test, a car was parked on the side of a house, opposite the direction of the oncoming blast. The house was completely destroyed, yet the car that was directly next to it sustained almost no damage.

Explosives and Incendiary Weapons

Explosives are the most common weapon used by terrorists today 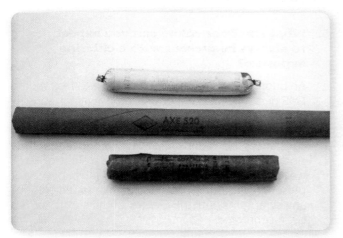 Figure 50-17 . Although terrorists are sometimes able to obtain and use military explosive weapons, **improvised explosive devices (IEDs)** are far more widely used. IEDs, or "homemade bombs" are explosive devices built from unrestricted and often common equipment. Although IEDs can be produced in almost any size, and for a variety of functions and delivery methods, they typically fall into three categories: package IEDs, vehicle-borne IEDs, and suicide bombs. IEDs may use military-grade or homemade explosive components and may be triggered by a variety of means, including timers, pressure switches, tripwires, motion triggers, sound triggers, radio remote control, and cell phones.

Incendiary weapons involve agents and chemicals used to start fires. Incendiary agents, such as acetone, can be combined with chemicals to produce explosives capable of massive destruction. Ranging from suicide bombings on public buses to trucks loaded with explosives set to go off in underground parking garages of government buildings, these explosions can be destructive.

▶ Package IEDs

Package IEDs can come in the form of pipe bombs, such as those used in the 1996 Atlanta Centennial Olympic Park bombing and in abortion clinic bombings; pressure cooker bombs, such as those used in the 2013 Boston Marathon bombings; and even simple bags stuffed with explosives, such as those used in the 2004 Madrid train bombings. Package IEDs are often packed with "enhancements," such as nuts, bolts, marbles, ball bearings, and other items, that can act as projectiles and penetrating objects. Other enhancements may include chemical or

radioactive agents. Package IEDs have also been known to be used as secondary weapons.

▶ Vehicle-Borne IEDs

IEDs can be made both larger and more mobile by packing a vehicle with explosives and driving it to the site of the terrorist attack. **Ammonium nitrate** is used commonly as an industrial-grade fertilizer and is not in itself dangerous to handle or transport, yet when it is mixed with fuel oil or diesel fuel and other easily acquired components, it forms an extremely explosive compound. In 1993, Al Qaeda attacked the World Trade Center using an ammonium nitrate and fuel oil (ANFO) bomb, killing 6 people and wounding more than 1,000. Similarly, the 1995 attack on the Alfred P. Murrah Federal Building in Oklahoma City (one of the deadliest terrorist attacks in the United States) involved a homemade explosive device made from an ANFO mixture. The perpetrators of that incident packed a van with 7,000 pounds (3,200 kg) of ANFO to destroy the Alfred P. Murrah Federal Building and severely damage most buildings in the immediate vicinity. In Israel, even ambulances have been used to disguise vehicle-born IEDs.

▶ Suicide Bombs

Suicide bombs merge the destructive power of military-grade explosives with the timing and accuracy of human guidance and triggering Figure 50-18 . They are a low-cost,

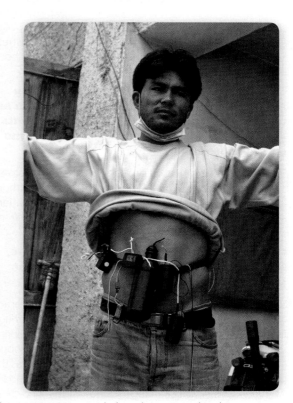

Figure 50-17 Every year, thousands of pounds of explosives are stolen.
© Jones & Bartlett Learning.

Figure 50-18 A suicide bomb merges the destructive power of explosives with human guidance and triggering.
© Musadeq Sadeq/AP Photo.

low-technology, and highly effective weapon of terror. Suicide bombs are easily concealed, carried, and delivered with accuracy to a selected target. Recruits for suicide bomb terrorism are readily available; they require little training and are generally deeply committed to killing others as well as themselves. In addition to men, women and children have acted as **suicide bombers**, making these acts even more difficult to prevent. Suicide bombers rely on the element of surprise and familiarity with the targeted area.

In addition to their tactical advantages, suicide bombers' attacks are occasionally recorded by the terrorist organization as propaganda and to perpetuate fear in the population. Outside of the United States, media outlets exhibit little self-censorship and often broadcast graphic terrorist attacks and videos made by terrorists. These broadcasts help to spread the message of terror.

Words of Wisdom

Two of the most common blast injuries are tympanic membrane rupture and barotraumas (damage to the structures of the inner ear).[12] These types of injures make it difficult or impossible to communicate with patients who have been near a bomb blast because they may be disoriented from vertigo (as a result of inner ear damage) or have greatly diminished or absent hearing. You will need to be aware of such impairments when triaging and treating these patients. The most common fatal blast injury is "blast lung," a barotrauma characterized by the clinical triad of apnea, bradycardia, and hypotension.[12]

YOU are the Paramedic   SUMMARY

1. What are some clues that might help you treat your patient?

Pay close attention to the information being provided from dispatch before you arrive as well as from on-scene communications and your own observations when you arrive. In this case, you know there was an explosion and some kind of toxic substance released into the air. Your assessment reveals a patient in acute respiratory distress but without significant bleeding or apparent signs of shock.

2. Chemical agents may be obtained easily and combined with other weapons such as explosives. What types of chemical agents may be likely to cause this patient's signs and symptoms?

This patient is exhibiting confusion, respiratory distress, and increased work of breathing, and he wheezes without any other significant changes in circulation. This patient appears to have signs and symptoms of a pulmonary agent.

3. On the basis of the information you have, to what agent do you think your patient was exposed?

The information that you have so far can be indicative of any one of several pulmonary agents that enter the body through inhalation and have immediate physiologic effects. Chlorine is the most commonly available pulmonary agent and would align with the early reports of a bleach smell as well as the patient's signs and symptoms of difficulty breathing and airway irritation, including burning eyes, nose, throat, and chest.

4. What should be the focus of your initial treatment?

As with any patient, initial treatment should focus on identifying and correcting any problems related to airway, breathing, and circulation. The patient's primary presenting problem is respiratory distress, so oxygen therapy is an appropriate place to start. Because the airway appears to be irritated, advanced airway management should be considered even though the patient can still maintain his own airway for now. As work of breathing increases, total airway and breathing control may be necessary in the near future. Consider consulting with incident command to see if the chemical can be positively identified, and consult with hazardous materials specialists or poison control to decide if additional treatment is indicated.

5. What smells or colors can you expect to always be present with a chlorine exposure?

An odor may not always be noticeable to responding EMS personnel. It is important to be aware of sensory clues, including smells, sights, and colors, but you should not rely on them solely for identification of toxic substances. Many substances may produce the same sights and smells. Also, just because a sight or smell was not noticed does not mean the substance is not present or hazardous. Treat the patient based on signs and symptoms until the identity of the substance has been confirmed.

6. What is the treatment of choice for a patient with chlorine gas exposure?

As with treatment for any other toxic exposure, patient decontamination and appropriate protective equipment for EMS providers are the first priorities.

No antidotes exist for exposure to chlorine gas. The key to treatment is high-quality supportive care, focusing especially on where the chlorine will cause the most damage, the airway and respiratory systems. As with any severe illness or injury, your assessment and treatment must stay ahead of the progress of the problem. As early signs and symptoms of airway irritation appear, prepare for and, as necessary, perform advanced airway management. Likewise, as respiratory distress increases, use oxygen therapy, continuous positive airway pressure, and bag-mask ventilation to alleviate the patient's work of breathing.

Remember, the toxic exposure itself may not be the only issue. Complete a thorough assessment and continue to monitor the patient, even if the primary issue has been found and is being managed.

Triage Tag
No. 35572009

Move the Walking Wounded	MINIMAL
No respirations after head tilt	EXPECTANT
☐ Respirations—over 30 or less than 10	IMMEDIATE
☐ Perfusion—capillary refill over 2 seconds	IMMEDIATE
☒ Mental status—unable to follow simple commands	IMMEDIATE
Otherwise	DELAYED

MAJOR INJURIES: *None*

HOSPITAL DESTINATION : *Southport*

ORIENTED ×☐   DISORIENTED ☒   UNRESPONSIVE ☐

TIME	PULSE	B/P	RESPIRATION
1055	112 beats/min	138/82 mm Hg	24 breaths/min
1100	112 beats/min	132/82 mm Hg	28 breaths/min, shallow; then ventilated at 12 breaths/min, wheezes
1105	108 beats/min	132/80 mm Hg	12 breaths/min ventilated

PERSONAL INFORMATION:

NAME: *Brett Murphy*

MALE ☒   FEMALE ☐   AGE: EST. 22   WEIGHT: EST. 83 lb (165 kg)

MEDICAL COMPLAINTS/HISTORY

Respiratory distress; chemical exposure

EXPECTANT   No   35572009

IMMEDIATE   No   35572009

© Jones & Bartlett Learning.

Prep Kit

▶ Ready for Review

- As a result of the increase in terrorist activity, it is possible that you could be called to respond to a terrorist event. You must be mentally and physically prepared for this possibility.
- The use of weapons of mass destruction (WMDs) further complicates the management of the terrorist incident. Maintain good situational awareness at all times, and elevate your awareness as the potential threat level increases.
- Terrorism is a violent act that is dangerous to human life, in violation of the criminal laws of the United States, to intimidate or coerce a government, the civilian population, or any segment thereof, in furtherance of political or social objectives.
- Terrorists are either international or domestic and can be categorized as state terrorists, religious extremists, issue-oriented terrorists, right-wing extremists, left-wing extremists, separatists, narcoterrorists, or pathologic terrorists.
- The National Terrorism Advisory System alerts responders to the potential for an attack, provides specifics of the threat if practical, and advises on measures to take for protection. The threat level can be elevated or imminent.
- On the basis of the current threat level, take appropriate actions and precautions. Be aware of established policies that your organization may have regarding the current threat level.
- Indicators that may give you clues as to whether the emergency is the result of an attack include the type of location, type of call, number of patients, patients' statements, and preincident indicators.
- If you suspect a terrorist or WMD event has occurred, ensure that the scene is safe. If you have any doubt that it may not be safe, do not enter. Wait for assistance.
- It is crucial to notify the dispatcher. Inform dispatch of the nature of the event, any additional resources that may be required, the estimated number of patients, and the upwind route of approach or optimal route of approach.
- Establish a staging area, where other units will converge. Be mindful of access and exit routes.
- Terrorists may set secondary devices to explode after the initial bomb to injure responders and secure media coverage. Constantly assess and reassess the scene for safety.
- A WMD is any weapon or agent designed to bring about mass death, casualties, and/or massive damage to property and infrastructure (bridges, tunnels, airports, and seaports). WMDs can be grouped into five major categories: chemical, biologic, radiologic, nuclear, and explosive, known collectively as CBRNE.
- Chemical agents include vesicants or blister agents, respiratory or choking agents, nerve agents, metabolic or blood agents, and irritating agents. When a patient has been exposed to one of these, decontamination is a necessary first step. Do not approach the patient until hazardous materials responders have declared that the patient is decontaminated. Treatment will usually include airway management, intravenous access, and rapid transport.
- Patients exposed to a nerve agent can be treated with an antidote. This is delivered as an auto-injector. Multiple doses may be needed. Follow your local protocols.
- Biologic agents include viruses such as smallpox and those that cause viral hemorrhagic fevers, bacteria such as those that cause anthrax and plague, and neurotoxins such as botulinum toxin and ricin.
- Standard precautions are extremely important when you treat patients who were potentially exposed to a biologic agent.
- Nuclear or radiologic weapons can create a massive amount of destruction. Radioactive material may be used in a radiologic dispersal device, or dirty bomb, but the majority of the damage from such a bomb is caused by the explosives, not from the radioactive material.
- As with exposure to chemical agents, patients who were potentially exposed to radioactive material must be decontaminated before you have any contact. Time, distance, and shielding are the best ways to protect yourself from radiation exposure.
- Explosives are the most common weapon used by terrorists. Incendiary weapons involve agents and chemicals used to start fires. Ammonium nitrate bombs and suicide bombers are two weapons commonly used by terrorists.

▶ Vital Vocabulary

alpha radiation A type of energy that is emitted from a strong radiologic source. It is the least harmful penetrating type of radiation and cannot travel fast or through most objects.

ammonium nitrate A commonly used industrial-grade fertilizer that is not in itself dangerous to handle or transport, but when mixed with fuel and other components, forms an extremely explosive compound.

anthrax A deadly bacterium (*Bacillus anthracis*) that lies dormant in a spore (protective shell); the germ is released from the spore when exposed to the optimal temperature and moisture. The route of entry is inhalational, cutaneous, or gastrointestinal (from consuming food that contains spores).

Prep Kit (continued)

apocalyptic violence A type of violence sought by some terrorists, such as violent religious groups and doomsday cults, in which they wish to bring about the end of the world.

bacteria Microorganisms that reproduce by binary fission. These single-cell creatures reproduce rapidly. Some can form spores (encysted variants) when environmental conditions are harsh.

beta radiation A type of energy that is emitted from a strong radiologic source. It is slightly more penetrating than alpha and requires a layer of clothing to stop it.

botulinum A very potent neurotoxin produced by bacteria; when introduced into the body, this neurotoxin affects the nervous system's ability to function and causes muscle paralysis.

buboes Enlarged lymph nodes (up to the size of tennis balls) that are characteristic of people infected with the bubonic plague.

bubonic plague An epidemic that spread throughout Europe in the Middle Ages, causing over 25 million deaths, also called the Black Death; transmitted by infected fleas and characterized by acute malaise, fever, and the formation of tender, enlarged, inflamed lymph nodes that appear as lesions, called buboes.

chlorine The first chemical agent ever used in warfare. It has a distinct odor of bleach and creates a green haze when released as a gas. Initially, it produces upper airway irritation and a choking sensation. Its military abbreviation is CL.

communicability The ease with which a disease spreads from one human to another human.

contact hazard A hazardous agent that gives off little or no vapors and typically enters the body through the skin; also called a skin hazard.

contagious The characteristic of being communicable from one person to another person.

covert An act in which the public safety community generally has no prior knowledge of the time, location, or nature of the attack.

cross-contamination Contamination of a person that results from coming into contact with another contaminated person, as opposed to coming into contact with the original source of contamination.

cyanide An agent that affects the body's ability to use oxygen. It is a colorless gas that has an odor similar to almonds. The effects begin on the cellular level and are very rapidly seen at the organ system level.

decay A natural process in which a material that is unstable attempts to stabilize itself by changing its structure.

dirty bomb A bomb that is used as a radiologic dispersal device (RDD).

disease vector An infected animal that spreads a disease to another animal.

dissemination The means with which a terrorist will spread a disease—for example, by poisoning the water supply or aerosolizing the agent into the air or ventilation system of a building.

domestic terrorism Terrorism that is carried out by native citizens against their own country.

DuoDote A nerve agent antidote kit that contains a single injection of both atropine (2 mg) and 2-PAM chloride (pralidoxime chloride; 600 mg).

elevated A threat level in which a terrorist event is suspected, but there is no specific information about its timing or location.

G agents Early nerve agents that were developed by German scientists in the period after World War I and into World War II. There are three such agents: sarin, soman, and tabun.

gamma radiation A type of energy that is emitted from a strong radiologic source that is far faster and stronger than alpha and beta rays. These rays easily penetrate the human body and require either several inches of lead or concrete to prevent penetration. Gamma rays share key characteristics with x-rays.

guerilla warfare A form of warfare in which a small group that is not part of the official military engages in combat that uses the element of surprise, such as raids and ambushes; sometimes used by terrorists to protect their training camps and bases of operation.

imminent A threat level in which a terrorist event is known to be impending or will occur very soon.

improvised explosive device (IED) An explosive device built from unrestricted and often common equipment.

incubation The period between the person's exposure to the agent and the onset of symptoms.

international terrorism Terrorism that is carried out by those not of the host's country; also known as cross-border terrorism.

ionizing radiation Energy that is emitted in the form of rays or particles.

LD_{50} The amount of an agent or substance that will kill 50% of people who are exposed to this level.

lewisite A blistering agent that has a rapid onset of symptoms and produces immediate intense pain and discomfort on contact. Its military abbreviation is L.

lymph node An area in the lymphatic system where infection-fighting cells are housed.

Prep Kit *(continued)*

lymphatic system A passive circulatory system that transports a plasma-like liquid called lymph, a thin fluid that bathes the tissues of the body.

MARK 1 A nerve agent antidote kit containing two auto-injector medications, atropine and 2-PAM chloride (pralidoxime chloride).

miosis Bilateral pinpoint constricted pupils.

National Terrorism Advisory System (NTAS) The US system for informing citizens of a potential terrorist threat; replaced the color-coded Homeland Security Advisory System.

nerve agents A class of chemicals called organophosphates that function by blocking an essential enzyme in the nervous system, which causes the body's organs to become overstimulated and burn out.

neurotoxins Biologic agents that are the most deadly substances known to humans. They include botulinum toxin and ricin.

neutron radiation A type of energy that is emitted from a strong radiologic source. It is the fastest moving and most powerful form of radiation. The particles easily penetrate lead and require several feet of concrete to stop them.

off-gassing The emitting of an agent after exposure—for example, from a person's clothes that have been exposed to the agent.

organophosphates A class of chemical found in many insecticides used in agriculture and in the home. Nerve agents fall into this class of chemicals.

patient collection point A location to which responders move patients to allow for safe assessment and treatment; also known as a casualty collection point.

patient generator The source that is causing people to become sick or injured.

persistency The length of time that a chemical agent will stay on a surface before it evaporates.

phosgene A pulmonary agent that is a product of combustion, such as might be produced in a fire at a textile factory or house or at the site of metalwork or burning Freon; a very potent agent that has a delayed onset of symptoms, usually hours. Its military abbreviation is CG.

phosgene oxime A blistering agent that has a rapid onset of symptoms and produces immediate intense pain and discomfort on contact. Its military abbreviation is CX.

pneumonic plague A lung infection, also known as plague pneumonia, that is the result of inhalation of plague bacteria.

point of distribution (POD) A strategically placed facility that has been preestablished for the mass distribution of antibiotics, antidotes, and vaccinations, along with other medications and supplies.

radioactive material Any material that emits radiation.

radiologic dispersal device (RDD) Any container that is designed to disperse radioactive material.

ricin A neurotoxin derived from mash that is left from pressing oil from a castor bean; causes pulmonary edema and respiratory and circulatory failure, leading to death.

route of exposure The manner by which a toxic substance enters the body.

sarin A nerve agent that is one of the G agents; a highly volatile colorless and odorless liquid that turns from liquid to gas within seconds to minutes at room temperature. Its military abbreviation is GB.

secondary device An additional explosive device used by terrorists that is set to explode after the initial bomb.

smallpox A highly contagious disease that may be spread in an aerosolized form as an act of warfare or terrorism. It is most contagious when blisters begin to form.

soman A nerve agent that is one of the G agents; twice as persistent as sarin and five times as lethal. It has a fruity odor as a result of the type of alcohol used in the agent and is both a contact and an inhalation hazard that can enter the body through skin absorption and through the respiratory tract. Its military abbreviation is GD.

special atomic demolition munition (SADM) A small suitcase-sized nuclear weapon that was designed to destroy individual targets, such as important buildings, bridges, tunnels, or large ships.

suicide bomber A terrorist who wears or carries a weapon, such as an explosive, and triggers its detonation, killing himself or herself in the process.

sulfur mustard A vesicant that is generally considered very persistent. It is a yellow-brown oily substance that has the distinct smell of garlic or mustard and, when released, is quickly absorbed into the skin and/or mucous membranes and begins an irreversible process of damaging the cells. Its military abbreviation is H.

syndromic surveillance The monitoring, usually by local or state health departments, of patients presenting to emergency departments and alternative care facilities, the recording of EMS call volume, and the use of over-the-counter medications.

tabun A nerve agent that is one of the G agents; 36 times more persistent than sarin and approximately half as lethal. It has a fruity smell and is unique because the components used to manufacture the agent are easy to acquire and the agent is easy to manufacture. Its military abbreviation is GA.

Prep Kit *(continued)*

terrorism A violent act dangerous to human life, in violation of the criminal laws of the United States or any segment to intimidate or coerce a government, the civilian population, or any segment thereof, in furtherance of political or social objectives.

VX nerve agent A nerve agent that is one of the G agents; over 100 times more lethal than sarin and extremely persistent. It is a clear, oily agent that has no odor and looks like baby oil.

vapor hazard An agent that enters the body through the respiratory tract.

vesicant A blister agent. The primary route of entry is through the skin.

viral hemorrhagic fevers (VHFs) A group of diseases that includes the Ebola, Rift Valley, and yellow fever viruses, among others. This group of viruses causes the blood in the body to seep out from the tissues and blood vessels.

virus A germ that requires a living host to multiply and survive.

volatility The length of time that a chemical agent will stay on a surface before it evaporates.

weapon of mass destruction (WMD) Any agent designed to bring about mass death, casualties, and/or massive damage to property and infrastructure (bridges, tunnels, airports, and seaports).

weaponization The creation of a weapon from a biologic agent generally found in nature and that causes disease. The agent is cultivated, synthesized, and/or mutated to maximize the target population's exposure to the germ.

worried well Generally health people who seek medical treatment because they are concerned that they are exhibiting symptoms associated with a particular illness or incident they recently learned about.

▶ References

1. Curtis K, Ramsden C. *Emergency and Trauma Care for Nurses and Paramedics*. New South Wales, Australia: Elsevier Health Sciences; 2011.
2. Prince R. 9/11 death toll rises as cancer cases soar among emergency workers. *The Telegraph* website. http://www.telegraph.co.uk/news/worldnews/northamerica/usa/10994227/911-death-toll-rises-as-cancer-cases-soar-among-emergency-workers.html. Published July 27, 2014. Accessed April 2, 2017.
3. White JR. *Terrorism and Homeland Security*. 9th ed. Boston, MA: Cengage Learning; 2016.
4. Federal Bureau of Investigation. *Terrorism 2002/2005*. Washington, D.C.: U.S. Department of Justice; 2006.
5. National Commission on Terrorist Attacks. *The 9/11 Commission Report: Final Report of the National Commission on Terrorist Attacks Upon the United States* (Authorized Edition). New York, NY: WW Norton & Company; 2011.
6. Rodgers L, Qurashi S, Connor S. *7 July London bombings: What happened that day?* BBC News. http://www.bbc.com/news/uk-33253598. Published July 3, 2015. Accessed April 7, 2017.
7. Bullock J, Haddow G, Coppola DP. *Introduction to Homeland Security*. Oxford, UK: Butterworth-Heinemann; 2015.
8. Phibbs WM, Snawder MA. Embracing the incident command system above and beyond theory. *FBI Law Enforcement Bulletin* website. https://leb.fbi.gov/2014/november/embracing-the-incident-command-system-above-and-beyond-theory. Published November 4, 2014. Accessed April 2, 2017.
9. Osaki T. Deadly sarin attack on Tokyo subway system recalled 20 years on. *The Japan Times* website. http://www.japantimes.co.jp/news/2015/03/20/national/tokyo-marks-20th-anniversary-of-aums-deadly-sarin-attack-on-subway-system/#.WOExcNLyuMo. Published March 20, 2015. Accessed April 2, 2017.
10. Management of patients with suspected viral hemorrhagic fever. *MMWR*. 1988;37(S-3);1-16. https://www.cdc.gov/mmwr/preview/mmwrhtml/00037085.htm. Accessed April 8, 2017.
11. Vaccines, blood and biologics: anthrax. US Food and Drug Administration website. https://www.fda.gov/BiologicsBloodVaccines/Vaccines/ucm061751.htm. Published June 17, 2015. Accessed April 2, 2017.
12. Explosions and blast injuries: a primer for clinicians. Centers for Disease Control and Prevention. http://emergency.cdc.gov/masscasualties/explosions.asp. Accessed April 8, 2017.

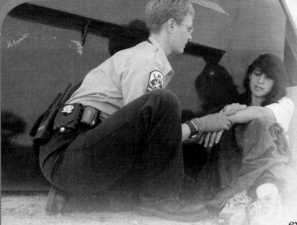

Assessment *in Action*

Local law enforcement has informed your EMS agency that they have received a credible threat that an ecoterrorist group has threatened to use a biologic agent to attack a local restaurant owned by a national chain with whose practices the group disagrees. Law enforcement states that at this time they do not have any further information at this time on the exact nature of the biologic agent the group intends to use.

1. Which of the following biologic agents would be most likely to contaminate a food supply?

   A. Pneumonic plague
   B. Botulinum toxin
   C. Viral hemorrhagic fever
   D. Smallpox

2. Which of the following biologic agents is considered highly communicable?

   A. Ricin
   B. Tabun
   C. Anthrax
   D. Smallpox

3. _____ affects the nervous system's ability to function and causes muscle paralysis.

   A. Tabun
   B. Botulinum
   C. Ricin
   D. Sarin

4. What is an indirect way through which a paramedic may help identify the use of a biologic agent?

   A. Blood testing
   B. Physical assessment
   C. Syndromic surveillance
   D. Delivery of vaccinations

5. The routes of entry for anthrax include all of the following EXCEPT:

   A. inhalation.
   B. cutaneous.
   C. gastrointestinal.
   D. sexual transmission.

6. The deadliest substances known to humans are:

   A. pulmonary agents.
   B. neurotoxins.
   C. organophosphates.
   D. vesicants.

7. Strategically placed facilities that have been preestablished for the mass distribution of antibiotics, antidotes, vaccinations, and other medications and supplies are called:

   A. strategic warehouses.
   B. points of distribution.
   C. rapid deployment units.
   D. central response centers.

8. While bombs and bullets have been frequently used for terrorist attacks in the United States, what other types of weapons might a paramedic expect to encounter at a terrorist attack?

9. What core EMS operations skills might a paramedic be called upon to use at a terrorist incident?

10. How might a paramedic manage a call for a worried well patient?

CHAPTER 51

Disaster Response

National EMS Education Standard Competencies

EMS Operations

Knowledge of operational roles and responsibilities to ensure patient, public, and personnel safety.

Mass-Casualty Incidents Due to Terrorism and Disaster

> Risks and responsibilities of operating on the scene of a natural or man-made disaster. (pp 2470-2487)

Knowledge Objectives

1. Define disaster, including the types of critical infrastructure that can be affected by a disaster. (p 2466)
2. Explain what is meant by an all-hazards approach to disaster planning. (p 2466)
3. Discuss preplanning questions to consider related to general items, such as geography, the infrastructure, and the population. (pp 2467-2469)
4. List items to consider when preplanning for a disaster of any sort. (pp 2467-2470)
5. Discuss preplanning considerations related to available emergency medical services (EMS) resources, such as mutual aid, fire, police, and hospitals. (pp 2468-2469)
6. Discuss other resources that should be considered when preplanning for a disaster event, such as nongovernmental organizations, disaster relief agencies, and local businesses. (p 2468)
7. Discuss other preplanning considerations for disaster planning, including communications, supplies, training, transportation, and media and legal concerns. (pp 2468-2469)
8. Describe early measures to take when responding to a disaster, including early preparation when a warning is received, inventory of supplies, mobilization of personnel, and command setup. (p 2470)
9. List items to consider when responding to a disaster emergency. (p 2470)
10. Discuss other general considerations for responding to a disaster, including personnel physical and mental needs, resupplying, surveillance, and media. (pp 2471-2473)
11. Discuss actions to take after responding to a disaster, including the after-action report, retraining, and reimbursement. (pp 2473-2474)
12. List items to consider after responding to a disaster. (p 2473)
13. Discuss concerns related to specific natural disasters, including natural fires, snow and ice storms, tornadoes, hurricanes, tsunamis, earthquakes, landslides, cave-ins, volcanic eruptions, flooding, sandstorms, drought, prolonged cold weather, heat wave, meteors, and pandemics. (pp 2474-2483)
14. Discuss concerns related to specific man-made disasters, including structural fires, construction failures, power failures, riots and stampedes, strikes, snipers and hostage situations, explosions, and technology disruptions. (pp 2483-2487)

Skills Objectives

There are no skills objectives for this chapter.

Introduction

The emergency medical services (EMS) system responds to small, medium, and large emergencies every hour, every day, and everywhere. A main function of EMS is responding to disasters. A **disaster** is a sudden, calamitous event, such as an accident or catastrophe, that causes great damage, loss, or destruction. A disaster can be man made or natural. Disasters overwhelm EMS and community resources because critical infrastructure has been damaged or destroyed **Figure 51-1**. **Critical infrastructure** includes the electrical power grid, communication systems, fuel for vehicles, drinkable water, sewage removal, food, hospitals, and transportation systems. In smaller, rural services, anything that overwhelms the capabilities of EMS and community resources may also be classified as a disaster. Two critical patients with only one ambulance crew responsible for their care can be classified as a disaster if not handled properly. **Disaster management** requires planners to take a broad look at preparedness, planning, training, response, and after-action review.

This chapter covers the general rules that should apply to all EMS responses to disasters, such as planning, and also covers specific man-made and natural emergencies. Chapter 47, *Incident Management and Mass-Casualty Incidents*; Chapter 49, *Hazardous Materials*; and Chapter 50, *Terrorism Response*, address those specific emergencies; therefore they are not discussed here. Refer to those chapters for specific information on those particular incidents.

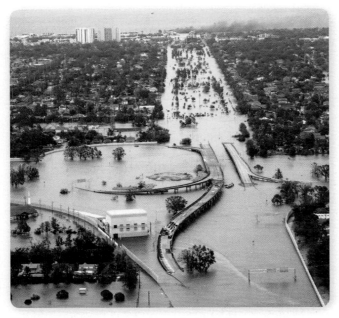

Figure 51-1 Disasters can overwhelm EMS resources and can damage critical infrastructure.

Courtesy of Petty Officer 2nd Class Kyle Niemi/U.S. Coast Guard. Photo courtesy of U.S. Army.

Disaster Response Planning

Federal, state, and local governments have plans in place to manage disasters. Large and small companies also have plans, as do military, educational, and similar institutions. EMS agencies are, or should be, no different. Plans should be suited to the geography, population, and potential risks specific to the area. The best way to plan for a disaster is to think, "What could happen here?" and "What plans do we have in place for this possibility?"

The key for any EMS response unit or provider when responding to a disaster is planning. The act of conducting comprehensive preplanning for all types of disasters is called an **all-hazards approach**. Before addressing specific issues particular to the disaster, general considerations that apply to any disaster must be addressed, such as the number of personnel needed, equipment required, and the hospital or hospitals to which patients are transported.

▶ Phases of a Disaster Response Plan

Disaster response by EMS is improving and changing as threats and knowledge about threats evolve. The key to any disaster response is planning. The key to planning is thinking, meeting, and brainstorming. A good motto to remember is that preparation prevents poor performance. With the right plans and mindset, EMS will be ready. The three phases of any plan of response are before the event (preplanning), during the event, and after the event.

YOU are the Paramedic   PART 1

You and your partner have been working in the aftermath of a major storm that caused a large amount of damage in your response area. You have been on duty for the past 24 hours with no end in sight and have seen many patients who were injured because of the storm. Currently, you and your partner are assigned to a large-scale incident at an apartment complex that collapsed during the storm.

1. What is the definition of a disaster?
2. What does the term *all-hazards approach* mean in disaster planning?

Before the Event

Preplanning is the process in which EMS agencies prepare for a potential event. **Table 51-1** lists some of the main items to consider when preplanning for a disaster. Depending on a responder's position within an EMS organization, certain questions will come to mind during the preplanning process. This section does not address every issue, but it should give you an idea of what to consider before an event occurs. Management considerations for specific disasters are discussed in the latter half of this chapter.

While no disaster is predictable, some events are more likely to occur than others. For example, an EMS agency in the Northeast may preplan for a snowstorm, whereas an agency in the Midwest may develop a response plan in the event of a tornado. However, natural disasters such as the tornado that landed in Springfield, Massachusetts, in 2011, and the earthquake centered in Virginia in the same year have proven that unlikely events do occur. General disaster preplanning with an all-hazards approach will put your agency in the best position to handle any disaster that may befall your area.

Geography of Response Area. Your area may be prone to a particular type of natural disaster (eg, flood, earthquake, tornado). During the preplanning process, hazards and life threats associated with a particular type of natural disaster can be identified. Advance knowledge of factors that can affect response, including obstacles (eg, flooded roads) as well as terrain features (eg, hills, rivers) that can hinder access for equipment and entry into a facility, helps to prepare responders for a more successful response. Consider how particular factors such as snow, ice, or smoke may impact your response **Figure 51-2**. For example, in the event of flooding, you should be familiar with secondary routes identified by your agency to avoid obstacles such as impassable bridges and blocked roads. Remember, as a paramedic, especially in times of disaster, you could easily become the lead EMS worker. Knowledge of your response area and its hazards is essential to preparation.

Population. It is beneficial to know whether a community's population is dynamic in relation to geography or time. Is the population spread out, densely packed, or mixed? Is the daytime population the same as the nighttime population? For example, many cities have as much as six times more people present during business hours than at night because businesses and shops are open primarily during daytime hours. There may be language differences or cultural aspects to consider during preplanning. Your area may include different types of facilities (eg, retirement community, handicapped facilities, prisons) that may be of special concern to EMS agencies because they present

Table 51-1	Disaster Response Preplanning Considerations
Geography of response area	
Population (urban, rural, mixed, special needs)	
Available EMS resources (mutual aid, medical supplies, transportation, maps)	
Mutual aid agreements and compacts	
Partnerships with private businesses	
Nongovernmental organizations (eg, Red Cross) and disaster relief agencies (eg, FEMA)	
Law enforcement resources	
Fire and rescue resources	
Training standards	
Infrastructure	
Internal communication	
Hospitals and health care resources	
Partnerships with media organizations	
Incident escalation	
Medical history of personnel	
Sheltering and protection	
Animal control	

Abbreviations: EMS, emergency medical services; FEMA, Federal Emergency Management Agency

© Jones & Bartlett Learning.

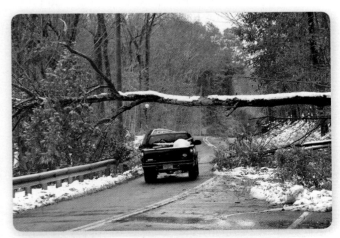

Figure 51-2 Considering the geography of your response area can help you to anticipate potential obstacles that could occur in a disaster.

© Gina Jacobs/Shutterstock.

numerous hazards, evacuation issues, and the condition of the people residing within these facilities may vary greatly. Special equipment (eg, special medications, special moving devices, power sources for ventilators) and training may be needed to care for these populations in the event of a disaster.

EMS Resources. Preplanning allows for the designation, acquisition, and movement of items needed to respond effectively and efficiently to an incident. Resources may include additional staff or personnel, specialized staff (eg, critical transport personnel), medical supplies, and equipment to handle tasks. Your agency must be able to cover its area of responsibility even if resources are dispatched to other communities to assist in a disaster response. Some important resources are mutual aid agreements, supplies on hand, transportation assets, and maps.

Mutual aid agreements (MAAs), sometimes called automatic fill-in/send-up policies, formally define the relationships between two or more agencies or municipalities and the support that those organizations will provide to each other when requested. EMS is normally accustomed to MAAs that allow EMS agencies and fire departments in neighboring jurisdictions to cover emergency calls.

Your agency may have a "disaster stash" (supplies on hand specifically for emergencies). It is important to keep your agency's inventory up to date, including tracking expiration dates of items, if applicable. The inventory list should be a living document whose quantities and items can be changed based on the threat. Who in your agency is responsible for predicting inventory needs (eg, extra supply of gloves and air purifying respirators for a predicted pandemic)? Who is the person responsible for ordering these? Many agencies have a designated supply officer or an inventory stored electronically with minimum stock lows and highs for disaster items.

Your agency may have access to special transportation equipment that can be used for a particular type of disaster situation. For example, if you are in a flood-prone zone, your agency may have access to boats or other water vehicles. It is important that drivers are trained and familiar with specialized vehicles and how to operate them in difficult conditions.

Emergency vehicles may be equipped with a global positioning device (GPS); however, in the event of satellite loss, you may need to use a laptop or paper maps. These maps should be updated to include information such as road closures and flood paths and the means to secure them. EMS personnel must be able to read maps, use compasses, and use protractors.

Partnerships With Private Businesses. Businesses in your area may be able to help your agency in a disaster (eg, a local lumber company may be able to supply wood for additional makeshift backboards). Your agency can determine what expertise is available to you from the private sector in your response area (eg, mechanics, electricians) and may have written agreements with local businesses that include information regarding how to contact business personnel after hours if a disaster occurs.

Nongovernmental Organizations and Disaster Relief Agencies. Nongovernmental organizations and disaster relief agencies such as the Salvation Army or Red Cross may also have the capability to provide support during a disaster. Your agency will determine the best method for contacting these organizations. You may be required to attend training programs offered by these organizations or your agency may invite them to your planning sessions.

Law Enforcement Resources. Your disaster response plans must also take into account state, regional or county, and local law enforcement resources and their goals and objectives in disaster operations. As with other agencies and organizations, your agency should outline how to contact, coordinate, and cooperate with them.

Fire and Rescue Resources. Your agency's disaster response plan will outline fire and rescue response during an event **Figure 51-3**. Plans should include a rehabilitation area for firefighters, paramedics, and other personnel. Command of an incident through structured interaction of major response organizations, which may include law enforcement, fire, rescue, and EMS organizations, is referred to as the **unified command system** within the **incident command system (ICS)**. Unified command may be formed when multiple jurisdictions or agencies are involved in a single incident. These agencies may involve services with different functional responsibilities such as law enforcement, fire, rescue, and EMS, or organizations from different geographic jurisdictions. Unified command is not a committee. It allows representatives from multiple jurisdictions to share command authority and responsibility, allowing the key players to contribute their perspectives and expertise, thereby working together as

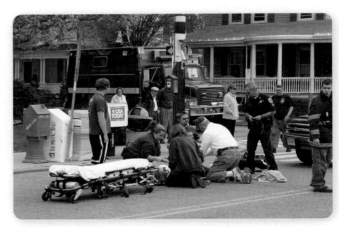

Figure 51-3 Emergency plans must be coordinated with those of local fire and police departments, as you will likely all be working together at a disaster scene.

© Larry St. Pierre/Shutterstock.

an incident command team. Before a disaster strikes, it is important to have an understanding of how your agency will work within a unified command structure.

Training Standards. One of the benefits of preplanning is that it helps organizations to learn from prior events and use that knowledge for disaster risk reduction. The preplanning is the "think about it" phase, the policy creation is the "write about it" phase, and training is the "do it" phase. Training is usually done in stages that follow progress from individual tasks, to crew tasks, to agency training, and then to interagency collaboration. Your agency will frequently train and update EMS providers on procedures to follow during a disaster, including personal protective equipment (PPE) protocols, safety procedures, and operation of new and specialized equipment.

Such preplanning and training proved critical for responders to be part of the successful control of the influenza outbreak that initially caused 240 deaths in Texas between 2009 and 2010.[1] Likewise, emergency response training proved crucial in supporting the response to the devastation of Hurricane Sandy in 2012.[2]

Infrastructure. It is important to be familiar with your agency's communication backup plan to be prepared when telephone landlines are down, when cell phones are overwhelmed, and when power grids fail. The backup plan will also include information about other backup procedures, such as how vehicles will be refueled if fuel pumps do not have electricity for operation and how cellular towers will operate once their backup generators have gone without refueling.

Internal Communication. Your agency's plan must include a way to maintain communication with all of its members (those at base camp, those off base camp, and those working with other agencies such as the fire or police departments) as well as backup methods of communication with all involved parties. Vehicles may be equipped to communicate with each other or specific radio frequencies and cell phones may be reserved for such use. It is imperative that any radio frequency changes be shared between agencies immediately to maintain communication.

Hospitals and Health Care Systems. You must be familiar with the level of care available in your area. Local hospitals may have limitations on the number and types (pediatric, trauma, burns, etc) of patients they can accept during a disaster. Your agency might participate with local hospitals during disaster drills, and there may be an agreement in place between your agency and local hospitals to provide personnel to your agency or vice versa.

Partnerships With Media Organizations. Your agency should have a designated public information officer who is trained to use the media to your agency's advantage. This person should be familiar with the *Standards for Privacy of Individually Identifiable Health Information*, also known as

the Privacy Rule under the Health Insurance Portability and Accountability Act (HIPAA).[3] Every agency should have a backup public information officer, because disasters may last many days, or the primary public information officer may not be immediately available.

Incident Escalation. It is important for members of your agency to know when and how to contact the next higher level of authority. Your agency and dispatch system should have a list of contacts at the state and federal levels, and those contacts should be verified on a regular basis. Redundancy is built into the plan to ensure that all necessary parties remain informed as an incident evolves. Has the system been tested at least semiannually? It should be clear what steps should be taken to ensure that higher levels of authority know who you are, where you are, and what you are going to do.

Immunizations of Personnel. Your agency requires that its members' immunization records be on file and up to date. Titers to verify immunization status are an option your agency can consider. This file should be forwarded to the agency's medical director and accessible to your agency's infection control officer. It is important to familiarize yourself with your agency's plan for inoculations pursuant to a specific emergency. For example, personnel may receive immunizations against typhoid fever or hepatitis A during emergencies where there is an increased risk of transmission.

Sheltering and Protection. Your agency's disaster plan should include procedures for sheltering members of the community as well as on-duty and off-duty personnel **Figure 51-4**. In addition, your agency may have an adult supervision plan for children of personnel or patients who cannot be cared for due to duty or incapacitation. Methods of providing food, water, proper waste disposal, and bathroom facilities for personnel and patients should be outlined in the plan as well.

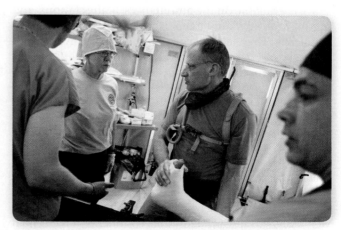

Figure 51-4 Emergency plans must include plans for sheltering patients as well as EMS personnel.
© Dina Rudick/*The Boston Globe*/Getty.

Animal Control. If your agency plans to assist in evacuations, your plan should address animals such as pets that must be left behind and service animals that must accompany patients. If you are in a rural area, precautions must be in place to manage carcasses. If there are zoos, wildlife refuges, or veterinary facilities in your area, it is important for your agency to plan for concerns related to these facilities. For example, your agency may identify a need for access to rabies prophylaxis for patients and personnel.

Special Populations

What is your agency's policy regarding pets? When involved in an evacuation, many patients will not leave without their pets, or at least some confirmation of the pet's security. Will pets be allowed at a makeshift field hospital? Now is the time to get these procedures written into your disaster plans.

During the Event

Once a disaster strikes, it is best to stick to the plan if possible, but remember that changing conditions and oversights in preplanning may require modifying the initial plan. Plans are not written in stone; they are guidelines to help EMS provide care in the safest and most efficient manner **Table 51-2**.

You may have advance warning of the upcoming event, such as a tornado or ice storm. If you do, the advance notice may be long or it may be incredibly brief. You must use this time to your advantage to "fine tune" your plan to the specific disaster predicted. Make sure you stay updated on the latest information.

Inventory. During the alert or preparation period, take immediate inventory of supplies on hand. For a snowstorm, put shovels as well as some rock salt in the ambulance. For a cold-weather emergency, pack extra blankets. Try to anticipate what you will need; determine how much space is available on the ambulances, at the stations, and at supply dumps; and prepare for the worst, mentally and physically. Then take a deep breath, take an inventory of yourself and your crew, and remember the emergency rule: "You can only do what you can do safely."

Mobilization of Personnel. Another important step is to gather the crew and activate the notification system. Personnel must be briefed and notified of changes to the plans as soon as possible and as often as needed. Agencies will assign jobs as needed, making sure that everyone realizes that assignments can change based on the circumstances as they unfold. The agency will also start an ICS-211 form to track personnel, noting who reported, when and where they were assigned, and any additional comments. It is essential to have a constant and continual inventory of where people are and what they are doing. Finally, each paramedic must have the necessary credentials on his or her person.

Table 51-2	Considerations During a Disaster
Inventory	
Mobilization of personnel	
Command setup or response	
Unification of command	
Personal protective and safety equipment	
Equipment resupply	
Triage and classification	
Patient tracking	
Assignment of personnel	
Personnel physical needs	
Personnel mental needs	
Hospital updates	
Providing and accepting relief	
Surveillance	
Weather conditions	
Media	
Legal issues	
Unit leadership reinforcement	

© Jones & Bartlett Learning.

Command Setup or Response. As a paramedic, you will either be setting up a command or reporting to a command. In either case, command must be visible (the incident commander and the location of incident command must be easily identifiable; for example, the incident commander should wear a command vest and helmet, and the command post as well as specific areas such as triage and treatment should be marked with panels or flags) and all responding personnel must be assimilated into the ICS properly.

Unification of Command. Command unity is essential to optimize operations effectiveness and to reduce problems such as potential miscommunication at responses to incidents. Fire, police, EMS, and other agencies should all be represented in the command structure with a lead agency directing the efforts. The lead agency can change many times depending on the course of events during an emergency. Cooperation is essential; egos must be checked at the door. In major disasters, a state or federal government entity usually leads the command structure.

Personal Protective and Safety Equipment. PPE and safety gear can wear out during a crisis. PPE must be replaced immediately; measures must be in place to replace gear as needed. This is both a command and a personal responsibility. Personnel must not take shortcuts or neglect to wear the gear assigned to them for their protection.

Equipment Resupply. Like PPE, equipment gets worn out, broken, or expended during the crisis. Resupply of disposables and recharging of battery-operated equipment are just a few examples of gear that must be resupplied during the event. The command structure should have plans in place or formulated for equipment resupply. Keep in mind that new, incoming personnel might not use exactly the same equipment as the assisted agency, so plans for either similar equipment or on-the-spot training should be enacted.

Triage and Classification. Patient classification may be disaster-dependent in some cases. For example, in a pandemic situation, patients who need ventilators would receive much more intense care than would patients who need palliative care or basic support. Triage and classification will be a constant and ongoing process, depending not only on patient needs, but also on availability, safety, and sustainability of EMS providers Figure 51-5 . As discussed in Chapter 47, *Incident Management and Mass-Casualty Incidents*, methods of triage include Simple Triage And Rapid Treatment (START) triage and Sort, Assess, Lifesaving interventions, and Treatment and/or Transport (SALT) triage.

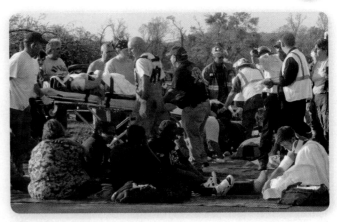

Figure 51-5 Patient triage is a constant, ongoing process that will occur throughout the disaster.
© Roger Nomer/AP Photo.

Patient Tracking. During the event, you must make a record for every patient you see or assist. This is typically done with a triage tag. If you are involved in transporting patients, you must complete a patient care report for the patients you transported. The transportation supervisor must maintain a log of all patients and the hospitals to which they are transported. Some areas use innovative methods for tracking patients, such as using bar-coded tags. Information you may collect includes patient names, their injury categories, which units transported, and where the patient was transported. This information should be listed, updated, and given to the incident commander. The incident commander can disclose this information to the proper authorities. This information is not a violation of HIPAA.

YOU are the Paramedic PART 2

You arrive at the staging area and check in. You are immediately assigned to transport one priority yellow patient to a local receiving hospital. You report to the transportation supervisor and she directs you to the yellow tarp. You take a report on a 24-year-old woman from the paramedic caring for the patients in the yellow area.

Recording Time: 1 Minute	
Appearance	Awake
Level of consciousness	Alert (oriented to person, place, time, and event)
Airway	Open
Breathing	Adequate
Circulation	Adequate

3. What is pre-event planning, and how can an event be predicted in advance?
4. Why are preplanned mutual aid agreements essential to your operation?

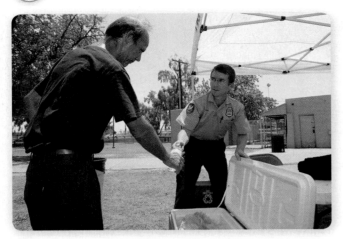

Figure 51-6 Plan for food, drink, and bathroom facilities to be supplied for patients and personnel working at disasters.
© Ross D. Franklin/AP Photo.

Assignment of Personnel. Assessment of new resource personnel must be done before they begin working, preferably in the staging areas, especially when receiving aid from other communities. The choice of appropriate personnel for patient care will depend on several factors, such as the level of training of EMS workers, the duration of event, and the amount of stress related to the event.

Personnel Physical Needs. Patients and personnel need to eat, drink, and use bathroom facilities **Figure 51-6**. In long-lasting emergencies, personnel will require sleep areas, access to their medications for chronic diseases, and a way to communicate with loved ones. It is imperative that the plan address methods of supplying the basic and fundamental needs of patients and EMS providers during a disaster.

Personnel Mental Health Needs. Disaster response is hard work! People become stressed, tired, aggravated, and burned-out. Use a buddy system approach to monitor these problems. In a long-lasting event, agencies should provide some downtime and an area where the EMS workers can unwind. EMS providers should be encouraged to talk about their experiences. Remember that light humor and a constant supply of information are often helpful. Be alert for mental health issues and incident fatigue in yourself and among your coworkers.

Hospital Updates. It is important to maintain communication with your destination hospitals. You need to know whether they can take more patients, and if so, what kind. For example, is your local hospital out of beds in their intensive care unit? This would necessitate transporting critical patients to another facility. Hospitals may be able to resupply your equipment and supplies. Do they need some of your agency's personnel or could your agency use some of theirs? You must keep the hospitals updated on field conditions so that they can readjust their priorities,

if necessary. Your help may be needed to set up an offsite hospital.

Providing and Accepting Relief. If your agency is providing relief, it must ensure that it has enough coverage in its home area of responsibility. If a crew is sent to another area, it may need to be self-sustaining for 48 to 72 hours. Before you go, make sure your equipment is compatible. For example, your radios will need to be able to work on the same frequencies as other radios at the scene. Your electrocardiogram (ECG) monitors may require adaptors to be used in another setting, and ECG leads need to be able to be switched from one machine to another, because the crew that transports the patient may be different than the crew that treated the patient. A phone call to the asset-requesting agency is a good way to double-check this information. If your agency is accepting relief, the rules for providing relief apply in reverse. Also, the credentials of the incoming personnel must be checked, and the agency accepting relief must ensure that these personnel have the proper PPE.

Surveillance. Depending on the incident, your observations and field updates could make all the difference in the progression of an event. In a terrorism event, as discussed in Chapter 50, *Terrorism Response*, suspicious people or packages should be reported. In a flooding environment, EMS providers can assist with disease monitoring by reporting on evolving trends in their patients such as diarrhea, vomiting, and rashes not normally encountered. Each agency should keep its personnel attuned to exactly what they should be on the lookout for.

Weather Conditions. Weather is the cause of many disaster events. It can significantly affect the ability of EMS to provide care during and after an event, which may affect a wide geographic area. Extreme weather not only hinders EMS operations, events such as heat waves and hurricanes can worsen medical illness and increase traumatic injuries. Monitoring of such events may be done through a variety of sources, ranging from state emergency operations centers to apps on mobile electronic devices. Such monitoring is crucial for the proper deployment, operation, and protection of EMS responders. Key items to consider include the time for the event to develop, the predicted duration of the event, the area significantly affected, the population affected, and any special hazards that may be triggered by the event.

Evidence-Based Medicine

There has been a trend of increasing frequency and severity of extreme weather-related events, including heat waves, droughts, wildfires, extreme rainfall, winter precipitation, hurricanes, tornadoes, and floods. This trend is expected to continue for the foreseeable future.[4]

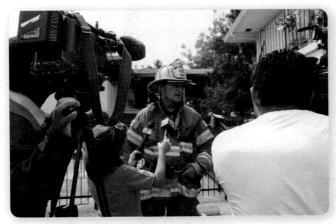

Figure 51-7 The public information officer or another responder must be trained in how to speak appropriately with the media regarding emergencies.

© Karin Hildebrand Lau/Shutterstock.

Table 51-3	Considerations After the Event
Accountability	
Resupply and repair	
Inventory	
Stress reaction review	
Physical examination of personnel	
Brainstorm	
After-action report	
Finance and reimbursement	
Acknowledgment	

© Jones & Bartlett Learning.

Media. Your agency will need to determine if there is a need for it to supply a public information officer **Figure 51-7**. Members of your agency may be trained to respond to questions from the press and to put measures in place to control rumors. It might be necessary to set up a press area and to direct questioners to this area. Your agency should use the press and social media to its advantage; for example, inform the public to stay indoors or to provide self-care in non-emergent cases or until help can be sent to them. Consider a press briefing location and provide prompt briefing so all the facts that you are allowed to release about the incident can be communicated through the media.

Legal Issues. Proper documentation during a crisis is essential; it is the best way to describe any events or issues that arise during an event. Most legal issues will be resolved long after the event, but eyewitness testimony and patient care issues are almost always helped by clear, concise write-ups. During a disaster, all patients who are transported should have a patient care report written, in addition to the triage tag.

Unit Leadership Reinforcement. During the crisis, if possible, it is best if a commander or supervisor performs occasional field checks to stay aware of conditions, complaints, and concerns. A strong, concerned unit commander can do a lot to bolster morale by listening to the field pulse. Many issues can be resolved with the early intervention of a concerned supervisor.

After the Event

There are specific measures to take after the event has occurred. These are listed in **Table 51-3**. The time period after the event can be very useful: personnel can recover, supplies can be restocked, reimbursements can occur, and training needs can be identified.

Accountability. Your agency must account for every worker and patient who was involved in an event. Duty rosters must be completed for each EMS provider to include: dates and times worked, duties, and any additional comments. A patient care report is required for every patient seen, transported, or assisted.

Resupply and Repair. All equipment used during the event must be replaced. All equipment that was not used must be checked to see if it was weathered or contaminated during the response. Finally, have equipment repaired and have vehicles that were used during the event serviced.

Inventory. After resupply and repair, a complete inventory of all physical assets should be done. This may be the time to reconsider equipment carried based on lessons learned during the crisis. The complete inventory will probably help in determining the reimbursement.

Stress Reaction Review. Posttraumatic stress disorder is being diagnosed more frequently. Your agency may consider using critical incident stress management teams, especially for long-term events or those with a high mortality rate. As you work with colleagues, note any changes in behavior in your coworkers, such as changes in mood or appetite. Any concerns should be immediately reported to your supervisor for further professional evaluation, in line with your agency's employee assistance program or critical incident stress debriefing (CISD) program plans. Open communication should be encouraged, and your agency should provide a receptive environment for those exposed to tragedy. If someone from your agency approaches you with concerns about your reaction to an incident, you should consider scheduling an unbiased, professional evaluation.

Physical Examination of Personnel. A physician should examine all injured personnel. This examination is useful for future workers' compensation claims in the event of claimed disability. Physicians' comments should be maintained with the protected personnel records. The EMS provider should be notified of test results as soon as they are received. Also, counseling services should be made available, if requested or required. Agencies can consider having a waiver for uninjured personnel to avoid illegitimate claims.

Brainstorm. Your agency should solicit input from its staff when evaluating the agency's response to a disaster. This process has a twofold benefit. The first is that EMS providers have a chance to share their observations and requests, making them stakeholders in the event. The second is that this feedback provides input for the after-action review. This process should occur as soon as possible after a disaster to keep the events fresh in responders' memories. Journals or notes made by responding personnel during the event are helpful for recalling events accurately.

After-action Report. The **after-action report (AAR)** is your official internal report of the entire event. It should contain a chronologic and accurate description of the facts of the incident. On the basis of this report, an agency can review the incident in its entirety. The AAR and all accumulated anecdotal evidence can be used to provide a basis for retraining in specific areas. On the basis of the AAR, EMS crews may become aware of areas of deficiency or skills that need to be refreshed. A plan for reinforcement of skills and knowledge should be prepared based on this data.

Finance and Reimbursement. In large incidents, monies spent on equipment, personnel, and losses may be covered by government organizations or insurance. This is one of the reasons why a "declaration of a disaster" is important and may open the door to state or federal disaster relief funds and low-interest loans. The key to reimbursement is accurate and specific documentation. It is also possible that some monies may be owed; again, itemization is the key.

Acknowledgment. New paramedics may not be accustomed to being in a supervisory role, but may be the most senior person in times of a prolonged disaster. Good performance should be praised so that EMS providers feel their services have not gone unnoticed. Learn to praise often, immediately, and honestly. Awards dinners and plaques are justified in this selfless profession and do wonders to increase morale and retention of trained personnel.

Up until this point, we have discussed concerns that apply to every emergency response. The next sections will discuss specific disaster responses.

◼ Natural Disasters

There are two types of disasters: natural and man made. Some disasters are a combination of both types. For example, riots and looting may occur after a hurricane.

Natural disasters can have a variety of significant impacts on emergency operations. For example, it is important that drivers of emergency vehicles understand the braking differences and the traction problems when driving in inclement conditions. Remember that you may have four-wheel drive vehicles, but you do not have four-wheel brakes; four-wheel drive will not help once your vehicle is in a skid.

Other important points to remember when working in natural disasters include the following:

- EMS may be represented in the **emergency operations center (EOC)** or in the unified command center. This means having a physical presence as well as communications capability with those in the field.
- EMS may be initially deployed to assist in evacuation efforts.
- During and after a natural disaster, roads will likely be damaged or cut off. Stay in touch with your local EOC and keep up with conditions in your response area.
- Consider coordinating emergency response with your local or state department of transportation or public works agencies to get you there safely. Many times they will be able to reprioritize their tasks based on your needs.
- After a natural disaster hits, landmarks may be gone; use lights to direct displaced people toward emergency services. You might be gathering uninjured patients and bringing them to collection points. In the case of many casualties, casualty collection points can be set up to pick up lightly treated, stable patients using buses and trucks.
- It is likely that radio communication and cell phones will not be reliable. Be prepared to act independently based on your preplanning, by identifying and utilizing amateur **radio operators** and communication experts who can "patch" through a temporary communication setup during a disaster.
- As in many big disasters, dignitaries may visit the site of the incident for various reasons. This will present issues such as crowd control and EMS protection for the visitors.
- EMS duties may be expanded from standard practice to deliver or administer medications or perform other related public health services.
- Your agency may need to plan to set up a temporary morgue site to accommodate patients who are beyond EMS help.

Table 51-4 lists some examples of natural disasters. There are certain general actions to take before, during, and after every event. However, actions related to specific natural disasters, must be considered as well. These actions should be prepared for during the preplanning phase.

Table 51-4	Examples of Natural Disasters
Forest and brush fires	
Snow and ice storms	
Tornadoes	
Hurricanes	
Tsunamis	
Earthquakes	
Landslides, avalanches, mudslides	
Cave-ins	
Volcanic eruptions	
Flooding	
Sandstorms and dust storms	
Drought	
Prolonged cold weather	
Heat wave	
Meteors and space debris	
Epidemics and pandemics	

© Jones & Bartlett Learning.

▶ Forest and Brush Fires

The response to forest and brush fires should be considered differently than the response to structural fires Figure 51-8. The following considerations apply to forest, brush, and lightning strike fires; some of these considerations apply to structural fires as well (discussed later).

- As a paramedic, remember that your role is not to fight fire. You will be directed to a staging or treatment area.
- Lightning is dangerous. Remain inside your vehicle or in another safe spot at any time when strikes are predicted in the area.
- Try to predict which kind of injuries you will be treating. Firefighters will most likely need care for smoke inhalation, exhaustion, and burns. Civilians will need care for exposure, physical and mental trauma, burns, exhaustion, and smoke inhalation.
- PPE should include proper gear in addition to infection control gear, such as bunker

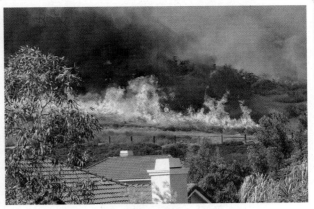

A

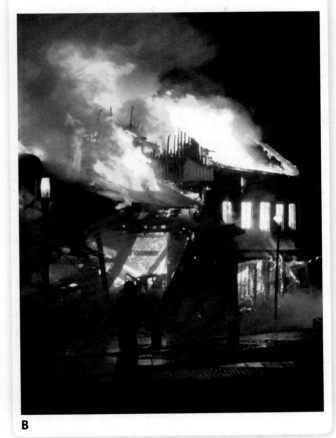

B

Figure 51-8 A. Most naturally occurring fires are forest or brush fires. **B.** Most man-made fires are structural.

A: © Peter Weber/Shutterstock; B: © Harald Høiland Tjøstheim/Shutterstock.

gear, air-purifying respirator (APR) masks, and heavy-duty gloves. Make sure you have extinguishers and protective blankets on board.
- Follow the directions of fire command and stay in touch at all times with the command post. Be prepared to move away immediately and have a couple of preplanned routes to safety.
- Firefighting is taxing; expect cardiac events, even in firefighters who appear young and healthy.

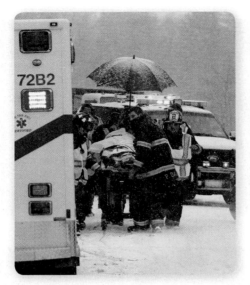

Figure 51-9 Working in a snow or ice storm requires proper gear and presents challenges when driving.

© Frank Becerra Jr./*The Journal News*/AP Photo.

▶ Snow and Ice Storms

The northern regions of the United States experience snow and ice storms regularly; however, these storms can occur in many areas Figure 51-9 . Personnel may have to adapt to changing conditions in a short period. It is important to make sure that your agency's vehicles are "snow ready." This includes using snow tires, possibly studded, or equipped with drop-down or freestanding chains. Also, be sure to check the vehicle's antifreeze and coolant levels. Cold weather motor oil should be used in vehicles.

Put a couple of snow shovels in the back of the ambulance just in case you need to dig a path through the snow. Clay kitty litter, calcium chloride crystals, and rock salt should also be on board to provide traction. Some important points to remember when working in snow and ice storms include the following:

- Clothing should be weather ready. Prepare for the conditions. You will need an extra supply of clothes, warm coats, gloves, boots, and hats.
- Your agency may have ancillary equipment such as snowmobiles, snow blowers, and plows. EMS providers should receive training on the equipment they may need to use during snow or ice storms.
- Take your time. Stretchers do not roll well in snow. You might not be able to park close to the scene; therefore, you may have to carry the patient farther. Plastic basket stretchers (Stokes litters) will be helpful. Make sure your crew has enough people.
- Look at the roof before entering a structure. EMS and fire personnel have been killed by snow and ice slides.
- If your company is on a standby status, prepare portable warm-up shelters for access to coffee, water, and hot chocolate.

▶ Tornadoes

Tornadoes can and do occur anywhere in the country. Most commonly, they occur in the Midwest and South. The warnings may be timely or there may be none. If possible, maintain supplies in tornado-proof shelters to avoid destruction of these supplies if they are in the tornado's path. Whenever possible, store vehicles in storm-proof shelters until the storm has passed. During the tornado and until it is declared safe, keep your crews in tornado-proof shelters, preferably underground. After the tornado passes through, be ready to stage in a **directed area** to await instructions. A directed area is an area considered by engineering expertise to be a safe place to stage until directed otherwise.

Important points to remember when working in tornadoes include the following:

- Remember, helicopters and air assets probably will not be available. Air currents, **thermals** (changes in temperature and wind speed in the air), and rain make flying dangerous or impossible. Calling for medevac will not be an option during the initial aftermath.
- Consider leaving landmarks in the field in place of street signs that have been blown over. These landmarks can include spray-painted directions on curbs and flags planted on street corners.
- You may need to help set up field hospitals and first aid stations at **casualty collection points**.

▶ Hurricanes

Hurricanes (ie, cyclones), can occur anywhere, but tend to happen in the southern states and in coastal regions. Usually, but not always, there is some type of warning.

Words of Wisdom

Hurricane Katrina and the response, or lack of response, to it has become the new standard for the EMS world in terms of lessons learned. EMS and hospital communities did truly heroic things during the hurricane, but that does not prevent criticism. All levels of emergency response and disaster preparedness—local, state, and federal—were put to the test after Hurricane Katrina and the subsequent flooding that occurred after the storm. The necessity of a coordinated response plan that includes preplanning and training was realized.[5] One lesson learned during and after Hurricane Katrina was that people's frustration can lead to feelings of fear or abandonment, which in turn can lead them to resort to violence to secure medical resources. If the situation is possibly dangerous to EMS worker (and personal) safety, do not go out without a security presence. If the situation is serious enough, the National Guard, Coast Guard, or State Police may be available to assist.

These warnings should always be taken seriously. Hurricanes come in five categories, ranging from category 1 (winds 74 to 95 mph; minimal damage expected) up to a category 5 (winds greater than 155 mph; severe damage expected). It is a good idea to plan on at least one level higher than the worst prediction.

Safety is first, always. You cannot help if you are injured or stranded. You will only add to the current problem if your response is not well thought out. If you are told to "hunker down," do it. Is your staging site hurricane proof? You may be able to use the time before the storm hits to fill sandbags and restock equipment. In addition to PPE, make sure you have wet weather gear, personal flotation devices, and access to boats and other specialized equipment.

Most patient care will come after the storm. Make sure to stay aware of post-storm updates, such as levees that are overcome, tidal surges, as well as bridges and roads that are flooded **Figure 51-10**. Your agency must have a means to communicate these changing developments with field personnel.

If you do not know the depth of the water, do not drive through it. You might want to consider high-axle vehicles such as ambulances as opposed to "fly car" sedans (for example, if you are meeting a basic life support crew at a scene) that may sit too low for water driving.

► Tsunamis

Tsunamis (also called tidal waves) are large waves with major destructive power. Tsunamis can travel thousands of miles, and can hit the shore at speeds of 500 to 600 mph.[6]

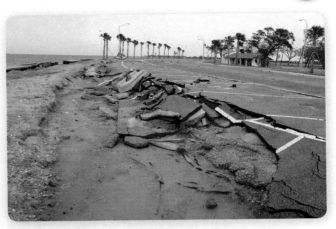

Figure 51-10 It is important to stay updated on post-storm failures such as levees that are overcome and bridges and roads that are flooded or washed out.
© Mike Smith/Dreamstime, LLC.

In 2011, the tsunami disaster in Japan showed the world the destructive power of a tidal wave and its potential for local annihilation **Figure 51-11**. Tsunamis and storm surges have the potential to occur in coastal areas of the continental United States and in Alaska, Hawaii, Puerto Rico, and other US territories. Unlike hurricanes, these events cannot always be predicted with the same amount of accuracy. There can be very little time, if any, for advance preparation.

Remember that your personal safety is essential. If you know a tsunami is coming, get out of the way. Move

YOU are the Paramedic — PART 3

Your patient fell from a second-floor window when she tried to escape from her collapsed apartment. She is responsive and able to speak with you. She has obvious fractures of the left lower leg and right ankle that have been splinted. There is an intravenous lock in place. You move the patient to your stretcher and then to your unit. The transportation supervisor reports that you will transport your patient to Regional Hospital.

Recording Time: 5 Minutes	
Respirations	18 breaths/min
Pulse	96 beats/min
Skin	Cool, dry, pink
Blood pressure	140/86 mm Hg
Oxygen saturation (Spo₂)	98% on room air
Pupils	PERRLA

5. How does the transportation supervisor know which hospital you should transport to?
6. What additional patient assessment should you accomplish en route to the hospital?

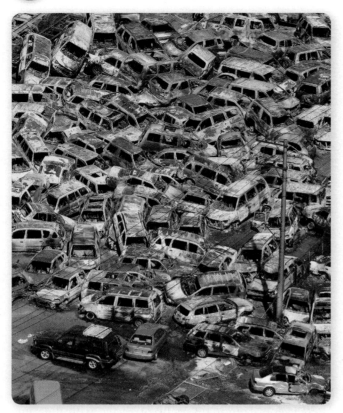

Figure 51-11 Tsunamis can cause local annihilation.
© Atsushi Taketazu/AP Photo.

inland and get uphill. Your work will begin after the event. It is safe to assume that nothing that the water hits will survive. Bring all of your vehicles uphill and inland, and bring as many supplies as you can with you. If items need to be secured, plans should be made for tie-down stakes or for the use of tents or safes to secure supplies and drugs.

Tsunamis can come in a series. Even if subsequent events are less severe, your first-line defenses have probably been overwhelmed. If subsequent events are even more intense, you may need to move farther inland and onto higher elevation. Buildings will have a hard time sustaining that kind of an impact, which may be successive in nature.

Some important points relating to EMS response to tsunamis include the following:

- Pay strict attention to the warning systems in place and comply with instructions. Monitor systems at all times and have a backup receiving system in place. There should be someone, preferably in the EOC or command post, keeping up with current changes.
- It may seem like your initial patients would be drowning victims, but those who drowned will likely already be dead by the time EMS can reach them. Instead, you should primarily prepare for trauma patients who have been struck by or entangled in debris. Exposure will also become problematic, especially as time goes on.

Remember that you cannot respond until the tsunami has done its damage. Until the danger has passed, resources and personnel must be kept safe. Patient care and cleanup begin once the safety of EMS personnel can be ensured. Your response will depend on what kind of access you will have once the tsunami has passed.

▶ Earthquakes

On August 23, 2011, a magnitude 5.8 earthquake struck Mineral, Virginia, affecting major population centers in the entire northeastern United States. This was a rare occurrence and despite the minimal damage and very few injuries that resulted, it demonstrates that no region of the country is safe from earthquake damage. As in other disasters, there may be little or no warning. Earthquakes, depending on their size, duration, and strength can cause thousands of deaths and billions of dollars of damage within minutes. Aftershocks will occur regularly after the initial earthquake and can be substantial. In some cases, they can last for days.

The biggest immediate danger resulting from an earthquake comes from structural collapse. Older buildings, not having been subject to newer building codes, are the most problematic. Also, severed gas and electrical power lines as well as propane tanks and fuel trucks contribute to fires during and after the event.

Important points related to EMS response to earthquakes include the following:

- If you have advance warning, or if you are in an area along an earthquake fault line, your building and vehicle contents should be secured. Straps, springs, and bungee cords can be used to secure contents. Look at your buildings and imagine something shaking them violently from the outside, then think about what you could do to secure items so that they do not fall or become damaged.
- A phenomenon known as **dust suffocation** can occur during the quake. This is caused by particles of dust and debris loosened and released into the air. These produce both a toxic and hypoxic atmosphere. Breathing will be difficult, and face masks, at the very least, should be worn during the recovery efforts.
- If you are responding to patients at the scene of a building collapse, leave the rescue to personnel who are trained in confined-space rescue. If a patient is outside the building and easy to reach, make sure your footing is good and that the patient platform is stable. When in doubt, do not go out! Your weight and that of your crew could make the bearing structure untenable.
- Rescuers will need ongoing rehabilitation. It is easy for personnel in these situations to develop tunnel vision and not recognize situations dangerous to them, such as fatigue, dehydration, and posttraumatic stress disorder.

- If possible, have extra food and water available. This is not just for you and your crew, but also for civilians, patients, and other rescuers. It will take time for authorities to get food and water delivery services up and running.
- Call your local hospitals and find out if they are able to receive patients. Find out whether the hospitals sustained damage. They may need you to set up a field hospital or assist a **forward surgical team** (a team, usually staffed with physicians, nurses, and EMS providers, that performs minor surgical procedures and débridements in the field, taking some of the load from the hospital facility).
- When you are out in the field, take note of hazards such as unstable buildings and severed gas lines. Make a list and report these to the EOC as soon as possible. This will, at the least, make others aware of the danger and help to get repairs scheduled.

Finally, if your local hospitals, schools, businesses, government offices, or fire departments participate in regular earthquake drills, try to become a part of them.

▶ Landslides, Avalanches, and Mudslides

There are many reasons for landslides, avalanches, and mudslides based on natural occurrences throughout the country. These include severe winter storms, heavy rainfall, wildfires and past wildfires, flash flooding, major and minor earthquakes, hurricanes, and intentional landslides performed to clear massive vegetation for urbanization. This happens because the surface tension in the earth and bedrock changes drastically. Southern California experiences earthquakes almost every year. Many western ski resorts have daily patrols and experience avalanches numerous times throughout the winter season. With the possible exception of some states with a low elevation, any place with a hill can be subject to landslides, avalanches, and mudslides.

Important points related to EMS response to landslides, avalanches, and mudslides include the following:

- Cliffs, high hills, and anything in the gravity path of a landslide, avalanche, or mudslide would obviously be in the danger area. If time permits, consider moving out of the target area and stage at a safer location.
- When a landslide occurs, it can cause such a buildup of soil and vegetation that it can block a stream or river, causing a lake to be formed. You may need to consider putting water rescue procedures in place.
- Underground pipes for drinking water and sewage, conduit for electrical lines, and telephone lines can be damaged. Plan for alternate water delivery and waste systems;

generators and cell phones may need to be employed, as well.
- Mudslides or mudflows are similar to a river of concrete. Do not venture into these or into the potential path either on foot or in vehicles. Indeed, you may treat people who were trapped in cars that were swept away by the mud.
- The intense heat of brushfires seals the soil surface, making mudslides, avalanches, and landslides move even faster over terrain. Consider the history of the area when preplanning. Past landslide events predict what could happen again; review past incident reports as a normal part of preplanning.
- Equipment that may be planned for in advance should include backhoes and earth movers.

▶ Cave-ins

Cave-ins occur naturally for the same reasons that landslides, mudslides, and avalanches occur. However, in cave-ins, the bedrock is not as important a consideration as is the actual soil composition. Cave-ins can be caused by rapid freezing and thawing, heavy rain, or excess vibration such as that associated with earthquakes and tremors **Figure 51-12A** .

Considerations for EMS response during a cave-in include the following:

- If a cave-in occurs in your response area, check with your local utility company to make sure power lines are not severed or unstable **Figure 51-12B** . Remember, underground mining can cause overhead lines to fail.
- Be watchful for loose rock in the collapse area. In cave-ins, EMS personnel are under the command of trench rescue responders. They will identify safe zones based on shoring and sloping techniques.
- In a cave-in there will almost always be accumulation of water. Expect that patients will have been trapped in water, and be prepared to treat the patient or patients for hypothermia. Pumping out accumulated water can cause further damage in the area of collapse; therefore, keep an eye on the run-off if the pump is still in service at the scene. If you are pumping out water, make sure the water that is being pumped is not degrading the area you are working on.
- There are three ways to secure the area of excavation: sloping, benching, and shoring **Figure 51-12C** . Unless you are qualified in these techniques, do not enter an area of collapse or potential collapse.
- The atmosphere in cave-ins is generally toxic. You can assume that any patient brought out of a cave-in has been in an oxygen-deficient atmosphere.

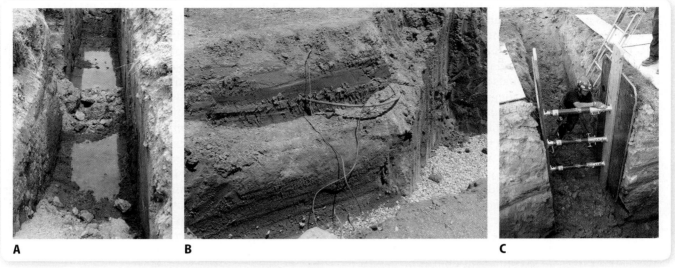

A **B** **C**

Figure 51-12 Cave-ins are associated with many dangers and require specially trained rescue personnel. Do not enter a cave-in scene until directed to do so by the incident commander. **A.** The presence of water can make a cave-in more likely. **B.** Electrical wires must be secured before entering the area. **C.** Walls must be secured with specialty techniques such as sloping, benching, and shoring. This photo shows a top shore being installed.

A and B: Courtesy of Cecil V. "Buddy" Martinette, Jr.; **C:** © Jones & Bartlett Learning. Courtesy of MIEMSS.

- If the patient care area is located in the collapse area, continuous monitoring of the lower explosive limit, carbon monoxide (CO), hydrogen sulfide gas, and oxygen levels is essential.
- Cave-ins can release sewer and chemical gases. After atmosphere security, consider positive-pressure ventilation in the patient care area.

▶ Volcanic Eruptions

It may surprise you to learn that the United States follows only Japan and Indonesia in having the highest number of volcanic eruptions in the world. Ten percent of the world's eruptions take place in the United States, and they occur primarily in Alaska, Hawaii, and the Pacific Northwest **Figure 51-13** . The primary emergencies come from **pyroclastic explosions**, which are the explosions that occur in the bubbling magma. These are associated with release of hot ash and gas emissions. Lava flow is rarely a problem as its course is slow and predictable.

Since volcanic eruptions usually occur at a height, rescue workers may be affected by secondary problems, including melting ice and snow and the resultant water flows. Landslides may also occur with mudflows.

During preplanning, identify buildings that are "volcano proof" (ie, made of fire-retardant construction materials), including your squad buildings. Are there warning systems in place? EMS crews should be trained to respond based on the projected timeline.

Consider the following when responding to a volcanic eruption:

- If a population is located close to an eruption and the warning is late or nonexistent, panic may spread. Evacuation will become the prime concern.
- Expected injuries include burns, respiratory problems, and crush trauma injuries. Respiratory problems will be continuous and serious. Acid rain and acid-based debris will also contribute to respiratory, eye, and skin problems.
- **Ashfall** is the residue left behind from the eruption. This can cause inhalation issues. Masks should be issued to everyone (crews and patients) in downrange positions. Ingestion also becomes a problem because ash gets into the food and water supply chains. Packaged food and water must be provided. The weight of ashfall can cause roofs to collapse. Try to shovel the ash to keep your agency's roofs clear, and clean the ash from windshields to make driving less difficult. Drive carefully because ash can make roads slippery.
- Try to make the public aware of the importance of wearing respiratory protection, even after the initial danger is resolved.

▶ Flooding

Although the flooding associated with Hurricane Katrina in 2005 was well publicized, severe flooding happens annually all over the United States. For example, flooding from Hurricane Sandy covered most of the eastern seaboard of the United States in 2012. It was devastating in terms of the economy (more than $50 billion in damage), lives lost (147 direct deaths), and number of people injured.[7] Never underestimate the power of water.

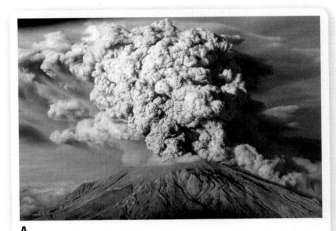

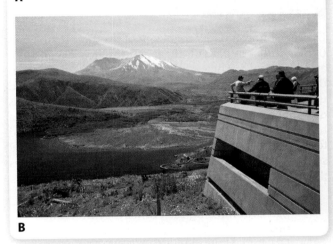

Figure 51-13 In 1980, Mount St Helens in Washington state experienced the most devastating volcanic eruption recorded in US history. **A.** The explosion. **B.** Regrowth of the area almost 30 years after the eruption.

A: © Jack Smith/AP Photo; B: © David Falconer/AP Photo.

Most preparations for flooding occur during pre-planning. Typically, the regions that will be affected can be predicted; therefore, during the preplanning process, agencies should identify the amount of time needed to execute response plans. Long-term consequences of flooding cannot be judged as easily.

Floods can significantly increase the incidence of disease. This can result from drinking water contamination and the spread of water-borne diseases, and the increase of vector-borne diseases such as those fostered by mosquitos and dead bodies that are inaccessible due to flood damage.[8]

Issues to watch for during EMS response to flooding are **overtopping** (reservoirs overflowing their borders); slow degradation of levees and banks; and debris flow, which contains large debris such as logs or cars and has a greater impact force than water that does not contain such debris. Also watch for sudden catastrophic degradation of levees, which tend to cause a "chain reaction" destructive effect. As one section of sandbags fails, the flow washes away the remaining bags.

Additional considerations for flood response include the following:

- Wear proper wet weather gear, and use personal flotation devices as well as **tag lines** (safety ropes tied around rescuers so they can be pulled to safety) when necessary.
- Driving through water can be challenging. Make sure you use only high-axle vehicles, such as ambulances, fire trucks, fire engines, and sport utility vehicles, not cars. Moving water as low as 2 inches (5 cm) can easily move a car.
- Walking in moving water that is over 6 inches (15 cm) deep may result in a fall that can cause you to be swept away. Make sure that you and your team members are connected with tag lines or at least link arms when walking through moving water.

Damage can be surveyed after the flood and when the water starts to recede. This is also when the contaminants and residue left behind by the floods can cause serious health problems. Cleanup is essential and should start as soon as practical.

▶ Sandstorms and Dust Storms

Sandstorms and dust storms are common in arid and semiarid regions of the country, especially after a prolonged period of drought. For the EMS provider, most of the problems associated with these storms are directly related to the abrasive and visual effects of the storm. Considerations for responding to a sandstorm or dust storm include the following:

- During a sandstorm sensory input becomes difficult. You may lose your orientation and should consider **shelter-in-place** until the storm subsides.
- Eye protection should be worn. It should cover the entire eye area because sand will come in from the side of standard EMS goggles.
- Do not rub your eyes, nose, or skin during a storm. Sand is an abrasive (like sandpaper) and can cause permanent injury, specifically to the eyes.
- Respiratory protection should be worn. Properly fitted APRs and N-95 masks will seal out more of the fine particles of sand than will a standard surgical mask.
- Lip balm as well as some kind of a cloth barrier over your whole head is a good idea during the storm.
- Driving is a challenge, even during a minor event. If you employ your windshield washer fluid, you will create a muddy windshield. Be prepared to stop and manually clean the windshield if you cannot see (ensure that you have windshield cleaner and a squeegee in your vehicle). Before heading out, you may

wish to consider applying one of the chemical spray-on appliques available that will make the windshield more slippery, which can prevent sand from accumulating as quickly. Vehicles need to be protected from sand getting into their engines.

- Objects may be hidden by the blowing sand. Keep low and be aware.

▶ Drought

Drought is caused by a lack of water available to the public. It is primarily based on a lack of precipitation over a length of time. Drought causes myriad problems for the medical community. Heat injuries are more common during droughts, and dust storms and wildfires, with their concurrent problems, occur more frequently. Snakes migrate from dry areas into irrigated back yards where people live, increasing the risk of snakebite injuries. Finally, both water quality and quantity are significantly reduced. Infections increase, as does the possibility of surface water contamination, because the remaining standing pools are more highly concentrated with bacteria and sediment from human waste.

Your agency may have to secure its working water supply. Civil unrest could spread if townspeople think EMS crews have water. EMS could require protection and security from police.

▶ Prolonged Cold Weather

Prolonged cold weather is relative; EMS workers in some regions of the country such as the northern states are used to working in cold conditions and have relatively little trouble adapting. What is cold to a person from Georgia compared with a Minnesota native might be dramatically different. In areas that do not regularly get a lot of cold weather, especially for a long period of time, EMS response can become challenging.

People who are exposed to cold weather for long periods of time, even though sheltered, can develop a condition called **cold stress**. This is similar to **seasonal affective disorder (SAD)** and can take a serious psychologic toll on EMS crews. EMS providers and management should monitor each other for changes in personality and work habits. The cold weather itself is taxing to EMS providers.

If maintenance or repair issues can wait until warmer weather, let them. If repairs must be done, try to make them during the warmest part of the day. Things like washing the vehicles may not be necessary, unless there are decontamination problems. Try to limit physical demands, if possible. For example, it is not a good idea to shovel snow or chop ice for hours and then have to respond to an EMS call.

Additional considerations for working in prolonged cold weather include the following:

- Dress loosely and in layers. Avoid tight clothing that can restrict blood flow. Have dry, clean replacement clothes with you, especially boots and socks. Hats and good gloves are important, as well.
- If you have to do standbys, try to switch crews frequently. If possible, have warm-up tents or sheds set up on a long scene. Hot liquids should be placed on the vehicles or delivered to field crews.
- Keep an eye on older EMS providers—for example, those older than 55 years. They may not handle the cold as well as younger workers. Also watch crew members who may have medical issues such as cardiac or pulmonary diseases or who are pregnant.

▶ Heat Wave

EMS personnel are very cognizant of the three main types of heat injury in patients: heat cramps, heat exhaustion, and heatstroke. They are less familiar with working in these conditions every day. A heat wave in 2011 subjected the citizens of Dallas, Texas, to 71 nonconsecutive days of temperatures greater than 100°F (38°C).[9] In 2016, a heat wave in the southwestern United States had recorded temperatures of over 120°F (49°C).[10] The following are some of the problems and potential solutions to issues that occur during a heat wave:

- Vigilance is the key. If possible, work in pairs, monitoring each other for heat-related problems.
- Do not wait until you feel thirsty to consume water. Hydrate regularly, but do not overhydrate. Be aware that you may not sweat noticeably in particularly arid climates. Small, constant sips of water throughout the day are best. You may also consider some electrolyte fluid replacement in addition to the water.
- Small, more frequent meals are better than large ones. Eat foods that are heavy in fluids, such as vegetables, fruits, and salads.
- Set up "water trains." As you empty your water bottles, have them refilled. Your agency must ensure that it has a good, clean source of water. Use of **water buffalo trailers** (500-gallon [1,893-L] water containers on trailers), **lister bags** (40-gallon [151-L] canvas bags that can be hung from trees), and portable water backpacks is advisable.
- If you have air conditioning in your buildings or vehicles, use it!
- Wet towels placed on the head or on the body can help reduce body temperature.
- Try to break up work schedules during the hottest part of the day. Take frequent rest breaks, in a cool, shady place, if possible. Schedule manual labor for evening or morning shifts if possible.

▶ Meteors and Space Debris

Meteors, asteroids, space debris, and **space junk** are not just in science fiction novels. Meteors regularly hit the earth, though mostly in desert areas. As meteors and asteroids approach earth's atmosphere, they become micrometeoroids and, for the most part, burn up. Space debris (natural materials, such as micrometeoroids) or space junk (man-made items), also burn up when entering the atmosphere.

Most space debris and large meteors coming from space can be detected. The problem is ascertaining just where they will land and how great the impact will be.

Other things can fall from the sky, such as spent bullets and waste products from aircraft. There is really no way to be prepared for them all. Keep an open mind when a patient has a history of sudden sharp pain with local bruising.

▶ Pandemics

An **epidemic** is an illness or disease that affects or tends to affect a disproportionately large number of people within a specific population, community, or region at the same time. A **pandemic** is an illness or disease that affects a high proportion of the population over a broad or potentially worldwide geographic area. The H1N1 influenza outbreak of 2009 is a good example of a pandemic. Not all pandemics are influenza. The bubonic plague of the 16th century and various diseases such as severe acute respiratory syndrome (SARS) and acquired immunodeficiency syndrome (AIDS) were also considered pandemics.

The most important consideration during these situations will always be personal protection from the disease. Gloves and goggles may not be enough. You may need N-95 or APR-type respiratory protection as well as gowns. Handwashing and sanitizing is the best first line of defense. In addition, prophylaxis such as vaccination should be administered free of charge to all health care workers in the crew (EMS providers as well as other health care workers, and their families, if possible). If vaccination is not available, after-care medicine should be provided.

The best method of detecting disease in workers is direct observation and reports from crew members. If someone appears to be sick, that person should be pulled from duty. Sick EMS providers should be sent to the hospital.

The **6-feet rule** should be applied. A person can transmit a sneeze or cough from a distance of 6 feet (2 m). Try to stay out of this area. Even though you should be wearing a mask, the patient may not be. Staying more than 6 feet (2 m) away becomes particularly challenging in the back of an ambulance, if not impossible. In those cases, maintain as much distance as possible.

Realize that in a pandemic situation, the full work force may not be present. They may be sick or caring for sick loved ones. Your agency's **continuity of operations plan (COOP)** should be in effect.

The public should be instructed via 9-1-1 dispatch, your public information officer, EOC, phone, or radio on how to care for sick people in place. In conjunction with your medical director, your agency should set specific guidelines for which emergencies you will respond to, and which calls will have to wait until more serious cases have been handled.

Your agency may have to set up field hospitals or care stations. Your agency may be called on to become a **point of distribution (POD)** for medicine or vaccination with minimal additional training provided. A POD is a temporary supply and inoculation or medicine distribution area.

■ Man-Made Disasters

Humans cause many types of disasters. Several examples are listed in ⟨ Table 51-5 ⟩. The next section discusses these, with the exception of weapons of mass destruction and hazardous materials incidents, which are discussed in Chapter 50, *Terrorism Response*, and Chapter 49, *Hazardous Materials*, respectively. Remember that as with natural disasters, general actions must be taken before, during, and after every event.

▶ Structural Fires

Wildland fires are horrendous, but structural fires, whether intentional or accidental, have a much higher death and injury rate ⟨ Figure 51-14 ⟩. Structural fires are different from forest and brush fires in that structural fires occur in populated areas and involve products of combustion that can be explosive, toxic, fast-spreading, and very unpredictable. In addition, if an arsonist set a structural fire, he or she may be strategically planning to entrap firefighters.

Table 51-5	**Examples of Man-Made Disasters**
Structural fires	
Construction failures and building collapse	
Power failures or disruptions	
Riots, civil disturbances, and stampedes	
Strikes and labor disputes	
Sniper, shooter, and hostage situations	
Explosions (intentional and unintentional)	
Information technology (cyber) disruptions	
Incidents involving weapons of mass destruction	
Hazardous materials incidents	

© Jones & Bartlett Learning.

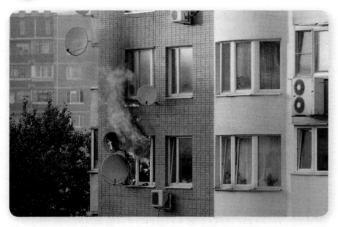

Figure 51-14 Structural fires have a much higher death and injury rate than wildland fires.
© Sergey Toronto/Shutterstock.

Remember to let the firefighters fight the fire. EMS crews probably do not have the proper bunker gear, training, or expertise to contain the conflagration or to rescue people from a burning building. Personnel must be staged properly at a safe, visible distance from the scene where vehicles or equipment will not interfere with firefighting operations or apparatus placement. Your agency must ensure that it has a representative in the unified command as the event materializes.

Additional key points for EMS response to structural fires include the following:

- Watch for falling or collapsing items. Roofs can collapse, and people, ice, or severed power lines can fall rapidly from above.

- Prepare to treat burns and respiratory problems. Injuries to firefighters will include exhaustion, heat injuries, cold injuries, CO poisoning, and trauma.
- Stay upwind. Smoke from artificial resins carries many toxins and carcinogens. You cannot always see the products of complete and incomplete combustion (CO and cyanide). At a minimum, wear a surgical mask; APRs provide even more protection.
- Be prepared to evacuate your position quickly. Fires double in size every minute if unchecked. Plan a few routes away from the scene, just in case.
- Be ready for cardiac events. These are the number one killer of firefighters at the scene of fires. CO and cyanide poisoning can cause ECG abnormalities such as T-wave aberrancies.

▶ Construction Failures and Building Collapse

In September 2015, a construction crane collapsed through the roof of the Grand Mosque in Mecca 10 days before the start of the Hajj, killing 107 people and injuring more than 200.[11] Many lessons can be learned from this type of mass-casualty disaster, especially regarding the role of triage. EMS crews and agencies must be prepared to handle engineering failures.

As part of preplanning, evaluate the new construction in your area. Buildings or other large structures are most dangerous while under construction. Review the site and

YOU are the Paramedic — PART 4

You assess the patient's legs for pulses, motor function, and sensation, and all appear grossly intact. The patient's vital signs remain stable. The intravenous lock is accessible and flushes easily. Your partner reports that there is a large stretch of damaged roadway between your current location and the hospital.

Recording Time: 10 Minutes	
Respirations	18 breaths/min
Pulse	96 beats/min
Skin	Warm, pink, dry
Blood pressure	140/84 mm Hg
Oxygen saturation (Spo₂)	98% on room air
Pupils	PERRLA

7. What actions should be taken after a disaster to ensure your well-being?

8. What is the purpose of the AAR?

preplan access and egress routes. Note conditions and placement of equipment such as cranes. Update these plans frequently. Your agency should remain in communication with construction personnel and share all information, especially potential hazards, with members of your organization.

While considering EMS care at these sites, consider what special PPE you might need, such as helmets, steel-toe safety boots, eye protection, knee pads, and heavy-duty work gloves **Figure 51-15**.

Considerations when responding to construction failures and building collapses include the following:

- If there is a lock out/tag out information sheet on site, review it. This sheet contains information regarding the number of people and conditions in the danger zone. In addition, all fixed buildings are required to have a current

Material Safety Data Sheet on file at the site and the local building department or fire department. This will tell you the quantities and types of materials on-site.

- During a response, particularly responses to large collapses, you may be called on to do a perimeter search for patients. Include all areas where patients may have wandered or been directed, but not the collapse area. Once you find these victims, escort them to a safe area and start both the accountability and triage processes. Use your sector tags and flags to prevent confusion.
- When victims are brought to triage, collect as much information as possible, such as patient position within the disaster area, potential hazardous exposure, initial patient complaints, and level of consciousness. If you have time, document this information on the patient care report or triage tag and include the names of rescuers who brought the patient to you.
- You may need to supply backboards, straps, and Stokes baskets to the rescuers. Make sure they know how to use the equipment and, if possible, rig it in advance to make it easier for rescuers to use.
- Careful thought is required to find the safest area for triaging and treatment. This area should be located in a cold zone.

▶ Power Failures or Disruptions

Power failures and electrical disruptions can be life threatening, especially if they occur for a prolonged period of time. These are common events that happen in all parts of the country, and they frequently occur during both man-made and natural disasters.

If your squad building has electric locks on its doors or equipment rooms, your agency should consider getting a manual override device. Remember that agency refrigerators and heaters will not be working. If fluids and medications are stored in there, your agency should have an alternate source for heating or cooling (eg, in its vehicles).

Backup generators must be checked on a regular basis, and they should be operated monthly. Fuel must be topped off and there should be an ample supply of fuel stored in a flameproof container. The operating manuals should be kept near the device. During Hurricane Sandy, the Northeast lost electrical power, causing gasoline pumps to be inoperable.

Make sure battery-powered devices, such as suction units, are fully charged. Have an ample supply of batteries (all types) available. Crew members may have their own flashlights, cell phones, and headlamps, which may take batteries that you do not normally use. Stock up on the common types needed to power these devices.

Make a list of all patients in your community who use electrically powered medical devices, such as ventilators,

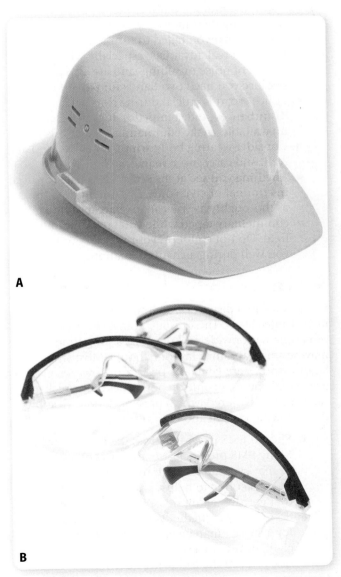

A

B

Figure 51-15 A. An ANSI Z89.1-Type 1 helmet. **B.** ANSI Z87.1 eye protection.

A: © cloki/Shutterstock; B: © mihalec/Shutterstock.

at home. Your organization can anticipate responding to these patients before equipment failure.

Computers will be down, so you will not be able to download electronic patient care reports. Make sure you have a printed version of the patient care report or triage tags to use as a substitute. Because cell phones and GPS may be out of service, be ready to use radios and paper maps.

▶ Riots, Civil Disturbances, and Stampedes

Emergency medical technicians (EMTs) and paramedics are accustomed to being exposed to dangers such as violent patients, cars speeding past on the freeway, family hysteria, and verbal and physical abuse. In the case of a riot or civil disturbance, these dangers are multiplied when people are in a state of panic. Even peaceful protests can turn into civil unrest, such as the events in Ferguson, Missouri, in 2014 **Figure 51-16** .

Before and during the response, collect as much information as possible from dispatch, police, or command about the scene you are entering. It is crucial to stay updated and maintain communication with these organizations. These events can change quickly. You do not want to get into a situation that is potentially dangerous.

Considerations during an EMS response to riots, civil disturbances, and stampedes include the following:

- Once a safe route is transmitted to you, do not report to or set up a staging area until you are sure the scene is safe or that you will have physical police presence. Ascertain the location of the command post and establish communications with it. Frequent updates are the key to safety.
- Determine what is currently happening, and consider potential complications. For example, if tear gas or pepper spray has been used, you

need to protect yourselves from the gas and you will need water for eye irrigation to treat a large number of patients. Rocks or other missiles are a potential cause of head trauma.

- Consider vehicle safety. Do not drive over broken glass, and if the crowd is still there, consider using a ground guide to walk in front of the slow-moving vehicle. Is there smoke from protestors burning tires and bonfires? Make sure you have respiratory protection and be prepared for limited visibility.
- Your situational awareness is paramount. The chaotic scene may not be familiar to you. Use the buddy system; do not split up. Make sure you always have a 360° view of the scene. GPS could be necessary if you need assistance. Most handheld GPS devices can identify your location to within 33 feet (10 meters). You must have a working radio. Do not make the mistake of thinking your radio is very quiet, only to discover that you failed to turn it on. Headsets become a real advantage especially when there is a lot of noise or yelling, and are also helpful because you need two hands for patient care.
- Police escort is crucial during riots, civil disturbances, and stampedes. If police escort is unavailable, make command aware of this fact.
- Consider wearing body armor, a helmet, and an APR, and carry more than one flashlight.
- Anything you see at the scene could later be used in criminal or civil court. Document everything as thoroughly as you can, or have a running commentary taped while you are out in the field. Do not count on your memory to serve you well during a chaotic situation.

▶ Strikes and Labor Disputes

Strikes and labor disputes are another everyday occurrence in the United States. These disputes can involve large groups of people nationwide and may last a long time. Others may be small and may last only hours. Most strikes and labor disputes are generally peaceful. However, even in peaceful disputes, people on both sides of the picket line can get sick or injured, which presents EMS with some of the following tactical and ethical considerations:

- Should EMS providers cross the picket line? Many EMS providers are members of a union or may sympathize with the strikers. Crossing the picket line to help a patient does not mean that you are taking sides. Remember that you do not know whether you are responding for a striker, management, or an uninvolved civilian. You are there to care for the patient. Ask yourself the following question, "What is in the best interest of the patient?" and follow that answer. However, this does not mean that you should sacrifice your safety in any way.

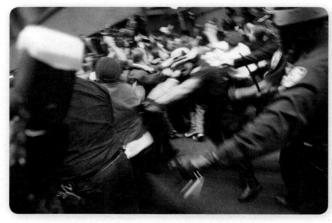

Figure 51-16 Protests can quickly degenerate into violent confrontations, as did this protest in Ferguson, Missouri, in 2014.

© Spencer Platt/Getty.

Secure police escort and get away from a violent situation immediately. Remember that failure to cross a picket line to care for an ill or injured patient simply because you support the cause of the strikers constitutes abandonment, gross negligence, and represents grounds for suit and grounds for disciplinary action relative to your license or certification.

- If the patient is ambulatory, he or she might be safely brought to you.
- Television coverage of an event, especially a volatile one, can act as a deterrent to verbal or physical attacks on EMS providers in front of a large audience. This may be a false security, but should give you something to think about. You may be able to use this to your advantage.
- Again, document and record all your findings, particularly if participants on either side of the labor action appeared to have delayed EMS response or patient care.

▶ Sniper, Shooter, and Hostage Situations

In all shooter and sniper scenarios, EMS should be staged out of gun range (the kill zone). You need to be out of the line of fire. In an indirect fire situation such as mortar or a rocket, you need to be out of the effective range. If gunshot victims are still exposed, do not go to help them. Trained people will either get them under cover or eliminate the threat. If you can see or hear about their wounds, you can tell a police officer or special weapons and tactics (SWAT) member how to stop bleeding by applying a tourniquet or how to open an airway.

In a hostage situation, the perpetrators may want EMS to examine or treat a hostage or a fellow perpetrator. Entering such a situation is very dangerous. Any such activity is at the direction of the law enforcement incident commander only and is unlikely unless you are a law enforcement paramedic.

The press and news media will probably be located near you in a safe area. Do not say anything to the press about the incident. Refer them to the public information officer at the scene. Be careful if they are listening to updates on your radio. You are responsible for communications security on your end. They may praise and compliment you in an effort to win your trust to get you to say something "off the record." This will come back to haunt you and could jeopardize the scenario. During a long standoff, do not lose your sense of urgency regarding communication security.

▶ Explosions

Explosions can be intentional or unintentional. The end result is the same: predictable injuries. Explosions were covered in Chapter 29, *Trauma Systems and Mechanism of Injury*, but here are a few additional considerations:

- Secondary and tertiary explosives may have been placed. The first bomb may have been set to draw in responders. Improvised explosive devices (IEDs) and vehicle-borne improvised explosive devices (VBIEDs) have been used in new waves of explosive attacks. One example is the Boston Marathon Bombing in April 2013. Law enforcement thought that the intended victims of the second bomb were responding personnel; however, the second bomb detonated seconds after the first explosion. These devices can be concealed in cars, trash containers, or anywhere near the safe zone. Keep your eyes open and stay alert.
- When you begin treating patients, carefully record anything a seriously injured patient has to say. This patient may not recover, and the information could prove valuable to the investigators.
- Ear injuries are common. Remember to speak loudly and face the patient.
- Air particles are probably contaminated. Wear your APR during patient care.
- Your agency may consider setting up a field hospital at the scene because local hospitals may be overwhelmed. Physicians, physician assistants, nurse practitioners, EMS providers, and security personnel from your mass-casualty incident plan can staff this facility.

▶ Information Technology (Cyber) Disruptions

Internet technology has helped EMS in many ways. In the field, you can transmit ECGs and can send real-time, visual patient presentations to hospitals thousands of miles away. However, there is a downside: hackers can penetrate EMS security to access secure patient information. EMS agencies must remain vigilant and use the latest security software. Every agency should have an information technology (IT) professional available to update and test the system regularly. Because technology is changing so rapidly, the task of updating your organization's security software should be delegated to a designated IT professional.

Use of your computer system should be limited to your agency. Limit access to those fields necessary; for example, a person who does basic life support does not need computer access to see what controlled substances are in stock. Protect systems with passwords, and change passwords frequently.

Finally, should you recognize a cyber threat, immediately report it to your supervisor and stop using the threatened browser or program.

1. **What is the definition of a disaster?**

   A disaster is a sudden, calamitous event, such as an accident or catastrophe, that causes great damage, loss, or destruction. A disaster can be natural or man made. Disasters overwhelm EMS and community resources.

2. **What does the term *all-hazards approach* mean in disaster planning?**

   The act of conducting comprehensive preplanning for a disaster is called an all-hazards approach. Before addressing specifics particular to the disaster that has occurred, general considerations that apply to any disaster must be addressed, such as the number of personnel and equipment needed and which hospital or hospitals to transport to.

3. **What is pre-event planning, and how can an event be predicted in advance?**

   Pre-event planning is the stage in which EMS providers prepare for any potential event. While no disaster is predictable, some events are more likely to occur than others. General disaster preplanning with an all-hazards approach will put your agency in the best position to handle any disaster that may befall your area.

4. **Why are preplanned mutual aid agreements essential to your operation?**

   Mutual aid agreements describe how your agency will access help from other areas when needed. It is important to identify the person who will request additional resources and the person who has the authority to grant permission to release resources. All parties should be aware of and train frequently on the plan.

5. **How does the transportation supervisor know which hospital you should transport to?**

   This determination must be made in advance of a disaster; a preplanning assessment of your area hospitals is essential! Preplanning includes knowing the level of care available in your area, the limitations on patient numbers at your local hospitals, which personnel local hospitals can supply to your agency, and vice versa.

6. **What additional patient assessment should you accomplish en route to the hospital?**

   Because the patient's legs were splinted prior to patient contact, you must continually reassess pulses, motor function, and sensation en route to the hospital. You should also check the patency of the intravenous lock. Your regular 5-minute serial assessments should continue as normal.

7. **What actions should be taken after a disaster to ensure your well-being?**

   You should be assessed physically as well as emotionally. Posttraumatic stress disorder is a real occurrence. Although it is not known definitively if CISD works, CISD teams should be considered, especially for long-term events or those with a high mortality rate. Be alert for behavioral changes in yourself and your coworkers. Open communication should be encouraged, and your agency should provide a receptive environment for those exposed to tragedy. A physician should check all personnel. Also, counseling services should be made available, if requested or required.

8. **What is the purpose of the AAR?**

   The AAR is your official internal report of the entire event. It should contain the facts of the incident reflected in a chronologic, accurate manner. Based on this report, an agency can review the incident in its totality. The AAR and all anecdotal evidence can be accumulated to provide a basis for additional training in areas that need scrutiny. Also, based on the incident, EMS crews may notice areas of deficiency or skills that need to be refreshed. An outline for reinforcement of skills and knowledge should be prepared based on this data.

YOU are the Paramedic SUMMARY (continued)

EMS Patient Care Report (PCR)

Date: 11-06-18	**Incident No.:** 2456		**Nature of Call:** Leg fractures		**Location:** Dawn Apartment Complex
Dispatched: N/A	**En Route:** N/A	**At Scene:** 2041	**Transport:** 2046	**At Hospital:** 2105	**In Service:** 2130

Patient Information

Age: 24 **Sex:** F **Weight (in kg [lb]):** 59 kg (130 lb)	**Allergies:** Denies **Medications:** Denies **Past Medical History:** Denies **Chief Complaint:** Bilateral leg fractures

Vital Signs

Time: 2046	**BP:** 140/86	**Pulse:** 96	**Respirations:** 18	**Spo$_2$:** 98% on room air
Time: 2051	**BP:** 140/84	**Pulse:** 96	**Respirations:** 18	**Spo$_2$:** 98% on room air

EMS Treatment (circle all that apply)

Oxygen @ _____ L/min via (circle one): NC NRM **Bag-mask device**	**Assisted Ventilation**	**Airway Adjunct**	**CPR**
Defibrillation	**Bleeding Control**	(**Bandaging**) (**Splinting**)	**Other:**

Narrative

Arrived from the Dawn Apartment staging area to the Priority Yellow treatment area for this pt. Pt is a 24-year-old woman who fell from a second-story window when the apartment building partially collapsed. Pt was triaged, moved, splinted, bandaged, and an IV lock was started prior to our pt contact. Pt report from the yellow sector treatment supervisor states the pt has an obvious fx of left tib/fib and a fx of her right ankle. All PMS assessments are reported acceptable. Pt moved to our stretcher for transport to Regional Hospital as directed by the transportation supervisor. Reassessment shows no change in pt condition. Pt remained comfortable and stable throughout the remainder of the transport. Report to charge nurse Mary on arrival at Regional Hospital.**End of report**

Prep Kit

► Ready for Review

- A disaster is a sudden, calamitous event bringing great damage, loss, or destruction.
- Disaster management requires planners to take a broad look at preparedness, planning, training, response, and after-action reporting.
- Emergency medical services agencies must have comprehensive plans in place to address all potential disasters. The act of conducting comprehensive preplanning that will address any disaster situation is called an all-hazards approach.
- The three phases of any plan of response are before the event (preplanning), during the event, and after the event.
- Preplanning is a crucial stage in disaster management. Preplanning should take into account general, predictable factors, such as the local geography, makeup of the population, EMS resources and supplies on hand, infrastructure, places to shelter, and potential assets that can be used.
- During a disaster, it is best to stick to the preplanned measures, if possible. Items to consider during the event include warnings, inventory, mobilization of personnel, personnel needs, command structure, equipment, hospital capabilities, surveillance, and media concerns, among others.
- Specific measures to take after a disaster event include ensuring accountability, resupply, repair, considering stress reaction review, retraining, reimbursement, the after-action report, and acknowledging EMS providers.
- A disaster can be man made or natural. Natural disasters include forest and brush fires; earthquakes; landslides; cave-ins; tsunamis; flooding; sandstorms; weather events such as tornadoes, hurricanes, snowstorms, cold weather, heat waves, and droughts; and pandemics.
- Examples of man-made disasters include structural fires, construction failures, building collapses, power failures, riots, civil disturbances, strikes, sniper and hostage situations, explosions, information technology disruptions, and hazardous materials incidents.
- Natural and man-made disasters should be handled with the all-hazards measures identified during preplanning, with additional measures used as needed based on the nature of the specific event.

► Vital Vocabulary

6-feet rule A guideline to follow regarding the distance to place between oneself and a person who sneezes or coughs, to avoid exposure to germs.

after-action report (AAR) The official internal report of the entire event, such as a disaster, which should contain the facts of the incident reflected in a chronologic, accurate manner.

all-hazards approach The act of conducting comprehensive preplanning that will apply to any disaster.

ashfall The residue left behind from a volcanic eruption.

casualty collection points Areas where slightly injured or noninjured displaced people can be gathered together and transported by bus or truck for further treatment.

cold stress A psychologic condition that can develop in people who are exposed to cold weather for long periods of time, even if sheltered.

continuity of operations plan (COOP) The detailed plan describing the functioning of the agency in situations that disrupt normal operations.

critical infrastructure The external foundation in communities made up of structures and services critical in the day-to-day living activities of humans: energy sources, fuel, water, sewage removal, food, hospitals, and transportation systems.

directed area An area away from the command post or emergency operations center, considered by engineering expertise to be a safe place to stage until directed otherwise.

disaster A sudden, calamitous event, such as an accident or catastrophe, that causes great damage, loss, or destruction.

disaster management A planned, coordinated response to a disaster that involves cooperation of multiple responders and agencies and enables effective triage and provision of care according to triage decisions.

dust suffocation A phenomenon that can occur during an earthquake, in which particles of dust and debris are loosened and released into the air, producing a toxic and hypoxic atmosphere.

emergency operations center (EOC) A central command and control facility, found at all government levels, responsible for strategic overview; tactical decisions are left to incident commanders.

epidemic An illness or disease that affects or tends to affect a disproportionately large number of people within a specific population, community, or region at the same time.

forward surgical team A team, usually staffed with physicians, nurses, and EMS providers, that performs minor surgical procedures and débridements in the field, taking some of the load from the hospital facility.

incident command system (ICS) A system implemented to manage disasters and mass-casualty incidents in which section chiefs, including operations, finance, logistics, and planning, report to the incident commander.

Prep Kit (continued)

lister bags Heavy canvas bags that can be hung from trees containing water in amounts from 40 to 100 gallons (151 to 379 L).

mutual aid agreements (MAAs) Documents that pre-plan how you will access help from other areas when needed.

overtopping A situation in which a reservoir overflows its borders.

pandemic An illness or disease that affects a high proportion of the population over a broad or potentially worldwide geographic area.

point of distribution (POD) A strategically placed facility that has been preestablished for the mass distribution of antibiotics, antidotes, and vaccinations, along with other medications and supplies.

pyroclastic explosions Blasts from flowing or standing lava that can have a wide dispersal circumference, spewing ash and magma.

radio operators Amateur radio operators who have a formal emergency communications set of standard operating procedures. Most are licensed by the Federal Communications Commission.

seasonal affective disorder (SAD) Depression that can affect people in long periods of bad weather, usually winter.

shelter-in-place A method of safeguarding oneself or others' position during an emergency event or event involving a hazardous material; includes measures such as remaining in a safe atmosphere, usually inside structures, or other simple measures such as shutting the windows, going to the cellar, or turning off the heating and air conditioning systems.

space junk Debris from satellites and other man-made objects that reenter the earth's atmosphere.

tag lines Rope or cord tied to a person who is entering a dangerous environment. Used for quick retrieval, usually in conjunction with a harness.

thermals Differing temperatures and swirling patterns of moving air with changes in wind speed.

unified command system A command system used in larger incidents in which there is a multiagency response or multijurisdictional response to coordinate decision making and cooperation among the agencies.

water buffalo trailers Portable trailers that contain from 500 to 3,000 gallons (1,893 to 11,356 L) of water.

▶ References

1. Texas A&M University—Training and Education Collaborative System Preparedness & Emergency Response Learning Center (TECS—PERLC). *Building community capacity for pandemic influenza*. Centers for Disease Control and Prevention website. https://www.cdc.gov/phpr/perlc/flu.htm. Accessed April 3, 2017.
2. Columbia University and University of Albany—Preparedness & Emergency Response Learning Center (PERLC). *On the front lines of a response: PERLC support during Hurricane Sandy*. Centers for Disease Control and Prevention website. https://www.cdc.gov/phpr/perlc/sandy.htm. Accessed April 3, 2017.
3. Summary of the HIPAA privacy rule. U.S. Department of Health & Human Services website. http://www.hhs.gov/hipaa/for-professionals/privacy/laws-regulations/. Accessed February 21, 2017.
4. US Environmental Protection Agency, Climate Change Science. *Understanding the link between climate change and extreme weather*. https://www.epa.gov/climate-change-science/understanding-link-between-climate-change-and-extreme-weather. Accessed April 3, 2017.
5. The White House. President George W. Bush. 2006. *The Federal Response to Hurricane Katrina: Lessons Learned*. https://georgewbush-whitehouse.archives.gov/reports/katrina-lessons-learned/chapter5.html. Accessed April 18, 2017.
6. Pacific Tsunami Warning Center. Frequently asked questions. NOAA's National Weather Service website. http://ptwc.weather.gov/faq.php. Updated November 25, 2009. Accessed February 21, 2017.
7. Blake ES, Kimberlain TB, Berg RJ, Cangialosi JP, Beven JL II. National Hurricane Center website. *Tropical cyclone report Hurricane Sandy* (AL182012), 22-29 October 2012. http://www.nhc.noaa.gov/data/tcr/AL182012_Sandy.pdf. Published February 12, 2013. Accessed March 6, 2017.
8. Flood waters or standing waters. *Water, sanitation, & hygiene (WASH)-related emergencies & outbreaks*. Centers for Disease Control and Prevention website. https://www.cdc.gov/healthywater/emergency/extreme-weather/floods-standingwater.html. Updated March 8, 2017. Accessed April 3, 2017.
9. Buchman H. *Dallas breaks record for most 100-degree days in a year*. AccuWeather website. http://www.accuweather.com/en/weather-news/dallas-breaks-record-for-most/55022. Published September 17, 2011. Accessed April 3, 2017.
10. Di Liberto T. *Scorching heat bakes the Southwest in mid-June 2016*. NOAA Climate website. https://www.climate.gov/news-features/event-tracker/scorching-heat-bakes-southwest-mid-june-2016. Published June 22, 2016. Accessed April 3, 2017.
11. Karimi F, Ellis R, Hanna J. CNN website. Crane collapse kills 107 people at mosque in Mecca days before Hajj. http://www.cnn.com/2015/09/12/middleeast/saudi-arabia-mecca-crane-collapse/. Accessed April 3, 2017.

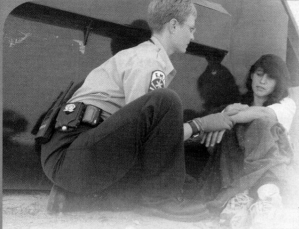

Assessment
in Action

You and your coworkers have received a notice that a major storm is expected in your response area in 24 hours and that a state of emergency is being issued. Your department has informed you to prepare to report to work with supplies for 72 hours. As you are packing for the deployment, you review your agency's policy, procedures, and definitions.

1. Any sudden, calamitous event bringing great damage, loss, or destruction is called a(n):

   A. event.
   B. disaster.
   C. mass-casualty incident.
   D. terrorism.

2. All of the following are items to consider during preplanning, and should have been addressed in preplanning for an event such as this storm, EXCEPT:

   A. geography.
   B. sheltering of personnel.
   C. specific personnel assignments.
   D. immunizations.

3. Your supervisor indicates that fire, police, and EMS will be operating together to form a command during this response. This is called:

   A. unified command.
   B. command structure.
   C. incident command.
   D. joint powers command.

4. You see your supervisor filling out an ICS-211 form. What is this form used for?

   A. Ordering supplies
   B. Tracking personnel
   C. Tracking patients
   D. Changing command

5. Two days later, when your agency's response to this storm is complete, your supervisor meets with you and your crew to discuss the official report of the entire event. This report is called an:

   A. incident command system report.
   B. end-of-shift report.
   C. after-event report.
   D. after-action report.

6. The two types of disasters are:

   A. natural and man made.
   B. biologic and chemical.
   C. terrorism and natural.
   D. natural and nuclear.

7. Examples of natural disasters include all of the following, EXCEPT:

   A. tornadoes.
   B. ice storms.
   C. civil disturbance.
   D. pandemic.

8. Discuss five considerations to take while you are working during a disaster.

9. What agencies might coordinate to form a unified command?

10. What are some common considerations across all natural disasters?

Crime Scene Awareness

National EMS Education Standard Competencies

EMS Operations

Knowledge of operational roles and responsibilities to ensure patient, public, and personnel safety.

Knowledge Objectives

1. Understand the significance of potential violence that can occur on an emergency medical services call, including the settings in which violence is more likely to occur. (pp 2493-2494)
2. Discuss practical measures paramedics should take to reduce the likelihood of becoming a victim on the scene, including uniform style and body armor. (pp 2494-2495)
3. Describe factors to assess during scene size-up that can help determine whether the scene is safe, including specific indicators of violence. (pp 2495-2496)
4. Discuss the role of standard operating procedures at a potentially violent incident. (p 2496)
5. Describe how to park and position your emergency vehicle when responding to a call involving another motor vehicle. (pp 2496-2497)
6. Describe the safest way to approach a passenger-style motor vehicle. (pp 2497-2498)
7. Describe the safest way to approach a van. (pp 2498-2499)

8. Describe how to retreat from danger. (p 2499)
9. Describe how to approach a residence safely. (p 2499)
10. Discuss primary and secondary types of exits. (pp 2499-2500)
11. List items that can potentially be used as a weapon. (p 2500)
12. Discuss techniques to use when responding to a call involving potential domestic violence. (p 2500)
13. Discuss concerns related to clandestine drug laboratories. (pp 2500-2501)
14. Discuss concerns related to gang territories and the measures paramedics can take to work safely in these areas. (pp 2501-2503)
15. Discuss the procedures paramedics should follow at mass shootings and at scenes involving active shooters or snipers. (pp 2503-2504)
16. Define cover and concealment; include and example of each. (pp 2504-2508)
17. Describe the measures paramedics should take to increase safety in a hostage situation. (pp 2505-2506)
18. Discuss the role self-defense can play in the practice of paramedicine. (pp 2508-2509)
19. Discuss the measures paramedics should take to preserve evidence at a crime scene, while still providing optimal patient care. (pp 2509-2511)

Skills Objectives

There are no skills objectives for this chapter.

■ Introduction

Within the past few years, emergency medical services (EMS) has become increasingly more dangerous for providers. From violent calls involving mass shootings to paramedics becoming the victim while treating a patient under the influence of psychoactive substances, there is a real danger to prehospital professionals. There is no such thing as a "normal" call, and you may find yourself in dangerous situations if you do not maintain situational awareness **Figure 52-1**. There is no way to anticipate every scenario you may encounter. You may encounter violent protestors while tending to an injured person at a rally. A confused individual who has access to a gun at his bedside may feel the need to protect himself from someone entering his residence to check on him. From reading the many cautions in this textbook about potentially

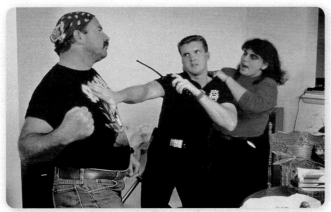

Figure 52-1 The most routine call can quickly turn violent.

From *When Violence Erupts: A Survival Guide for Emergency Responders*, courtesy of Dennis R. Krebs.

violent and dangerous scenes, remember, paramedics have been severely injured or killed in violent incidents while attempting to reach and treat sick and injured people. According to *Injuries and Fatalities among Emergency Medical Technicians and Paramedics in the United States*, more than 540 prehospital providers were injured during the 4-year period that data were being collected.[1] It is reasonable to assume this number is grossly underreported. There are many assaults that do not result in serious injury or lost time and, subsequently, are not reported. While the reporting of occupational injuries related to EMS personnel has recently surged and research used to help assist identifying injuries may still leave something to be desired, most studies suggest that EMS work is on par with other hazardous occupations including firefighting and law enforcement. A quick search of media sources reveals several recent, tragic stories about EMS providers who were seriously injured or killed in the line of duty. Some of these stories involve malicious attacks that were sprung after luring providers into a trap, while others involve patients who were confused and attacked their would-be rescuers.

As an educated and effective health care provider, you need to know how to avoid violence when possible and how to protect yourself when violence erupts. Because all EMS agencies respond to potentially life-threatening situations daily, you should actively seek out and encourage your organization to offer self-protection courses that are geared specifically toward EMS providers. Sound survival skills training will help you identify and avoid potentially dangerous situations. Once you recognize a violent situation, your goal is to retreat to a safe location and await the assistance of law enforcement personnel.

Awareness

At some point in your education, you likely have heard various accounts of violence against EMS providers. You may have first-hand experience of a dangerous situation. Throughout your career, you will respond to an infinite number of different scenarios, all with dynamic qualities, requiring a well-tuned sense of situational awareness. Violence is not isolated to one socioeconomic class and does not live in only one neighborhood.

Proper awareness begins when you are dispatched to a call. Look for information in the call notes or radio transmissions from your dispatch center that might raise a red flag, such as a report of a loud party, the address is a known crack house, or the address has known previous underage drinking violations . This is one situation where you must trust your gut instinct. If you feel uneasy about the information surrounding the call, there is likely a valid reason, even if you aren't able to identify exactly what it is. If you do not feel the scene is safe, request law enforcement personnel to secure the scene. You will not be able to assist anyone if you rush into an unsafe scene or become injured.

▶ Paramedics Mistaken for Law Enforcement Personnel

In some departments, the uniforms of EMS professionals and law enforcement personnel are very similar. The general public may have difficulty distinguishing among law enforcement personnel, EMS personnel, and fire department personnel. This can lead to unintentional violence toward you and your partner, since some violent outbursts are specifically targeted toward police officers.

YOU are the Paramedic   PART 1

You and your partner are dispatched to a single-family residence for an unknown problem. As you are responding, the dispatcher informs you the call was made by a neighbor who heard several loud voices shouting and a woman screaming for help in the house next door. The dispatcher also states attempts are being made to get more information from the caller, and a request has been made for law enforcement personnel. While responding to the call, your partner checks the map and informs you the house is at the end of a long street and there are no other streets leading away from the house.

1. On the basis of the limited amount of information available, do you have any concerns about entering this scene?
2. Considering the location of the residence, what information should cause you to carefully design your response and staging plan?

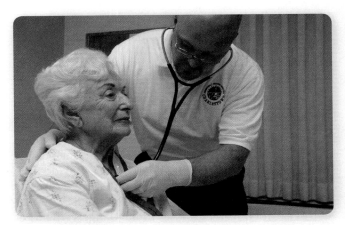

Figure 52-2 Some emergency medical services (EMS) agencies have adopted unique uniforms for their members that are not only more comfortable, but can help clearly identify the wearer as an EMS provider and not a law enforcement officer.

© Jones & Bartlett Learning. Courtesy of MIEMSS.

You should evaluate your services' uniforms and advocate for easily identifiable characteristics like unique colors or having them clearly marked "EMS" Figure 52-2 .

▶ Body Armor

EMS systems have witnessed a rise in violence toward their providers, which has prompted many agencies to provide some form of body armor for their personnel. Speak with local law enforcement officials or subject matter experts with a strong understanding of ballistics to learn about the details of body armor.

Various types of body armor may be resistant to different things. From a general awareness standpoint, it is important to remember a few key points. You should know what type of body armor your service provides. What caliber handgun is your vest effective against? What type of weapon is it not effective against? Bulletproof vests can help absorb some of the impact and decrease the risk of a bullet penetrating your armor, but there are weapons available today that will penetrate some of the most resilient vests. There are "stab proof" vests that may protect you from a knife or blade attack. There are "spike proof" vests that will offer some protection from screwdrivers, ice picks, and needles. Take the time to understand exactly what your body armor is designed to do. Again, local law enforcement agencies may be the best resource to answer your questions.

Take time to ensure your body armor fits you properly. For example, agencies will commonly purchase body armor to keep on the unit. These pieces will be a generic size. Take the time to adjust the fit of the armor before you attempt to wear it. Take the time during your check off at the start of the shift to adjust the fit of the body armor to your body. You do not want to find yourself in a violent situation with loose fitting body armor; it could be a fatal mistake. Body armor serves no purpose if not worn or worn properly; however, just because you have body armor on, you should *not* be entering areas that you would not normally enter without law enforcement.

▶ Indicators of Violence

Violence can sometimes be predicted based on the nature of the call. You would anticipate an increased potential

YOU ⟩ are the Paramedic   PART 2

As you arrive at the staging area, dispatch informs you the caller says she just heard one loud boom and sees two women huddled in the front yard crying. The caller says she still does not know what has happened, but she believes the scene is safe. The caller says there is no more violent shouting or screaming, only two women heard quietly crying. Law enforcement officers have not made it on scene. Dispatch instructs you to stage until law enforcement arrives and determines it is safe for you to proceed in to the scene.

Recording Time: 1 Minute	
Appearance	Unknown
Level of consciousness	Unknown
Airway	Unknown
Breathing	Unknown
Circulation	Unknown

3. Is the scene safe to enter?
4. Should you enter the scene prior to the arrival of law enforcement personnel?

for violence when you are dispatched to a shooting or stabbing. However, you should maintain a heightened sense of awareness even when responding to a sick or injured person. The patient may be upset, confused, or combative. Family members have been known to become extremely emotional when they see their loved one has been severely injured or killed. Your actions or lack of action (as in the case of a person who is already deceased upon your arrival) may be enough to trigger a violent outburst from family or bystanders. Remember to expect the unexpected, and do your best to identify any potential indicators of violence, such as abnormal behavior, body positioning, or harsh language. It may be as obvious as someone walking around with clenched fists who is shouting curse words at you and your partner; however, when you are focused on treating a patient who is gravely injured from a car crash it can be difficult to recognize the potential danger of others at the scene. You must not become so completely involved with patient care that you fail to see the possibility of physical harm to the patient or other EMS providers. Experts call this **tunnel vision**.

Despite your best efforts, you must understand there are times when there are almost no obvious signs of danger as responders approach the scene. This could be a calculated measure by a person who is intent on harming others. A person could call responders to a dark alley with the intent of shooting them as they arrive on scene. In other cases, it may be the last ditch effort of a person desperate to escape after committing a crime. Regardless of the scenario, tragic events have taught us that we must be vigilant and always do what we can to maintain the highest level of safety.

Words of Wisdom

When you enter a scene that has been secured by law enforcement, do not assume it will remain secure. Violent crimes often involve dynamic scenes where the perpetrator may return to the scene. Always keep your egress routes in mind, carry a radio, and watch each other's back.

▶ Standard Operating Procedures

Some agencies or regions have developed standard operating procedures (SOPs) for dealing with potentially violent incidents. Specific procedures for response to methamphetamine labs, civil disturbances, and hostage or barricade incidents provide paramedics with specific steps to be taken at such scenes. There may be information regarding what types of scenes require you to wear your body armor or how far away to stage for a barricaded subject. Much like standing orders for patient care, SOPs and policies will not be able to cover every single possible scenario. Always use them as the basis for your approach

to the scene or patient care, but be prepared to modify them if they interfere with the preservation of you or your partner's life.

■ Highway and Rural Road Incidents

In a study published in 2013, 86% of fatalities involving EMS were transportation related.[1] Law enforcement dashboard cameras mounted in vehicles have provided the public a rare view of the dangers routinely faced by law enforcement officers when approaching vehicles on the side of the road. You may face similar dangers whenever you walk to the door of a motor vehicle. Calls to a "man slumped over the steering wheel" or an "unresponsive person in a vehicle" can be disastrous for an unsuspecting paramedic. Several tragic stories exist where first responders were the target of malicious attacks while responding to an incident. Not only must you be mindful of the obvious hazards posed by fast-moving vehicles and curious drivers gawking at the incident, but you must also still be aware of potentially violent patients. The motor vehicle crash that you respond to may not be just a routine incident, but rather could be the culmination of a number of circumstances such as armed robbery, drug use, stolen vehicles, or perpetrators fleeing the scene of a violent crime.

▶ Approach and Vehicle Positioning

For your maximum safety when you are arriving at incidents with a single vehicle and you are the first vehicle to respond, your vehicle should be positioned a minimum of 21 feet (6 m) behind the stopped vehicle at a 10° angle to the driver's side facing the shoulder **Figure 52-3**. The front wheels should be turned all the way to the

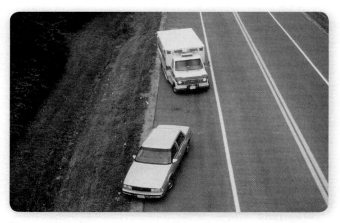

Figure 52-3 When you are the first vehicle to respond, position the unit a minimum of 21 feet (6 m) behind the stopped vehicle at a 10° angle to the left if you are the only emergency vehicle on the scene. Then call for law enforcement and set some flares if they will be delayed.

From *When Violence Erupts: A Survival Guide for Emergency Responders*, courtesy of Dennis R. Krebs.

left. In this position, the wheels and the motor block will provide limited protection in the event of gunfire. If you are not the first vehicle to arrive at the scene, ask the incident commander (IC) where he or she would like you to park your vehicle or try to park downstream of the incident. Law enforcement vehicles and fire engines are often placed behind the vehicle that was involved in the crash. They can help to provide a buffer in the event that someone inadvertently drives into a stopped vehicle. At an incident with law enforcement on scene, EMS usually park downstream unless told otherwise by the IC.

Your agency may have specific policies regarding the use of light after dark. For example, you may use your vehicle's high beams and spotlights to illuminate the interior and exterior of the patient's vehicle. Bright light will also conceal you as you approach the vehicle; however, you should be aware that your bright lights may impair the vision of drivers traveling in the opposite direction. Do not walk between the spotlight and the vehicle because you will provide a silhouette in the patient's rearview mirror and alert any responsive occupants to your position.

Do not approach a vehicle if you have an uneasy feeling about it. If law enforcement is not present and there is any potential that the scene is not safe, request them and remain in your vehicle until they declare the scene safe.

If you do approach a vehicle with no law enforcement on scene yet, consider notifying the dispatcher of the situation, your location, and the license plate number and state of the motor vehicle. If something happens to you and your partner, a record of the motor vehicle will now exist. This information will allow your agency to react quickly.

▶ Approaching the Motor Vehicle

A systematic approach to a motor vehicle is usually not required by EMS personnel. If you arrive at the scene of a rollover crash to find a vehicle on its side, you can approach the vehicle with a standard method. However, if you are responding to an unknown problem with a vehicle parked at the end of a boat ramp, you may consider a more strategic approach.

When there are two or more paramedics in the unit, the person riding in the right front seat, the IC of the emergency vehicle, makes the approach. All other members of the emergency response team remain with the ambulance or medical unit in the event there is a problem.

Proceed to the rear passenger-side trunk area **Figure 52-4** . Consider whether there may be people hiding in the trunk of a motor vehicle, and check the trunk lid to ensure it is properly closed. If the trunk is open, retreat to your vehicle. Using a belly-in movement, proceed to the C post on the passenger side of the motor vehicle **Figure 52-5** . Moving belly-in toward the motor vehicle creates as small an image as possible for the occupants of the motor vehicle to see.

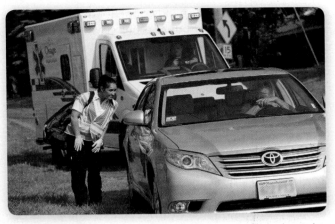

Figure 52-4 The incident commander moves from the right front of the unit directly to the right rear-trunk area of the vehicle.
© Jones & Bartlett Learning. Photographed by Glen E. Ellman.

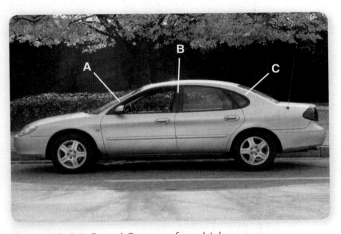

Figure 52-5 A, B, and C posts of a vehicle.
© Jones & Bartlett Learning. Courtesy of MIEMSS.

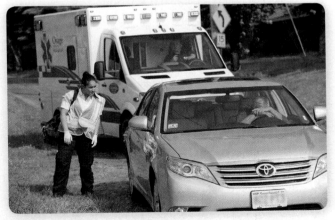

Figure 52-6 Stop at the right C post and look in the rear and side windows.
© Jones & Bartlett Learning. Photographed by Glen E. Ellman.

Stop at the right C post and look in the rear and side windows **Figure 52-6** . Notice the number of people in the vehicle. Pay particular attention to the location of their hands. Any attempt to stab, strike, or shoot will be accomplished using the hands. Look for deadly weapons such as guns or knives, but also objects such as baseball bats, beer bottles, tire iron, or pieces of pipe. If you see or suspect a deadly weapon, retreat to a safe location and call for law enforcement assistance. Officers are trained to retrieve and secure weapons; you are not. *Never* attempt to unload a weapon. Although you will not retreat every time you see a bat or pipe, your awareness that an object is within reach of the people in the vehicle gives you time to react if that object becomes a weapon. It is that awareness that will provide you with the time needed to escape a violent scene.

If the back seat is occupied, do not pass the C post. If you pass the C post, the back-seat passengers will be behind you. You will have to divide your attention between the front and rear seats.

If there are no passengers in the back seat, move forward to the B post with the same belly-in movement **Figure 52-7** . As with the C post, the B post will conceal you from the front-seat passengers of the vehicle. Examine the front-seat area. Where are the occupants' hands? What are the occupants doing? Are any weapons visible? When you are ready to let the driver know you are there, do so without moving past the B post into the driver's door area. Law enforcement personnel refer to this area as the kill zone. Tap lightly on the window of the vehicle to get the driver's attention and announce yourself: "Paramedic. Do you need help?"

Words of Wisdom

Weapon locations:
- Glove box
- Under the front dash
- Arm rest
- Under either side of the seat
- In the center console
- In side-door pockets
- Next to driver's right thigh

After the IC declares the incident scene is safe and determines the occupants of the motor vehicle need medical or other assistance, you should follow the SOPs for your department.

Keep your flashlight off until you need it. Hold the light at arms-length and away from your body before you turn it on **Figure 52-8** . Illuminate the scene for only a few seconds during each use.

Take special precautions when you approach vans. Vans can carry many types of cargo, and your inability to see that cargo is a danger. A van can carry a large number of people or a large quantity of weapons.

A safe approach to a van is modified from the approach made to the passenger side of a standard motor vehicle. When you exit the unit with the jump kit, move 10 to 15 feet (3 to 5 m) away from the passenger side of the van. If you are belly-in to the van, an occupant may suddenly open the side door and grab you. Instead, remain clear of the side door of the van throughout the approach **Figure 52-9** . From this distance, walk parallel to the van

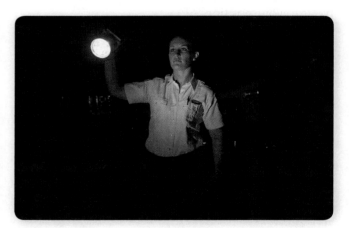

Figure 52-8 Because a light makes a good target, hold a flashlight away from your body when illuminating an area.
© Jones & Bartlett Learning. Photographed by Glen E. Ellman.

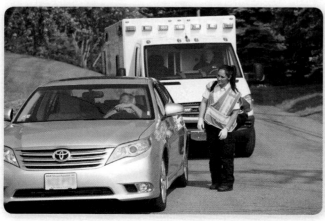

Figure 52-7 At this stage of the approach, do not move past the B post for any reason.
© Jones & Bartlett Learning. Photographed by Glen E. Ellman.

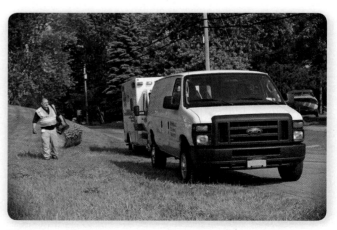

Figure 52-9 Until you are at a 45° angle forward of the A post, maintain 10 to 15 feet (3 to 5 m) distance between yourself and the passenger side of the van.
© Jones & Bartlett Learning. Photographed by Glen E. Ellman.

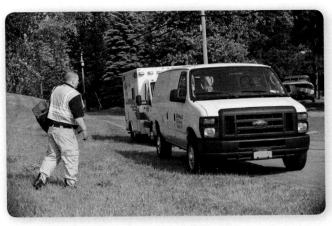

Figure 52-10 Position yourself at a 45° angle forward of the A post before making contact with the occupants of a van.

© Jones & Bartlett Learning. Photographed by Glen E. Ellman.

until you are approximately at a 45° angle forward of the A post. This position gives you the greatest visibility inside of the van but keeps you at a safe distance until you can determine the situation is secure **Figure 52-10** .

▶ Retreating from Danger

You will be in situations in which unsafe circumstances dictate your retreat to a safe area. The safest means of retreat is to back away and call for law enforcement assistance. If your partner is injured while approaching a motor vehicle, the best way to ensure help will arrive quickly is to back away and call for assistance yourself. The minimum amount of information recommended for this call for help should include your unit identifier or ambulance number and your current location. That way, if you are unable to get out any other information, the dispatcher has at least identified your unit and can dispatch immediate assistance. Back away from the danger zone, remain in your vehicle if able, and provide the dispatcher with all the needed information. This would include:

- Your unit identifier or ambulance number
- Your location and location of the injured
- The number of aggressors involved
- The number and types of injuries
- The number and types of weapons involved
- The make, color, body style, and license number of the vehicle involved
- The direction of travel if the vehicle leaves the scene before the law enforcement personnel arrive

In addition, ensure you document in detail why you had to leave the scene.

■ Residential Incidents

▶ Warning Signs

Emergency response personnel are frequently called to residential areas to assist someone injured in an assault,

domestic dispute, shooting, or stabbing. These calls require an obvious level of caution. But many routine calls have the potential for violent outcomes. A patient who has just suffered a seizure may be confused and pull a handgun from under his or her pillow. An intoxicated family member may be upset about a loved one's illness and become aggressive when you are treating the patient.

Your standard procedure for responding to any call involving violence should allow for law enforcement officers to secure the scene and make it safe enough for you to enter. You must continually reevaluate the situation while providing patient care.

Remember, sometimes the warning sign will be your gut instinct. Is there something suspicious about the dispatch information? Is there something in the call notes that raises a red flag?

▶ Approaching a Residence

Information provided to dispatchers may be limited, and a complete picture of the circumstances at the scene may not be available to paramedics. Keep in mind that all calls have a potential for violence. If you and your partner are approaching a residence, one of you should approach the house while the other stays a short distance away. This would allow for one person to call for help if violence erupts. When you are arriving at a residence, listen for loud, threatening voices. Glance through available windows for anything suspicious. In addition, look for visible weapons. After a quick evaluation, you can make a decision about the relative safety of the scene. Any time you perceive danger, back away to your vehicle. Call for law enforcement assistance, and wait for the officers to arrive.

▶ Entering a Residence

The front door to a residence can be a point of extreme danger. Many law enforcement officers have been shot and killed while standing in front of a door waiting to gain entry. Most bullets pass easily through all but the heaviest doors. Use an alternative path while approaching, rather than using the path to the front door. Once at the front door, you should stand to the doorknob side of the door when you are preparing to knock **Figure 52-11** . If you stand on the hinged side of the door, any person in the room can observe you by opening the door only slightly, and you would have a limited view of conditions inside the room. Knock on the door and announce: "Paramedics," "Fire department," or "Rescue squad." In doing so, you will not be mistaken for a law enforcement officer. Ask whomever answers the door to lead you to the patient. If you do this, you will not only get to the patient quickly, but the person who leads you acts as a shield for you and gives you a few extra moments to react if the situation deteriorates. If there are no lights on, have whomever leads you to the patient put on the lights so you are not at a disadvantage in low light.

When you are entering any type of structure, you should pick a **primary exit** and a **secondary exit**. Your primary exit

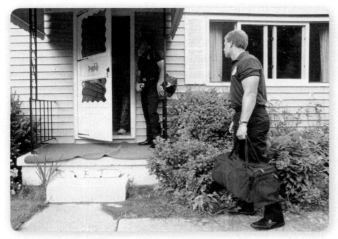

Figure 52-11 Stand on the doorknob side of the entrance when announcing your arrival.

From *When Violence Erupts: A Survival Guide for Emergency Responders*, courtesy of Dennis R. Krebs.

is the main means of escape if violence erupts, usually the door that was used to enter the building. A secondary exit is any other means of egress. This might be a rear door or a window. Whenever you are in a building, try to keep at least one means of escape accessible at all times.

As you arrive at the patient's location, scan the room for weapons. If there is a gun or knife, back your way out of the residence and call for law enforcement assistance. Many people keep loaded firearms in the house for personal protection. A nightstand, a dresser drawer, and a table next to a comfortable chair are popular locations to conceal these weapons. However, there could also be weapons under pillows or behind doors. Be aware of objects like ashtrays, scissors, bottles, fireplace pokers, and knitting needles that can be used as weapons. Move any potential weapon out of the patient's reach.

▶ Domestic Violence

Domestic disturbances are among the most dangerous situations faced by paramedics. You must be aware of the dangers involved and handle these incidents with extreme caution.

If a violent or physical dispute is in progress when you arrive at a residence, wait for law enforcement assistance before you enter. Remember, these types of scenes typically involve heightened emotions that have already reached a boiling point prior to your arrival; avoid confrontational actions or words that will reignite those emotions. Use good communication skills in conjunction with eye contact and appropriate body language to help defuse the situation and keep tempers from flaring. Your voice is the most effective tool you can use to keep out of trouble in a dispute. Use proper tone, pace, and pitch when speaking with the patient, family members, and bystanders. Maintain a professional and respectful tone to help ease tensions and facilitate a safe environment in which you may treat the patient.

If you find yourself attempting to defuse a heated situation, remember not to "return fire" by escalating your own emotional response. Remind yourself that the person who may be shouting at or insulting you does not know you personally. These verbal attacks are often designed to produce an emotional response from you. Do not give in. Remain calm and approach the situation with a level head. Show the person respect even if he or she is not giving it to you. This will help you to defuse the situation.

You may also use a technique known as **contact and cover**, which will be described in greater depth later in the chapter. One aspect of the technique involves one paramedic making contact with the patient to provide care. The second paramedic obtains patient information, and more important, gauges the level of tension and warns his or her partner at the first sign of trouble.

Your most important mandate is to conduct yourself as a professional when you are providing patient care. Your duty is to act in a professional manner, no matter how unpleasant or difficult the situation.

Most paramedics are not trained as marriage counselors, psychologists, psychiatrists, or clergy. At times, patients may ask you difficult questions regarding a failed relationship, abusive partner, or substance abuse. Do not be afraid to tell the patient you do not know the answer. Crisis intervention is not part of your job and should be left to the professionals. If law enforcement is not already involved, you may be required by law to report certain conditions such as domestic violence or child abuse to local authorities. Be sure to check your state's statutes and your community's laws to learn your mandatory reporting duties.

■ Violence on the Streets

The increase in gang activity and the prevalence of clandestine drug laboratories pose unique challenges to paramedics. Active shooter situations have become an unfortunate reality. These situations pose a huge risk to all responders.

▶ Clandestine Drug Laboratories

Clandestine drug laboratories are a growing problem. The most popular substance manufactured in clandestine labs is methamphetamine, known on the street as meth, speed, and crank. With a little bit of cash and some supplies, it does not take much for a "cook" to begin manufacturing methamphetamine.

Clandestine drug laboratories are incredibly dangerous to paramedics. There are several toxic chemicals involved in the manufacturing process. These chemicals may also undergo exothermic reactions that can ignite a fire. When a lab is found, you must evacuate immediately and request appropriate personnel to respond. Remember, personnel who have been involved in the manufacturing process

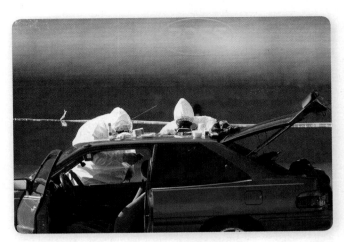

Figure 52-12 Some methamphetamine labs may resemble a high school chemistry laboratory or can even be simply stowed inside the trunk of a car. Do not touch anything!

© *The Sun News*, Janet Blackmon Morgan/AP Photo.

will require decontamination before you can provide treatment and transport.

Although some methamphetamine "cooking" operations may look like a typical high school chemistry laboratory, others are much harder to recognize. Large quantities of over-the-counter cold remedies containing ephedrine or pseudoephedrine, gallon containers of camping fuel, and sulfuric acid in the form of lye may be the only signs of methamphetamine production. Almost every chemical involved is a hazardous material.

There has been a rise in the number of "mobile meth labs" which involve motor vehicles and even mopeds **Figure 52-12** . These scenarios raise the danger level because you may not realize that the dangerous chemicals are present when you respond to a car fire, motor vehicle crash, or unknown problem in a parking lot.

In addition to the chemical hazards found at clandestine labs, some cookers use booby traps to safeguard their operations. These may include fragmentation and incendiary devices, animal traps, and impaling stakes.

Once a clandestine laboratory is identified, it is your job to remain clear of the area until the scene is secured by trained law enforcement personnel and hazardous materials specialists. As you evacuate the scene, remove patients from the scene only if you are able to do so without contaminating yourself.

▶ Gangs

Gangs pose an increasing threat in communities across the nation. What was once a problem only in major cities is now a problem in smaller suburban and rural communities. In 2012, the National Gang Center estimated there were approximately 32,000 gangs with almost one million members.[2] Gang activity has migrated from the cities into suburban and rural areas, in part to evade law enforcement and other gangs, as well as to extend their influence, recruit new members, and promote drug trafficking into virgin territories. The FBI estimates almost

every community across the nation either has some level of gang activity or is affected by gang activity. Today's gangs operate from the lowest level of retail or street drug sales, all the way up to major drug trafficking, rivaling the activity of international drug cartels.

Words of Wisdom

Youths usually join gangs for the following reasons:
- Identity
- Respect
- Recognition
- Love
- Belonging
- Money
- Fear

Gangs predominantly survive through the drug trade. Whereas they thrive on the drug trade, they also earn money through robbery, extortion, human trafficking, gun-running, prostitution rings, and identity theft. There are different types of gangs, including street gangs, prison gangs, and motorcycle gangs. All operate differently with rules on sex, age, race, religion, and national origin, but all have similar codes with regard to committing violence. They recruit young children from schools, and are a growing cause of school violence and drug proliferation. While many people are familiar with the "gang signs" **Figure 52-13** , most gang communication is far more sophisticated, using multiple prepaid cell phones that are easily discarded, text messaging, email, and even

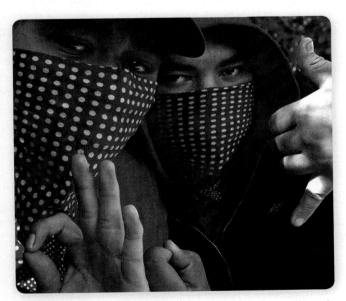

Figure 52-13 This form of hand communication is still used today, although gangs employ more sophisticated means of communicating such as the Internet and satellite phones.

© Nzgmw2788/Dreamstime.com.

satellite communications in more remote areas. Like many of us, gang members use Internet social networks. Gang membership is so pervasive that, according to the FBI, numerous gangs have representation in the US Armed Forces, with the intent on receiving military weapons and tactics training to pass on to other members, as well as to spread their influence.[3]

Knowing this, you should contact your local law enforcement to ask about and be aware of known gang territories. Many gangs have literally carved out sections of the map where they operate, and that no other gangs may enter **Figure 52-14** . When you enter these areas, you must always be mindful of the threat of gang violence and the types of activities in which the local gangs are involved. Often local law enforcement has a "gang unit" that keeps its finger on the pulse of gang activity. These resources can be an invaluable source of information that could help keep you safe. You should encourage your service or agency to work with local law enforcement to share information such as new gangs that may be entering the area and looking to make a name for themselves, which areas you should expect potential retaliation to come from, and illegal activities that are on the rise. You and your agency need to concern yourselves with these issues because when you are responding to an incident in a gang's territory. Knowledge is power. Knowledge can keep you and your partner safe. Remember: the last thing a rival gang wants to see is the paramedics coming to rescue the person that they just shot or stabbed. In all potentially violent situations, the paramedic's best and

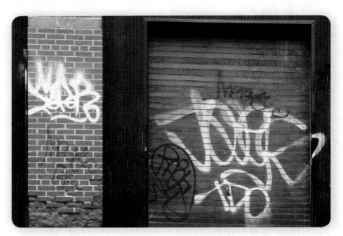

Figure 52-14 Many gangs use graffiti to mark off their territories. It is imperative that paramedics be aware of when they are entering a gang's area.
© iStockphoto/Thinkstock/Getty.

YOU are the Paramedic PART 3

Ten minutes after multiple police vehicles rush past your location, your dispatch informs you the scene has been secured by law enforcement officers and it is safe for you to proceed. They also request you to expedite your response because they have one patient who was shot in the head. As you arrive on scene, a police officer approaches you and tells you an adult male has shot himself in the head with a shotgun. The officer informs you there was a family argument that preceded the patient grabbing the weapon and shooting himself in the head. There are no other patients at this time, and the family is screaming and crying in the front yard. After grabbing your equipment, you follow the police officer inside the residence. You find a 50-year-old man with an obvious, severe head wound lying prone next to a dining room table. There is a shotgun lying approximately 3 feet (approximately 1 m) away from the patient next to the wall. As you approach, you see a large pool of blood around his head, and you do not see any spontaneous respirations. You ask the police officer to secure the weapon and then inform him that you need to roll the patient over to assess the patient and determine the need for resuscitation.

Recording Time: 10 Minutes	
Respirations	0 breaths/min, apneic
Pulse	Absent peripheral pulses
Skin	Cool and mottled
Blood pressure	Not applied
Oxygen saturation (Spo$_2$)	Not applied
Pupils	Unknown due to patient being prone

5. Should you have the officer move the weapon from its current location?
6. What special considerations should you have while moving the patient to determine the need for resuscitation?

often only defense is **situational awareness**. That means knowing your surroundings, the people and groups in your environment, and the climate of violence or strife that may exist. Having good situational awareness will help you make an effective decision when you are forced to react in a destabilized scene.

▶ Mass Shootings, Active Shooters, and Snipers

The last decade has been especially violent with regard to mass shootings Table 52-1 . You, as the paramedic, are an integral part of emergency operations at these scenes. Paramedics must prepare, plan, and train for these complex and difficult violent incidents. Unfortunately, mass shootings are on the rise, and show no signs of tapering off. Mass shootings garner a tremendous amount of media coverage and, as such, afford those persons an opportunity to be infamous. Some mass shootings have been protracted events, associated with long standoffs and hostage-taking. However, many of the most recent shootings have been rapidly developing, dynamic events that leave a lot of killed and wounded while challenging those responding to the event. As such, you may find yourself on the scene with an **active shooter**—a gunman who has begun to fire on people and is still at large. These scenes are especially tense because people who appear to be released hostages could in fact be the perpetrators or

their accomplices. Domestic terrorism has come into the spotlight in recent years with radical people using large, violent events to make a statement about their personal beliefs. What is dispatched as a simple call may quickly escalate into a mass-casualty incident as more information comes in to responding units.

Paramedics must take direction from law enforcement personnel on the scene and may even be instructed as to *whom* to treat and *when* a victim can be treated (but never *how* to treat). This situation is largely based on the safety of the location of the patients and not on physical injuries. This is not your normal triage situation because law enforcement has absolute control of the scene, and they may dictate that you initiate or withhold treatment not based on medical necessity, but rather on safety. For example, you may be asked to proceed past patients who are potentially salvageable because that area has not been secured or there are concerns regarding a secondary shooter or improvised explosive device. Ensure that you carefully document any deviation from your guidelines or special circumstances that you encountered.

This is a situation where you may have ethical or moral questions about whom to treat. You may be directed to leave someone that may be medically salvageable but is not in a secure area. However, the time to dispute the ethics of what is being asked of you is not while there is an active shooter at large. You may be unable to contact on scene supervisors due to the fast-paced nature of the

Table 52-1		Mass Shootings (2012–2016)
Year	**Month**	**Incident**
2012	July	A young man entered a movie theater during the premiere of a popular movie in Aurora, Colorado. He killed 12 people and injured another 58 before being apprehended outside of the theater.
2012	December	A gunman entered the Sandy Hook Elementary School in Newtown, Connecticut and killed 20 first-grade students and 6 adults. The gunman committed suicide at the scene. It was also discovered the gunman had murdered his mother at home, prior to his shooting rampage.
2013	September	A Navy contractor entered the Washington Navy Yard in Washington, DC, and began a shooting spree that claimed the lives of 12 people. The shooter was shot and killed by authorities.
2014	May	In a premeditated attack, a young man in a small community in Isla Vista, California, killed 6 people and wounded 7 others before turning the gun on himself.
2015	June	A young Caucasian man entered a historic African American church in Charleston, South Carolina. He sat with the prayer group before he opened fire and killed 9 members of the congregation. He was later apprehended in North Carolina after an extensive manhunt.
2016	June	The worst mass shooting in US history occurred in Orlando, Florida. A gunman entered a gay nightclub and opened fire on the crowd. The final toll for the shooting stood at 50 killed and 53 injured. The gunman was killed by a SWAT team after taking hostages following his initial assault.

event, but it may be reasonable during longer events to contact them to discuss your concerns. Otherwise, it is a crime scene, and you *must* follow the directives of law enforcement personnel until the scene has been secured.

EMS and law enforcement should train together in active shooter drills to better understand each other's roles. Most law enforcement personnel who have received training carry tourniquets to stop life-threatening external bleeding.

As with any other shooting or stabbing incident, responding paramedic units should remain in the staging area until the scene is secured by law enforcement personnel.

Words of Wisdom

During a mass shooting or active shooter situation, law enforcement is the lead agency, and you must follow their instructions at all times for your safety and that of your partner and the public.

Words of Wisdom

The Hartford Consensus[4]

The American College of Surgeons (ACS), in collaboration with the medical community, representatives from governmental and nongovernmental agencies, and various emergency medical response organizations, among others, developed a national protocol to maximize survivability from active shooter and other mass-casualty incidents. These recommendations, called the Hartford Consensus, emphasize a continuum of care from initial response to definitive care that involves the seamless integration of hemorrhage control intervention. An integrated active shooter response should include the critical actions contained in the acronym THREAT:

- **T**hreat suppression
- **H**emorrhage control
- **R**apid **E**xtrication to safety
- **A**ssessment by medical providers
- **T**ransport to definitive care

Life-threatening bleeding from extremity wounds is best controlled initially through use of tourniquets, while internal bleeding resulting from penetrating wounds to the chest and trunk is best addressed through immediate transport to a medical facility.

The *Stop the Bleed* campaign, initiated by the US government in partnership with various organizations including ACS, emphasizes the need for the public to act as immediate responders who stem bleeding at an emergency scene, even before emergency responders arrive. This campaign aims to raise awareness of how quickly a person can die from life-threatening bleeding, and teaches bleeding control principles to empower laypeople.[5]

Recent events have led to discussion of rescue task forces entering a scene that has been made "safe enough" to evacuate medical casualties. With a rescue task force, EMS can move forward with law enforcement officers to minimize the time before injured personnel receive initial treatment. Patients with penetrating trauma may benefit from early hemorrhage control or simple airway maneuvers. Rescue task forces allow paramedics to deploy to forward locations under the protection of law enforcement officers during an active shooter event. Rescue task forces may have some simple body armor but little tactical training, if any. Remember your situational awareness as you move toward a forward location. You will not be armed, and you will need to rely on your law enforcement officers to provide safety and threat suppression if necessary. Follow your local policies and guidelines. If you believe your life is in immediate danger, remain staged in a safe area.

Staging, treatment, and triage areas may need to be ½ to 1 mile (2 km) away from the actual scene. Line-of-sight and, thus, line-of-fire from windows must be avoided when you are establishing these sites. Although parking lots or playing fields at schools may seem to be ideal locations for staging, they could allow an assailant a wide field of fire, causing a chaotic situation to deteriorate even further **Figure 52-15** .

Paramedics who respond to a mass or active shooting scene need to know how to use **cover** and **concealment**. You need to know the difference between objects that provide cover and those that offer concealment only **Figure 52-16** . Cover objects, such as trees, utility poles, mail collection boxes, dumpsters, curbs, vehicles, and depressions in the ground are obstacles that are difficult or impossible for bullets to penetrate. Tall grass, shrubbery, and dark shadows are areas of concealment. When cover is not readily available, use concealment to help you from being seen while you assess your position. Your job at that point is to find cover until either the scene is secure, or until you can retreat to a position of safety. Remember, people are going to need your help. Do not do anything that could get you or your partner injured.

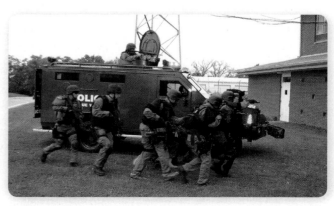

Figure 52-15 At a shooting or stabbing incident, a SWAT team may be employed. Remain in your safe staging area and follow all instructions from law enforcement.

Courtesy of John Wipfler.

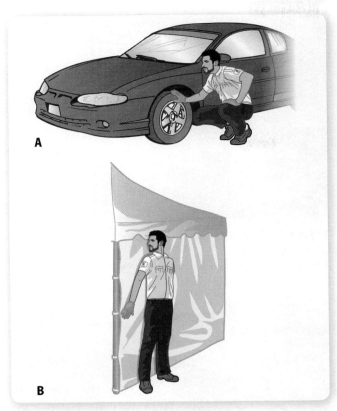

Figure 52-16 Examples of cover **(A)** and concealment **(B)**.
© Jones & Bartlett Learning.

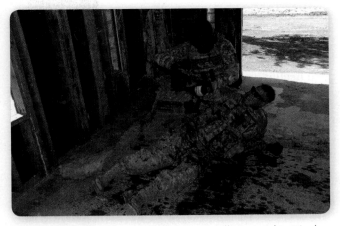

Figure 52-17 Many systems have specially trained tactical paramedics who can render care in violent and dangerous situations.
Courtesy of Lawrence Heiskell.

Paramedics should consider having a training session with local police on how to assess the police officer who has been shot, to address specific topics such as the removal of full-body armor and the officer's duty belt. The protocol for who removes the officer's weapons, and how, should be established before a potential incident. Remember, an injured officer who is panicking or has an altered mental status should be disarmed by another officer. A confused officer who is unsure of whether he or she is still in danger could be a threat to you if another officer has not appropriately removed the weapons.

Many services are using **tactical paramedics** in mass shootings and other scenes where there is actual violence or the potential for violence. Tactical paramedics are specially trained medics who provide medical care for SWAT/mobile response team members conducting operations, barricaded patients, patients being held hostage, and other special operations. Tactical paramedics are a critical link in providing medical care in hostile situations, including mass shootings. Training in this newly emerging subspecialty is widely available from reputable training centers **Figure 52-17**.

In your local area, there is likely some form of active shooter training exercise that is conducted with emergency responders. These events are excellent training opportunities where multiple agencies can practice their response plans to identify their strengths and weaknesses. As mentioned, there is ongoing discussion about the role of the paramedic in an active shooter response. Should paramedics respond

when the scene is "safe enough" or wait for the all clear? There are fire and EMS agencies that have placed paramedics in the forward areas (areas where there may still be the possibility of an active threat) of an active shooter with police personnel. As injured personnel can die from external hemorrhage or tension pneumothorax, well-placed paramedics could make a significant impact in treating the wounded. This means a decreased time to point of medical care for the injured patients inside of an event, but it does come with an increased risk to the providers.

You should become active with your local law enforcement agencies to plan the best approach for you and your fellow responders. Whether it is placing tactical paramedics at the front lines with a SWAT team or planning where your ambulance will stage during an active shooter event, practicing your response and coordinating with local agencies will make a difference. Having an active shooter plan that you have practiced during exercises can help you save lives when the inevitable happens.

▶ Hostage Situations

EMS personnel sometimes arrive on a scene before it is secure. Once again, hostage situations are under the jurisdiction of law enforcement until the scene is secure. Have you considered what you would do if you met an armed adversary? Because no hard and fast rules apply, you should take additional training about handling armed people in the field. The possibility of being taken hostage is extremely remote, but it exists. Your behavior can greatly enhance your chances of surviving the ordeal.

Hostages are usually held as a form of human collateral to ensure compliance with a promise. If you are taken hostage, you can increase your chances of survival if you can anticipate the feelings and actions of the hostage taker and the negotiators.

The psychologic results of being held hostage are of greater concern than physical problems. Even if you are physically unharmed, you may experience strong psychologic reactions during the incident. A person who has been held hostage can develop posttraumatic stress disorder (PTSD). It is often wise to seek professional counseling after your release, even if you do not think you need it, to prevent long-term problems later. Knowing what to expect if you are held hostage can help you keep your psychologic equilibrium during the situation and help you deal with the psychologic stress that often accompanies your release.

If you are taken hostage, manage yourself and your personal environment. Do not do anything that will attract unwanted attention, and do not stare at your captors. If the hostage takers believe you are in their way or you irritate them, they may kill you. Remember, any one of your captors can walk in and kill you at any time. Your only chance for survival is to maintain your role as a bargaining chip.

Because you are wearing a uniform, other hostages may look to you for guidance and strength. Your captors may consider this image of authority as a threat. Anything that draws attention to you increases the possibility of violence. Make every effort to be inconspicuous. Develop a nonthreatening image by removing the badge, collar pins, and patches from your uniform, or turn your uniform shirt inside out so these items are not visible. Ask to treat the wounded, if possible, even for minor injuries. This will serve to help you gauge the intentions of your captors, as well as make you seem less threatening. It will also keep your mind sharp, by performing tasks that you are used to doing as opposed to sitting around like the other captives, and hopefully offer the other captives some comfort. You may also consider offering to treat the injuries of any captors. This may seem ethically inconceivable, but not only is it consistent with your code of ethics and training (paramedics do not discriminate nor withhold treatment, regardless of the circumstances), but it may also help your captors perceive you as less of a threat, and make you more valuable.

Cover and Concealment

In any violent situation, you must never assume you will not be harmed because you are clearly identified as a paramedic. Always assume the person with a gun will shoot anyone in sight. If you see law enforcement personnel seeking cover, remain in the immediate vicinity.

Remember the difference between objects that provide cover and those that offer concealment only. You should make your body conform to the shape of the object as much as possible **Figure 52-18**.

People shooting from a higher position than you (such as in an upper floor window or on a roof) can usually see the upper part of your torso or head over the top of your cover, especially if you are using a wall or motor vehicle as cover **Figure 52-19**. If this occurs, use the engine block and wheel area of a motor vehicle as cover. Avoid the area near the fuel tank, and do not use the area between the wheels as cover **Figure 52-20**.

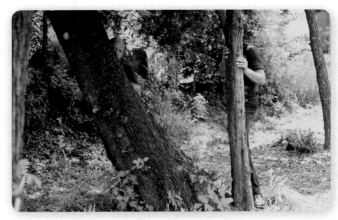

Figure 52-18 Choose a tree that is large enough to conceal all of your body.
From *When Violence Erupts: A Survival Guide for Emergency Responders*, courtesy of Dennis R. Krebs.

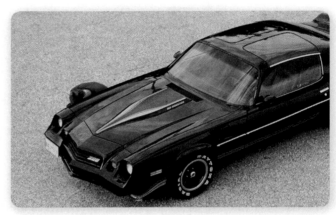

Figure 52-19 A sniper who is shooting from a higher position than you can see part of your body from above your position of cover.
From *When Violence Erupts: A Survival Guide for Emergency Responders*, courtesy of Dennis R. Krebs.

Select a fire hydrant as cover only if you cannot immediately find larger objects. You will soon become uncomfortable trying to match your body to the small hydrant. There is a real possibility in such a situation that you could be shot in the arm, knee, or shoulder. However, your central body mass vital organs will be protected. If this is the only cover available, it is better than remaining in the open.

If you are not outdoors, items inside a structure and the structure itself can provide cover or concealment, depending on their construction. Furniture and appliances, such as a solid oak desk or a refrigerator, can be used for cover because they may stop or deflect a bullet. If you position yourself behind a sofa or a stuffed chair, you have concealed yourself but you are not protected by cover.

▶ Using Walls as Cover

You cannot assume a wall will provide safe cover—many provide only concealment. For your safety and survival, you must determine whether the type of wall you have chosen gives you cover or only concealment. For example,

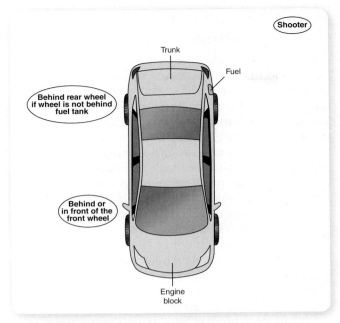

Figure 52-20 The engine block and the wheel area of a motor vehicle can be used as cover when shooting is occurring from overhead, but avoid the area near the fuel tank and the area between the wheels.

© Jones & Bartlett Learning.

brick and concrete block walls are much safer than cinder block walls. The porous nature of cinder blocks will not absorb the bullet's energy and stop it. However, most interior walls are constructed with wood or aluminum studs and covered with drywall or siding. They may conceal you but they are not good cover because they are not impenetrable. If your only protection is behind a frame wall, try to stand near the door or window frames. These areas are usually constructed with extra framing materials and contain more wood than other areas of the wall.

▶ Evasive Tactics

Change locations only if the new location is better cover, farther from the hostile atmosphere, and can be reached without revealing yourself to the attacker. Do not change your position of cover just for the sake of changing. Before changing locations, quickly look out from your cover several times. Look from a different height and angle each time. Use this "quick-peek" technique to evaluate the advisability of changing locations. Always return to cover as quickly as possible.

If you decide you would be safer in another location, do not run directly away from the assailant's position; run in a zigzag pattern. You have less chance of being hit if your movement takes you across the assailant's field of view.

YOU are the Paramedic   PART 4

With your partner's assistance, the patient has been rolled into a supine position. There is a severe head wound noted with exposed brain matter present. The patient is pulseless and apneic. The cardiac monitor displays asystole in more than one lead. In accordance with your protocol, you contact medical control and relay your findings. The online physician pronounces the patient dead. You then inform the police officer and your dispatch center that the patient has been pronounced dead by online medical control. You carefully gather your equipment and proceed outside of the house. With a heavy heart, you stop to speak with the family of the patient realizing the sensitive nature of the scene.

Recording Time: 12 Minutes	
Respirations	0 breaths/min, apneic
Pulse	Central and peripheral pulses absent
Skin	Cool and mottled
Cardiac monitor	Asystole in all leads
Oxygen saturation (Spo$_2$)	Not applied
Pupils	7 mm, fixed and dilated

7. What questions will you likely be asked as more law enforcement officers and crime scene investigators arrive?
8. How would you document the circumstances of this event in your patient care report? Are there any special considerations regarding the documentation of your actions and assessment?

▶ Concealment Techniques

Tall grass, shrubbery, and dark shadows are considered areas of concealment. When cover is not readily available, use concealment to provide some protection while you assess your position and seek cover.

Areas of concealment are more common after dark than during daylight hours. If you are involved in a violent situation at night, move into the darkness or shadows and stand still. The assailant cannot see you and may not shoot. If the assailant fires shots at random, chances are you will not be hit.

In rural areas, tall grass or a cornfield can conceal you whether it is day or night. Remain motionless so the foliage does not move and you do not make any noise. After you finish analyzing the situation, move toward cover.

■ Self-Defense

Recognize the potential for violence when you arrive on the scene to give yourself time to request support and protection from law enforcement officers. Their presence may offer you the protection you need to safely treat your patient after the scene is secure. However, you must also consider what to do if the violence is ongoing or breaks out while you are providing care. Remember to expect the unexpected on every scene. Defensive moves may allow you to resolve the situation or allow you time to retreat to a safe area. Self-defense must be physically practiced to be learned effectively; consider taking a self-defense course to learn techniques that can help you on the job.

If someone prevents you from reaching your patient, identify yourself and inform him or her that you are there to help. Instruct the person to move away. Inform the person you will not be able to help the patient if you are not allowed access to the patient. Remember, this may be the goal of the person blocking your path. If the person blocking your way moves, contact your dispatcher and request law enforcement personnel respond just in case the person becomes uncooperative again. If the person does not move, take a side step and repeat the request to be granted access to the ill person. Keep in mind, however, a verbal challenge or threats to summon law enforcement may only further anger any opposition.

You cannot control when an unexpected attack will occur, but you can improve your ability to think on your feet. Again, it's about situational awareness. Always ensure your exit path is not blocked, and you can easily retreat the way you came. If this exit has been blocked, search for a back door or window to exit through. Use household objects to try to obstruct the assailant's path toward you as you retreat. Stretchers and equipment are also excellent obstructions, and you should be ready to leave them behind if you need to make a swift escape.

▶ Self-Defense in Armed Encounters

Distraction techniques are useful in breaking the chain of events (turn, locate, focus, and fire) in a shooting incident and in preventing attacks with knives or other sharp objects. Again, the purpose of the distraction is to increase your chances of survival by giving you time to escape. The distraction does not have to be elaborate.

When you see something is coming at you, your initial instinct is to blink or flinch. Consider what happens when you are driving during a heavy rain and a passing vehicle splashes water on your vehicle's windshield. Even though you know the water is not going to hit you, you still blink or flinch when the water strikes the windshield. This is the reaction you want to provoke.

Throwing a lightweight object may elicit the desired response. It does not have to be accurate to interrupt the chain of events long enough to permit you to get out of the line of fire and run to safety.

If the patient takes aggressive action during your initial interview, one technique is to throw a light object directly at the aggressor's nose. A soft or lightweight object will not cause undue harm, and may already be in your hand. A roll of tape or blood pressure cuff may be enough to distract your attacker and remove his focus from you. A hard or heavy object such as a metal clipboard, laptop computer, or portable radio may cause needless (and permanent) injuries. While a heavier object may be preferred in a situation where there is an imminent life threat, a lighter object may be more reasonable when facing most attackers.

After you throw the object, do not wait for a reaction. As soon as it is out of your hand, turn toward your vehicle, get out of the possible line of fire, and run to safety.

Put as much distance as possible between you and the aggressor. If it is possible, run to your vehicle **Figure 52-21** . You can call for help or drive to a safer location. If you are cut off from the ambulance, evaluate the surrounding area for the best possible cover and concealment.

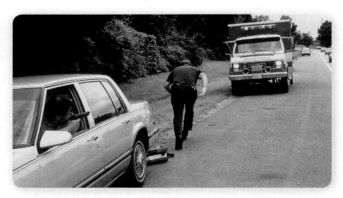

Figure 52-21 While the aggressor flinches and attempts to refocus, run toward the unit.

From *When Violence Erupts: A Survival Guide for Emergency Responders*, courtesy of Dennis R. Krebs.

Use physical force as a defensive technique, not an aggressive motion. Properly executed defensive motions can be as effective as physical strikes and are easier to defend if you face civil liability charges.

The amount of defensive force needed to protect yourself varies with each incident. If you believe your life is in imminent danger, any action that gets you out of the situation is a reasonable level of force.

Words of Wisdom

Undoubtedly, you will encounter situations where things unexpectedly get out of hand. Having a heightened sense of awareness, knowing your escapes routes, and being able to effectively use cover, concealment, and evasive techniques may be the difference between you getting hurt and being able to get away without injury.

Crime Scenes

As a paramedic, you will respond to assist the victims of violent crime. Your first responsibility is your own safety, then your partner's safety, then the patient's safety, and then bystander safety. However, you also have a responsibility to the community at large. By assisting law enforcement personnel to maintain the integrity of the crime scene, you increase the probability that a suspect will be captured and convicted.

▶ Preserving Evidence

Generally, there are two types of evidence: testimonial and real or physical. **Testimonial evidence** is the oral documentation by a witness of a criminal act. Real or **physical evidence** ties a suspect or victim to a crime. It may include materials on the body, objects, and impressions. You should be acutely concerned with not disturbing, damaging, or potentially altering physical evidence at the scene. Small blood stains on the wall or floor unperceivable to the untrained eye can yield critical forensic information that can be used to apprehend the perpetrator **Figure 52-22**. Unnecessary cutting or removal of clothes can potentially destroy or dislodge fibers, hair, or other evidence deposited by the perpetrator **Figure 52-23**.

When using trauma shears to remove clothing necessary to assess and treat the patient, ensure you avoid any bullet holes or knife marks in the clothing. If it is possible, cut along the seams of the clothing so the larger surfaces remain intact. Once the clothes are removed, do not shake them because valuables, including valuable trace evidence, may fall from the pockets to the floor. Do your best not to leave any of

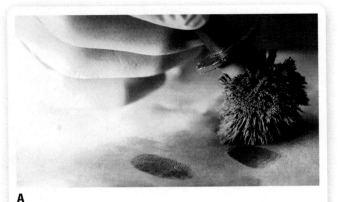

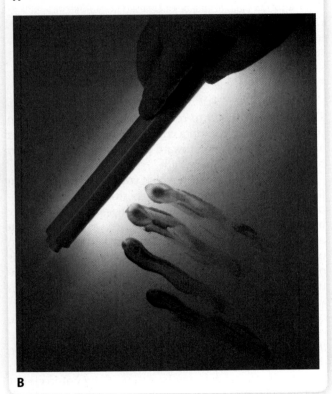

Figure 52-22 Fingerprints can be left on the scene in a variety of mediums. **A.** Some fingerprint marks can be dusted with a powder that adheres to residue on the print. **B.** Ultraviolet light can be used in other cases; this example shows a bloody fingerprint smear.

A: © Jochen Tack/Alamy; B: © Olivier Le Queinec/Shutterstock.

your own equipment on scene. Do your best to collect gloves or medical waste or sharps containers that may have been placed next to the patient during the initial resuscitation.

Law enforcement personnel should collect evidence. If you must remove a piece of evidence (for example, clothing) to treat the patient, place each piece of evidence into a brown paper bag. If the item is saturated, then place the paper bag into a plastic bag for biohazard control.

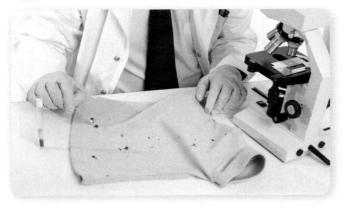

Figure 52-23 Hair, fibers, or body fluid containing DNA (blood, sweat, semen) can be found and analyzed in articles of clothing months to years after the transfer has occurred.
© Leah-Anne Thompson/Shutterstock.

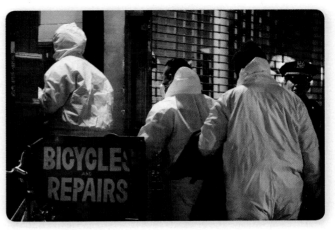

Figure 52-24 This joint New York City Crime Scene Investigation team comprises various agencies, whose members use suits that prevent them from depositing their own false evidence on the scene and also prevents them from collecting any on their body.
© Stephen Chernin/AP Photo.

This may be difficult to remember while performing an intense resuscitation on a critical patient, but remember any extra consideration toward evidence preservation may benefit the investigation.

There are situations in which you must recognize that life-saving efforts are futile, and the initiation of a resuscitation is not medically indicated. Your response may involve high levels of emotions and adrenaline. Do not get caught up in the emotions of a call and attempt a full resuscitation on a patient who is not salvageable. Futile efforts like this may appear heroic, but they can often damage evidence unnecessarily. While you are focused on providing life-saving treatment to critically injured patients, you also need to recognize that the best thing you can do for some patients may be to do nothing at all. Consider the evidence that may be destroyed during futile efforts that could be the only physical evidence available to identify and catch the perpetrator. There may be times, if law enforcement officers believe the patient is obviously dead, when only one provider is asked to enter into the crime scene to determine if the patient is dead based on predetermined criteria. Always follow local protocols, which may include contacting medical control for direction regarding termination of resuscitation efforts or the initiation of resuscitation efforts in the context of obvious death of the patient. Remember, this may be appropriate in an attempt to minimize the amount of evidence that could be disturbed by limiting the amount of people entering the scene.

Follow law enforcement direction when you are asked to park in a specific area or to avoid a certain location. Officers may be attempting to safeguard tire imprints, bullet casings, or blood. The number of EMS personnel entering the scene should be limited to only those who are necessary. Crime scene investigators commonly wear full-body Tyvek suits Figure 52-24. This is because every time they enter a crime scene, not only do they deposit evidence (in the form of DNA), but evidence can collect on their clothes and damage the evidence or make it less useful.

You should also keep these principles in mind whenever you enter a crime scene. Every interaction with a space or surface entails the deposition of your DNA onto that area. Limit your time and interaction (what you touch) with the crime scene and *always* wear gloves when entering. First responders are typically the first to enter a crime scene and view it in its most pristine condition. Once you enter the scene, regardless of how careful you are to preserve evidence, that scene is inexorably altered. This is often why paramedics are called to speak with investigators and prosecutors and appear at trials and pretrial hearings (ie, grand jury). These people will want to know exactly what you saw, what you touched, what you smelled, what you heard (television or other electronic device, fan, alarm clock), and what you did while you were there. You must not clean up the scene, alter items, or move bodies unless doing so is essential to establish the need for resuscitation. Be mindful of bullet casings, weapons, blood spatter, and puddles. Whenever possible, walk around such evidence Figure 52-25. Do not pick up expended cartridge casings to determine the caliber; that is irrelevant to rendering patient care. Do not use telephones, flush toilets, or turn on water in a sink. In each case, valuable evidence can be lost.

Because it is likely you will be called to provide testimonial evidence in court regarding what you saw or heard at the scene of a crime, it is imperative that the incident be properly documented. A significant amount of time may pass before you are asked to testify about every detail of the scene and the events that transpired. It could be a few months or even years. During that time, you will likely have responded to several other crime scenes. Details of the various scenes may become blurred in your mind; therefore, it is imperative whenever you encounter a crime scene that you properly document what you find. This document may be read by dozens of people

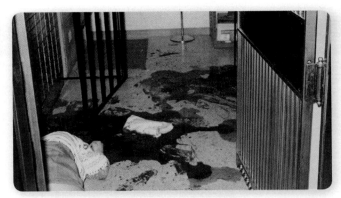

Figure 52-25 Do not disturb bullet casings, and avoid stepping in blood spatter and puddles.

From *When Violence Erupts: A Survival Guide for Emergency Responders*, courtesy of Dennis R. Krebs.

(and potentially a jury), and the quality of your report will speak volumes to your level of professionalism and credibility. More practically, the better your documentation is of the scene, the more likely that you will recall years later what you witnessed when all you have is your patient care report to refresh your memory.

The following are the elements of proper documentation: document what you saw; what you heard; what you were told; what you smelled (if there were any odors); what you moved, altered, or disturbed; and the chain of custody of any items that were presented to you, or that you found on the patient or decedent. Documentation should include a description of the scene. How many patients or decedents? Was the victim supine or prone? Where was the weapon? Were any characteristics of the scene noteworthy? Do not draw conclusions or overstate facts. Any statements made by the patient during transfer to a medical facility should be documented.

Documentation & Communication

Your report should answer the following questions:

What did you see?	■ Overturned or damaged furniture ■ Weapons ■ Position of victim and other persons at the scene
What did you hear?	■ Arguing or screams ■ Weapons being chambered or talk of the use of a weapon ■ Incriminating statements by persons on the scene ■ Television or other electronic device ■ Alarm clock or timer
What did you smell?	■ Gunpowder or smoke ■ Rotten food or garbage ■ Putrefaction (decomposition) ■ Chemical odors
What were you told?	■ By the patient ■ By police or fire personnel ■ By bystanders or neighbors ■ By family members or caregivers
What was done with evidence or personal effects taken from the victim?	■ Clothing (left with the emergency department staff) ■ Weapons (law enforcement personnel should secure weapons whenever possible) ■ Medications (brought to the emergency department) ■ Identification/wallet or purse (best to give to law enforcement)
What did you alter or disturb?	■ Where you went (and where you did not go) ■ What you had to move to get to or assess the patient ■ What you looked in (refrigerator, medicine cabinet, or drawer) ■ For what purpose you moved, altered, or disturbed something ■ Document your use of gloves and any other personal protective equipment that you wore that would prevent the spread of your DNA throughout the crime scene

As always, print legibly!

YOU ▶ are the Paramedic SUMMARY

1. **On the basis of the limited amount of information available, do you have any concern for entering this scene?**

   You should have concern for your safety and your crew's safety any time there is limited information for a call that may indicate violence. It is not usual for screams to come from a residence that are loud enough for a neighbor to be concerned. Listen to your instincts and if something does not sound safe or indicates a potential for violence, request assistance from law enforcement personnel.

2. **Considering the location of the residence, what information should cause you to carefully design your response and staging plan?**

   The fact that there is only one street to access the patient should cause you to pause and consider the circumstances. You do not know what has happened here. You will likely want to stage for law enforcement to secure the scene. Consider where you will stage your ambulance. You do not want to stage on the street where the scene is located. If there is an assailant or someone attempting to flee the scene, you do not want them to have to pass your ambulance on the way out of the scene. This may provide someone with an opportunity to cause you harm or prevent the people on scene from receiving medical attention.

3. **Is the scene safe to enter?**

   Based on the information you have, you cannot determine whether the scene is safe to enter. While there may be no active threats to you or your partner's safety, there is no way for you to guarantee that based on the limited information relayed from dispatch. There are several red flags: screams for help, a loud boom, and people crying in the yard. These red flags should tell you that staging for law enforcement would be the prudent decision.

4. **Should you enter the scene prior to the arrival of law enforcement personnel?**

   Your standard procedure for responding to any call involving violence should be to allow law enforcement personnel to arrive and secure the scene before your entry. Securing a scene demands more than the simple presence of a law enforcement officer at the scene. Responding paramedics must ensure the scene is safe before going in to provide patient care.

5. **Should you have the officer move the weapon from its current location?**

   Always ask law enforcement if the weapon has been secured prior to your arrival. This should help prevent anyone else from successfully using the weapon on themselves or others. However, if you are unsure if the weapon has been secured, it is reasonable to ask the police officer to confirm the scene is safe. You may also have to consider the circumstances of the scene. Law enforcement officials may not wish to move the firearm again if they have already cleared the weapon and placed it in its current location.

6. **What special considerations should you have while moving the patient to determine the need for resuscitation?**

   In this situation, you must quickly determine the need for resuscitation. You are likely to have a high index of suspicion that the patient is already deceased, but you may be required to perform a rapid assessment to confirm the patient is not salvageable. While moving this patient, you should consider what is near the patient and where you could easily move him. Do not move the patient into a position that would be more difficult to work with in case the patient is salvageable and requires an aggressive resuscitation. However, you also do not want to disturb the surrounding area or evidence on or around the patient if he is deceased.

7. **What questions will you likely be asked of you as more law enforcement officers and crime scene investigators arrive?**

   As mentioned in the chapter, you may be asked to account for everywhere you went and everything you did from the time you arrived at the scene to the time you left the scene. You may be asked to recall the exact path you took walking into the house and toward the patient. How was the patient positioned inside of the room? Did you move the patient? And, if so, where did you touch the patient as you rolled him over? Where else did you go once you left the patient's side? All of these are potential questions that you may be asked by investigators.

8. **How would you document the circumstances of this event in your patient care report?**

   Documentation of what you received in the dispatch information may be important to include because if may illustrate why you staged for law enforcement to secure the scene. Include as much information as you feel is appropriate in this report. From what you saw as you walked into the house to the patient's initial position to the application of the cardiac monitor, all of this information is pertinent. Remember, if you are called to testify about anything regarding the call, a significant length of time may have elapsed since the event. Your documentation may be the only information that can help to refresh your memory.

EMS Patient Care Report (PCR)

Date: 10-10-18	Incident No.: 2786		Nature of Call: Unknown		Location: 1 Ashley River Manor
Dispatched: 1958	**En Route:** 1959	**At Scene:** 2012	**Transport:** N/A	**At Hospital:** N/A	**In Service:** 2112

Patient Information

Age: 50 **Sex:** M **Weight (in kg [lb]):** 100 kg (220 lb)	**Allergies:** None **Medications:** None **Past Medical History:** Depression **Chief Complaint:** Gunshot wound to head

Vital Signs

Time: 2022	BP: N/A	Pulse: 0	Respirations: 0	Spo$_2$: N/A
Time: 2024	BP: N/A	Pulse: 0	Respirations: 0	Spo$_2$: N/A
Time:	BP:	Pulse:	Respirations:	Spo$_2$:

EMS Treatment (circle all that apply)

Oxygen @ _____ L/min via (circle one): NC NRM **Bag-mask device**	Assisted Ventilation	Airway Adjunct	CPR
Defibrillation	**Bleeding Control**	**Bandaging**	**Splinting**	**Other:** Cardiac monitor

Narrative

Staged for law enforcement to secure scene due to possible violent circumstances on scene. After 10 minutes, scene declared safe. Entered to find 50-year-old male prone on the ground in a dining room next to a table. Black shotgun noted to be lying approximately 3 feet to the patient's side by the wall. Large pool of blood surrounding the patient's head. Obvious gunshot wound to the head with exposed brain matter present. Unable to appropriately assess patient due to positioning. Patient rolled from prone position over his right side to the supine position. Patient found to be pulseless and apneic. The cardiac monitor is applied and asystole is noted to be present in all leads. Medical control contacted, findings relayed, and online physician pronounced the patient dead at 2025. Dispatch notified that the patient is deceased as well as time of death as pronounced by medical control. Request was made to notify the coroner. EMS is escorted out of the residence by law enforcement. Chaplains requested for family members on scene. Wife able to provide a history of recent events. The patient's wife reports a recent argument regarding their daughter's boyfriend. The argument escalated as the night progressed. The wife reports the patient was visibly upset and had voiced suicidal ideations. The wife reports a brief struggle occurred when she saw the patient attempting to retrieve a shotgun from their closet. She states she attempted to get her daughter away from the patient as he walked into the dining room with the gun. She reports she heard a loud boom as they reached the front yard. She reports that she screamed for someone to call an ambulance, but she reports she did not go back inside of the residence.
EMS provided a brief statement to law enforcement. Medic 21 returned to service.**End of report**

Prep Kit

▶ Ready for Review

- Emergency medical services (EMS) can be a dangerous profession. Always remember your mission, beyond providing optimal patient care, is to return safely at the end of each shift. An injured paramedic cannot care for patients.
- No community, socioeconomic group, race, or religion is immune to violence. The use of good situational awareness will reduce the potential for you to fall victim to an act of violence while on an emergency medical call.
- Before performing patient care, perform a scene size-up for indicators of potential violence and escape routes. If you feel a scene is not safe, retreat to your ambulance and wait for law enforcement personnel to secure the scene.
- Obvious indicators of violence include calls for shootings, stabbings, or attempted suicides; body language such as clenched fists; and use of profane language or yelling.
- Be aware of the possibility that secondary violence can occur during a call, even if indicators of violence were not present at the outset.
- Familiarize yourself with your agency's standard operating procedures for dealing with potentially violent incidents, and ensure you follow them.
- When you are responding to a vehicle on a road, park your vehicle a minimum of 21 feet (6 m) behind the stopped vehicle, at a 10° angle to the driver's side facing the shoulder of the road. Turn your front wheels all the way to the left; this provides limited protection in the event of gunfire.
- When you approach a standard motor vehicle, turn on your vehicle's high beam light, but do not walk in the spotlight. Approach the vehicle with your abdomen facing the vehicle. Consider whether there may be people hiding in the trunk of the motor vehicle or inside the vehicle before reaching the B post. If the back seat is occupied, do not proceed past the C post.
- As you approach a van, remain clear of the side door of the van. Walk parallel to the van until you are at an approximately 45° angle forward of the A post.
- When a dangerous situation develops, retreat from the scene and alert your dispatcher of the situation, including details such as the number of aggressors involved.
- When you approach a residence, stand to the side of the entry door. Do not stand on the hinged side;

this will provide a view of you as the person inside opens the door.

- When you enter a structure, always identify a primary exit as well as a secondary exit, should the primary exit become inaccessible.
- Clandestine drug laboratories are extremely hazardous. Once such a site is identified, remain clear of it until trained law enforcement and hazardous materials specialists have secured it.
- Gang activity can present hazards to EMS crews. Work with local law enforcement so you are aware of gang-affiliated areas.
- In situations involving an active shooter or sniper, follow law enforcement's direction, even if it means a patient cannot receive care immediately.
- Use cover and concealment if a scene becomes dangerous. Cover includes objects or areas that are difficult or impossible for bullets to penetrate. Concealment includes objects or areas where it is difficult or impossible for you to be seen, but that could still be penetrated by bullets.
- Consider taking a self-defense course to help increase your ability to survive should dangerous situations develop.
- When you are working at a crime scene, make every attempt not to disturb, damage, or potentially alter the scene or physical evidence. Properly and thoroughly document these scenes and the actions you performed.

▶ Vital Vocabulary

active shooter A gunman who has begun to fire on people and is still at large.

clandestine drug laboratories Locations where illegal drugs such as methamphetamine, lysergic acid diethylamide (LSD), ecstasy, and phencyclidine hydrochloride (PCP) are manufactured.

concealment Protection from being seen.

contact and cover A technique that involves one paramedic making contact with the patient to provide care, while the second paramedic obtains patient information, gauges the level of tension, and warns his or her partner at the first sign of trouble.

cover Obstacles that are difficult or impossible for bullets to penetrate.

physical evidence The evidence that ties a suspect or victim to a crime. It may include body materials, objects, and impressions.

primary exit The main means of escape should violence erupt. This is usually the door you used to enter the building.

secondary exit Any other means of egress, including windows and rear doors.

Prep Kit *(continued)*

situational awareness Knowing your surroundings, the people and groups in your environment, and the climate of violence or strife.

tactical paramedics Specially trained paramedics who provide medical care for SWAT team members conducting operations, barricaded patients, patients being held hostage, and other special operations.

testimonial evidence The oral documentation by a witness of his or her perceived facts of a criminal act.

tunnel vision A situation in which a paramedic becomes so completely involved with patient care that he or she fails to see the possibility of physical harm to the patient or other care providers.

▶ References

1. Maguire BJ, Smith S. *Injuries and Fatalities among Emergency Medical Technicians and Paramedics in the United States.* Cambridge Core website. https://www.cambridge.org/core/journals/prehospital-and-disaster-medicine/article/injuries-and-fatalities-among-emergency-medical-technicians-and-paramedics-in-the-united-states/50afa4d33a190aaeb7b48a0637c3c4e3. Published May 9, 2013. Accessed September 25, 2016.
2. National Youth Gang Survey Analysis. *Measuring the Extent of Gang Problems.* https://www.nationalgangcenter.gov/survey-analysis/measuring-the-extent-of-gang-problems. Accessed September 25, 2016.
3. Federal Bureau of Investigation. *2011 National Gang Threat Assessment—Emerging Trends.* https://www.fbi.gov/stats-services/publications/2011-national-gang-threat-assessment. Accessed April 13, 2017.
4. American College of Surgeons. *The Hartford Consensus.* https://www.facs.org/about-acs/hartford-consensus. Accessed April 13, 2017.
5. Stop the Bleed. U.S. Department of Homeland Security website. https://www.dhs.gov/stopthebleed. Published October 11, 2016. Accessed May 18, 2017.

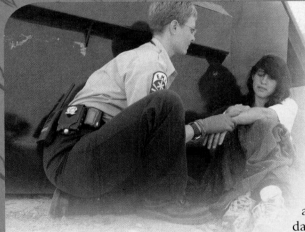

Assessment in Action

You are dispatched to a subdivision for a victim of a fight. The dispatcher informs you there were reports of four to five people fighting in the street. Two of them got into a vehicle that crashed into a pole across the street from the address you are given. The other people went into the home. As you arrive, you look at the front of the vehicle and see moderate damage to the front of the driver's side A post. Inside the vehicle are two occupants who are actively yelling at each other. You look at the residence and find the front door is open. There are two large windows and you see no one is inside. Law enforcement personnel are arriving on scene right behind you.

1. If you get distracted by the vehicle's occupants that are shouting at one another, you run the risk of:

   A. concentration.
   B. tunnel vision.
   C. exclusionary.
   D. concealment.

2. When you approach the vehicle, which post on a standard passenger vehicle should you approach first?

   A. A
   B. B
   C. C
   D. D

Assessment *in Action* (continued)

3. When you enter this residence, the door you enter through is called the:

    A. primary exit.
    B. secondary exit.
    C. front exit.
    D. back exit.

4. After you enter the house, you hear a large commotion from behind you that is moving toward the front door of the house. You realize you may have to exit through the side window. This would be referred to as using a(n):

    A. engaging tactic.
    B. secondary exit.
    C. concealment.
    D. diversion.

5. When you return to the vehicle, you assess the patients in the vehicle. What is the most effective tool you can use to keep out of trouble in a dispute?

    A. Your vehicle
    B. Your partner
    C. Your radio
    D. Your voice

6. If your partner has been standing closer to the ambulance, he may be able to contact help or notify others of increasing tension and a threat of violence. What technique is this called?

    A. Contact and cover
    B. Contact and assess
    C. Concealment and cover
    D. Cover and call

7. You see someone emerging from the residence with a gun and pointing it in your general direction. Your first reaction should be to find:

    A. concealment.
    B. contact.
    C. cover.
    D. shadows.

8. What is the difference between testimonial evidence and physical evidence?

9. In what types of situations would a rescue task force be beneficial?

10. What can you do to help yourself maintain good situational awareness when operating around a crime scene?

Career Development

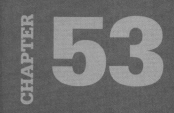
Career Development

National EMS Education Standard Competencies

There are no National EMS Education Standard Competencies for this chapter.

Knowledge Objectives

1. Explain the role of emergency medical technicians (EMTs) and paramedics as described by the Bureau of Labor Statistics. (p 2519)
2. Identify future job growth for EMTs and paramedics as predicted by the Bureau of Labor Statistics. (pp 2519-2520, 2521-2524)
3. Explain the importance of career development. (pp 2520-2521)
4. List the nontraditional specialties that paramedics may need in the future to fill evolving roles in the health care system. (pp 2521-2522)
5. Describe the changes occurring in the US health care system that impact the role and potential job growth of the paramedic. (p 2524)
6. Identify the role that the paramedic can play in the evolving US health care system. (p 2525)
7. Describe at least five strategies from industry leaders for developing a long-term career as a paramedic. (pp 2521, 2524, 2526)

Skills Objectives

There are no skills objectives for this chapter.

▎ Introduction

Your achievement as a paramedic starts the first chapter of the rest of your career—a career with unlimited possibilities in the fields of health care and public safety. The US Bureau of Labor Statistics reported 244,960 emergency medical technician (EMT) and paramedic positions in 2016.[1] This number is projected to grow 24% from 2014 to 2024, which is faster than any other occupation.[2] According to the Bureau, the top five industries with the highest levels of employment include (1) other ambulatory health care services (eg, ambulance services), (2) local government, (3) general medical and surgical hospitals, (4) other support services, and (5) outpatient care centers.[1] As of May 2016, states with the highest employment level of emergency medical services (EMS) providers included (1) Texas, (2) California, (3) New York, (4) Illinois, and (5) Pennsylvania.[1]

Examples of factors influencing the continued need for paramedics include the following:

- Growth in the middle-aged and older adult population and age-related health emergencies in these age groups.
- The increased lifespan for patients with special heath care needs including patients with chronic or debilitating conditions who are living at home and who are dependent on technology.
- The increased demonstrated success of advanced life support providers in administering life-saving interventions in the prehospital environment. Previously, prehospital providers were less able to intervene in meaningful ways to improve health and save lives.
- The increase in the roles, responsibilities, and education levels of prehospital providers and the increase in the number of conditions

in which they can effectively intervene, creating an increased need for providers with a higher level of education, preparation, and training.

- The increasing number of specialized medical facilities and the need for transport and transfer of patients with specific conditions to these facilities for ongoing care.
- The creation of nontraditional roles for paramedics. Some of these roles are within the larger health care system (eg, emergency departments [EDs], urgent care clinics) while others are in locations such as cruise ships, Hollywood movie sets, oil rigs, and schools.
- The increase in the number of suicides, the increase in the availability of lethal drugs on the streets, and the rise in violent crimes and terrorist activities.

As a paramedic, your future can take many paths. This chapter will help you embark on a career in the amazing field of EMS career opportunities.

Words of Wisdom

"We have seen individuals move on in many different positions from Vice President of Oil companies to a Director of Safety and Compliance at a major sporting venue. Current needs in departments and companies are EMS/Emergency Operations Center Liaisons, Homeland Security Liaisons, EMS Planner for Operations and Special Events, Community Outreach, Public Information Officer, Clinical Officer (Quality Improvement), Program Manager or Specialist, EMS Chief of Staff, Human Resource or Compliance Officer, Logistics Director, Finance Director, Hospital/Public Safety/Administrative Liaison."

Carl A. Flores
EMS Chief, City of New Orleans
New Orleans, Louisiana

The Importance of Career Development

A career plan that includes your short- and long-term goals and the steps you need to take to achieve those goals is important.[3] You may have already achieved one of your goals as a newly certified paramedic. Are other goals in your plan? Do you want to specialize your training and become a flight paramedic? Do you want to pursue an advanced degree to lead your EMS organization? A career plan will help ensure a long and fulfilling career in EMS. Only you can determine your personal goals and create a plan to achieve them.

The four components of career development include: self-assessment, career exploration, career identification, and creating an action plan.[4] Of these four components, self-assessment and creating an action plan are key for dedicated EMS professionals.

▶ Self-assessment

You'll need to assess your current skills honestly to know where to begin making decisions about your personal career development, which may include enlisting opinions and advice from friends and mentors. Are there areas that you want to improve? For example, would you like to be able to communicate more effectively in front of a large audience? Self-assessment, however, is not only about targeting areas of personal improvement. You also need to determine your strengths, your interests, and your values. Your initial ideas from your self-assessment will help you structure your goals.

▶ Your Action Plan

Achieving goals requires action. Make a list of achievable short- and long-term goals and the steps you want to take to achieve your personal goals. Determine the organizations that can provide you with help in areas of your interest Table 53-1. Periodically reevaluate these goals and change them to keep the goals personal and

Table 53-1	Contact Organizations for EMS Providers for Career Development

- National Association of Emergency Medical Technicians (www.naemt.org)
- National Association of State EMS Officials (www.nasemso.org)
- National Association of EMS Educators (www.naemse.org)
- Association for Critical Care Transport (www.acctforpatients.org)
- National Association of Tactical Medics (www.naotm.com)
- International Association of Flight & Critical Care Paramedics (www.iafccp.org)
- Wilderness Medical Society (https://wms.org)
- National EMS Management Association (www.nemsma.org)
- National Emergency Management Association (www.nemaweb.org)
- International Police Mountain Bike Association (www.ipmba.org)
- Health Industry Representatives Association (www.hira.org)

relevant. The growth in career opportunities in EMS will make updating your action plan an exciting part of your journey.

Words of Wisdom

"I made a decision early in life to make EMS my career. I never perceived it as a job, but a calling, a highly skilled hobby I wanted to master, a passion for the ability to impact lives (patients and providers) and save a few people (patients and providers) along the way. My father was an EMS innovator who never saw a limit to what he could design, achieve, or affect. He was my first, and best role model. My best advice for students and new graduates is to adopt a role model, never rely on machines alone to make clinical decisions, and stay hungry for education and continue that education constantly in this amazing (and ever-changing) field, because no two patients present exactly the same way, new challenges will always confront you, and those challenges can only be confronted, analyzed, and defeated if you are constantly ahead of the curve. Some of your ability comes from experience, but most of it comes from constant learning and muscle memory."

A.J. Heightman, MPA, EMT-P
Editor-in-Chief, Journal of Emergency
Medical Services

Words of Wisdom

"Your learning has just commenced and not ended with completion of the paramedic program. Competence and relevance have expiration dates. Make it your life's mission to learn something new every day. It could be in medicine, response strategies, finance, management, or art history . . . take the opportunity to learn and expand your horizons and professional prowess daily. After several years in the discipline it is easy to become complacent and believe you have earned a street PhD, but remember your advancement within this very diverse discipline could be helped or hurt by a college degree. Pursue the completion of your baccalaureate degree to help you round out the body of knowledge and capabilities you will acquire. Maybe consider continuing your education at the graduate and doctoral levels. Each of these accomplishments will provide you the next step in the long road of this great profession."

Paul Maniscalco
Dep. Chief / Paramedic FDNY (ret.)
President Emeritus International Association
of EMS Chiefs
Past President National Association of EMTs

Growth and Opportunities in EMS

Specialty roles within the EMS service delivery model offer avenues of growth within the system. The following specialties are examples of career development opportunities.

▶ Mobile Integrated Health Care Providers/Community Paramedics

The role of **mobile integrated health care providers/community paramedics (MIHPs/CPs)** differs from the traditional role of the paramedic because the MIHP/CP's focus is on working with the patient in the home to prevent conditions from escalating into threats requiring emergency care **Figure 53-1**. MIHP/CP programs across the United States have grown exponentially over the past few years, due primarily to issues such as reducing preventable ED visits, reducing preventable hospital readmissions, and the safe navigation of patients to destinations more suitable for medical care than EDs.[5] Ultimately, the primary goal of an MIHP/CP is to get the right patient to the right resource and right treatment with the right tools at the right time. An MIHP/CP is essential for providing patient-centered

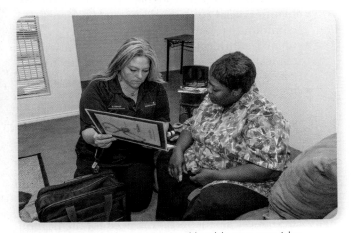

Figure 53-1 A mobile integrated health care provider assisting a patient in her home.
© Bob Strickland Photography.

care and must develop a plethora of knowledge as well as a high skill base to treat the patient directly or navigate the patient to the appropriate resource. This new professional role is exciting and continuing to grow internationally!

While the training requirements are still evolving, MIHPs/CPs generally undergo additional training, either through a college-based MIHP/CP training program or other specially designed educational curricula by local agencies. The training focuses primarily on pathophysiology, public health, social assessment needs, and preventive medicine. A career as an MIHP/CP takes a special type of individual who is able to communicate with patients and with a wide range of professionals within the health care community. The MIHP/CP can identify, address, treat, or navigate all aspects of a patient's needs—nutritional, social, clinical, and psychologic. The CP-C certification is offered from the international board of specialty certification.

The general responsibilities of an MIHP/CP are to:

- Function as a field paramedic, performing direct advanced-life-support care activities
- Be team oriented and able to communicate and work effectively and efficiently with other members of the health care team to coordinate care for enrolled patients
- Function in nontraditional settings and provide nonemergency care with a preventive and long-term focus
- Monitor and manage chronic disease in the home setting
- Provide wellness checks
- Obtain patient medication inventory and determine adherence to recommended guidelines.
- Communicate with multiple agencies to facilitate continuity of care
- Participate in data collection and research
- Identify clinical barriers that a patient may have in navigating health care needs
- Identify social barriers and navigate patients to community resources for assistance
- Identify nutritional needs and refer client to clinical dietitians to further assist in daily intake needs
- Identify psychologic needs; provide navigation to resources therefore eliminating barriers the patient may encounter

The primary role of an MIHP/CP is to assist patients, such as those who frequently use the EMS system for health care needs that can be managed outside the ED, in managing their health care needs more effectively. An MIHP/CP generally helps patients access and use primary care, educates patients on the need for medication and diet adherence, and assists patients in managing chronic illness. In addition to these roles, the MIHP/CP may also be credentialed to provide point-of-care blood testing and relay findings to the patient's physician while modifying the patient care plan based on the results. The MIHP/CP may implement treatment modalities such as in-home diuresis for patients in heart failure, antibiotic administration, breathing treatments for patients with chronic obstructive pulmonary disease, or dextrose administration for patients with diabetes. The MIHP/CP may also modify a patient's blood pressure medications with guidance of a physician and change supplements and diets after working with a clinical dietitian. The MIHP/CP may work with a variety of specialists, including cardiologists, psychiatrists/psychologists, clinical dietitians, case managers, nephrologists, neurologists, and orthopaedic

surgeons. After in-home treatment is completed, the patient is referred for definitive care with a physician's office or at a clinic, avoiding an unnecessary visit to the ED. The use of MIHPs/CPs for patient assessments and treatment coordination with the patient's physician can effectively reduce the need for ambulance transports or ED visits. In some parts of the country, MIHPs/CPs arrange for patient transportation to physician or clinics visits and help staff at fixed site clinics or even roving mobile clinics, bringing valuable primary or specialty care to areas that lack this resource. MIHP/CP programs address the specific needs of the community. The career positions in some areas are fully comprehensive care providers whereas in other areas the positions provide navigational capacities. Knowledge of the MIHP/CP principles are essential as you move up your career ladder. Mobile integrated healthcare may involve teams of physicians, pharmacists, physician assistants, nurse practitioners, nurse case managers, social workers, and paramedics. Understanding the growth potential and broad knowledge base is essential to understanding a full patient-centered outcome in mobile integrated healthcare.

MIHP/CPs may also serve as an adjunct member of an agency's disaster response team. These team members are valuable to the large-scale disaster response team and have an understanding of the long-term patient needs to be addressed acutely and subacutely during the response.

▶ Critical Care Paramedic

One of the most common specialty roles for paramedics, the **critical care paramedic (CCP)**, is sometimes referred to as a critical care transport professional (CCTP). Although the recommended educational qualifications for CCTPs vary, they must be able to provide care at the same level and in most cases, at a higher level, than their noncritical care or emergent transport counterparts. In addition, CCTPs must be educated and proficient in advanced practice procedures, which may include the following:

- Advanced airway management with mechanical ventilators
- Administration of vasoactive intravenous medications
- Hemodynamic monitoring
- Monitoring of chest tubes and intracranial pressure monitors
- Interpretation of laboratory data
- Management of patients on intra-aortic balloon pumps or heart bypass machines
- Management of neonatal patients
- Utilization of sonography and medical diagnostic tools

Training programs typically consist of a formal course of study, clinical internships, and a certification exam administered either by a national certification agency, such as the International Board of Specialty Certification or other local regulatory bodies. Some agencies are using CCTPs in addition to 9-1-1 team responses for highly critical incidents.

These paramedics, with their expanded scope of knowledge, are providing the highest level of clinical critical care in the field. Recently there have been agencies utilizing CCTPs to assist with mobile stroke units, and some are performing extracorporeal membrane oxygenation in the field.[6,7] These paramedics must undergo significant amounts of additional training and continuing education to keep the proficiency of their skills to par with the physicians that perform these skills/procedures on a daily basis in the hospital setting. Agencies also utilize CCTPs as a dual or additional member of the MIHP/CP team. For example, CCTPs may provide episodic nonscheduled responses to navigate patients to the appropriate care or treatment team.

▶ Flight Paramedic

Flight paramedics work as part of an air rescue team that provides either on-scene care in remote field settings or interfacility transports from one clinical setting to another **Figure 53-2**. Typically, flight paramedics are thought of as working helicopter EMS programs, but flight paramedics also work on jet aircraft and other fixed-wing aircraft that transport patients over great distances. A career as a flight paramedic may require the following skills:

- Aircraft fundamentals, safety, and survival
- Flight physiology
- Trauma management
- Advanced airway management
- Neurologic emergency management
- Critical cardiac care
- Pediatric/neonatal management
- Toxic exposure management

Flight paramedics and CCTPs undergo many of the same training and clinical continuing education hours. The difference in their training is the understanding of flight physiology and survival.

Helicopter paramedics in Maryland provide police intercept.[8] Paramedics or troopers in this agency must gain

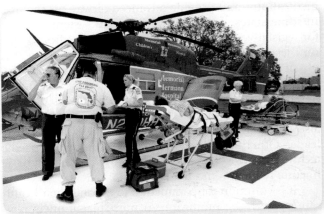

Figure 53-2 A flight paramedic may provide emergency medical care to patients who need to be transported quickly over short distances.
Courtesy of Ed Edahl/FEMA.

experience as a ground trooper prior to being accepted as part of the helicopter flight crew. Another important part of a flight paramedic's education includes learning how to rescue and survive without resources for up to 48 hours or longer if the aircraft has to land or is unable to fly because of inclement weather. Flight paramedics must be able to not only provide high levels of critical care but also be able to provide these services in austere environments.

▶ Bicycle Emergency Response Paramedic

Bicycle paramedics provide EMS standby assistance to events with large crowds or where standard ambulances or transport capability is not possible.

Bicycle emergency response teams have the following skills:

- Basic nutrition and physical fitness
- Bicycle maintenance/repairs
- Cycling fundamentals of all terrains
- Public safety cycling response

Bicycle emergency response is crucial to the success of a first response in areas where vehicles cannot be used. Bicycle paramedics undergo a significant amount of training, including working with other bicycle professionals such as bicycle police units. A bicycle paramedic must be in good physical condition and able to maintain long-term physical fitness. Training and certification is provided by the International Police Mountain Bike Association. In addition to providing emergency care at special events, bicycle emergency response teams can work full time in agencies that provide care in metropolitan downtown areas or large parks.

▶ Tactical Paramedic

Tactical paramedics have undergone additional training to learn how to practice medicine while in the "hot" zone. These paramedics generally train with and work as members of a specialty trained team that includes law enforcement officers. They are able to provide rapid basic and advanced life support to officers or patients when the situation is considered unsafe for traditional paramedics.

Tactical paramedics have gained skills and credentialing pertaining to:

- Combat casualty assessment
- Stabilization and evacuation of patients in hostile and austere environments
- Tactical principles, triage, and operational medicine
- Weapons training and management
- Rescue techniques
- Body armor and tactical specialty

Tactical paramedics may work in military combat settings or civilian settings as part of special response teams such as Special Weapons and Tactics (SWAT) teams. In some cases, law enforcement personnel who are cross-trained as EMS providers can serve in this role. In other models, EMS personnel may receive specialty training from local law enforcement officials and become part of the special response law enforcement team. Many paramedics are highly sought after in law enforcement capacity. Due to the recent increase in violence and terrorist activity, law enforcement agencies find a need to fill their ranks with certified and experienced health care professionals. These paramedics also have specialty equipment, such as combat tourniquets, to enable rapid treatment of the injuries sustained in combat.

Tactical paramedics may also serve as training instructors for the law enforcement agency in areas such as "self-care" and "buddy-care." Some agencies also have employed these combat-trained paramedics to specialty units as in Fort Worth, TX where they have EMT/paramedic-trained officers to deploy for any incident, even if SWAT is not deployed.

▶ Wilderness Paramedic

Wilderness paramedics provide trauma care and other emergency services in remote and frontier areas. This role may not only be clinically demanding due to the extended length of time between injury and illness and definitive care, but could also be physically demanding. Wilderness paramedics must apply the principles and concepts of urban and traditional emergency medicine in an austere environment, for an extended period of time, and with limited resources.

Responsibilities of a wilderness paramedic may include:

- Tropical and travel medicine
- High-altitude and mountaineering medicine
- Expedition medicine
- Safety, rescue, and evacuation
- Preventive medicine, field sanitation, and hygiene
- General environmental medicine
- Improvised medicine
- Survival skills
- Disaster and humanitarian assistance

Wilderness EMS is one of the most exciting yet challenging parts of an EMS career. Wilderness paramedics must be able to adapt and overcome challenges in any environment. Training for wilderness EMS may take place in the most austere environments, such as in high-elevation mountainous regions of the country or deserts, under all weather conditions. Wilderness paramedics may learn how to manufacture a splint and transport device for a patient who has suffered a traumatic injury while backpacking. The paramedic must be able to stabilize the patient, secure the patient, transport the patient, and deliver the patient to another responding agency with only the resources in a backpack and from nature. Physical and mental endurance is critical. Some wilderness guides obtain certification to enhance their marketability. These invaluable skills are truly the difference between life, death, and suffering in the remote environment.

■ Growth and Opportunities in the Larger Health Care System

▶ Clinical

The changing dynamics of the health care system have created additional career opportunities for paramedics. While it is true that EMTs and paramedics have often worked in hospitals and clinics, in the past these roles have been generally limited to a technician role, such as an emergency department technician, who provided basic assessments, vital signs, and patient transport within the facility. However, the need for clinical care in an era of managing scarce resources has led hospitals and health care systems to move paramedics into clinical roles. Paramedics in the ED can start intravenous lines, administer medications, and provide advanced airway procedures. In some states, such as Texas, hospital systems pushed for legislative changes that allowed paramedics to take on these new clinical roles under the supervision of a physician.[9] This clinical role for paramedics in Texas not only applies to hospitals, but any medical facility such as freestanding EDs, urgent care centers, and clinics, opening an entire new career path for paramedics. Some agencies also add the additional responsibilities of being a code leader. Others allow paramedics to become orthopaedic technicians, who are able to perform sutures and basic fracture reduction in the ED.

It is common for paramedics to expand their health care careers by becoming nurses, nurse practitioners, physician assistants, or even physicians. In many EMS systems, paramedics continue their education to become physicians while still maintaining their paramedic licensure, returning to the EMS profession as medical directors. In fact, physician assistants originated as navy hospital corpsmen, similar to paramedics, who underwent considerable medical training while serving in the military.[10] Clinical experience is a highly valued skill on applications to medical school.

▶ Health Care Administration

Hospital EMS Coordinator

Hospital and health care systems are rapidly becoming more aware of the need for enhanced relationships with EMS providers. They often recruit paramedics to serve as EMS coordinators for their health care system—a vital link between the hospital and the EMS community. EMS coordinators typically serve as a bridge in communication and relationships by offering patient outcome feedback, learning what EMS may desire from this hospital system, resolving any conflict between EMS and the hospital, as well as offering continuing education to EMS providers in the area **Figure 53-3**. These providers take the experience they have gained in the field to create a level of communication that is invaluable to the EMS agencies they serve. Programs in some areas are able to provide clinical rotations for continuing education such as rotations in a cardiac catheterization lab and interventional radiology labs.

Emergency Management Coordinator

EMS professionals are often tapped for roles as emergency management coordinators. As hospitals have become more involved in the mitigation of major disasters, the need for a position dedicated to emergency management within the hospital has become more apparent. Emergency management coordinators assist hospitals with disaster planning, drills, and training on the concepts of a hospital incident command system.[11] The same is true for local jurisdictions such as cities or counties. The unique skill set derived by paramedics in the EMS setting often translates well into emergency preparedness positions in hospitals and local government. These professionals utilize Federal Emergency Management Agency standards, which are similar to those in incident command systems. A local school of public health may value the experience paramedic educators can bring by involving them in an annual interdisciplinary, interagency response training exercise training future public health professionals on the effects of, for example, a pandemic.

Transportation Coordinator

Hospitals and health care systems face increasing need to navigate patients within the system. Navigation often includes being able to transport patients effectively from one facility to another within the system in the safest, least expensive way possible. An EMT or paramedic with experience in patient transportation and EMS care is an ideal candidate to serve as a transportation coordinator. Many hospital systems have developed extensive transport coordination centers to receive patient transfer requests from all system participants. These coordination centers review the clinical needs of the patient during transfer, determine the most appropriate method of transfer, and contact the best provider for the transport.

Job Description—Hospital EMS Coordinator

Position Summary

Acme Medical Center EMS liaison serves as a liaison between the hospital, EMS workers, fire departments, and other providers of emergency services. The primary responsibility of this role is to develop a business plan, driving service line growth, and improving operations in terms of quality process. In addition, this position is responsible for ensuring collaboration across all care settings within the facility as it relates to EMS and disaster preparedness. Job may include direct supervision of students at the discretion of the area supervisor. Direct supervision means the primary caregiver is readily available to the student throughout the shift.

Qualifications/Position Requirements

- **Licensure/Certification/Registration:** BLS required. ACLS, PALS, and Certified Paramedic (National Registry and/or local) preferred.
- **Education:** A bachelor's degree in a health-related field such as nursing or emergency medical services is preferred.
- **Experience:** Experience working in a hospital emergency department as well as familiarity with other local emergency resources, agencies, and services is crucial to this position.
- **Knowledge, Skills, Abilities and/or Other Attributes:** Strong interpersonal and relationship-building skills, team facilitation, and project management. Needs good organization and time-management skills.

Figure 53-3 Sample position description for a hospital EMS coordinator.

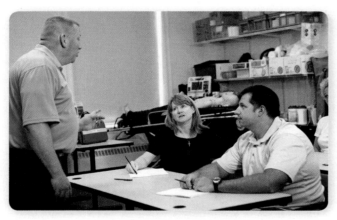

Figure 53-4 Emergency medical technicians and paramedics may be credentialed to teach didactic and practical skills in the classroom.

© Jones & Bartlett Learning.

▶ EMS Educator

The growth in the need for EMTs and paramedics will require education and certification programs to train EMTs and paramedics to meet this demand. Paramedics with a passion for teaching will find many opportunities as an EMS educator **Figure 53-4**. Many EMT and paramedic courses are college-based. Other educational programs may be taught at a local EMS agency. In addition to the entry-level courses, EMTs and paramedics may become credentialed instructors for many of the specialty certification courses.

Institutions of higher education may value paramedic assistance with the education of future physician assistants and physicians. Students are assigned to an MIHP/CP program where they learn about effective patient communication, how to identify patient barriers to health care, and health care navigation skills as well as the business model of mobile integrated health care.

Other opportunities as an educator include being able to author textbooks and present at conferences. One of the best ways to maintain interest in your profession is to train and educate others to provide the same level of care you provide. Also, while writing and preparing for conference presentations, you must stay on top of trends in EMS and in the field of medicine.

Regardless of the course setting, the demand for effective EMS instructors will continue to be strong.

▶ EMS Agency Leader

Career advancement within EMS is also prevalent. Paramedics in EMS-based fire departments often move up the ranks to Lieutenant, Captain, EMS Chief, and even Fire Chief positions. The same advancement occurs in nonfire agencies as well. It is not unusual to trace the roots of many EMS Agency CEOs back to field EMS positions as EMTs or paramedics. To prepare for advancement, set personal goals and understand the steps needed to achieve these goals. Many current agency leaders encourage field providers interested in advancement within the agency to seek higher education degrees, such as a bachelor's degree or even master's degree. Other educational opportunities are provided internally at many agencies. If components of EMS management interest you, seek a mentor to learn how he or she achieved success in the field.

Many EMS agency leaders also serve on various community boards and task forces. Participation presents an opportunity for the EMS agency to help evaluate, develop, advocate, coordinate, and deliver public health needs to the community. Interagency collaboration to develop community programs helps prevent injury and illness, which is probably one of the reasons you have chosen being a paramedic.

▶ EMS Researcher

The EMS delivery system has only sporadically conducted peer-reviewed research to prove the efficacy of clinical modalities, deployment strategies, or even whether or not "EMS" makes a demonstrable difference in patient outcomes. This type of research is invaluable to furthering your chosen profession. Perhaps one of the reasons there is such limited peer-reviewed publications is that EMTs and paramedics are not well prepared to conduct clinical research. Becoming an EMS researcher requires a specific skill set, but one that you can achieve through attending conferences to learn how to conduct EMS research and by partnering with research teams from institutions of higher learning or health care systems that have research divisions. These professionals are given the opportunity to publish research, participate on institutional review boards, and evaluate the effectiveness of EMS and clinical care. The integration of EMS into the institutes of higher learning keeps EMS at the forefront of health care internationally.

▶ EMS and Health Care Sales Representative

Training and experience in the field of EMS as a paramedic exposes you to countless products, devices, and even medications that have significant benefit to providers and the patients they serve. One of the career paths you may choose may involve medical sales. Some paramedics are sales reps for manufacturers of automated external defibrillators, ambulances, ambulance stretchers, or even pharmaceuticals. These paramedics utilize their experience to develop a relationship with EMS agencies to bring state of the art technology and products to the EMS forefront. Some of these professionals also have the ability to work with research and development teams of their agency to make products more effective for the EMS provider. Sales representatives may serve as a liaison from the company to the EMS providers to learn about EMS trends and needs, therefore allowing the company to develop technology, tools, and devices that bring value to patient care.

■ Making EMS a Lifelong Career

This chapter has mentioned only some of the many important roles you can pursue within EMS and the broader health care system. Other areas beyond those discussed here, into which a paramedic's career can develop, include the roles of patient advocate, prevention specialist, driving instructor, and writer or editor, among others. Visualize and strategize your career dreams in EMS. Make plans to achieve your goals and motivate yourself daily to make them a reality. Seek out peers who inspire you to take on new challenges.

Regardless of the career path you choose, you will gain invaluable career skills as a paramedic. Understanding how to remain calm in chaotic environments, understanding emergency management and preparedness, how to effectively communicate, and self-care will elevate you to becoming the best at who you want to become. There is no limit to the number of skills and amount of experience you can gain as a paramedic. Your chance of lifelong success and job satisfaction during your career in EMS relies on you.

Prep Kit

▶ Ready for Review

- The US Bureau of Labor Statistics reported 244,960 emergency medical technician and paramedic positions in 2016. The number of paramedic positions is projected to grow 24% from 2014 to 2024, which is faster than any other occupation.
- A career plan that includes your short- and long-term goals and the steps you need to take to achieve those goals is important.
- The four components of career development include: self-assessment, career exploration, career identification, and creating an action plan. Of these four components, self-assessment and creating an action plan are key for dedicated emergency medical services (EMS) professionals.
- Growth and opportunities in EMS can be found in the following specialty areas: mobile integrated health care provider/community paramedic, critical care paramedic, flight paramedic, tactical paramedic, bicycle paramedic, and wilderness paramedic.

- Growth and opportunities in the larger health care system include the following: clinical roles in the emergency department, health care administration, emergency management coordinator, EMS educator, EMS agency leader, EMS researcher, and health care sales representative.
- EMS can be a rewarding, lifelong career if you develop a career plan with your personal goals in mind.

▶ Vital Vocabulary

critical care paramedic (CCP) A specialty role for paramedics, in which the paramedic is trained to provide advanced care and transport for critically injured or ill patients; also called a critical care transport professional (CCTP).

flight paramedics Paramedics who work as part of an air rescue team that provides either on-scene care in remote field settings or interfacility transports from one clinical setting to another.

mobile integrated health care providers/community paramedics (MIHPs/CPs) Paramedics whose primary role is to assist patients, such as those who frequently use the EMS system for health care needs that can

Prep Kit *(continued)*

be managed outside the emergency department, in managing their health care needs more effectively.

tactical paramedics Paramedics who may work in military combat settings or civilian settings as part of special response teams such as special weapons and tactics (SWAT) teams.

wilderness paramedics Paramedics who provide trauma care and other emergency services in remote and frontier areas.

► References

1. Occupational employment statistics: Occupational employment and wages, May 2016 29-2041 Emergency Medical Technicians and Paramedics. US Department of Labor, Bureau of Statistics website. https://www.bls.gov/oes/current/oes292041.htm. Updated March 31, 2017. Accessed April 28, 2017.
2. Occupational outlook handbook, 2016-17 edition, EMTs and paramedics. U.S. Department of Labor, Bureau of Labor Statistics website. http://www.bls.gov/ooh/healthcare/emts-and-paramedics.htm. Accessed April 28, 2017.
3. Cebollero C. How to attain your EMS career goals. EMS1 website. https://www.ems1.com/ems-management/articles/2078390-How-to-attain-your-EMS-career-goals/. Published January 9, 2015. Accessed April 12, 2017.
4. The career planning process. Career Profiles website. http://www.careerprofiles.info/the-career-planning-process.html. Accessed April 5, 2017.
5. Iezzoni LI, Dorner SC, Ajayi T. Community paramedicine—addressing questions as programs expand. *N Engl J Med.* 2016;374(12):1107-1109.
6. Arlt M, Philipp A, Voelkel S, et al. Out-of-hospital extracorporeal life support for cardiac arrest: a case report. *Resuscitation.* 2011;82(9):1243-1245.
7. Peek GJ. Community extracorporeal life support for cardiac arrest: when should it be used? *Resuscitation.* 2011;82(9):1117.
8. State trooper/flight paramedic. Maryland State Police website. http://mdsp.maryland.gov/Careers/Pages?TrooperMedic.aspx. Accessed May 8, 2017.
9. Health—emergency services and personnel. Texas Legislature Online website. http://www.capitol.state.tx.us/BillLookup/History.aspx?LegSess=84R&Bill=HB2020. Accessed April 14, 2017.
10. US Navy hospital corpsmen. Physician Assistant History Society website. https://pahx.org/gallery/+US-navy-hospital-corpsmen/. Accessed May 8, 2017.
11. Emergency management. FEMA Center for Domestic Preparedness website. https://cdp.dhs.gov/find-training/emergency-management. Accessed April 14, 2017.

Glossary: Volume 2

6-feet rule A guideline to follow regarding the distance to place between oneself and a person who sneezes or coughs, to avoid exposure to germs.

6 Ps of musculoskeletal assessment Pain, Paralysis, Parasthesias, Pulselessness, Pallor, and Pressure.

abandonment Termination of medical care for the patient without giving the patient sufficient opportunity to find another suitable health care professional to take over his or her medical treatment; in the context of abuse and neglect, a type of child maltreatment in which a parent or guardian physically leaves a child without regard to the child's health, safety, or welfare.

abortion Expulsion of the fetus, from any cause, before 20 weeks' gestation.

abrasion An injury in which a portion of the body is denuded of the epidermis by scraping or rubbing.

abruptio placenta A premature separation of the placenta from the wall of the uterus.

absence seizures A type of seizure characterized by a brief lapse of attention during which the patient may stare and not respond; formerly known as a petit mal seizure.

absorption The process by which the molecules of a substance are moved from the site of entry or administration into systemic circulation; in the context of decontamination, a type of decontamination that is done with large pads that the hazardous materials team uses to soak up liquid and remove it from the patient.

acceleration (a) The rate of change in velocity; speeding up.

accountability system A method of accounting for all personnel at an emergency incident and ensuring only those with specific assignments are permitted to work within the various zones.

acrocyanosis A decrease in the amount of oxygen delivered to the extremities. The hands and feet turn blue because of narrowing (constriction) of small arterioles (tiny arteries) toward the end of the arms and legs.

active compression-decompression CPR A manual technique that involves compressing the chest and then actively pulling it back up to its neutral position or beyond (decompression); may increase the amount of blood that returns to the heart and, thus, the amount of blood ejected from the heart during the compression phase.

active shooter A gunman who has begun to fire on people and is still at large.

acute angle-closure glaucoma (AACG) Increased intraocular pressure that leads to ocular pain and decreased visual acuity. Sudden onset is a medical emergency.

acute lung injury A condition in which lung tissue is damaged, characterized by hypoxemia, low lung volume, and pulmonary edema.

acute mountain sickness (AMS) An altitude illness characterized by headache plus at least one of the following: fatigue or weakness, gastrointestinal symptoms (nausea, vomiting, or anorexia), dizziness or light-headedness, or difficulty sleeping.

acute radiation syndrome The clinical course that usually begins within hours of exposure to a radiation source. Symptoms include nausea, vomiting, diarrhea, fatigue, fever, and headache. The long-term symptoms are dose related and are hematopoietic and gastrointestinal in nature.

adnexa The surrounding structures and accessories of an organ; for the eye, these parts include the eyelids, lashes, and lacrimal structures.

adult protective services (APS) An organization that investigates cases involving abuse and neglect and provides case management services in some cases.

aerobic metabolism Metabolism that can proceed only in the presence of oxygen.

after-action report (AAR) The official internal report of the entire event, such as a disaster, which should contain the facts of the incident reflected in a chronologic, accurate manner.

afterdrop Continued fall in core body temperature after a victim of hypothermia has been removed from a cold environment, due at least in part to the return of cold blood from the body surface to the body core.

afterload The pressure gradient in the aorta against which the left ventricle of the heart must pump; an increase in this pressure can decrease cardiac output.

aircraft transport Fixed-wing aircraft and helicopters that have been modified for medical care; used to evacuate and transport patients with life-threatening injuries to treatment facilities.

all-hazards approach The act of conducting comprehensive preplanning that will apply to any disaster.

alpha radiation A type of energy that is emitted from a strong radiologic source. It is the least harmful penetrating type of radiation and cannot travel fast or through most objects.

alternative power vehicle A vehicle powered by energy other than petroleum-based fuel, or a vehicle that relies on a combination of petroleum and another fuel or energy source for power.

altitude illnesses Conditions caused by the effects from hypobaric (low atmospheric pressure) hypoxia on the central nervous system and pulmonary systems as a result of unacclimatized people ascending to altitude; range from acute mountain sickness to high-altitude cerebral edema and high-altitude pulmonary edema.

alveoli The air sacs at the end of the bronchioles in the lungs, in which the exchange of oxygen and carbon dioxide takes place; also, small pits or cavities, such as the bony sockets for the teeth that reside in the mandible and maxilla; (singular, *alveolus*).

Alzheimer disease A progressive organic condition in which neurons die, causing dementia.

ammonium nitrate A commonly used industrial-grade fertilizer that is not in itself dangerous to handle or transport, but when mixed with fuel and other components, forms an extremely explosive compound.

amniotic fluid A clear, slightly yellow, watery fluid that surrounds the fetus and provides it a weightless environment in which to develop during pregnancy; contained in the amniotic sac.

amniotic fluid embolism An extremely rare, life-threatening condition that occurs when amniotic fluid and fetal cells enter the pregnant woman's pulmonary and circulatory system through the placenta via the umbilical veins, causing an exaggerated allergic response from the woman's body.

amniotic sac The fluid-filled, baglike membrane in which the fetus develops.

amputation An injury in which part of the body is completely or partially severed.

anaerobic metabolism Metabolism that occurs in the absence of oxygen.

anaphylactic shock A severe hypersensitivity reaction that involves bronchoconstriction and cardiovascular collapse.

anatomic snuffbox The region at the base of the thumb where the scaphoid may be palpated.

anchoring bias A type of bias in which an initial reference point distorts your estimates.

angioedema Recurrent large areas of subcutaneous edema of sudden onset, usually disappearing within 24 hours, which is seen mainly in young women, frequently as a result of allergy to food or drugs.

angle of impact The angle at which an object hits another; this characterizes the force vectors involved and has a bearing on patterns of energy dissipation.

angulation The presence of an abnormal angle or bend in an extremity.

anterior chamber The anterior area of the globe between the lens and the cornea, which is filled with aqueous humor.

anterior cord syndrome A condition that occurs with flexion injuries or fractures, resulting in the displacement of bony fragments into the anterior portion of the spinal cord. Findings include paralysis below the level of the insult and loss of pain, temperature, and touch perception.

anterograde (posttraumatic) amnesia Loss of memory of events that occurred after an injury.

anthrax A deadly bacterium (*Bacillus anthracis*) that lies dormant in a spore (protective shell); the germ is released from the spore when exposed to the optimal temperature and moisture. The route of entry is inhalational, cutaneous, or gastrointestinal (from consuming food that contains spores).

Apgar scoring system A scoring system for assessing the status of a newborn 1 and 5 minutes after birth, that assigns a number value to each of five areas of assessment, for a total score ranging from 0 to 10.

apocalyptic violence A type of violence sought by some terrorists, such as violent religious groups and doomsday cults, in which they wish to bring about the end of the world.

appendicular skeleton The portion of the skeletal system made up of the upper extremities, shoulder girdle, pelvic girdle, and lower extremities.

apraxia A neurologic impairment in which the brain is intermittently unable to carry out the command for speech or other tasks.

arachnoid The middle membrane of the three meninges that enclose the brain and spinal cord.

arterial air embolism Air bubbles in the arterial blood vessels.

arterial gas embolism (AGE) The resultant gaseous emboli from the forcing of gas into the vasculature from barotrauma.

arthritis Inflammation of the joints.

ashfall The residue left behind from a volcanic eruption.

asphyxia Condition of severely deficient supply of oxygen to the body leading to end organ damage.

asphyxiant Any gas that displaces oxygen from the atmosphere; can be deadly if exposure occurs in a confined space.

associated fractures Musculoskeletal injuries that commonly occur together.

asynchronous In cardiopulmonary resuscitation, when two rescuers perform ventilations and compressions individually; ventilations are not timed and do not require waiting for the other rescuer to pause.

ataxia Alteration in the ability to perform coordinated motions such as walking.

atelectasis Alveolar collapse that prevents use of that portion of the lungs for ventilation and oxygenation.

atmosphere absolute (ATA) A measurement of ambient pressure; the weight of air at sea level, equivalent in pressure to 33 feet of seawater (fsw; 10 m).

atrial septal defect A hole in the atrial septal wall that allows oxygenated and deoxygenated blood to mix; patients with this hole have a higher incidence of stroke.

auditory neuropathy A condition characterized by normal function of the structures of the ear without a corresponding stimulation of auditory centers of the brain; also called auditory dyssynchrony.

authority having jurisdiction (AHJ) An organization, office, or person responsible for enforcing the requirements of a code or standard, or for approving equipment, materials, an installation, or a procedure.

autism A developmental disorder characterized by impairments of social interaction; may include severe behavioral problems, repetitive motor activities, and impairment in verbal and nonverbal skills.

autism spectrum disorder A group of complex disorders of brain development, characterized by difficulties in social interaction, repetitive behaviors, and verbal and nonverbal communication.

automated external defibrillator (AED) A defibrillator that can analyze the patient's heart rhythm and determine whether a defibrillating shock is needed to terminate ventricular fibrillation or ventricular tachycardia, and which can guide the user through the resuscitation effort via voice commands.

automatic transport ventilator (ATV) A portable mechanical ventilator attached to a control box that allows the variables of ventilation (such as rate and tidal volume) to be set.

autonomic dysreflexia A late, life-threatening complication of spinal cord injury in which stimulation of the sympathetic nervous system below the level of injury generates a massive, uninhibited, uncompensated cardiovascular response; also known as autonomic hyperreflexia.

autoregulation An increase in mean arterial pressure to compensate for decreased cerebral perfusion pressure; compensatory physiologic response that occurs in an effort to shunt blood to the brain; manifests clinically as hypertension.

avascular necrosis Tissue death resulting from the loss of blood supply.

avulsing A tearing away or forcible separation.

avulsion An injury that leaves a piece of skin or other tissue partially or completely torn away from the body.

avulsion fracture A fracture that occurs when a piece of bone is torn free at the site of attachment of a tendon or ligament.

awareness The first level of rescue training provided to all responders; emphasizes recognizing hazards, securing the scene, and calling for appropriate assistance. There is no use of actual rescue skills.

axial skeleton The portion of the skeleton made up of the skull, spinal column, and thoracic cage.

axon A long, slender extension of a neuron (nerve cell) that conducts electrical impulses away from the nerve cell body to adjacent cells.

Babinski reflex Upward movement of the toe(s) in response to stimulation to the sole of the foot. Under normal circumstances, the toe(s) move downward.

bacteria Small organisms that can grow and reproduce outside the human cell in the presence of the needed temperature and nutrients and cause disease by invading and multiplying in the tissues of the host.

bacterial tracheitis An acute bacterial infection of the subglottic area of the upper airway that is complicated by copious thick, pus-filled secretions.

ballistics The study of nonpowered objects in flight; most often associated with rifle or handgun bullet travel.

bandage Material used to secure a dressing in place.

bariatrics The medical specialty dedicated to prevention and treatment of obesity.

barometric energy The energy that results from sudden changes in pressure as may occur in a diving accident or sudden decompression in an airplane.

baroreceptors Nerve endings that are stimulated by pressure changes, including increased arterial blood pressure; they are located in the aortic arch and carotid sinuses, and the kidneys.

barotrauma Injury resulting from pressure disequilibrium (too much pressure) across body surfaces, for example in the lungs.

basal metabolic rate (BMR) The heat energy produced at rest from normal body metabolic reactions; the rate at which nutrients are consumed in the body; determined mostly by the liver and skeletal muscles.

basilar skull fracture Fracture generally resulting from the extension of a linear fracture into the base of the skull; usually occurs after a diffuse impact to the head (as in a fall or motor vehicle crash) and can be difficult to diagnose, even with radiography.

Battle sign Bruising over the mastoid bone behind the ear, which may indicate a basilar skull fracture; also called retroauricular ecchymosis or raccoon eyes.

belay A technique used to control a rope as it is fed out to climbers.

belt noise A chirping or squealing sound, synchronous with engine speed.

bereavement Sadness from loss; grieving.

beta radiation A type of energy that is emitted from a strong radiologic source. It is slightly more penetrating than alpha and requires a layer of clothing to stop it.

bill of lading A document carried by drivers of commercial vehicles that should provide specific information about what is carried on the vehicle.

biomechanics The study of the physiology and mechanics of a living organism using the tools of mechanical engineering.

Biot (ataxic) respirations Irregular pattern, rate, and depth of respirations with intermittent periods of apnea; result from increased intracranial pressure.

blast front The leading edge of the shock wave.

blastocyst The term for an oocyte once it has been fertilized and multiplies into cells.

blind spot An area of the road that is blocked from your sight by your own vehicle or mirrors.

blood The fluid tissue that is pumped by the heart through the arteries, veins, and capillaries; it consists of plasma and formed elements or cells, such as red blood cells, white blood cells, and platelets.

bloody show A plug of mucus, sometimes mixed with blood, that is expelled from the dilating cervix and discharged from the vagina.

blow-by technique A method of delivering oxygen by holding a face mask or similar device near an infant's or a child's face; used when a nonrebreathing mask is not tolerated.

blowout fracture A fracture to the floor of the orbit, usually caused by a blow to the eye.

blunt trauma An impact on the body by objects that cause injury without penetrating soft tissues or internal organs and cavities.

botulinum A very potent neurotoxin produced by bacteria; when introduced into the body, this neurotoxin affects the nervous system's ability to function and causes muscle paralysis.

box crib A pallet like framework used to shore up a heavy load.

boxer's fracture A fracture of the head of the fifth metacarpal that usually results from striking an object with a clenched fist.

Boyle's law A gas law that demonstrates that as pressure increases, volume decreases; at a constant temperature, the volume of a gas is inversely proportional to its pressure (if the pressure on a gas is doubled, then its volume is halved); written as $PV = K$, where P = pressure, V = volume, and K = a constant.

brainstem The area of the brain between the spinal cord and cerebrum that contains the midbrain, pons, and medulla; controls functions that are necessary for life, such as breathing.

brake fade A sensation that an emergency vehicle has lost its power brakes.

brake pull A sensation that when an operator depresses the brake pedal, the steering wheel is being pulled to the left or the right.

breath-hold diving Also called free diving, this type of diving does not require any equipment, except sometimes a snorkel.

breech presentation A delivery in which the buttocks come out first.

brief resolved unexplained event (BRUE) An unexpected sudden episode of color change, tone change, or apnea that requires mouth-to-mouth resuscitation or vigorous stimulation; formerly known as apparent life-threatening event.

brisance The shattering effect of a shock wave and its ability to cause disruption of tissues and structures.

bronchiolitis A condition seen in children younger than 2 years, characterized by dyspnea and wheezing.

bronchopulmonary dysplasia A spectrum of lung conditions found in premature neonates who require long periods of high-concentration oxygen and ventilator support, ranging from mild reactive airway to debilitating chronic lung disease.

Brown-Séquard syndrome A condition associated with penetrating trauma and characterized by hemisection of the spinal cord and complete damage to all spinal tracts on the involved side.

buboes Enlarged lymph nodes (up to the size of tennis balls) that are characteristic of people infected with the bubonic plague.

bubonic plague An epidemic that spread throughout Europe in the Middle Ages, causing over 25 million deaths, also called the Black Death; transmitted by infected fleas and characterized by acute malaise, fever, and the formation of tender, enlarged, inflamed lymph nodes that appear as lesions, called buboes.

buckle fracture A common incomplete fracture in children in which the cortex of the bone fractures from an excessive compression force; also called a torus fracture.

buddy splinting Securing an injured digit to an adjacent uninjured one to allow the intact digit to act as a splint.

bursitis Inflammation of a bursa.

CAMEO Computer-Aided Management of Emergency Operations; a tool to help predict downwind concentrations of hazardous materials based on the input of environmental factors into a computer model.

cancellous bone Trabecular or spongy bone.

cancer Excessive growth and division of abnormal cells within the body that can occur in many body systems, tissues, and organs and that can progress rapidly and cause death in a relatively short period.

capacitance vessels The smallest venules.

carbon monoxide A chemical asphyxiant that results in a cellular respiratory failure; this gas ties up hemoglobin to the extent that oxygen in the blood becomes inaccessible to the cells.

carboy A glass, plastic, or steel nonbulk storage container, ranging in volume from 5 to 15 gallons (19 to 600 L).

cardiac output (CO) The amount of blood pumped by the heart per minute; calculated by multiplying the stroke volume by the pulse rate per minute.

cardiac tamponade A pathologic condition characterized by restriction of cardiac contraction, falling cardiac output, and shock as a result of pericardial fluid accumulation.

cardiogenic shock A condition caused by loss of 40% or more of the functioning myocardium; the heart is no longer able to circulate sufficient blood to maintain adequate oxygen delivery.

cardiovascular collapse Failure of the heart and blood vessels; shock.

cargo tank Bulk packaging that is permanently attached to or forms a part of a motor vehicle, or is not permanently attached to any motor vehicle, and that, because of its size, construction, or attachment to a motor vehicle, is loaded or unloaded without being removed from the motor vehicle.

carpal tunnel syndrome Compression of the median nerve at the wrist where it passes through the carpal canal, causing numbness and tingling in the hand, and possibly pain.

casualty collection points Areas where slightly injured or noninjured displaced people can be gathered together and transported by bus or truck for further treatment.

cauda equina The location where the spinal cord separates; composed of nerve roots.

cauda equina syndrome A neurologic condition caused by compression of the bundle of nerve roots located at the end of the spinal cord.

cavitation Cavity formation; shock waves that push tissues in front of and lateral to the projectile and may not necessarily increase the wound size or cause permanent injury but can result in cavitation.

cellulitis An acute inflammation in the skin caused by a bacterial infection.

central auditory processing disorder (CAPD) A disorder in which patients have difficulty interpreting speech and differentiating it from other sounds that are present.

central cord syndrome A condition resulting from hyperextension injuries to the cervical area that damage the dorsal column of the spinal cord; characterized by hemorrhage or edema. Findings include greater loss of function in the upper extremities, with variable sensory loss of pain and temperature.

central cyanosis Blue discoloration of the skin due to the presence of deoxygenated hemoglobin in blood vessels near the skin surface.

central neurogenic hyperventilation Deep, rapid respirations; similar to Kussmaul, but without an acetone breath odor; commonly seen after brainstem injury.

central shock A type of shock caused by central pump failure, including cardiogenic shock and obstructive shock (Weil-Shubin classification).

central venous catheter A catheter inserted into the vena cava to permit intermittent or continuous monitoring of central venous pressure and to facilitate obtaining blood samples for chemical analysis.

cephalopelvic disproportion A situation in which the head of the fetus is larger than the woman's pelvis; in most cases, cesarean section is required for such a delivery.

cerebellum Area of the brain involved in fine and gross muscle coordination; responsible for interpretation of actual movement and correction of any movements that interfere with coordination and the body's position.

cerebral concussion Injury that occurs when the brain is jarred around in the skull; a mild diffuse brain injury that does not result in structural damage or permanent neurologic impairment.

cerebral contusion A focal brain injury in which brain tissue is bruised and damaged in a defined area.

cerebral cortex The largest portion of the cerebrum; outer covering of gray matter that covers the cerebral hemispheres; regulates voluntary skeletal movement and plays an important role in one's level of awareness.

cerebral edema Excessive fluid in the brain; swelling of the brain.

cerebral palsy (CP) A developmental condition in which damage is done to the brain. It presents during infancy as a delay in walking or crawling and can take on a spastic form in which muscles are in a nearly constant state of contraction.

cerebral perfusion pressure (CPP) The pressure inside the cerebral arteries and an indicator of brain perfusion; calculated by subtracting intracranial pressure from mean arterial pressure.

cerebrospinal fluid (CSF) Fluid produced in the ventricles of the brain that flows in the subarachnoid space and bathes the meninges.

cerebrospinal fluid shunt (CSF shunt) A tube placed in the body to relieve pressure by drawing excess cerebrospinal fluid away from the brain or spinal cord.

cerebrum The largest part of the brain, responsible for higher functions such as reasoning; made up of several lobes that control movement, hearing, balance, speech, visual perception, emotions, and personality; divided into right and left hemispheres; also called gray matter.

cervical canal The interior of the cervix.

chemical asphyxiant A substance that interferes with the use of oxygen at the cellular level.

chemical energy The energy released as a result of a chemical reaction.

chemoreceptors Sense organs that monitor the levels of oxygen and carbon dioxide and the pH of cerebrospinal fluid and blood and provide feedback to the respiratory centers to modify the rate and depth of breathing based on the body's needs at any given time.

chemotactic factors The factors that cause cells to migrate into an area.

CHEMTREC (Chemical Transportation Emergency Center) A resource available to emergency responders via telephone on a 24-hour basis.

Cheyne-Stokes respirations A gradually increasing rate and depth of respirations followed by a gradual decrease with intermittent periods of apnea; associated with brainstem insult.

chilblains Itchy red and purple swollen lesions that occur primarily on the extremities, due to longer exposure to temperatures just above freezing or sudden rewarming after exposure to cold.

child abuse Any improper or excessive action that injures or otherwise harms a child or infant; includes physical abuse, sexual abuse, neglect, and emotional abuse.

child protective services (CPS) The community-based legal organization responsible for protection, rehabilitation, and prevention of child maltreatment and neglect. This agency has the legal authority to temporarily remove children from homes if there is reason to believe they are at risk for injury or neglect and to secure foster placement.

chlorine The first chemical agent ever used in warfare. It has a distinct odor of bleach and creates a green haze when released as a gas. Initially, it produces upper airway irritation and a choking sensation. Its military abbreviation is CL.

choanal atresia A narrowing or blockage of the nasal airway by membranous or bony tissue; a congenital condition, meaning it is present at birth.

cholestasis A disease of the liver that occurs only during pregnancy, in which hormones affect the gallbladder by slowing down or blocking the normal bile flow from the liver; the most common symptom is profuse, painful itching, particularly of the hands and feet.

chronic hypertension A blood pressure that is equal to or greater than 140/90 mm Hg, which exists prior to pregnancy, occurs before the 20th week of pregnancy, or persists postpartum.

circumferential burn A burn on the neck or chest, which may compress the airway, or on an extremity, which might act like a tourniquet.

clandestine drug laboratories Locations where illegal drugs such as methamphetamine, lysergic acid diethylamide (LSD), ecstasy, and phencyclidine hydrochloride (PCP) are manufactured.

classic heatstroke Also called passive heatstroke, this is a serious heat illness that usually occurs during heat waves and is most likely to strike very old, very young, or bedridden people.

clavicle An S-shaped bone, also called the collarbone, that articulates medially with the sternum and laterally with the shoulder.

cleaning The process of removing dirt, dust, blood, or other visible contaminants from a surface.

cleft lip An abnormal defect or fissure in the upper lip that failed to close during development. It is often associated with cleft palate.

cleft palate A fissure or hole in the palate (roof of the mouth) that forms a communicating pathway between the mouth and nasal cavities.

closed fracture A fracture in which the skin is not broken.

closed incident A contained incident in which patients are found in one focal location and the situation is not expected to produce more patients than are initially present.

closed wound An injury in which damage occurs beneath the skin or mucous membrane but the surface remains intact.

coagulation necrosis Cell death typically caused by ischemia or infarction.

coarctation of the aorta Pinching or narrowing of the aorta that obstructs blood flow from the heart to the systemic circulation.

code team leader The code team member who has the responsibility for managing the rescuers or team members during a cardiac arrest, as well as choreographing the effort of the group.

code team member A member of the resuscitation team trying to revive the patient.

cold diuresis Secretion of large amounts of urine in response to cold exposure and the consequent shunting of blood volume to the body core.

cold stress A psychologic condition that can develop in people who are exposed to cold weather for long periods of time, even if sheltered.

cold zone A safe area for agencies involved in a rescue operation; the incident commander, command post, EMS providers, and other necessary support functions should be located in the cold zone.

cold-protective response A phenomenon associated with cold-water immersion in which the body reflexively lowers its metabolic rate in an effort to preserve basic bodily functions.

collagen A protein that gives tensile strength to the connective tissues of the body.

colostomy The surgical establishment of an opening between the colon and the surface of the body for the purpose of providing drainage of the bowel.

colostomy bag A plastic pouch or bag attached over a colostomy to collect stool.

comfort care Medical treatment aimed at symptom relief and providing comfort for the patient.

command In incident command, the position that oversees the incident, establishes the objectives and priorities, and from there develops a response plan.

comminuted fracture A fracture in which the bone is broken into three or more pieces.

commotio cordis An event in which an often-fatal cardiac dysrhythmia is produced by a sudden blow to the thoracic cavity.

communicability The ease with which a disease spreads from one human to another human.

compartment syndrome An increase in tissue pressure in a closed fascial space or compartment that compromises the circulation to the nerves and muscles within the involved compartment.

compensated shock The early stage of shock, in which the body can still compensate for blood loss. The systolic blood pressure and brain perfusion are maintained.

complete abortion Expulsion of all products of conception from the uterus.

complete fracture A fracture in which the bone is broken into two or more completely separate pieces.

complete spinal cord injury Total disruption of all spinal cord tracts, with permanent loss of all cord-mediated functions below the level of injury.

complex access Complicated entry requiring special tools, advanced training, and the use of force, such as breaking windows.

complex febrile seizures An unusual form of seizure that occurs in association with a rapid increase in body temperature.

complex partial seizures A type of seizure characterized by alteration of consciousness with or without complex focal motor activity.

compression fraction An indication of how well the team is minimizing pauses in cardiopulmonary resuscitation; it is calculated by dividing the amount of time compressions are delivered by the amount of time compressions are indicated.

concealment Protection from being seen.

conduction Transfer of heat to a solid object or a liquid by direct contact.

conductive hearing loss A type of hearing impairment due to problems with the middle ear bones' ability to conduct sounds from the outer ear to the inner ear.

confined space A space that is not meant for continuous occupancy and to which access is limited or restricted, such as a manhole, well, or tank.

confirmation bias A type of bias that occurs with the tendency to gather and rely on information that confirms your existing views and to avoid or downplay information that does not conform to your preexisiting hypothesis or field diagnosis.

congenital adrenal hyperplasia (CAH) Inadequate production of cortisol and aldosterone by the adrenal gland.

congenital heart disease (CHD) The most common birth defect; associated with hypoxia in the newborn period requiring intervention during the first months of life.

conjunctiva A thin, transparent membrane that covers the sclera and internal surfaces of the eyelids.

conjunctivitis An inflammation of the conjunctivae that usually is caused by bacteria, viruses, allergies, or foreign bodies; should be considered highly contagious if infectious in origin; also called pinkeye.

Consensus formula A formula that recommends giving 2–4 mL of lactated Ringer solution for each kilogram of body weight, multiplied by the percentage of total body surface area burned; sometimes used to calculate fluid needs during lengthy transport times; formerly called the Parkland formula.

contact and cover A technique that involves one paramedic making contact with the patient to provide care, while the second paramedic obtains patient information, gauges the level of tension, and warns his or her partner at the first sign of trouble.

contact burn A burn produced by touching a hot object.

contact hazard A hazardous agent that gives off little or no vapors and typically enters the body through the skin; also called a skin hazard.

contagious The characteristic of being communicable from one person to another person.

container Any vessel or receptacle that holds material, including storage vessels, pipelines, and packaging.

continuity of operations plan (COOP) The detailed plan describing the functioning of the agency in situations that disrupt normal operations.

contusion A bruise; an injury that causes bleeding beneath the skin but does not break the skin.

convection The mechanism by which body heat is picked up and carried away by moving air currents.

conversion disorder A psychologic condition in which stress or mental conflict is converted into physical complaints.

core body temperature (CBT) The temperature in the part of the body comprising the heart, lungs, brain, and abdominal viscera.

cornea The transparent anterior portion of the eye that overlies the iris and pupil.

corpus luteum The remains of a follicle after an oocyte has been released, and which secretes progesterone.

corrosives A class of chemicals with either high or low pH levels. Exposure can cause severe soft-tissue damage.

coup-contrecoup injury Dual impacting of the brain into the skull. Coup injury occurs at the point of impact; contrecoup injury occurs on the opposite side of impact, as the brain rebounds.

cover Obstacles that are difficult or impossible for bullets to penetrate.

covert An act in which the public safety community generally has no prior knowledge of the time, location, or nature of the attack.

cranial vault The bones that encase and protect the brain, including the parietal, temporal, frontal, occipital, sphenoid, and ethmoid bones; the roof of the skull (cranium).

craniofacial disjunction A Le Fort III fracture that involves a fracture of all of the midfacial bones, which separates the entire midface from the cranium.

crepitus A grating, grinding, or crackling sensation made when two pieces of broken bone rub together or subcutaneous emphysema is palpated.

cribbing A type of basic physical support, such as blocks or short lengths of wood, used to stabilize a vehicle during a rescue operation.

critical care paramedic (CCP) A specialty role for paramedics in which the paramedic is trained to provide advanced care and transport for critically injured or ill patients; also called a critical care transport professional.

critical incident stress management (CISM) A process which utilizes trained counselors who confront responses to critical incidents and help to defuse them, directing emergency services personnel toward physical and emotional equilibrium.

critical infrastructure The external foundation in communities made up of structures and services critical in the day-to-day living activities of humans: energy sources, fuel, water, sewage removal, food, hospitals, and transportation systems.

critical minimum threshold Minimum cerebral perfusion pressure required to adequately perfuse the brain; 60 mm Hg in the adult.

critical patient A patient who is in premorbid condition, has experienced major trauma, or is in the peri arrest period.

cross-contamination Contamination of a person that results from coming into contact with another contaminated person, as opposed to coming into contact with the original source of contamination.

croup A common disease of infancy and childhood caused by upper airway obstruction and characterized by stridor, hoarseness, and a barking cough.

crown The part of the tooth that is external to the gum.

crowning The appearance of the newborn's body part (usually the head) at the vaginal opening at the beginning of labor.

crush syndrome A condition that arises after a body part that has been compressed for a significant period is released, leading to the entry of potassium and other metabolic toxins into the systemic circulation.

cubital tunnel syndrome Compression of the ulnar nerve at the tunnel along the outer edge of the elbow, causing numbness, tingling, and possible partial loss of function of the little finger and medial aspect of the ring finger.

curative care Medical treatment aimed at curing an illness.

Cushing triad Hypertension (with a widening pulse pressure), bradycardia, and irregular respirations; classic trio of findings associated with increased intracranial pressure.

cushion of safety A safe distance maintained between your vehicle and other vehicles on any side of you.

cusps Points at the top of a tooth.

cyanide An agent that affects the body's ability to use oxygen. It is a colorless gas that has an odor similar to almonds; exposure can occur from by-products of combustion at structure fires. The effects begin on the cellular level and are very rapidly seen at the organ system level.

cylinder A portable, nonbulk, compressed gas container used to hold liquids and gases. Uninsulated compressed gas containers of this sort are used to store substances such as nitrogen, argon, helium, and oxygen. They have a range of sizes and internal pressures.

cystic fibrosis (CF) A genetic disorder of the endocrine system that makes it difficult for chloride to move through cells; primarily targets the respiratory and digestive systems.

cytomegalovirus (CMV) A herpesvirus that can produce the symptoms of prolonged high fever, chills, headache, malaise, extreme fatigue, and an enlarged spleen.

Dalton's law Each gas in a mixture exerts the same partial pressure that it would exert if it were alone in the same volume, and the total pressure of a mixture of gases is the sum of the partial pressures of all the gases in a mixture.

decay A natural process in which a material that is unstable attempts to stabilize itself by changing its structure.

deceleration A negative acceleration—that is, slowing down.

decerebrate (extensor) posturing Abnormal posture of the arms and legs, in which the arms are extended with rotation of the wrists and the toes are pointed; indicates pressure on the brainstem.

decompensated (hypotensive) shock The late stage of shock, when blood pressure is falling.

decompression illness (DCI) A term for decompression sickness and air gas embolism.

decompression sickness (DCS) A broad range of signs and symptoms caused by nitrogen bubbles in blood and tissues coming out of solution on ascent.

decontaminate To remove or neutralize radiation, chemical, or other hazardous material from clothing, equipment, vehicles, and personnel.

decontamination corridor A controlled area within the warm zone where decontamination takes place.

decorticate (flexor) posturing Abnormal posture of the arms and legs, in which the arms are flexed toward the chest the toes are pointed; this finding indicates lower cerebral damage.

deep frostbite A type of frostbite in which the affected part looks white, yellow-white, or mottled blue-white and is hard, cold, and without sensation.

deep vein thrombosis (DVT) The formation of a blood clot within the larger veins of an extremity, typically following a period of prolonged stabilization.

defibrillation The use of an unsynchronized direct current electric shock to terminate ventricular fibrillation or pulseless ventricular tachycardia.

degloving A traumatic injury that results in the soft tissue of a part of the body being drawn downward like a glove being removed.

delirium An acute confusional state characterized by global impairment of thinking, perception, judgment, and memory.

dementia The slow, progressive onset of disorientation, shortened attention span, and loss of cognitive function.

demobilization The process of directing responders to return to their facilities when work at a disaster or mass-casualty incident has finished, at least for the particular responders.

dentin The principal mass of the tooth, which is made up of a material that is much denser and stronger than bone.

depressed skull fracture Fracture caused by high-energy direct trauma applied to a small surface area of the skull with a blunt object (such as a baseball bat striking the head); commonly accompanied by bony fragments driven into the brain, causing further injury.

depression fracture A fracture in which the broken region of the bone is pushed deeper into the body than the remaining intact bone.

dermatome An area of the skin supplied by a specific sensory spinal nerve.

dermis The inner layer of skin, containing hair follicle roots, sweat glands, blood vessels, nerve endings, and sebaceous glands.

desquamation The continual shedding of the dead cells on the surface of the skin.

devascularization The loss of blood to a part of the body.

developmental delay A broad term that describes an infant or child's failure to reach a particular developmental milestone by the expected time.

developmental disability Insufficient development of a portion of the brain, resulting in some level of dysfunction or impairment.

diaphragmatic hernia Passage of loops of bowel with or without other abdominal organs, through a developmental defect in the diaphragm muscle; occurs as the bowel from the abdomen "herniates" upward through the diaphragm into the chest (thoracic) cavity.

diastasis An increase in the distance between the two sides of a joint.

differential diagnosis The process of weighing the probability of one disease versus other diseases by comparing clinical findings that could account for a patient's illness; also refers to the list of possible conditions considered based on the patient's signs and symptoms.

diffuse axonal injury (DAI) Diffuse brain injury that is caused by stretching, shearing, or tearing of nerve fibers with consequent axonal damage.

diffuse brain injury Any injury that affects the entire brain.

diffusion The process of particles moving from an area of higher concentration to an area of lower concentration along a concentration gradient until equilibrium is achieved.

dilated cardiomyopathy A condition in which the heart becomes weakened and enlarged, making it less efficient and causing a negative impact to the pulmonary, hepatic, and other systems.

dilution A type of decontamination method that uses copious amounts of water to flush the contaminant from the skin or eyes.

diplopia Double vision.

directed area An area away from the command post or emergency operations center, considered by engineering expertise to be a safe place to stage until directed otherwise.

dirty bomb A bomb that is used as a radiologic dispersal device (RDD).

disaster A sudden, calamitous event, such as an accident or catastrophe, that causes great damage, loss, or destruction; a situation declared by a locale, or by the county, state, or federal government for the purposes of providing additional resources and funds to those in need.

disaster management A planned, coordinated response to a disaster that involves cooperation of multiple responders and agencies and enables effective triage and provision of care according to triage decisions.

disease vector An infected animal that spreads a disease to another animal.

disentanglement Use of specialized tools and advanced techniques to free a patient from the area or object in which he or she is trapped.

disinfection The killing of pathogenic agents by direct application of chemicals.

dislocation The displacement of a bone from its normal position within a joint.

displaced fracture A break in which the ends of the fractured bone move out of their normal positions.

disposal A type of decontamination in which as much clothing and equipment as possible is disposed of to reduce the magnitude of the problem.

dissemination The means with which a terrorist will spread a disease—for example, by poisoning the water supply or aerosolizing the agent into the air or ventilation system of a building.

distraction injury An injury that results from a force that tries to increase the length of a body part or separate one body part from another.

distributive shock The type of shock caused by widespread dilation of the resistance vessels (small arterioles), the capacitance vessels (small venules), or both.

domestic terrorism Terrorism that is carried out by native citizens against their own country.

dorsiflex To bend the foot or hand backward.

dose effect The principle that the longer a hazardous material is in contact with the body or the greater the concentration, the greater the effect will most likely be.

DOT KKK 1822 Federal standards that regulate the design and manufacturing guidelines of emergency medical vehicles.

Down syndrome A genetic chromosomal defect that can occur during fetal development and that results in intellectual disability and certain physical characteristics, such as a round head with a flat occiput and slanted, wide-set eyes.

dressing Material used to directly cover a wound.

drift A finding that when the operator lets go of the steering wheel, a vehicle consistently wanders left or right.

drowning The process of experiencing respiratory impairment from submersion or immersion in liquid.

drum A barrel-like nonbulk storage vessel used to store a wide variety of substances, including food-grade materials, corrosives, flammable liquids, and grease. Drums may be constructed of low-carbon steel, polyethylene, cardboard, stainless steel, nickel, or other materials.

dry bulk cargo tank A tank designed to carry dry bulk goods such as powders, pellets, fertilizers, or grain. Such tanks are generally V-shaped with rounded sides that funnel toward the bottom.

due regard Driving with awareness and responsibility for other drivers on the roadways when you are operating an emergency vehicle in the emergency mode, and making sure that other drivers are aware of your approach.

DUMBELS A mnemonic that stands for diarrhea, urination, miosis/muscle weakness, bradycardia/bronchospasm/bronchorrhea, emesis, lacrimation, seizures/salivation/sweating, which are the signs and symptoms that can be produced by exposure to organophosphate and carbamate pesticides or other nerve-stimulating agents.

DuoDote A nerve agent antidote kit that contains a single injection of both atropine (2 mg) and 2-PAM chloride (pralidoxime chloride; 600 mg).

dura mater The outermost layer of the three meninges that enclose the brain and spinal cord; the toughest meningeal layer.

dust suffocation A phenomenon that can occur during an earthquake, in which particles of dust and debris are loosened and released into the air, producing a toxic and hypoxic atmosphere.

dysarthria A speech disorder caused by neuromuscular disturbance that causes speech to become slow and slurred.

dysconjugate gaze Paralysis of gaze or lack of coordination between the movements of the two eyes.

dysphagia Pain, discomfort, or difficulty in swallowing.

ecchymosis Localized bruising or collection of blood within or under the skin.

eclampsia Seizures that result from severe hypertension in a pregnant woman.

ectopic pregnancy A pregnancy in which the fertilized oocyte implants somewhere other than the uterus, typically in a fallopian tube.

effacement Thinning and shortening of the cervix; a normal process that occurs as the uterus contracts.

ejection fraction (EF) The percentage of blood that leaves the heart each time it contracts.

elastin A protein that gives the skin its elasticity.

elective abortion Intentional expulsion of the fetus.

electrical energy Energy delivered in the form of high voltage.

elevated A threat level in which a terrorist event is suspected, but there is no specific information about its timing or location.

emergency decontamination The process of removing the bulk of contaminants from a person without regard for containment. It is used in potentially life-threatening situations, without the formal establishment of a decontamination corridor.

emergency operations center (EOC) A central command and control facility, found at all government levels, responsible for strategic overview; tactical decisions are left to incident commanders.

emotional abuse A form of abuse that may be verbal (such as ridicule, threats, blaming, or humiliation) or nonverbal (such as caregiver ignoring the victim or isolating the victim from others). The abuse causes a substantial change in the victim's behavior, emotional response, or cognitive function, or may manifest as a variety of mental illnesses.

entrance wound The point at which a penetrating object enters the body.

entrapment A circumstance in which a patient is unable to extricate himself or herself from an impediment, such as debris or soil.

envenomation The injecting of venom via a bite or sting.

environmental emergencies Medical conditions caused or exacerbated by the weather, terrain, or unique atmospheric conditions such as high altitude or underwater.

epidemic An illness or disease that affects or tends to affect a disproportionately large number of people within a specific population, community, or region at the same time.

epidermis The outermost layer of the skin.

epidural hematoma An accumulation of blood between the skull and dura.

epiglottitis Inflammation of the epiglottis.

episiotomy An incision in the perineal skin made to prevent tearing during childbirth.

epistaxis Nosebleed.

epithelialization The formation of fresh epithelial tissue to heal a wound.

Erb palsy Lack of movement at the shoulder due to nerve injury resulting from the stretching of the cervical nerve roots (C5 and C6 most commonly) during delivery of the newborn's head during birth. The effect is usually transient, but can be permanent.

erythema Reddening of the skin.

escharotomy A surgical cut through the eschar or leathery covering of a burn injury to allow for swelling and minimize the potential for development of compartment syndrome in a circumferentially burned limb or the thorax.

evacuation The removal or relocation of people who may be affected by an approaching release of a hazardous material.

evaporation The conversion of a liquid to a gas.

evisceration Displacement of an organ outside the body.

exercise-associated hyponatremia (EAH) A condition due to prolonged exertion in hot environments coupled with excessive hypotonic fluid intake that leads to nausea, vomiting, and, in severe cases, mental status changes and seizures (also known as exertional hyponatremia or exercise-induced hyponatremia).

exertional heatstroke A serious type of heatstroke usually affecting young and fit people exercising in hot and humid conditions.

exit wound The point at which a penetrating object leaves the body, which may or may not be in a straight line from the entry wound.

exophthalmos Protrusion of the eyes from the normal position within the socket.

exsanguination The loss of the total blood volume, resulting in death.

external ear One of the three anatomic parts of the ear; it contains the pinna, the ear canal, and the external portion of the tympanic membrane.

extrication task force leader In incident command, the person appointed to determine the type of equipment and resources needed for a situation involving extrication or special rescue; also called the rescue task force leader.

facet joint The joint on which each vertebra articulates with adjacent vertebrae.

false lumen An area that a device was not intended to be inserted into—for example, a tracheostomy tube inserted into an area other than the trachea.

fascia A sheet or band of tough, fibrous connective tissue that covers, supports, and separates muscles, and which also covers arteries, veins, tendons, and ligaments.

fasciitis Inflammation of the fascia.

fatigue fracture A fracture that results from multiple compressive loads.

feet of seawater (fsw) An indirect measure of pressure under water, equal to one atmosphere absolute.

femoral shaft fracture A break in the diaphysis of the femur.

fenestrated Having perforations, holes, or openings.

fetal macrosomia A situation in which a fetus is large, usually defined as weighing more than 4,500 grams (almost 9 pounds); also known as "large for gestational age."

fetal transition The process through which the fluid in the fetal lungs is replaced with air, the ductus arteriosus constricts, and the newborn begins adequate oxygenation of its own blood.

fetus The developing, unborn infant inside the uterus.

Fick principle A principle that states the movement and use of oxygen in the body are dependent on an adequate concentration of inspired oxygen, appropriate movement of oxygen across the alveolar-capillary membrane into the arterial bloodstream, adequate number of red blood cells to carry the oxygen, proper tissue perfusion, and efficient offloading of oxygen at the tissue level.

finance section chief In incident command, the position in an incident responsible for accounting of all expenditures.

first stage of labor The stage of labor that begins with the onset of regular labor pains (crampy abdominal pains), during which the uterus contracts and the cervix effaces.

fistula A surgically created connection between an artery and a vein, usually in the arm, for dialysis access; an abnormal connection between two cavities.

flail chest An injury that involves two or more adjacent ribs fractured in two or more places, allowing the segment between the fractures to move independently of the rest of the thoracic cage.

flame burn A thermal burn caused by flames touching the skin.

flammable range An expression of a fuel-air mixture, defined by upper and lower limits, that reflects an amount of flammable vapor mixed with a given volume of air.

flange The part of a tracheostomy tube that is used to stabilize the tube to the patient's neck.

flash burn An electrothermal injury caused by arcing of electric current.

flash point The minimum temperature at which a liquid or a solid releases sufficient vapor to form an ignitable mixture with air.

flexion injury A type of injury that results from forward movement of the head, typically as the result of rapid deceleration, such as in a vehicle crash, or with a direct blow to the occiput.

flexor tenosynovitis of the hand A closed-space infection of the hand.

flight paramedics Paramedics who work as part of an air rescue team that provides either on-scene care in remote field settings or interfacility transports from one clinical setting to another.

focal brain injury A specific, grossly observable brain injury.

follicle-stimulating hormone (FSH) A hormone produced by the anterior pituitary gland that is important in the menstrual cycle.

foramen ovale An opening in the septum of the heart that closes after birth.

forward surgical team A team, usually staffed with physicians, nurses, and EMS providers, that performs minor surgical procedures and débridements in the field, taking some of the load from the hospital facility.

fracture A break or rupture in the bone.

free-flow oxygen Oxygen administered via oxygen tube and a cupped hand on the patient's face.

freelancing When individual units or different organizations make independent and often inefficient decisions about the next appropriate action.

frontal lobe The portion of the brain that is important in voluntary motor actions and personality traits.

frostbite Localized damage to tissues resulting from prolonged exposure to extreme cold.

frostnip Early frostbite, characterized by numbness and pallor without significant tissue damage.

full-thickness burn A burn that extends through the epidermis and dermis into the subcutaneous tissues beneath; previously called a third-degree burn.

G agents Early nerve agents that were developed by German scientists in the period after World War I and into World War II. There are three such agents: sarin, soman, and tabun.

gamma radiation A type of energy that is emitted from a strong radiologic source that is far faster and stronger than alpha and beta rays. These rays easily penetrate the human body and require either several inches of lead or concrete to prevent penetration. Rays of this type share key characteristics with x-rays.

gangrene An infection commonly caused by *Clostridium perfringens*. The result is tissue destruction and gas production that may lead to cell death.

gastroesophageal reflux A condition in which stomach acid rises into the esophagus on a regular or frequent basis, potentially causing irritation and damage; a common cause of vomiting.

gastrostomy tube (G-tube) A tube that is surgically placed directly into the patient's stomach through the skin to provide nutrition or medications.

generalized seizures A type of seizure characterized by manifestations that indicate involvement of both cerebral hemispheres.

geriatrics The assessment and treatment of disease in someone 65 years or older.

gestational hypertension High blood pressure that develops after the 20th week of pregnancy in women with previously normal blood pressures, and that resolves spontaneously in the postpartum period; formerly known as pregnancy-induced hypertension.

gestation Period of time from conception to birth. For humans, the full period is normally 9 months (or 40 weeks).

gestational period The time that it takes for the fetus to develop in utero, normally 38 weeks.

glenoid fossa The socket in the scapula in which the head of the humerus rotates.

globe The eyeball.

glomerular filtration The process by which the kidneys filter the blood, removing excess wastes and fluids.

gout A painful disorder characterized by the crystallization of uric acid within a joint.

granulocytes Cells that contain granules.

gravidity The total number of times a woman has been pregnant, including the current pregnancy.

gravity (g) The acceleration of a body by the attraction of the earth's gravitational force, normally 32.2 ft/sec^2 (9.8 m/sec^2).

greenstick fracture A type of fracture occurring most frequently in children in which there is incomplete breakage of the bone.

grunting A short, low-pitched sound at the end of exhalation, present in children with moderate to severe hypoxia. It reflects poor gas exchange because of fluid in the lower airways and air sacs.

guerilla warfare A form of warfare in which a small group that is not part of the official military engages in combat that uses the element of surprise, such as raids and ambushes; sometimes used by terrorists to protect their training camps and bases of operation.

habitual abortion Three or more consecutive pregnancies that end in miscarriage.

hand tool Any tool or piece of equipment operated by human power.

hangman's fracture The most classic distraction injury, which occurs when a person is hanged by the neck. Bending and fractures occur at the C1 to C2 region, which quickly tear the spinal cord.

hard palate The bony anterior part of the palate that is supported by bone (primarily maxillary bone) and forms the roof of the mouth.

hazardous material Any substance that is toxic, poisonous, radioactive, flammable, or explosive and causes injury or death with exposure.

HAZWOPER (HAZardous Waste OPerations and Emergency Response) The federal OSHA regulation that governs hazardous materials waste site and response training. Specifics can be found in Title 29, standard number 1910.120. Subsection (q) is specific to emergency response.

head injury A traumatic insult to the head that may result in injury to soft tissue of the scalp and bony structures of the head and skull, not including the face.

head trauma A general term that includes both head injuries and traumatic brain injuries.

heat cramps Acute and involuntary muscle pains, usually in the lower extremities, the abdomen, or both, that occur because of profuse sweating and subsequent sodium losses in sweat.

heat exhaustion A clinical syndrome characterized by volume depletion and heat stress that is thought to be a milder form of heat illness and on a continuum leading to heatstroke.

heat illness The increase in core body temperature due to inadequate thermolysis.

heat syncope An orthostatic or near-syncopal episode that typically occurs in nonacclimated people who may be under heat stress.

heatstroke The least common and most deadly heat illness, caused by a severe disturbance in thermoregulation, usually characterized by a core temperature of more than 104°F (40°C) and altered mental status.

heavy-duty emergency vehicle An extra–heavy-duty transport vehicle.

hematemesis Vomit with blood; can either look like coffee grounds, indicating the presence of partially digested blood, or contain bright red blood, indicating active bleeding.

hematochezia The passage of stool in which bright red blood can be distinguished; caused by lower gastrointestinal bleeding.

hematocrit The proportion of red blood cells in the total blood volume.

hematoma A mass of blood in the soft tissues beneath the skin; it indicates bleeding into soft tissues and may be the result of a minor or a severe injury; a potential complication of IV therapy.

hematuria The presence of blood in the urine.

hemodynamic monitoring Monitoring and measurement of blood movement, volume, and pressure.

hemoperitoneum The presence of extravasated blood in the peritoneal cavity.

hemophilia A bleeding disorder that is primarily hereditary, in which clotting does not occur or occurs insufficiently.

hemopneumothorax A collection of blood and air in the pleural cavity.

hemoptysis Coughing up blood in the sputum.

hemorrhage Bleeding.

hemorrhagic shock A condition in which volume is lost in the form of blood.

hemostasis The body's natural blood-clotting mechanism; involves the steps of blood vessel spasm, platelet plug formation, and blood clotting.

hemothorax The collection of blood within the normally closed pleural space.

Henry's law A law of gas that states that the amount of a gas in a solution varies directly with the partial pressure of a gas over a solution.

heparinized solution A saline solution mixed with heparin, an anticoagulant used to prevent blood clots from forming.

herniation A process in which tissue is forced out of its normal position, such as when the brain is forced from the cranial vault, either through the foramen magnum or over the tentorium.

herpes zoster Shingles; a contagious condition caused by the reactivation of the varicella virus on nerve roots.

high-altitude cerebral edema (HACE) An altitude illness in which there is a change in mental status and/or ataxia in a person with acute mountain sickness or the presence of mental status changes and ataxia in a person without acute mountain sickness.

high-altitude pulmonary edema (HAPE) An altitude illness characterized by at least two of the following: dyspnea at rest, cough, weakness or decreased exercise performance, or chest tightness or congestion. Also, at least two of the following signs: central cyanosis, audible crackles or wheezing in at least one lung field, tachypnea, or tachycardia.

high-angle operation A rope rescue operation in which the angle of the slope is greater than 45°. Rescuers depend on life safety rope rather than working from a fixed support surface, such as the ground.

high-level disinfection The killing of pathogenic agents by using potent means of disinfection.

high-pressure injection injuries Types of injuries that occur when a foreign material is forcefully injected into soft tissue.

homeostasis A tendency to constancy or stability in the body's internal environment; processes that balance the supply and demand of the body's needs.

hospice An organization that provides end-of-life care to patients with terminal illnesses and their families.

hospital surge capacity The capabilities of a receiving hospital to handle a large number of unexpected emergency patients, such as those seen in a mass-casualty incident.

hot zone The area that directly surrounds an incident site and is considered immediately dangerous to life and health. All personnel working in the hot zone must wear all appropriate protective clothing and equipment. Entry requires approval by the incident commander or a designated sector officer. Complete backup, rescue, and decontamination teams must be in place at the perimeter before operations begin.

human immunodeficiency virus (HIV) The virus that may lead to acquired immunodeficiency syndrome; cells in the immune system are killed or damaged so that the body is unable to fight infections and certain cancers.

hydramnios A condition in which there is too much amniotic fluid; also known as polyhydramnios.

hydrocephalus A medical condition in which there is an abnormal buildup of cerebrospinal fluid in the ventricles of the brain; this can be acquired (occurring after birth) or congenital (developing before birth).

hydroplaning A condition in which the tires of a vehicle may be lifted off the road surface as water "piles up" under them, making the vehicle feel as though it is floating.

hyoid bone A bone at the base of the tongue that supports the tongue and its muscles.

hypercapnia Increased carbon dioxide levels in arterial blood.

hyperemesis gravidarum A condition of persistent nausea and vomiting during pregnancy.

hyperesthesia Hyperacute pain to touch.

hyperextension Extension of a limb or other body part beyond its usual range of motion.

hyperkalemia An abnormally elevated level of potassium in the blood.

hyperphosphatemia An abnormally elevated level of phosphate in the blood; often associated with decreased calcium. Normal levels are between 0.81 and 1.45 mmol/L.

hyperpyrexia A high body temperature.

hyperthermia Unusually elevated body temperature.

hypertrophic cardiomyopathy A condition in which the heart muscle wall is unusually thick, requiring the heart to pump harder to eject blood from the left ventricle.

hypertrophic scar An abnormal scar with excess collagen that does not extend over the wound margins.

hyperuricemia High levels of uric acid in the blood.

hyphema Bleeding into the anterior chamber of the eye; results from direct ocular trauma.

hypoperfusion A condition that occurs when the level of tissue perfusion decreases below that needed to maintain normal cellular functions; also called shock.

hypopituitarism A condition in which the pituitary gland does not produce normal amounts of some or all of its hormones. It can be congenital; occur secondary to tumors, infection, or stroke; or develop after trauma or radiation therapy.

hypoplastic left heart syndrome Underdevelopment of the aorta, aortic valve, left ventricle, and mitral valve; this defect involves the entire left side of the heart.

hypothalamus An area of the diencephalon that is the primary link between the endocrine system and the nervous system; responsible for control of many body functions, including heart rate, digestion, sexual development, temperature regulation, emotion, hunger, thirst, and regulation of the sleep cycle.

hypothermia Condition in which the core body temperature is significantly below normal.

hypotonia Low or poor muscle tone (floppiness).

hypovolemic shock A condition that occurs when the circulating blood volume is inadequate to deliver adequate oxygen and nutrients to the body; also referred to as *burn shock*, the shock or hypoperfusion caused by a burn injury and the tremendous loss of fluids; capillaries leak, resulting in intravascular fluid volume oozing out of the circulation and into the interstitial spaces, and cells take in increased amounts of salt and water.

hypoxemia A decrease in arterial oxygen level.

hypoxic-ischemic encephalopathy Damage to cells in the central nervous system (the brain and spinal cord) from inadequate oxygen.

ignition temperature The minimum temperature at which a fuel, when heated, will ignite in air and continue to burn; also called the autoignition temperature.

ileus Disruption or loss of normal gastrointestinal motility.

immediately dangerous to life and health (IDLH) An atmospheric concentration of any toxic, corrosive, or asphyxiant substance that poses an immediate threat to life, or could cause irreversible or delayed adverse health effects, or serious interference for a team member attempting to escape from the dangerous atmosphere; there are three general types: toxic, flammable, and oxygen-deficient. A respirator is mandatory when working in such an environment.

imminent A threat level in which a terrorist event is known to be impending or will occur very soon.

imminent abortion A spontaneous abortion that cannot be prevented.

impacted fracture A broken bone in which the cortices of one bone become wedged into another bone, as could be the case in a fall from a significant height.

implosion A bursting inward.

improvised explosive device (IED) An explosive device built from unrestricted and often common equipment.

inborn errors of metabolism (IEMs) A group of congenital conditions that cause either accumulation of toxins or disorders of energy metabolism in the neonate. These conditions are characterized by an infant's failure to thrive and by vague signs such as poor feeding.

incident action plan (IAP) An oral or written plan stating general objectives reflecting the overall strategy for managing an incident.

incident command system (ICS) A system implemented to manage disasters and mass-casualty incidents in which section chiefs, including operations, finance, logistics, and planning, report to the incident commander.

incident commander (IC) The overall leader of the incident command system to whom commanders or leaders of the incident command system divisions report.

incision A wound usually made deliberately, as in surgery; a clean cut, as opposed to a laceration.

incomplete abortion Expulsion of the fetus that results in some products of conception remaining in the uterus.

incomplete fracture A fracture in which the bone does not fully break.

incomplete spinal cord injury Spinal cord injury in which there is some degree of cord-mediated function. Initial dysfunction may be temporary and there may be potential for recovery.

incubation The period between the person's exposure to the agent and the onset of symptoms.

index of suspicion Anticipating the possibility of specific types of injury.

indirect injury An injury that results from a force that is applied to one region of the body but leads to an injury in another area.

infantile hypertrophic pyloric stenosis (IHPS) Marked hypertrophy and hyperplasia of the two (circular and longitudinal) muscular layers of the pylorus, resulting in the pylorus becoming thick and obstructing the end of the stomach.

inhibin A protein that plays a key role in the menstrual cycle by triggering release of follicle-stimulating hormone.

inner cannula The inner tube that is inserted into the outer cannula of a tracheostomy tube.

inner ear One of the three anatomic parts of the ear; it consists of the cochlea and semicircular canals.

integument The skin.

intellectual disability A primarily cognitive disorder that appears during childhood and is accompanied by lack of adaptive behaviors, such as the ability to live and function independently or interact successfully with others; generally defined as an intelligence quotient below 70; formerly called mental retardation.

intermodal tank A bulk container that serves as both a shipping and a storage vessel. Such tanks hold between 5,000 and 6,000 gallons (18,900 to 22,700 L) of product and can be pressurized or nonpressurized. Intermodal tanks may be shipped by all modes of transportation.

international terrorism Terrorism that is carried out by those not of the host's country; also known as cross-border terrorism.

intertrochanteric fracture A fracture that occurs in the region between the lesser and greater trochanters.

intestinal atresia A congenital condition in which part of the bowel does not develop.

intestinal stenosis A congenital condition in which part of the bowel is narrow.

intra-aortic balloon pump A balloon that is inserted into the aorta and connected to a pump via a catheter. This therapy helps to increase the blood flow to the coronary arteries during diastole (inflation) and decrease afterload of blood from the left ventricle (deflation).

intracerebral hematoma Bleeding within the brain tissue (parenchyma) itself; also called an intraparenchymal hematoma.

intracranial pressure (ICP) The pressure within the cranial vault; normally 0 to 15 mm Hg in adults.

intuition Pattern recognition and pattern matching, based on your own past experiences.

intussusception An event where one part of the intestine folds into another part of the intestines, leading to a blockage.

ionizing radiation Energy that is emitted in the form of rays or particles.

iris The colored portion of the eye.

irreversible shock The point at which shock has progressed to a terminal stage, resulting in death.

joint information center (JIC) An area designated by the incident commander, or a designee, in which public information officers from multiple agencies disseminate information about the incident.

Joule's law A description of the relationship between heat production, current, and resistance.

jugular venous distention (JVD) The visible bulging of the jugular veins when a patient is in semi-Fowler or full Fowler position, due to increased volume or increased pressure within the central venous system or the thoracic cavity; indicates inadequate blood movement through the heart and/or lungs.

JumpSTART triage A sorting system for pediatric patients younger than 8 years or weighing less than 100 pounds (45 kg). There is a minor adaptation for infants and children (including those with special needs) who cannot ambulate on their own.

Kehr sign Left shoulder pain that may indicate a ruptured spleen.

keloid scar An abnormal scar commonly found in people with darkly pigmented skin. It extends over the wound margins.

kinetic energy (KE) The energy associated with bodies in motion, expressed mathematically as half the mass times the square of the velocity.

kinetics The study of the relationship among speed, mass, vector direction, and physical injury.

Klumpke paralysis An injury of childbirth affecting the spinal nerves C8 to T1 of the brachial plexus. It can be contrasted to Erb palsy, which affects C5 and C6.

label A type of signage at least 3.9 inches (9.9 cm) on each side that is often required on all four sides of individual packages and boxes that are being transported.

labor The mechanism by which the fetus and the placenta are expelled from the uterus.

laceration A wound made by tearing or cutting tissues.

lamina Posterior arch of the vertebral bone; arises from the posterior pedicles and fuses to form the posterior spinous processes.

laminated glass A type of window glazing that incorporates a sheeting material to keep the glass from breaking into shards. This kind of glass, often used for windshields, resists even deliberate breakage.

landing zone A designated location for the landing of aircraft.

language-based learning disability A type of disability in which difficulties with reading, spelling, or writing cause a person to fall behind expectations for a given age.

laryngospasm Severe constriction of the larynx in response to allergy, noxious stimuli, or illness.

lateral compression A force that is directed from the side toward the midline of the body.

law of conservation of energy The law of physics that states energy can be neither created nor destroyed; it can only change form.

LD$_{50}$ The amount (lethal dose) of an agent or substance that will kill 50% of people who are exposed to this level.

Le Fort fractures Maxillary fractures that are classified into three categories based on their anatomic location.

lethal concentration (LC) The concentration of a material in air that, on the basis of laboratory tests (inhalation route), is expected to kill a specified number of the group of test animals when administered over a specified period.

lethal dose (LD) A single dose that causes the death of a specified number of the group of test animals exposed by any route other than inhalation.

level A ensemble The highest level of protective suit worn by hazardous materials personnel; may also be referred to as fully encapsulating because the suit covers everything, including the breathing apparatus.

level B ensemble Personal protective equipment that is one step less protective than level A, but provides for a high level of respiratory protection.

level C ensemble A level of personal protective equipment that provides splash protection.

level D ensemble A level of personal protective equipment worn by support personnel working in the cold zone at a hazardous materials incident, or when there is little or no threat posed by the released substance; includes little to no respiratory protection.

lewisite A blistering agent that has a rapid onset of symptoms and produces immediate intense pain and discomfort on contact. Its military abbreviation is L.

liaison officer (LNO) In incident command, the person who relays information, concerns, and requests among responding agencies.

lightening In pregnancy, a feeling of relief of pressure in the upper abdomen; a premonitory sign of labor.

limbic system Structures within the cerebrum and diencephalon that influence emotions, motivation, mood, and sensations of pain and pleasure.

linear fracture A fracture that runs parallel to the long axis of a bone.

linear skull fracture A fracture that usually occurs in the temporal-parietal region of the skull; not associated with skull deformity; accounts for 80% of skull fractures; also called nondisplaced skull fracture.

liquefaction necrosis A form of necrosis that results from the transformation of tissue into a liquid viscous mass (pus).

lister bags Heavy canvas bags that can be hung from trees containing water in amounts from 40 to 100 gallons (151 to 379 L).

local effect An effect of a hazardous material on the body that is limited to the area of contact.

lochia The vaginal discharge of blood and mucus that occurs following delivery of a newborn; it usually lasts several days and then gradually decreases over the weeks following delivery.

logistics section In incident command, the section that helps procure and stockpile equipment and supplies during an incident.

low-angle operation A rope rescue operation carried out on a mildly sloping surface (less than 45°) or on level ground.

The ground is the rescuer's primary means of support, and the rope system is the secondary means of support.

lower flammable limit (LFL) The minimum amount of gaseous fuel that must be present in the air for the air-fuel mixture to be flammable or explosive.

loxoscelism A potentially fatal condition resulting from a brown recluse spider bite that begins with a painful, inflamed vesicle that may progress to a gangrenous sloughing of the skin.

Lund-Browder chart A detailed version of the rule of nines chart that takes into consideration the changes in total body surface area that occur with growth.

luxation A complete dislocation.

lymph nodes Round or bean-shaped structures interspersed along the course of the lymph vessels, which filter the lymph and serve as a source of lymphocytes.

lymphangitis Inflammation of a lymph channel.

lymphatic system A network of capillaries, vessels, ducts, nodes, and organs that helps to maintain the fluid environment of the body by producing lymph and transporting it through the body.

malignant hyperthermia A condition that can result from common anesthesia medications (notably succinylcholine) and present with hyperthermia, muscular rigidity, altered mental status, and a hyperdynamic state.

mallet finger An avulsion fracture of the extensor tendon of the distal phalynx caused by jamming a finger into an object.

malocclusion Misalignment of the teeth.

malrotation A congenital anomaly of rotation of the midgut, the small bowel is found predominantly on the right side of the abdomen. Results in increased incidence of intestinal volvulus.

malrotation with volvulus A condition that occurs when there is a twisting of the bowel around its mesenteric attachment to the abdominal wall.

mandatory reporter A category of professional required by some states to report suspicions of child maltreatment. Prehospital professionals may be included.

mandible The movable lower jaw bone.

manual defibrillation A mode available on automated external defibrillators, allowing the paramedic to interpret the cardiac rhythm and determine whether defibrillation is indicated (rather than the monitor making the determination).

MARK 1 A nerve agent antidote kit containing two auto-injector medications, atropine and 2-PAM chloride (pralidoxime chloride).

mass-casualty incident (MCI) An emergency situation that can place great demand on the equipment or personnel of the EMS system or has the potential to overwhelm available resources.

mass decontamination The physical process of reducing or removing surface contaminants from large numbers of victims in potentially life-threatening situations in the fastest time possible.

MC-306/DOT 406 flammable liquid tanker A vehicle that typically carries between 6,000 and 10,000 gallons (22,700 to 37,900 L) of a product such as gasoline or other flammable and combustible materials. The tank is nonpressurized.

MC-307/DOT 407 chemical hauler A tanker with a rounded or horseshoe-shaped tank capable of holding 6,000 to 7,000 gallons (22,700 to 26,500 L) of flammable liquid, mild corrosives, and poisons. The tank has a high internal working pressure.

MC-312/DOT 412 corrosive tanker A tanker that often carries aggressive (highly reactive) acids such as concentrated sulfuric and nitric acid. It is characterized by several heavy-duty reinforcing rings around the tank and holds approximately 6,000 gallons (22,700 L) of product.

MC-331 pressure cargo tanker A tanker that carries materials such as ammonia, propane, Freon, and butane. This type of tank is commonly constructed of steel and has rounded ends and a single open compartment inside. The liquid volume inside the tank varies, ranging from the 1,000-gallon (3,800-L) delivery truck to the full-size 11,000-gallon (41,600-L) cargo tank.

MC-338 cryogenic tanker A low-pressure tanker designed to maintain the low temperature required by the cryogens it carries. A boxlike structure containing the tank control valves is typically attached to the rear of the tanker.

mean arterial pressure (MAP) The blood pressure required to sustain organ perfusion; the average (or mean) pressure against the arterial wall during a cardiac cycle; roughly 60 mm Hg in the average person.

mechanical energy The energy that results from motion (kinetic energy) or that is stored in an object (potential energy).

mechanism of injury (MOI) The series of events that result in traumatic injuries; the forces that act on the body to cause injury.

Meckel diverticulum One of the most common congenital malformations of the small intestines, which presents with painless rectal bleeding.

meconium A dark green-black material in the amniotic fluid that indicates fetal distress, and that can be aspirated into the fetus's lungs during delivery; the fetus's first bowel movement.

medevac Medical or trauma evacuation of a patient by helicopter.

mediastinitis Inflammation of the mediastinum, often a result of the gastric contents leaking into the thoracic cavity after esophageal perforation.

medical incident command A group of operations in a unified command system, whose three designated sector positions are triage, treatment, and transport.

medical monitoring The process of assessing the health status of hazardous materials team members before and after entry to a hazardous materials incident site.

melena Dark, tarry, malodorous stools caused by upper gastrointestinal bleeding.

meninges A set of three tough membranes—the dura mater, arachnoid, and pia mater—that encloses the entire brain and spinal cord.

meningitis An inflammation of the meningeal coverings of the brain and spinal cord; usually caused by a virus or bacterium; the viral type is not communicable and is less severe than the bacterial type, which can result in brain damage, hearing loss, learning disability, or death.

mesentery A membranous double fold of tissue in the abdomen that attaches various organs to the body wall.

middle ear One of the three anatomic parts of the ear; it consists of the inner portion of the tympanic membrane and the ossicles.

miosis Bilateral pinpoint constricted pupils.

missed abortion A situation in which a fetus has died during the first 20 weeks of gestation, but has remained in utero.

missile fragmentation A primary mechanism of tissue disruption from certain rifles in which pieces of the projectile break apart, allowing the pieces to create their own separate paths through tissues.

mobile integrated health care providers/community paramedics (MIHPs/CPs) Paramedics whose primary role is to assist patients, such as those who frequently use the EMS system for health care needs that can be managed outside the emergency department, in managing their health care needs more effectively.

morgue unit leader In incident command, the person who works with area medical examiners, coroners, and law enforcement agencies to coordinate the disposition of dead victims.

mottling A blotchy pattern on the skin, caused by vasoconstriction or inadequate perfusion; a typical finding in states of severe protracted hypoperfusion and shock.

mucopolysaccharide gel One of the complex materials found, along with the collagen fibers and elastin fibers, in the dermis of the skin.

multifocal seizure Seizure activity that involves more than one site, is asynchronous, and is usually migratory.

multiple-casualty incident Any situation with more than one patient, but which will not overwhelm available resources.

multiple-organ dysfunction syndrome (MODS) A progressive condition usually characterized by combined failure of several organs, such as the lungs, liver, and kidneys, along with some clotting mechanisms, which occurs after severe illness or injury.

multisystem trauma Trauma caused by generalized mechanisms which affect numerous body systems.

muscular dystrophy A broad term that describes a category of incurable genetic diseases that cause a slow, progressive degeneration of the muscle fibers.

mutual aid agreements (MAAs) Documents that preplan how you will access help from other areas when needed.

mutual aid response An agreement between neighboring EMS systems to respond to mass-casualty incidents or disasters in each other's region when local resources are insufficient to handle the response.

myalgia Muscle pain.

myasthenia gravis A condition in which the body generates antibodies against its own acetylcholine receptors, causing muscle weakness, often in the face.

myasthenic crisis A complication of myasthenia gravis in which weakened respiratory muscles lead to respiratory failure.

myelomeningocele A developmental anomaly in which a portion of the spinal cord or meninges protrudes outside the spinal column or even outside the body, usually in the area of the lumbar spine (the lower third of the spine); also called spina bifida.

myocardial contractility The ability of the heart to contract.

myocardial contusion Blunt force injury to the heart that results in capillary damage, interstitial bleeding, and cellular damage in the area.

myocardial rupture An acute traumatic perforation of the ventricles, atria, intraventricular septum, intra-atrial septum, chordae, papillary muscles, or valves.

myocarditis Inflammation of the myocardium.

myometrium The middle layer of tissue in the uterus.

myositis Inflammation of the muscle, usually caused by infection.

myotome A region of the body innervated by the motor components of spinal nerves.

National Incident Management System (NIMS) A Department of Homeland Security system designed to enable federal, state, and local governments and private sector and nongovernmental organizations to effectively and efficiently prepare for, prevent, respond to, and recover from domestic incidents, regardless of cause, size, or complexity, including acts of catastrophic terrorism.

National Terrorism Advisory System (NTAS) The US system for informing citizens of a potential terrorist threat; replaced the color-coded Homeland Security Advisory System.

necrotizing fasciitis Death of tissue from bacterial infection, caused by more than one infecting organism—most commonly, *Staphylococcus aureus* and hemolytic streptococci; this condition has a high mortality rate.

needle decompression Also referred to as a needle thoracentesis, this procedure introduces a needle or angiocath into the pleural space in an attempt to relieve a tension pneumothorax.

negative wave pulse The phase of an explosion in which pressure from the blast is less than atmospheric pressure.

neglect Refusal or failure on the part of the caregiver to provide life necessities. Compare to emotional abuse, which involves a lack of emotional support by the caregiver.

neonate Infant during the first month after birth.

neovascularization Development of new blood vessels to aid in healing injured soft tissue.

nerve agents A class of chemicals called organophosphates that function by blocking an essential enzyme in the nervous system, which causes the body's organs to become overstimulated and burn out.

nerve root injury Injury to a nerve at the level of the spinal cord.

neurogenic shock A type of shock in which circulatory failure is caused by paralysis of the nerves that control the size of the blood vessels, leading to widespread dilation; seen in patients with spinal cord injuries.

neuroleptic malignant syndrome (NMS) A condition caused by antipsychotic and even common antiemetic medications that presents with hyperthermia, muscular rigidity, altered mental status, and a hyperdynamic state.

neuronal soma The body of a neuron (nerve cell).

neurotoxins Biologic agents that are the most deadly substances known to humans. They include botulinum toxin and ricin.

neurovascular compromise The loss of sensation blood supply, or both to a region of the body, typically distal to a site of injury; characterized by alterations in sensation.

neutralization A type of decontamination that uses one chemical to change the hazardous material into two less harmful substances; rarely used by hazardous materials teams.

neutron radiation A type of energy that is emitted from a strong radiologic source. It is the fastest moving and most powerful form of radiation. The particles easily penetrate lead and require several feet of concrete to stop them.

newborn Infant within the first few hours after birth.

Newton's first law of motion The law of motion that states a body at rest will remain at rest unless acted on by an outside force.

Newton's second law of motion The law of motion that states the force that an object can exert is the product of its mass times its acceleration.

nitrogen narcosis A state resembling alcohol intoxication produced by nitrogen gas dissolved in the blood at high ambient pressure; also called rapture of the deep.

nonbulk storage vessel Any container other than a bulk storage container, such as drums, bags, compressed gas cylinders, and cryogenic containers; these hold commonly used commercial and industrial chemicals such as solvents, cleaners, and compounds.

nondisplaced fracture A break in which the bone remains aligned in its normal position.

nonhemorrhagic shock Shock that occurs as a result of fluid loss contained within the body, such as in dehydration, burn injury, crush injury, and anaphylaxis.

nuchal cord A situation in which the umbilical cord is wrapped around the fetus's neck; cord compression may occur during labor, causing the fetal heart rate to slow and resulting in fetal distress.

nuchal rigidity A stiff or painful neck; commonly associated with meningitis.

nursemaid's elbow The subluxation of the radial head that often results from pulling on an outstretched arm.

obesity A condition in which a person's body mass index is greater than 30 kilograms per meters squared (kg/m^2).

oblique fracture A fracture that travels diagonally from one side of the bone to the other.

obstructive shock The type of shock that occurs when there is a block to blood flow in the heart or great vessels, causing an insufficient blood supply to the body's tissues.

obturator A solid plug at the end of a tracheostomy tube.

occipital lobe The portion of the brain responsible for processing visual information.

ocular myasthenia gravis An autoimmune disorder in which the extraocular muscles become weakened and are fatigued.

oculomotor nerve The third cranial nerve; it innervates the muscles that cause motion of the eyeballs and upper eyelid.

odynophagia Painful swallowing.

off-gassing The emitting of an agent after exposure—for example, from a person's clothes that have been exposed to the agent.

Ohm's law The formula that describes the relationship between voltage and resistance: Current (I) = Voltage (V) divided by Resistance (R).

old-age dependency ratio A formula used to determine the number of older people in a society as compared with the number of potential workers who are theoretically capable of providing resources to sustain the whole population. It is the number of older people (65 years and older) for every 100 adults (potential caregivers) between the ages of 18 and 64 years.

olecranon The proximal bony projection of the *ulna* at the elbow; the part of the ulna that constitutes the "funny bone."

oligohydramnios Decreased volume of amniotic fluid during a pregnancy; a risk factor associated with abnormalities of the urinary tract, postmaturity (birth after a prolonged pregnancy), and intrauterine growth retardation.

open fracture Any break in a bone in which the overlying skin has been damaged.

open incident An ongoing or uncontained incident in which rescuers will have to search for patients and then triage or treat them. The situation may produce more patients. Examples include school shootings, tornadoes, a hazardous materials release, and rising floodwaters.

open pneumothorax The result of a defect in the chest wall that allows air to enter the thoracic space.

open wound An injury in which there is a break in the surface of the skin or the mucous membrane, exposing deeper tissue to potential contamination.

open-book pelvic fracture A life-threatening fracture of the pelvis caused by a force that displaces one or both sides of the pelvis laterally and posteriorly.

operations The technical rescue training level geared toward working in the warm zone of an incident. Training at this level allows responders to directly assist those conducting the rescue operation and to use certain rescue skills and procedures.

operations section In incident command, the section that is responsible for managing the tactical operations, including standard triage, treatment, and transport of patients.

optic nerve Either of the second cranial nerves that enter the eyeball posteriorly, through the optic foramen.

optic nerve hypoplasia A congenital condition characterized by failure of the optic nerve to completely develop, possibly resulting in optic nerve atrophy over time.

orbits Bony cavities in the frontal part of the skull that enclose and protect the eyes.

organophosphates A class of chemical found in many insecticides used in agriculture and in the home. Nerve agents fall into this class of chemicals.

orthostatic hypotension A fall in blood pressure that occurs when moving from a recumbent to a sitting or standing position.

ossification center An area where cartilage is transformed through calcification into a new area of bone.

osteoarthritis (OA) The degeneration of a joint surface caused by wear and tear that lead to pain and stiffness.

osteoporosis A condition characterized by decreased bone mass and density and increased susceptibility to fractures.

outer cannula The larger (outer) tube of a tracheostomy tube.

overriding The overlap of a bone that occurs from the muscle spasm that follows a fracture, leading to a decrease in the length of the bone.

overtopping A situation in which a reservoir overflows its borders.

ovum A mature oocyte.

packaging The act of preparing a patient for movement as a unit by means of a backboard or similar stabilization device.

palliative care A type of medical care intended to provide comfort and relief from pain, for example in terminally ill patients.

pandemic An illness or disease that affects a high proportion of the population over a broad or potentially worldwide geographic area.

panhypopituitarism The inadequate production or absence of the pituitary hormones, including adrenocorticotropic hormone, cortisol, thyroxine, luteinizing hormone, follicle-stimulating hormone, estrogen, testosterone, growth hormone, and antidiuretic hormone.

paraplegia Paralysis of the lower extremities.

parasympathetic nervous system Subdivision of the autonomic nervous system; involved in control of involuntary, vegetative functions; mediated largely by the vagus nerve through the chemical acetylcholine.

paresthesia An abnormal sensation such as burning, numbness, or tingling.

parietal lobe The portion of the brain that receives and evaluates most sensory information, except smell, hearing, and vision.

parity The number of live births a woman has had.

Parkinson disease A neurologic condition in which the portion of the brain responsible for production of dopamine has been damaged or overused, resulting in tremors.

paronychia Infection of the area around the fingernail bed.

partial pressure The amount of the total pressure contributed by various gases in solution.

partial seizures A type of seizure that involves only one part of the brain.

partial-thickness burn A burn that involves the epidermis and part of the dermis, characterized by pain and blistering; previously called a second-degree burn.

patent ductus arteriosus A situation in which the ductus arteriosus, which assists in fetal circulation, does not transition as it should after birth to become the ligamentum arteriosum; the result is that the connection between the pulmonary artery and the aorta remains, allowing some oxygenated blood to move back into the heart rather than all of it moving out of the aorta and into the systemic circulation.

pathologic fracture A fracture that occurs when normal forces are applied to abnormal bone structures, such as a weakened bone.

pathway expansion The tissue displacement that occurs as a result of low-displacement shock waves that travel at the speed of sound in tissue.

patient collection point A location to which responders move patients to allow for safe assessment and treatment; also known as a casualty collection point.

patient generator The source that is causing people to become sick or injured.

peak load A time of day or day or week in which the call volume is at its highest.

pectoral girdle The shoulder girdle.

Pediatric Assessment Triangle (PAT) An assessment tool that allows rapid formation of a general impression of the type and level of illness or injury in an infant or child without touching him or her; consists of assessing appearance, work of breathing, and circulation to the skin.

pedicles Thick lateral bony struts that connect the vertebral body with the spinous and transverse processes and make up the lateral and posterior portions of the spinal foramen; a narrow strip of tissue by which an avulsed piece of tissue remains connected to the body.

pelvic girdle The large bone that arises in the area of the last nine vertebrae and sweeps around to form a complete ring.

penetrating trauma Injury caused by objects that pierce the surface of the body, such as knives and bullets, and damage internal tissues and organs.

perfusion The delivery of oxygen and nutrients to the cells, organs, and tissues of the body; also involves the removal of wastes.

peri-arrest period The period either just before or just after cardiac arrest when the patient is critical and care must be taken to prevent progression or regression into cardiac arrest.

pericardial sac The potential space between the layers of the pericardium.

pericardiocentesis A procedure in which a needle or angiocath is introduced into the pericardial sac to relieve cardiac tamponade.

perimetrium The outer protective layer of tissue in the uterus.

periorbital ecchymosis Bruising under or around the orbits that is commonly seen after a basilar skull fracture; also called raccoon eyes.

peripheral nerve injury Injury to a nerve anywhere in the body outside the spinal cord.

peripheral shock Shock caused by peripheral circulatory abnormalities; includes hypovolemic shock and distributive shock (Weil-Shubin classification).

peritoneal cavity The area in the abdomen encased in the peritoneum. It consists of an upper and a lower part. The upper portion contains the diaphragm, liver, spleen, stomach, gallbladder, and transverse colon. The lower portion contains the small bowel, sigmoid colon, parts of the descending and ascending colon, and, in women, the internal reproductive organs.

peritoneum A double-layered serous membrane that lines the abdominal cavity, encasing the liver, spleen, diaphragm, stomach, and transverse colon.

peritonitis Inflammation of the peritoneum, the protective membrane that lines the abdominal and pelvic cavities.

periumbilical Pertaining to the area around the umbilicus.

permanent cavity The path of crushed tissue produced by a missile traversing part of the body.

permissible exposure limit (PEL) The maximum concentration of a chemical that a person may be exposed to under OSHA regulations.

persistency The length of time that a chemical agent will stay on a surface before it evaporates.

persistent pulmonary hypertension Delayed transition from fetal to neonatal circulation.

personal flotation device (PFD) Also known as a life vest, a water rescue device that allows the body to float.

pertussis An acute communicable, infectious disease characterized by a catarrhal stage, followed by a paroxysmal cough that ends in a whooping inspiration; also called whooping cough.

petechial Characterized by small purple, nonblanching spots on the skin.

petechial hemorrhage A pinpoint red dot in the sclera of the eye.

phagocytosis The process in which one cell "eats" or engulfs a foreign substance to destroy it; a form of endocytosis.

phonologic process disorders A category of disorders that impact a person's ability to produce sounds that combine into spoken words.

phosgene A pulmonary agent that is a product of combustion, such as might be produced in a fire at a textile factory or house or at the site of metalwork or burning Freon; a very potent agent that has a delayed onset of symptoms, usually hours. Its military abbreviation is CG.

phosgene oxime A blistering agent that has a rapid onset of symptoms and produces immediate intense pain and discomfort on contact. Its military abbreviation is CX.

physical abuse A form of abuse that involves an intentional act such as throwing, striking, hitting, kicking, burning, or biting a vulnerable person.

physical evidence The evidence that ties a suspect or victim to a crime. It may include body materials, objects, and impressions.

pia mater The innermost and thinnest of the three meninges that enclose the brain and spinal cord; rests directly on the brain and spinal cord.

Pierre Robin sequence A condition present at birth marked by a small lower jaw (micrognathia). The tongue tends to fall back and downward (glossoptosis), and there is a cleft soft palate.

pinna A formation of cartilage within the inner ear that protects the ear and collects sounds into the ear canal, while allowing some perception of the direction from which the sound comes; also called the auricle.

placard A type of signage at least 10.8 inches (27 cm) on each side that is often required to be on all four sides of transport vehicles identifying the hazardous contents of the vehicle.

placenta The tissue attached to the uterine wall that nourishes the fetus through the umbilical cord.

placenta previa A condition in which the placenta develops in the lower part of the uterus, near or over the cervix.

planning section In incident command, the component that ultimately produces a plan to resolve any incident.

plantarflex To bend the foot toward the ground.

plasma A component of blood, made of 92% water, 6% to 7% proteins, and electrolytes, clotting factors, and glucose; plasma accounts for 55% of the total blood volume; this watery, yellow fluid carries the blood cells and nutrients and transports cellular waste material to the organs of excretion.

platelets Formed elements of the blood that function in blood clotting; also called thrombocytes.

plexus A cluster of nerve roots that permits peripheral nerve roots to rejoin and function as a group.

pneumonia An inflammation of the lungs caused by bacterial, viral, or fungal infections or infections with other microorganisms.

pneumonic plague A lung infection, also known as plague pneumonia, that is the result of inhalation of plague bacteria.

pneumothorax The collection of air within the normally closed pleural space.

point of distribution (POD) A strategically placed facility that has been preestablished for the mass distribution of antibiotics, antidotes, and vaccinations, along with other medications and supplies.

point tenderness The tenderness that is sharply localized at the site of the injury, found by gently palpating along the bone with the tip of one finger.

poliomyelitis A viral infection that attacks and destroys nerve axons, especially motor axons; the disease can cause weakness, paralysis, and respiratory arrest; the development of an effective vaccine has made its incidence rare.

polycythemia An overabundance or overproduction of red blood cells, white blood cells, and platelets, making the blood thick; a characteristic of people with chronic lung disease and chronic hypoxia.

polyhydramnios An excessive amount of amniotic fluid. May cause preterm labor.

polyneuropathy A type of disorder in which multiple nerves become dysfunctional.

polypharmacy The use of multiple medications.

positive wave pulse The phase of the explosion in which there is a pressure front with a pressure higher than atmospheric pressure.

posterior cord syndrome A condition associated with extension injuries in which there is isolated injury to the dorsal portion of the spinal cord. The condition is characterized by decreased sensation to light touch, proprioception, and vibration. Most other motor and sensory functions are unaffected.

posting The placement of an emergency vehicle at a specific geographic location to cover larger areas of territory and reduce response times.

postpartum The period of time after a woman has given birth.

postpolio syndrome The death of nerve fibers as a late consequence of poliomyelitis; characterized by swallowing difficulties, weakness, fatigue, and breathing problems.

postterm Any pregnancy that lasts more than 42 weeks.

potential energy The amount of energy stored in an object, the product of mass, gravity, and height, that is converted into kinetic energy and results in injury, such as from a fall.

preductal oxygen saturation The pulse oximetry value obtained during neonatal resuscitation, which evaluates the oxygenation status of blood from the brachiocephalic artery, prior to the ductus arteriosus. Tissues perfused with blood from the brachiocephalic artery better reflect the oxygenation status of the heart and brain. This value is best obtained from the right hand or earlobe.

preeclampsia A condition of late pregnancy that involves gradual onset of hypertension, headache, visual changes, and swelling of the hands and feet; also called pregnancy-induced hypertension or toxemia of pregnancy.

preload The precontraction pressure in the heart, which increases as the volume of blood builds up, stretching the cardiac muscle; the pressure of blood that is returned to the heart (venous return).

premature Underdeveloped; the condition of an infant born too soon. Refers to infants delivered before 37 weeks from the first day of the last menstrual period.

premorbid condition A condition preceding the onset of disease.

prenatal The state of the pregnant woman before birth.

presbycusis Progressive hearing loss, particularly in the high frequencies, along with lessened ability to discriminate between a particular sound and background noise.

pressure ulcer An ulcer that occurs when pressure is applied to body tissue, resulting in a lack of perfusion and ultimately necrosis.

preterm Describes an infant delivered at less than 37 completed weeks.

primary apnea Apnea caused by oxygen deprivation; usually corrected with stimulation, such as drying or slapping the newborn's feet; typically preceded by an initial period of rapid breathing.

primary brain injury Injury to the brain and its associated structures that is a direct result of impact to the head.

primary contamination An exposure that occurs with direct contact with the hazardous material.

primary exit The main means of escape should violence erupt. This is usually the door you used to enter the building.

primary spinal cord injury Injury to the spinal cord that is a direct result of trauma (eg, spinal cord transection from penetrating trauma or displacement of ligaments and bone fragments, resulting in cord compression).

primary triage A type of patient sorting used to rapidly categorize patients; the focus is on speed in locating all patients and determining an initial priority as their condition warrants.

primigravida First pregnancy.

prolapsed cord When the umbilical cord presents itself outside of the uterus while the fetus is still inside; an obstetric emergency during pregnancy or labor that acutely endangers the life of the fetus; can happen when the amniotic sac breaks and with the gush of amniotic fluid the cord comes along.

prolapsed umbilical cord A situation in which the umbilical cord comes out of the vagina before the newborn.

proprioception The ability to perceive the position and movement of one's body or limbs.

psychogenic shock A sudden reaction of the nervous system that produces a temporary, generalized vascular dilation, resulting in syncope (vasovagal syncope).

public information officer (PIO) In incident command, the person who keeps the public informed and relates any information to the press.

pulmonary blast injuries Pulmonary trauma resulting from short-range exposure to the detonation of high explosives.

pulmonary contusion Injury to the lung parenchyma that results in capillary hemorrhage into the tissue.

pulmonary embolism Obstruction of a pulmonary artery or arteries by solid, liquid, or gaseous material, such as a blood clot or foreign matter, which is swept through the right side of the heart into the lungs and becomes trapped within the pulmonary circulation.

pulmonary hypertension Elevated blood pressure in the pulmonary arteries from constriction; causes problems with the blood flow in the lungs, and makes the heart work harder.

pulmonary overpressurization syndrome (POPS) Also called burst lung, this diving emergency can occur during rapid ascent and can cause pneumothorax, mediastinal and subcutaneous emphysema, alveolar hemorrhage, and the lethal arterial gas embolism.

pulmonary stenosis Narrowing of the pulmonary valve.

pulp Specialized connective tissue within the cavity of a tooth.

pulse pressure The difference between the systolic blood pressure and the diastolic blood pressure.

pulsus paradoxus A drop in the systolic blood pressure of 10 mm Hg more during inspiration; characteristic of conditions that cause profound pressure changes in the thorax; commonly seen in patients with cardiac tamponade or severe asthma.

puncture wound An injury resulting from a piercing object, such as a nail or a knife; also referred to as a penetrating wound.

pupil The circular opening in the center of the eye through which light passes to the lens.

purpuric Pertaining to bruising of the skin.

pyloric stenosis Hypertrophy (enlargement) of the pyloric sphincter of the stomach; ultimately leads to intestinal obstruction, often in infants.

pyroclastic explosions Blasts from flowing or standing lava that can have a wide dispersal circumference, spewing ash and magma.

quadriplegia Paralysis of the upper and lower extremities.

rabid Describes an animal that is infected with rabies.

raccoon eyes Bruising under or around the orbits that is commonly seen after a basilar skull fracture; also called periorbital ecchymosis.

radiation Emission of heat from an object into surrounding, colder air.

radioactive material Any material that emits radiation.

radiologic dispersal device (RDD) Any container that is designed to disperse radioactive material.

radio operators Amateur radio operators who have a formal emergency communications set of standard operating procedures. Most are licensed by the Federal Communications Commission.

range of motion (ROM) The arc of movement of an extremity at a joint in a particular direction; the full distance that a joint can be moved.

rappelling The act of descending from a height on a fixed rope.

rehabilitation group leader In incident command, the person who establishes an area that provides protection for responders from the elements and the situation.

rescue task force leader In incident command, the person appointed to determine the type of equipment and resources needed for a situation involving extrication or special rescue; also called the extrication task force leader.

resistance vessels The smallest arterioles.

respiratory arrest The absence of respirations with detectable cardiac activity.

respiratory distress A clinical state characterized by increased respiratory rate, effort, and work of breathing.

respiratory failure A clinical state of inadequate oxygenation, ventilation, or both.

respiratory syncytial virus (RSV) A virus that affects the upper and lower respiratory tracts. Disease—namely, pneumonia and bronchiolitis—is more prevalent in the lower respiratory tract.

reticular activating system (RAS) Group of specialized neurons in the brainstem; involved in sleep and wake cycles; maintains consciousness, specifically one's level of arousal.

retina A delicate 10-layered structure of nervous tissue located in the rear of the interior of the globe of the eye; it receives light and generates nerve signals that are transmitted to the brain through the optic nerve; the inner layer of the eye wall, including the visual receptors.

retinal detachment Separation of the inner layers of the retina from the underlying choroid, the vascular membrane that nourishes the retina.

retinopathy Any eye disorder in which the retina becomes diseased, leading to partial or total vision loss.

retinopathy of prematurity A disease of the eye that affects premature infants, thought to be caused by disorganized growth of retinal blood vessels resulting in scarring and retinal detachment; can lead to blindness in serious cases.

retractions A sign of respiratory distress characterized by skin pulling inward between and around the ribs and clavicles during inhalation.

retrograde amnesia Loss of memory of events that occurred before the injury.

retroperitoneal space The area in the abdomen containing the aorta, vena cava, pancreas, kidneys, ureters, and portions of the duodenum and large intestine.

return of spontaneous circulation (ROSC) The return of spontaneous heart beat and blood pressure during the resuscitation of a patient in cardiac arrest.

Revised Trauma Score (RTS) A scoring system used for patients with head trauma.

Rh factor An antigen found on the red blood cells of most people; when a woman without this protein is impregnated by a man with this protein, the woman's body can create antibodies against the protein and attack future pregnancies.

rhabdomyolysis The destruction of muscle tissue leading to a release of potassium and myoglobin.

rheumatoid arthritis (RA) An inflammatory disorder that affects the entire body and leads to degeneration and deformation of joints.

ricin A neurotoxin derived from mash that is left from pressing oil from a castor bean; causes pulmonary edema and respiratory and circulatory failure, leading to death.

rotation-flexion injury A type of injury typically resulting from high acceleration forces; can result in a stable unilateral facet dislocation in the cervical spine.

route of exposure The manner by which a toxic substance enters the body.

rule of nines A system that assigns percentages to sections of the body, allowing for calculation of the amount of total body surface area burned.

rule of palms A system that estimates the total body surface area burned by comparing the affected area with the size of the patient's palm, which is roughly equal to 1% of the patient's total body surface area; also called rule of ones.

sacral edema Swelling that presents around the sacral region of the spinal column.

safety data sheet (SDS) A document that provides a detailed product description and that is kept on site at workplaces for every potentially hazardous chemical at the workplace.

safety officer In incident command, the person who gives the "go ahead" to a plan or who may stop an operation when rescuer safety is an issue.

sarin A nerve agent that is one of the G agents; a highly volatile colorless and odorless liquid that turns from liquid to gas within seconds to minutes at room temperature. Its military abbreviation is GB.

saturation diving A type of diving in which the diver remains at depth for prolonged periods.

scald burn A burn produced by hot liquids.

scaphoid A concave shape of the abdomen; can be caused by evisceration; in the context of anatomy, the wrist bone that is found just beyond the most distal portion of the radius.

scar revision A surgical procedure to improve the appearance of a scar, reestablish function, or correct disfigurement from soft-tissue damage, surgical incision, or lesion.

sclera The white, fibrous outer layer of the eyeball.

scrambling A cross between hill climbing and rock climbing used to ascend rocky surfaces and ridges.

search and rescue (SAR) The process of locating a lost or overdue person and removing him or her from a hostile environment.

seasonal affective disorder (SAD) Depression that can affect people in long periods of bad weather, usually winter.

second stage of labor The stage of labor in which the newborn's head enters the birth canal, during which contractions become more intense and more frequent.

secondary apnea When asphyxia continues after primary apnea, the infant responds with a period of gasping respirations, falling pulse rate, and falling blood pressure. Positive pressure ventilation is indicated to reverse secondary apnea.

secondary brain injury The aftereffects of the primary injury; includes abnormal processes such as cerebral edema, increased intracranial pressure, cerebral ischemia and hypoxia, and infection. Onset is often delayed after the primary brain injury.

secondary collapse A collapse that occurs after the primary trench, excavation, or structural collapse.

secondary containment An engineered method to control spilled or released product if the main containment vessel fails.

secondary contamination Exposure to a hazardous material by contact with a contaminated person or object.

secondary device An additional explosive device used by terrorists that is set to explode after the initial bomb.

secondary exit Any other means of egress, including windows and rear doors.

secondary spinal cord injury Injury to the spinal cord, thought to be the result of multiple factors that result in a progression of inflammatory responses from primary spinal cord injury.

secondary triage A type of patient sorting used in the treatment sector that involves retriage of patients.

segmental fracture A bone that is broken in more than one place.

self-contained underwater breathing apparatus The expansion of the acronym SCUBA for specialized underwater breathing equipment.

self-rescue position A position used by a swift-water rescuer to avoid objects below the surface; the rescuer rolls into a faceup arched position, with the lower back higher than the feet (which are held together and face in the direction of travel—that is, feet first) and the arms at the sides.

semantic-pragmatic disorder A condition characterized by delayed language developmental milestones, resulting in the person repeatedly using irrelevant phrases out of context, confusing word pairs, and having trouble following conversations.

sensitization Developing a sensitivity to a substance that initially caused no allergic reaction.

sensorineural hearing loss A permanent lack of hearing caused by a lesion or damage of the inner ear.

sepsis A disease state of life-threatening organ dysfunction that results from the presence of invading microorganisms or their toxic products in the bloodstream; usually occurs in a febrile patient.

septic abortion A life-threatening emergency in which the uterus becomes infected following any type of abortion.

septic arthritis Inflammation of a joint based on a bacterial or fungal infection.

septic shock The type of shock that occurs as a result of widespread infection, usually bacterial; untreated, the result is multiple organ dysfunction syndrome and often death.

sexual abuse A form of abuse that involves a vulnerable person being forced into unwanted sexual acts, or into involvement in sexual activities such as pornography.

sexual exploitation A form of abuse that involves forcing a vulnerable person to perform or be involved in sexual acts, or to be involved in sexual activities such as pornography, in return for something they need or want, such as money, food, or shelter.

shallow water blackout A diving emergency that occurs when a person hyperventilates just before submerging underwater and becomes unresponsive before resurfacing due to hypoxemia and cerebral vasoconstriction.

shearing An applied force or pressure exerted against the surface and layers of the skin as tissues slide in opposite but parallel planes.

shelter-in-place A method of safeguarding oneself or others' position during an emergency event or event involving a hazardous material; includes measures such as remaining in a safe atmosphere, usually inside structures, or other simple measures such as shutting the windows, going to the cellar, or turning off the heating and air conditioning systems.

shim A slim, low-profile, wedgelike object used to snug loose cribbing under a load or to fill a void.

shock An abnormal state associated with inadequate oxygen and nutrient delivery to the metabolic apparatus of the cell; also called hypoperfusion.

shoring A hydraulic, pneumatic, or wood system to support a trench wall or reinforce building components such as walls, floors, or ceilings to prevent collapse.

shoulder dystocia A complication of delivery in which there is difficulty delivering the shoulders of a newborn; the shoulder cannot get past the woman's symphysis pubis.

sickle cell disease A disease that causes red blood cells to be misshapen, resulting in poor oxygen-carrying capability and potentially resulting in lodging of the red blood cells in blood vessels or the spleen.

silver fork deformity The dorsal deformity of the forearm that results from a Colles fracture.

simple access Access easily achieved with the use of simple hand tools or application of force.

simple febrile seizures A brief, self-limited, generalized seizure in a previously healthy child between ages 6 months and 6 years that is associated with the onset of or sudden increase in fever.

simple partial seizures A type of seizure that involves focal motor jerking or sensory abnormality in a patient who remains conscious.

single command system A command system in which one person is in charge, generally used with small incidents that involve only one responding agency or one jurisdiction.

situational awareness Knowing your surroundings, the people and groups in your environment, and the climate of violence or strife.

slipped capital femoral epiphysis (SCFE) A dislocation of the epiphyseal end of the femur, usually found in children and adolescents.

small for gestational age An infant whose size and weight are considerably less than the average for infants of the same age.

smallpox A highly contagious disease that may be spread in an aerosolized form as an act of warfare or terrorism. It is most contagious when blisters begin to form.

SMART A mnemonic used to describe the objectives of a community-based program to improve the survival of patients in out-of-hospital cardiac arrest: Specific, Measurable, Attainable and Achievable, Realistic and Relevant, and Timely.

sniffing position An upright position in which the patient's head and chin are thrust slightly forward to keep the airway open; the patient appears to be sniffing when in this position.

solvent The fluid that dissolves a solute, or the substance in which a solute is dissolved or mixed.

soman A nerve agent that is one of the G agents; twice as persistent as sarin and five times as lethal. It has a fruity odor as a result of the type of alcohol used in the agent and is both a contact and an inhalation hazard that can enter the body through skin absorption and through the respiratory tract. Its military abbreviation is GD.

somatic pain Pain caused by the activation of pain receptors in the body's superficial tissues, such as the skin, bones, muscles, and joints, usually felt deeply, that represents irritation or injury to tissue; in contrast to visceral pain, this is generally more intense and more precisely localized.

space junk Debris from satellites and other man-made objects that reenter the earth's atmosphere.

span of control In incident command, the subordinate positions under the commander's direction to which the workload is distributed; the supervisor-to-worker ratio.

spastic paralysis A chronic form of paralysis in which the affected muscles experience continued spasm.

spastic tetraplegia A form of cerebral palsy in which all fours limbs are affected.

special atomic demolition munition (SADM) A small suitcase-sized nuclear weapon that was designed to destroy individual targets, such as important buildings, bridges, tunnels, or large ships.

special weapons and tactics (SWAT) team A specialized law enforcement tactical unit.

specific gravity The measure that indicates whether a hazardous material will sink or float in water.

sphincters Muscles arranged in circles that are able to decrease the diameter of tubes. Examples are found within the rectum, bladder, and blood vessels.

spina bifida A developmental anomaly in which a portion of the spinal cord or meninges protrudes outside the spinal column or even outside the body, usually in the area of the lumbar spine (the lower third of the spine); also called myelomeningocele.

spinal clearance The act of declaring that a spinal injury is not present.

spinal shock The temporary local neurologic condition that occurs immediately after spinal trauma. Spinal cord swelling and edema begin immediately after injury, causing severe pain and possible paralysis.

spinal stenosis Narrowing of the spinal canal, causing compression of exiting nerve roots and pain radiating into the legs or arms.

spiral fracture A break in a bone that appears like a spring on a radiograph.

spoil pile The pile of dirt unearthed from an excavation. The pile may be unstable and prone to collapse.

spondylosis A degenerative condition resulting in decreased mobility of vertebral joints and compression of neural elements.

spontaneous abortion Expulsion of the fetus that occurs naturally; also called miscarriage.

spotter A person who assists a driver in backing up an emergency vehicle to compensate for blind spots at the back of the vehicle.

sprain An injury, including a stretch or a tear, to the ligaments of a joint that commonly leads to pain and swelling.

staging area manager In incident command, the person who locates an area to stage equipment and personnel and tracks unit arrival and deployment from the staging area.

START triage Simple Triage And Rapid Treatment; a patient sorting process that uses a limited assessment of the patient's ability to walk, respiratory status, hemodynamic status, and neurologic status.

status epilepticus A condition in which a seizure lasts longer than 4 to 5 minutes, or consecutive seizures without a return to consciousness between seizures.

steam burn A burn that has been caused by direct exposure to hot steam exhaust, as from a broken pipe.

steering play A sensation of looseness or sloppiness in a vehicle's steering.

steering pull A drift that is persistent enough that an operator can feel a tug on the steering wheel.

step chock A specialized cribbing assembly of wood or plastic blocks arranged in a step configuration.

sterilization A process, such as heating, that removes microbial contamination.

stoma In the context of the airway, the resultant orifice of a tracheostomy that connects the trachea to the outside air; located in the midline of the anterior part of the neck.

straddle fracture A fracture of the pelvis that results from landing on the peroneal region.

strain Stretching or tearing of a muscle or tendon by excessive stretching or overuse.

strategic deployment The staging of emergency vehicles to strategic locations within a service area to allow for coverage of emergency calls.

stress fracture A fracture that results from exaggerated stress on the bone caused by unusually rapid muscle development.

stroke volume (SV) The amount of blood that the left ventricle ejects into the aorta per contraction.

subarachnoid hemorrhage Bleeding into the subarachnoid space, where the cerebrospinal fluid circulates.

subconjunctival hematoma The collection of blood within the sclera of the eye, presenting as a bright red patch of blood over the sclera but not involving the cornea.

subcutaneous emphysema A physical finding of air within the subcutaneous tissue.

subdural hematoma An accumulation of blood beneath the dura but outside the brain.

subgaleal hemorrhage Bleeding between the periosteum of the skull and the galea aponeurosis.

subglottic Located below the glottic opening, as in the lower airway structures.

subglottic space The narrowest part of the pediatric airway.

subluxation A partial or incomplete dislocation.

sudden infant death syndrome (SIDS) The sudden death of an infant younger than 1 year that cannot be explained after a thorough investigation is conducted, including a complete autopsy, examination of the death scene, and a review of the clinical history.

suicide bomber A terrorist who wears or carries a weapon, such as an explosive, and triggers its detonation, killing himself or herself in the process.

sulfur mustard A vesicant that is generally considered very persistent. It is a yellow-brown oily substance that has the distinct smell of garlic or mustard and, when released, is quickly absorbed into the skin and/or mucous membranes and begins an irreversible process of damaging the cells. Its military abbreviation is H.

superficial burn A burn involving only the epidermis, which produces very red, painful skin; previously called a first-degree burn.

superficial frostbite A type of frostbite characterized by altered sensation (numbness, tingling, or burning) and white, waxy skin that is firm to palpation, but the underlying tissues remain soft.

supine hypotensive syndrome Low blood pressure resulting from compression of the inferior vena cava by the weight of the pregnant uterus when the woman is supine.

supplemental restraint system A system of specialized devices, such as airbags and seat belt pretensioners, used to restrain a driver or passenger in the protected passenger compartment of a motor vehicle during a crash.

supracondylar fracture A fracture of the distal humerus that occurs just proximal to the elbow.

supragaleal hematoma Bleeding between the subgaleal area of the skull and the galea aponeurosis.

supraglottic Located above the glottic opening, as in the upper airway structures.

surface-tended diving A type of diving in which air is piped to the diver through a tube from the surface.

surrogate decision maker A person legally authorized to make health care decisions on behalf of a patient who is incapable of making or communicating the decision on his or her own.

sympathetic eye movement The movement of both eyes in unison.

sympathetic nervous system Subdivision of the autonomic nervous system that governs the body's fight-or-flight reactions by inducing smooth muscle contraction or relaxation of the blood vessels and bronchioles.

synchronized cardioversion The use of a synchronized direct current (DC) electric shock to convert a tachydysrhythmia (such as atrial fibrillation or supraventricular tachycardia) to a normal sinus rhythm.

syndromic surveillance The monitoring, usually by local or state health departments, of the number and nature of medical cases against the expected volume of these cases at a given time and place in the community; can include the recording of EMS call volume, and the monitoring of the use of over-the-counter medications.

systemic effect A physiologic effect on the entire body or one of the body's systems.

systemic vascular resistance The resistance that blood must overcome to be able to move within the blood vessels; related to the amount of dilation or constriction in the blood vessel; present in all blood vessels except the pulmonary vessels.

tabun A nerve agent that is one of the G agents; 36 times more persistent than sarin and approximately one-half as lethal. It has a fruity smell and is unique because the components used to manufacture the agent are easy to acquire and the agent is easy to manufacture. Its military abbreviation is GA.

tactical paramedics Specially trained paramedics who provide medical care for SWAT team members conducting operations, barricaded patients, patients being held hostage, and other special operations.

tactical situation A high-risk situation involving the potential for physical violence or armed combat typically involving law enforcement teams interacting with potentially dangerous criminal suspects.

tag lines Rope or cord tied to a person who is entering a dangerous environment. Used for quick retrieval, usually in conjunction with a harness.

talus The bone of the foot that articulates with the tibia.

targeted temperature management (TTM) A procedure intended to lower body temperature in patients who are in a coma after return of spontaneous circulation; ideally performed in the hospital setting; formerly called therapeutic hypothermia.

technical decontamination A multistep process of carefully scrubbing and washing contaminants from a person or object, collecting runoff water, and collecting and properly handling all items.

technical rescue incident (TRI) A complex rescue requiring specially trained personnel and sophisticated equipment and involving vehicle extrication; rescue from water, ice, or confined spaces; rescue following trench, structural, or other collapse; high-angle rescue; response to hazardous materials incidents; or wilderness search and rescue.

technical rescue team A group of rescuers expertly trained in the various disciplines of technical rescue.

technician The level of training necessary for a rescuer directly involved in a rescue operation; indicates a high level of competency in technical or hazardous materials rescue.

tempered glass A type of glass that is heat-treated so that it breaks into small, relatively dull pieces.

temporal lobe The portion of the brain that has an important role in hearing and memory.

temporomandibular joint (TMJ) The joint between the temporal bone and the posterior condyle that allows for movements of the mandible.

tendinitis Inflammation of a tendon that most commonly results from overuse.

tension lines The pattern of tautness of the skin, which is arranged over body structures and affects how well wounds heal.

tension pneumothorax A life-threatening collection of air within the pleural space; the volume and pressure have both collapsed the involved lung and caused a shift of the mediastinal structures to the opposite side.

tenting A condition in which the skin slowly retracts after being pinched and pulled away slightly from the body; a sign of dehydration.

tentorium A horizontal projection of the dura that separates the cerebellum from the cerebrum.

term Describes a newborn delivered at 38 to 42 weeks of gestation.

terminal illness A disease that a patient cannot be cured of. Death is imminent.

termination of command The end of the incident command structure when an incident draws to a close.

terrorism A violent act dangerous to human life, in violation of the criminal laws of the United States or any segment to intimidate or coerce a government, the civilian population, or any segment thereof, in furtherance of political or social objectives.

testimonial evidence The oral documentation by a witness of his or her perceived facts of a criminal act.

tetanus A disease caused by spores that enter the body through a puncture wound contaminated with animal feces, street dust, or soil or that can enter through contaminated street drugs; signs and symptoms include pain at the wound site and painful muscle contractions in the neck and trunk muscles.

tetralogy of Fallot A cardiac anomaly that consists of four defects: a ventricular septal defect, pulmonary stenosis, right ventricular hypertrophy, and an overriding aorta.

thermal burn An injury caused by radiation or direct contact with a heat source on the skin.

thermal energy Energy transferred from sources that are hotter than the body, such as a flame, hot water, steam.

thermals Differing temperatures and swirling patterns of moving air with changes in wind speed.

thermogenesis The production of heat in the body.

thermolysis The liberation of heat from the body.

thermoregulation The process by which the body maintains temperature through a combination of heat gain by metabolic processes and muscular movement and heat loss through respiration, evaporation, conduction, convection, and perspiration.

third stage of labor The stage of labor in which the placenta is expelled.

Thompson test Squeezing of the calf muscle to evaluate for plantar flexion of the foot to determine whether the Achilles tendon is intact.

thoracic inlet The superior aspect of the thoracic cavity, this ring like opening is created by the first vertebral vertebra, the first rib, the clavicles, and the manubrium.

threatened abortion Expulsion of the fetus that is attempting to take place but has not occurred yet; usually occurs in the first trimester.

threshold limit value (TLV) The concentration of a substance that is supposed to be safe for exposure no more than 8 hours per day and 40 hours per week.

threshold limit value/ceiling (TLV/C) The maximum concentration of hazardous material to which a worker should not be exposed, even for an instant.

threshold limit value/short-term exposure limit (TLV-STEL) The concentration of a substance that a worker can be exposed to for up to 15 minutes but no more than four times per day with at least 1 hour between each exposure.

threshold limit value/skin The concentration at which direct or airborne contact with a material could result in possible and significant exposure from absorption through the skin, mucous membranes, and eyes.

thrombocytopenia A reduction in the number of platelets in the blood.

thromboembolic disease The condition in which a patient has a deep vein thrombosis or pulmonary embolism.

thrombosis The development of a blood clot.

tonic-clonic seizures A type of seizure that features rhythmic back-and-forth motion of an extremity and body stiffness.

TORCH syndrome Infections that occur in neonates as a result of organisms passing through the placenta from the woman to the fetus; includes toxoplasmosis, other agents, rubella, cytomegalovirus, and herpes simplex.

torus fracture *See* buckle fracture.

total anomalous pulmonary venous return A rare congenital defect in which the four pulmonary veins do not connect to the left atrium; instead, the pulmonary veins connect to the right atrium, resulting in diminished oxygen and an increased load on the right ventricle.

toxic products of combustion Hazardous chemical compounds that are released when a material decomposes under heat.

toxoplasmosis An infection caused by a parasite that pregnant women may get from handling or eating contaminated food or exposure from handling cat litter; the fetus can become infected.

tracheal transection Traumatic separation of the trachea from the larynx.

tracheostomy tube A plastic tube placed within the tracheostomy site (stoma).

traffic incident management (TIM) The process of coordinating different partner agencies to detect, respond to, and clear traffic incidents as quickly as possible to reduce the impacts of incidents on safety and congestion, while protecting the safety of on-scene responders and the traveling public.

transducer A device that converts energy or pressure into electrical signals.

transfer of command In incident command, when an incident commander turns over command to someone with more experience in a critical area.

transportation unit leader In incident command, the person who coordinates transportation and distribution of patients to appropriate receiving hospitals.

transposition of the great arteries A defect in which the great vessels are reversed; the aorta is connected to the right ventricle, and the pulmonary artery is connected to the left ventricle.

transverse fracture A fracture that runs in a straight line from one edge of the bone to the other and that is perpendicular to each edge.

transverse presentation A delivery in which the fetus lies crosswise in the uterus; one hand may protrude through the vagina.

trauma Acute physiologic and structural change (injury) that occurs in a person's body as a result of the rapid dissipation of energy delivered by an external source.

trauma lethal triad A combination of hypothermia, coagulopathy (poor blood clotting), and acidosis that is a major contributor to death in patients with severe traumatic bleeding.

trauma score A score that relates to the likelihood of patient survival with the exception of a severe head injury. It is calculated on a scale from 1 to 16, with 16 being the best possible score. It takes into account the Glasgow Coma Scale score, respiratory rate, respiratory expansion, systolic blood pressure, and capillary refill.

traumatic aortic disruption Dissection or rupture of the aorta.

traumatic asphyxia A pattern of injuries seen after a severe force is applied to the thorax, forcing blood from the great vessels and back into the head and neck.

traumatic brain injury (TBI) An impairment of brain function caused by an external force that may involve physical, intellectual, emotional, social, and vocational changes.

treatment unit leader In incident command, the person responsible for locating, setting up, and supervising the treatment area.

trench foot A process similar to frostbite but caused by prolonged exposure to cool, wet conditions.

triage To sort patients based on the severity of their conditions and prioritize them for care accordingly.

triage unit leader The person in charge of prioritizing patients, whose primary duty is to ensure that every patient receives initial triage.

tricuspid atresia The absence of a tricuspid valve, which normally separates the right atrium and the right ventricle.

tripoding An abnormal position that a person assumes to keep the airway open; involves leaning forward onto two arms stretched forward.

trismus The involuntary contraction of the mouth resulting in clenched teeth; occurs during seizures and head injuries.

truncus arteriosus A condition in which the pulmonary artery and the aorta are combined into one.

tube trailer A high-volume transportation device made up of several individual compressed gas cylinders banded together and affixed to a trailer. Tube trailers carry compressed gases such as hydrogen, oxygen, helium, and methane. One trailer may carry several different gases in individual tubes.

tunnel vision A situation in which a paramedic becomes so completely involved with patient care that he or she fails to see the possibility of physical harm to the patient or other care providers; focusing on or considering only one aspect of a situation without first taking into account all possibilities.

twisting injury An injury that commonly occurs during athletic activities in which an extremity rotates around a planted foot or hand.

tympanic membrane The eardrum; a thin, semitransparent membrane in the middle ear that transmits sound vibrations to the internal ear by means of the auditory ossicles.

type I emergency medical vehicle Conventional, truck-cab chassis with a modular body that can be transferred to a new chassis as needed.

type II emergency medical vehicle Standard van, forward-control integral cab-body.

type III emergency medical vehicle Specialty van, forward-control integral cab-body.

umbilical cord The conduit connecting the pregnant woman to the fetus via the placenta; it contains two arteries and one vein.

umbilical vein The blood vessel in the umbilical cord used to administer emergency medications.

unibody construction A vehicle design with no formal frame structure. The body and frame are one piece, which is considered to be the structural integrity of the vehicle.

unified command system A command system used in larger incidents in which there is a multiagency or multijurisdictional response to coordinate decision making and cooperation among the agencies.

upper flammable limit (UFL) The maximum amount of gaseous fuel that can be present in the air if the air-fuel mixture is to be flammable or explosive.

urostomy A surgically constructed opening for the urinary system.

uterine cavity The interior of the body of the uterus.

uterine inversion A potentially fatal complication of childbirth in which the placenta fails to detach properly and results in the uterus turning inside out.

vapor density The weight of an airborne concentration (vapor or gas) as compared with an equal volume of dry air.

vapor hazard An agent that enters the body through the respiratory tract.

vapor pressure For the purpose of this chapter, the pressure associated with liquids held inside any type of closed container.

velocity (V) The distance an object travels per unit time.

ventricular septal defect A hole in the septum separating the ventricles, allowing blood from the left ventricle to flow into the right ventricle.

ventricular shunt A surgically inserted tube draining cerebrospinal fluid from the cerebral ventricles into a body cavity, often the peritoneal cavity or the right atrium.

vertebral body Anterior weight-bearing structure in the spine made of cancellous bone and surrounded by a layer of hard, compact bone that provides support and stability.

vertical compression A type of injury typically resulting from a direct blow to the crown of the head or rapid deceleration from a fall, with the force moving through the feet, legs, and pelvis, possibly causing a burst fracture or disk herniation.

vertical shear The type of pelvic fracture that occurs when a massive force displaces the pelvis superiorly.

vesicant A blister agent. The primary route of entry is through the skin.

viral hemorrhagic fevers (VHFs) A group of diseases that includes the Ebola, Rift Valley, and yellow fever viruses, among others. This group of viruses causes the blood in the body to seep out from the tissues and blood vessels.

virus A germ that requires a living host to multiply and survive.

visceral pain Crampy, aching, deep pain caused by activation of pain receptors in internal areas of the body that are enclosed within a cavity, such as the chest, abdomen, or pelvis; common with genitourinary problems.

vitreous humor A jellylike substance found in the posterior compartment of the eye between the lens and the retina; helps the globe maintain its shape without distorting light.

volar Pertaining to the palm or sole; referring to the flexor surfaces of the forearm, wrist, or hand.

volatility The length of time that a chemical agent will stay on a surface before it evaporates.

Volkmann ischemic contracture Contraction of the fingers and sometimes the wrist following severe injury around the elbow joint; characterized by loss of muscular power and rapid onset of death and resultant contracture of the forearm musculature.

von Willebrand disease A bleeding disorder in which the patient is missing the von Willebrand factor (a protein essential for platelet adhesion), preventing the blood from clotting well.

VX nerve agent A nerve agent that is one of the G agents; over 100 times more lethal than sarin and extremely persistent. It is a clear, oily agent that has no odor and looks like baby oil.

Waddell triad A pattern of vehicle versus pedestrian injuries in children and people of short stature in which (1) the bumper hits pelvis and femur, (2) the chest and abdomen hit the grille or low hood, and (3) the head strikes the ground.

warm ischemic time The amount of time that specific tissues of the body are deprived of oxygen typically as a result of an injury or arterial occlusion.

warm zone The area located between the hot and cold zones at an incident. Decontamination stations are located in the warm zone.

water buffalo trailers Portable trailers that contain from 500 to 3,000 gallons (1,893 to 11,356 L) of water.

water reactive A property that indicates that a material will undergo a chemical reaction (for example, explosion) when mixed with water.

water soluble A property that indicates a material can be dissolved in water.

waybill A cargo document kept by the conductor of a train; also referred to as a consist.

weapon of mass destruction (WMD) Any agent designed to bring about mass death, casualties, and/or massive damage to property and infrastructure (bridges, tunnels, airports, and seaports).

weaponization The creation of a weapon from a biologic agent generally found in nature and that causes disease. The agent is cultivated, synthesized, and/or mutated to maximize the target population's exposure to the germ.

wedge A tapered shaft of wood or other material used to snug loose cribbing.

wheel bounce A vibration, synchronous with road speed, that can be felt in the steering wheel.

wheel wobble A common finding at low speeds when a vehicle has a bent wheel.

whiplash An injury to the cervical vertebrae or its supporting ligaments and muscles, usually resulting from hyperextension caused by sudden acceleration or deceleration; can be difficult to differentiate from injuries that involve cervical bony structures and the spine.

wilderness paramedics Paramedics who provide trauma care and other emergency services in remote and frontier areas.

wind-chill factor A measurement that takes into account the temperature and wind velocity in calculating the effect of a given ambient temperature on living organisms.

working diagnosis The one diagnosis from a differential list used to base the patient's treatment plan.

worried well Generally health people who seek medical treatment because they are concerned that they are exhibiting symptoms associated with a particular illness or incident they recently learned about.

zone of coagulation The reddened area surrounding the leathery and sometimes charred tissue that has sustained a full-thickness burn.

zone of hyperemia In a thermal burn, the area that is least affected by the burn injury; an area of increased blood flow where the body is attempting to repair injured but otherwise viable tissue.

zone of stasis The peripheral area surrounding the zone of coagulation that has decreased blood flow and inflammation; it can undergo necrosis within 24 to 48 hours after the injury, particularly if perfusion is compromised due to burn shock.

Index: Volume 2